Primer on the Metabolic Bone Diseases and Disorders of Mineral Metabolism

Fifth Edition

An Official Publication of the American Society for Bone and Mineral Research

Primer on the Metabolic Bone Diseases and Disorders of Mineral Metabolism

Fifth Edition

EDITOR

Murray J. Favus, M.D.
Department of Medicine
The University of Chicago Medical Center
Chicago, Illinois

ASSOCIATE EDITORS

Sylvia Christakos, Ph.D.
University of Medicine and Dentistry of New Jersey
New Jersey Medical School
Newark, New Jersey

Pamela Gehron Robey, Ph.D.
National Institute of Dental Research
National Institutes of Health
Bethesda, Maryland

Steven R. Goldring, M.D.
Beth Israel Deaconess Medical Center
Boston, Massachusetts

Michael F. Holick, Ph.D., M.D.
Boston University School of Medicine
Boston, Massachusetts

Frederick S. Kaplan, M.D.
University of Pennsylvania
School of Medicine
Philadelphia, Pennsylvania

Michael Kleerekoper, M.D., F.A.C.E.
Wayne State University
Detroit, Michigan

Nancy Lane, M.D.
University of California
San Francisco, California

Craig B. Langman, M.D.
Northwestern University Medical School
Children's Memorial Hospital
Chicago, Illinois

Jane B. Lian, Ph.D.
University of Massachusetts
Medical School
Worcester, Massachusetts

Elizabeth Shane, M.D.
Columbia University
College of Physicians and Surgeons
New York, New York

Dolores M. Shoback, M.D.
Veterans Affairs Medical Center
University of California
San Francisco, California

Andrew F. Stewart, M.D.
University of Pittsburgh School of Medicine
Pittsburgh, Pennsylvania

Michael P. Whyte, M.D.
Shriners Hospital for Children
St. Louis, Missouri

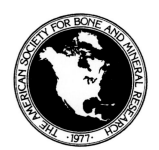

Published by the American Society for Bone and Mineral Research
Washington, D.C.

Cover Designer: Christopher Coleman
Printer: Cadmus Professional Communications

©2003 by American Society for Bone and Mineral Research. Published by:

American Society for Bone and Mineral Research
2025 M Street, NW, Suite 800
Washington, DC 20036-3309
www.asbmr.org

Printed in the USA

Library of Congress Cataloging-in-Publication Data

Primer on the metabolic bone diseases and disorders of mineral metabolism / editor, Murray J. Favus ; associate editors, Sylvia Christakos ... [et al.].-- 5th ed.
p. ; cm.
Includes bibliographical references and index.
ISBN 0-9744782-0-2 (alk. paper)
1. Bones--Metabolism--Disorders. 2. Mineral metabolism--Disorders.
3. Bones--Diseases.
[DNLM: 1. Bone Diseases, Metabolic. 2. Bone and Bones--metabolism.
3. Minerals--metabolism. WE 250 P953 2003] I. Favus, Murray J. II.
American Society for Bone and Mineral Research.

RC931.M45P75 2003
616.7'16--dc22

2003058328
CIP

Care has been taken to confirm the accuracy of the information presented and to describe generally accepted practices. However, the authors, editors and publisher are not responsible for errors or omissions or for any consequences from application of the information in this book and make no warranty, expressed or implied, with respect to the currency, completeness, or accuracy of the contents of the publication. Application of this information in a particular situation remains the professional responsibility of the practitioner. The authors, editors and publisher have sought to ensure that drug selection and dosage set forth in this text are in accordance with current recommendations and practice at the time of publication. However, in view of ongoing research, changes in government regulations, and the constant flow of information relating to drug therapy and drug reactions, the reader is urged to check the package insert for each drug for any change in indications and dosage and for added warnings and precautions. This is particularly important when the recommended agent is a new or infrequently employed drug. Some drugs and medical devices presented in this publication have Food and Drug Administration (FDA) clearance for limited use in restricted research settings. It is the responsibility of the health care provider to ascertain the FDA status of each drug or device planned for use in their clinical practice.

Contents

Contributing Authors

John S. Adams, M.D.
Andrew Arnold, M.D.
Jane E. Aubin, Ph.D.
Daniel T. Baran, M.D.
M. Janet Barger-Lux, M.S.
Roland Baron, D.D.S., Ph.D.
Paolo Bianco, M.D.
Daniel D. Bikle, M.D., Ph.D.
John P. Bilezikian, M.D.
Christopher M. Bono, M.D.
Adele L. Boskey, Ph.D.
Alan Boyde, Ph.D.
Arthur E. Broadus, M.D., Ph.D.
Edward M. Brown, M.D.
David B. Burr, Ph.D.
David A. Bushinsky, M.D.
Ernesto Canalis, M.D.
Thomas O. Carpenter, M.D.
Di Chen, M.D., Ph.D.
Charles H. Chesnut III, M.D.
Gregory A. Clines, M.D., Ph.D.
Jack W. Coburn, M.D.
Frederick L. Coe, M.D.
Adi Cohen, M.D.
David E.C. Cole, M.D., Ph.D.
Michael T. Collins, M.D.
Gary J.R. Cook, M.B.B.S., M.R.C.P., F.R.C.R.
Cyrus Cooper, M.A., D.M., F.R.C.P.
Gilbert J. Cote, Ph.D.
Bess Dawson-Hughes, M.D.
Leonard J. Deftos, M.D., J.D.
Pierre D. Delmas, M.D., Ph.D.
Robert W. Downs Jr., M.D.
Richard Eastell, M.D., F.R.C.P.
Peter R. Ebeling, M.D., F.R.A.C.P.
Thomas A. Einhorn, M.D.
Murray J. Favus, M.D.
Ignac Fogelman, M.D., F.R.C.P.
Robert F. Gagel, M.D.
J. Christopher Gallagher, M.D.
Harry K. Genant, M.D.
Vicente Gilsanz, M.D.
David L. Glaser, M.D.
Francis H. Glorieux, M.D., Ph.D.
Lauren H. Golden, M.D.
Steven R. Goldring, M.D.
David Goltzman, M.D.

William G. Goodman, M.D.
Susan L. Greenspan, M.D.
Theresa A. Guise, M.D.
Robert P. Heaney, M.D., F.A.C.P., F.A.I.N.
Martin Hewison, Ph.D.
Michael F. Holick, M.D., Ph.D.
Mara J. Horwitz, M.D.
Keith A. Hruska, M.D.
Karl L. Insogna, M.D.
Suzanne M. Jan de Beur, M.D.
Marjorie K. Jeffcoat, D.M.D.
Michael Jergas, M.D.
Sheila J. Jones, Ph.D.
Harald Jüppner, M.D.
John A. Kanis, M.D.
Frederick S. Kaplan, M.D.
Sundeep Khosla, M.D., F.A.C.P.
Douglas P. Kiel, M.D., M.P.H.
Samuel C. Kim, M.D.
Michael Kleerekoper, M.D., F.A.C.E.
Christopher S. Kovacs, M.D., F.R.C.P.C.
Paul H. Krebsbach, D.D.S., Ph.D.
Henry M. Kronenberg, M.D.
Ramsay L. Kuo, M.D.
Rajiv Kumar, M.D.
Joseph M. Lane, M.D.
Craig B. Langman, M.D.
Meryl S. LeBoff, M.D.
Eleanor D. Lederer, M.D.
Jacob Lemann Jr., M.D.
Mary B. Leonard, M.D.
Michael A. Levine, M.D.
Jane B. Lian, Ph.D.
Uri A. Liberman, M.D., Ph.D.
Julie T. Lin, M.D.
James E. Lingeman, M.D.
Marjorie M. Luckey, M.D.
Barbara P. Lukert, M.D.
Stephen J. Marx, M.D.
Katharine H. Mikulec, M.D.
David G. Monroe, Ph.D.
Gregory R. Mundy, M.D.
Elizabeth R. Myers, Ph.D.
Dorothy A. Nelson, Ph.D.
Robert A. Nissenson, Ph.D.
Michael E. Norman, M.D.
Bjorn R. Olsen, M.D., Ph.D.

Eric S. Orwoll, M.D.
Babatunde O. Oyajobi, Ph.D., M.B.B.Ch.
Joan H. Parks, M.B.A.
Ryan F. Paterson, M.D.
John M. Pettifor, M.B.B.Ch., Ph.D.
Peter J. Polverini, D.D.S., D.M.Sc.
Anthony A. Portale, M.D.
Richard L. Prince, M.D.
L. Darryl Quarles, M.D.
Robert R. Recker, M.D., F.A.C.P., F.A.C.E.
Jonathan Reeve, D.M., D.Sc., F.R.C.P.
Ian R. Reid, M.D., F.R.A.C.P.
Pamela Gehron Robey, Ph.D.
G. David Roodman, M.D., Ph.D.
Clifford J. Rosen, M.D.
Robert K. Rude, M.D.
Isidro B. Salusky, M.D.
Elizabeth Shane, M.D.
Dolores M. Shoback, M.D.
Eileen M. Shore, M.D.

Richard M. Shore, M.D.
Shonni J. Silverberg, M.D.
Stuart L. Silverman, M.D.
Ethel S. Siris, M.D.
Peter M. Sklarin, M.D.
Eduardo Slatopolsky, M.D.
Everett L. Smith, Ph.D.
Thomas C. Spelsburg, Ph.D.
Stuart M. Sprague, D.O.
Gary S. Stein, Ph.D.
Andrew F. Stewart, M.D.
Gordon J. Strewler, M.D.
Peter J. Tebben, M.D.
Rajesh V. Thakker, M.D., F.R.C.P.
Charles H. Turner, Ph.D.
Marjolein C.H. van der Meulen
Jean Wactawski-Wende, Ph.D.
Nelson B. Watts, M.D.
Michael P. Whyte, M.D.
John J. Wysolmerski, M.D.

Preface to the Fifth Edition

The ASBMR *Primer on the Metabolic Bone Diseases and Disorders of Bone and Mineral Metabolism* was created to serve as a comprehensive educational source for practitioners and investigators in the field and for those graduate students and post-graduate trainees with an interest in bone disease. The subject of the Fifth Edition of the *Primer* is the core knowledge of bone biology, mineral metabolism, action of hormones on bone and mineral metabolism, and the clinical disorders that involve these complex systems. The study of bone structure and its function provides insight into the pathogenesis of the many disorders that affect bone and mineral. New knowledge of the basic science of bone offers our best opportunity to develop novel approaches to treat and reverse these disorders. This edition is the first to be published independently by ASBMR, which underscores the Society's commitment to promoting excellence in bone and mineral research, fostering integration of clinical and basic science, and facilitating the translation of bone and mineral science to health care and clinical practice.

The diseases referred to as metabolic bone diseases and mineral disorders comprise a collection of rare and unusual diseases admixed with very common conditions. Rapid expansion of osteoporosis research has led to many insights into the pathogenesis of this disease, to new assays, procedures, and therapies that may benefit the millions of people affected. Many other bone and mineral diseases that affect people of all ages have also experienced important advances in recent years. The identification of genes that encode molecules that mediate osteoblast-osteoclast interaction has led to the discovery of mutations of these genes and the genetic disorders that result.

This new knowledge is incorporated into the revised chapters as well as the chapters that are new to the Fifth Edition. The new chapters reflect advances on topics of growing interest including: osteogenic growth factors, the skeletal physiology of the fetus and neonate, and the calcium sensing receptor. The substantial problem of osteoporosis is reflected in the large number of chapters on this topic. Important advances in the genetic basis of bone and mineral disorders are contained in several of the revised chapters and in the Appendix, in which a new table contains all of the known mutations that result in human disease.

The *Primer* offers a concise yet thorough discussion of the basic information needed to become familiar with the diseases, the underlying pathophysiology, and the basic sciences that provide an understanding for the basis of the disorders. The book is directed towards clinicians, basic scientists, students and residents in general practice, internal medicine, pediatrics, gynecology, orthopaedics, radiology and nuclear medicine. A number of subspecialty groups will be particularly interested in the *Primer*, including endocrinology, genetics, rheumatology, nephrology, nutrition, gastroenterology and geriatrics. Basic scientists and clinical investigators interested in bone will find the *Primer* useful at all levels of inquiry, including molecular biology, cell biology, biochemistry, physiology, genetics, pathology, immunology and nutrition.

Research in this field advances at a rapid rate and its direct benefits are appreciated in the clinical sciences. The *Primer* continues to evolve as a result, and I welcome readers' comments and suggestions as to how to present this field in the most useful and informative way.

Murray J. Favus, M.D.
University of Chicago

Acknowledgement

The editorial board's efforts to bring out the Fifth Edition of the *Primer* faced challenges similar to that of any far-flung group attempting to work. The Fifth Edition is a product of the electronic era in communications and publishing - talk between editors, authors and staff conducted by e-mail, and chapters submitted, reviewed and transmitted via the internet. The Fifth Edition is also the first attempt by the American Society for Bone and Mineral Research to independently publish the *Primer*. This Herculean effort was skillfully performed by the ASBMR editorial staff in North Carolina. We are grateful to the American Society for Bone and Mineral Research for committing staff time and resources to the publication of the *Primer*.

Of course, it was the collaborative work of the editorial board that once again resulted in a successful edition. I thank Sylvia Christakos, Steven R. Goldring, Michael F. Holick, Frederick S. Kaplan, Nancy Lane, Michael Kleerekoper, Craig B. Langman, Jane P. Lian, Pamela Gehron Robey, Elizabeth Shane, Dolores M. Shoback, Andrew F. Stewart and Michael P. Whyte for their enthusiasm, dedication and selfless work.

Murray J. Favus, M.D.
University of Chicago

The American Society for Bone and Mineral Research

We are delighted to publish the 5th edition of the American Society for Bone and Mineral Research *Primer on the Metabolic Bone Diseases and Disorders of Mineral Metabolism.* Launched in 1990, this highly regarded teaching tool presents and defines core knowledge in bone and mineral research. For its existence we are indebted to all contributors and editors, but most centrally to the vision, persistence and dedication of Dr. Murray J. Favus.

In 1987 Murray began chairing the ASBMR Education Committee and quickly recognized the need for a text that would illuminate the field of bone and mineral metabolism for interested scientists, physicians and students. Beyond that, he was willing to do the work to create such a book: convincing Council leadership of the need for the project, raising funds for the production of the book and, most important, shepherding authors and editors through the arduous process of writing, editing and revising *Primer* chapters.

Just as significantly, Murray has taken on the duty of overseeing four subsequent editions of the *Primer*, insuring that the Society continues to present information that reflects the most important advances in our field and provides an important educational resource for those already working in the bone field as well as young investigators learning about bone and mineral disorders. At the time this edition went to press more than 100,000 copies of this book were already in circulation, making the *Primer* one of the most widely used sources of information on metabolic bone and mineral disorders.

Integrating and disseminating scientific knowledge in accessible fashion is no easy task; that the *Primer* accomplishes this so successfully is due to the leadership of Dr. Favus and to the editors and authors who have committed their time and expertise to this effort.

Clifford J. Rosen
President
American Society for Bone and Mineral Research

Anatomy and Biology of Bone Matrix and Cellular Elements

Chapter 1.   General Principles of Bone Biology

Roland Baron

Departments of Orthopedics and Cell Biology, Yale University, School of Medicine, New Haven, Connecticut

INTRODUCTION

Bone is a specialized connective tissue that makes up, together with cartilage, the skeletal system. These tissues serve three functions: (1) mechanical, as support and site of muscle attachment for locomotion; (2) protective, for vital organs and bone marrow; and (3) metabolic, as a reserve of ions, especially calcium and phosphate, for the maintenance of serum homeostasis, which is essential to life.

In bone, as in all connective tissues, the fundamental constituents are the cells and the extracellular matrix. The latter is particularly abundant in this tissue and is composed of collagen fibers and noncollagenous proteins. In bone, cartilage, and the tissues forming the teeth, however, unlike in other connective tissues, the matrices have the unique ability to become calcified (or have lost the ability to prevent calcification).

BONE AS AN ORGAN: MACROSCOPIC ORGANIZATION

Anatomically, two types of bones can be distinguished in the skeleton: flat bones (skull bones, scapula, mandible, and ileum) and long bones (tibia, femur, humerus, etc.). These two types are derived by two distinct types of development, intramembranous and endochondral, although the development and growth of long bones actually involve both types of processes.

External examination of a long bone (Fig. 1) shows two wider extremities (the epiphyses), a more or less cylindrical tube in the middle (the midshaft or diaphysis), and a developmental zone between them (the metaphysis). In a growing long bone, the epiphysis and the metaphysis, which originate from two independent ossification centers, are separated by a layer of cartilage, the *epiphyseal cartilage* (also called growth plate). This layer of proliferative cells and expanding cartilage matrix is responsible for the longitudinal growth of bones; it becomes entirely calcified and remodeled and replaced by bone by the end of the growth period. The external part of the bones is formed by a thick and dense layer of calcified tissue, the *cortex* (compact bone), which, in the diaphysis, encloses the medullary cavity where the hematopoietic bone marrow is housed. Toward the metaphysis and the epiphysis, the cortex becomes progressively thinner, and the internal space is filled with a network of thin, calcified trabeculae; this is the *cancellous bone*, also named spongy or *trabecular bone*. The spaces enclosed by these thin trabeculae are also filled with hematopoietic bone marrow and are in continuity with the medullary cavity of the diaphysis. The bone surfaces at the epiphyses that take part in the joint are covered with a layer of articular cartilage that does not calcify.

There are consequently two bone surfaces at which the bone is in contact with the soft tissues (Fig. 1): an external surface (the periosteal surface) and an internal surface (the endosteal surface). These surfaces are lined with osteogenic cells organized in layers, the periosteum and the endosteum. Cortical and trabecular bone are made of the same cells and the same matrix elements, but there are structural and functional differences. The primary structural difference is quantitative: 80–90% of the volume of compact bone is calcified, whereas only 15–25% of the trabecular bone is calcified (the remainder being occupied by bone marrow, blood vessels, and connective tissue). The result is that 70–85% of the interface with soft tissues is at the endosteal bone surface, which leads to the functional difference: the cortical bone fulfills mainly (but not exclusively) a mechanical and protective function and the trabecular bone a metabolic function.

BONE AS A TISSUE

Microscopic Organization

Bone Matrix and Mineral. Bone is formed by collagen fibers (type I, 90% of the total protein), usually oriented in a preferential direction, and noncollagenous proteins. Spindle- or plate-shaped crystals of hydroxyapatite $[3Ca_3(PO_4)_2(OH)_2]$ are found on the collagen fibers, within them, and in the ground substance. They tend to be oriented in the same direction as the collagen fibers. The ground substance is primarily composed of glycoproteins and proteoglycans. These highly anionic complexes have a high ion-binding capacity and are thought to play an important

---

The author has no conflict of interest.

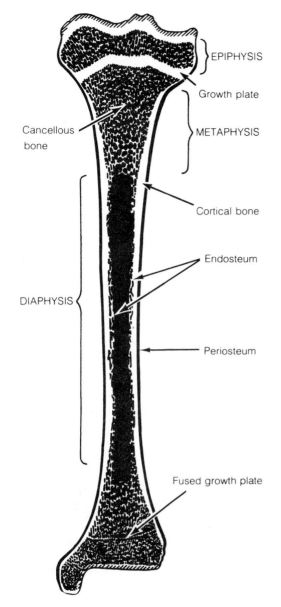

EPIPHYSIS

Growth plate

METAPHYSIS

Cancellous bone

Cortical bone

Endosteum

DIAPHYSIS

Periosteum

Fused growth plate

FIG. 1. Schematic view of a longitudinal section through a growing long bone. (Reproduced with permission from Jee WSS 1983 The skeletal tissues. In: Weiss L, ed. Histology, Cell and Tissue Biology. Elsevier Biomedical, New York, NY, USA, pp. 200–255.)

part in the calcification process and the fixation of hydroxyapatite crystals to the collagen fibers.

Numerous noncollagenous proteins present in bone matrix have recently been purified and sequenced, but their role has been only partially characterized. Most of these proteins are synthesized by bone-forming cells, but not all: a number of plasma proteins are preferentially absorbed by the bone matrix, such as HS-glycoprotein, which is synthesized in the liver.

The preferential orientation of the collagen fibers alternates in adult bone from layer to layer, giving to this bone a typical lamellar structure, best seen under polarized light or by electron microscopy. This fiber organization allows the highest density of collagen per unit volume of tissue.

The lamellae can be parallel to each other if deposited along a flat surface (trabecular bone and periosteum), or concentric if deposited on a surface surrounding a channel centered on a blood vessel (haversian system, Fig. 2). However, when bone is being formed very rapidly (during development and fracture healing, or in tumors and some metabolic bone diseases), there is no preferential organization of the collagen fibers. They are not as tightly packed and found in somewhat randomly oriented bundles; this type of bone is called woven bone, as opposed to lamellar bone.

Cellular Organizations Within the Bone Matrix: Osteocytes. The calcified bone matrix is not metabolically inert, and cells (osteocytes) are found embedded deep within the bone in small osteocytic lacunae (25,000/mm^3 of bone) (Figs. 2 and 3). They were originally bone-forming cells (osteoblasts), which became trapped in the bone matrix that they produced and later became calcified. They nevertheless express some specific membrane proteins. These cells have numerous and long cell processes rich in microfilaments, which are in contact with cell processes from other osteocytes (there are frequent gap junctions), or with processes from the cells lining the bone surface (osteoblasts or flat lining cells in the endosteum or periosteum). These processes are organized during the formation of the matrix and before its calcification; they form a network of thin canaliculi permeating the entire bone matrix (Fig. 2).

Between the osteocyte plasma membrane and the bone matrix itself is the periosteocytic space. This space exists both in the lacunae and in the canaliculi, and it is filled with extracellular fluid (ECF).

The physiological significance of this system is readily demonstrated by some numbers. The total bone surface area of the canaliculate and lacunae is 1000–5000 m^2 in an adult (compared with a surface area of 140 m^2 for lung capillaries); the volume of bone ECF is 1.0–1.5 liters; and the surface calcium contained on bone mineral crystals is approximately 5–20 g, which accounts for a significant percentage of the total exchangeable bone calcium. The fact that the calcium concentration in the bone ECF (0.5 mM) is lower than in plasma (1.5 mM) suggests that there is a constant flow of calcium ions out of the bone.

The morphology of the osteocytes varies according to their age and functional activity. A young osteocyte has most of the ultrastructural characteristics of the osteoblast from which it was derived, except that there has been a decrease in cell volume and in the importance of the organelles involved in protein synthesis (rough endoplasmic reticulum, Golgi). An older osteocyte, located deeper within the calcified bone, shows these decreases further accentuated, and in addition, there is an accumulation of glycogen in the cytoplasm. These cells have been shown to be able to synthesize new bone matrix at the surface of the osteocytic lacunae, which can subsequently calcify. Although historically they have been considered able to resorb calcified bone from the same surface, this point has recently been disputed. The fate of the osteocytes is to be phagocytized and digested, together with the other components of bone, during osteoclastic bone resorption. These cells may also

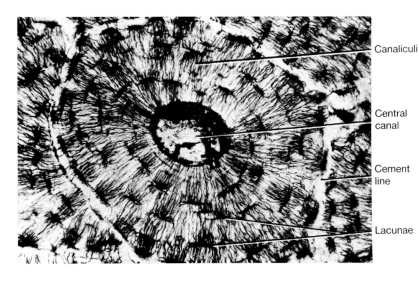

Canaliculi

Central canal

Cement line

Lacunae

FIG. 2. Cross-sectional view of a haversian system in cortical bone, showing the lamellar organization of collagen in mature bone matrix, and the morphology and canalicular organization of osteocytes. (Reproduced with permission from Jee WSS 1983 The skeletal tissues. In: Weiss L, ed. Histology, Cell and Tissue Biology. Elsevier Biomedical, New York, NY, USA, pp. 200–255.)

play a role as mechanosensors and in the local activation of bone turnover (remodeling).

Bone Surface

Most of the bone tissue turnover occurs at the bone surfaces, mainly at the endosteal surface where it interfaces with bone marrow. This surface is morphologically heterogeneous, reflecting the various specific cellular activities involved in remodeling and turnover.

Osteoblast and Bone Formation. The osteoblast is the bone lining cell responsible for the production of the matrix constituents (collagen and ground substance) (Fig. 3). It originates from a local mesenchymal stem cell (bone marrow stromal stem cell or connective tissue mesenchymal stem cell) under the influence of local growth factors such as fibroblast growth factors (FGFs), bone morphogenetic proteins (BMPs), and Wnt proteins and requires the transcription factors Runx2 and Osterix. These precursors undergo proliferation and differentiate into preosteoblasts and then into mature osteoblasts. Osteoblasts never appear or function individually but are always found in clusters of cuboidal cells along the bone surface (~100–400 cells per bone-forming site). At the light microscope level, the osteoblast is characterized by a round nucleus at the base of the cell (opposite to the bone surface), a strongly basophilic cytoplasm, and a prominent Golgi complex located between the nucleus and the apex of the cell, reflecting the high biosynthetic and secretory activity of these cells. Osteoblasts are always found lining the layer of bone matrix that they are producing, before it is calcified (called, at this point, osteoid tissue). Osteoid tissue exists because of a time lag between matrix formation and its subsequent calcification (the osteoid maturation period), which is approximately 10 days in humans. Behind the osteoblast can usually be found one or two layers of cells: activated mesenchymal cells and preosteoblasts. At the ultrastructural level, the osteoblast is characterized by (1) the presence of an extremely well-developed rough endoplasmic reticulum with dilated cisternae and a dense granular content and (2) the

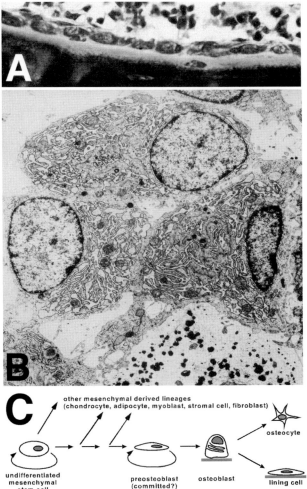

FIG. 3. Osteoblasts and osteoid tissue. (A and B) Light and electron micrograph of a group of osteoblasts (top) covering a layer of mineralizing osteoid tissue (bottom) with a newly embedded osteocyte (arrow). Basal nuclei, prominent (C) Golgi, and endoplasmic reticulum, and characteristics of active osteoblasts. Schematic representation of the life cycle of the osteoblast, differentiating from a mesenchymal cell, into preosteoblasts and osteoblasts and later into either osteocytes or bone lining cells. (Reproduced with permission from Sims NA, Baron R 2002 Bone: Structure, function, growth, and remodeling. In Fitzgerald RH Jr, Kaufer H, Malkani AL (eds.) Orthopaedics. Mosby, Elsevier Science, St. Louis, MO, USA, pp. 147–159.)

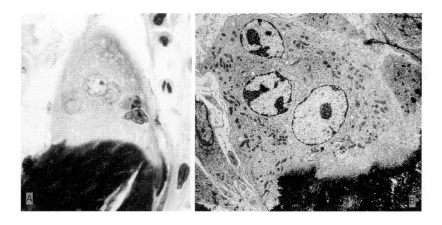

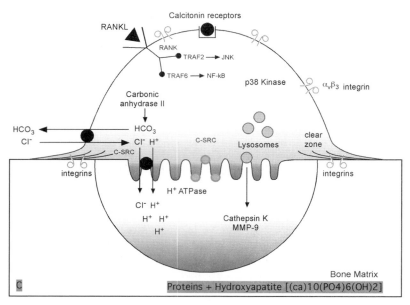

FIG. 4. Osteoclast. Section of an osteoclast in light microscopy (A) or electron microscopy (B). The osteoclast contains multiple nuclei, an endoplasmic reticulum where lysosomal enzymes are synthesized, and prominent Golgi stacks around each nucleus. The cell is attached to bone matrix (bottom) and forms a separate compartment underneath itself, limited by the sealing zone. The plasma membrane of the cell facing this compartment is extensively folded and forms the ruffled border, with pockets of extracellular space between the folds. Multiple small vesicles in the cytoplasm transport enzymes toward the bone matrix and internalize partially digested bone matrix. (C) Schematic representation of a polarized active osteoclast including the main molecular players in the process of bone resorption (see text).

presence of a large circular Golgi complex comprising multiple Golgi stacks. Cytoplasmic processes on the secreting side of the cell extend deep into the osteoid matrix and are in contact with the osteocyte processes in their canaliculi. Junctional complexes (gap junctions) are often found between the osteoblasts. The plasma membrane of the osteoblast is characteristically rich in alkaline phosphatase (whose concentration in the serum is used as an index of bone formation) and has been shown to have receptors for parathyroid hormone and prostaglandins but not for calcitonin. Osteoblasts also express steroid receptors for estrogens and vitamin D_3 as well as several adhesion molecules (integrins) and receptors for cytokines. They also express cytokines in their membrane, and in particular, colony-stimulating factor 1 (CSF-1) and RANKL, which can be cleaved to activate osteoclastogenesis in a local, paracrine manner. They also secrete osteoprotegerin, a decoy RANK receptor capable of inhibiting osteoclast formation. Toward the end of the secreting period, the osteoblast becomes either a flat lining cell or an osteocyte.

Osteoclast and Bone Resorption. The osteoclast is the bone lining cell responsible for bone resorption (Fig. 4).

Morphology. The osteoclast is a giant multinucleated cell, containing 4–20 nuclei. It is usually found in contact with a calcified bone surface and within a lacuna (Howship's lacunae) that is the result of its own resorptive activity. It is possible to find up to four or five osteoclasts in the same resorptive site, but there usually are only one or two. Under the light microscope, the nuclei appear to vary within the same cell; some are round and euchromatic, and some are irregular in contour and heterochromatic, possibly reflecting the asynchronous fusion of mononuclear precursors. The cytoplasm is "foamy," with many vacuoles. The zone of contact with the bone is characterized by the presence of a ruffled border with dense patches on each side (the sealing zone).

Characteristic ultrastructural features of this cell are the abundant Golgi complexes characteristically disposed around each nucleus, the mitochondria, and the transport vesicles loaded with lysosomal enzymes. The most prominent features of the osteoclast are, however, the deep foldings of the plasma membrane in the area facing the bone matrix: the ruffled border in the center is surrounded by a ring of actin (sealing zone) that serves to attach the cell to the bone surface, thus sealing off the subosteoclastic bone-resorbing compartment. The attachment of the cell to the

Key Factors Regulating the Differentiation and Activity of Osteoclasts

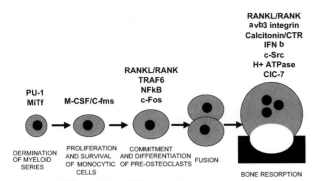

Steps in the Differentiation of Osteoclasts

FIG. 5. Schematic representation of the factors regulating the differentiation and activity of osteoclasts (top) and the corresponding steps that they control in the process (bottom).

matrix is performed through integrin receptors (mostly αv $\beta 3$, αv $\beta 5$, and $\alpha 2$ $\beta 1$), which bind to specific sequences in matrix proteins and require several specific signaling molecules to ensure adhesion and cell motility (c-Src, Pyk2, Cbl, gelsolin). The plasma membrane in the ruffled border area contains proteins that are also found at the limiting membrane of lysosomes and related organelles and a specific type of electrogenic proton ATPase as well as a specific chloride channel (ClC 7) responsible for acidification of the extracellular bone resorbing compartment. The basolateral plasma membrane of the osteoclast is highly and specifically enriched in Na^+,K^+ ATPase (sodium-potassium pumps), HCO_3^-/Cl^- exchangers, and Na^+/H^+ exchangers, as well as several ion channels. This membrane is also expressing RANK, the receptor for RANKL, and the macrophage-colony stimulating factor (M-CSF) receptor, both of which are responsible for osteoclast differentiation, as well as the calcitonin receptor, capable of inactivating rapidly the osteoclast.

Mechanisms of Bone Resorption. Lysosomal enzymes (TRACP, cathepsin K, etc.) are actively synthesized by the osteoclast and are found in the endoplasmic reticulum, Golgi, and many transport vesicles. The enzymes are secreted, through the ruffled border, into the extracellular bone-resorbing compartment; they reach a sufficiently high extracellular concentration because this compartment is sealed off. The transport and targeting of these enzymes for secretion at the apical pole of the osteoclast involves mannose-6-phosphate receptors. Furthermore, the cell secretes several metalloproteases such as collagenase and gelatinase.

The osteoclast acidifies the extracellular compartment by secreting protons across the ruffled-border membrane (by proton pumps). Recent genetic evidence show that the electrogenic proton-pump ATPase is related to, but different from, that of the kidney-tubule-acidifying cells or lysosomes. The protons are provided to the pumps by the enzyme carbonic anhydrase, and they are highly concentrated in the cytosol of the osteoclast; ATP and CO_2 are provided by the mitochondria. Apical chloride channels

(ClC-7) in the ruffled border membrane serve to prevent the hyperpolarization created by the massive extrusion of positively charged protons by the V-ATPase. The basolateral membrane activity exchanges bicarbonate for chloride, thereby avoiding an alkalinization of the cytosol and providing chloride for the ruffled-border channels. The basolateral sodium pumps might be involved in secondary active transport of calcium and/or protons in association with a Na^+/Ca^{2+} exchanger and/or a Na^+/H^+ antiport. This cell could therefore function in a manner similar to that of kidney tubule or gastric parietal cells, which also acidify lumens.

The extracellular bone-resorbing compartment is therefore the functional equivalent of a secondary lysosome, with (1) a low pH, (2) lysosomal enzymes, and (3) the substrate, that is, the bone matrix. First, the hydroxyapatite crystals are mobilized by digestion of their link to collagen (the non-collagenous proteins) and dissolved by the acid environment. Then, the residual collagen fibers are digested either by the activation of latent collagenase or by the action of cathepsins at low pH. The enzymes, now at optimal pH, degrade the matrix components; the residues from this extracellular digestion are internalized, transported across the cell (by transcytosis) and released at the basolateral domain, or released during periods of relapse of the sealing zone, possibly induced by a calcium sensor responding to the rise of extracellular calcium in the bone-resorbing compartment.

Clinically, this explains why (1) bone resorption helps to maintain calcium and inorganic phosphate levels in the plasma, and (2) the concentrations of hydroxyproline and N-terminal or C-terminal collagen peptides in the serum or the urine are used as indirect measurements of bone resorption in humans (collagen type I is highly enriched in hydroxyproline and pyridinoline links).

Origin and Fate of the Osteoclast. The osteoclast derives from cells in the mononuclear/phagocytic lineage (Fig. 5). Their differentiation requires the transcription factors PU-1 and MiTf at early stages, committing the precursors into the

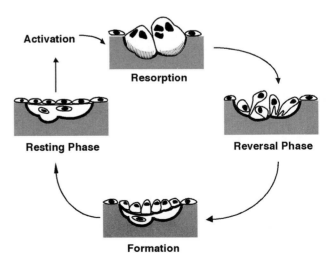

FIG. 6. Bone remodeling. The bone remodeling sequence as it occurs in trabecular bone. (The same principles apply to haversian remodeling; see text.)

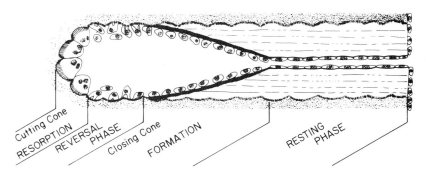

FIG. 7. The bone-remodeling activity in cortical bone as seen in longitudinal sequence. Osteoclasts dig out a tunnel, creating a "cutting cone." Subsequently new bone is formed in the area of the "closing cone," leading to the creation of a new bone structural unit (i.e., the haversian system).

myeloid lineage. M-CSF is then required to engage the cells in the monocyte lineage and ensure their proliferation and the expression of the RANK receptor. At that stage, the cells require the presence of RANKL, produced by stromal cells, to truly commit to the osteoclast lineage and progress in their differentiation program. This step also requires expression of TRAF6, NFκB and c-*Fos*, all downstream effectors of RANK signaling. Although this differentiation occurs at the early promonocyte stage, monocytes and macrophages already committed to their own lineage might still be able to form osteoclasts under the right stimuli.

Despite its mononuclear/phagocytic origin, the osteoclast membrane express distinct markers: it is devoid of Fc and C_3 receptors, as well as of several other macrophage markers; like mononuclear phagocytes, however, the osteoclast is rich in nonspecific esterases, synthesizes lysozyme, and expresses CSF-1 receptors. Monoclonal antibodies have been produced that recognize osteoclasts but not macrophages. The osteoclast, unlike macrophages, also expresses, millions of copies of the RANK, calcitonin, and vitronectin (integrin $\alpha_v\beta3$) receptors. Whether it expresses receptors for parathyroid hormone, estrogen, or vitamin D is still controversial. Recent evidence suggest that the osteoclast undergoes apoptosis after a cycle of resorption, a process favored by estrogens and possibly explaining the increased bone resorption after gonadectomy or menopause.

BONE REMODELING

The previously described activity of bone cells is performed along the surfaces of bone, mainly the endosteal surface, and it results in bone remodeling, a process involved in bone growth and turnover. Bone formation and bone resorption do not, however, occur along the bone surface at random; they are either part of the process of bone development and growth or part of the turnover mechanism by which old bone is replaced by new bone. In the normal adult skeleton (i.e., after the period of development and growth), bone formation occurs for the most part only where bone resorption has previously occurred. The sequence of events at the remodeling site (Figs. 6 and 7) is the activation-resorption-formation (ARF) sequence, first described by H. Frost. During the intermediate phase between resorption and formation (the reversal phase), some macrophage-like, uncharacterized mononuclear cells are observed at the site of the remodeling, and a cement line is formed, which marks the limit of resorption and acts to cement together the old and the new bone. The duration of these various phases has been measured (Fig. 7): the complete remodeling cycle at each microscopic site takes about 3–6 months. Although cortical bone is anatomically different, its remodeling follows the same biological principles (Fig. 8). Lamellar bone being formed within such a system gives the characteristic structure of an haversian system when seen in cross-section (see Fig. 2).

BONE DEVELOPMENT AND GROWTH

There are two types of processes involved in bone development: intramembranous ossification (flat bones) and endochondral ossification (long bones) (Fig. 9). The main difference between them is the presence of a cartilaginous phase in the latter.

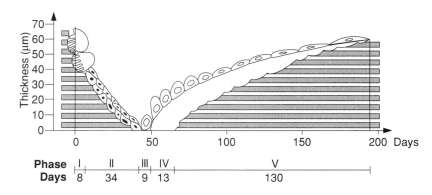

FIG. 8. Duration and depth of the various phases of the normal cancellous bone remodeling sequence, calculated from histomorphometric analysis of bone biopsy samples obtained from young individuals. Note the balance between the erosion depth and the mean wall thickness. (Reproduced with permission from Eriksen EF, Axelrod DW, Melsen F 1994 Bone Histomorphometry. Raven Press, New York, NY, USA, pp. 13–20.)

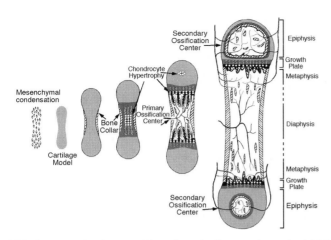

FIG. 9. Bone development. The schematic diagram shows the initial stages of endochondral ossification. Bone development begins with mesenchymal condensation to form a cartilage model of the bone to be formed. After chondrocyte hypertrophy and cartilage matrix mineralization, osteoclast activity and vascularization result in the formation of the primary and secondary ossification centers. In mature adult bones, the growth plate is fully resorbed so that one marrow cavity extends the full length of the bone. See text for details. (Reproduced with permission from Sims NA, Baron R 2002 Bone: Structure, function, growth, and remodeling. In Fitzgerald RH Jr, Kaufer H, Malkani AL (eds.) Orthopaedics. Mosby, Elsevier Science, St. Louis, MO, USA, pp. 147–159.)

Intramembranous Ossification

In intramembranous ossification, a group of mesenchymal cells, under the influence of local growth factors (FGFs, BMPs, Hedgehogs, PTHrP, and the transcription factors

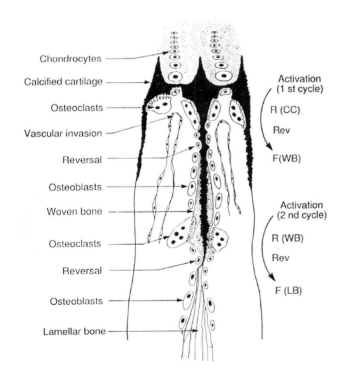

FIG. 10. Bone growth and remodeling at the epiphyseal plate. Schematic representation of the cellular events occurring at the growth plate in long bones. R, resorption; Rev, reversal; F, formation; CC, calcified cartilage; WB, woven bone; LB, lamellar bone.

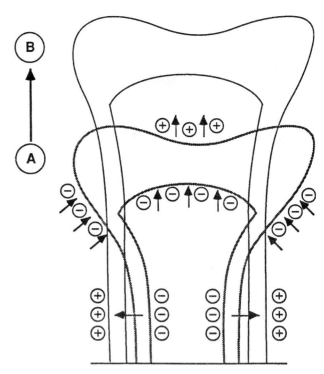

FIG. 11. Resorption (−) and formation (+) activities during the longitudinal growth of bones. During growth from A to B, the cortex in the diaphysis must be resorbed inside and reformed outside (bottom). The growth plate moves upward (see Fig. 10), and the wider parts of the bone must be reshaped into a diaphysis. (Reproduced with permission from Jee WSS 1983 The skeletal tissues. In: Weiss L, ed. Histology, Cell and Tissue Biology. Elsevier Biomedical, New York, NY, USA, pp. 200–255.)

Runx2 and Osterix), forms a condensation within a highly vascularized area of the embryonic connective tissue by proliferating and differentiate directly into preosteoblasts and then into osteoblasts. These cells synthesize a bone matrix with the following characteristics: (1) the collagen fibers are not preferentially oriented but appear as irregular bundles, (2) the osteocytes are large and extremely numerous, and (3) calcification is delayed and does not proceed in an orderly fashion but in irregularly distributed patches. This type of bone is called woven bone. At the periphery, mesenchymal cells continue to differentiate, following the same steps. Blood vessels incorporated between the woven bone trabeculae will form the hematopoietic bone marrow. Later, this woven bone is remodeled following the ARF sequence, and it is progressively replaced by mature lamellar bone.

Endochondral Ossification

Formation of a Cartilage Model. Within the abovementioned condensations and probably under a different ratio of the same local growth factors, mesenchymal cells proliferate and differentiate into prechondroblasts and then into chondroblasts instead of osteoblasts. These cells secrete the cartilaginous matrix. Like the osteoblasts, the chondroblasts become progressively embedded within their own matrix, where they lie within lacunae; they are then called chondrocytes. However, unlike the osteocytes, they continue to proliferate for some time, this being allowed in part by the gel-like consistency of cartilage. At the periphery of this cartilage (the perichondrium), the mesenchymal cells continue to proliferate and differentiate. This is called appositional growth. Another type of growth is observed in the cartilage by synthesis of new matrix between the chondrocytes (interstitial growth). In the growth plate, the cells appear in regular columns called isogenous groups, each clonally derived from a single chondroblast. Later on, the chondrocytes enlarge progressively, become hypertrophic, and undergo programmed cell death (apoptosis). The key molecules involved in the regulation of chondrocyte differentiation and in the formation and expansion of the growth plate have recently been identified as being mostly Indian Hedgehog and PTHrP. In this model, Ihh coordinates chondrocyte proliferation and differentiation as well as osteoblast differentiation. It is synthesized by prehypertrophic chondrocytes and induces the production of PTHrP by perichondrial cells. In turn, PTHrP acts on proliferating chondrocytes to keep them proliferating. When PTHrP levels decrease in more differentiated chondrocytes, this allows the production of Ihh, allowing progression to hypertrophy, and in turn, closing the loop by inducing PTHrP production at the ends of bones.

Vascular Invasion and Longitudinal Growth (Remodeling). The embryonic cartilage is avascular (Figs. 9 and 10). During its early development, a ring of woven bone is formed by intramembranous ossification in the future midshaft area under the perichondrium (which is then a periosteum). Just after the calcification of this woven bone, and under the influence of VEGF, blood vessels (preceded by osteoclasts) penetrate the cartilage, bringing the blood supply that will form the hematopoietic bone marrow.

The growth plate in a growing long bone shows, from the epiphyseal area to the diaphyseal area, the following cellular events (Fig. 10). In a proliferative zone, chondroblasts divide actively under the influence of PTHrP, forming isogenous groups and actively synthesizing the matrix as well as producing ihh. These cells become progressively larger, enlarging their lacunae in the hypertrophic zone, and then they undergo programmed cell death (apoptosis). At this level of the epiphyseal plate, the matrix of the longitudinal cartilage septa selectively calcifies (zone of provisional calcification). Once calcified, the cartilage matrix is resorbed, but only partially, by osteoclasts, (although the concept of a specific chondroclast is also considered now) and blood vessels appear in the zone of invasion. After resorption, osteoblasts differentiate and form a layer of woven bone on top of the cartilaginous remnants of the longitudinal septa.

Thus, the first ARF sequence is complete: the cartilage has been remodeled and replaced by woven bone. The resulting trabeculae are called the primary spongiosa. Still lower in the growth plate, this woven bone is subjected to further remodeling (a second ARF sequence), in which the woven bone and the cartilaginous remnants are replaced with lamellar bone, resulting in the mature state of trabecular bone called secondary spongiosa (Fig. 10).

Growth in Diameter and Shape Modification (Modeling). Growth in the diameter of the shaft is the result of a deposition of new membranous bone beneath the periosteum that will continue throughout life. In this case, resorption does not immediately precede formation. The midshaft is narrower than the metaphysis, and the growth of a long bone progressively destroys the lower part of the metaphysis and transforms it into a diaphysis, accomplished by continuous resorption by osteoclasts beneath the periosteum (Fig. 11).

The following chapters in this section of the Primer will detail these various aspects of bone biology.

SUGGESTED READINGS

1. Aubin JE, Triffitt JT 2002 Mesenchymal stem cells and osteoblast differentiation. In: Principles of Bone Biology, 2nd ed., vol. 1. Academic Press, pp. 59–81.
2. Ducy P, Schinke T, Karsenty G 2000 The osteoblast: A sophisticated fibroblast under central surveillance. Science **289**:1501–1504.
3. Karaplis AC 2002 Embryonic development of bone and the molecular regulation of intramembranous and endochondral bone formation. In: Principles of Bone Biology, 2nd ed., vol. 1. Academic Press, pp. 33–58.
4. Marks SC, Odgren PR 2002 Structure and development of the skeleton. In: Principles of Bone Biology, 2nd ed., vol. 1. Academic Press, pp. 3–15.
5. Rodan GA, Martin TJ 2000 Therapeutic approaches to bone diseases. Science **289**:1508–1514.
6. Takahashi N, Udagawa N, Takami M, Suda T 2002 Cells in bone, osteoclast generation. In: Principles of Bone Biology, 2nd ed., vol. 1. Academic Press, San Diego, CA, USA, pp. 109–126.
7. Teitelbaum SL 2000 Bone resorption by osteoclasts. Science **289**:1504–1508.
8. Kronenberg HM 2003 Developmental regulation of the growth plate. Nature **423**:332–336.
9. Boyle WJ, Simonet WS, Lacey DL 2003 Osteoclast differentiation and activation. Nature **423**:337–342.
10. Harada S-I, Rodan GA 2003 Control of osteoblast function and regulation of bone mass. Nature **423**:349–355.

Chapter 2. Bone Morphogenesis and Embryological Development

Bjorn R. Olsen

Department of Cell Biology, Harvard Medical School, and Department of Oral and Developmental Biology, Harvard School of Dental Medicine, Boston, Massachusetts

INTRODUCTION

The cells that make up the vertebrate skeleton are derived from three lineages. Neural crest cells give rise to the branchial arch derivatives of the craniofacial skeleton, paraxial mesoderm contributes to the craniofacial skeleton and forms most of the axial skeleton (through the sclerotome division of the somites), and cells in the lateral plate mesoderm contribute to the skeleton of the limbs. In areas where bones are formed, mesenchymal cells from these sources condense and form regions of high cell density that represent outlines of future skeletal elements. During this condensation process, important changes take place in the extracellular matrix between the cells allowing cells to establish contact with each other and activate signaling pathways that regulate cell differentiation. Classical experiments have demonstrated that by the time mesenchymal condensations appear the cells within them have already acquired properties that give them positional identity. Mechanisms that ensure the development of a complex skeleton with elements of unique size, shape, and anatomical identity can therefore be traced back to molecular and cellular events in precondensed mesenchyme.

CARTILAGE MODELS OF DEVELOPING BONES

As mesenchymal cells within condensations differentiate, they can follow one of two paths. They can either differentiate into bone forming cells, osteoblasts, or they can differentiate into chondrocytes and secrete the characteristic extracellular matrix of hyaline cartilage. Differentiation into osteoblasts, regulated by the transcription factors CBFA1/RUNX2 and osterix (OSX),[1-4] occurs in areas of membranous ossification, such as in the calvarium of the skull, the maxilla, and the mandible, and in the subperiosteal bone-forming layer of long bones. Differentiation into chondrocytes, regulated by the transcription factor SOX9 and other members of the SOX-family,[5] occurs in the remaining skeleton where cartilage models of the future bones are formed. These models, frequently described by their German term anlagen, are subsequently replaced by bone in a process called endochondral ossification. The differentiation of chondrocytes and the formation of cartilage starts with cells becoming large and round in the center of mesenchymal condensations. They develop organelles for high level synthesis and secretion of proteins (endoplasmic reticulum and Golgi complex) and switch from production of an extracellular matrix containing collagens I and III to a matrix containing the cartilage-specific collagens II, IX, and

XI. The cartilage anlagen grow by interstitial and appositional growth so that they over time come to resemble the future bones in shape and size. While they normally are replaced by bone through endochondral ossification, they can grow into shapes that resemble the final bones even in the absence of bone formation. This is dramatically seen in mice that carry two inactivated alleles of the gene for the transcription factor CBFA1/RUNX2.[2,3] This factor is required for osteoblastic differentiation[1] and in mice without functional CBFA1 no osteoblasts are formed. In these mice, the cartilaginous anlagen are not ossified; yet they form a nearly complete "skeleton" of the correctly shaped elements, consisting entirely of cartilage. The patterning of the endochondral skeleton therefore depends on processes that regulate the spatial differentiation and growth of cartilage. In humans, heterozygosity for loss-of-function mutations in CBFA1/RUNX2 are associated with cleidocranial dysplasia.[6] Affected individuals exhibit short stature, hypoplasia/aplasia of the clavicle, hypoplasia of the pelvis, delayed ossification and closure of cranial sutures, and defects in tooth eruption and tooth number (supernumerary teeth in the permanent dentition).

REGULATION OF MESENCHYMAL CONDENSATION AND CHONDROCYTE DIFFERENTIATION IN THE AXIAL SKELETON

During the fourth week of human development, cells of the paraxial mesoderm condense to the segmented structures called somites on either side of the neural tube and the notochord (Fig. 1). Within the somites cells undergo transition from a mesenchymal to an epithelial phenotype, and this is followed by transition back to mesenchyme and migration of cells in the most ventral region of the somites into an area surrounding the notochord (Fig. 1). These cells form the sclerotomes.

Sclerotome cells differentiate into chondrocytes that form the anlagen of vertebral bodies. The notochord subsequently disappears within the vertebral bodies but remains as the nucleus pulposus within intervertebral discs. The neural arches of the vertebrae are formed by sclerotome cells that migrate dorsally around the neural tube, while sclerotome cells that migrate laterally form the rib anlagen in the thoracic region. In the anterior body wall, mesenchymal cell condensations on each side of the midline form the sternal anlagen. Cells within these condensations form two cartilaginous bars that later fuse into the sternum. Condensations above the sternum give rise to the manubrium and pairs of lateral condensations form the anterior cartilaginous portions of the ribs that are connected with the sternum.

The condensation, segmentation, and mesenchymal-epithelial transformation of paraxial mesoderm cells to somites is controlled in part by signaling between neigh-

Dr. Olsen has served as a consultant for Proskelia—an Aventis Pharma Subsidiary.

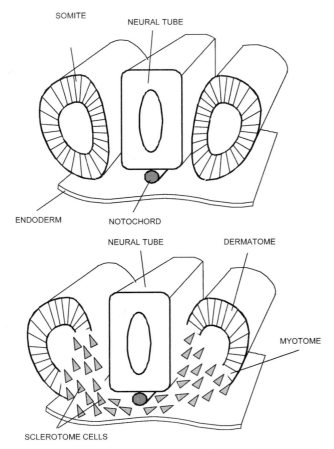

FIG. 1. Diagrams showing differentiation of somites in the trunk region of the embryo. (A) The ectoderm has been removed to reveal the somites adjacent to the neural tube. At this stage, the cells of the somites have an epithelial organization. (B) Later cells from the medial region of the somites migrate toward the notochord and form the sclerotomes. The remainder differentiate into dermatome (skin) and myotome (striated muscle). (Adapted with permission from Hogan B, Beddington R, Costantini F, Lacy E 1994 Manipulating the Mouse Embryo—A Laboratory Manual, 2nd ed. Cold Spring Harbor Laboratory Press, Cold Spring Harbor, MA, p.77.)

boring cells involving the cell surface receptor Notch1 and ligands that bind to it.[7,8] Notch1 is a large transmembrane protein with several repeated amino acid sequence domains. The ligands that bind to Notch1 and activate signaling pathways that are downstream of Notch1 are themselves transmembrane molecules with signaling potential.[9] The interactions between Notch1 and its ligands therefore require cell-cell contact. In mice carrying inactivated alleles for a mouse homolog of the Drosophila Notch ligand Delta,[10] and in mice with inactivated *Notch1* genes,[5] early defects in the condensation and patterning of somites lead to defects in the vertebral column. Also, genes that control the expression of Notch1 or are controlled by Notch1 have been shown to be important for early stages of vertebral column development.[11,12] In humans, loss-of-function mutations in the Notch ligand δ-like 3 (DLL3) cause the recessive form of spondylocostal dysostosis, characterized by short stature, vertebral abnormalities in the form of semivertebrae, and deletions and fusions of ribs.[13] Mutations resulting in haploinsufficiency of the Notch ligand Jagged 1 (JAG1) are

associated with Alagille syndrome.[14,15] Affected individuals have abnormally shaped vertebral bodies (butterfly vertebrae) and abnormalities of the liver, heart, eye, and facial structures.

Differentiation of cells within sclerotomes to cartilage-producing chondrocytes is also under complex regulation. A master regulator of sclerotome cell differentiation and therefore of vertebral column formation is the secreted cytokine sonic hedgehog.[16] Sonic hedgehog is produced by the notochord as a protein that undergoes proteolytic self-cleavage and gets a cholesterol residue attached before it becomes an active cytokine.[17,18] That its signaling activity is absolutely required for sclerotome differentiation is evident from the phenotype of mice that carry inactivated sonic hedgehog alleles.[19] Such mice develop without a vertebral column and the posterior portions of the ribs. They do, however, form a sternum and the anterior portions of ribs, the shoulder, and pelvic girdles, showing that the anlagen for those portions of the skeleton are not controlled by sonic hedgehog. Another important regulator is the transcription factor PAX1, which is, at least in part, induced by sonic hedgehog. A mutation in PAX1 in humans causes a neural tube defect,[20] and mutations in mice lead to defective sclerotome differentiation and abnormalities in the vertebral column.[21]

SKELETAL MORPHOGENESIS IN THE LIMB

Skeletal development in the limb starts with formation of limb buds, outgrowths of the lateral body wall, appearing early in the second month of human development as a result of proliferation of mesenchymal cells from the lateral plate mesoderm. A group of tall, specialized epithelial cells, called the apical ectodermal ridge (AER), caps the limb bud. As the limb bud grows and cartilage anlagen of future bones develop within it, the developing limb is patterned along three axes (Fig. 2): a proximal to

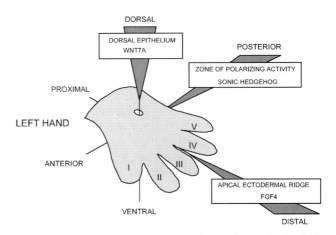

FIG. 2. Diagram showing the three axes of patterning for the developing (left) hand. Key regulatory molecules that play important roles in these patterning processes are indicated in the boxed areas under their cellular sources. Thus, the secreted molecule *Wnt7a* produced by dorsal epithelial cells is important for dorsal-ventral patterning; *sonic hedgehog*, produced by cells in the zone of polarizing activity, is important for establishing the pattern along the posterior-anterior axis; *FGF4* is one of the fibroblast growth factors produced by cells of the apical ectodermal ridge that control limb outgrowth and proximal-distal patterning.

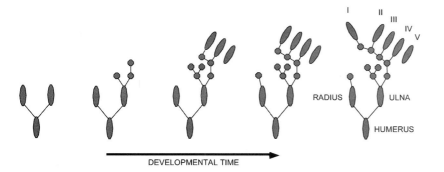

FIG. 3. Diagram showing branching and segmentation of mesenchymal condensations during limb development. As the limb bud grows (indicated by the horizontal arrow from left to right) the condensations develop in a distinct sequence to form the cartilage anlagen of the future bones (humerus, radius, ulna, carpal bones, and metacarpal bones for the five fingers (I-V).

distal axis, a dorsal to ventral axis, and a posterior to anterior axis.

Patterning along the proximal to distal axis is largely controlled by factors produced by the AER.[22] These include fibroblast growth factors that are important for stimulating proliferation and patterning of the underlying mesenchyme.[23,24] They are therefore essential for normal limb outgrowth. As the limb grows out, mesenchymal cells condense in the center to form the cartilage anlagen of the limb bones. The anlagen develop in a proximal to distal direction, and their development can be described as a series of bifurcations and segmentations that follow an axis along the humerus, through the ulna and the distal carpal (or tarsal in the foot) anlagen (Fig. 3).[25]

In the lower arm (leg) and hands (feet) the patterning of the anlagen from one side to the other is regulated by a cascade of signaling molecules and transcription factors. The most important of these include sonic hedgehog, secreted by a small group of cells (called the zone of polarizing activity) located at the posterior (ulnar) aspect of the developing limb bud, homeobox transcription factors, and members of the TGFβ-superfamily of signaling molecules.[26] How all these and many other molecules are working together as an orchestrated system to generate the normal limb skeletal pattern is not known in detail, but recent studies are rapidly filling in the missing pieces.

Mutations in many of these genes result in striking abnormalities in the limb skeleton. For example, mutations involving expansions of a polyalanine stretch in the transcription factor HOXD13 cause polysyndactyly (extra fingers) in humans[27]; other polysyndactyly syndromes have been shown to be caused by mutations in an intracellular, downstream target of sonic hedgehog signaling, a transcription factor called GLI3.[28,29] Mutations in a TGFβ-homolog (CDMP1) cause abnormal shortening of distal limb bones, perhaps as a result of a defect in formation of joints between bones.[30] Mutations in Noggin, an extracellular molecule that binds and inactivates CDMP1 and other members of the TGFβ superfamily of molecules, are associated with proximal symphalangism, characterized by fusion of proximal joints between digits and early onset conductive deafness, and multiple dysostoses syndrome, including fusion of multiple joints in hands and feet, elbows, and hips and of intervertebral joints.[31]

Several studies also provide insights into mechanisms that ensure patterning along the dorsal-ventral axis. As a consequence of such studies, the basis for the Nail-patella syndrome in humans, characterized by dysplasia of nails and absent or hypoplastic patellae, has been found to be mutations in a transcription factor called LMX1B.[32]

Molecules and signaling pathways controlling the formation of digits in hands and feet are rapidly being identified from studies of human brachydactylies, a group of disorders characterized by shortening of fingers and toes. Five different clinical subtypes of brachydactyly are recognized; heterozygous mutations in the cytokine Indian hedgehog (see below), receptor tyrosine kinase ROR2, and CDMP1 have been described in subtypes A1, B, and C, respectively.[30,33,34]

CHONDROCYTE PROLIFERATION AND DIFFERENTIATION IN GROWTH PLATES

During endochondral ossification, the cartilage anlagen are replaced by bone marrow and bone. In this process, epiphyseal growth plates are formed. A sequence of chondrocyte proliferation, differentiation to hypertrophy, and cell death (apoptosis) within growth plates results in longitudinal bone growth, and thus, the final steps in bone morphogenesis. Proliferation and differentiation of growth plate chondrocytes are controlled in several ways. An important brake on chondrocyte proliferation is local signaling through fibroblast growth factor (FGF; most likely Fgf18[35]) interaction with the cell surface tyrosine kinase receptor FGFR3. Activating mutations in FGFR3 cause decreased bone growth in achondroplasia and hypochondroplasia in humans.[36,37] The cytokine parathyroid hormone-related peptide (PTHrP) has an inhibitory effect on chondrocyte differentiation to hypertrophy,[38] and both activating and loss-of-function mutations in the PTHrP receptor (a cell-surface G-protein–coupled receptor) cause decreased bone growth and distinct forms of dwarfism due to either inhibition of chondrocyte hypertrophy (Jansen's metaphyseal chondrodysplasia) or accelerated chondrocyte hypertrophy (Blomstrand's chondrodysplasia) in growth plates.[39,40] Signaling from the PTHrP receptor involves an inhibitory effect on the expression of a secreted signaling molecule called Indian hedgehog.[38] Indian hedgehog is homologous to sonic hedgehog and acts on cells through the same type of receptor as sonic hedgehog. Indian hedgehog induces expression of PTHrP so the two molecules seem to be involved in a self-regulating feed-back loop within growth plates.[38] In addition, Indian hedgehog is a positive regulator of chondrocyte proliferation and induces (directly or indirectly) osteoblastic differentiation in the perichondrium (the bone collar) during endochondral ossification.[41]

Chondrocyte hypertrophy leads to the synthesis of an extracellular matrix that is significantly different from that of the rest of growth plate cartilage. This hypertrophic matrix is readily degraded and permits ingrowth of blood vessels and osteoblasts (in part because of CBFA1/RUNX2-dependent expression of vascular endothelial growth factor [VEGF] by hypertrophic chondrocytes[42]) from the underlying bone marrow. Loss-of-function mutations in collagen X, a unique extracellular matrix component made by hypertrophic chondrocytes,[43] cause a distinct form of dwarfism, Schmid type metaphyseal chondrodysplasia, in humans.[44]

REFERENCES

1. Ducy P, Zhang R, Geoffroy V, Ridall AL, Karsenty G 1997 Osf2/Cbfa1: A transcriptional activator of osteoblast differentiation. Cell **89:**747–754.
2. Otto F, Thornell AP, Crompton T, Denzel A, Gilmour KC, Rosewell IR, Stamp GW, Beddington RS, Mundlos S, Olsen BR, Selby PB, Owen MJ 1997 Cbfa1, a candidate gene for cleidocranial dysplasia syndrome, is essential for osteoblast differentiation and bone development. Cell **89:**765–771.
3. Komori T, Yagi H, Nomura S, Yamaguchi A, Sasaki K, Deguchi K, Shimizu Y, Bronson RT, Gao YH, Inada M, Sato M, Okamoto R, Kitamura Y, Yoshiki S, Kishimoto T 1997 Targeted disruption of Cbfa1 results in a complete lack of bone formation owing to maturational arrest of osteoblasts. Cell **89:**755–764.
4. Nakashima K, Zhou X, Kunkel G, Zhang Z, Deng JM, Behringer RR, de Crombrugghe B 2002 The novel zinc finger-containing transcription factor osterix is required for osteoblast differentiation and bone formation. Cell **108:**17–29.
5. Akiyama H, Chaboissier MC, Martin JF, Schedl A, de Crombrugghe B 2002 The transcription factor Sox9 has essential roles in successive steps of the chondrocyte differentiation pathway and is required for expression of Sox5 and Sox6. Genes Dev **16:**2813–2828.
6. Mundlos S, Otto F, Mundlos C, Mulliken JB, Aylsworth AS, Albright S, Lindhout D, Cole WG, Henn W, Knoll JHM, Owen MJ, Zabel BU, Mertelsmann R, Olsen BR 1997 Mutations involving the transcription factor CBFA1 cause cleidocranial dysplasia. Cell **89:**773–779.
7. Gossler A, Hrabe de Angelis M 1998 Somitogenesis. Curr Top Dev Biol **38:**225–287.
8. Conlon RA, Reaume AG, Rossant J 1995 Notch1 is required for the coordinate segmentation of somites. Development **121:**1533–1545.
9. Lendahl U 1998 A growing family of Notch ligands. Bioessays **20:**103–107.
10. Kusumi K, Sun ES, Kerrebrock AW, Bronson RT, Chi DC, Bulotsky MS, Spencer JB, Birren BW, Frankel WN, Lander ES 1998 The mouse pudgy mutation disrupts Delta homologue Dll3 and initiation of early somite boundaries. Nat Genet **19:**274–278.
11. Wong PC, Zheng H, Chen H, Becher MW, Sirinathsinghji DJ, Trumbauer ME, Chen HY, Price DL, Van der Ploeg LH, Sisodia SS 1997 Presenilin 1 is required for Notch1 and DII1 expression in the paraxial mesoderm. Nature **387:**288–292.
12. Saga Y, Hata N, Koseki H, Taketo MM 1997 Mesp2: A novel mouse gene expressed in the presegmented mesoderm and essential for segmentation initiation. Genes Dev **11:**1827–1839.
13. Bulman MP, Kusumi K, Frayling TM, McKeown C, Garrett C, Lander ES, Krumlauf R, Hattersley AT, Ellard S, Turnpenny PD 2000 Mutations in the human Delta homologue DLL3, cause axial skeletal defects in spondylocostal dysostosis. Nat Genet **24:**438–441.
14. Oda T, Elkahloun AG, Pike BL, Okajima K, Krantz ID, Genin A, Piccoli DA, Meltzer PS, Spinner NB, Collins FS, Chandrasekharappa SC 1997 Mutations in the human Jagged1 gene are responsible for Alagille syndrome. Nat Genet **16:**235–242.
15. Li L, Krantz ID, Deng Y, Genin A, Banta AB, Collins CC, Qi M, Trask BJ, Kuo WL, Cochran J, Costa T, Pierpont ME, Rand EB, Piccoli DA, Hood L, Spinner NB 1997 Alagille syndrome is caused by mutations in human Jagged1, which encodes a ligand for Notch1. Nat Genet **16:**243–251.
16. Johnson RL, Laufer E, Riddle RD, Tabin C 1994 Ectopic expression of Sonic hedgehog alters dorsal-ventral patterning of somites. Cell **79:**1165–1173.
17. Porter JA, von Kessler DP, Ekker SC, Young KE, Lee JJ, Moses K, Beachy PA 1995 The product of hedgehog autoproteolytic cleavage active in local and long-range signalling. Nature **374:**363–366.
18. Porter JA, Young KE, Beachy PA 1996 Cholesterol modification of hedgehog signaling proteins in animal development. Science **274:**255–259.
19. Chiang C, Litingtung Y, Lee E, Young KE, Corden JL, Westphal H, Beachy PA 1996 Cyclopia and defective axial patterning in mice lacking Sonic hedgehog gene function. Nature **383:**407–413.
20. Hol FA, Geurds MP, Chatkupt S, Shugart YY, Balling R, Schrander-Stumpel CT, Johnson WG, Hamel BC, Mariman EC 1996 PAX genes and human neural tube defects: An amino acid substitution in PAX1 in a patient with spina bifida. J Med Genet **33:**655–660.
21. Wilm B, Dahl E, Peters H, Balling R, Imai K 1998 Targeted disruption of Pax1 defines its null phenotype and proves haploinsufficiency. Proc Natl Acad Sci USA **95:**8692–8697.
22. Robertson KE, Tickle C 1997 Recent molecular advances in understanding vertebrate limb development. Br J Plast Surg **50:**109–115.
23. Niswander L, Jeffrey S, Martin GR, Tickle C 1994 A positive feedback loop coordinates growth and patterning in the vertebrate limb. Nature **317:**609–612.
24. Crossley PH, Minowada G, MacArthur CA, Martin GR 1996 Roles for FGF8 in the induction, initiation, and maintenance of chick limb development. Cell **84:**127–136.
25. Shubin NH, Alberch P 1986 A morphogenetic approach to the origin and basic organization of the tetrapod limb. Evol Biol **20:**319–387.
26. Johnson RL, Tabin CJ 1997 Molecular models for vertebrate limb development. Cell **90:**979–990.
27. Muragaki Y, Mundlos S, Upton J, Olsen BR 1996 Altered growth and branching patterns in synpolydactyly caused by mutations in HOXD13. Science **272:**548–551.
28. Wild A, Kalff-Suske M, Vortkamp A, Bornholdt D, Konig R, Grzeschik KH 1997 Point mutations in human GLI3 cause Greig syndrome. Hum Mol Genet **6:**1979–1984.
29. Kang S, Graham JM Jr, Olney AH, Biesecker LG 1997 GLI3 frameshift mutations cause autosomal dominant Pallister-Hall syndrome. Nat Genet **15:**266–268.
30. Polinkovsky A, Robin NH, Thomas JT, Irons M, Lynn A, Goodman FR, Reardon W, Kant SG, Brunner HG, van der Burgt I, Chitayat D, McGaughran J, Donnai D, Luyten FP, Warman ML 1997 Mutations in CDMP1 cause autosomal dominant brachydactyly type C. Nat Genet **17:**18–19.
31. Gong Y, Krakow D, Marcelino J, Wilkin D, Chitayat D, Babul-Hirji R, Hudgins L, Cremers CW, Cremers FP, Brunner HG, Reinker K, Rimoin DL, Cohn DH, Goodman FR, Reardon W, Patton M, Francomano CA, Warman ML 1999 Heterozygous mutations in the gene encoding noggin affect human joint morphogenesis. Nat Genet **21:**302–304.
32. Dreyer SD, Zhou G, Baldini A, Winterpacht A, Zabel B, Cole W, Johnson RL, Lee B 1998 Mutations in LMX1B cause abnormal skeletal patterning and renal dysplasia in nail patella syndrome. Nat Genet **19:**47–50.
33. McCready ME, Sweeney E, Fryer AE, Donnai D, Baig A, Racacho L, Warman ML, Hunter AG, Bulman DE 2002 A novel mutation in the IHH gene causes brachydactyly type A1: A 95- year-old mystery resolved. Hum Genet **111:**368–375.
34. Oldridge M, Fortuna AM, Maringa M, Propping P, Mansour S, Pollitt C, DeChiara TM, Kimble RB, Valenzuela DM, Yancopoulos GD, Wilkie AO 2000 Dominant mutations in ROR2, encoding an orphan receptor tyrosine kinase, cause brachydactyly type B. Nat Genet **24:**275–278.
35. Ohbayashi N, Shibayama M, Kurotaki Y, Imanishi M, Fujimori T, Itoh N, Takada S 2002 FGF18 is required for normal cell proliferation and differentiation during osteogenesis and chondrogenesis. Genes Dev **16:**870–879.
36. Shiang R, Thompson LM, Zhu YZ, Church DM, Fielder TJ, Bocian M, Winokur ST, Wasmuth JJ 1994 Mutations in the transmembrane domain of FGFR3 cause the most common genetic form of dwarfism, achondroplasia. Cell **78:**335–342.
37. Bellus GA, McIntosh I, Smith EA, Aylsworth AS, Kaitila I, Horton WA, Greenhaw GA, Hecht JT, Francomano CA 1995 A recurrent mutation in the tyrosine kinase domain of fibroblast growth factor receptor 3 causes hypochondroplasia. Nat Genet **10:**357–359.
38. Vortkamp A, Lee K, Lanske B, Segre GV, Kronenberg HM, Tabin CJ

1996 Regulation of rate of cartilage differentiation by Indian hedgehog and PTH-related protein. Science **273**:613–622.

39. Schipani E, Langman CB, Parfitt AM, Jensen GS, Kikuchi S, Kooh SW, Cole WG, Juppner H 1996 Constitutively activated receptors for parathyroid hormone and parathyroid hormone-related peptide in Jansen's metaphyseal chondrodysplasia. N Engl J Med **335**:708–714.

40. Jobert AS, Zhang P, Couvineau A, Bonaventure J, Roume J, Le Merrer M, Silve C 1998 Absence of functional receptors for parathyroid hormone and parathyroid hormone-related peptide in Blomstrand chondrodysplasia. J Clin Invest **102**:34–40.

41. Long F, Zhang XM, Karp S, Yang Y, McMahon AP 2001 Genetic manipulation of hedgehog signaling in the endochondral skeleton

reveals a direct role in the regulation of chondrocyte proliferation. Development **128**:5099–5108.

42. Zelzer E, Glotzer DJ, Hartmann C, Thomas D, Fukai N, Shay S, Olsen BRT 2001 Tissue specific regulation of VEGF expression by Cbfa1/Runx2 during bone development. Mech Dev **106**:97–106.

43. Linsenmayer TF, Eavey RD, Schmid TM 1988 Type X collagen: A hypertrophic cartilage-specific molecule. Pathol Immunopathol Res **7**:14–19.

44. Warman ML, Abbott MH, Apte SS, Hefferon T, McIntosh I, Cohn DH, Hecht JT, Olsen BR, Francomano CA 1993 A type X collagen mutation causes Schmid metaphyseal chondrodysplasia. Nat Genet **5**:79–82.

Chapter 3.   Bone Formation: Maturation and Functional Activities of Osteoblast Lineage Cells

Jane B. Lian,[1] Gary S. Stein,[1] and Jane E. Aubin[2]

[1]*Department of Cell Biology and Cancer Center, University of Massachusetts Medical School, Worcester, Massachusetts; and*
[2]*Department of Medical Genetics and Microbiology, University of Toronto, Toronto, Ontario, Canada*

INTRODUCTION

Bone is a dynamic connective tissue, comprised of an exquisite assembly of functionally distinct cell populations that are required to support the structural, biochemical, and mechanical integrity of bone and its central role in mineral homeostasis. The responsiveness of bone to mechanical forces and metabolic regulatory signals that accommodate requirements for maintaining the organ and connective tissue functions of bone are operative throughout life. As such, bone tissue undergoes remodeling, a continual process of resorption and renewal. The principal cells that mediate the bone forming processes of the mammalian skeleton are the following: *osteoprogenitor cells* that contribute to maintaining the osteoblast population and bone mass; *osteoblasts* that synthesize the bone matrix on bone forming surfaces; *osteocytes*, organized throughout the mineralized bone matrix that support bone structure; and the protective bone surface *lining cells* (Fig. 1). The fidelity of bone tissue structure and metabolic functions necessitates exchange of regulatory signals among these cell populations. Current concepts for understanding molecular and cellular mechanisms regulating the progression of osteoblast differentiation and functional activities of distinct cell populations will be presented with emphasis on the signaling pathways, regulatory proteins, and transcription factors that contribute to the maturation of osteoblast lineage cells. Within this context, a basis can be provided for improved diagnosis of skeletal disease and treatment that is targeted to specific cells in bone tissue.

DISTINCT AND INTERACTING REGULATORY PATHWAYS INFLUENCE OSTEOBLAST GROWTH AND DIFFERENTIATION

The progression of osteoblast maturation requires a sequential activation and suppression of genes that encode the phenotypic and functional proteins of the osteoblast populations. Signaling proteins, transcription factors, and regulatory proteins support the temporal expression of genes that characterize stages of osteoblast differentiation and bone formation (Figs. 2 and 3). Factors playing key roles in the growth, commitment, and differentiation of mesenchymal stem cells to the osteochondrogenic lineage and osteoblasts, as well as their functional activities and lifetime, have been identified by several approaches. These include expression studies in bone tissue by in situ analyses, functional studies using null mice lacking the gene and transgenic mouse models overexpressing proteins to reveal skeletal defects, and characterization of gene abnormalities in human skeletal disorders. Examples are shown in Table 1 for those genes affecting bone development and osteoblast differentiation.

Table 1 is organized by functional categories and includes specific proteins characterized in vivo for their effects on osteogenesis and osteoblast maturation. A spectrum of signaling factors that contribute to skeletogenesis, affecting osteoblast differentiation, include fibroblast growth factors (FGFs) and their receptors,[1,2] parathyroid hormone (PTH) and PTH-related protein (PTHrP) receptor, Indian hedgehog, the bone morphogenetic protein (BMP)/TGFβ superfamily, the Wnt pathway,[3] and members of the growth hormone(GH)/insulin-like growth factor (IGF)-1 axis; all provide the early developmental cues that indirectly mediate the initial cascade of gene expression for bone development and osteoblast differentiation. Specific Wnt pathway components with key roles in osteoblasts are being identified.[3] Identification of the human mutation activating LRP5, a Wnt co-receptor protein, as the high bone mass trait gene has intensified research in this area. BMP-2, BMP-4, and BMP-7 (also designated OP-1) are potent inducers of osteogenesis in vivo and in vitro.[4,5] Because of the early embryonic lethality of BMP null mutants, elucidation of their precise functions in osteoblastogenesis and bone formation is being approached through analysis of deficiencies and mutations of their receptors and intracellular SMAD

The authors have no conflict of interest.

© 2003 American Society for Bone and Mineral Research

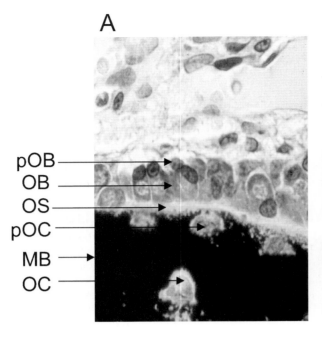

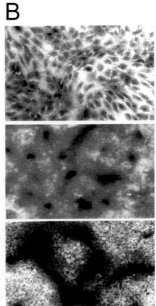

pOB
OB
OS
pOC
MB
OC

FIG. 1. Osteoblast differentiation (A) in vivo and (B) in vitro. (A) Cellular organization of bone formation: OP, osteoprogenitors; OB, osteoblasts; OS, osteoid; preOC, preosteocytes; MB, mineralized bone matrix; OC, osteocyte. (B) Recapitulation of osteoblast differentiation in cultured cells isolated from fetal rat calvarial bone. Proliferating osteoprogenitors (top), post-proliferative osteoblasts in nodules expressing alkaline phosphatase activity (middle), amd mineral deposition (von Kossa stain) of the ECM (bottom).

signaling components.[6] Novel BMP gene targets that will likely contribute to osteoblast maturation are also being identified through microarray gene profiling.[7–9]

How regulatory factors transduce their signals through intracellular pathways is now being facilitated from in vitro studies with specific pathway inhibitors and characterization of human disorders. These studies have demonstrated that the protein kinase C pathway mediates the bone anabolic effects of FGF and IGF,[10,11] while PTH mediates many of its effects in bone cells through protein kinase A.[12] Tyrosine kinases have been identified for their role in bone through study of null mouse models.[13,14] It is also important to recognize that many of these pathways are integrated through inductive signals and feedback loops for highly regulated control of osteogenesis. It should be emphasized that within osteoblast lineage cells, subpopulations can respond selectively to any of these physiologic signals. Studies show that osteoblasts from axial and appendicular bone exhibit different responses to physiologic, mechanical, and development cues (Table 1[15,16]). Whether this reflects the local, cellular, and tissue environment or inherent properties of the cells selected at an early stage during osteoblast differentiation remains to be determined. Subtle yet important differences may reflect selective responses of osteoblasts that relate to either homeostatic functions or the establishment and maintenance of bone structure.

Osteoprogenitor Cells: Provide for Bone Growth

Osteoprogenitor cells will arise under the appropriate stimulus from stem cells occurring in many tissues. Stem cells by definition have self-renewal capacity, generate cell lineages, and repopulate in a tissue environment.[17] The lack of unique identifying markers for the multipotential stem cells that give rise to a number of mesenchymal tissues including bone, fat, and cartilage has necessitated that their existence and presence be defined by a variety of pheno-

typic and functional or retrospective outcome assays. The bone marrow stroma contains cells with robust proliferative activity that will form single colonies (CFU-Fs). These are mesenchyme-derived stem cells (most commonly referred

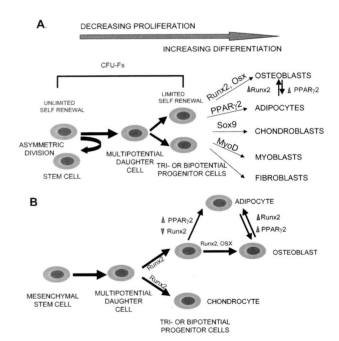

FIG. 2. Stem cell commitment to mesenchymal phenotypes. A schematic of stem cell commitment through either (A) a single step process or (B) a multistep hierarchical process with increasing lineage restriction to various end-stage mesenchymal cell types. Stem cells have unlimited self-renewal through asymmetric divisions with daughter cells assuming properties of a pluripotent progenitor cell (CFU-Fs). Some of the known transcription factors playing key regulatory roles in the mesenchymal lineages are indicated. Also depicted is apparent plasticity between osteoblasts and adipocytes.

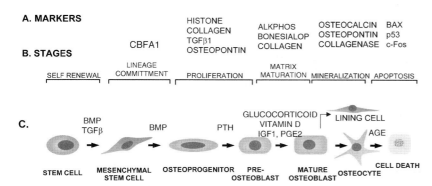

A. MARKERS

		HISTONE		ALKPHOS	OSTEOCALCIN	BAX
CBFA1		COLLAGEN		BONESIALOP	OSTEOPONTIN	p53
		TGFβ1		COLLAGEN	COLLAGENASE	c-Fos
		OSTEOPONTIN				

B. STAGES

| SELF RENEWAL | LINEAGE COMMITMENT | PROLIFERATION | MATRIX MATURATION | MINERALIZATION | APOPTOSIS |

C. STEM CELL — BMP TGFβ → MESENCHYMAL STEM CELL — BMP → OSTEOPROGENITOR — PTH → PRE-OSTEOBLAST — GLUCOCORTICOID VITAMIN D IGF1, PGE2 → MATURE OSTEOBLAST → LINING CELL / OSTEOCYTE — AGE → CELL DEATH

FIG. 3. Growth and differentiation of osteoblasts. Schematic illustration of (A) frequently used markers of (B) osteoblast maturation stages. (C) The bone morphogenetic proteins (BMP2/4/7) are required for lineage direction. At each stage of maturation, cells are responsive to steroid and polypeptide hormones that promote their further differentiation, as well as mediating their functional activities (e.g., PGE$_2$, IGF-1). Selected examples of regulatory factors are shown.

to as mesenchymal stem cells [MSCs]) and are distinguished from the hematopoietic stem cell lineage.

Postnatal bone marrow stroma contains cells that have both significant proliferative capacity and the capacity to form bone, cartilage, adipocytes, and fibrous tissue when transplanted in vivo in diffusion chambers.[18] All the tissues can arise from transplanted single colonies or colony forming units-fibroblasts (CFU-Fs).[19–21] The in vivo analyses of stromal cells have been augmented by functional assays in vitro that show formation of a range of differentiated cell phenotypes that includes not only osteoblasts, chondrocytes, and adipocytes, but also muscle cells, and have led many to identify stromal populations as MSCs or adult stem cells. What is already clear is that stromal populations grown in vitro under currently available protocols are heterogeneous with respect to differentiation capacity.[22,23] However, more studies remain to be done to address whether marrow stroma contains a classically defined stem cell, that is, a cell with unlimited self-renewal capacity and ability to repopulate all the appropriate differentiated lineages.[24] It is estimated that only a low percentage (15%) of all CFU-Fs have stem cell-like properties,[18,19] and only a proportion of CFU-Fs are bone colony-forming cells.[25,26] These data are consistent with the view that CFU-Fs belong to a lineage hierarchy in which only some of the cells are multipotential stem or primitive progenitors, while others have more limited differentiation capacity[27] (Fig. 2). Numerous studies using cell lines with various culture conditions have established a hierarchy of primitive progenitors, multipotential stem cells, or more restricted osteochondroprogenitors that differentiate into pre-osteoblasts.[28] Two different kinds of events have been proposed to underlie MSC commitment. The first is a non-random, single step process in which multipotential progenitors become restricted to a single mesenchymal lineage by culture conditions or particular environmental cues (e.g., soluble inducers, different substrates, and/or cell density; Fig. 2A). This is consistent with CFU-F heterogeneity with respect to phenotype and function, supporting a second model comprising a stochastic process with an expanding hierarchy of increasingly restricted progeny (Fig. 2B).

Identifying markers for isolation of stem cell populations has been challenging, particularly with the need for such cells in treating genetic disorders, tissue engineering, and reconstruction of bone tissue. Immunoselection and flow cytometry procedures have been applied for enrichment of osteoprogenitor lineage cells from whole marrow.[29,30] His-

torically, the STRO-1 antibody identified the CFU population in human bone marrow.[31,32] Other antibodies include SP-10, a monoclonal antibody generated from human MSCs, which detects marrow stromal cells and osteoprogenitors, but not mature osteoblasts.[33] SP-10 was later identified as an activated leukocyte cell adhesion molecule (ALCAM), which is the ligand for CD6 antigen present in lymphoid tissue.[34,35] The SH2 antibody, which immunoprecipitates CD105 (endoglin, TGFβ-3),[36] and the HOP-26 antibody, which recognizes CD-63, the cell surface lysosomal enzyme member of the tetraspan glycoprotein family,[37,38] also detect the more primitive cells of the osteogenic lineage, but are also present on nonosseous phenotypes. Thus, while a specific osteoprogenitor lineage marker has not been identified, these antibodies are useful for enriching osteoprogenitor populations from marrow and for monitoring phenotypic changes when such cell populations require manipulation in vitro before therapeutic applications. For MSC-based therapeutic applications, maintaining the undifferentiated stem-cell like properties is an important factor for engraftment and repopulation of a tissue by these cells in vivo,[39,40] as well as for maintained expression of infected gene constructs.

Commitment of MSCs to tissue-specific cell types is orchestrated by transcriptional regulators that serve as "master switches" (Fig. 2). The BMP2/4/7 proteins induce transcription factors that mediate commitment of early progenitors (stem-cell like) toward the osteogenic lineage. Potency of these factors is reflected by their ability to transdifferentiate to other phenotypes through forced expression of a transcriptional regulator, for example, by expressing either peroxisome proliferation-activated receptor γ2 (PPARγ2) or Runx2 in osteoblasts and adipocytes, respectively, their phenotype can be changed[41–44] (Fig. 2). Committed phenotypes from MSCs may dedifferentiate during proliferation and post-mitotically assume a different phenotype dependent on the local cellular environment.[45] In this manner, pericytes can also be induced into the osteogenic lineage.[46] Such observations and their cellular and molecular basis have led to considerable interest in the concept of "plasticity" of stromal and other adult stem and precursor cell types.[47–52] Among MSC progeny, precursor cells have been identified as bipotential adipocyte-osteoblast precursors.[53,54] It has been suggested that the inverse relationship sometimes seen between expression of the osteoblast and adipocytic phenotypes in marrow stroma (e.g., in osteoporosis) may reflect the ability of single or combinations of

Table 1. Regulatory Factors Supporting Bone Formation and Osteoblast Growth and Differentiation

Regulatory protein	Mouse/human defect	References
Developmental Factors: Regulate chondrocyte maturation for endochondral bone growth; promote stem cell and osteoprogenitor growth		
FGF R1	Pfeiffer syndrome	(196)
FGF R2} Effectors of cranio-facial development	Crouzon syndrome	(197,198)
FGF R3	Skeletal dysplasias, dwarfism	(199,200)
PTH/PTHrP-R	Mouse targeted inactivation: premature HC differentiation	(201,202)
	Mouse activating mutation: delays HC differentiation	(203)
	Jansen chondrodysplasia	(204)
Ihh	Null mouse: no bone collar	(180,205,206)
	Chimeric Ihh$^{-/-}$ and PTH/PTHrp$^{-/-}$ mice: studies define Ihh as a signal for osteoblast differentiation	
Signaling Proteins: Promote osteoblast differentiation; support phenotypic properties		
BMP2/4/7	Osteoinductive in numerous models	(6)
BMP3 (antagonist of BMPs)	Null mice: trabecular bone increased 2-fold	(207)
TGFβ	TGFβ2 targeted expression: increased OB differentiation, but low bone mass	(208)
	TGFβ3 binding protein null mouse: ectopic ossification in skull; older mice develop osteosclerosis and OA	(209)
Tob (inhibitor of BMP2/TGFβ signaling)	Null mice: Increased numbers of osteoblasts and bone formation rate	(210)
Noggin (BMP antagonist)	Null mice: joint fusion of the appendicular skeleton	(211)
	Transgenic mouse: osteopenia and fractures; impaired osteoblast function;	(212)
	misexpression in calvarium prevents suture fusion	(213)
C type natrinertic peptide (CNN)	Null mice: impaired endochondral ossification, dwarfism	(214)
PDGF-Rα	Patch mutant mice; targeted null mutation; apoptosis; attenuations due to ribs, vertebrae and sternum myotome formation	(215)
LRP5 (Wnt co-receptor)	Null mouse: osteopenia, similar to human osteoporosis-pseudoglioma syndrome	(216,217)
	Activating mutation: high bone mass trait	(218,219)
GH-R	Null mouse: decreased BMD in post-natal	(220)
Osteo-testicular Tyrosine Kinase	Null mouse: calcification defect in distal limbs	(221,222)
c-Src non receptor tyrosine kinase	Null mouse: osteopetrosis and accelerated osteoblast differentiation	(13,14)
Notch 1	Transmembrane protein stimulates osteoblast differentiation	(223)
IGF1-R	Osteoblast specific knock-out: decreased cancellous bone volume and mineralization	(224)
	Null mouse: decreased BF rate	(225)
	Double knockout IGF1/GH: decreased linear growth and ossification	(226)
IGF-BP1	Tg mouse: growth retardation, mineralization defect	(227)
Retinoic Acid Orphan Receptor (RORα)	Mouse mutant staggerer: thin bones; osteopenia	(228,229)
	Null mutant: defects in bone formation	(230)
	Human disorders: Brachydactly B and recessive Robinow syndrome	(228,231)
Cyclooxygenase 2	Null mouse: undifferentiated mesenchyme increased, reduced osteoblastogenesis	(232)
Homeobox Genes: Involved in pattern formation; stimulates growth of pre-osteoblasts; marks cells for apoptosis; mutations associated with craniofacial disorders; most often transcriptional repressors of osteoblast genes		
Hoxa-2	Tg mouse: inhibits intramembranous BF	(233)
Msx1	Null mutant: absence of teeth and alveolar bone	(234)
	Tg knock-in mouse: shows Msx1 involved in skeletal growth and remodeling	(140)
	Witkop Syndrome	(235)
Msx2	Loss of function: decreased parietal ossification	(236,237)
	Tg mouse: increased bone growth	(238)
	Gain of function human mutation: craniosynostosis	(238,239)
Dlx2	Null mouse: altered morphogenesis of proximal skeletal elements	(240)
Dlx5	Null mouse: delayed skull formation and endochondral ossification	(241,242)
Dlx5/6	Null mouse: craniofacial and limb abnormalities	(243,244)
	Split hand/foot malformations	
BAPX1	Null mouse: axial skeleton malformations	(245–247)

TABLE 1. (CONTINUED)

Regulatory protein	Mouse/human defect	References
Transcription Factors: General activators of gene expression; can also repress or attenuate transcription through interactions with co-regulatory proteins		
Twist (Helix-Loop-Helix proteins)	Saethe-Chotzen syndrome; important for skull development	(81,248–250)
Runx2/Cbfa1 (runt homology domain protein)	Null mouse: absence of bone	(146,251,252)
	Loss of function; C terminal mutation: absence of bone	(176)
	Cleidocranial dysplasia	(251–253)
	Promotes OB differentiation	(152,254)
Osterix (an SP 1-like family member)	Null mouse: absence of bone	(145)
ATF2 (activating transcription factor 2)	Null mouse: chondrodysplasia	(255)
	Role in osteoblasts	(256)
C/EBPβ, δ (CAAT enhancer binding protein)	Positive regulator of OB differentiation and OB specific genes	(144,257,258)
CREB (cAMP responsive element binding protein)	Dominant negative mutant: delayed endochondral bone development; dwarfisms	(259)
	Oasis; expressed in osteoblasts in vivo	(260)
p53	Regulates cell cycle and cell survival;	(261)
	Null mouse: similar to WT;	
	Mouse activating mutation: osteoporosis	(262)
p27	Cell cycle inhibitor	(88)
	Null mouse: larger size, increased osteoprogenitor numbers	
Activator Proteins: Members of the ZIP family; mediate growth factor and hormone responses; support both growth & differentiation; activation or repression of transcription dependent on heterodimer complex and target gene		
FOSB	Null mouse: normal BF	(263)
cFOS	Tg mouse: osteosarcoma	(264)
	Null mouse: osteopetrosis	(265,266)
Fra1	Tg mouse: osteosclerosis; OB proliferation and differentiation increased	(267)
ΔFOSβ, mutant protein lacking activator domain similar to Fra1	Tg: osteosclerosis independent of reduced adipogenesis	(268)
Adhesion Molecules: Involved in cell-cell and cell-matrix interactions to promote osteoblast differentiation; establish communication among osteoblast populations		
Integrin β1 (α1β1, α2β1, α3β1)	Tg mouse: dominant negative-β1 in osteoblasts reduced bone mass	(269)
Integrin α5β1 Selective FN receptor	Blocking antibodies impair osteoblast differentiation and lead to osteoblast apoptosis	(270,271)
Periostin	Expressed in osteoprogenitor cells; promotes cell motility; associated with bone metastasis	(272,273)
Ig Superfamily	N-CAM: expressed during osteogenesis; may mediate osteoblast differentiation	(34,274,275)
	AL-CAM: antigen for SB-10, an osteoprogenitor marker	(33)
Galectin 3	Null mouse: reduced number of HC, apoptosis in the chondrovascular junction	(276)
	Expression regulated by Runx2 in osteoprogenitors	(151)
Cadherins	Cad 11 null mouse; reduced calcification and bone density	(277)
	N-cadherin dominant negative mutant in vitro: inhibits OB differentiation	(278)
Connexin 43	Null mouse: skeletal malformations, delayed mineralization, osteoblast differentiation	(117)
Others		
Pleiotrophin/OSF-1, a heparin binding protein	Tg mice: Increased intramembranous BF and continual growth rate; encroachment of subchondral bone into articular cartilage	(77,279,280)
	In vitro induction of osteoprogenitor migration, growth and differentiation	(77)
Alkaline phosphatase, membrane bound enzyme	Null mice: rachitic bone, osteopenia, fractures	(281,282)
	Infantile hypophosphatasia	(283)
Sca-1	Null mice: normal development	(75)
	Aging mice: osteoporosis	
OF45 (MEPE), a bone specific ECM	Null mice: increased bone mass and osteoblast number; resistant to age-associated bone loss	(284)

Abbreviations: BMD, bone mineral density; BF, bone formation; Tg, transgenic mouse; HC, hypertrophic chondrocytes; OA, osteoarthritis; CAM, cell adhesion molecules.

agents to alter the commitment or at least the differentiation pathway these bipotential cells will transit.[54,55] In some cases, individual colonies are seen in which both osteoblast and adipocyte markers are present simultaneously.[56] However, whether a clearly distinguishable bipotential adipo-osteoprogenitor exists or other developmental paradigms such as plasticity or transdifferentiation underlie expression in these two and the other mesenchymal lineages needs to be further analyzed. Recent reports indicate that at least some of what has been heralded as intrinsic plasticity may actually reflect fusion of donor and recipient cells.[57–61]

The issue of stem cells in the adult organism (adult stem cells) is currently receiving enormous attention for most lineages, including those of the skeleton. However, most studies have not addressed or demonstrated whether a single tissue-specific stem cell differentiates into functional cells of multiple tissues.[62] Multipotent adult progenitor cells (MAPCs), which copurify with MSCs, have extremely high proliferative capacity in vitro and differentiate, at the single cell level, not only into mesenchymal cells,[63,64] but also into cells with visceral mesoderm, neuroectoderm, and endoderm characteristics in vitro. Single MAPCs in vivo contribute to most, if not all, somatic cell types.[64] Cells with features similar to adult bone marrow MSCs have also been isolated from adult peripheral blood,[65,66] fetal cord blood,[67] fetal liver, blood, and bone marrow,[68] and tooth pulp.[69,70] Muscle satellite cells have also recently been found to be multipotential, undergoing myogenic, osteogenic, and adipogenic differentiation in vitro.[71] Cells with MSC-like properties, including capacity for osteo-chondrogenic differentiation in vitro, have also been isolated from extramedullary adipose tissue,[72,73] including the inguinal fat pad.[74] The relationship of these cells to each other developmentally, phenotypically, and functionally must be investigated further, but the fact that seemingly diverse populations of cells exist with apparently similar regenerative and developmental potential is important for development of cell and gene therapy approaches in the skeleton.

Factors maintaining the undifferentiated state of osteoprogenitors are being characterized and allow for approaches to expand a potential mesenchymal stem cell and osteoprogenitor population. Among these factors includes leukemia inhibitory factor (LIF), a cytokine that will stimulate osteoprogenitor growth only in low-density undifferentiated adherence to normal cells. Sca-1/LY-6A has recently been identified as being required for self-renewal of mesenchymal progenitor cells,[75] and interleukin-18 has been characterized as a mitogen for both osteogenic and chondrogenic cells.[76] In general, factors promoting proliferation of the MSC will be inhibitory to the final differentiation stages. Other factors such as osteoblast stimulating factor-1/pleiotrophin[77] are chemotactic for osteoprogenitors and will stimulate colony formation increasing representation of phenotypically alkaline phosphatase positive cells. IGF-1 has been reported to stimulate proliferation only in MSCs,[78] as well as osteoblast differentiation markers in osteoblasts. The connective tissue growth factor[79] also functions in stimulating cell proliferation, as well as differentiation. Of clinical significance, inactivation of Menin-1, the product of the multiple endocrine neoplasia type-I genes, has been shown to inhibit the commitment of pluripotent mesenchymal stem cells to the osteoblast lineage.[80] Finally, transcriptional regulators, such as members of helix-loop-helix (HLH) family, have been proposed as mediators in maintaining the osteoprogenitor population.[81] The bone microenvironment supports continued growth and differentiation of osteoblasts lineage cells by extracellular matrix (ECM) accumulation of circulating and osteoblast synthesized cytokines, growth factors, non-collagenous proteins, and other molecules that cooperatively function to recruit progenitor cells and induce their maturation.

Osteoblasts: Synthesize the Bone Matrix

Committed preosteoblasts in a nondividing state are recognizable near the bone by their proximity to surface osteoblasts and by histochemical detection of alkaline phosphatase enzyme activity, one of the earliest markers of the osteoblast phenotype. The active osteoblast distinguishes itself on the bone surface by its morphological and ultra-structural properties, which are typical of a cell engaged in secretion of a connective tissue matrix, having a large nucleus, enlarged Golgi, and extensive endoplasmic reticulum. The osteoblast is highly enriched in alkaline phosphatase and vectorially secretes type I collagen and specialized bone matrix proteins as unmineralized osteoid toward the bone-forming front. On quiescent bone surfaces, single layers of flattened osteoblasts or bone lining cells are observed. These inactive lining cells form either the endosteum separating bone from the marrow or they underlie the periosteum directly on the mineralized surfaces.

The osteoblasts and lining cells are in close contact with each other, joined by adhering junctions. Cadherins are calcium-dependent transmembrane proteins that are an integral part of the adherence junctions and together with tight junctions and desmosomes join cells by anchorage through their cytoskeleton. The changes in relative abundance of the different cadherins in mesenchymal cells seems to define their differentiation pathway.[82] Major cadherins expressed in osteoblasts include N-cadherin and caderin-11, which are critical for embryonic limb development (Table 1). N-cadherin is important for cell-cell adhesion mediated by BMP2,[83] promoting differentiation of the early osteoprogenitor and osteoblast survival.[84]

Bone matrix synthesis by the osteoblast supports both cell-cell and cell-matrix interactions that are mediated by transmembrane proteins (e.g., Notch-1; Table 1) and several classes of adhesion proteins (Table 1 and reviewed in ref. 85). Integrins, which couple the extracellular matrix to the cytoskeleton's structural proteins, mediate signals to modulate cell differentiation, cytoskeletal organization, cell adhesion, cell shape change, and cell spreading. The $\beta 1$ integrins ($\alpha 1 \beta 1$, $\alpha 1 \beta 2$, $\alpha 3 \beta 1$, $\alpha 2 \beta 1$) play key roles in early bone development and during osteoblast differentiation by binding various collagens and inducing signals that lead to expression of osteoblast phenotypic genes. Osteoblast differentiation is accelerated by interaction of the type I collagen matrix with $\alpha 1 \beta 1$ or $\alpha 2 \beta 1$ integrins, which activate the MAPK signaling pathway. This intracellular pathway is emerging as a key regulator of osteoblast differentiation. Of significance, α1 integrin increases expression of the Cbfa1/ Runx2, a transcription factor essential for osteogenesis, and the MAPK pathway phosphorylates Runx2 and induces its activity.[86] Thus, multiple signaling pathways converge to regulate osteoblast differentiation.

The temporal expression of proteins involved in extracellular matrix biosynthesis and matrix mineralization provides a panel of osteoblast phenotypic markers that reflect stages of osteoblast differentiation (Fig. 3). Based on bone nodule formation in vitro, the process has been subdivided into three stages: (1) proliferation, (2) extracellular matrix development and maturation, and (3) mineralization, with characteristic changes in gene expression at each stage; some apoptosis can also be seen in mature nodules. In many studies, it has been found that genes associated with proliferative stages (e.g., histones, proto-oncogenes such as c-*fos* and c-*myc*) characterize the first phase, while certain cyclins (e.g., cyclins B and E) are upregulated postproliferatively.[87] Cell cycle inhibitors, such as p27 and p21, promote osteochondroprogenitor cell differentiation.[88,89] Expression of the most frequently assayed osteoblast-associated genes collagen type I (COLLI), alkaline phosphatase (ALP), osteopontin (OPN), osteocalcin (OCN), bone sialoprotein (BSP), and PTH/PTHrP receptor (PTH1R) is asynchronously upregulated, acquired, and/or lost as the progenitor cells differentiate and matrix matures and mineralizes.[27,87] In general, ALP increases then decreases when mineralization is well progressed; OPN peaks twice, during proliferation and then again later but before certain other matrix proteins including BSP and OCN; BSP is transiently expressed very early and then upregulated again in differentiated osteoblasts forming bone; and OCN appears approximately concomitantly with mineralization.[27]

The developmental sequence of gene expression observed by in vitro osteoblasts can be visualized at the single cell level in bone tissue by in situ methods.[90,91] When the preosteoblast ceases to proliferate, a key signaling event occurs for development of the large cuboidal differentiated osteoblast on the bone surface from the spindle shaped osteoprogenitor. Synthesis of the ECM contributes to cessation of cell growth leading to a "matrix maturation" stage when induced expression of ALP and specialized bone proteins renders the ECM competent for mineral deposition. Mineralization results in upregulated expression of several non-collagenous enriched proteins, thereby providing markers of the mature osteoblast (e.g., OCN, OPN, BSP). These calcium and phosphate binding proteins may function in regulating the ordered deposition of mineral, amount of the hydroxyapatite crystals, or crystal size. High throughput screening analyses and microarray gene profiling approaches are identifying an increasing number of regulatory factors and signature genes for specific stages of osteoblast maturation.[7,92,93] While Fig. 3 presents only three major stages of maturation, additional stages of maturation are becoming apparent with newer methodologies.[94] Furthermore, variations in levels of gene products are observed dependent on the maturation of the cell and reflected by its location in bone tissue.[90]

There is growing evidence from both in vitro and in vivo observations that somewhat different gene expression profiles for both proliferation and differentiation regulatory markers may underlie developmental and maturational events among osteoblasts.[90,95] It has been evident for some time that not all osteoblasts associated with bone nodules in vitro are identical.[96–99] That extensive diversity in expressed gene repertoires is not a consequence or an artifact of the in vitro environment. This has been confirmed by analysis of osteoblastic cells in vivo where individual osteoblasts differentially express various osteoblast-associated molecules at both mRNA and protein levels.[90,100–103] The observed differences in mRNA and protein expression repertoires in different osteoblasts may contribute to the heterogeneity in trabecular microarchitecture seen at different skeletal sites,[104] to site-specific differences in disease manifestation such as seen in osteoporosis[105,106] and to regional variations in the ability of osteoblasts to respond to therapeutic agents.

Osteocytes: Mechanotransduction Properties Support Bone Structure and Function

The osteocyte is the terminal differentiation stage of the osteoblast supporting bone structure and metabolic functions. Osteocytes develop by forming numerous cytoplasmic connections with adjacent cells to ensure their viability as the mineralizing osteoid renders the ECM impermeable. A distinguishing morphological feature of osteocytes is the location of each osteocyte in a lacunae and the numerous cellular extensions of filapodial processes that lie in canaliculi. The osteocyte, when isolated directly from bone tissue, retains this morphologic feature in vitro.[107–110] In bone, it appears negative for ALP, but produce large amounts of OCN,[111] galectin-3,[29] and CD44, a cell adhesion receptor for hyaluronate and several bone matrix proteins that may be involved in cellular extensions.[112–114] Osteocytes have the capacity to synthesize certain matrix molecules to support cellular adhesive properties and regulate the deposition of mineral to maintain the necessary surrounding barrier of bone fluid in their lacunae and canalicular network for diffusion of physiological elements. They also function in osteolysis and contain lysosomal vacuoles and other features of phagocytic cells.

Osteocytes within the mineralized matrix are in direct communication with each other and surface osteoblasts through their cellular processes. They form a continuum by connection at the tip of their cell processes through gap junctions. Connexins are the integral membrane proteins that form the gap junctions between cells to allow direct communications through intercellular channels. Osteocytes are metabolically and electrically coupled through gap junction protein complexes principally comprised of Connexin 43[115] (Table 1). Gap junction formation is essential for osteocyte maturation, activity, and survival.[116,117] The primary function of the osteoblast (or lining cell)–osteocyte continuum is considered to be mechanosensory, by transducing stress signals (stretching, bending) to biological activity. The flow of extracellular fluid in response to mechanical forces throughout the canalicular induces a spectrum of cellular responses in osteocytes.[107] Rapid fluxes of bone calcium across these junctions are thought to facilitate transmission of information between osteoblasts on the bone surface and osteocytes within the structure of bone itself.[118,119] Signaling pathways mediating the mechanotransducing properties of osteocytes from the extracellular matrix through the cytoskeleton and finally to the nucleus to modulate gene transcription are beginning to be characterized. They involve prostaglandin (PGE_2) and cyclooxygenase 2, kinases, Cbfa1/Runx2, and nitrous oxide–mediated responsiveness of the bone to systemic factors and mechanical forces.[120–123]

Osteocytes can reside for long periods, even decades, in healthy bone that is not turned over. In aging bone, empty lacunae are observed, suggesting osteocytes may undergo apoptosis.[124,125] Disruption of intercellular communication systems, as gap junctions or cell-matrix interactions, will lead to apoptosis and nonviable bone that will be resorbed. Apoptosis or programmed cell death is important for skeletal development, as well as the growth and maintenance of bone tissue. The timely apoptosis of mesenchymal cells is required for digit formation, and apoptosis of hypertrophic chondrocytes is necessary for endochondral bone formation, while osteoclast apoptosis is one control mechanism for the regulation of bone resorption. However, osteocyte apoptosis may be deleterious to bone structure. In vivo quantitation of apoptotic cells in the mouse and mouse models of accelerated aging and osteopenic bone induced by ovariectomy or glucocorticoid treatment confirm that programmed cell death contributes to active bone loss.[126–128] Recently, bisphosphonates, which inhibit bone resorption and are used to treat osteoporosis, have been found to inhibit osteoblast and osteocyte apoptosis.[129] Importantly, mechanical loading of bone in a physiologic range in the rat reduces osteocyte apoptosis.[130] In summary, the organization of osteocytes in direct contact with osteoblasts or surface lining cells is consistent with the concept that bone cells support bone structure and responses to physiological signals and can communicate their responses for bone formation and resorption.

Transcriptional Mechanisms Control Osteoblastogenesis

Many classes of DNA binding proteins have been shown to regulate the transcription and required expression levels of bone phenotypic genes during the development of bone tissue. For example, steroid receptors, the homeodomain proteins (Msx-2, Dlx-2, Dlx-5, BAPX1), and classes of other transcription factors shown in Table 1 are among the early regulators of transcription in osteoprogenitors. Transcription factors further interact with coregulatory proteins that can provide the necessary control for either activating or repressing gene expression dependent on the maturation stage of the osteoblasts or its physiologic responsiveness at a particular bone site.[131–133] Knowledge of these regulatory factors provides a basis for understanding bone-related disorders. A recent example is how the osteopenia associated with diabetes results from inadequate expression of bone-related transcriptional regulators.[134]

The developmental expression levels of transcription factors during osteoblast maturation reflects their roles as key determinants of osteoblast differentiation. The HLH proteins (Id, Twist, Dermo), are expressed at peak levels in proliferating progenitor cells and important for expansion of osteoprogenitors. HLH proteins repress genes representing the mature bone phenotype and are negative regulators of osteoblast differentiation. They must be downregulated for osteoblast differentiation to proceed.[135,136] Among the family of activating proteins (AP) that form complexes at AP-1 recognition sites, c-fos is expressed in osteoprogenitor cells and periosteal tissues, and if overexpressed, will result in osteosarcomas. C-fos is not detected in mature osteoblasts,[137] whereas fra-2 is abundant and increases expression of bone specific genes.[138] The homeodomain class of transcription factors comprise critical determinants of craniofacial and limb development (Table 1). During bone formation in vivo and osteoblast differentiation in vitro, Msx-2 is expressed maximally in the mesenchymal/osteoprogenitor population and subsequently downregulated in the mature bone forming cells.[139] Msx-1 must be turned off in periosteal progenitors for progression of osteoblast differentiation in vivo.[140] In vitro, Dlx-5 appears in the postproliferative osteoblast and increases during mineralization.[141] Relatively few of the homeodomain proteins and other critical regulators of the early stage of skeletal formation (e.g., see in Table 1 the δ-like3 gene) have been studied directly in osteoblasts.

The runt homology domain Runx2/Cbfa1/AML3/PEBPα1 and the zinc finger protein Osterix, C/EBPβ, C/EBPδ, and others that exhibit increased mRNA protein or DNA binding activity during osteoblast differentiation are actively contributing to the differentiation process through activation of genes expressed in mature osteoblasts.[142–147] Requirements for Runx2 and Osterix in bone formation have been demonstrated by the inhibition of bone tissue formation and perinatal lethality in null mouse mutants. Runx2 is also important for chondrocyte maturation to the hypertrophic phenotype, mineralization of the cartilage,[148] endothelial cell migration,[149] and for vascular invasion, directly upregulating vascular endothelial growth factor.[150] Runx2 target genes include those contributing not only to bone formation (osteocalcin, osteopontin, bone sialoprotein, galectin, TGFB receptor I, and dentin sialophosphoprotein-1),[143,151–155] but to bone turnover also (collagenase 3, osteoprotegrin, and RANKL).[156–158] Because Runx2 expression occurs earlier than Osterix (i.e., it is unaltered in Osterix$^{-/-}$ mice), these two factors may represent a temporal sequence of regulation essential for the final stages of osteoblast differentiation and bone formation.[145] Indeed, studies in transgenic mice overexpressing Runx2 in osteoblasts or chondrocytes exhibit osteoblast maturational defects, osteopenia, and fractures, indicating that Runx2 expression levels may be more important for induction of the bone phenotype and must be tightly controlled in mature osteoblasts.[159]

Runx2 has been studied extensively and new paradigms have been established for understanding its properties as a master gene switch.[160] Runx2 will induce the osteoblast phenotype in nonosseous progenitor cells and can convert an adipocyte into a cell expressing bone-related genes.[161] Runx2 interacts with numerous coregulatory proteins for gene activation and repression including factors that remodel chromatin and integrate key signaling pathways for osteogenesis.[132,162,163] These coregulators include CBFβ1, which increases DNA binding (see Table 1),[164,165] histone deacetylases,[166] the Wnt pathway regulator LEF-1,[167] AP-1 factors,[168,169] TGFβ/BMP responsive SMAD proteins,[170–172] FGF/PKC,[173] the cSrc responsive proteins, YAP,[174] and the WW domain protein TAZ.[175] A key property of Runx factors is a specific nuclear matrix signal that targets Runx2 to subnuclear domains, facilitating the formation of mulitmeric complexes with Runx2 partner proteins. Abrogation of this targeting function and interactions with coregulatory proteins result in severe bone abnormalities in the mouse[176] and accounts for several of the cleidocranial dysplasia disorders (CCD) variants.[177,178] The central role of Runx2 in regulating bone formation and turnover is becoming more evident as an increasing number of target genes are discovered, and its increased functional activity in response to developmental, hormonal, and mechanical signals better understood.

Hormonal Regulation of Osteoblast Differentiation

Steroid and polypeptide hormones contribute to the growth of osteoprogenitors and/or their progression to mature osteoblasts. PTH stimulates growth of osteoprogenitor populations, while PTHrP functions as a local cytokine regulating cell growth for differentiation during development.[179] Numerous mouse genetic models (Table 1) have defined the role of this pathway, integrated with other developmental regulators, such as Indian hedgehog (IHH), in the control of chondrocyte proliferation and maturation for endochondral bone formation and osteoblast differentiation.[180] Glucocorticoids promote the differentiation of human and rat marrow mesenchymal cells to osteoblasts in vitro, but when used therapeutically, they can have negative effects on bone formation and can contribute to osteoporosis by inducing cell apoptosis.[181–183] Vitamin D [1,25(OH)$_2$D$_3$] is a potent regulator of gene transcription, increasing or decreasing expression of numerous osteoblasts phenotypic genes that are consistent with more differentiated osteoblasts, (e.g., enhanced osteocalcin synthesis).[184] The sex steroids have anabolic effects on bone and osteoblasts. Retinoic acid has a well-established role in skeletal development of the embryo; recently, an orphan receptor for retinoic acid has been recognized for contributing to bone formation in the postnatal mouse (Table 1). Andrenomedullin increases cellular proliferation in cultured calvariae, suggesting stimulated osteoblast growth.[185] Leptin is secreted largely by adipose tissue but also by human osteoblasts at the mineralization stage.[186,187] It was characterized as a systemic factor that could contribute to decreased bone mass in a null mouse model acting through the hypothalamus.[188,189] More recent studies show exogenously added leptin has anabolic effects on osteoblasts and stromal cells promoting their differentiation in vitro[186,190] and in vivo.[191] Furthermore, positive correlations between circulating leptin levels and bone mineral density (BMD) in postmenopausal and nonobese women have been reported.[192] However, leptin was also found to induce apoptosis in human bone marrow stromal cells.[193] It is thus apparent that leptin is an important regulator of bone cell function but seems to control bone growth and osteoblast activities through several distinct mechanisms.[194,195]

Functional Activities of Osteoblast Lineage Cells

The functional properties and regulated activity of bone cells evolve during progression of osteoblast differentiation. As described above, they form the structural components of bone, producing a mineralized matrix and a cellular syncytium to respond to physiologic and mechanical demands on the skeleton. An equally important function of osteoblasts, the pre-osteoblasts that lie in close proximity, and osteocytes is their responsiveness to endocrine factors and the production of paracrine and autocrine factors for the recruitment of osteoprogenitors, the growth of preosteoblasts, and the regulation of osteoclastic resorption of the mineralized bone matrix.

The bone microenvironment seems to be essential for two components of osteoclastogenesis: (1) maturation and fusion of the mononuclear precursor to the multinucleated osteoclast and (2) activation and regulation of the activity of the functional osteoclast. The requirement for stromal osteoprogenitors or osteoblasts in mediating osteoclast differentiation is linked to the role of osteotrophic hormones and cytokines in regulating development of pre-osteoclasts and the multinucleated phenotype. Osteoblast lineage cells secrete osteoprotegerin, a soluble inhibitor of osteoclastogenesis and have receptors for RANKL, PTH, and 1,25(OH)$_2$D$_3$, which will promote osteoclast activity and bone turnover. Osteoblasts are the major source of the colony-stimulating factor 1 (CSF1) and also secrete some cytokines, which participate in osteoclastogenesis. Prostaglandins produced by bone cells, a potent stimulator of bone formation, as well as resorption, exemplifies the complexity of cellular responses in bone. The regulation of bone resorption and coupling of osteoblast and osteoclast activities is detailed elsewhere.

REFERENCES

1. Ornitz DM, Marie PJ 2002 FGF signaling pathways in endochondral and intramembranous bone development and human genetic disease. Genes Dev **16**:1446–1465.
2. Iseki S, Wilkie AO, Morriss-Kay GM 1999 Fgfr1 and Fgfr2 have distinct differentiation- and proliferation-related roles in the developing mouse skull vault. Development **126**:5611–5620.
3. Moon RT, Bowerman B, Boutros M, Perrimon N 2002 The promise and perils of Wnt signaling through beta-catenin. Science **296**:1644–1646.
4. Hoffmann A, Gross G 2001 BMP signaling pathways in cartilage and bone formation. Crit Rev Eukaryot Gene Expr **11**:23–45.
5. Ebara S, Nakayama K 2002 Mechanism for the action of bone morphogenetic proteins and regulation of their activity. Spine **27**:S10–S15.
6. Goumans MJ, Mummery C 2000 Functional analysis of the TGF beta receptor/Smad pathway through gene ablation in mice. Int J Dev Biol **44**:253–265.
7. Harris SE, Harris MA 2001 Gene expression profiling in osteoblast biology: Bioinformatic tools. Mol Biol Rep **28**:139–156.
8. Vaes BLT, Dechering KJ, Feijen A, Hendriks JMA, Lefevre C, Mummery C, Olijve W, Van zoelen EJ, Steegenga WT 2002 Comprehensive microarray analysis of bone morphogenetic protein 2-induced osteoblast differentiation resulting in the identification of novel markers for bone development. J Bone Miner Res **17**:2106–2118.
9. Balint E, Lapointe D, Drissi H, Van Der Meijden C, Young DW, Van Wijnen AJ, Stein JL, Stein GS, Lian JB 2003 Phenotype discovery by gene expression profiling: Mapping of biological processes linked to BMP-2-mediated osteoblast differentiation. J Cell Biochem **89**:401–426.
10. Kim HJ, Kim JH, Bae SC, Choi JY, Kim HJ, Ryoo HM 2003 The

protein kinase C pathway plays a central role in the fibroblast growth factor-stimulated expression and transactivation activity of Runx2. J Biol Chem **278:**319–326.

11. McCarthy TL, Ji C, Casinghino S, Centrella M 1998 Alternate signaling pathways selectively regulate binding of insulin-like growth factor I and II on fetal rat bone cells. J Cell Biochem **68:**446–456.

12. Swarthout JT, D'Alonzo RC, Selvamurugan N, Partridge NC 2002 Parathyroid hormone-dependent signaling pathways regulating genes in bone cells. Gene **282:**1–17.

13. Soriano P, Montgomery C, Geske R, Bradley A 1991 Targeted disruption of the c-src proto-oncogene leads to osteopetrosis in mice. Cell **64:**693–702.

14. Marzia M, Sims NA, Voit S, Migliaccio S, Taranta A, Bernardini S, Faraggiana T, Yoneda T, Mundy GR, Boyce BF, Baron R, Teti A 2000 Decreased c-Src expression enhances osteoblast differentiation and bone formation. J Cell Biol **151:**311–320.

15. Stein MS, Packham DK, Wark JD, Becker GJ 1999 Response to parathyroidectomy at the axial and appendicular skeleton in renal patients. Clin Nephrol **52:**172–178.

16. Suwanwalaikorn S, van Auken M, Kang MI, Alex S, Braverman LE, Baran DT 1997 Site selectivity of osteoblast gene expression response to thyroid hormone localized by in situ hybridization. Am J Physiol **272:**E212–E217.

17. Caplan AI 1991 Mesenchymal stem cells. J Orthop Res **9:**641–650.

18. Friedenstein AJ 1980 Stromal mechanisms of bone marrow: Cloning in vitro and retransplantation in vivo. Haematol Blood Transfus **25:**19–29.

19. Friedenstein AJ 1990 Osteogenic stem cells in the bone marrow. In: Heersche JNM, Kanis JA (eds.) Bone and Mineral Research, 7th ed. Elsevier Science Publishers B. V. (Biomedical Division), New York, NY, USA, pp. 243–270.

20. Bianco P, Riminucci M, Kuznetsov S, Robey PG 1999 Multipotential cells in the bone marrow stroma: Regulation in the context of organ physiology. Crit Rev Eukaryot Gene Expr **9:**159–173.

21. Owen ME 1998 The marrow stromal cell system. In: Beresford JN, Owen ME (eds.) Marrow Stromal Stem Cells in Culture. Cambridge University Press, Cambridge, UK, pp. 88–110.

22. Kuznetsov SA, Krebsbach PH, Satomura K, Kerr J, Riminucci M, Benayahu D, Robey PG 1997 Single-colony derived strains of human marrow stromal fibroblasts form bone after transplantation in vivo. J Bone Miner Res **12:**1335–1347.

23. Pittenger MF, Mackay AM, Beck SC, Jaiswal RK, Douglas R, Mosca JD, Moorman MA, Simonetti DW, Craig S, Marshak DR 1999 Multilineage potential of adult human mesenchymal stem cells. Science **284:**143–147.

24. Morrison SJ, Shah NM, Anderson DJ 1997 Regulatory mechanisms in stem cell biology. Cell **88:**287–298.

25. Aubin JE 1999 Osteoprogenitor cell frequency in rat bone marrow stromal populations: Role for heterotypic cell-cell interactions in osteoblast differentiation. J Cell Biochem **72:**396–410.

26. Wu X, Peters JM, Gonzalez FJ, Prasad HS, Rohrer MD, Gimble JM 2000 Frequency of stromal lineage colony forming units in bone marrow of peroxisome proliferator-activated receptor-alpha-null mice. Bone **26:**21–26.

27. Aubin JE 1998 Bone stem cells. J Cell Biochem Suppl **30–31:**73–82.

28. Malaval L, Aubin JE 2001 Biphasic effects of leukemia inhibitory factor on osteoblastic differentiation. J Cell Biochem **81:**63–70.

29. Aubin JE, Gupta AK, Bhargava U, Turksen K 1996 Expression and regulation of galectin 3 in rat osteoblastic cells. J Cell Physiol **169:**468–480.

30. van Vlasselaer P, Falla N, Snoeck H, Mathieu E 1994 Characterization and purification of osteogenic cells from murine bone marrow by two-color cell sorting using anti-Sca-1 monoclonal antibody and wheat germ agglutinin. Blood **84:**753–763.

31. Simmons PJ, Torok-Storb B 1991 Identification of stromal cell precursors in human bone marrow by a novel monoclonal antibody, STRO-1. Blood **78:**55–62.

32. Gronthos S, Graves SE, Ohta S, Simmons PJ 1994 The STRO-1+ fraction of adult human bone marrow contains the osteogenic precursors. Blood **84:**4164–4173.

33. Bruder SP, Horowitz MC, Mosca JD, Haynesworth SE 1997 Monoclonal antibodies reactive with human osteogenic cell surface antigens. Bone **21:**225–235.

34. Bruder SP, Ricalton NS, Boynton RE, Connolly TJ, Jaiswal N, Zaia J, Barry FP 1998 Mesenchymal stem cell surface antigen SB-10 corresponds to activated leukocyte cell adhesion molecule and is involved in osteogenic differentiation. J Bone Miner Res **13:**655–663.

35. Bowen MA, Aruffo AA, Bajorath J 2000 Cell surface receptors and their ligands: In vitro analysis of CD6-CD166 interactions. Proteins **40:**420–428.

36. Barry FP, Boynton RE, Haynesworth S, Murphy JM, Zaia J 1999 The monoclonal antibody SH-2, raised against human mesenchymal stem cells, recognizes an epitope on endoglin (CD105). Biochem Biophys Res Commun **265:**134–139.

37. Zannettino AC, Harrison K, Joyner CJ, Triffitt JT, Simmons PJ 2003 Molecular cloning of the cell surface antigen identified by the osteoprogenitor-specific monoclonal antibody, HOP-26. J Cell Biochem **89:**56–66.

38. Joyner CJ, Bennett A, Triffitt JT 1997 Identification and enrichment of human osteoprogenitor cells by using differentiation stage-specific monoclonal antibodies. Bone **21:**1–6.

39. Prockop DJ 1997 Marrow stromal cells as stem cells for nonhematopoietic tissues. Science **276:**71–74.

40. Hou Z, Nguyen Q, Frenkel B, Nilsson SK, Milne M, van Wijnen AJ, Stein JL, Quesenberry P, Lian JB, Stein GS 1999 Osteoblast-specific gene expression after transplantation of marrow cells: Implications for skeletal gene therapy. Proc Natl Acad Sci USA **96:**7294–7299.

41. Jeon MJ, Kim JA, Kwon SH, Kim SW, Park KS, Park SW, Kim SY, Shin CS 2003 Activation of peroxisome proliferator-activated receptor-gamma inhibits the Runx2-mediated transcription of osteocalcin in osteoblasts. J Biol Chem **278:**23270–23277.

42. Lecka-Czernik B, Gubrij I, Moerman EJ, Kajkenova O, Lipschitz DA, Manolagas SC, Jilka RL 1999 Inhibition of Osf2/Cbfa1 expression and terminal osteoblast differentiation by PPARgamma2. J Cell Biochem **74:**357–371.

43. Skillington J, Choy L, Derynck R 2002 Bone morphogenetic protein and retinoic acid signaling cooperate to induce osteoblast differentiation of preadipocytes. J Cell Biol **159:**135–146.

44. Nuttall ME, Patton AJ, Olivera DL, Nadeau DP, Gowen M 1998 Human trabecular bone cells are able to express both osteoblastic and adipocytic phenotype: Implications for osteopenic disorders. J Bone Miner Res **13:**371–382.

45. Park SR, Oreffo RO, Triffitt JT 1999 Interconversion potential of cloned human marrow adipocytes in vitro. Bone **24:**549–554.

46. Doherty MJ, Ashton BA, Walsh S, Beresford JN, Grant ME, Canfield AE 1998 Vascular pericytes express osteogenic potential in vitro and in vivo. J Bone Miner Res **13:**828–838.

47. Vescovi AL, Snyder EY 1999 Establishment and properties of neural stem cell clones: Plasticity in vitro and in vivo. Brain Pathol **9:**569–598.

48. Williams JH, Klinken SP 1999 Plasticity in the haemopoietic system. Int J Biochem Cell Biol **31:**1237–1242.

49. Hole N 1999 Embryonic stem cell-derived haematopoiesis. Cells Tissues Organs **165:**181–189.

50. Bianco P, Cossu G 1999 Uno, nessuno e centomila: Searching for the identity of mesodermal progenitors. Exp Cell Res **251:**257–263.

51. Seale P, Rudnicki MA 2000 A new look at the origin, function, and "stem-cell" status of muscle satellite cells. Dev Biol **218:**115–124.

52. Hodge CJ Jr, Boakye M 2001 Biological plasticity: The future of science in neurosurgery. Neurosurgery **48:**2–16.

53. Aubin JE, Heersche JNM 1997 Vitamin D and osteoblasts. In: Feldman D, Glorieux FH, Pike JW (eds.) Vitamin D. Academic Press, San Diego, CA, pp. 313–328.

54. Nuttall ME, Gimble JM 2000 Is there a therapeutic opportunity to either prevent or treat osteopenic disorders by inhibiting marrow adipogenesis? Bone **27:**177–184.

55. Gimble JM, Robinson CE, Wu X, Kelly KA 1996 The function of adipocytes in the bone marrow stroma: An update. Bone **19:**421–428.

56. Rickard DJ, Kassem M, Hefferan TE, Sarkar G, Spelsberg TC, Riggs BL 1996 Isolation and characterization of osteoblast precursor cells from human bone marrow. J Bone Miner Res **11:**312–324.

57. Ying QL, Nichols J, Evans EP, Smith AG 2002 Changing potency by spontaneous fusion. Nature **416:**545–548.

58. Terada N, Hamazaki T, Oka M, Hoki M, Mastalerz DM, Nakano Y, Meyer EM, Morel L, Petersen BE, Scott EW 2002 Bone marrow cells adopt the phenotype of other cells by spontaneous cell fusion. Nature **416:**542–545.

59. Wang X, Willenbring H, Akkari Y, Torimaru Y, Foster M, Al Dhalimy M, Lagasse E, Finegold M, Olson S, Grompe M 2003 Cell fusion is the principal source of bone-marrow-derived hepatocytes. Nature **422:**897–901.

60. Vassilopoulos G, Wang PR, Russell DW 2003 Transplanted bone marrow regenerates liver by cell fusion. Nature **422**:901–904.
61. Wurmser AE, Gage FH 2002 Stem cells: Cell fusion causes confusion. Nature **416**:485–487.
62. Orkin SH, Zon LI 2002 Hematopoiesis and stem cells: Plasticity versus developmental heterogeneity. Nat Immunol **3**:323–328.
63. Reyes M, Lund T, Lenvik T, Aguiar D, Koodie L, Verfaillie CM 2001 Purification and ex vivo expansion of postnatal human marrow mesodermal progenitor cells. Blood **98**:2615–2625.
64. Jiang Y, Jahagirdar BN, Reinhardt RL, Schwartz RE, Keene CD, Ortiz-Gonzalez XR, Reyes M, Lenvik T, Lund T, Blackstad M, Du J, Aldrich S, Lisberg A, Low WC, Largaespada DA, Verfaillie CM 2002 Pluripotency of mesenchymal stem cells derived from adult marrow. Nature **418**:41–49.
65. Huss R, Lange C, Weissinger EM, Kolb HJ, Thalmeier K 2000 Evidence of peripheral blood-derived, plastic-adherent CD34(-/low) hematopoietic stem cell clones with mesenchymal stem cell characteristics. Stem Cells **18**:252–260.
66. Kuznetsov SA, Mankani MH, Gronthos S, Satomura K, Bianco P, Robey PG 2001 Circulating skeletal stem cells. J Cell Biol **153**:1133–1140.
67. Erices A, Conget P, Minguell JJ 2000 Mesenchymal progenitor cells in human umbilical cord blood. Br J Haematol **109**:235–242.
68. Campagnoli C, Roberts IA, Kumar S, Bennett PR, Bellantuono I, Fisk NM 2001 Identification of mesenchymal stem/progenitor cells in human first-trimester fetal blood, liver, and bone marrow. Blood **98**:2396–2402.
69. Shi S, Gronthos S 2003 Perivascular niche of postnatal mesenchymal stem cells in human bone marrow and dental pulp. J Bone Miner Res **18**:696–704.
70. Miura M, Gronthos S, Zhao M, Lu B, Fisher LW, Robey PG, Shi S 2003 SHED: Stem cells from human exfoliated deciduous teeth. Proc Natl Acad Sci USA **100**:5807–5812.
71. Asakura A, Komaki M, Rudnicki M 2001 Muscle satellite cells are multipotential stem cells that exhibit myogenic, osteogenic, and adipogenic differentiation. Differentiation **68**:245–253.
72. Gronthos S, Franklin DM, Leddy HA, Robey PG, Storms RW, Gimble JM 2001 Surface protein characterization of human adipose tissue-derived stromal cells. J Cell Physiol **189**:54–63.
73. Zuk PA, Zhu M, Mizuno H, Huang J, Futrell JW, Katz AJ, Benhaim P, Lorenz HP, Hedrick MH 2001 Multilineage cells from human adipose tissue: Implications for cell-based therapies. Tissue Eng **7**:211–228.
74. Huang JI, Beanes SR, Zhu M, Lorenz HP, Hedrick MH, Benhaim P 2002 Rat extramedullary adipose tissue as a source of osteochondrogenic progenitor cells. Plast Reconstr Surg **109**:1033–1041.
75. Bonyadi M, Waldman SD, Liu D, Aubin JE, Grynpas MD, Stanford WL 2003 Mesenchymal progenitor self-renewal deficiency leads to age-dependent osteoporosis in Sca-1/Ly-6A null mice. Proc Natl Acad Sci USA **100**:5840–5845.
76. Cornish J, Gillespie MT, Callon KE, Horwood NJ, Moseley JM, Reid IR 2003 Interleukin-18 is a novel mitogen of osteogenic and chondrogenic cells. Endocrinology **144**:1194–1201.
77. Yang X, Tare RS, Partridge KA, Roach HI, Clarke NM, Howdle SM, Shakesheff KM, Oreffo RO 2003 Induction of human osteoprogenitor chemotaxis, proliferation, differentiation, and bone formation by osteoblast stimulating factor-1/pleiotrophin: Osteoconductive biomimetic scaffolds for tissue engineering. J Bone Miner Res **18**:47–57.
78. Thomas T, Gori F, Spelsberg TC, Khosla S, Riggs BL, Conover CA 1999 Response of bipotential human marrow stromal cells to insulin-like growth factors: Effect on binding protein production, proliferation, and commitment to osteoblasts and adipocytes. Endocrinology **140**:5036–5044.
79. Safadi FF, Xu J, Smock SL, Kanaan RA, Selim AH, Odgren PR, Marks SC Jr, Owen TA, Popoff SN 2003 Expression of connective tissue growth factor in bone: Its role in osteoblast proliferation and differentiation in vitro and bone formation in vivo. J Cell Physiol **196**:51–62.
80. Sowa H, Kaji H, Canaff L, Hendy GN, Tsukamoto T, Yamaguchi T, Miyazono K, Sugimoto T, Chihara K 2003 Inactivation of menin, the product of the multiple endocrine neoplasia type 1 gene, inhibits the commitment of multipotential mesenchymal stem cells into the osteoblast lineage. J Biol Chem **278**:21058–21069.
81. Lee MS, Lowe GN, Strong DD, Wergedal JE, Glackin CA 1999 TWIST, a basic helix-loop-helix transcription factor, can regulate the human osteogenic lineage. J Cell Biochem **75**:566–577.
82. Shin CS, Lecanda F, Sheikh S, Weitzmann L, Cheng SL, Civitelli R 2000 Relative abundance of different cadherins defines differentiation of mesenchymal precursors into osteogenic, myogenic, or adipogenic pathways. J Cell Biochem **78**:566–577.
83. Hay E, Lemonnier J, Modrowski D, Lomri A, Lasmoles F, Marie PJ 2000 N- and E-cadherin mediate early human calvaria osteoblast differentiation promoted by bone morphogenetic protein-2. J Cell Physiol **183**:117–128.
84. Marie PJ 2002 Role of N-cadherin in bone formation. J Cell Physiol **190**:297–305.
85. Bennett JH, Moffatt S, Horton M 2001 Cell adhesion molecules in human osteoblasts: Structure and function. Histol Histopathol **16**:603–611.
86. Franceschi RT, Xiao G 2003 Regulation of the osteoblast-specific transcription factor, Runx2: Responsiveness to multiple signal transduction pathways. J Cell Biochem **88**:446–454.
87. Stein GS, Lian JB, Stein JS, van Wijnen AJ, Frenkel B, Montecino M 1996 Mechanisms regulating osteoblast proliferation and differentiation. In: Bilezikian JP, Raisz LG, Rodan GA (eds.) Principles of Bone Biology. Academic Press, San Diego, CA, USA, pp. 69–86.
88. Drissi H, Hushka D, Aslam F, Nguyen Q, Buffone E, Koff A, van Wijnen A, Lian JB, Stein JL, Stein GS 1999 The cell cycle regulator p27kip1 contributes to growth and differentiation of osteoblasts. Cancer Res **59**:3705–3711.
89. Beier F, Taylor AC, LuValle P 1999 The Raf-1/MEK/ERK pathway regulates the expression of the p21(Cip1/Waf1) gene in chondrocytes. J Biol Chem **274**:30273–30279.
90. Candeliere GA, Liu F, Aubin JE 2001 Individual osteoblasts in the developing calvaria express different gene repertoires. Bone **28**:351–361.
91. Aubin JE, Liu F, Candeliere GA 2002 Single-cell PCR methods for studying stem cells and progenitors. Methods Mol Biol **185**:403–415.
92. Seth A, Lee BK, Qi S, Vary CP 2000 Coordinate expression of novel genes during osteoblast differentiation. J Bone Miner Res **15**:1683–1696.
93. Beck GR Jr, Zerler B, Moran E 2001 Gene array analysis of osteoblast differentiation. Cell Growth Differ **12**:61–83.
94. Liu F, Malaval L, Aubin JE 2003 Global amplification polymerase chain reaction reveals novel transitional stages during osteoprogenitor differentiation. J Cell Sci **116**:1787–1796.
95. Aubin JE, Triffitt JT 2002 Mesenchymal stem cells and osteoblast differentiation. In: Bilezikian JP, Raisz LG, Rodan GA (eds.) Principles of Bone Biology, 2nd ed. Academic Press, San Diego, CA, USA, pp. 59–82.
96. Liu F, Malaval L, Gupta AK, Aubin JE 1994 Simultaneous detection of multiple bone-related mRNAs and protein expression during osteoblast differentiation: Polymerase chain reaction and immunocytochemical studies at the single cell level. Dev Biol **166**:220–234.
97. Malaval L, Modrowski D, Gupta AK, Aubin JE 1994 Cellular expression of bone-related proteins during in vitro osteogenesis in rat bone marrow stromal cell cultures. J Cell Physiol **158**:555–572.
98. Pockwinse SM, Stein JL, Lian JB, Stein GS 1995 Developmental stage-specific cellular responses to vitamin D and glucocorticoids during differentiation of the osteoblast phenotype: Interrelationship of morphology and gene expression by in situ hybridization. Exp Cell Res **216**:244–260.
99. Liu F, Malaval L, Aubin JE 1997 The mature osteoblast phenotype is characterized by extensive plasticity. Exp Cell Res **232**:97–105.
100. Heersche JNM, Reimers SM, Wrana JL, Waye MMY, Gupta AK 1992 Changes in expression of alpha 1 type 1 collagen and osteocalcin mRNA in osteoblasts and adontoblasts at different stages of maturity as shown by in situ hybridization. Proc Finn Dent Soc **88**:173–182.
101. Bianco P, Riminucci M, Bonucci E, Termine JD, Robey PG 1993 Bone sialoprotein (BSP) secretion and osteoblast differentiation: Relationship to bromodeoxyuridine incorporation, alkaline phosphatase, and matrix deposition. J Histochem Cytochem **41**:183–191.
102. Ingram RT, Clarke BL, Fisher LW, Fitzpatrick LA 1993 Distribution of noncollagenous proteins in the matrix of adult human bone: Evidence of anatomic and functional heterogeneity. J Bone Miner Res **8**:1019–1029.
103. Ikeda T, Nagai Y, Yamaguchi A, Yokose S, Yoshiki S 1995 Age-related reduction in bone matrix protein mRNA expression in rat bone tissues: Application of histomorphometry to in situ hybridization. Bone **16**:17–23.
104. Amling M, Herden S, Posl M, Hahn M, Ritzel H, Delling G 1996 Heterogeneity of the skeleton: Comparison of the trabecular microarchitecture of the spine, the iliac crest, the femur, and the calcaneus. J Bone Miner Res **11**:36–45.

105. Byers RJ, Denton J, Hoyland JA, Freemont AJ 1997 Differential patterns of osteoblast dysfunction in trabecular bone in patients with established osteoporosis. J Clin Pathol **50**:760–764.

106. Riggs BL, Khosla S, Melton LJ III 1998 A unitary model for involutional osteoporosis: Estrogen deficiency causes both type I and type II osteoporosis in postmenopausal women and contributes to bone loss in aging men. J Bone Miner Res **13**:763–773.

107. Nijweide PJ, Burger EH, Klein-Nulend J 2002 The osteocyte. In: Bilezikian JP, Raisz LG, Rodan GA (eds.) Principles of Bone Biology, 2nd ed. Academic Press, San Diego, CA, USA, pp. 93–107.

108. Nijweide PJ, Burger EH, Klein-Nulend J, van der Plas A 1996 The osteocyte. In: Bilezikian JP, Raisz LG, Rodan GA (eds.) Principles of Bone Biology. Academic Press, San Diego, CA, USA, pp. 115–126.

109. van der Plas A, Aarden EM, Feijen JH, de Boer AH, Wiltink A, Alblas MJ, de Leij L, Nijweide PJ 1994 Characteristics and properties of osteocytes in culture. J Bone Miner Res **9**:1697–1704.

110. Bonewald LF 1999 Establishment and characterization of an osteocyte-like cell line, MLO-Y4. J Bone Miner Metab **17**:61–65.

111. Mikuni-Takagaki Y, Kakai Y, Satoyoshi M, Kawano E, Suzuki Y, Kawase T, Saito S 1995 Matrix mineralization and the differentiation of osteocyte-like cells in culture. J Bone Miner Res **10**:231–242.

112. Kato Y, Windle JJ, Koop BA, Mundy GR, Bonewald LF 1997 Establishment of an osteocyte-like cell line, MLO-Y4. J Bone Miner Res **12**:2014–2023.

113. Jamal HH, Aubin JE 1996 CD44 expression in fetal rat bone: *in vivo* and *in vitro* analysis. Exp Cell Res **223**:467–477.

114. Bodine PVN, Vernon SK, Komm BS 1996 Establishment and hormonal regulation of a conditionally-transformed preosteocytic cell line from adult human bone. Endocrinology **137**:4592–4604.

115. Civitelli R, Beyer EC, Warlow PM, Robertson AJ, Geist ST, Steinberg TH 1993 Connexin43 mediates direct intercellular communication in human osteoblastic cell networks. J Clin Invest **91**:1888–1896.

116. Schiller PC, D'Ippolito G, Brambilla R, Roos BA, Howard GA 2001 Inhibition of gap-junctional communication induces the trans-differentiation of osteoblasts to an adipocytic phenotype in vitro. J Biol Chem **276**:14133–14138.

117. Furlan F, Lecanda F, Screen J, Civitelli R 2001 Proliferation, differentiation and apoptosis in connexin43-null osteoblasts. Cell Commun Adhes **8**:367–371.

118. Rubin CT, Lanyon LE 1987 Osteoregulatory nature of mechanical stimuli: Function as a determinant for adaptive bone remodeling. J Orthop Res **5**:300–310.

119. Jorgensen NR, Teilmann SC, Henriksen Z, Civitelli R, Sorensen OH, Steinberg TH 2003 Activation of L-type calcium channels is required for gap junction-mediated intercellular calcium signaling in osteoblastic cells. J Biol Chem **278**:4082–4086.

120. Jiang JX, Cheng B 2001 Mechanical stimulation of gap junctions in bone osteocytes is mediated by prostaglandin E2. Cell Commun Adhes **8**:283–288.

121. Reher P, Harris M, Whiteman M, Hai HK, Meghji S 2002 Ultrasound stimulates nitric oxide and prostaglandin E2 production by human osteoblasts. Bone **31**:236–241.

122. Wang FS, Wang CJ, Sheen-Chen SM, Kuo YR, Chen RF, Yang KD 2002 Superoxide mediates shock wave induction of ERK-dependent osteogenic transcription factor (CBFA1) and mesenchymal cell differentiation toward osteoprogenitors. J Biol Chem **277**:10931–10937.

123. Ziros PG, Gil AP, Georgakopoulos T, Habeos I, Kletsas D, Basdra EK, Papavassiliou AG 2002 The bone-specific transcriptional regulator Cbfa1 is a target of mechanical signals in osteoblastic cells. J Biol Chem **277**:23934–23941.

124. Noble BS, Stevens H, Loveridge N, Reeve J 1997 Identification of apoptotic changes in osteocytes in normal and pathological human bone. Bone **20**:273–282.

125. Boyce BF, Xing L, Jilka RJ, Bellido T, Weinstein RS, Parfitt AM, Manolagas SC 2002 Apoptosis in bone cells. In: Bilezikian JP, Raisz LG, Rodan GA (eds.) Principles of Bone Biology, 2nd ed. Academic Press, San Diego, CA, USA, pp. 151–168.

126. Bellido T, Huening M, Raval-Pandya M, Manolagas SC, Christakos S 2000 Calbindin-D$_{28K}$ is expressed in osteoblastic cells and suppresses their apoptosis by inhibiting caspase-3 activity. J Biol Chem **275**:26328–26332.

127. Lynch MP, Capparelli C, Stein JL, Stein GS, Lian JB 1998 Apoptosis during bone-like tissue development in vitro. J Cell Biochem **68**:31–49.

128. Gohel A, McCarthy MB, Gronowicz G 1999 Estrogen prevents glucocorticoid-induced apoptosis in osteoblasts in vivo and in vitro. Endocrinology **140**:5339–5347.

129. Plotkin LI, Manolagas SC, Bellido T 2002 Transduction of cell survival signals by connexin-43 hemichannels. J Biol Chem **277**:8648–8657.

130. Noble BS, Peet N, Stevens HY, Brabbs A, Mosley JR, Reilly GC, Reeve J, Skerry TM, Lanyon LE 2003 Mechanical loading: Biphasic osteocyte survival and targeting of osteoclasts for bone destruction in rat cortical bone. Am J Physiol Cell Physiol **284**:C934–C943.

131. Stein GS, Lian JB, Stein JL, van Wijnen AJ, Montecino M, Pratap J, Choi J, Zaidi SK, Javed A, Gutierrez S, Harrington K, Shen J, Young D 2003 Intranuclear organization of RUNX transcriptional regulatory machinery in biological control of skeletogenesis and cancer. Blood Cells Mol Dis **30**:170–176.

132. Lian JB, Stein JL, Stein GS, van Wijnen AJ, Montecino M, Javed A, Gutierrez S, Shen J, Zaidi SK, Drissi H 2003 Runx2/Cbfa1 functions: Diverse regulation of gene transcription by chromatin remodeling and co-regulatory protein interactions. Connect Tissue Res **44**:141–148.

133. McKenna NJ, Xu J, Nawaz Z, Tsai SY, Tsai MJ, O'Malley BW 1999 Nuclear receptor coactivators: Multiple enzymes, multiple complexes, multiple functions. J Steroid Biochem Mol Biol **69**:3–12.

134. Lu H, Kraut D, Gerstenfeld LC, Graves DT 2003 Diabetes interferes with the bone formation by affecting the expression of transcription factors that regulate osteoblast differentiation. Endocrinology **144**:346–352.

135. Ogata T, Noda M 1991 Expression of Id, a negative regulator of helix-loop-helix DNA binding proteins, is down-regulated at confluence and enhanced by dexamethasone in a mouse osteoblastic cell line, MC3T3E1. Biochem Biophys Res Commun **180**:1194–1199.

136. Glackin CA, Lee M, Lowe G, Morales S, Wergedal J, Strong D 1997 Overexpressing human TWIST in high SaOS (HSaOS) cells results in major differences in cellular morphology, proliferation rates, and ALP activities. Knocking out human Id-2 greatly reduces the expression of all TWIST family members, indicating that Id-2 may regulate TWIST during osteoblast differentiation. J Bone Miner Res **12**:S154–S154.

137. Machwate M, Jullienne A, Moukhtar M, Marie PJ 1995 Temporal variation of c-fos proto-oncogene expression during osteoblast differentiation and osteogenesis in developing bone. J Cell Biochem **57**:62–70.

138. McCabe LR, Banerjee C, Kundu R, Harrison RJ, Dobner PR, Stein JL, Lian JB, Stein GS 1996 Developmental expression and activities of specific fos and jun proteins are functionally related to osteoblast maturation: Role of fra-2 and jun D during differentiation. Endocrinology **137**:4398–4408.

139. Sumoy L, Wang CK, Lichtler AC, Pierro LJ, Kosher RA, Upholt WB 1995 Identification of a spatially specific enhancer element in the chicken Msx-2 gene that regulates its expression in the apical ectodermal ridge of the developing limb buds of transgenic mice. Dev Biol **170**:230–242.

140. Orestes-Cardoso S, Nefussi JR, Lezot F, Oboeuf M, Pereira M, Mesbah M, Robert B, Berdal A 2002 Msx1 is a regulator of bone formation during development and postnatal growth: In vivo investigations in a transgenic mouse model. Connect Tissue Res **43**:153–160.

141. Ryoo H-M, Hoffmann HM, Beumer TL, Frenkel B, Towler DA, Stein GS, Stein JL, van Wijnen AJ, Lian JB 1997 Stage-specific expression of Dlx-5 during osteoblast differentiation: Involvement in regulation of osteocalcin gene expression. Mol Endocrinol **11**:1681–1694.

142. Ji C, Chen Y, Centrella M, McCarthy TL 1999 Activation of the insulin-like growth factor-binding protein-5 promoter in osteoblasts by cooperative E box, CCAAT enhancer-binding protein, and nuclear factor-1 deoxyribonucleic acid-binding sequences. Endocrinology **140**:4564–4572.

143. Javed A, Barnes GL, Jassanya BO, Stein JL, Gerstenfeld L, Lian JB, Stein GS 2001 *Runt* homology domain transcription factors (Runx, Cbfa, and AML) mediate repression of the bone sialoprotein promoter: Evidence for promoter context-dependent activity of Cbfa proteins. Mol Cell Biol **21**:2891–2905.

144. Gutierrez S, Javed A, Tennant D, van Rees M, Montecino M, Stein GS, Stein JL, Lian JB 2002 CCAAT/enhancer-binding proteins (C/EBP) β and δ Activate osteocalcin gene transcription and synergize with Runx2 at the C/EBP element to regulate bone-specific expression. J Biol Chem **277**:1316–1323.

145. Nakashima K, Zhou X, Kunkel G, Zhang Z, Deng JM, Behringer RR, de Crombrugghe B 2002 The novel zinc finger-containing transcription factor osterix is required for osteoblast differentiation and bone formation. Cell **108**:17–29.

146. Komori T, Yagi H, Nomura S, Yamaguchi A, Sasaki K, Deguchi K,

Shimizu Y, Bronson RT, Gao Y-H, Inada M, Sato M, Okamoto R, Kitamura Y, Yoshiki S, Kishimoto T 1997 Targeted disruption of *Cbfa1* results in a complete lack of bone formation owing to maturational arrest of osteoblasts. Cell **89**:755–764.

147. Shui C, Spelsberg TC, Riggs BL, Khosla S 2003 Changes in Runx2/Cbfa1 expression and activity during osteoblastic differentiation of human bone marrow stromal cells. J Bone Miner Res **18**:213–221.

148. Stricker S, Fundele R, Vortkamp A, Mundlos S 2002 Role of runx genes in chondrocyte differentiation. Dev Biol **245**:95–108.

149. Sun L, Vitolo M, Passaniti A 2001 Runt-related gene 2 in endothelial cells: Inducible expression and specific regulation of cell migration and invasion. Cancer Res **61**:4994–5001.

150. Zelzer E, Glotzer DJ, Hartmann C, Thomas D, Fukai N, Soker S, Olsen BR 2001 Tissue specific regulation of VEGF expression during bone development requires Cbfa1/Runx2. Mech Dev **106**:97–106.

151. Stock M, Schafer H, Stricker S, Gross G, Mundlos S, Otto F 2003 Expression of galectin-3 in skeletal tissues is controlled by Runx2. J Biol Chem **278**:17360–17367.

152. Ducy P, Zhang R, Geoffroy V, Ridall AL, Karsenty G 1997 Osf2/Cbfa1: A transcriptional activator of osteoblast differentiation. Cell **89**:747–754.

153. Ji C, Casinghino S, Chang DJ, Chen Y, Javed A, Ito Y, Hiebert SW, Lian JB, Stein GS, McCarthy TL, Centrella M 1998 CBFa(AML/PEBP2)-related elements in the TGF-beta type I receptor promoter and expression with osteoblast differentiation. J Cell Biochem **69**:353–363.

154. Sato M, Morii E, Komori T, Kawahata H, Sugimoto M, Terai K, Shimizu H, Yasui T, Ogihara H, Yasui N, Ochi T, Kitamura Y, Ito Y, Nomura S 1998 Transcriptional regulation of osteopontin gene in vivo by PEBP2alphaA/CBFA1 and ETS1 in the skeletal tissues. Oncogene **17**:1517–1525.

155. Chen S, Gu TT, Sreenath T, Kulkarni AB, Karsenty G, MacDougall M 2002 Spatial expression of Cbfa1/Runx2 isoforms in teeth and characterization of binding sites in the DSPP gene. Connect Tissue Res **43**:338–344.

156. Thirunavukkarasu K, Halladay DL, Miles RR, Yang X, Galvin RJ, Chandrasekhar S, Martin TJ, Onyia JE 2000 The osteoblast-specific transcription factor Cbfa1 contributes to the expression of osteoprotegerin, a potent inhibitor of osteoclast differentiation and function. J Biol Chem **275**:25163–25172.

157. Geoffroy V, Kneissel M, Fournier B, Boyde A, Matthias P 2002 High bone resorption in adult aging transgenic mice overexpressing cbfa1/runx2 in cells of the osteoblastic lineage. Mol Cell Biol **22**:6222–6233.

158. Jimenez MJ, Balbin M, Lopez JM, Alvarez J, Komori T, Lopez-Otin C 1999 Collagenase 3 is a target of Cbfa1, a transcription factor of the runt gene family involved in bone formation. Mol Cell Biol **19**:4431–4442.

159. Liu W, Toyosawa S, Furuichi T, Kanatani N, Yoshida C, Liu Y, Himeno M, Narai S, Yamaguchi A, Komori T 2001 Overexpression of Cbfa1 in osteoblasts inhibits osteoblast maturation and causes osteopenia with multiple fractures. J Cell Biol **155**:157–166.

160. Lian JB Stein GS 2003 The temporal and spatial subnuclear organization of skeletal gene regulatory machinery: Integrating multiple levels of transcriptional control. Calcif Tissue Int (in press).

161. Gori F, Thomas T, Hicok KC, Spelsberg TC, Riggs BL 1999 Differentiation of human marrow stromal precursor cells: Bone morphogenetic protein-2 increases OSF2/CBFA1, enhances osteoblast commitment, and inhibits late adipocyte maturation. J Bone Miner Res **14**:1522–1535.

162. Westendorf JJ, Hiebert SW 1999 Mammalian runt-domain proteins and their roles in hematopoiesis, osteogenesis, and leukemia. J Cell Biochem Suppl**32–33**:51–58.

163. Sierra J, Villagra A, Paredes R, Cruzat F, Gutierrez S, Arriagada G, Olate J, Imschenetzky M, van Wijnen AJ, Lian JB, Stein GS, Stein JL, Montecino M 2003 Regulation of the bone-specific osteocalcin gene by p300 Requires Runx2/Cbfa1 and the Vitamin D3 Receptor but not p300 Intrinsic Histone Acetyl Transferase Activity. Mol Cell Biol **23**:3339–3351.

164. Kundu M, Chen A, Anderson S, Kirby M, Xu L, Castilla LH, Bodine D, Liu PP 2002 Role of Cbfb in hematopoiesis and perturbations resulting from expression of the leukemogenic fusion gene Cbfb-MYH11. Blood **100**:2449–2456.

165. Miller J, Horner A, Stacy T, Lowrey C, Lian JB, Stein G, Nuckolls GH, Speck NA 2002 The core-binding factor beta subunit is required for bone formation and hematopoietic maturation. Nat Genet **32**:645–649.

166. Westendorf JJ, Zaidi SK, Cascino JE, Kahler R, van Wijnen AJ, Lian JB, Yoshida M, Stein GS, Li X 2002 Runx2 (Cbfa1, AML-3) interacts with histone deacetylase 6 and represses the p21(CIP1/WAF1) promoter. Mol Cell Biol **22**:7982–7992.

167. Kahler RA, Westendorf JJ 2003 Lymphoid enhancer factor-1 and beta-catenin inhibit Runx2-dependent transcriptional activation of the osteocalcin promoter. J Biol Chem **278**:11937–11944.

168. D'Alonzo RC, Selvamurugan N, Karsenty G, Partridge NC 2002 Physical interaction of the activator protein-1 factors c-fos and c-jun with cbfa1 for collagenase-3 promoter activation. J Biol Chem **277**:816–822.

169. Hess J, Porte D, Munz C, Angel P 2001 AP-1 and Cbfa/Runt physically interact and regulate PTH-dependent MMP13 expression in osteoblasts through a new OSE2/AP-1 composite element. J Biol Chem **276**:20029–20038.

170. Zaidi SK, Sullivan AJ, van Wijnen AJ, Stein JL, Stein GS, Lian JB 2002 Integration of runx and smad regulatory signals at transcriptionally active subnuclear sites. Proc Natl Acad Sci USA **99**:8048–8053.

171. Derynck R, Zhang Y, Feng XH 1998 Smads: Transcriptional activators of TGF-beta responses. Cell **95**:737–740.

172. Zhang YW, Yasui N, Ito K, Huang G, Fujii M, Hanai J, Nogami H, Ochi T, Miyazono K, Ito Y 2000 A RUNX2/PEBP2αA/CBFA1 mutation displaying impaired transactivation and Smad interaction in cleidocranial dysplasia. Proc Natl Acad Sci USA **97**:10549–10554.

173. Xiao G, Jiang D, Gopalakrishnan R, Franceschi RT 2002 Fibroblast growth factor 2 induction of the osteocalcin gene requires MAPK activity and phosphorylation of the osteoblast transcription factor, Cbfa1/Runx2. J Biol Chem **277**:36181–36187.

174. Zaidi K, Sullivan AJ, Yagi R, Ito Y, van Wijnen AJ, Stein JL, Lian JB, Stein GS 2000 Targeting of the Yes-associated protein (YAP), a coregulator of Runx/Cbfa function, to nuclear matrix associated Cbfa sites requires interaction with Runx2/Cbfa1. J Bone Miner Res **15**:S498–S498.

175. Cui CB, Cooper LF, Yang X, Karsenty G, Aukhil I 2003 Transcriptional coactivation of bone-specific transcription factor Cbfa1 by TAZ. Mol Cell Biol **23**:1004–1013.

176. Choi J-Y, Pratap J, Javed A, Zaidi SK, van Wijnen AJ, Lian JB, Stein JL, Jones SN, Stein GS 2000 In vivo replacement of the Runx2/Cbfa1 gene with a mutant gene lacking a subnuclear targeting signal and transcriptional regulatory functions results in severe skeletal abnormalities. J Bone Miner Res **15**:S157–S157.

177. Otto F, Kanegane H, Mundlos S 2002 Mutations in the RUNX2 gene in patients with cleidocranial dysplasia. Hum Mutat **19**:209–216.

178. Zhang YW, Bae SC, Takahashi E, Ito Y 1997 The cDNA cloning of the transcripts of human PEBP2alphaA/CBFA1 mapped to 6p12.3-p21.1, the locus for cleidocranial dysplasia. Oncogene **15**:367–371.

179. Karaplis AC, Goltzman D 2000 PTH and PTHrP effects on the skeleton. Rev Endocr Metab Disord **1**:331–341.

180. Chung UI, Schipani E, McMahon AP, Kronenberg HM 2001 Indian hedgehog couples chondrogenesis to osteogenesis in endochondral bone development. J Clin Invest **107**:295–304.

181. Kream BE, Lukert BP 2002 Clinical and basic aspects of glucocorticoid action in bone. In: Bilezikian JP, Raisz LG, Rodan GA (eds.) Principles of Bone Biology, 2nd ed. Academic Press, San Diego, CA, USA, pp. 723–740.

182. Weinstein RS, Jilka RL, Parfitt AM, Manolagas SC 1998 Inhibition of osteoblastogenesis and promotion of apoptosis of osteoblasts and osteocytes by glucocorticoids. Potential mechanisms of their deleterious effects on bone. J Clin Invest **102**:274–282.

183. Noble BS, Reeve J 2000 Osteocyte function, osteocyte death and bone fracture resistance. Mol Cell Endocrinol **159**:7–13.

184. Van Leeuwen JP, van Driel M, van den Bemd GJ, Pols HA 2001 Vitamin D control of osteoblast function and bone extracellular matrix mineralization. Crit Rev Eukaryot Gene Expr **11**:199–226.

185. Cornish J, Callon KE, Coy DH, Jiang NY, Xiao L, Cooper GJ, Reid IR 1997 Adrenomedullin is a potent stimulator of osteoblastic activity in vitro and in vivo. Am J Physiol **273**:E1113–E1120.

186. Gordeladze JO, Drevon CA, Syversen U, Reseland JE 2002 Leptin stimulates human osteoblastic cell proliferation, de novo collagen synthesis, and mineralization: Impact on differentiation markers, apoptosis, and osteoclastic signaling. J Cell Biochem **85**:825–836.

187. Reseland JE, Syversen U, Bakke I, Qvigstad G, Eide LG, Hjertner O, Gordeladze JO, Drevon CA 2001 Leptin is expressed in and secreted from primary cultures of human osteoblasts and promotes bone mineralization. J Bone Miner Res **16**:1426–1433.

188. Ducy P, Amling M, Takeda S, Priemel M, Schilling AF, Beil FT, Shen J, Vinson C, Rueger JM, Karsenty G 2000 Leptin inhibits bone

formation through a hypothalamic relay: A central control of bone mass. Cell **100**:197–207.

189. Takeda S, Elefteriou F, Levasseur R, Liu X, Zhao L, Parker KL, Armstrong D, Ducy P, Karsenty G 2002 Leptin regulates bone formation via the sympathetic nervous system. Cell **111**:305–317.

190. Thomas T, Gori F, Khosla S, Jensen MD, Burguera B, Riggs BL 1999 Leptin acts on human marrow stromal cells to enhance differentiation to osteoblasts and to inhibit differentiation to adipocytes. Endocrinology **140**:1630–1638.

191. Burguera B, Hofbauer LC, Thomas T, Gori F, Evans GL, Khosla S, Riggs BL, Turner RT 2001 Leptin reduces ovariectomy-induced bone loss in rats. Endocrinology **142**:3546–3553.

192. Pasco JA, Henry MJ, Kotowicz MA, Collier GR, Ball MJ, Ugoni AM, Nicholson GC 2001 Serum leptin levels are associated with bone mass in nonobese women. J Clin Endocrinol Metab **86**:1884–1887.

193. Kim GS, Hong JS, Kim SW, Koh JM, An CS, Choi JY, Cheng SL 2003 Leptin induces apoptosis via ERK/cPLA2/cytochrome c pathway in human bone marrow stromal cells. J Biol Chem **278**:21920–21929.

194. Whitfield JF, Morley P, Willick GE 2002 The control of bone growth by parathyroid hormone, leptin, & statins. Crit Rev Eukaryot Gene Expr **12**:23–51.

195. Amling M, Pogoda P, Beil FT, Schilling AF, Holzmann T, Priemel M, Blicharski D, Catala-Lehnen P, Rueger JM, Ducy P, Karsenty G 2001 Central control of bone mass: Brainstorming of the skeleton. Adv Exp Med Biol **496**:85–94.

196. Muenke M, Schell U, Hehr A, Robin NH, Losken HW, Schinzel A, Pulleyn LJ, Rutland P, Reardon W, Malcolm S 1994 A common mutation in the fibroblast growth factor receptor 1 gene in Pfeiffer syndrome. Nat Genet **8**:269–274.

197. Reardon W, Winter RM, Rutland P, Pulleyn LJ, Jones BM, Malcolm S 1994 Mutations in the fibroblast growth factor receptor 2 gene cause Crouzon syndrome. Nat Genet **8**:98–103.

198. Graham JM Jr, Braddock SR, Mortier GR, Lachman R, Van Dop C, Jabs EW 1998 Syndrome of coronal craniosynostosis with brachydactyly and carpal/tarsal coalition due to Pro250Arg mutation in FGFR3 gene. Am J Med Genet **77**:322–329.

199. Colvin JS, Bohne BA, Harding GW, McEwen DG, Ornitz DM 1996 Skeletal overgrowth and deafness in mice lacking fibroblast growth factor receptor 3. Nat Genet **12**:390–397.

200. Iwata T, Chen L, Li C, Ovchinnikov DA, Behringer RR, Francomano CA, Deng CX 2000 A neonatal lethal mutation in FGFR3 uncouples proliferation and differentiation of growth plate chondrocytes in embryos. Hum Mol Genet **9**:1603–1613.

201. Karaplis AC, Luz A, Glowacki J, Bronson RT, Tybulewicz VL, Kronenberg HM, Mulligan RC 1994 Lethal skeletal dysplasia from targeted disruption of the parathyroid hormone-related peptide gene. Genes Dev **8**:277–289.

202. Lanske B, Karaplis AC, Lee K, Luz A, Vortkamp A, Pirro A, Karperien M, Defize LHK, Ho C, Mulligan RC, Abou-Samra AB, Juppner H, Segre GV, Kronenberg HM 1996 PTH/PTHrP receptor in early development and Indian hedgehog-regulated bone growth. Science **273**:663–666.

203. Schipani E, Lanske B, Hunzelman J, Luz A, Kovacs CS, Lee K, Pirro A, Kronenberg HM, Juppner H 1997 Targeted expression of constitutively active receptors for parathyroid hormone and parathyroid hormone-related peptide delays endochondral bone formation and rescues mice that lack parathyroid hormone-related peptide. Proc Natl Acad Sci USA **94**:13689–13694.

204. Schipani E, Langman CB, Parfitt AM, Jensen GS, Kikuchi S, Kooh SW, Cole WG, Juppner H 1996 Constitutively activated receptors for parathyroid hormone and parathyroid hormone-related peptide in Jansen's metaphyseal chondrodysplasia. N Engl J Med **335**:708–714.

205. St Jacques B, Hammerschmidt M, McMahon AP 1999 Indian hedgehog signaling regulates proliferation and differentiation of chondrocytes and is essential for bone formation. Genes Dev **13**:2072–2086.

206. Vortkamp A, Lee K, Lanske B, Segre GV, Kronenberg HM, Tabin CJ 1996 Regulation of rate of cartilage differentiation by Indian hedgehog and PTH-related protein. Science **273**:613–622.

207. Daluiski A, Engstrand T, Bahamonde ME, Gamer LW, Agius E, Stevenson SL, Cox K, Rosen V, Lyons KM 2001 Bone morphogenetic protein-3 is a negative regulator of bone density. Nat Genet **27**:84–88.

208. Erlebacher A, Derynck R 1996 Increased expression of TGF-beta 2 in osteoblasts results in an osteoporosis-like phenotype. J Cell Biol **132**:195–210.

209. Dabovic B, Chen Y, Colarossi C, Obata H, Zambuto L, Perle MA, Rifkin DB 2002 Bone abnormalities in latent TGF-[beta] binding protein (Ltbp)-3-null mice indicate a role for Ltbp-3 in modulating TGF-[beta] bioavailability. J Cell Biol **156**:227–232.

210. Yoshida Y, Tanaka S, Umemori H, Minowa O, Usui M, Ikematsu N, Hosoda E, Imamura T, Kuno J, Yamashita T, Miyazono K, Noda M, Noda T, Yamamoto T 2000 Negative regulation of BMP/Smad signaling by Tob in osteoblasts. Cell **103**:1085–1097.

211. Brunet LJ, McMahon JA, McMahon AP, Harland RM 1998 Noggin, cartilage morphogenesis, and joint formation in the mammalian skeleton. Science **280**:1455–1457.

212. Devlin RD, Du Z, Pereira RC, Kimble RB, Economides AN, Jorgetti V, Canalis E 2003 Skeletal overexpression of noggin results in osteopenia and reduced bone formation. Endocrinology **144**:1972–1978.

213. Warren SM, Brunet LJ, Harland RM, Economides AN, Longaker MT 2003 The BMP antagonist noggin regulates cranial suture fusion. Nature **422**:625–629.

214. Chusho H, Tamura N, Ogawa Y, Yasoda A, Suda M, Miyazawa T, Nakamura K, Nakao K, Kurihara T, Komatsu Y, Itoh H, Tanaka K, Saito Y, Katsuki M, Nakao K 2001 Dwarfism and early death in mice lacking C-type natriuretic peptide. Proc Natl Acad Sci USA **98**:4016–4021.

215. Soriano P 1997 The PDGF alpha receptor is required for neural crest cell development and for normal patterning of the somites. Development **124**:2691–2700.

216. Kato M, Patel MS, Levasseur R, Lobov I, Chang BH, Glass DA, Hartmann C, Li L, Hwang TH, Brayton CF, Lang RA, Karsenty G, Chan L 2002 Cbfa1-independent decrease in osteoblast proliferation, osteopenia, and persistent embryonic eye vascularization in mice deficient in Lrp5, a Wnt coreceptor. J Cell Biol **157**:303–314.

217. Gong Y, Slee RB, Fukai N, Rawadi G, Roman-Roman S, Reginato AM, Wang H, Cundy T, Glorieux FH, Lev D, Zacharin M, Oexle K, Marcelino J, Suwairi W, Heeger S, Sabatakos G, Apte S, Adkins WN, Allgrove J, Arslan-Kirchner M, Batch JA, Beighton P, Black GC, Boles RG, Boon LM, Borrone C, Brunner HG, Carle GF, Dallapiccola B, De Paepe A, Floege B, Halfhide ML, Hall B, Hennekam RC, Hirose T, Jans A, Juppner H, Kim CA, Keppler-Noreuil K, Kohlschuetter A, LaCombe D, Lambert M, Lemyre E, Letteboer T, Peltonen L, Ramesar RS, Romanengo M, Somer H, Steichen-Gersdorf E, Steinmann B, Sullivan B, Superti-Furga A, Swoboda W, van den Boogaard MJ, van Hul W, Vikkula M, Votruba M, Zabel B, Garcia T, Baron R, Olsen BR, Warman ML 2001 LDL receptor-related protein 5 (LRP5) affects bone accrual and eye development. Cell **107**:513–523.

218. Little RD, Carulli JP, Del Mastro RG, Dupuis J, Osborne M, Folz C, Manning SP, Swain PM, Zhao SC, Eustace B, Lappe MM, Spitzer L, Zweier S, Braunschweiger K, Benchekroun Y, Hu X, Adair R, Chee L, FitzGerald MG, Tulig C, Caruso A, Tzellas N, Bawa A, Franklin B, McGuire S, Nogues X, Gong G, Allen KM, Anisowicz A, Morales AJ, Lomedico PT, Recker SM, Van Eerdewegh P, Recker RR, Johnson ML 2002 A mutation in the LDL receptor-related protein 5 gene results in the autosomal dominant high-bone-mass trait. Am J Hum Genet **70**:11–19.

219. Van Wesenbeeck L, Cleiren E, Gram J, Beals RK, Benichou O, Scopelliti D, Key L, Renton T, Bartels C, Gong Y, Warman ML, de Vernejoul MC, Bollerslev J, van Hul W 2003 Six novel missense mutations in the ldl receptor-related protein 5 (lrp5) gene in different conditions with an increased bone density. Am J Hum Genet **72**:763–771.

220. Sjogren K, Bohlooly YM, Olsson B, Coschigano K, Tornell J, Mohan S, Isaksson OG, Baumann G, Kopchick J, Ohlsson C 2000 Disproportional skeletal growth and markedly decreased bone mineral content in growth hormone receptor-/- mice. Biochem Biophys Res Commun **267**:603–608.

221. Takeuchi S, Takeda K, Oishi I, Nomi M, Ikeya M, Itoh K, Tamura S, Ueda T, Hatta T, Otani H, Terashima T, Takada S, Yamamura H, Akira S, Minami Y 2000 Mouse Ror2 receptor tyrosine kinase is required for the heart development and limb formation. Genes Cells **5**:71–78.

222. Nomi M, Oishi I, Kani S, Suzuki H, Matsuda T, Yoda A, Kitamura M, Itoh K, Takeuchi S, Takeda K, Akira S, Ikeya M, Takada S, Minami Y 2001 Loss of mRor1 enhances the heart and skeletal abnormalities in mRor2-deficient mice: Redundant and pleiotropic functions of mRor1 and mRor2 receptor tyrosine kinases. Mol Cell Biol **21**:8329–8335.

223. Tezuka K, Yasuda M, Watanabe N, Morimura N, Kuroda K, Miyatani S, Hozumi N 2002 Stimulation of osteoblastic cell differentiation by Notch. J Bone Miner Res **17**:231–239.

224. Zhang M, Xuan S, Bouxsein ML, von Stechow D, Akeno N, Faugere MC, Malluche H, Zhao G, Rosen CJ, Efstratiadis A, Clemens TL 2002 Osteoblast-specific knockout of the insulin-like growth factor (IGF) receptor gene reveals an essential role of IGF signaling in bone matrix mineralization. J Biol Chem 277:44005–44012.

225. Bikle D, Majumdar S, Laib A, Powell-Braxton L, Rosen C, Beamer W, Nauman E, Leary C, Halloran B 2001 The skeletal structure of insulin-like growth factor I-deficient mice. J Bone Miner Res 16:2320–2329.

226. Lupu F, Terwilliger JD, Lee K, Segre GV, Efstratiadis A 2001 Roles of growth hormone and insulin-like growth factor 1 in mouse post-natal growth. Dev Biol 229:141–162.

227. Ben Lagha N, Menuelle P, Seurin D, Binoux M, Lebouc Y, Berdal A 2002 Bone formation in the context of growth retardation induced by hIGFBP-1 overexpression in transgenic mice. Connect Tissue Res 43:515–519.

228. Meyer T, Kneissel M, Mariani J, Fournier B 2000 In vitro and in vivo evidence for orphan nuclear receptor RORalpha function in bone metabolism. Proc Natl Acad Sci USA 97:9197–9202.

229. Steinmayr M, Andre E, Conquet F, Rondi-Reig L, Delhaye-Bouchaud N, Auclair N, Daniel H, Crepel F, Mariani J, Sotelo C, Becker-Andre M 1998 Staggerer phenotype in retinoid-related orphan receptor alpha-deficient mice. Proc Natl Acad Sci USA 95:3960–3965.

230. Dussault I, Fawcett D, Matthyssen A, Bader JA, Giguere V 1998 Orphan nuclear receptor ROR alpha-deficient mice display the cerebellar defects of staggerer. Mech Dev 70:147–153.

231. DeChiara TM, Kimble RB, Poueymirou WT, Rojas J, Masiakowski P, Valenzuela DM, Yancopoulos GD 2000 Ror2, encoding a receptor-like tyrosine kinase, is required for cartilage and growth plate development. Nat Genet 24:271–274.

232. Zhang X, Schwarz EM, Young DA, Puzas JE, Rosier RN, O'Keefe RJ 2002 Cyclooxygenase-2 regulates mesenchymal cell differentiation into the osteoblast lineage and is critically involved in bone repair. J Clin Invest 109:1405–1415.

233. Kanzler B, Kuschert SJ, Liu YH, Mallo M 1998 Hoxa-2 restricts the chondrogenic domain and inhibits bone formation during development of the branchial area. Development 125:2587–2597.

234. Chen Y, Bei M, Woo I, Satokata I, Maas R 1996 Msx1 controls inductive signaling in mammalian tooth morphogenesis. Development 122:3035–3044.

235. Jumlongras D, Bei M, Stimson JM, Wang WF, DePalma SR, Seidman CE, Felbor U, Maas R, Seidman JG, Olsen BR 2001 A nonsense mutation in MSX1 causes Witkop syndrome. Am J Hum Genet 69:67–74.

236. Satokata I, Ma L, Ohshima H, Bei M, Woo I, Nishizawa K, Maeda T, Takano Y, Uchiyama M, Heaney S, Peters H, Tang Z, Maxson R, Maas R 2000 Msx2 deficiency in mice causes pleiotropic defects in bone growth and ectodermal organ formation. Nat Genet 24:391–395.

237. Wilkie AO, Tang Z, Elanko N, Walsh S, Twigg SR, Hurst JA, Wall SA, Chrzanowska KH, Maxson RE Jr 2000 Functional haploinsufficiency of the human homeobox gene MSX2 causes defects in skull ossification. Nat Genet 24:387–390.

238. Liu YH, Tang Z, Kundu RK, Wu L, Luo W, Zhu D, Sangiorgi F, Snead ML, Maxson RE 1999 Msx2 gene dosage influences the number of proliferative osteogenic cells in growth centers of the developing murine skull: A possible mechanism for MSX2-mediated craniosynostosis in humans. Dev Biol 205:260–274.

239. Jabs EW, Muller U, Li X, Ma L, Luo W, Haworth IS, Klisak I, Sparkes R, Warman ML, Mulliken JB, Snead ML, Maxson R 1993 A mutation in the homeodomain of the human MSX2 gene in a family affected with autosomal dominant craniosynostosis. Cell 75:443–450.

240. Qiu M, Bulfone A, Ghattas I, Meneses JJ, Christensen L, Sharpe PT, Presley R, Pedersen RA, Rubenstein JL 1997 Role of the Dlx homeobox genes in proximodistal patterning of the branchial arches: Mutations of Dlx-1, Dlx-2, and Dlx-1 and -2 alter morphogenesis of proximal skeletal and soft tissue structures derived from the first and second arches. Dev Biol 185:165–184.

241. Ferrari D, Kosher RA 2002 Dlx5 is a positive regulator of chondrocyte differentiation during endochondral ossification. Dev Biol 252:257–270.

242. Acampora D, Merlo GR, Paleari L, Zerega B, Postiglione MP, Mantero S, Bober E, Barbieri O, Simeone A, Levi G 1999 Craniofacial, vestibular and bone defects in mice lacking the distal-less-related gene dlx5. Development 126:3795–3809.

243. Robledo RF, Rajan L, Li X, Lufkin T 2002 The Dlx5 and Dlx6 homeobox genes are essential for craniofacial, axial, and appendicular skeletal development. Genes Dev 16:1089–1101.

244. Crackower MA, Scherer SW, Rommens JM, Hui CC, Poorkaj P, Soder S, Cobben JM, Hudgins L, Evans JP, Tsui LC 1996 Characterization of the split hand/split foot malformation locus SHFM1 at 7q21.3-q22.1 and analysis of a candidate gene for its expression during limb development. Hum Mol Genet 5:571–579.

245. Tribioli C, Lufkin T 1999 The murine Bapx1 homeobox gene plays a critical role in embryonic development of the axial skeleton and spleen. Development 126:5699–5711.

246. Akazawa H, Komuro I, Sugitani Y, Yazaki Y, Nagai R, Noda T 2000 Targeted disruption of the homeobox transcription factor Bapx1 results in lethal skeletal dysplasia with asplenia and gastroduodenal malformation. Genes Cells 5:499–513.

247. Lettice LA, Purdie LA, Carlson GJ, Kilanowski F, Dorin J, Hill RE 1999 The mouse bagpipe gene controls development of axial skeleton, skull, and spleen. Proc Natl Acad Sci USA 96:9695–9700.

248. Yousfi M, Lasmoles F, Lomri A, Delannoy P, Marie PJ 2001 Increased bone formation and decreased osteocalcin expression induced by reduced Twist dosage in Saethre-Chotzen syndrome. J Clin Invest 107:1153–1161.

249. Jabs EW 2001 A TWIST in the fate of human osteoblasts identifies signaling molecules involved in skull development. J Clin Invest 107:1075–1077.

250. Rice DP, Aberg T, Chan Y, Tang Z, Kettunen PJ, Pakarinen L, Maxson RE, Thesleff I 2000 Integration of FGF and TWIST in calvarial bone and suture development. Development 127:1845–1855.

251. Mundlos S, Otto F, Mundlos C, Mulliken JB, Aylsworth AS, Albright S, Lindhout D, Cole WG, Henn W, Knoll JHM, Owen MJ, Mertelsmann R, Zabel BU, Olsen BR 1997 Mutations involving the transcription factor CBFA1 cause cleidocranial dysplasia. Cell 89:773–779.

252. Otto F, Thornell AP, Crompton T, Denzel A, Gilmour KC, Rosewell IR, Stamp GWH, Beddington RSP, Mundlos S, Olsen BR, Selby PB, Owen MJ. Cbfa1, a candidate gene for cleidocranial dysplasia syndrome, is essential for osteoblast differentiation and bone development. Cell 89:765–771, 1997.

253. Zhou G, Chen Y, Zhou L, Thirunavukkarasu K, Hecht J, Chitayat D, Gelb BD, Pirinen S, Berry SA, Greenberg CR, Karsenty G, Lee B 1999 CBFA1 mutation analysis and functional correlation with phenotypic variability in cleidocranial dysplasia. Hum Mol Genet 8:2311–2316.

254. Banerjee C, McCabe LR, Choi J-Y, Hiebert SW, Stein JL, Stein GS, Lian JB 1997 Runt homology domain proteins in osteoblast differentiation: AML-3/CBFA1 is a major component of a bone specific complex. J Cell Biochem 66:1–8.

255. Reimold AM, Grusby MJ, Kosaras B, Fries JW, Mori R, Maniwa S, Clauss IM, Collins T, Sidman RL, Glimcher MJ, Glimcher LH 1996 Chondrodysplasia and neurological abnormalities in ATF-2-deficient mice. Nature 379:262–265.

256. Zayzafoon M, Botolin S, McCabe LR 2002 P38 and activating transcription factor-2 involvement in osteoblast osmotic response to elevated extracellular glucose. J Biol Chem 277:37212–37218.

257. Umayahara Y, Ji C, Centrella M, Rotwein P, McCarthy TL 1997 CCAAT/enhancer-binding protein delta activates insulin-like growth factor-I gene transcription in osteoblasts. Identification of a novel cyclic AMP signaling pathway in bone. J Biol Chem 272:31793–31800.

258. Pereira RC, Delany AM, Canalis E 2002 Effects of cortisol and bone morphogenetic protein-2 on stromal cell differentiation: Correlation with CCAAT-enhancer binding protein expression. Bone 30:685–691.

259. Long F, Schipani E, Asahara H, Kronenberg H, Montminy M 2001 The CREB family of activators is required for endochondral bone development. Development 128:541–550.

260. Nikaido T, Yokoya S, Mori T, Hagino S, Iseki K, Zhang Y, Takeuchi M, Takaki H, Kikuchi S, Wanaka A 2001 Expression of the novel transcription factor OASIS, which belongs to the CREB/ATF family, in mouse embryo with special reference to bone development. Histochem Cell Biol 116:141–148.

261. Sakai A, Sakata T, Tanaka S, Okazaki R, Kunugita N, Norimura T, Nakamura T 2002 Disruption of the p53 gene results in preserved trabecular bone mass and bone formation after mechanical unloading. J Bone Miner Res 17:119–127.

262. Tyner SD, Venkatachalam S, Choi J, Jones S, Ghebranious N, Igelmann H, Lu X, Soron G, Cooper B, Brayton C, Hee PS, Thomp-

son T, Karsenty G, Bradley A, Donehower LA 2002 p53 mutant mice that display early ageing-associated phenotypes. Nature **415**:45–53.

263. Gruda MC, van Amsterdam J, Rizzo CA, Durham SK, Lira S, Bravo R 1996 Expression of FosB during mouse development: Normal development of FosB knockout mice. Oncogene **12**:2177–2185.

264. Grigoriadis AE, Schellander K, Wang Z-Q, Wagner EF 1993 Osteoblasts are target cells for transformation in *c-fos* transgenic mice. J Cell Biol **122**:685–701.

265. Johnson RS, Spiegelman BM, Papaioannou V 1992 Pleiotropic effects of a null mutation in the c-fos proto-oncogene. Cell **71**:577–586.

266. Wang Z-Q, Ovitt C, Grigoriadis AE, Mohle-Steinlein U, Ruther U, Wagner EF 1992 Bone and haematopoietic defects in mice lacking *c-fos*. Nature **360**:741–745.

267. Jochum W, David JP, Elliott C, Wutz A, Plenk H Jr, Matsuo K, Wagner EF 2000 Increased bone formation and osteosclerosis in mice overexpressing the transcription factor Fra-1. Nat Med **6**:980–984.

268. Sabatakos G, Sims NA, Chen J, Aoki K, Kelz MB, Amling M, Bouali Y, Mukhopadhyay K, Ford K, Nestler EJ, Baron R 2000 Overexpression of DeltaFosB transcription factor(s) increases bone formation and inhibits adipogenesis. Nat Med **6**:985–990.

269. Zimmerman D, Jin F, Leboy P, Hardy S, Damsky C 2000 Impaired bone formation in transgenic mice resulting from altered integrin function in osteoblasts. Dev Biol **220**:2–15.

270. Globus RK, Doty SB, Lull JC, Holmuhamedov E, Humphries MJ, Damsky CH 1998 Fibronectin is a survival factor for differentiated osteoblasts. J Cell Sci **111**:1385–1393.

271. Moursi AM, Globus RK, Damsky CH 1997 Interactions between integrin receptors and fibronectin are required for calvarial osteoblast differentiation in vitro. J Cell Sci **110**:2187–2196.

272. Horiuchi K, Amizuka N, Takeshita S, Takamatsu H, Katsuura M, Ozawa H, Toyama Y, Bonewald LF, Kudo A 1999 Identification and characterization of a novel protein, periostin, with restricted expression to periosteum and periodontal ligament and increased expression by transforming growth factor beta. J Bone Miner Res **14**:1239–1249.

273. Sasaki H, Yu CY, Dai M, Tam C, Loda M, Auclair D, Chen LB, Elias A 2003 Elevated serum periostin levels in patients with bone metastases from breast but not lung cancer. Breast Cancer Res Treat **77**:245–252.

274. Tanaka Y, Morimoto I, Nakano Y, Okada Y, Hirota S, Nomura S, Nakamura T, Eto S 1995 Osteoblasts are regulated by the cellular adhesion through ICAM-1 and VCAM-1. J Bone Miner Res **10**:1462–1469.

275. Fang J, Hall BK 1995 Differential expression of neural cell adhesion molecule (NCAM) during osteogenesis and secondary chondrogenesis in the embryonic chick. Int J Dev Biol **39**:519–528.

276. Colnot C, Sidhu SS, Balmain N, Poirier F 2001 Uncoupling of chondrocyte death and vascular invasion in mouse galectin 3 null mutant bones. Dev Biol **229**:203–214.

277. Kawaguchi J, Azuma Y, Hoshi K, Kii I, Takeshita S, Ohta T, Ozawa H, Takeichi M, Chisaka O, Kudo A 2001 Targeted disruption of cadherin-11 leads to a reduction in bone density in calvaria and long bone metaphyses. J Bone Miner Res **16**:1265–1271.

278. Cheng SL, Lecanda F, Davidson MK, Warlow PM, Zhang SF, Zhang L, Suzuki S, St. John T, Civitelli R 1998 Human osteoblasts express a repertoire of cadherins, which are critical for BMP-2-induced osteogenic differentiation. J Bone Miner Res **13**:633–644.

279. Imai S, Kaksonen M, Raulo E, Kinnunen T, Fages C, Meng X, Lakso M, Rauvala H 1998 Osteoblast recruitment and bone formation enhanced by cell matrix-associated heparin-binding growth-associated molecule (HB-GAM). J Cell Biol **143**:1113–1128.

280. Tare RS, Oreffo RO, Sato K, Rauvala H, Clarke NM, Roach HI 2002 Effects of targeted overexpression of pleiotrophin on postnatal bone development. Biochem Biophys Res Commun **298**:324–332.

281. Fedde KN, Blair L, Silverstein J, Coburn SP, Ryan LM, Weinstein RS, Waymire K, Narisawa S, Millan JL, MacGregor GR, Whyte MP 1999 Alkaline phosphatase knock-out mice recapitulate the metabolic and skeletal defects of infantile hypophosphatasia. J Bone Miner Res **14**:2015–2026.

282. Narisawa S, Frohlander N, Millan JL 1997 Inactivation of two mouse alkaline phosphatase genes and establishment of a model of infantile hypophosphatasia. Dev Dyn **208**:432–446.

283. Whyte MP 1994 Hypophosphatasia and the role of alkaline phosphatase in skeletal mineralization. Endocr Rev **15**:439–461.

284. Gowen LC, Petersen DN, Mansolf AL, Qi H, Stock JL, Tkalcevic GT, Simmons HA, Crawford DT, Chidsey-Frink KL, Ke HZ, McNeish JD, Brown TA 2003 Targeted disruption of the osteoblast/osteocyte factor 45 gene (OF45) results in increased bone formation and bone mass. J Biol Chem **278**:1998–2007.

Chapter 4.   Osteogenic Growth Factors

Ernesto Canalis

Department of Research, Saint Francis Hospital and Medical Center, Hartford, Connecticut

INTRODUCTION

Growth factors are polypeptides with effects on the replication and differentiation of undifferentiated cells, resulting in an increase or decrease of a specific cell population. Growth factors also can enhance or suppress the differentiated function of a mature cell and thus play a central role in bone remodeling. Bone remodeling is a complex process involving a number of cellular functions directed toward the coordinated resorption and formation of new bone. The continuous turnover of bone is regulated by systemic hormones and by local factors, which affect cells of the osteoclast and osteoblast lineages.[1] The factors present in the bone microenvironment include growth factors, cytokines, and prostaglandins, and they have distinct functions in specific cells.[1] Growth factor activity can be regulated by different agents and mechanisms, including synthesis, activation, receptor binding, and binding proteins. Bone is a rich source of growth factors, with important actions in the regulation of bone formation and bone resorption. Frequently, these local factors are synthesized by bone-forming cells, although some cytokines are secreted by stromal cells and by cells of the immune or hematological system, and as such, they are present in the bone microenvironment. Growth factors may be present in the circulation and act as systemic regulators of skeletal metabolism. This review will address classic skeletal growth factors and their function in the bone microenvironment.

INSULIN-LIKE GROWTH FACTORS

Insulin-like growth factors (IGFs) are polypeptides with a molecular mass (Mr) of 7600.[2] Two IGFs have been characterized: IGF-I and IGF-II. These peptides are present in the systemic circulation and are synthesized by multiple tissues, including bone, where they act as local regulators of

The author has no conflict of interest.

cell metabolism. Systemic IGF-I is secreted by the liver, and its synthesis is growth hormone-dependent, whereas the synthesis of IGF-I in peripheral tissues is regulated by diverse hormones.[2] In the circulation, IGFs are bound to IGF binding proteins (IGFBPs) and to an acid-labile subunit.[2,3] The most abundant IGFBP in serum is IGFBP-3, which also is growth hormone-dependent. IGF-I and IGF-II have similar biological activities, but IGF-I is more potent than IGF-II. IGFs have modest mitogenic activity for cells of the osteoblastic lineage and enhance the function of the mature osteoblast, increasing bone matrix synthesis.[4] In addition, IGFs prevent osteoblastic apoptosis, maintaining a larger population of mature osteoblasts.[5] IGFs increase type I collagen transcription and decrease the transcription of collagenase 3 or matrix metalloproteinase (MMP)-13, a collagen-degrading protease.[6] As a consequence of a decrease in collagenase levels, IGFs inhibit bone collagen degradation. This dual effect, an increase in collagen synthesis and a decrease in its degradation, is central to the maintenance of bone matrix and bone mass. In vivo experiments have confirmed IGF actions in vitro. IGF-I null mice have decreased bone formation, and transgenic animals overexpressing IGF-I under the control of the osteocalcin promoter have increased bone formation.[7,8] Infusions of IGF-I to humans cause a generalized anabolic effect and an increase in bone remodeling.[9] IGFs play a role in the maintenance of cortical bone in rodents, and low IGF-I levels correlate with a decrease in bone mineral density (BMD) in elderly women and in patients with anorexia nervosa.[9–11]

IGFs can be modified by changes in their synthesis, receptor binding and IGF binding proteins (IGFBPs). The synthesis of skeletal IGF-I is regulated by hormones and growth factors. Parathyroid hormone (PTH) is a major inducer of IGF-I synthesis in osteoblasts, and IGF-I is required to observe the anabolic effect of PTH in bone.[7] Growth hormone plays a modest role in enhancing IGF-I production in bone, although growth hormone receptor null mice have decreased bone formation, which is normalized by IGF-I administration.[12] Glucocorticoids inhibit IGF-I expression, and this is an important mechanism that contributes to the decreased bone formation observed after glucocorticoid exposure.[13] The molecular mechanism of this effect involves the regulation of CCAAT-enhancer binding proteins (C/EBP), a family of transcription factors critical to cell differentiation and function.[14] Glucocorticoids induce C/EBPs β and δ and inhibit IGF-I transcription through a C/EBP binding site next to the third start site of transcription in the IGF-I promoter.[15] Skeletal growth factors with mitogenic properties inhibit the synthesis of IGF-I and IGF-II by the osteoblast, an effect that correlates with a decrease in the differentiated function of this cell.[16]

Bone cells also secrete the six known IGFBPs, which may prolong the half-life of IGF, neutralize or enhance its biological activity, or be involved in the transport of IGF to its target cells.[3] Some binding proteins, such as IGFBP-4, have inhibitory activity. Others, such as IGFBP-5, were reported to be stimulatory. However, recent work demonstrated that transgenic animals overexpressing IGFBP-5 under the control of the osteocalcin promoter develop osteopenia caused by decreased bone formation.[17] The synthesis of

IGFBPs is regulated by specific agents and mechanisms, and their degradation by specific and nonspecific proteases including serine proteases and MMPs.[18]

BONE MORPHOGENETIC PROTEINS

Bone morphogenetic proteins (BMPs) are members of the transforming growth factor β (TGF β) superfamily of polypeptides, which includes TGF βs, activins, and inhibins.[19] The proteins display extensive conservation among species having seven characteristic cysteine knot domains, which participate in the formation of an interchain disulfide bond between two monomers to form a dimeric precursor protein. Mature proteins have a Mr of 20,000 to 30,000. BMPs are synthesized by skeletal and extraskeletal tissues, and BMP-2, -4, and -6 are synthesized by osteoblasts and play an autocrine role in osteoblastic function.[20] BMPs are unique and induce the differentiation of cells of the osteoblastic lineage, increasing the pool of mature cells, and enhance the differentiated function of the osteoblast.[21,22] A consequence of their effects on osteoblast differentiation is increased osteoclastogenesis, a process tightly coordinated with osteoblastogenesis. BMPs induce terminal osteoblastic differentiation, and this process is associated with apoptosis, an ultimate fate of a mature cell.[23] BMPs also induce endochondral ossification and chondrogenesis acting in conjunction with Indian/Sonic hedgehog.[24]

BMPs initiate signaling from the cell surface by interacting with two distinct serine/threonine kinase receptors. After receptor activation, BMPs, TGF β, and activin signal through Smads.[25–27] At least eight Smads have been isolated in mammals and two additional Smads in lower species. There are three classes of Smads: (1) receptor-regulated Smads that can be BMP activated, such as Smad 1, 5, and 8, or TGF β- and activin-activated, such as Smad 2 and 3; (2) common TGF β and BMP mediator Smads, Smad 4; and (3) inhibitory Smads, Smad 6 and 7.[27] After BMP exposure, Smad 1/5 are phosphorylated at serine residues and translocated to the nucleus after heterodimerization with Smad 4, a common partner with TGF β signaling, to regulate transcription by interacting with other nuclear factors and DNA sequences. The effect of BMPs on osteoblastic differentiation and targeting of Smads to specific cellular fractions requires interactions of Smads with Runx-2/Cbfa-1.[28] BMPs and TGF β also can activate Smad-independent pathways, such as those dependent on Ras/MAP kinase signaling.[29]

BMP activity can be suppressed by a variety of mechanisms including (1) dominant negative nonsignaling pseudoreceptors; (2) inhibitory Smads 6 and 7; (3) intracellular Smad binding proteins, Tob and Ski; (4) ubiquitination and degradation of signaling Smads by Smurf 1 and 2; and (5) extracellular specific antagonist BMP binding proteins, including the components of the Spemann organizer, noggin, chordin, and follistatin, members of the Dan/Cerberus family, and twisted gastrulation.[19] The existence of these BMP antagonists reveal a need to temper the activity of BMPs and possibly of growth factors in general.

Wnt AND LOW DENSITY LIPOPROTEIN RECEPTOR-RELATED PROTEIN 5

Wnts have similar activities to those of BMPs and induce cell differentiation.[30] By inhibiting a glycogen-synthase 3, Wnts prevent the degradation of β catenin, which after nuclear translocation, associates with members of the lymphoid enhancer binding factor/T cell specific factor (LEF/TCF) transcription factor family and targets specific genes. β catenin and LEF/TCF can form a complex with Smad 4, and as such, have the potential to regulate BMP and TGF β signaling.[31] Low-density lipoprotein receptor–related protein 5 (LRP 5) is a coreceptor for Wnt and signals through the canonical Wnt signaling pathway, resulting in β catenin accumulation.[32] LRP 5 is expressed by osteoblasts and stromal cells and its expression is stimulated by BMPs.[33] LRP 5 is required for optimal Wnt signaling in osteoblasts, and LRP 5 null mice are osteopenic.[34] In humans, mutations inactivating LRP 5 result in decreased bone mass, and mutations resulting in an LRP 5 resistant to inactivation cause increased bone mass.[33,35]

TGF β

TGF β is a polypeptide with a Mr of 25,000.[36] Three isoforms of mammalian TGF β, with similar biological activities, have been described and are synthesized by bone cells. They are TGF β1, β2, and β3. TGF β stimulates the replication of preosteoblasts, bone collagen synthesis, and inhibits bone resorption by inducing osteoclastic apoptosis.[36] However, TGF β opposes the effect of BMPs on osteoblastic cell differentiation and transgenic mice overexpressing TGF β under the control of the osteocalcin promoter are osteopenic, suggesting a predominant negative effect on bone formation.[37,38] The levels of TGF β can be modified by activation and by changes in synthesis. The gene elements responsible for regulation of TGF β1, β2, and β3 expression are different, leading to their differential regulation by hormones and various factors. TGF β is released in an inactive form bound to a precursor and to a binding protein, and bone resorbing agents activate and induce the release of TGF β from this tissue, becoming available to modulate bone remodeling.[36] Like BMPs, TGF β binds to two distinct serine-threonine kinase receptors, which after dimerization, activate Smad 2 and 3 and these bind to Smad 4 to regulate transcription.[27,29]

FIBROBLAST GROWTH FACTORS

Fibroblast growth factor (FGF) 1 and 2 are polypeptides with a Mr of 17,000.[39] FGFs are members of a large family of related genes. FGFs have angiogenic properties and are considered important for neovascularization, wound healing, and bone repair. FGF 1 and 2 stimulate bone cell replication, which results in an increased bone cell population capable of synthesizing bone collagen.[40,41] Bones treated with FGF synthesize greater amounts of collagenous matrix secondary to an increased number of collagen-synthesizing cells, but FGFs do not enhance the differentiated function of the osteoblast directly. In vivo FGF is important in the maintenance of bone mass and FGF null

mice have decreased osteoblast number and bone formation.[42] FGFs play a minor role in bone resorption, and increase the expression of MMP-13, indicating a possible function in bone collagen degradation and remodeling. The systemic administration of FGF 2 increases the number of preosteoblasts that eventually mature and form bone.[43] Similarly, FGF 2 accelerates the healing of fractures. TGF β and FGF increase FGF expression in osteoblasts, indicating a local control of its synthesis. There are four related FGF receptors (FGFR) termed FGFR-1 to -4. FGFR-1, -2, and -3 mediate the mitogenic response to FGF, and the pattern of FGFR expression differs during skeletal development.[39,40] FGFR signaling is essential for skeletal and limb development and for chondrogenesis, and mutations of FGFR-1, -2, and -3 result in serious skeletal abnormalities. An activating mutation of FGFR-3 results in achondroplasia, a common cause of dwarfism, and early closure of cranial sutures.[44]

PLATELET-DERIVED GROWTH FACTOR

Platelet-derived growth factor (PDGF), a polypeptide with a Mr of 30,000, was initially isolated from blood platelets and was considered important in the early phases of wound repair.[45] Normal and neoplastic tissues also synthesize PDGF, indicating that it may act as a systemic or local regulator of tissue growth. PDGF is a dimer of the products of two genes, PDGF-A and -B, so that mature peptides can exist as PDGF-AA or -BB homodimers or as PDGF-AB heterodimers. PDGF-AB and -BB are the predominant isoforms present in the systemic circulation. Osteoblasts express the PDGF-A and -B genes.[46] PDGF has activities similar to those described for FGF. It stimulates bone cell replication, and as a consequence of an increased number of cells, PDGF stimulates bone collagen synthesis. However, PDGF does not have a direct stimulatory effect on the differentiated function of the osteoblast and inhibits bone mineral apposition rates.[47] PDGF-BB also stimulates bone resorption increasing osteoclast number and induces the expression of MMP-13 by the osteoblast.[46] PDGF-A expression is enhanced by TGF β and PDGF, and PDGF-B expression by TGF β. There are two PDGF receptors, α and β, and the activity of PDGF can be regulated by changes in receptor binding. There are no specific binding proteins for PDGF, but PDGF-B chains bind to osteonectin (SPARC), a matrix protein essential for the maintenance of bone structure.[48] PDGF acts as a systemic agent, and when released by the aggregating platelet, it may increase the replication of cells critical for the process of fracture and wound repair.

In conclusion, skeletal growth factors play diverse roles in the differentiation and activity of cells of the osteoblastic lineage and in the maintenance of bone structure and function.

REFERENCES

1. Margolis RN, Canalis E, Partridge NC 1996 Anabolic hormones in bone: Basic research and therapeutic potential. J Clin Endocrinol Metab 81:872–877.
2. Jones JL, Clemmons DR 1995 Insulin-like growth factors and their binding proteins: Biological actions. Endocr Rev 16:3–34.
3. Hwa V, Oh Y, Rosenfeld RG 1999 The insulin-like growth factor-binding protein (IGFBP) superfamily. Endocr Rev 20:761–787.

4. Hock JM, Centrella M, Canalis E 1998 Insulin-like growth factor I (IGF-I) has independent effects on bone matrix formation and cell replication. Endocrinology **122**:254–260.

5. Hill PA, Tumber A, Meikle MC 1997 Multiple extracellular signals promote osteoblast survival and apoptosis. Endocrinology **138**:3849–3858.

6. Canalis E, Rydziel S, Delany A, Varghese S, Jeffrey J 1995 Insulin-like growth factors inhibit interstitial collagenase synthesis in bone cell cultures. Endocrinology **136**:1348–1354.

7. Bikle DD, Sakata T, Leary C, Elalieh H, Ginzinger D, Rosen CJ, Beamer W, Majumdar S, Halloran BP 2002 Insulin-like growth factor I is required for the anabolic actions of parathyroid hormone on mouse bone. J Bone Miner Res **17**:1570–1578.

8. Zhao G, Monier-Gaugere MC, Langub MC, Geng Z, Nakayama T, Pike JW, Chernausek SD, Rosen CJ, Donahue L-R, Malluche HH, Fagin JA, Clemens TL 2000 Targeted overexpression of insulin-like growth factor I to osteoblasts of transgenic mice: Increased trabecular bone volume without increased osteoblast proliferation. Endocrinology **141**:2674–2682.

9. Grinspoon S, Thomas L, Miller K, Herzog D, Klibanski A 2002 Effects of recombinant human IGF-I and oral contraceptive administration on bone density in anorexia nervosa. J Clin Endocrinol Metab **87**:2883–2891.

10. Barrett-Connor E, Goodman-Gruen D 1998 Gender differences in insulin-like growth factor and bone mineral density association in old age: The Rancho Bernardo study. J Bone Miner Res **13**:1343–1349.

11. Rosen CJ, Dimai HP, Vereault D, Donahue LR, Beamer WG, Farley J, Linkhart S, Linkhart T, Mohan S, Baylink DJ 1997 Circulating and skeletal insulin-like growth factor-I (IGF-I) concentrations in two inbred strains of mice with different bone mineral densities. Bone **21**:217–223.

12. Sims NA, Clement-Lacroix P, Da Ponte F, Bouali Y, Binart N, Moriggl R, Goffin V, Coschigano K, Gaillard-Kelly M, Kopchick J, Baron R, Kelly PA 2000 Bone homeostasis in growth hormone receptor-null mice is restored by IGF-I independent of Stat5. J Clin Invest **106**:1095–1103.

13. Canalis E, Giustina A 2001 Glucocorticoid-induced osteoporosis: Summary of a workshop. J Clin Endocrinol Metab **86**:5681–5685.

14. Hanson RW 1998 Biological role of the isoforms of C/EBP minireview series. J Biol Chem **273**:28543.

15. Delany AM, Durant D, Canalis E 2001 Glucocorticoid suppression of IGF I transcription in osteoblasts. Mol Endocrinol **15**:1781–1789.

16. Gangji V, Rydziel S, Gabbitas B, Canalis E 1998 Insulin-like growth factor II promoter expression in cultured rodent osteoblasts and adult rat bone. Endocrinology **139**:2287–2292.

17. Devlin RD, Du Z, Buccilli V, Jorgetti V, Canalis E 2002 Transgenic mice overexpressing insulin-like growth factor binding protein-5 display transiently decreased osteoblastic function and osteopenia. Endocrinology **143**:3955–3962.

18. Conover CA 1995 Insulin-like growth factor binding protein proteolysis in bone cell models. Prog Growth Factor Res **6**:301–309.

19. Canalis E, Economides AN, Gazzerro E 2003 Bone morphogenetic proteins, their antagonists and the skeleton. Endocr Rev **24**:218–235.

20. Pereira RC, Rydziel S, Canalis E 2000 Bone morphogenetic protein-4 regulates its own expression in cultured osteoblasts. J Cell Physiol **182**:239–246.

21. Thies RS, Bauduy M, Ashton BA, Kurtzberg L, Wozney JM, Rosen V 1992 Recombinant human bone morphogenetic protein-2 induces osteoblastic differentiation in W-20–17 stromal cells. Endocrinology **130**:1318–1324.

22. Hughes FJ, Collyer J, Stanfield M, Goodman SA 1995 The effects of bone morphogenetic protein-2, -4, and -6 on differentiation of rat osteoblast cells *in vitro*. Endocrinology **136**:2671–2677.

23. Hay E, Lemonnier J, Fromigue O, Marie PJ 2001 Bone morphogenetic protein-2 promotes osteoblast apoptosis through a Smad-independent, protein kinase C-dependent signaling pathway. J Biol Chem **276**:29028–29036.

24. Zeng L, Kempf H, Murtaugh CL, Sato ME, Lassar AB 2002 Shh establishes an Nkx3.2/Sox9 autoregulatory loop that is maintained by BMP signals to induce somatic chondrogenesis. Genes Dev **16**:1990–2005.

25. Kretzschmar M, Massague J 1998 Smads: Mediators and regulators of TGF-β signaling. Curr Opin Genet Dev **8**:103–111.

26. Yamashita H, ten Dijke P, Heldin C-H, Miyazono K 1996 Bone morphogenetic protein receptors. Bone **19**:569–574.

27. Derynck R, Zhang Y, Feng X-H 1998 Smads: Transcriptional activators of TGF-β responses. Cell **95**:737–740.

28. Zaidi SK, Sullivan AJ, van Wijnen AJ, Stein JL, Stein GS, Lian JB 2002 Integration of Runx and Smad regulatory signals at transcriptionally active subnuclear sites. Proc Natl Acad Sci USA **99**:8048–8053.

29. Attisano L, Wrana J 2002 Lignal transduction by the TGF-β superfamily. Science **296**:1646–1647.

30. Moon RT, Bowerman B, Boutros M, Perrimon N 2002 The promise and perils of Wnt signaling through β-catenin. Science **296**:1644–1646.

31. Nishita M, Hashimoto MK, Ogata S, Laurent MN, Ueno N, Shibuya H, Cho KWY 2000 Interaction between Wnt and TGF-β signalling pathways during formation of Spemann's organizer. Nature **403**:781–784.

32. Mao J, Wang J, Liu B, Pan W, Farr GH III, Flynn C, Yuan H, Takada S, Kimelman D, Li L, Wu D 2001 Low-density lipoprotein receptor-related protein-5 binds to Axin and regulates the canonical Wnt signaling pathway. Mol Cell **7**:801–809.

33. Gong Y, Slee RB, Fukai N, Rawadi G, Roman-Roman S, Reginato AM, Wang H, Cundy T, Glorieux FH, Lev D, Zacharin M, Oexle K, Marcelino J, Suwairi W, Heeger S, Sabatakos G, Apte S, Adkins WN, Allgrove J, Arslan-Kirchner M, Batch JA, Beighton P, Black GCM, Boles RG, Boon LM, Borrone C, Brunner HG, Carle GF, Dallapiccola B, De Paepe A, Floege B, Halfhide ML, Hall B, Hennekam RC, Hirose T, Jans A, Juppner H, Kim CA, Keppler-Noreuil K, Kohlschuetter A, LaCombe D, Lambert M, Lemyre E, Letteboer T, Peltonen L, Ramesar RS, Romanengo M, Somer H, Steichen-Gersdorf E, Steinmann B, Sullivan B, Superti-Furga A, Swoboda W, van den Boogaard M-J, Van Hul W, Vikkula M, Votruba M, Zabel B, Garcia T, Baron R, Olsen BR, Warman ML 2001 LDL receptor-related protein 5 (LRP5) affects bone accrual and eye development. Cell **107**:513–523.

34. Kato M, Patel MS, Levasseur R, Lobov I, Chang BH-J, Glass DA, Hartmann C, Li L, Hwang T-H, Brayton CF, Lang RA, Karsenty G, Chan L 2002 Cbfa1-independent decrease in osteoblast proliferation, osteopenia, and persistent embryonic eye vascularization in mice deficient in Lrp5, a Wnt coreceptor. J Cell Biol **157**:303–314.

35. Boyden LM, Mao J, Belsky J, Mitzner L, Farhi A, Mitnick MA, Wu D, Insogna K, Lifton RP 2002 High bone density due to a mutation in LDL-receptor-related protein 5. N Engl J Med **346**:1513–1521.

36. Centrella M, McCarthy TL, Canalis E 1991 Transforming growth factor-beta and remodeling of bone. J Bone Joint Surg Am **73**:1418–1428.

37. Spinella-Jaegle S, Roman-Roman S, Faucheu C, Dunn F-W, Dawai S, Gallea S, Stiot V, Blanchet AM, Courtois B, Baron R, Rawadi G 2001 Opposite effects of bone morphogenetic protein-2 and transforming growth factor-β1 on osteoblast differentiation. Bone **29**:323–330.

38. Erlebacher A, Derynck R 1996 Increased expression of TGF-β2 in osteoblasts results in an osteoporosis-like phenotype. J Cell Biol **132**:195–210.

39. Baird A, Ornitz DM 2000 Fibroblast growth factors and their receptors. In: Canalis E (ed.) Skeletal Growth Factors. Lippincott Williams & Wilkins, Philadelphia, PA, USA, pp. 167–178.

40. Marie PJ, Lomri A, Debiais F, Lemonnier J 2000 Fibroblast growth factors and osteogenesis. In: Canalis E (ed.) Skeletal Growth Factors. Lippincott Williams & Wilkins, Philadelphia, PA, USA, pp. 179–196.

41. Canalis E, Centrella M, McCarthy T 1998 Effects of basic fibroblast growth factor on bone formation in vitro. J Clin Invest **81**:1572–1577.

42. Montero A, Okada Y, Tomita M, Ito M, Tsurukami H, Nakamura T, Doetschman T, Coffin JD, Hurley MM 2000 Disruption of the fibroblast growth factor-2 gene results in decreased bone mass and bone formation. J Clin Invest **105**:1085–1093.

43. Nakamura T, Hanada K, Tamura M, Sibanushi T, Nigi H, Tagawa M, Fukumoto S, Matsumoto T 1995 Stimulation of endosteal bone formation by systemic injections of recombinant basic fibroblast growth factor in rats. Endocrinology **136**:1276–1284.

44. Shiang R, Thompson LM, Zhu YZ, Church DM, Fielder TJ, Bocian M, Winokur ST, Wasmuth JJ 1994 Mutations in the transmembrane domain of FGFR3 cause the most common genetic form of dwarfism, achondroplasia. Cell **78**:335–342.

45. Lowe HC, Rafty LA, Collins T, Khachigian LM 2000 Biology of platelet-derived growth factor. In: Canalis E (ed.) Skeletal Growth Factors. Lippincott Williams & Wilkins, Philadelphia, PA, USA, pp. 129–151.

46. Canalis E, Ornitz DM 2000 Platelet-derived growth factor – Skeletal actions and regulation. In: Canalis E (ed.) Skeletal Growth Factors. Lippincott Williams & Wilkins, Philadelphia, PA, USA, pp. 153–165.

47. Hock JM, Canalis E 1994 Platelet-derived growth factor enhances bone cell replication but not differentiated function of osteoblasts. Endocrinology **134**:1423–1428.

48. Delany AM, Amling M, Priemel M, Howe CC, Baron R, Canalis E 2000 Osteopenia and decreased bone formation in osteonectin-deficient mice. J Clin Invest **105**:915–923.

Chapter 5.   Gonadal Steroids and Receptors

David G. Monroe and Thomas C. Spelsberg

Department of Biochemistry and Molecular Biology, Mayo Clinic and Foundation, Rochester, Minnesota

INTRODUCTION

Since steroid hormones were discovered in the early 1900s, studies of their molecular actions have extended from the whole body, to the target organs, to specific functions within those target tissues, to the specific cells, and finally to specific genes and their protein products. It is well accepted that sex steroids play an important role in bone cell metabolism, including the regulation of osteoblast and osteoclast activities and reinforcing the coupling between these cells through paracrine factors. The overall function of the gonadal steroids in bone is to maintain a steady state in bone metabolism to prevent the loss of bone mass in humans. Type I osteoporosis is believed to be an acceleration of the rapid phase of bone loss during the first 5–10 years after menopause. Estrogen replacement therapy reinstates the homeostasis between the osteoblasts and osteoclasts and prevents bone loss, thereby supporting the role of estrogen deficiency in osteoporosis. This chapter presents a brief overview of the structure and function of gonadal steroid hormones, their receptors, receptor coregulators, and the mechanisms by which they regulate gene expression and cell function.

STEROID HORMONES

There are three categories of steroid hormones: glucocorticoids, mineralocorticoids, and the gonadal steroids (estrogens, androgens, and progesterone), each with different functions in the human body. Sex steroids are synthesized in response to signals from the brain. Certain signals from the central nervous system initiate a stimulus from the hypothalamus to the pituitary gland, which releases peptide hormones that target the reproductive organs. These peptide hormones, luteinizing hormone and follicle-stimulating hormone, stimulate the synthesis of progesterone and estrogens in the female ovaries and testosterone in the male testes. Comprehensive reviews on these processes are available.[1–3] Traditionally, sex steroids were thought to only regulate activity in reproductive organs, but the discovery of steroid hormone receptors throughout the body has implicated varied patterns of functionality in many other tissues.

Biosynthesis of Steroid Hormones

The synthesis of steroid hormones from cholesterol involves pathways with 10 or more enzymes (Fig. 1A). The level of steroid hormones in the bloodstream is primarily controlled by its rate of synthesis, because little steroid is stored. The increase of these hormones in the serum takes from hours to days, so cellular responses are delayed but last longer than the effects mediated by the peptide hormones.

In ovulating women and during pregnancy, progesterone is secreted by the ovaries. Progesterone not only exhibits biological activity, but as shown in Fig. 1A, also serves as a precursor for all other steroid hormones.

Estrone and estradiol are formed from androstenedione and testosterone, respectively (Fig. 1A). This reaction is mediated by the enzyme aromatase, a cytochrome P-450 enzyme present in the ovary, as well as the testis, adipocytes, and bone cells. Estradiol and estrone are in reversible equilibrium caused by hepatic and intestinal 17β-hydroxysteroid dehydrogenases. The major circulating estrogen in postmenopausal women is estrone, which in turn, follows two main pathways of metabolism into 16α-hydroxyestrone and 2-hydroxyestrone. The balance in the ratio of these hydroxylated estrones has been implicated as playing a role in several disease states, including breast cancer, osteoporosis, systemic lupus erythematosis, and liver cirrhosis.

The steroidogenic pathway is essentially the same in the testes as in the ovaries, with the exception that testosterone is the major secretory product, although small amounts of estradiol are also secreted. Testosterone is converted to more active metabolites in target tissues, including the gonads, brain, and bone. This modification is accomplished by two enzymes: 5α-reductase and aromatase. As depicted in Fig. 1A, the 5α-reductase irreversibly converts testosterone to dihydroxytestosterone, which then cannot be aromatized to estrogens. Conversely, aromatase irreversibly converts testosterone into estrogenic molecules.

Transport Through the Bloodstream

The major sex steroids in circulation are androgens and estrogens (estradiol and estrone). Because their chemical structure makes them fat soluble, most are bound to specific carrier proteins for transportation through the bloodstream to hormone receptors, which reside in the cells of target tissues. Only 1–3% of the total circulating sex steroids are free in solution. Both the free steroid and the albumin-bound fraction (35–55%) can enter target tissues, thereby representing the "bioavailable" steroid pool. The remaining fraction, bound to sex hormone-binding globulin, is unable to enter the cells. The sex steroids enter all cells by simple diffusion through the cell membrane and then, in target cells, bind to specific receptor molecules in the nucleus to regulate gene transcription.

Selective Estrogen Receptor Modulators

Steroid analogs have been developed to elicit tissue-specific rather than systemic effects, avoiding common side effects of steroid replacement therapy. One particular class of these compounds is called selective estrogen receptor modulators (SERMs), because they bind to estrogen receptors as a ligand, but can act as an agonist, antagonist, or even have no apparent effect, depending on the cell/tissue-type

The authors have no conflict of interest.

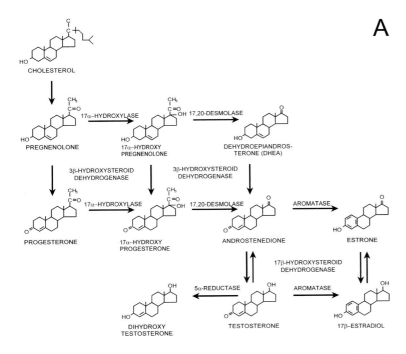

A

B

TAMOXIFEN

RALOXIFENE

DIETHYLSTIL
BESTROL

ICI 182,780

RU 486
(MIFEPRISTONE)

FLUTAMIDE

FIG. 1. (A) Pathways of steroid hormones biosynthesis from cholesterol. The initiation of steroid hormone synthesis involves the hydrolysis of cholesterol esters and the uptake of cholesterol into mitochondria of cells in the target organ. Dehydrogenation of pregnenolone produces progesterone, which serves as a precursor molecule for the generation of all other gonadal steroid hormones. (Adapted from Dynamics of Bone and Cartilage Metabolism, Seibel M, Robins S, Bilezikian J, Sex steroid effects on bone metabolism, pp. 233–245, 1999 with permission from Elsevier.) (B) Chemical structures of common steroid analogs.

(Fig. 1B). For example, the SERM, tamoxifen, is an antagonist in reproductive tissues with little effect on bone, and raloxifene is an agonist in bone with little effect in reproductive tissues. Diethylstilbestrol is not a steroid but mimics estrogen action in reproductive and bone tissues. The synthetic steroid, ICI 182,780, is a pure antiestrogen, with no estrogenic activity in any tissue investigated to date. Similarly, both RU 486 and flutamide are synthetic antagonists of progesterone and testosterone, respectively. Further studies with SERM analogs will provide new alternatives to steroid replacement therapy.[3]

STEROID HORMONE RECEPTORS

Steroid hormones generate their intracellular signaling by binding to steroid-specific proteins called receptors. There are three steps in the general mechanism of action for steroid receptors: (1) binding of the steroid ligand to the receptor in the nucleus, (2) translocation of the steroid receptor complex to a specific site on the DNA, and (3) the regulation of gene transcription.

Specific receptors exist for each of the steroid hormones, because of their unique structure that allows them to differentiate between the diverse species of steroid and nonsteroid molecules. As shown in Fig. 2, steroid receptor proteins have multiple "domains," each of which has specific functions. All steroid receptor species share significant homology in terms of their sequence and their functional domains along the protein molecules. There are currently two sites, located in domains I and IV, identified as having transcriptional activation functions (TAFs). These domains are responsible for activation of gene transcription, once the steroid receptor complex interacts with the regulatory regions of genes. In addition, a sequence of basic amino acids near the second zinc finger in domain III represents a nuclear localization sequence, which directs the receptor to the nucleus. Additional nuclear localization signals have been identified in the hormone-binding domain (IV), and these have been shown to be hormone-dependent.[4,5] As shown in Fig. 2B, the receptor domains have been further expanded/divided into six domains (A/B, C, D, E, and F) based on molecular structure and functions.

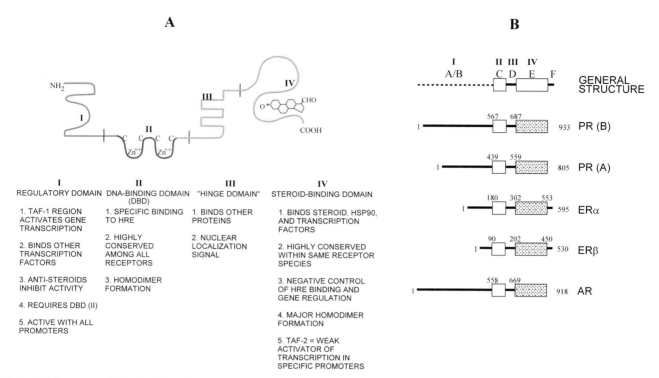

FIG. 2. (A) Structure and functional domains of steroid hormone receptors. Proceeding in the N-terminal to C-terminal direction, the receptors contain a variable domain (I or A/B), thought to be involved in cell type-specific regulation of gene transcription, a DNA binding domain (II or C) of 66–68 amino acids, which shows a high degree of homology among members of the steroid receptor family, a "hinge" domain (III or D), a steroid binding domain (IV or E), showing some homology, and variable regions (V or F) with little homology that somehow contribute to optimal function of the receptor. (B) Structural homology among sex steroid receptor family members. The sex steroid receptors range in size from 530 amino acids for the estrogen receptor β to 933 amino acids for the progesterone receptor. Human progesterone receptors exist in two isoforms, A and B, generated by the same gene through differential promoters. The estrogen receptor also exists in two forms (ERα and ERβ); however, they arise from different genes, each with unique domains that allow for tissue- and ligand-specific functions. TAF, transcriptional activation function; DBD, DNA binding domain; HRE, hormone response element. (Adapted from Osteoporosis, Marcus R, Feldman D, Kelsey J, Regulation of bone cell function by gonadal steroids, pp. 237–260, 1996 with permission from Elsevier.)

It should be mentioned that most classes of steroid receptors have two receptor isoforms (species) coded from the same or different genes (see Fig. 2B). In fact, some isoforms have been shown to include several species or "variants" of each isoform. One of the two isoforms of progesterone, estrogen, and glucocorticoids acts as a primary acting receptor (gene regulator) and the other as an antagonist to this action.

exhibit absolute ligand specificity (e.g., gonadal steroids can bind to more than one class of receptor) if the steroid ligands are at high concentrations that encourages lower affinity interactions. This lack of steroid specificity among receptors is not unexpected in view of the significant homology among their ligand binding domains. The primary

Heat Shock Proteins

In their inactive state (i.e., steroid unbound), steroid receptors exist as part of a large complex in association with other nonsteroid-binding proteins within cells not exposed to the steroid, as depicted in Fig. 3. One of these nonsteroid-binding proteins, a 90-kDa heat shock protein (hsp90), is also called a molecular chaperone. It assists in other proteins to become active, and it is needed to create a functional receptor.[6] While the role of these associated proteins in steroid receptor function is not fully understood, it is believed that they play a role in some aspect of receptor transport, stability, and/or transformation.

Receptor Activation

Each receptor reversibly binds its respective steroid with high affinity and specificity. However, few steroid receptors

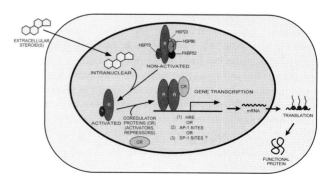

FIG. 3. Activation of steroid hormone receptors by ligand binding. The inactive receptor protein is complexed to several heat-shock proteins (hsp). On binding of the steroid hormone, a conformational change in the receptor allows for transcriptional regulation by binding to HREs on DNA. In many cases, hsp90 may function as a protein "chaperone," which regulates and directs the assembly of receptor/coregulator protein complexes. It has been suggested that these hsp proteins are required for signal transduction or that they may function in the general maintenance of the cell.

effect of ligand binding to domain IV is to "activate" the receptor molecule by inducing a conformational change in the whole protein, so that it can interact with DNA. This conformational change in the receptor caused by ligand binding seems to be conserved across steroid family members.

CONTROL OF GENE EXPRESSION

The mechanism by which steroid hormone receptors exert their effect is fundamentally different from that for receptors of other types of hormones. Once bound by their specific ligand, cell surface (membrane) receptors initiate signal transduction cascades that eventually alter the activities of select transcription factors. In contrast, the activated sex steroid receptors are capable of interacting either directed with a specific response DNA sequence, called a hormone response element (HRE), or indirectly through specific transcription factors, as shown in Fig. 3. Once bound to the gene promoters, the steroid receptor complex is then bound by steroid receptor coregulators (activators or repressors), which in turn, bind to the transcriptional machinery (including RNA polymerase) to initiate gene transcription (see Fig. 3).[7]

Receptor Binding to DNA Elements

The DNA binding domain of the receptor contains two "zinc fingers," looped structures involving chelated metal ions, which are responsible for the binding to the HREs of target genes. A characteristic hexanucleotide inverted palindromic repeat allows the receptor to bind the DNA as a dimer. The orientation, sequence, and space between the hexanucleotide repeats are unique for each steroid hormone. Similarity among the steroid receptor superfamily results in cross-reactivity between ligands, receptors, and DNA sequences.[8,9]

General Coregulator Function—Coactivators and Corepressors

Steroid hormone receptor coactivators are involved in enhancing the transcriptional signal of the steroid hormone receptors after ligand binding.[7] Steroid receptor coactivator-1 (SRC1), the founding member of the SRC family (also called the p160 family), was originally identified as an interacting protein with the progesterone receptor (PR) ligand binding domain (LBD).[10] Further analysis demonstrated that SRC1 exhibits transcriptional coactivation properties not only with the PR but also with nearly all type I nuclear hormone receptors. Two additional members of the p160 family of coactivators, SRC2 and SRC-3, were also identified which interact with and coactivate numerous nuclear hormone receptors.[11,12]

The p160 family of proteins mediate the interactions with steroid hormone receptors through a centrally located receptor interaction domain (RID) of the p160 protein, which contains three α-helical LXXLL motifs necessary for interaction with steroid hormone receptors.[13] Binding of ligand to the receptor induces a conformational change that allows

association of the RID domain with the LBD/AF-2 function of the steroid hormone receptor. Mutation or deletion of the SRC RID domains disrupts physical interaction with the steroid receptor LBD and thus abolishes the transcriptional coactivation potential of the SRC molecule and the steroid receptor.

The p160 family of coactivators contains intrinsic transcriptional activation domains that contribute to the overall transcriptional activation elicited by the ligand-bound steroid hormone receptor. These domains function to recruit other molecules involved in activating transcription such as CBP/p300 (see Fig. 4 for a model of this action). One interesting domain found in both SRC1 and SRC3 is the histone acetyltransferase (HAT) domain. This domain functions to modulate a condensed chromatin structure into a conformation permissive to transcriptional activation. HAT activity serves to transfer acetyl groups to specific lysines in histones and is thought to "loosen" the histone's grip on DNA, facilitating the entry of other transcription factors (or the basal transcriptional machinery itself) to activate transcription. Thus, the various coactivators serve numerous functions in the processes of transcriptional activation.

Transcriptional repression by steroid hormone receptors is mediated by the recruitment of corepressors that function by competing with coactivators for the ligand-bound LBD of steroid receptors. The recently discovered corepressor, REA (repressor of estrogen action), functions in this manner by directly competing with SRC1 in binding to the LBD.[14] Other transcriptional corepressors bind the LBD either in the absence of ligand or in the presence of steroid receptor antagonists such as tamoxifen or ICI 182,780.

A. COACTIVATORS (STEROID RECEPTOR BOUND WITH STEROID AGONIST)

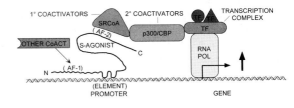

B. COREPRESSORS (STEROID RECEPTOR BOUND WITH ANTAGONIST)

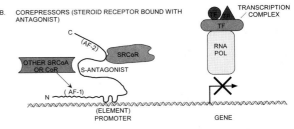

FIG. 4. Effects of coactivator/corepressor binding in response to either an agonist or an antagonist on transcription. (A) Binding of an agonist causes a conformational change to occur in the ligand binding domain (LBD) of the steroid receptor followed by recruitment of primary coactivators (SRCoA), such as the SRC family of coactivators. This in turn, recruits other transcription factors (sometimes called "secondary" coactivators), such as p300/CBP, allowing for recruitment of the basal transcription complex and culminating in a productive transcriptional response. (B) Binding of an antagonist, on the other hand, produces a conformational change in the LBD of the steroid receptor which may recruit specific steroid receptor corepressors (SRCoR) that cannot recruit the transcription factors necessary for a productive transcriptional response.

The structure of corepressors in many ways mirrors that of coactivators. Certain corepressors contain histone deactylation interacting domains that appear to antagonize transcriptional activation by recruiting factors involved in histone deactylation, called HDACs[15,16]. Thus, the activities of corepressors and coactivators target similar processes in opposing manners (e.g., HAT activity versus HDAC activity). The regulation of coactivators and corepressor function is a major component in determining the activation state of a gene. Figure 4 describes the sequence of events that may occur when either a coactivator or a corepressor is bound to the steroid receptor.

Chronology of Steroid Hormone Action

The chronological order in which genes are regulated by steroids is important to both the physiological and mechanistic responses to steroid treatments, as depicted in Fig. 5. In animals, the diffusion of steroids into cells and the nuclear binding of the steroid-receptor complex occurs within minutes after injection. This is followed by "early" gene transcription and translation of regulatory proteins, which activate "late" gene expression within 2–10 h through the cascade model of steroid action.[17,18] The late genes code for other proteins including enzymes and cytokines that trigger cell proliferation and in turn act as paracrine factors to regulate neighboring cells. The major physiological effects of steroids in cells are usually observed 24–48 h after steroid treatment.[19,20]

NONGENOMIC EFFECTS

There is a growing body of evidence that steroids can alter cell metabolism by nongenomic effects (i.e., without interaction with DNA). These effects have been characterized by rapid responses ranging from seconds to minutes, involving steroid interaction with membrane receptors or steroid receptor activation in the absence of ligand.[21] Non-genomic estrogen effects signal through the activation of cell surface receptors, leading to alterations in cyclic adenosine monophosphate (cAMP) levels, calcium influx, and direct channel gating. Covalent modification of the steroid receptor, such as a change in phosphorylation state, is also thought to be responsible for activation by nonsteroid effectors.[19,20,22,23]

PHYSIOLOGY OF STEROID EFFECTS ON BONE

The two major types of cells in bone that are responsible for the maintenance of normal bone density are osteoblasts (OB) and osteoclasts (OCL). Normal bone remodeling processes involve bone resorption by OCL and bone formation by OB, which are tightly coupled to prevent a net loss of bone mass. Many factors that influence bone resorption can either act directly on the OCL or indirectly through the OB. Some of these factors are local regulators, including interleukins, tumor necrosis factor, prostaglandins, and transforming growth factor-β (TGF-β), or systemic factors, including parathyroid hormone, vitamin D_3, calcitonin, glucocorticoid, and the sex steroid hormones.

Estrogens

Estrogen has been shown to play an important role in maintaining bone mass. The major effect of estrogen is on reducing bone resorption indirectly by inhibiting osteoclastogenesis and directly by inhibiting OCL function. In postmenopausal women, there is an increase in bone remodeling activity in which resorption is no longer coupled to equal bone formation, resulting in a net loss of bone. Estrogen deficiency is recognized as the most important factor in the pathogenesis of postmenopausal bone loss, since estrogen replacement therapy has been shown to be effective in preventing and treating osteoporosis. The identification of estrogen receptors in human OB and OCL implicated estrogen as a direct effector on these bone cells, as opposed to

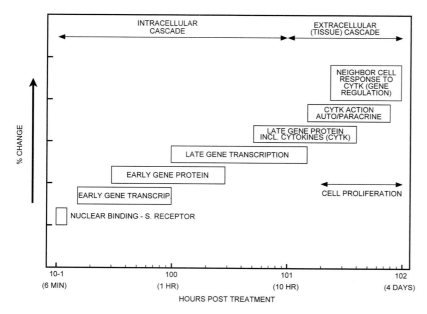

FIG. 5. Chronology of events in steroid action on target cells. After the steroid-receptor complex formation (1–4 minutes) is the binding of this complex to the specific "acceptor" sites on the promoter of the gene (2–5 minutes). The resulting regulation of gene transcription occurs within minutes for "early" genes but not until several hours for "late" genes. The late genes, in turn, code for enzymes and cytokines within 10 h, which act as paracrine/autocrine factors to regulate neighboring cells for 12–24 h and beyond. (Adapted with permission from Robinson and Spelsberg.[18])

previous theories that other calcitropic hormones were the primary mediators of the skeletal effects of estrogen deficiency.[18–20] Estrogens have recently been shown to play an important role in the selected physiology of men.[24] As outlined in Fig. 5, many of the late effects of steroid receptors are generated as secondary effects through the steroid regulated production of growth factors/cytokines, which in turn, can affect these target cells.

Progesterone

At menopause, there is a decrease in circulating levels of progesterone as well as estrogens, which implicates progesterone in postmenopausal bone loss. However, in contrast to the abundance of work on the effects of estrogens on bone metabolism, there is little evidence of direct effects of progesterone on bone.[25] Clinical studies suggest that the effects of progesterone treatment on postmenopausal women are similar to those of estrogen, but combined estrogen and progesterone treatment has effects that differ from those of treatment with either steroid alone. Because of the adverse side effects of estrogen-alone therapy, alternative therapies, such as the combined estrogen and progesterone treatments, are being pursued. Although estrogen is usually required to induce their synthesis, progesterone receptors have been identified in human OB cells, so progesterone could exert direct effects on bone through its own receptor. Another possible mechanism for progesterone action is through interaction with glucocorticoid receptor. Progesterone displaces glucocorticoids from their receptors without activating the receptor, effectively blocking glucocorticoid responses.

Androgens

Like estrogens, androgens influence bone development and metabolism with dramatic clinical manifestations. Decreased androgen levels have been linked to lower bone density in men, and there is a strong correlation between hypogonadism in elderly men and hip fracture and spinal osteoporosis. Clinical studies also show that treatment of osteoporosis with androgens is effective in increasing bone density in both men and women. Human bone cells have androgen receptor concentrations similar to estrogen receptors and 5α-reductase and aromatase activity, for the conversion of testosterone to dihydroxytestosterone and estrogen, respectively. Androgens decrease bone resorption by acting directly on human OCL cells. In addition, androgens also regulate the production of a number of bone-resorbing factors by mature OB or by marrow stromal cells, which contain OB progenitor cells. As with progesterone, further studies are needed to determine the complete role of androgens on bone metabolism.[26]

SUMMARY

The steroid receptors are cyto-nuclear transcription factors, whose structures are altered by steroid ligand binding, such that the transcription activating domains of the receptor molecule are free to regulate gene transcription. The binding of steroid analogs to these receptors can alter the receptor structure, thereby modulating which protein factors are bound to the receptor and which TAF region is active. The types and relative amounts of steroid receptors in a cell determines the response as much as the circulating hormone levels, for example, $ER\alpha$ and $ER\beta$ in different ratios can modulate a particular cell type response to a steroid and have identified new target cells for estrogens. The interaction of steroids with membrane receptors and the activation of steroid receptors in the absence of ligand by phosphorylation events can cause alternative biological/physiological responses. In addition to the well known steroid receptor gene promoter processes described above, other processes which modulate the steroid effects on target cells are (1) the ratio of the receptor isoforms and possibly the levels of their isoform variants, (2) the activity of the nongenomic and membrane steroid receptor pathway, and (3) the activity of the nonligand-dependent, receptor activation by phosphorylation signals. These molecular discoveries are explaining the physiological actions of steroid hormones and their select steroid receptor modulators.

REFERENCES

1. Wilson JD, Foster DW, Kronenberg HM, Larsen PR 1998 Principles of endocrinology. In: Wilson JD, Foster DW, Kronenberg HM, Larsen PR (eds.) Williams Textbook of Endocrinology, 9th ed. WB Saunders, Philadelphia, PA, USA, pp. 1–10.
2. Parl FF 2000 Estrogen synthesis and metabolism. In: Parl FF (ed.) Estrogens, Estrogen Receptor and Breast Cancer. IOS Press, Amsterdam, The Netherlands, pp. 21–55.
3. Lobo RA 1997 The postmenopausal state and estrogen deficiency. In: Lindsay R, Demster DW, Jordan VC (eds.) Estrogens and Antiestrogens: Basic and Clincal Aspects. Lippincott-Raven, Philadelphia, PA, USA, pp. 63–74.
4. Ing NH, O'Malley BW 1995 The steroid hormone receptor superfamily: Molecular mechanisms of action. In: Weintraub BD (ed.) Molecular Endocrinology: Basic Concepts and Clinical Correlations. Raven Press, New York, NY, USA, pp. 195–215.
5. Vegeto E, Wagner BL, Imhof MO, McDonnell DP 1996 The molecular pharmacology of ovarian steroid receptors. Vitam Horm **52:**99–128.
6. Pratt WB, Toft DO 2003 Regulation of signaling protein function and trafficking by the hsp90/hsp70-based chaperone machinery. Exp Biol Med **228:**111–133.
7. Edwards DP 1999 Coregulatory proteins in nuclear hormone receptor action. In: Litwack G (ed.) Vitamins and Hormones, vol. 55. Academic Press, San Diego, CA, USA, pp. 165–218.
8. Rastinejad F 1998 Structure and function of the steroid and nuclear receptor DNA binding domain. In: Freeman LP (ed.) Molecular Biology of Steroid and Nuclear Hormone Receptors. Birkhauser, Boston, MA, USA, pp. 105–132.
9. Jensen EV 1991 Overview of the nuclear receptor family. In: Parker MG (ed.) Nuclear Hormone Receptors: Molecular Mechanisms, Cellular Functions, Clinical Abnormalities. Academic Press, London, UK, pp. 1–13.
10. Onate SA, Tsai SY, Tsai MJ, O'Malley BW 1995 Sequence and characterization of a coactivator for the steroid hormone receptor superfamily. Science **270:**1354–1357.
11. Voegel JJ, Heine MJ, Zechel C, Chambon P, Gronemeyer H 1996 TIF2, a 160 kDa transcriptional mediator for the ligand-dependent activation function AF-2 of nuclear receptors. EMBO J **15:**3667–3675.
12. Li H, Gomes PJ, Chen JD 1997 RAC3, a steroid/nuclear receptor-associated coactivator that is related to SRC-1 and TIF2. Proc Natl Acad Sci USA **94:**8479–8484.
13. Heery DM, Kalkhoven E, Hoare S, Parker MG 1997 A signature motif in transcriptional coactivators mediates binding to nuclear receptors. Nature **387:**733–736.
14. Montano MM, Ekena K, Delage-Mourroux R, Chang W, Martini P, Katzenellenbogen BS 1999 An estrogen receptor-selective coregulator

that potentiates the effectiveness of antiestrogens and represses the activity of estrogens. Proc Natl Acad Sci USA **96**:6947–6952.

15. Heinzel T, Lavinsky RM, Mullen TM, Soderstrom M, Laherty CD, Torchia J, Yang WM, Brard G, Ngo SD, Davie JR, Eisenman RN, Rose DW, Glass CK, Rosenfeld MG 1997 A complex containing N-CoR, mSin3 and histone deacetylases mediates transcriptional repression. Nature **387**:43–48.

16. Nagy L, Kao HY, Chakravarti D, Lin RJ, Hassig CA, Ayer DE, Schreiber SL, Evans RM 1997 Nuclear receptor repression mediated by a complex containing SMRT, mSin3A, and histone deacetylase. Cell **89**:373–380.

17. Landers JP, Spelsberg TC 1991 Updates and new models for steroid hormone action. Ann NY Acad Sci **637**:26–55.

18. Robinson JA, Spelsberg TC 1997 Mode of action at the cellular level with specific reference to bone cells. In: Lindsay R, Dempster DW, Jordan VC (eds.) Estrogens and Antiestrogens: Basic and Clinical Aspects. Lippincott-Raven Publishers, Philadelphia, PA, USA, pp. 43–62.

19. Oursler MJ, Kassem M, Turner R, Riggs BL, Spelsberg TC 1996 Regulation of bone cell function by gonadal steroids. In: Marcus R,

Feldman D, Kelsey J (eds.) Osteoporosis. Academic Press, San Diego, CA, USA, pp. 237–260.

20. Khosla S, Spelsberg TC, Riggs BL 1999 Sex steroid effects on bone metabolism. In: Seibel M, Robins S, Bilezikian J (eds.) Dynamics of Bone and Cartilage Metabolism. Academic Press, San Diego, CA, USA, pp. 233–245.

21. Monroe DG, Spelsberg TC 2003 A case for estrogen receptors on cell membranes and nongenomic actions of estrogen. Calcif Tissue Int **72**:183–184.

22. Moss RL, Gu Q, Wong M 1997 Estrogen: Nontranscriptional signaling pathways. Recent Progr Horm Res **52**:33–69.

23. Weigel NL 1996 Steroid hormone receptors and their regulation by phosphorylation. Biochem J **319**:657–667.

24. Khosla S, Melton LJ, Riggs BL 2002 Clinical review 144: Estrogen and the male skeleton. J Clin Endocrinol Metab **87**:1443–1450.

25. Prior JC 1990 Progesterone as a bone-trophic hormone. Endocr Rev **11**:386–398.

26. Vanderschueren D, Bouillon R 1995 Androgens and bone. Calcif Tissue Int **56**:341–346.

Chapter 6. Extracellular Matrix and Biomineralization of Bone

Pamela Gehron Robey[1] and Adele L. Boskey[2]

[1]Craniofacial and Skeletal Diseases Branch, National Institute of Dental and Craniofacial Research, National Institutes of Health, Department of Health and Human Services, Bethesda, Maryland; and [2]Research Division, Hospital for Special Surgery, and Department of Biochemistry, Weill Medical College of Cornell University Medical and Graduate Medical Schools, New York, New York

INTRODUCTION

Bone composes the largest proportion of the body's connective tissue mass. Unlike most other connective tissue matrices, bone matrix is physiologically mineralized and is unique in that it is constantly regenerated throughout life as a consequence of bone turnover. Information on the gene and protein structure and potential function of bone extracellular matrix (ECM) constituents has exploded during the last two decades. This information has been described in great detail in several recent reviews,[1,2] to which the reader is referred for specific references, which are too numerous to be listed adequately here. This chapter summarizes salient features of the classes of bone matrix proteins, and the tables list specific details for the individual components.

COLLAGEN

This basic building block of the bone matrix fiber network is type I collagen, which is a triple-helical molecule containing two identical α1(I) chains and a structurally similar, but genetically different, α2(I) chain (reviewed in ref. 3; Table 1). Collagen α chains are characterized by a Gly-X-Y repeating triplet (where X is usually proline and Y is often hydroxyproline) and by several post-translational modifications including (1) hydroxylation of certain lysyl or hydroxylysyl residues with glucose or galactose residues or

both, and (2) formation of intra- and intermolecular covalent cross-links that differ from those found in soft connective tissues. Measurement of these bone-derived collagen cross-links in urine have proved to be good measures of bone resorption.[4] Bone matrix proper consists predominantly of type I collagen; however, trace amounts of type III, V, and FACIT collagens may be present during certain stages of bone formation and may regulate collagen fibril diameter (Table 1).

NONCOLLAGENOUS PROTEINS

Noncollagenous proteins (NCPs) compose 10–15% of the total bone protein content. Approximately one-fourth of the total NCP content is exogenously derived. This fraction is largely composed of serum-derived proteins, such as albumin and α2-HS-glycoprotein (Table 2), which are acidic in character and bind to bone matrix because of their affinity to hydroxyapatite. Although these proteins are not endogenously synthesized, they may exert effects on matrix mineralization, and α2-HS-glycoprotein, which is the human analog of fetuin, also may regulate bone cell proliferation. The remainder of this exogenous fraction is composed of growth factors and a large variety of other molecules present in trace amounts, which also may influence local bone cell activity (see ref. 2 for review).

Bone-forming cells synthesize and secrete as many molecules of NCP as of collagen, on a mole-to-mole basis. These molecules can be broken down into four general (and

The authors have no conflict of interest.

Table 1. Characteristics of Collagen-Related Genes and Proteins Found in Bone Matrix

Protein/gene	Function	Disease/animal model
Type I—17q21.23, 7q21.3-22 [α1(I)$_2$α2(I)] [α1(I)$_3$]	Most abundant protein in bone matrix (90% of organic matrix), serves as scaffolding, binds and orients other proteins that nucleate hydroxyapatite deposition.	Osteogenesis imperfecta (m); oim mouse (m); mov 14 mouse (m); knock-in mouse; bones mechanically weak; mineral crystals small; some mineral outside collagen
Type X—6q21-22.3 [α1(x)$_3$]	Present in hypertrophic cartilage but does not appear to regulate matrix mineralization	Human mutations—Schmid metaphyseal chondrodysplasia knockout mouse—no apparent skeletal phenotype
Type III—2q24.3-31 [α1(III)$_3$]	Present in bone in trace amounts, may regulate collagen fibril diameter, their paucity in bone may explain the large diameter size of bone collagen fibrils	Human mutations—different forms of Ehlers-Danlos syndrome
Type V—9q34.2-34.3; 2q24.3-31, 9q34.2-34.3 [α1(V)$_2$α2(V)] [α1(V)α2(V)α3(V)]		

sometimes overlapping) groups: (1) proteoglycans, (2) glycosylated proteins, (3) glycosylated proteins with potential cell-attachment activities, and (4) γ-carboxylated (gla) proteins. The physiological roles for individual bone protein constituents are not well defined; however, they may participate not only in regulating the deposition of mineral, but also in the control of osteoblastic and osteoclastic metabolism.

PROTEOGLYCANS, LEUCINE RICH REPEAT PROTEINS, AND HYALURONAN

Proteoglycans are macromolecules that contain acidic polysaccharide side chains (glycosaminoglycans) attached to a central core protein, and bone matrix contains several members of this family.[5] During initial stages of bone formation, the large chondroitin sulfate proteoglycan, versican, and the glycosaminoglycan, hyaluronan (which is not attached to a protein core), are produced and may delineate areas that will become bone (Table 3). With continued osteogenesis, versican is replaced by two small chondroitin sulfate proteoglycans, decorin and biglycan, composed of tandem repeats of a leucine-rich repeat sequence (LRR). Decorin has been implicated in the regulation of collagen fibrillogenesis and is distrib-

uted predominantly in the ECM space of connective tissues and in bone, whereas biglycan tends to be found in pericellular locales. Although their exact physiological functions are not known, they are assumed to be important for the integrity of most connective tissue matrices. One function might rise from their ability to bind and modulate the activity of the TGF-β family members in the extracellular space, thereby influencing cell proliferation and differentiation. Recently it was determined that deletion of the biglycan gene in transgenic animals leads to a significant decrease in the development of trabecular bone, indicating that it is a positive regulator of bone formation.[6] Other LRRs (which may or may not bear glycosaminoglycans), such as fibromodulin, osteoglycin, osteoadherin, lumican, and asporin are found in bone matrix but at lower levels than decorin and biglycan and may function in other aspects of bone metabolism[7] (Table 4).

GLYCOPROTEINS

One of the hallmarks of bone formation is the synthesis of high levels of alkaline phosphatase (Table 5). This enzyme, primarily bound to the cell surface through a phosphoinositol linkage, can be cleaved from the cell surface and found within

Table 2. Gene and Protein Characteristics of Serum Proteins Found in Bone Matrix

Protein/gene	Function	Disease/animal model
Albumin—2q11-13 69-kDa, non-glycosylated, one sulfhydryl, 17 disulfide bonds, high affinity hydrophobic binding pocket	Inhibits hydroxyapatite crystal growth	
α2-HS glycoprotein—3q27-29 Precursor protein of, cleaved to form A and B chains that are disulfide linked, Ala-Ala and Pro-Pro repeat sequences, N-linked oligosaccharides, cystatin-like domains	Promotes endocytosis, has opsonic properties, chemoattractant for monocytic cells, bovine analog (fetuin) is a growth factor	Knockout mouse—adult ectopic calcification

TABLE 3. GENE AND PROTEIN CHARACTERISTICS OF GLYCOPROTEINS IN BONE MATRIX

Glycoproteins	Function	Disease/animal models
Alkaline phosphatase (bone-liver-kidney isozyme)—1p34-36.1		
Two identical subunits of ~80 kDa, disulfide bonded, tissue specific post translational modifications	Potential Ca^{2+} carrier, hydrolyzes inhibitors of mineral deposition such as pyrophosphates	Hypophosphatasia (decreased activity), TNAP knockout mouse—growth impaired; decreased mineralization
Osteonectin—5q31-33		
~35–45 kDa, intramolecular disulfide bonds, α helical amino terminus with multiple low affinity Ca^{2+} binding sites, two EF hand high affinity Ca^{2+} sites, ovomucoid homology, glycosylated, phosphorylated, tissue specific modifications	May mediate deposition of hydroxyapatite, binds to growth factors, may influence cell cycle, positive regulator of bone formation	Knockout mouse—decreased trabecular connectivity; decreased mineral content; increased crystal size
Tetranectin—3p22-p21.3		
21 kDa protein composed of four identical subunits of 5.8 kDa, sequence homologies with asialoprotein receptor and G3 domain of aggrecan	Binds to plasminogen, may regulate matrix mineralization	Knockout mouse—no long bone phenotype, spinal deformity, increased mineralization in implant model
Tenascin-C—9q33		
Hexameric structure, six identical chains of 320 kDA, Cys rich, EGF-like repeats, FN type III repeats	Interferes with cell-FN interactions	Knockout mouse—no apparent skeletal phenotype

mineralized matrix. The function of alkaline phosphatase in bone cell biology has been the matter of much speculation, and remains undefined.[8] The most abundant NCP produced by bone cells is osteonectin, a phosphorylated glycoprotein accounting for ~2% of the total protein of developing bone in most animal species. Osteonectin is transiently produced in non-bone tissues that are rapidly proliferating, remodeling, or undergoing profound changes in tissue architecture and is found constitutively in certain types of epithelial cells, cells associated with the skeleton, and in platelets. Its function(s) in bone may be multiple, with potential association with osteoblast growth, proliferation, or both, as well as with matrix mineralization.[2,9] A transgenic mouse deficient in osteonectin exhibits a defect in bone formation.[10] Tetranectin and tenascin also have been found in bone matrix, but their function is not yet known.

SIBLINGS AND OTHER GLYCOPROTEINS WITH CELL ATTACHMENT ACTIVITY

All connective tissue cells interact with their extracellular environment in response to stimuli that direct or coordinate (or both) specific cell functions, such as migration, proliferation, and differentiation (Table 6). These particular interactions involve cell attachment through transient or stable focal adhesions to extracellular macromolecules, which are mediated by cell-surface receptors that subsequently transduce intracellular signals. Bone cells synthesize at least nine proteins that may mediate cell attachment: members of the SIBLING (small integrin-binding ligand, N-glycosylated proteins) family (osteopontin, bone sialoprotein, dentin matrix protein-1) (Table 4), type I collagen, fibronectin, thrombospondin(s) (predominantly TSP-2 with lower levels of TSP1,3,4 and

COMP), vitronectin, fibrillin, BAG-75 (Table 5), and osteoadherin (which is also a proteoglycan).[1,5,11,12] Many of these proteins are phosphorylated and/or sulfated, and all contain RGD (Arg-Gly-Asn), the cell-attachment consensus sequence that binds to the integrin class of cell-surface molecules. However, in some cases, cell attachment seems to be independent of RGD, indicating the presence of other sequences or mechanisms of cell attachment. Thrombospondin(s), fibronectin, vitronectin, fibrillin, and osteopontin are expressed in many tissue systems, whereas bone sialoprotein is virtually specific to the skeleton, and its appearance is tightly correlated with the appearance of mineral. Both osteopontin and bone sialoprotein are known to anchor osteoclasts to bone and in addition to supporting cell attachment, bind Ca^{2+} with extremely high affinity through polyacidic amino acid sequences. It is not immediately clear why there are such a plethora of RGD-containing proteins in bone; however, the pattern of expression varies from one RGD protein to another, as does the pattern of the different integrins that bind to these proteins. This variability indicates that cell-matrix interactions change as a function of maturational stage, suggesting that they also may play a role in osteoblastic maturation.[2,13]

GLA-CONTAINING PROTEINS

Three bone-matrix NCPs, matrix gla protein (MGP), osteocalcin (bone gla-protein [BGP]), both of which are made endogenously, and protein S (made primarily in the liver but also made by osteogenic cells), are post-translationally modified by the action of vitamin K–dependent γ-carboxylases[2,14] (Table 6). The production of di-

TABLE 4. GENE AND PROTEIN CHARACTERISTICS GLYCOSAMINOGLYCAN-CONTAINING MOLECULES, LEUCINE RICH REPEAT PROTEINS (LRRs), AND HYALURONAN

Protein/gene	Function	Disease/animal model
Aggrecan—15q26.1 ~2.5 × 10^6 intact protein, ~180–370,000 core, ~100 CS chains of 25 kDa, and some KS chains of similar size, G1, G2 and G3 globular domains with hyaluronan binding sites, EGF and CRP-like sequences	Matrix organization, retention of water and ions, resilience to mechanical forces	Brachymorphic mouse (mutation), accelerated growth plate calcification, nanomelic chick (mutation)—abnormal bone shape
Versican (PG-100)—5112-14 ~1 × 10^6 intact protein, ~360 kDa core, ~12 CS chains of 45 kDa, G1 and G3 globular domains with hyaluronan binding sites, EGF and CRP-like sequences	May "capture" space that is destined to become bone	
Decorin (Class 1 LRR)—12q21-23 ~130 kDa intact protein, ~38–45 kDa core with 10 leucine rich repeat sequences, 1 CS chain of 40 kDa	Binds to collagen and may regulate fibril diameter, binds to TGF-β and may modulate activity, inhibits cell attachment to fibronectin	Knockout—no apparent skeletal phenotype, DCN/BGN double knockout—progeroid form of Ehler's-Danlos syndrome
Biglycan (Class 1 LRR)—Xq27 ~270 kDa intact protein, ~38–45 kDa core protein with 12 leucine rich repeat sequences, 2 CS chains of 40 kDa	May bind to collagen, may bind to TGF-β, peri-cellular environment, a genetic determinant of peak bone mass	Knockout mouse, Turner's syndrome—osteopenia; thin bones, decreased mineral content, increased crystal size; short stature, thin bones; Kleinfelder's disease—excessive height
Asporin (Class 1 LRR)—9q22 67 kDa, most likely not GAG chains		
Fibromodulin (Class 2 LRR)—1q32 59 kDa intact protein, 42 kDa core protein, one N-linked KS chain	Binds to collagen, may regulate fibril formation, binds to TGF-β	Fibromodulin/biglycan double knockout—joint laxity and formation of supernumery sesmoid bones
Osteoadherin (Class 2 LRR) 85 kDa intact protein, 47 kDa core protein, RGD sequence	May mediate cell attachment	
Lumican (Class 2 LRR)—12q21.3-q22 70–80 kDa intact protein, 37 kDa core protein	Binds to collagen, may regulate fibril formation	Lumican/fibromodulin double knockout mouse—ectopic calcification
Osteoglycin/Mimecan (Class 3 LRR)—9q22 299 aa precursor, 105 aa mature protein, no GAG in bone, keratan sulfate in other tissues.	Binds to TGF-β	
Hyaluronan—multi-gene complex Multiple proteins associated outside of the cell, structure unknown	May work with versican molecule to capture space destined to become bone	

carboxylic glutamyl (gla) residues enhances calcium binding. MGP is found in many connective tissues, whereas osteocalcin is bone specific. The physiological role of both of these proteins is still somewhat unclear; however, they may function in the inhibition of mineral deposition. MGP-deficient mice develop calcification in extraskeletal sites such as in the aorta.[15] Osteocalcin-deficient mice are reported to have increased bone mineral density (BMD) compared with normal mice.[16] In human bone, osteocalcin is concentrated in osteocytes, and its release may be a signal in the bone turnover cascade. Osteocalcin measurements in serum have proved valuable as a marker of bone turnover in metabolic disease states.

BONE MINERALIZATION

The composition of bone enables it to perform its unique mechanical, protective, and homeostatic functions. While this composition varies with age, anatomic location, diet, and health status, in general, mineral accounts for 50–70% of adult mammalian bone, the organic matrix for 20–40%, water for 5–10%, and lipids for less than 3%. The mineral, a calcium- and hydroxide-deficient analog of the geologic mineral, hydroxyapatite [$Ca_{10}(PO_4)_6(OH)_2$], provides mechanical rigidity and load bearing strength to the bone composite. In contrast to large geologic hydroxyapatite crystals, bone mineral crystals are extremely small (~200 Å

TABLE 5. GENE AND PROTEIN CHARACTERISTICS OF SIBLINGS (SMALL INTEGRIN-BINDING LIGANDS, *N*-GLYCOSYLATED PROTEINS)

Protein/gene	Function	Disease/animal models
Osteopontin—4q21		
~44–75 kDa, polyaspartyl stretches, no disulfide bonds, glycosylated, phosphorylated, RGD located ⅔ from the N-terminal	Binds to cells, may regulate mineralization, may regulate proliferation, inhibits nitric oxide synthase, may regulate resistance to viral infection	Knockout mouse—decreased crystal size; increased mineral content; not subject to osteoclast remodeling
Bone Sialoprotein—4q21		
~46–75 kDa, polyglutamyl stretches, no disulfide bonds, 50% carbohydrate, tyrosine-sulfated, RGD near the C terminus	Binds to cells, may initiate mineralization	Knockout mouse—no published data on phenotype
DMP-1—4q21		
513 amino acids predicted; acidic, RGD ⅔ from N-terminus	Possible cell attachment protein	Knockout mouse—craniofacial and growth plate abnormalities
Other SIBLINGs at 4q21—enamelin, MEPE, Dentin Sialophosphoprotein	Possible cell attachment proteins	MEPE—a candidate "phosphatonin" involved in tumor-induced osteomalacia

in their largest dimension). Bone mineral contains numerous impurities (carbonate, magnesium, acid phosphate) and vacancies (missing OH^-) and is usually referred to as a poorly crystalline, carbonate-substituted apatite.[17] These small imperfect crystals are more soluble than geologic apatite, enabling bone to act as a reservoir for calcium, phosphate, and magnesium ions.

The organic matrix, predominantly type I collagen, provides elasticity and flexibility to bone and also determines its structural organization. Both the collagen and the noncollagenous proteins associated with the collagen influence the way bone mineralization occurs and the way bone remodels. The cells responsible for bone formation, repair, and remodeling respond to hormonal, mechanical, and other extrinsic signals. Lipids, found in the membranes of these cells, control the flux of ions and also are directly involved mineralization. Water, found within the cells and in the extracellular matrix, is important for maintenance of tissue properties and nutrition.

Bone mineral is initially deposited at discrete sites in the collagenous matrix.[17] As bone matures, the mineral crystals become larger and more perfect (containing fewer impurities). The increase in crystal dimension is due both to the actual addition of ions to the crystals (crystal growth) and to aggregation of the crystals.[18,19] The initial sites of mineralization are the "hole" zones between the collagen fibrils.[17] There is still debate as to whether bone mineral forms concurrently in the protected environment of membrane bound bodies known as extracellular matrix vesicles, as it does in calcifying cartilage and mineralizing turkey tendons.[2] Because the body fluids are undersaturated with respect to apatite (i.e., apatite will not precipitate spontaneously), the bone matrix must contain one or more components that facilitate apatite deposition.

TABLE 6. GENE AND PROTEIN CHARACTERISTICS OF OTHER RGD-CONTAINING GLYCOPROTEINS

Protein/gene	Function	Disease/animal models
Thrombospondins (1–4, COMP)—15Q-1, 6q27, 1q21—24, 5q13, 19p13.1		
~450 kDa molecule, three identical disulfide linked subunits of ~150–180 kDa, homologies to fibrinogen, properdin, EGF, collagen, von Willebrand, *P. falciparum* and calmodulin, RGD at the C terminal globular domain	Cell attachment (but usually not spreading), binds to heparin, platelets, types I and V collagens, thrombin, fibrinogen, laminin, plasminogen and plasminogen activator inhibitor, histidine rich glycoprotein	TSP-2 knockout mouse—large collagen fibrils, thickened bones, spinal deformities
Fibronectin—2q34		
~400 kDa with 2 non-identical subunits of ~200 kDa, composed of type I, II, and III repeats, RGD in the 11th type III repeat ⅔ from N terminus	Binds to cells, fibrin heparin, gelatin, collagen	Knockout mouse—lethal prior to skeletal development
Vitronectin—17q11		
~70 kDa, RGD close to N terminus, homology to somatomedin B, rich in cysteines, sulfated, phosphorylated	Cell attachment protein, binds to collagen, plasminogen and plasminogen activator inhibitor, and to heparin	
Fibrillin 1 and 2—15q21.1, 5q23-q31		
350 kDa, EGF-like domains, RGD, cysteine motifs	May regulate elastic fiber formation	Fibrillin 1 mutations—Marfan's syndrome, Fibrillin 2 mutations—congenital contractural arachnodactyly

TABLE 7. Gene and Protein Characteristics of Gamma-Carboxy Glutamic Acid-Containing Proteins in Bone Matrix

Protein/gene	Function	Disease/animal model
Matrix Gla protein—12p ~15 kDa, five gla residues, one disulfide bridge, phosphoserine residues	May function in cartilage metabolism, a negative regulator of mineralization	Knockout mouse—excessive cartilage calcification, tiptoe walking Yoshimura mouse (mutation)—osteochondral lesions
Osteocalcin—1q25-31 ~5 kDa, one disulfide bridge, gla residues located in α helical region	May regulate activity of osteoclasts and their precursors, may mark the turning point between bone formation and resorption	Knockout mouse, osteopetrotic mouse (mutation)—thickened bones, decreased crystal size, increased mineral content
Protein S—3p11-q11.2 ~72 kDa	Primarily a liver product, but may be made by osteogenic cells	Deficiency in human—osteopenia

INITIAL MINERAL DEPOSITION

The membrane-bound extracellular bodies released from chondrocytes (and osteoblasts) known as "extracellular matrix vesicles" can facilitate initial mineral deposition by accumulating calcium and phosphate ions in a protected environment. Additionally, they provide enzymes that can degrade inhibitors of mineralization (e.g., ATP, pyrophosphate, proteoglycans) that are found in the surrounding matrix. They also contain a "nucleational core," consisting of proteins and a complex of acidic phospholipids, calcium, and inorganic phosphate, which can induce apatite formation.[2] Because these matrix vesicles are not directly associated with the collagen fibrils, the question of how mineral crystals form at discrete sites on the collagen fibrils remains. It is thought that there may be some association of vesicle mineral with the mineral in the collagen matrix or that the matrix vesicle mineral may serve as a source of calcium and phosphate ions to support initial collagen based mineralization.

In general, crystals form when the component ions of the crystal lattice, or clusters of those ions, come together with the proper orientation and with sufficient energy to generate the first stable crystal ("critical nucleus"). The formation of this miniature crystal, perhaps only one or two unit cells in size,[19] is the most energy-demanding step of crystallization. Nucleation is then followed by the addition of ions and ion clusters to the critical nucleus as the crystal grows. Growth may occur in one or more dimensions, or additional crystals may start to form at "kink" sites on the crystal in a fashion analogous to glycogen branching. This so-called "secondary nucleation" allows for exponential proliferation of crystals.

Macromolecules may facilitate the formation of the critical nucleus, sequester ions increasing the local concentrations, or bind one or more ions creating a structure on which "heterogenous nucleation" occurs. As crystals proliferate, the macromolecules may bind to crystal surfaces, blocking growth in one or more directions, thereby regulating the size, shape, or (if secondary nucleation is blocked) the number of crystals.

Several possible promoters (nucleators) of bone mineral formation have been identified based on solution studies and studies of animals in which the proteins have been ablated (knockouts), overexpressed (knock-ins), or mutated (transgenics) (see Tables 1–7 for specific proteins). Originally, collagen was thought to be the bone mineral nucleator,[20] but later studies demonstrated that removal of noncollagenous proteins from bone collagen matrices prevented these matrices from causing apatite formation.[21] Removal of protein phosphate from demineralized bones reduced their nucleational ability in a concentration-dependent fashion,[22] implying that one of the bone mineral nucleators was a phosphoprotein.

As discussed above, the phosphoproteins of bone include collagen itself, the SIBLINGs (osteopontin, bone sialoprotein [BSP], matrix extracellular phosphoglycoprotein [MEPE], dentin matrix protein–1 [DMP-1], osteonectin, and bone acidic glycoprotein-75 [BAG-75]).[2] Of these, to date, only BSP has been shown to act as an apatite nucleator in solution,[23] although DMP-1, when overexpressed in cell culture, accelerated mineralization.[24] Both osteopontin[25] and BSP[23,25] inhibit apatite proliferation and growth in solution. Table 8 lists the bone matrix proteins that have been shown to affect apatite formation and growth in cell-

TABLE 8. Effect of Bone Matrix Proteins on Mineralization In Vitro

Promote or support apatite formation	Inhibits mineralization	Dual function (nucleate and inhibit)	No known effect on mineralization
Type I collagen Proteolipid (matrix vesicle nucleational core)	Aggrecan α2-HS glycoprotein Matrix gla protein (MGP) Osteopontin Osteocalcin	Biglycan Osteonectin Fibronectin Bone sialoprotein	Decorin BAG-75 Lumican Tetranectin Osteoadherin Thrombospondin

free solution or in cell cultures. As can be seen from Table 8, most of these macromolecules are anionic and thus can bind Ca^{+2} in solution or on the apatite crystal surface.

Several enzymes that regulate phosphoprotein phosphorylation and dephosphorylation have also been associated with the mineralization process.[2] Of these, the phosphoprotein kinases, which regulate phosphoprotein phosphorylation, and alkaline phosphatase and other phosphoprotein phosphatases seem to be most important. Alkaline phosphatase hydrolyzes phosphate esters, increasing the local phosphate concentration and enhancing the rate and extent of mineralization. Blocking phosphoprotein phosphorylation in culture decreases rates of mineralization, and cells that lack alkaline phosphatase do not mineralize in certain culture systems unless transfected with that enzyme. Patients with hypophosphatasia, a deficiency of alkaline phosphatase, also show abnormal bone mineralization. Whether the function of alkaline phosphatase is simply to increase local phosphate concentrations; to remove phosphate containing inhibitors of apatite growth (such as ATP); or to modify phosphoproteins, thereby controlling their ability to act as nucleators, is still undetermined.

GROWTH, PROLIFERATION, AND MATURATION OF MINERAL CRYSTAL

The growth of bone mineral crystals is governed in part by the constraints of the collagen matrix on which the mineral is deposited. Noncollagenous proteins that bind to the mineral crystals can also regulate their size and shapes. These proteins are also important in recruiting bone resorbing cells (osteoclasts) to the apatite crystal surface.[2] As bone apatite crystals grow and mature, substances in addition to proteins and lipids can affect their fates. They may be introduced through the diet, given therapeutically, or may accumulate from dialysis fluids. For example, of the dietary cations, both Mg^{2+} and Sr^{2+} can be incorporated directly into the bone mineral, substituting for Ca^{2+} in the crystal lattice, and yielding mineral crystals that are smaller and less perfect than those formed in their absence. Cadmium (Cd^{2+}), a toxic pollutant, when ingested, has a similar effect on bone mineral. Carbonate (CO_3^-), part of the body fluids, is a common constituent impurity of bone mineral, substituting for both OH^- and PO_4^{-3}, as well as adsorbing onto the crystal surface. Citrate is another impurity that adsorbs onto the surface of bone mineral. With age, the total amount of carbonate increases, but the surface (labile) carbonate decreases with maturation of the mineral.[24]

While each of these impurities tend to make the crystals smaller, more imperfect, and more soluble, fluoride incorporation increases the size and therefore decreases the solubility of the apatite crystals.[26] This in part was the basis for fluoride supplementation in osteoporosis therapy, because larger crystals are more resistant to osteoclastic turnover. Another type of antiresorptive agent used in osteoporosis, the bisphosphonates, binds to the surface of apatite crystals and thereby blocks dissolution. Thus, bisphosphonate-treated crystals are stabilized and not apparently altered in size.[27,28] Tetracycline and other fluorescent compounds used to measure bone formation rates are Ca chelators that bind with high affinity to the surface of the most recently formed mineral. Because the newest formed crystals are small, their surface to volume ratios are very high, and the amount of label bound is similarly high.

EFFECTS OF MINERAL ALTERATION ON BONE PROPERTIES

While the inclusion of "foreign" ions into the bone apatite lattice can influence the properties of bone, cellular activities can also influence mineral properties. For example, where mineral deposition is retarded, for example, hypophosphatemic rickets, crystals tend to be larger than normal.[29] Crystals are smaller in osteopetrotic bone,[30] where remodeling is impaired, and the small crystals persist rather than being resorbed. In osteoporosis, where bone formation may be impaired and resorption accelerated, the larger crystals persist.[31] In skeletal fluorosis, and in general, as bone fluoride content increases, mineral content is increased, and crystals are increased in size.[27]

The size and distribution of mineral crystals in the bone matrix influences bone mechanical properties.[28,32] Bone strength is dependent on bone architecture, as well as numerous other factors. The mechanical strength of bone is correlated with "bone mineral density," (BMD)[33] a measurement that describes the amount of bone in a given area without providing information on architecture, mineral content, or crystal properties. However, there is not a 100% correlation between BMD and mechanical strength, and it is suggested that material properties (crystal size and composition, collagen maturity, etc.) may be important determinants.[28] It should be clear from the diseases mentioned above that if there are too few crystals, or crystals are too small, the mechanical strength will be compromised. Similarly, if there are too many crystals, or crystals are excessively large, as in the cases of skeletal fluorosis, bones many become brittle (unable to bear load). Thus, there is an optimal crystal size distribution, as well as an optimal amount of mineral.

MINERAL FORMATION IN CELL CULTURE

Osteoblasts in vitro synthesize an extracellular matrix that mineralizes in the presence of an exogenous phosphate source. Cell culture studies for the most part have focused on the factors controlling osteoblast differentiation and proliferation and sequence of expression of matrix proteins.[34,35] Few of these studies,[36–39] however, have demonstrated that the mineral formed was bone-like apatite. Numerous methods can be used to prove that bone-like apatite is present. The least rigorous are the histochemical stains (von Kossa for phosphate or alizarin red for calcium). The von Kossa silver stain gives positive reactions with anions that complex silver and all phosphate-containing materials. The alizarin red stain, specific for calcium, similarly cannot distinguish calcium complexed to the organic matrix from calcium bound to phosphate. Even when these two stains are colocalized, this does not prove that apatite is present. Similarly, more sophisticated electron microscopic methods such as microprobe analyses or chemical analyses of Ca and PO_4 contents cannot conclusively establish the presence of apatite. Electron micrographs showing the presence of thin plates or needles associated with collagen fibrils provide more convincing evidence of the presence of apatite, but morphology can be confusing, and calcium phosphates can take on other shapes (apatite in Greek means "deceiving"). Thus, the electron micrographs must be accompanied by electron diffraction analyses that provide definite structure verification or other diffraction methods (X-ray, synchrotron, or neutron) that provide unambiguous proof that the mineral phase examined is apatite.[36-38] Unambiguous identification of apatite can also be provided by nuclear magnetic resonance (NMR) and spectroscopic methods.[39-41] Infrared and Raman spectra also reveal the relative proportions and properties of the organic matrix, data not obtainable from diffraction methods.

Table 8 includes those bone matrix proteins that have been demonstrated to affect mineral deposition in culture, as well as in solution, and Tables 1–7 list animal models and human diseases in which the absence, modification, or overexpression of these proteins affects bone mineral properties. It thus should be apparent that the bone cells, the bone matrix, and the extracellular environment can influence mineralization, and in turn, because the mineral properties affect mechanical strength, the properties of bone.

REFERENCES

1. Gorski JP 1998 Is all bone the same? Distinctive distributions and properties of non-collagenous matrix proteins in lamellar vs. woven bone imply the existence of different underlying osteogenic mechanisms. Crit Rev Oral Biol Med **9:**201–223.
2. Gokhale JA, Robey PG, Boskey AL 2001 The biochemistry of bone. In: Marcus R, Feldman D, Kelsey A (eds.) Osteoporosis, vol. 1. Academic Press, San Diego, CA, USA, pp. 107–188.
3. Rossert J, de Crombrugghe B 2002 Type I collagen: Structure, synthesis and regulation. In: Bilezikian JP, Raisz LA, Rodan GA (eds.) Principles of Bone Biology, 2nd ed., vol. 1. Academic Press, San Diego, CA, USA, pp. 189–210.
4. Seibel MJ, Woitge HW 1999 Basic principles and clinical applications of biochemical markers of bone metabolism: Biochemical and technical aspects. J Clin Densitom **2:**299–321.
5. Robey PG 2002 Bone proteoglycans and glycoproteins. In: Bilezikian JP, Raisz LA, Rodan GA (eds.) Principles of Bone Biology. Academic Press, San Diego, CA, USA, pp. 225–238.
6. Xu T, Bianco P, Fisher LW, Longenecker G, Smith E, Goldstein S, Bonadio J, Boskey A, Heegaard AM, Sommer B, Satomura K, Dominguez P, Zhao C, Kulkarni AB, Robey PG, Young MF 1998 Targeted disruption of the biglycan gene leads to an osteoporosis-like phenotype in mice. Nat Genet **20:**78–82.
7. Hocking AM, Shinomura T, McQuillan DJ 1998 Leucine-rich repeat glycoproteins of the extracellular matrix. Matrix Biol **17:**1–19.
8. Henthorn PS 1996 Alkaline phosphatase. In: Bilezikian JP, Raisz LA, Rodan GA (eds.) Principles of Bone Biology. Academic Press, San Diego, CA, USA, pp. 197–216.
9. Brekken RA, Sage EH 2001 SPARC, a matricellular protein: At the crossroads of cell-matrix communication. Matrix Biol **19:**816–827.
10. Delany AM, Amling M, Priemel M, Howe C, Baron R, Canalis E 2000 Osteopenia and decreased bone formation in osteonectin-deficient mice. J Clin Invest **105:**915–923.
11. Denhardt DT, Noda M, O'Regan AW, Pavlin D, Berman JS 2001 Osteopontin as a means to cope with environmental insults: Regulation of inflammation, tissue remodeling, and cell survival. J Clin Invest **107:**1055–1061.
12. D'Souza RN, Cavender A, Sunavala G, Alvarez J, Ohshima T, Kulkarni AB, MacDougall M 1997 Gene expression patterns of murine dentin matrix protein 1 (Dmp1) and dentin sialophosphoprotein (DSPP) suggest distinct developmental functions in vivo. J Bone Miner Res **12:**2040–2049.
13. Robey PG, Bianco P 2002 The cell and molecular biology of bone formation. In: Coe FL, Favus MJ (eds.) Disorders of Mineral Metabolism. Williams & Wilkins, Philadelphia, PA, USA, pp. 199–226.
14. Ducy P, Karsenty G 1996 Skeletal gla proteins: Gene structure, egulation of expression and function. In: Bilezikian JP, Raisz LA, Rodan GA (eds.) Principles of Bone Biology. Academic Press, San Diego, CA, USA, pp. 183–196.
15. Luo G, Ducy P, McKee MD, Pinero GJ, Loyer E, Behringer RR, Karsenty G 1997 Spontaneous calcification of arteries and cartilage in mice lacking matrix GLA protein. Nature **386:**78–81.
16. Ducy P, Desbois C, Boyce B, Pinero G, Story B, Dunstan C, Smith E, Bonadio J, Goldstein S, Gundberg C, Bradley A, Karsenty G 1996 Increased bone formation in osteocalcin-deficient mice. Nature **382:**448–452.
17. Glimcher MJ 1998 The nature of the mineral phase in bone: Biological and clinical implications. In: Avioli LV, Krane SM (eds.) Metabolic Bone Disease and Clinically Related Disorders, 3rd ed. Academic Press, San Diego, CA, pp. 23–51.
18. Landis WJ 1995 The strength of a calcified tissue depends in part on the molecular structure and organization of its constituent mineral crystals in their organic matrix. Bone **16:**533–544.
19. Eppell SJ, Tong W, Katz JL, Kuhn L, Glimcher MJ 2001 Shape and size of isolated bone mineralites measured using atomic force microscopy. J Orthop Res **19:**1027–1034.
20. Glimcher MJ 1959 Molecular biology of mineralized tissues with particular reference to bone. Rev Mod Physics **31:**359–393.
21. Termine JD, Belcourt AB, Conn KM, Kleinman HK 1981 Mineral and collagen-binding proteins of fetal calf bone. J Biol Chem **256:**10403–10408.
22. Glimcher MJ 1989 Mechanism of calcification: Role of collagen fibrils and collagen-phosphoprotein complexes in vitro and in vivo. Anat Rec **224:**139–153.
23. Stubbs JT III, Mintz KP, Eanes ED, Torchia DA, Fisher LW 1997 Characterization of native and recombinant bone sialoprotein: Delineation of the mineral-binding and cell adhesion domains and structural analysis of the RGD domain. J Bone Miner Res **12:**1210–1222.
24. Rey C, Shimizu M, Collins B, Glimcher MJ 1991 Resolution-enhanced Fourier transform infrared spectroscopy study of the environment of phosphate ion in the early deposits of a solid phase of calcium phosphate in bone and enamel and their evolution with age: 2. Investigations in the $\nu_3 PO_4$ domain. Calcif Tissue Int **49:**383–388.
25. Boskey AL 1995 Osteopontin and related phosphorylated sialoproteins: Effects on mineralization. Ann NY Acad Sci **760:**249–256.
26. Grynpas MD 1990 Fluoride effects on bone crystals. J Bone Miner Res **5:**S1;S169–S175.
27. Fratzl P, Schreiber S, Roschger P, Lafage MH, Rodan G, Klaushofer K 1996 Effects of sodium fluoride and alendronate on the bone mineral in minipigs: A small-angle X-ray scattering and backscattered electron imaging study. J Bone Miner Res **11:**248–253.
28. Boskey AL Bone mineral crystal size. Osteoporos Int (in press).
29. Boskey AL, Gilder H, Neufeld E, Ecarot B, Glorieux FH 1991 Phospholipid changes in the bones of the hypophosphatemic mouse. Bone **12:**345–351.
30. Boskey AL, Marks SC Jr 1985 Mineral and matrix alterations in the bones of incisors-absent (ia/ia) osteopetrotic rats. Calcif Tissue Int **37:**287–292.
31. Paschalis EP, Betts F, DiCarlo E, Mendelsohn R, Boskey AL 1997 FTIR microspectroscopic analysis of human iliac crest biopsies from untreated osteoporotic bone. Calcif Tissue Int **61:**487–492.
32. Martin RB 1993 Aging and strength of bone as a structural material. Calcif Tissue Int **53:**34–40.
33. Currey JD, Brear K, Zioupos P 1996 The effects of ageing and changes in mineral content in degrading the toughness of human femora. J Biomech **29:**257–260.
34. Siggelkow H, Rebenstorff K, Kurre W, Niedhart C, Engel I, Schulz H, Atkinson MJ, Hufner M 1999 Development of the osteoblast phenotype in primary human osteoblasts in culture: Comparison with rat calvarial cells in osteoblast differentiation. J Cell Biochem **75:**22–35.
35. Ferrera D, Poggi S, Biassoni C, Dickson GR, Astigiano S, Barbieri O, Favre A, Franzi AT, Strangio A, Federici A, Manduca P 2002 Three-dimensional cultures of normal human osteoblasts: Proliferation and differentiation potential in vitro and upon ectopic implantation in nude mice. Bone **30:**718–725.
36. Ecarot-Charrier B, Glorieux FH, van der Rest M, Pereira G 1983 Osteoblasts isolated from mouse calvaria initiate matrix mineralization in culture. J Cell Biol **96:**639–643.
37. Gerstenfeld LC, Chipman SD, Kelly CM, Hodgens KJ, Lee DD, Landis WJ 1988 Collagen expression, ultrastructural assembly, and mineralization in cultures of chicken embryo osteoblasts. J Cell Biol **106:**979–989.

38. Rey C, Kim HM, Gerstenfeld L, Glimcher MJ 1996 Characterization of the apatite crystals of bone and their maturation in osteoblast cell culture: Comparison with native bone crystals. Connect Tissue Res **35**:343–349.
39. Kato Y, Boskey A, Spevak L, Dallas M, Hori M, Bonewald LF 2001 Establishment of an osteoid preosteocyte-like cell MLO-A5 that spontaneously mineralizes in culture. J Bone Miner Res **16**:1622–1633.
40. Kuhn LT, Wu Y, Rey C, Gerstenfeld LC, Grynpas MD, Ackerman JL, Kim HM, Glimcher MJ 2000 Structure, composition, and maturation of newly deposited calcium-phosphate crystals in chicken osteoblast cell cultures. J Bone Miner Res **15**:1301–1309.
41. Lin DL, Tarnowski CP, Zhang J, Dai J, Rohn E, Patel AH, Morris MD, Keller ET 2001 Bone metastatic LNCaP-derivative C4–2B prostate cancer cell line mineralizes in vitro. Prostate **47**:212–221.

Chapter 7.   Bone Remodeling

Gregory R. Mundy,[1,2] Di Chen,[1] and Babatunde O. Oyajobi[1]

[1]*Department of Cellular and Structural Biology and* [2]*Department of Orthopaedics, University of Texas Health Science Center at San Antonio, San Antonio, Texas*

INTRODUCTION

The adult skeleton is in a dynamic state, being continually broken down and reformed by the coordinated actions of osteoclasts and osteoblasts on trabecular (also called cancellous) bone surfaces and in Haversian systems. This turnover or remodeling of bone occurs in focal and discrete packets throughout the skeleton. The remodeling of each packet takes a finite period of time (estimated to be about 3–4 months, but differing in cortical and cancellous bone, and probably longer in cancellous bone). The remodeling that occurs in each packet (called a bone remodeling unit by Frost, who gave the first modern description of this sequence almost 40 years ago)[1] is geographically and chronologically separated from other packets of remodeling. This suggests that activation of the sequence of cellular events responsible for remodeling is locally controlled, most likely by local mechanisms in the bone microenvironment. The sequence is always the same activation of osteoclast precursors, and osteoclastic bone resorption is followed by osteoblastic bone formation to repair the defect. A diagram of the cellular events involved in bone remodeling is shown in Fig. 1. The new bone that is formed is called a bone structural unit (BSU).[1]

In this chapter, a review of the cellular events involved in remodeling, the disturbances in remodeling that occur in bone diseases, and the hypotheses that have been proposed for coordination of these cellular events will be outlined.

REMODELING IN DIFFERENT PARTS OF THE SKELETON

The bones of the adult skeleton consist either of cortical (or compact) bone and cancellous (or trabecular) bone. Current evidence indicates that cortical bone and cancellous bone do not change with age in exactly the same way; therefore, they probably should be considered as two separate functional entities. The proportions of cortical and cancellous bone differ at the different sites in the skeleton where osteoporotic fractures frequently occur (Fig. 2). Cancellous bone is relatively prominent in the vertebral column,

the most common site of fracture associated with osteoporosis. In the lumbar spine, cancellous bone comprises more than 66% of the total bone. In the intertrochanteric area of the femur, bone is comprised of 50% cortical and 50% cancellous. In the neck of the femur, the bone is 75% cortical and 25% cancellous. In contrast, in the mid-radius, more than 95% of the bone is cortical bone. The differences in behavior of bone at these different sites are most likely caused by the different environments of the bone cells in cortical or cancellous bone. Bone remodeling cells on cancellous bone surfaces are in intimate contact with the cells of the marrow cavity, which produce a variety of potent osteotropic cytokines. It is likely that the cells in cortical bone, which are more distant from the influences of these cytokines, are controlled more by the systemic osteotropic hormones such as parathyroid hormone (PTH) and 1,25 dihydroxyvitamin D_3 [1,25$(OH)_2D_3$]. Osteoclasts and osteoblasts on cancellous bone surfaces may be controlled primarily by factors produced by adjacent bone marrow cells. Similar cells that are present in Haversian systems of cortical bone are not in such close contact with the myriad of osteotropic cytokines that are produced by marrow mononuclear cells.

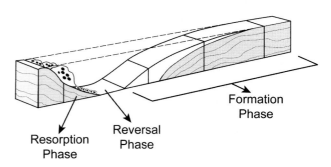

FIG. 1. Bone remodeling in cancellous bone as seen in longitudinal sequence and cross sections. Five different phases can be distinguished over time: (1) osteoclastic resorption, (2) reversal, (3) preosteoblastic migration and differentiation into osteoblasts, (4) osteoblastic matrix (osteoid) formation, and (5) mineralization. The end-product of remodeling in cancellous bone is the completed cancellous bone structural unit (BSU) covered by lining cells (6). (Modified from Eriksen EF, Axelrod DW, Melsen F 1994 Bone Histomorphometry. Raven Press, New York, NY, USA, pp. 3–124.)

The authors have no conflict of interest.

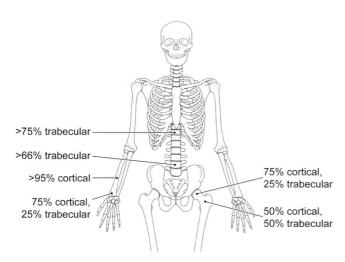

>75% trabecular

>66% trabecular

>95% cortical

75% cortical, 25% trabecular

75% cortical, 25% trabecular

50% cortical, 50% trabecular

FIG. 2. Relative proportions of cortical (compact) and trabecular (cancellous) bone in different parts of the skeleton.

Remodeling of Cortical Bone

Cortical bone is dense or compact bone. It comprises 85% of the total bone in the body and is relatively most abundant in the long bone shafts of the appendicular skeleton. The volume of cortical bone is regulated by the formation of periosteal bone, by remodeling within Haversian systems, and by endosteal bone resorption. Cortical bone is removed primarily by endosteal resorption and resorption within the Haversian canals. The latter leads to increased porosity of cortical bone. However, periosteal bone formation continues to increase the diameter of cortical bone throughout life. Cortical bone loss probably begins to occur after the age of 40 (according to most studies), and there is an acceleration of cortical bone loss that occurs for 5–10 years after menopause. This accelerated phase of cortical bone loss continues for 15 years and then gradually slows. There is irrefutable evidence that estrogen replacement therapy after the menopause preserves cortical bone. In later life, women with osteoporosis lose cortical bone at similar rates to those of premenopausal women. Loss of cortical bone is the major predisposing factor for fractures that occur at the hip and around the wrist. Cortical bone is particularly prone to increased resorption in patients with primary hyperparathyroidism.

Remodeling of Cancellous Bone

Although cancellous bone comprises only 15% of the skeleton, the changes that occur in this type of bone after the age of 30 largely determine whether spinal osteoporotic fractures will occur. Depending on the technique used, decline in cancellous bone mass begins in early adult life, occurring earlier than the decline in cortical bone mass.[2] Other studies have disagreed with these findings and suggested that the decline in cancellous bone mass begins later, after ovarian function ceases.[3] Riggs and Melton[4] have suggested that acceleration in cancellous bone loss occurring at the time of menopause is not as prominent as the accelerated loss of cortical bone mass that occurs at this time.

The loss of cancellous bone that occurs with aging is not due simply to a generalized thinning of the bone plates, but is rather caused by complete perforation and fragmentation of trabeculae.[5,6] Because cancellous bone has a broad surface area, resorption may be modulated by focal osteoclastic resorption regulated by local hormonal factors produced by cells in the bone marrow microenvironment, including marrow cells as well as other types of bone cells and accessory cells.

Osteoclast activation is the initial step in the remodeling sequence. Osteoclasts are activated in specific focal sites by mechanisms that are still not understood. The rate of bone remodeling is to a large degree dependent on the activation frequency of osteoclasts. The mechanism responsible for the initiation of bone remodeling is unknown. One possibility is that osteoclast precursors recognize a change in the mechanical properties of aging bone, which requires replacement with new bone for optimal structural integrity. This theoretical possibility could occur because other cells such as immune cells or osteocytes recognize a change in the bone surface and send signals to osteoclasts to activate them. However, the initial trigger for such activation of immune cells is unknown. The eventual activation of the osteoclast may occur because of interactions between integral membrane proteins (integrins) on osteoclast cell membranes with proteins in bone matrix, which contain RGD (arginine-glycine-asparagine) amino acid sequences (such as osteopontin).[7] The resorptive phase of the remodeling process has been estimated to last 10 days (Fig. 1). This period is followed by repair of the defect by a team of osteoblasts that are attracted to the site of the resorption defect and then presumably proceed to make new bone. This part of the process takes approximately 3 months. The initial events in the formation phase are possibly unidirectional migration (chemotaxis) of osteoblast precursors to the site of the defect followed by enhanced cell proliferation. The complete sequence of cellular events that occur at the bone surface during the remodeling process have been described in detail by Baron et al.,[8] from studies on the alveolar bone of the rat, and from Boyce et al.,[9] from the calvarial bone of the mouse. The cellular events that occur in these models are similar to those in adult human bone.

Coupling

In physiological as well as most pathological circumstances, the coupling of bone formation to previous bone resorption occurs faithfully. Packets of bone that are removed during resorption are replaced during formation. The cellular and humoral mechanisms that are responsible for mediating the coupling process (or disrupting it, as in the diseases described above) are still not clear. A number of theories have been proposed to account for coupling. Almost 30 years ago, Rasmussen and Bordier[10] suggested that the osteoclast, once it finishes the resorptive phase of the remodeling sequence, undergoes fission to form mononuclear cells, which are the precursors of osteoblasts. However, it is now widely accepted that osteoclasts and osteoblasts have different origins. Osteoclasts arise from hematopoietic stem cells or at least stem cells in the marrow environment that have the capacity to circulate. Osteoblasts, in contrast, arise from mesenchymal (stromal) stem cells. Many investigators have favored the notion that coupling is mediated locally by humoral factors acting through osteoblasts and other cells in the osteogenic lineage,[11] or that an osteoblast-stimulating factor (such as insulin growth factor [IGF]-I, IGF-II, or transforming growth factor [TGF]-β) is released from bone matrix during the process of osteoclastic bone resorption and that the stimulation of osteoblast activity leads to new bone formation.[12,13]

A variation on this humoral concept is that the factor, which stimulates resorption, also acts directly (but more slowly) on osteoblasts to cause their activation and subsequent new bone formation.[14] This notion suggests that coupling does not involve sequential signals released during the process of bone remodeling, but rather that secreted factors that work, for example, through the gp130 signal transduction mechanism, are responsible for simultaneous stimulation of osteoclast and osteoblast lineages. Alternatively, coupling may involve transcription factors expressed in osteogenic lineage cells such as the Runt-homology domain transcription factor, Runx2/Cbfa1, which is not only obligatory for bone formation but has also recently been shown to also regulate osteoclastogenesis.[15] More recently, it has been suggested that coupling, or at least the bone formation component of bone remodeling, may be systemically mediated by leptin acting on the hypothalamus to stimulate the sympathetic nervous system and lead to β2-adrenergic stimulation of cells in the osteoblast lineage to retard bone formation. An alternative to the humoral hypothesis for coupling (local, systemic, or both) is that, because osteoblasts normally line bone surfaces, once the phase of osteoclastic resorption is over and osteoclasts disappear from the resorption sites, osteoblasts and their precursors repopulate the resorption site and merely reline the bone surface. Possibly through cell surface molecules, they recognize the resorption site, and this stimulates their differentiation into mature bone-forming cells. They may thus repair the resorptive defect without the necessity for involvement of a humoral mediator that is specifically generated as a consequence of resorption.

Obviously, understanding this sequence of cellular events may lead to clarification of the mechanisms responsible for the decreased osteoblast activity that occurs in age-related bone loss and possibly the pathophysiology of osteoporosis, as well as the specific defects in osteoblast function that occur in malignancies such as myeloma, breast cancer, and prostate cancer.

Bone Remodeling and Disease

All diseases of bone are superimposed on this normal cellular remodeling sequence. In diseases such as primary hyperparathyroidism, hyperthyroidism, and Paget's disease, in which osteoclasts are activated, there is a compensatory and (relatively) balanced increase in the formation of new bone. However, there are also a number of well-described conditions in which osteoblast activity does not completely repair and replace the defect left by previous resorptive activity. One example is multiple myeloma, usually charac-

terized by punched-out lytic bone lesions with little new bone formation.[16] In myeloma, there appears to be a specific defect in osteoblast maturation.[17] There are probably increased numbers of osteoblasts around the edges of the lytic lesions, but the osteoblasts fail (in the great majority of patients) to synthesize more than thin osteoid seams. In solid tumors associated with malignancy, there is also a failure of bone formation to repair resorptive defects, especially in patients dying from their malignancy.[18] Cancellous bone is the type of bone lost predominantly in patients with osteolytic bone disease caused by malignancy. In this situation, the malignant cells lodge in the marrow cavity and produce local factors that stimulate adjacent osteoclasts on trabecular plates and on endosteal surfaces of cortical bone.[19]

In elderly patients with osteoporosis, there is a decrease in mean wall thickness, presumably reflecting the inability of osteoblasts to repair adequately the resorptive defects made during normal osteoclastic resorption.[20] It should also be stressed that progressive bone loss, beginning at about 35 years of age (depending on the bone) occurs in all humans, and is indicative of a "physiological" imbalance between resorption and formation.

Although bone formation usually occurs on sites of previous osteoclastic resorption in normal adult humans, there are several special situations in which osteoblasts may lay down new bone on surfaces not previously resorbed. Two examples are osteoblastic metastases associated with tumors such as carcinoma of the prostate and breast and during prolonged exposure to pharmacologic doses of fluoride therapy.

CELLULAR EVENTS INVOLVED IN THE RESORPTION PHASE

Osteoclast Origin and Cell Lineage

The origin and cell lineage of the osteoclast is discussed elsewhere. The first event during bone remodeling is osteoclast activation, followed by osteoclast formation, polarization, formation of a ruffled border, resorption, and ultimately apoptosis. Apoptosis occurring at the conclusion of the resorbing phase of the bone remodeling process is a recently observed phenomenon.[21] The morphologic characteristics of osteoclast apoptosis are condensation of the nuclear chromatin, darker staining of the osteoclast cytoplasm, loss of ruffled border and detachment from the mineralized bone matrix, and cessation of bone resorption. Observations by Hughes et al. suggest that osteoclast apoptosis is a common occurrence at reversal sites and may be precipitated by resorption inhibitors such as estrogen and bisphosphonates and also by TGF-β.[21,22] Regulation of the process of osteoclast apoptosis may be potentially important during bone remodeling, because this represents a step by which bone resorption could be regulated.

Regulation of Osteoclast Activity

Osteoclasts lie on bone surfaces in a bed of elliptical or fusiform spindle-shaped cells called lining cells, which are probably members of the osteoblast lineage. When exposed to a bone resorptive agent, the first response is that these lining cells retract and the osteoclasts insinuate an arm into the retracted area, a ruffled border forms, and bone is resorbed at the exposed surface.[23] Why lining cells retract at specific sites and what initiates osteoblast formation and activation are still unknown. The osteoclast is ultimately activated by a membrane-bound signal expressed by cells in the osteoblast lineage, recently discovered to be the ligand for RANK.

Many hormones and factors have not been shown to directly stimulate osteoclast activity. Their mechanisms of action differ. Osteoclastic resorption may be stimulated by factors that enhance proliferation of osteoclast progenitors, which cause differentiation of committed precursors into mature cells or activation of the mature multinucleated cell to resorb bone.[24] Similarly, osteoclasts could be inhibited by agents, which block proliferation of precursors, inhibit differentiation or fusion, or inactivate the mature multinucleated resorbing cell. Current evidence indicates that most factors that stimulate or inhibit osteoclasts act on at least two of these steps.

Systemic Hormones. The systemic hormones PTH, 1,25-$(OH)_2D_3$, and calcitonin all influence osteoclast activity.

PTH. PTH stimulates bone formation and osteoclastic bone resorption in vitro and in vivo depending on whether it is administered intermittently or continuously. However, the mechanism responsible for these differing effects is still unclear. Recent evidence suggests that the dual effects of PTH on bone are mediated through its regulation of Cbfa1 expression because the transcription factor is obligatory for bone formation and because Cbfa1 also regulates RANKL expression.[20,25] Thus, the effect of PTH on osteoclast formation is likely indirect, mediated through cells in the osteoblast lineage including lining cells, which express RANKL. However, mammalian osteoclasts express PTH receptors, and the possibility of direct activation of osteoclasts cannot be excluded.

PTH-related protein (PTHrP) has identical biphasic effects to those of PTH on bone, including enhancing osteoclastic activity in vitro and in vivo.

1,25 Dihydroxyvitamin D. $1,25(OH)_2D_3$ is a potent stimulator of osteoclastic bone resorption. Like PTH, it stimulates differentiation and fusion of osteoclast progenitors,[26] and this has now been shown to be mediated indirectly by osteoblast lineage cells in a RANKL-dependent fashion. $1,25(OH)_2D_3$ also has other effects on bone resorption that are direct as it activates mature preformed osteoclasts, possibly by a similar mechanism to that of PTH. $1,25(OH)_2D_3$ is also a potent immunoregulatory molecule.[27] It inhibits T-cell proliferation and the production of interleukin (IL)-2. Under some circumstances, it can enhance IL-1 production from monocyte-macrophages. Thus, the overall effects of $1,25(OH)_2D_3$ on bone resorption are multiple and complex.

Calcitonin. Calcitonin is a polypeptide hormone that is a potent inhibitor of osteoclastic bone resorption, but its effects are only transient. Osteoclasts escape from the inhibitory effects of calcitonin after continued exposure.[28] Thus, patients treated for hypercalcemia with calcitonin will respond for only a limited period of time before hypercalcemia recurs (usually 48–72 h). Even in Pagetic patients, the beneficial effects of calcitonin may eventually be lost with continued treatment. The "escape" phenomenon is likely caused by downregulation of mRNA for the receptor.[29] Calcitonin causes cytoplasmic contraction of the osteoclast cell membrane, which has been correlated with its capacity to inhibit bone resorption.[30] It also causes the dissolution of mature osteoclasts into mononuclear cells. However, it also inhibits osteoclast formation, inhibiting both proliferation of the progenitors and differentiation of the committed precursors. The effects of calcitonin on osteoclasts are mediated by cyclic AMP.

Local Hormones/Cytokines. Local hormones and cytokines may be more important than systemic hormones for the initiation of physiologic bone resorption and for the normal bone remodeling sequence. Because bone remodeling occurs in discrete and distinct packets throughout the skeleton, it seems probable that the cellular events are influenced by factors generated in the microenvironment of bone, as well as systemic factors. A number of potent local stimulators and inhibitors of osteoclast activity have recently been identified.

Osteoprotegrin/RANKL/RANK. It has become clear in the last few years that the tumor necrosis factor (TNF) ligand family member, RANK ligand, and its two known receptors RANK and osteoprotegerin (OPG) are the key regulators of osteoclastic bone resorption in vitro and in vivo.

OPG is a TNF receptor (TNFR) superfamily member that constitutively lacks a transmembrane domain and is thus secreted. When expressed, recombinant OPG was shown to inhibit both physiological and pathological bone resorption and hepatic overexpression of the *Opg* gene in mice resulted in severe osteopetrosis.[31] Independently, another group isolated a heparin-binding protein from conditioned media of human fibroblast cultures that profoundly inhibited osteoclast formation and was designated "osteoclastogenesis inhibitory factor" (OCIF).[32] Subsequently, OCIF was shown to be identical to OPG.[33] Other groups also independently cloned the same molecule as the TNF receptor-like molecule 1 (TR1), follicular dendritic cell-derived receptor I (FDCR-1).[34–36] As proposed by ASBMR, we will hereafter refer to the protein (including OCIF, FDCR-1, and TR1) as OPG.[37]

OPG has only two known ligands, RANKL and TRAIL, both of which are type II membrane-bound TNF homologs.[38–40] In contrast to most other TNF receptor family members, OPG is secreted and circulates in vivo.[31] There is now incontrovertible evidence that it acts as a nonsignaling decoy receptor for RANKL and thereby regulates bone turnover.[41–44] Although OPG can also bind to TRAIL, the significance of this is unknown. It is unlikely that the interaction between TRAIL and OPG influences bone remodeling because *Trail*-deficient mice have no skeletal abnormalities.[45] The relationship between circulating OPG levels and bone turnover remains unclear. The few studies investigating the relationship between circulating OPG levels and bone turnover in humans have yielded variable results.[46–48]

The effects of OPG on bone have been best shown in rodents. *Opg*-deficient mice produced by targeted disruption of the gene exhibit profound osteoporosis from birth caused by enhanced osteoclast formation and function as well as prolonged osteoclast survival. Histology reveals a destruction of growth plates, lack of trabeculae, and histomorphometric analyses revealed an increase in bone resorption indices in long bones of adult null mutant mice. This is accompanied by a marked decrease in the strength and mineral densities of their bones. Interestingly, osteoblast surface areas were also increased in *Opg*-deficient mice. OPG null mutant mice also develop calcification of the aorta and renal arteries.[49,50] These results indicate that OPG is a physiological humoral regulator of osteoclast-mediated bone resorption during postnatal bone growth. It also suggests that OPG might play a role in preventing calcification of larger arteries. In vivo, parenteral administration of OPG results in a marked increase in bone mineral density (BMD) and bone volume associated with a decrease in the number of active osteoclasts both in normal and ovariectomized rats.[51] Serum calcium concentration also decreased rapidly on parenteral administration of OPG, independent of any changes in urinary calcium excretion, in thyroparathyroidectomized rats whose serum calcium levels were raised acutely by PTH infusion.[52] This suggests that OPG, in addition to its effect on osteoclastogenesis, also affects the function and/or survival of mature osteoclasts.

In vitro, in the presence of M-CSF, RANKL induces osteoclast formation in the absence of osteoblasts/stromal cells, and adding OPG abrogates this.[41,42] OPG also strongly inhibits osteoclast formation induced by a range of osteotropic hormones and cytokines including $1,25(OH)_2$-D_3, PTH, PGE_2, IL-1, and IL-11 in cocultures of osteoblasts/stromal cells and hematopoietic osteoclast progenitors. Interestingly, almost all of the factors that stimulate RANKL expression conversely inhibit OPG production.[41–44] OPG also directly inhibits the bone-resorbing activity of isolated mature osteoclasts, in part, by suppressing osteoclast survival. In contrast, OPG gene expression and production in marrow stromal/osteoblastic cells is markedly enhanced by TGF-β,[43] and this likely explains the powerful effect of TGF-β to inhibit osteoclast formation and to enhance osteoclast apoptosis. Furthermore, TGF-β had no effect on OPG expression by human dental mesenchymal cells,[53] raising the possibility of tissue-specific regulation of OPG expression.

Evidence had accrued over a number of years pointing to the existence of a cell surface-associated factor on osteogenic cells obligatory for proliferation and differentiation of osteoclast precursors. This factor, termed osteoclast differentiation factor (ODF) and stromal cell-derived osteoclast formation activity (SOFA), was postulated to be inducible by cytokines and hormones known to regulate osteoclast differentiation. This factor is the TNF ligand superfamily member molecularly cloned by four independent groups and designated as RANKL,[38] TRANCE,[54] ODF,[55] and OPG ligand.[39] The expression of this molecule is obligatory for osteoclastic resorption and normal bone modeling and remodeling.[41–44] As proposed by ASBMR, this cytokine will be referred to hereafter as RANKL.[37]

RANKL is a type II membrane protein with a cytoplasmic N- and extracellular C-termini. Although the existence of a secreted form of RANKL representing the extracellular C-terminal domain has been alluded to in a number of studies,[39,56,57] there is as yet no unequivocal evidence that a soluble form of RANKL exists in vivo or is generated by proteolytic cleavage in the bone microenvironment. In addition, membrane-bound RANKL is more potent than an engineered soluble form.[58] RANKL expression in cells of the osteogenic lineage appears to be related to their differentiation state; more mature osteoblasts express RANKL constitutively, whereas its expression in immature osteoblasts and bone marrow stromal cells is largely inducible by osteotropic hormones and cytokines.[43,59] RANKL expression has also been detected on mature osteoclasts in vivo,[60] although the significance of this with regards to osteoclast differentiation and activation is still unclear.

As with OPG, our understanding of the role of RANKL in bone remodeling in vivo has increased tremendously with generation of RANKL knockout mice, which exhibit typical osteopetrosis with total occlusion of bone marrow space with endosteal bone. The bones of these RANKL null mutant mice lack osteoclasts, although they contain osteoclast progenitors that differentiate into functionally active osteoclasts when cocultured with normal osteoblasts/ stromal cells from wild-type littermates.[61] Administration of recombinant RANKL to mice increases blood ionized calcium and osteoclasts.[39,62] These results suggest that RANKL is an absolute requirement for osteoclast development.

RANKL, in the presence of M-CSF, induces osteoclast formation in all model systems presently available to study osteoclast ontogeny.[41–44] Treatment of stromal/ osteoblastic cells of human and murine origin with known stimulators of osteoclast formation, $1,25(OH)_2D_3$, PTH, PGE_2, IL-1β, TNF-α, IL-11, IL-6, and basic fibroblast growth factor (FGF) induces or enhances RANKL mRNA levels.[41,43] A recombinant soluble form of RANKL also stimulates bone resorption in organ cultures that was completely inhibited by OPG. Polyclonal antibodies against RANKL inhibited bone resorption in organ cultures induced by not only soluble RANKL but also by a variety of unrelated hormones and cytokines, clearly indicating that bone resorption induced by these osteotropic factors is mediated by RANKL. In cultures of isolated rat osteoclasts, devoid of stromal or osteoblastic cells and where there is no new osteoclast formation, recombinant RANKL markedly increases the bone-resorbing activity of mature osteoclasts as well as prolongs their survival.[41–44]

The TNFR superfamily member RANK is the only known signaling receptor for RANKL. RANK, a type I transmembrane protein, mediates all of the signals essential for osteoclast differentiation from hematopoietic progenitors as well as activation of mature osteoclasts.[62–65] Interestingly, overexpression of RANK in human embryonic kidney fibroblasts (293) cells induces ligand-independent

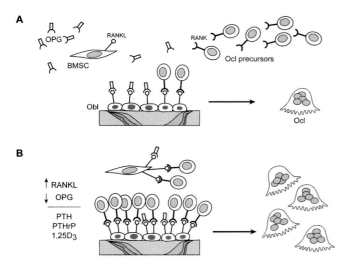

FIG. 3. Osteoblast and osteoclast coupling mediated through RANKL/RANK interactions. Osteoblasts (Obl) express RANKL constitutively on their cell surface, whereas RANKL expression in bone marrow stromal cells (BMSC) is largely inducible by various hormones and cytokines.[42,58] Interaction of RANKL with its cognate receptor RANK expressed on osteoclast (Ocl) precursors promotes osteoclast differentiation, and the interaction of the RANKL with RANK on mature Ocl results in their activation and prolonged survival. OPG, present in the bone microenvironment, is secreted primarily by BMSC/Obl, and in this milieu (and in conditioned media harvested from BMSC and Obl cultures), there is an excess of OPG. In vivo, OPG blocks the interaction of RANKL with its cognate receptor RANK on Ocl precursors as well as on mature Ocl's, thus acting as a physiological regulator of bone turnover.

NF-κB activation,[63] suggesting that pathological conditions associated with RANK overexpression or misexpression may result in increased osteoclast formation independent of RANKL. In accord with this notion, mutations in exon 1 of the RANK gene have been detected in familial expansile osteolysis (FEO), a condition characterized by osteolytic lesions and generalized osteopenia. The resulting mutant RANK proteins are constitutively active or exhibit increased NF-κB activation in vitro consistent with a gain-of-function mutation.[66,67] *Rank*-deficient mice have been generated,[64,65] and as expected, they exhibit severe osteopetrosis caused by complete absence of osteoclasts and lack of bone resorption. Although these RANK null mutant mice form incisors, there is complete failure of teeth eruption, thus confirming the absolute requirement of an intact RANKL/RANK pathway for osteoclastogenesis in vitro and in vivo.

A schematic of osteoblast and osteoclast coupling illustrating RANKL/RANK interactions and the role of OPG is shown in Fig. 3.

IL-1. There are two IL-1 molecules, IL-1α and β. Their effects on bone seem to be the same and are mediated through the same receptor. IL-1 is released by activated monocytes, but also by other types of cells, including osteoblasts and tumor cells. It is a potent stimulator of osteoclasts.[9] It works at all phases in the formation and activation of osteoclasts. Its effects are mediated through RANKL.[43]

IL-1 also stimulates osteoclastic bone resorption when

infused in vivo and causes a substantial increase in plasma calcium levels.[9,68] It has been implicated as a potential mediator of bone resorption and increased bone turnover in osteoporosis.[69] It may be responsible for the increase in bone resorption seen in some malignancies, as well as the localized bone resorption associated with collections of chronic inflammatory cells in diseases such as rheumatoid arthritis.

Lymphotoxin and TNF-α. Lymphotoxin and TNF-α are molecules that are related functionally to IL-1. Many of their biological properties overlap with those of IL-1.[70] They share the same receptor with each other, which is distinct from that of IL-1. Their effects on bone are synergistic with IL-1.

M-CSF. Colony-stimulating factor-1 (CSF-1), which was once thought to be specific for the monocyte-macrophage lineage, has recently been shown to be required for normal osteoclast formation in rodents during the neonatal period. In the *op/op* variant of osteopetrosis, there is impaired production of CSF-1, and the consequence is osteopetrosis because of decreased normal osteoclast formation. The disease can be cured by treatment with CSF-1.[71] CSF-1 is produced by stromal cells in the osteoclast microenvironment. Cells in the osteoclast lineage express the CSF-1 receptor (a receptor tyrosine kinase). CSF-1 works in conjunction with RANKL and TGF-β to cause osteoclastic bone resorption.

IL-6. IL-6 is a pleiotropic cytokine that has important effects on bone. It is expressed and secreted by normal bone cells in response to osteotropic hormones such as PTH, 1,25(OH)$_2$D$_3$, and IL-1.[72,73] The osteoclast is the most prodigious cell source of IL-6 so far described. IL-6 is a fairly weak stimulator of osteoclast formation and less powerful than other cytokines such as IL-1, TNF-α, and lymphotoxin.[73,74] It has been implicated in the bone loss associated skeletal metastases and with estrogen withdrawal (ovariectomy) in the mouse.[74,75] It is probable that related cytokines such as IL-11 and leukemia inhibitory factor (LIF) work through similar mechanisms.

FGF: Interferon-γ. Interferon-γ (IFN-γ) is a multifunctional lymphokine produced by activated T-lymphocytes. In contrast to the other immune cell products, it potently inhibits osteoclastic bone resorption.[76,77] Its major effect seem to be inhibition of differentiation of committed osteoclast precursors to mature cells through induction of degradation of TRAF components of the signaling pathway downstream of RANK.[77] It also has effects on osteoclast precursor proliferation, albeit much less potent. Unlike calcitonin, it does not cause cytoplasmic contraction of isolated osteoclasts.

TGF-β. TGF-β is a multifunctional polypeptide that is produced by immune cells but is also secreted by stromal cells/osteoblasts, sequestered in the bone matrix and released during resorption. TGF-β has unique and complex effects on osteoclasts, which may even differ in different species. For example, in one system, neonatal mouse calvariae, exogenous TGF-β stimulates prostaglandin generation, which in turn, leads to bone resorption, which is the opposite effect to that seen in the rat or human systems where exogenous TGF-β blocks osteoclast formation by inhibiting both proliferation and differentiation of osteoclast precursors.[78] However, more recent data implicate endogenous TGF-β as a stimulator of osteoclastogenesis in human model systems.[79] Because TGF-β has a powerful effect on osteoblasts (stimulates proliferation and synthesis of differentiated proteins, increases mineralized bone formation),[80] it may be a pivotal factor during bone turnover acting as a central component coupling bone formation to resorption during bone remodeling. For example, low levels of TGF-β in the bone microenvironment may stimulate osteoclastic differentiation and activation. However, with continued release from the matrix during the resorptive process, active TGF-β accumulates, and this high level of the growth factor may serve as a natural inhibitor of continued osteoclast activity. At the same time, working in conjunction with other bone factors, it may lead to osteoblast stimulation and the eventual formation of new bone. In mice with osteoblasts unresponsive to TGF-β, there is an age-dependent increase in trabecular bone mass most likely because of decreased osteoclastic bone resorption because osteoblast activity and the rate of osteoblastic bone formation was not significantly altered.[81]

IL-6, IL-15, IL-17, IL-18. IL-15 is an IL-2–like cytokine produced almost exclusively by T-cells and which binds the same receptor as IL-2.[82] IL-15 has recently been reported to stimulate the formation of TRACP$^+$, calcitonin receptor positive multinucleated osteoclast-like cells in rat bone marrow cultures that resorb calcified matrices.[83] Although IL-15 is a potent inducer of TNF-α, this effect to stimulate formation of osteoclast-like cells is not blocked by a specific anti-TNF neutralizing antibody. Although IL-15 and IL-2 also share some receptor components, IL-2 does not stimulate formation of osteoclast-like cells.

IL-17 is also a product of activated T-cells that stimulates osteoclastogenesis and bone resorption.[84] It induces production of IL-6 and prostaglandin E_2 by marrow stromal/osteoblastic cells that in turn stimulate RANKL expression.[84,85] Furthermore, although it had no effect on either basal or IL-1–induced bone resorption in bone organ cultures, IL-17 markedly enhanced TNF-α-induced osteoclastic bone resorption in fetal mouse long bones.[84]

IL-18 (IFN-γ−-inducing factor) is a pro-inflammatory cytokine homologous to IL-1. IL-18 was originally described as a product of activated macrophages but is also produced by marrow stromal/osteoblastic cells.[86,87] Unlike IL-15 and IL-17, IL-18 inhibits osteoclast formation in cocultures of murine spleen cells and osteoblasts, an effect likely mediated through T-cell produced GM-CSF, because neutralizing antibodies to GM-CSF abolished osteoclast formation.[87] However, despite its induction of IFN-γ production, the inhibitory effect of IL-18 on osteoclastogenesis and bone resorption seems to be independent of IFN-γ.[86] IL-18

signals by binding to IL-1 receptor type 1 (IL-1R) related protein I (IL-1RrP-1), which is in turn highly homologous to IL-1 receptor (IL-1R). Although both IL-1R and IL-1RrP-1 associate with IL-1R associated kinase (IRAK) and both recruit TRAF6 and activate NF-κB,[88] they elicit divergent downstream responses. The molecular basis of this difference remains unclear.

Other Factors. There are a number of other factors whose precise role in physiological and pathological bone resorption is still to be clearly delineated. These include:

- Retinoids: Vitamin A is the only fully characterized factor that has a direct stimulatory effect on osteoclasts.[89] Vitamin A excess eventually leads to increased bone resorption in vivo and hypercalcemia. It is unknown if the effects of vitamin A on osteoclasts have any physiological significance.
- TGF-α: TGF-α, like the related compound epidermal growth factor (EGF), is a powerful stimulator of osteoclastic bone resorption.[90–93] TGF-α is produced by many tumors and is likely involved in increased bone resorption associated with cancer. It is probably produced normally during embryonic life. It stimulates the proliferation of osteoclast progenitors and probably also acts on nonmature multinucleated cells. Its actions on osteoclasts are comparable with those of the colony-stimulating factors on other hematopoietic cells.[93] The effects of TGF-α on bone cells are mediated through the EGF receptor, although it is more potent than EGF on bone resorption. Injections or infusions of TGF-α increase the plasma calcium in vivo.[90]
- Inorganic Phosphate and Calcium: Inorganic phosphate inhibits osteoclast activity in organ cultures.[94] The precise mode of action is not clear. Phosphate is a useful form of therapy in patients with increased bone resorption and diseases such as cancer or primary hyperparathyroidism, although it may have other effects in addition to those of inhibiting bone resorption such as impairment of calcium absorption from the gut. High extracellular calcium concentrations also lead to decreased osteoclast activity associated with an increase in intracellular calcium concentrations.[95] This suggests another mechanism by which continued osteoclastic activity to resorb bone may be regulated by increased local calcium concentrations.

Prostaglandins. Prostaglandins have complex and multiple effects on osteoclasts depending on the species. Prostaglandins have been linked to the hypercalcemia and increased bone resorption associated with malignancy and chronic inflammation.[96] However, the effects of prostaglandins are confusing and depend on the assay system in which they are studied. Their overall effects on bone resorption in humans are still uncertain.

Leukotrienes. Leukotrienes, like prostaglandins, are arachidonic acid metabolites that have been linked to osteoclastic bone resorption.[97] They are produced by the metabolism of arachidonic acid by a 5-lipoxygenase enzyme. Several of these leukotrienes have been shown to activate osteoclasts in vitro[98] and may be related to the bone resorption that is seen in giant cell tumors of bone. Null mutant mice in which the *5-lipoxygenase* gene is nonfunctional have increased amounts of cortical bone.[99]

Thyroid Hormones. The thyroid hormones thyroxine and triiodothyronine stimulate osteoclastic bone resorption in organ cultures.[100] Some patients with hyperthyroidism have increased bone loss, increased osteoclast activity, and hypercalcemia. Thyroid hormones act directly on osteoclastic bone resorption, but their precise mode of action is unknown.

Glucocorticoids. Glucocorticoids inhibit osteoclast formation in vitro and inhibit osteoclastic bone resorption in organ cultures. Their efficacy depends on the stimulus to bone resorption. They are less effective in inhibiting bone resorption stimulated by PTH than they are in inhibiting bone resorption stimulated by cytokines such as IL-1.[101]

In vivo, glucocorticoid administration is associated with increased bone resorption. This is an indirect effect and is caused by the effects of glucocorticoids to inhibit calcium absorption from the gut. As a consequence, parathyroid gland activity is stimulated, and secondary hyperparathyroidism leads to a generalized increase in osteoclastic bone resorption.

Estrogens and Androgens. Estrogen lack is associated with increased osteoclastic bone resorption for approximately 10 years after the menopause.[102] The mechanisms are not entirely clear. Some reports have suggested estrogens may affect osteoclasts directly,[103] but in addition, estrogens may mediate their effects on osteoclasts indirectly by suppressing peripheral blood monocyte production of potent bone resorbing cytokines such as IL-1, TNF-α, and IL-6.[69,75,104]

Pharmacologic Agents. A number of pharmacologic agents have been used as inhibitors of bone resorption and are useful therapies in patients with diseases such as malignancy associated with hypercalcemia. These include plicamycin (mithramycin), gallium nitrate, and the bisphosphonates.[24] All of these agents inhibit osteoclastic activity, although their specific mechanism of action is unknown or controversial. In the case of the cytotoxic drugs plicamycin and gallium nitrate, it is possible that their actions are mediated through cytotoxic effects on osteoclasts or inhibition of proliferation of the osteoclast progenitors.

Bisphosphonates are very important inhibitors of osteoclastic bone resorption in vivo that are achieving increased use in diseases associated with increased bone resorption, particularly in osteoporosis, hypercalcemia of malignancy, Paget's disease of bone, and cancer-induced osteolytic bone diseases. Bisphosphonates ultimately cause osteoclast apoptosis[21,105] but do this in different ways depending on their structure. The nitrogen-containing bisphosphonates inhibit the enzyme farnesyl diphosphate synthase, which is in the mevalonate pathway, and inhibition of this enzyme causes changes in osteoclast function leading to apoptosis.[106] The non-nitrogen containing bisphosphonates are incorporated into cellular ATP and cause osteoclast apoptosis through this means. Whatever their target, it has recently been shown that the end result is osteoclast apoptosis.[106]

The mevalonate pathway seems to be very important for both bone formation and bone resorption. In addition to being the target of nitrogen-containing bisphosphonates in osteoclasts, drugs that inhibit the first step in this pathway in osteoblasts by inhibiting HMG CoA reductase such as statins enhance osteoblast differentiation by stimulating expression of the bone growth factor BMP-2.[107]

Sex hormone deficiency increases osteoclastic bone resorption. The mechanism is still unclear. Thus, estrogens or androgens may be used as therapy in postmenopausal women or hypogonadal males, respectively. Although relatively small numbers of estrogen receptors are present in osteoclasts,[103] it is likely that the main primary cellular target is not the osteoclast and that inhibitory effects on osteoclasts are mediated through accessory cells for bone resorption. Several cytokines have been implicated in the increased bone resorption associated with estrogen withdrawal, including IL-1, IL-6, TNF-α, and prostaglandins of the E series. As indicated earlier, evidence from in vivo studies suggest that both IL-1 and IL-6 may be involved.[69,75,104] Because the majority of patients will not take estrogens, drugs have been developed that have estrogen-like effects on bone and the cardiovascular system, but not the deleterious effects of estrogens on the breast and endometrium of the uterus. One member of this group of estrogen agonists/antagonists is raloxifene.[108] A newly discovered unrelated class of ligands have been identified that reverse bone loss caused by sex steroid withdrawal in mice through nongenotropic effects.[109]

Cellular Events Involved in the Formation Phase of the Remodeling Sequence

The specific cellular events that occur at sites of osteoclastic resorption are osteoclast apoptosis, followed by a series of sequential changes in cells in the osteoblast lineage, including osteoblast chemotaxis, proliferation, and differentiation, which in turn, are followed by formation of mineralized bone and cessation of osteoblast activity. The osteoblast changes are preceded by osteoclast apoptosis, which may be dependent on active TGF-β released from the resorbed bone.[22] This is followed by chemoattraction of osteoblasts or their precursors to the sites of the resorption defect. Chemotaxis of osteoblast precursors is also likely mediated by other local factors produced during the resorption process, because resorbing bone releases chemotactic factors for cells with osteoblast characteristics in vitro.[110,111] Structural proteins such as collagen or osteocalcin could also be involved, because type 1 collagen and osteocalcin and their fragments have the same chemotactic effects.[110,111] TGF-β, which is enriched in the bone matrix and released in active form as a consequence of bone resorption,[112,113] is also chemotactic for bone cells.[114] Platelet-derived growth factor (PDGF) is chemotactic for some mesenchymal cells,[115–117] and it is possible that a combination of chemotactic factors is responsible for attraction of osteoblast precursors to resorption sites.

Proliferation of osteoblast precursors is an important event at the remodeling site. This is also likely to be enhanced by local osteoblast growth factors released during the resorption process. Likely candidates include members of the TGF-β superfamily (TGF-βs I and II) and PDGF, which also causes proliferation of cells with osteoblast characteristics. IGFs-I and II as well as the heparin-binding FGFs also stimulate osteoblast proliferation. All of these factors are sequestered in the bone matrix.[118]

The next sequential event during the formation phase is the differentiation of the osteoblast precursors into mature, terminally differentiated cells. Several of the bone-derived growth factors induce appearance of markers of the differentiated osteoblast phenotype, including expression of alkaline phosphatase activity, type I collagen, and osteocalcin synthesis. Most prominent of these are IGF-I and BMP-2. Active TGFβ inhibits osteoblast differentiation in vitro, which suggests its role may be to "trigger" the process of bone formation by attracting a pool of committed and proliferating precursors to the right sites, after which it is removed or becomes inactivated, allowing this increased pool of precursors to undergo differentiation.

The final phase of the formation process is cessation of osteoblast activity. The resorption lacunae are usually repaired either completely or almost completely. It is not known how this level of time regulation is achieved. One possibility is that factors produced during osteoblast differentiation decrease osteoblast activity. One such factor could be TGF-β since active TGF-β decreases differentiated function in osteoblasts, and as noted above is expressed by osteoblasts as they differentiate.[118] Manolagas et al. have emphasized the importance of osteoblast life span and factors that regulate this such as PTH (which prolongs it) and glucocorticoids (which decrease it).[119]

OSTEOBLASTOTROPIC FACTORS WHICH MAY BE INVOLVED IN THE COUPLING PROCESS

Osteotropic factors that could be involved in the coupling phenomenon are TGF-β, BMPs, IGFs-I and II, PDGF, and FGFs (Fig. 4). This area has been reviewed by others.[118,120] These factors are likely to be released locally from bone as it resorbs or by bone cells activated as a consequence of the resorption process. They may then act in a sequential manner to regulate all of the cellular events required for the formation of bone.

The TGF-β superfamily may be particularly important in the coupling that links bone formation to prior bone resorption. Prolonged primary cultures of fetal rat calvarial osteoblasts show that the BMPs are expressed as these cells differentiate to form new bone in parallel with other differentiation markers such as osteocalcin and alkaline phosphatase. Transient exposure of these cells to TGF-β stimulates proliferation of the osteoblasts (continued exposure inhibits the formation of mineralized bone expression of differentiation markers). Addition of BMPs to culture leads to increased numbers of mature osteoblasts and mineralized bone nodules.

Recently, Wnt proteins have been identified that may play an important role in bone formation.[121] These proteins

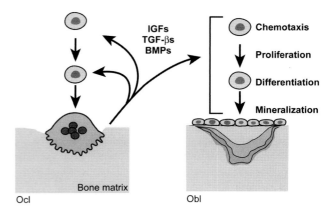

FIG. 4. Growth factor concept of coupling. This concept suggests that coupling of osteoblast (OBL) differentiation and bone formation is caused by growth factors such as TGF-β and related family members and other growth factors such as IGF-1 and the FGFs being released from bone in active form as a consequence of osteoclastic (Ocl) resorption.

bind to two classes of cell membrane proteins, the seven-transmembrane *Frizzled* proteins and the single-transmembrane LDL-receptor-related proteins 5 or 6 (LRP5/6) or Arrow. Activating single mutations in *LRP5* has been shown to cause high bone mass,[122] whereas inactivating mutations cause a form of osteoporosis.[123,124]

Ducy et al.[125] have also proposed a special role for the polypeptide hormone leptin in mediating the relationship between body weight and bone mass. These workers have studied two murine models of obesity in mice, the *ob/ob* and *db/db* mice, which are leptin- and leptin-receptor–deficient, respectively. Both types of mutant mice have increased bone formation rates and high bone mass. Although the authors could find no evidence of leptin receptors in osteoblasts, they did find that intracerebroventricular infusions of leptin induced bone loss in wild-type mice and reversed the high bone mass phenotype in *ob/ob* mice that were leptin deficient. Thus, they propose that leptin modulates bone mass indirectly by a central effect and link leptin deficiency to high bone mass. More recently, they have suggested that this effect is mediated in bone by β2-adrenergic receptors on osteoblasts, activated by the effects of leptin on the hypothalamus.[126] These results are potentially very important, but as yet, not all investigators agree that leptin does not have direct effects on bone cells,[127] and it is unknown if these results in mice are also applicable to humans. Irrespective of whether leptin has effects on bone cells directly, these studies emphasize the potential importance of leptin as a central regulator of bone formation.

The potential interactions between these factors are extraordinarily complex, possibly even as complex as the interactions between the colony-stimulating factors during hematopoiesis, but it will be essential to unravel them to understand the local and systemic controls responsible for bone formation. It is likely that the effects of systemic factors such as leptin and PTH superimposed on the complicated interactions between factors released locally in active form as a consequence of the resorption process are responsible for the carefully coordinated formation of new bone that occurs at recent resorption sites.

REFERENCES

1. Frost HM 1964 Dynamics of bone remodeling. In: Bone Biodynamics. Little and Brown, Boston, MA, USA, pp. 315.
2. Riggs BL, Wahner HW, Melton LJ III, Richelson LS, Judd HL, Offord KP 1986 Rates of bone loss in the axial and appendicular skeletons of women: Evidence of substantial vertebral bone loss prior to menopause. J Clin Invest 77:1487–1491.
3. Genant HK, Cann CE, Ettinger B, Gordan GS 1982 Quantitative computed tomography of vertebral spongiosa: A sensitive method for detecting early bone loss after oophorectomy. Ann Intern Med 97:699–705.
4. Riggs BL, Melton LJ III 1986 Involutional osteoporosis. N Engl J Med 314:1676–1686.
5. Parfitt AM, Mathews CHE, Villanueva AR, Kleerekoper M, Frame B, Rao DS 1983 Relationships between surface, volume, and thickness of iliac trabecular bone in aging and in osteoporosis: Implications for the microanatomic and cellular mechanisms of bone loss. J Clin Invest 72:1396–1409.
6. Kleerekoper M, Villanueva AR, Stanciu J, Rao DS, Parfitt AM 1985 The role of three dimensional trabecular microstructure in the pathogenesis of vertebral compression fractures. Calcif Tissue Int 37:594–597.
7. Miyauchi A, Alvarez J, Greenfield EM, Teti A, Grano M, Colucci S, Zambonin-Zallone A, Ross FP, Teitelbaum SL, Cheresh D 1991 Recognition of osteopontin and related peptides by an $\alpha v\beta 3$ integrin stimulates immediate cell signals in osteoclasts. J Biol Chem 266:20369–20374.
8. Baron R, Vignery A, Horowitz M 1984 Lymphocytes, macrophages and the regulation of bone remodeling. In: Peck WA (ed.) Bone Mineral Research. Elsevier, Amsterdam, The Netherlands, pp. 175–243.
9. Boyce BF, Aufdemorte TB, Garrett IR, Yates AJ, Mundy GR 1989 Effects of interleukin-1 on bone turnover in normal mice. Endocrinology 125:1142–1150.
10. Rasmussen H, Bordier P 1974 The Physiological and Cellular Basis of Metabolic Bone Disease. Williams and Wilkins, Baltimore, MD, USA.
11. Rodan GA, Martin TJ 1981 Role of osteoblasts in hormonal control of bone resorption: A hypothesis. Calcif Tissue Int 33:349–351.
12. Howard GA, Bottemiller BL, Turner RT, Rader JI, Baylink DJ 1981 Parathyroid hormone stimulates bone formation and resorption in organ culture: Evidence for a coupling mechanism. Proc Natl Acad Sci USA 78:3204–3208.
13. Locklin RM, Khosla S, Turner RT, Riggs BL 2003 Mediators of the biphasic responses of bone to intermittent and continuously administered parathyroid hormone. J Cell Biochem 89:180–190.
14. Manolagas SC, Jilka RL 1995 Mechanisms of disease: Bone marrow, cytokines, and bone remodeling—emerging insights into the pathophysiology of osteoporosis. N Engl J Med 332:305–311.
15. Enomoto H, Shiojiri S, Hoshi K, Furuichi T, Fukuyama R, Yoshida CA, Kanatani N, Nakamura R, Mizuno A, Zanma A, Yano K, Yasuda H, Higashio K, Takada K, Komori T 2003 Induction of osteoclast differentiation by Runx2 through RANKL and OPG regulation and partial rescue of osteoclastogenesis in Runx2-/- mice by RANKL transgene. J Biol Chem 278:23971–23977.
16. Snapper I, Kahn A 1971 Myelomatosis. Karger, Basel, Switzerland.
17. Valentin-Opran A, Charhon SA, Meunier PJ, Edouard CM, Arlot ME 1982 Quantitative histology of myeloma induced bone changes. Br J Haematol 52:601–610.
18. Stewart AF, Vignery A, Silvergate A, Ravin ND, LiVolsi V, Broadus AE, Baron R 1982 Quantitative bone histomorphometry in humoral hypercalcemia of malignancy: Uncoupling of bone cell activity. J Clin Endocrinol Metab 55:219–227.
19. Mundy GR, Luben RA, Raisz LG, Oppenheim JJ, Buell DN 1974 Bone-resorbing activity in supernatants from lymphoid cell lines. N Engl J Med 290:867–871.
20. Darby AJ, Meunier PJ 1981 Mean wall thickness and formation periods of trabecular bone packets in idiopathic osteoporosis. Calcif Tissue Int 33:199–204.
21. Hughes DE, Wright KR, Uy HL, Sasaki A, Yoneda T, Roodman GD, Mundy GR, Boyce BF 1995 Bisphosphonates promote apoptosis in murine osteoclasts *in vitro* and *in vivo*. J Bone Miner Res 10:1478–1487.
22. Hughes DE, Dai A, Tiffee JC, Li HH, Mundy GR, Boyce BF 1996 Estrogen promotes apoptosis of murine osteoclasts mediated by TGF-β. Nat Med 7:1132–1136.
23. Jones SJ, Boyde A, Ali NN 1985 A review of bone cell substratum interactions. Scanning 7:5–24.
24. Mundy GR, Roodman GD 1987 Osteoclast ontogeny and function. In: Peck WA (ed.) Bone Mineral Research. V. Elsevier, Amsterdam, The Netherlands, pp. 209–280.
25. Krishnan V, Moore TL, Ma YL, Helvering LM, Frolik CA, Valasek KM, Ducy P, Geiser AG 2003 Parathyroid hormone bone anabolic action requires Cbfa1/Runx2-dependent signaling. Mol Endocrinol 17:423–435.
26. Roodman GD, Ibbotson KJ, MacDonald BR, Kuehl TJ, Mundy GR 1985 1,25(OH)$_2$ vitamin D$_3$ causes formation of multinucleated cells with osteoclast characteristics in cultures of primate marrow. Proc Natl Acad Sci USA 82:8213–8217.
27. Tsoukas CD, Provvedini DM, Manolagas SC 1984 1,25-dihydroxyvitamin D$_3$: A novel immunoregulatory hormone. Science 224:1438–1440.
28. Wener JA, Gorton SJ, Raisz LG 1972 Escape from inhibition of resorption in cultures of fetal bone treated with calcitonin and parathyroid hormone. Endocrinology 90:752–759.
29. Takahashi S, Goldring S, Katz M, Hilsenbeck S, Williams R, Roodman GD 1995 Down regulation of calcitonin receptor mRNA expression by calcitonin during human osteoclast-like cell differentiation. J Clin Invest 95:167–171.
30. Chambers TJ, Magnus CJ 1982 Calcitonin alters the behavior of isolated osteoclasts. J Pathol 136:27–40.
31. Simonet WS, Lacey DL, Dunstan CR, Kelley M, Chang MS, Luthy R, Nguyen HQ, Wooden S, Bennett L, Boone T, Shimamoto G, DeRose M, Elliott R, Colombero A, Tan HL, Trail G, Sullivan J, Davy E, Bucay N, Renshaw-Gegg L, Hughes TM, Hill D, Pattison W, Campbell P, Boyle WJ 1997 Osteoprotegerin: A novel secreted protein involved in the regulation of bone density. Cell 89:309–310.
32. Tsuda E, Goto M, Mochizuki S, Yano K, Kobayashi F, Morinaga T, Higashio K 1997 Isolation of a novel cytokine from human fibroblasts that specifically inhibits osteoclastogenesis. Biochem Biophys Res Commun 234:137–142.
33. Yasuda H, Shima N, Nakagawa N, Yamaguchi K, Kinosaki M, Mochizuki S, Tomoyasu A, Yano K, Goto M, Murakami A, Tsuda E, Morinaga T, Higashio K, Udagawa N, Takahashi N, Suda T 1998 Osteoclast differentiation factor is a ligand for osteoprotegerin/osteoclastogenesis-inhibitory factor and is identical to TRANCE/RANKL. Proc Natl Acad Sci USA 95:3597–3602.
34. Tan KB, Harrop J, Reddy M, Young P, Terrett J, Emery J, Moore G, Truneh A 1997 Characterization of a novel TNF-like ligand and recently described TNF ligand and TNF receptor superfamily genes and their constitutive and inducible expression in hematopoietic and non-hematopoietic cells. Gene 204:35–46.
35. Kwon BS, Wang S, Udagawa N, Haridas V, Lee ZH, Kim KK, Oh KO, Greene J, Li Y, Su J, Gentz R, Aggarwal BB, Ni J 1998 TR1, a new member of the tumor necrosis superfamily, induces fibroblast proliferation and inhibits osteoclastogenesis and bone resorption. FASEB J 12:845–854.
36. Yun TJ, Chaudhary PM, Shu GL, Frazer JK, Ewings MK, Schwartz SM, Pascual V, Hood LE, Clark EA 1998 OPG/FDCR-1, a TNF receptor family member, is expressed in lymphoid cells and is upregulated by ligating CD40. J Immunol 161:6113–6121.
37. ASBMR President's Committee on Nomenclature 2000 Proposed standard nomenclature for new Tumor Necrosis Factor family members involved in the regulation of bone resorption. J Bone Miner Res 15:2293–2296.
38. Anderson DM, Maraskovsky E, Billingsley WL, Dougall WC, Tometsko ME, Roux ER, Teepe MC, DuBose RF, Cosman D, Galibert L 1997 A homologue of the TNF receptor and its ligand enhance T-cell growth and dendritic cell function. Nature 390:175–179.
39. Lacey DL, Timms E, Tan HL, Kelley MJ, Dunstan CR, Burgess T, Elliott R, Colombero A, Elliott G, Scully S, Hsu H, Sullivan J, Hawkins N, Davy E, Capparelli C, Eli A, Qian YX, Kaufman S, Sarosi I, Shalhoub V, Senaldi G, Guo J, Delaney J, Boyle WJ 1998 Osteoprotegerin ligand is a cytokine that regulates osteoclast differentiation and activation. Cell 93:165–176.
40. Emery JG, McDonnell P, Burke MB, Deen KC, Lyn S, Silverman C, Dul E, Appelbaum ER, Eichman C, DiPrinzio R, Dodds RA, James IE, Rosenberg M, Lee JC, Young PR 1998 Osteoprotegerin is a receptor for the cytotoxic ligand TRAIL. J Biol Chem 273:14363–14367.
41. Hofbauer LC, Heufelder AE 2001 Role of receptor activator of nuclear factor-kappaB ligand and osteoprotegerin in bone cell biology. J Mol Med 79:243–253.
42. Theill LE, Boyle WJ, Penninger JM 2002 RANK-L and RANK: T

cells, bone loss, and mammalian evolution. Annu Rev Immunol **20**:795–823.

43. Walsh MC, Choi Y 2003 Biology of the TRANCE axis. Cytokine Growth Factor Rev **14**:251–263.

44. Boyle WJ, Simonet WS, Lacey DL 2003 Osteoclast differentiation and activation. Nature **423**:337–342.

45. Sedger LM, Glaccum MB, Schuh JC, Kanaly ST, Williamson E, Kayagaki N, Yun T, Smolak P, Le T, Goodwin R, Gliniak B 2002 Characterization of the *in vivo* function of TNF-α-related apoptosis-inducing ligand, TRAIL/Apo2L, using TRAIL/Apo2L gene-deficient mice. Eur J Immunol **32**:2246–2254.

46. Yano K, Tsuda E, Washida N, Kobayashi F, Goto M, Harada A, Ikeda K, Higashio K, Yamada Y 1999 Immunological characterization of circulating osteoprotegerin/osteoclastogenesis inhibitory factor: Increased serum concentrations in post-menopausal osteoporosis. J Bone Miner Res **14**:518–527.

47. Rogers A, Saleh G, Hannon RA, Greenfield D, Eastell R 2002 Circulating estradiol and osteoprotegerin as determinants of bone turnover and bone density in postmenopausal women. J Clin Endocrinol Metab **87**:4470–4475.

48. Khosla S, Arrighi HM, Melton LJ III, Atkinson EJ, O'Fallon WM, Dunstan C, Riggs BL 2002 Correlates of osteoprotegerin levels in women and men. Osteoporos Int **13**:394–399.

49. Bucay N, Sarosi I, Dunstan CR, Morony S, Tarpley J, Capparelli C, Scully S, Tan HL, Xu W, Lacey DL, Boyle WJ, Simonet WS 1998 *Osteoprotegerin*-deficient mice develop early onset osteoporosis and arterial calcification. Genes Dev **12**:1260–1268.

50. Mizuno A, Amizuka N, Irie K, Murakami A, Fujise N, Kanno T, Sato Y, Nakagawa N, Yasuda H, Mochizuki S, Gomibuchi T, Yano K, Shima N, Washida N, Tsuda E, Morinaga T, Higashio K, Ozawa H 1998 Severe osteoporosis in mice lacking osteoclastogenesis inhibitory factor/osteoprotegerin. Biochem Biophys Res Commun **247**:610–615.

51. Akatsu T, Murakami T, Ono K, Nishikawa M, Tsuda E, Mochizuki SI, Fujise N, Higashio K, Motoyoshi K, Yamamoto M, Nagata N 1998 Osteoclastogenesis-inhibitory factor exhibits hypocalcemic effects in normal rats and in hypercalcemic nude rats carrying tumors associated with humoral hypercalcemia of malignancy. Bone **23**:495–498.

52. Yamamoto M, Murakami T, Nishikawa M, Tsuda E, Mochizuki S, Higashio K, Akatsu T, Motoyoshi K, Nagata N 1998 Hypocalcemic effect of osteoclastogenesis inhibitory factor/osteoprotegerin in the thyroparathyroidectomized rat. Endocrinology **139**:4012–4015.

53. Sakata M, Shiba H, Komatsuzawa H, Fujita T, Ohta K, Sugai M, Suginaka H, Kurihara H 1999 Expression of osteoprotegerin (osteoclastogenesis inhibitory factor) in cultures of human dental mesenchymal cells and epithelial cells. J Bone Miner Res **14**:1486–1492.

54. Wong BR, Rho J, Arron J, Robinson E, Orlinick J, Chao M, Kalachikov S, Cayani E, Bartlett FS III, Frankel WN, Lee SY, Choi Y 1997 TRANCE is a novel ligand of the tumor necrosis factor receptor family that activates c-jun N-terminal kinase in T cells. J Biol Chem **272**:25190–25194.

55. Yasuda H, Shima N, Nakagawa N, Mochizuki SI, Yano K, Fujise N, Sato Y, Goto M, Yamaguchi K, Kuriyama M, Kanno T, Murakami A, Tsuda E, Morinaga T, Higashio K 1998 Identity of osteoclastogenesis inhibitory factor (OCIF) and osteoprotegerin (OPG): A mechanism by which OPG/OCIF inhibits osteoclastogenesis *in vitro*. Endocrinology **139**:1329–1337.

56. Lum L, Wong BR, Josien R, Becherer JD, Erdjument-Bromage H, Schlondorff J, Tempst P, Choi Y, Blobel CP 1999 Evidence for a role of a tumor necrosis factor alpha (TNF-α)-converting enzyme-like protease in shedding of TRANCE, a TNF family member involved in osteoclastogenesis and dendritic cell survival. J Biol Chem **274**:13613–13618.

57. Wong BR, Josien R, Choi Y 1999 TRANCE is a TNF family member that regulates dendritic cell and osteoclast function. J Leukoc Biol **65**:715–724.

58. Fuller K, Wong B, Fox S, Choi Y, Chambers TJ 1998 TRANCE is necessary and sufficient for osteoblast-mediated activation of bone resorption in osteoclasts. J Exp Med **188**:997–1001.

59. Atkins GJ, Kostakis P, Pan B, Farrugia A, Gronthos S, Evdokiou A, Harrison K, Findlay DM, Zannettino ACW 2003 RANKL expression is related to the differentiation state of human osteoblasts. J Bone Miner Res **18**:1088–1098.

60. Kartsogiannis V, Zhou H, Horwood NJ, Thomas RJ, Hards DK, Quinn JM, Niforas P, Ng KW, Martin TJ, Gillespie MT 1999 Localization of RANKL (receptor activator of NF-κB ligand) mRNA and protein in skeletal and extraskeletal tissues. Bone **25**:525–534.

61. Kong Y-Y, Yoshida H, Sarosi I, Tan HL, Timms E, Capparelli C, Morony S, Oliveira-dos-Santos AJ, Van G, Itie A, Khoo W, Wakeham A, Dunstan CR, Lacey DL, Mak TW, Boyle WJ, Penninger JM 1999 OPGL is a key regulator of osteoclastogenesis, lymphocyte development and lymph node organogenesis. Nature **397**:315–323.

62. Burgess TL, Qian Y, Kaufman S, Ring BD, Van G, Capparelli C, Kelley M, Hsu H, Boyle WJ, Dunstan CR, Hu S, Lacey DL 1999 The ligand for osteoprotegerin (OPGL) directly activates mature osteoclasts. J Cell Biol **145**:527–538.

63. Hsu H, Lacey DL, Dunstan CR, Solovyev I, Colombero A, Timms E, Tan HL, Elliott G, Kelley MJ, Sarosi I, Wang L, Xia XZ, Elliott R, Chiu L, Black T, Scully S, Capparelli C, Morony S, Shimamoto G, Bass MB, Boyle WJ 1999 Tumor necrosis factor receptor family member RANK mediates osteoclast differentiation and activation induced by osteoprotegerin ligand. Proc Natl Acad Sci USA **96**:3540–3545.

64. Li J, Sarosi I, Yan XQ, Morony S, Capparelli C, Tan HL, McCabe S, Elliott R, Scully S, Van G, Kaufman S, Juan SC, Sun Y, Tarpley J, Martin L, Christensen K, McCabe J, Kostenuik P, Hsu H, Fletcher F, Dunstan CR, Lacey DL, Boyle WJ 1999 RANK is the intrinsic hematopoietic cell surface receptor that controls osteoclastogenesis and regulation of bone mass and calcium metabolism. Proc Natl Acad Sci USA **97**:1566–1571.

65. Dougall WC, Glaccum M, Charrier K, Rohrbach K, Brasel K, De Smedt T, Daro E, Smith J, Tometsko ME, Maliszewski CR, Armstrong A, Shen V, Bain S, Cosman D, Anderson D, Morrissey PJ, Peschon JJ, Schuh J 1999 RANK is essential for osteoclast and lymph node development. Genes Dev **13**:2412–2424.

66. Hughes AE, Ralston SH, Marken J, Bell C, MacPherson H, Wallace RG, van Hul W, Whyte MP, Nakatsuka K, Hovy L, Anderson DM 2000 Mutations in *TNFRSF11A*, affecting the signal peptide of RANK, cause familial expansile osteolysis. Nat Genet **24**:45–48.

67. Johnson-Pais TL, Singer FR, Bone HG, McMurray CT, Hansen MF, Leach RJ 2003 Identification of a novel tandem duplication in exon 1 of the TNFRSF11A gene in two unrelated patients with familial expansile osteolysis. J Bone Miner Res **18**:376–380.

68. Sabatini M, Boyce B, Aufdemorte T, Bonewald L, Mundy GR 1988 Infusions of recombinant human interleukin-1α and β cause hypercalcemia in normal mice. Proc Natl Acad Sci USA **85**:5235–5239.

69. Pacifici R, Rifas L, McCracken R, Vered I, McMurtry C, Avioli LV, Peck WA 1989 Ovarian steroid treatment blocks a postmenopausal increase in blood monocyte interleukin-1 release. Proc Natl Acad Sci USA **86**:2398–2402.

70. Tashjian AH Jr, Voelkel EF, Lazzaro M, Goad D, Bosma T, Levine L 1987 Tumor necrosis factor-α (cachectin) stimulates bone resorption in mouse calvaria via a prostaglandin-mediated mechanism. Endocrinology **120**:2029–2036.

71. Felix R, Cecchini MG, Fleisch H 1990 Macrophage colony stimulating factor restores in vivo bone resorption in the op/op osteopetrotic mouse. Endocrinology **127**:2592–2594.

72. Feyen JHM, Elford P, Dipadova FE, Trechsel U 1989 Interleukin-6 is produced by bone and modulated by parathyroid hormone. J Bone Miner Res **4**:633–638.

73. Ishimi Y, Miyaura C, Jin CH, Akatsu T, Abe E, Nakamura Y, Yamaguchi A, Yoshiki S, Matsuda T, Hirano T, Kishimoto T, Suda T 1990 IL-6 is produced by osteoblasts and induces bone resorption. J Immunol **145**:3297–3303.

74. Black K, Garrett IR, Mundy GR 1991 Chinese hamster ovarian cells transfected with the murine interleukin-6 gene cause hypercalcemia as well as cachexia, leukocytosis and thrombocytosis in tumor-bearing nude mice. Endocrinology **128**:2657–2659.

75. Jilka RL, Hangoc G, Girasole G, Passeri G, Williams DC, Abrams JS, Boyce B, Broxmeyer H, Manolagas SC 1992 Increased osteoclast development after estrogen loss: Mediation by interleukin-6. Science **257**:88–91.

76. Gowen M, Nedwin G, Mundy GR 1986 Preferential inhibition of cytokine stimulated bone resorption by recombinant interferon gamma. J Bone Miner Res **1**:469–474.

77. Takayanagi H, Ogasawara K, Hida S, Chiba T, Murata S, Sato K, Takaoka A, Yokochi T, Oda H, Tanaka K, Nakamura K, Taniguchi T 2000 T-cell-mediated regulation of osteoclastogenesis by signaling cross-talk between RANKL and IFN-γ. Nature **408**:600–605.

78. Chenu C, Pfeilschifter J, Mundy GR, Roodman GD 1988 Transforming growth factor β inhibits formation of osteoclast-like cells in long-term human marrow cultures. Proc Natl Acad Sci USA **85**:5683–5687.

79. Kaneda T, Nojima T, Nakagawa M, Ogasawara A, Kaneko H, Sato T, Mano H, Kumegawa M, Hakeda Y 2000 Endogenous production of

TGF-β is essential for osteoclastogenesis induced by a combination of receptor activator of NF-κB ligand and macrophage-colony-stimulating factor. J Immunol 165:4254–4463.

80. Noda M, Camilliere JJ 1989 In vivo stimulation of bone formation by transforming growth factor-beta. Endocrinology 124:2991–2994.

81. Filvaroff E, Erlebacher A, Ye J-Q, Gitelman S, Lotz J 1999 Inhibition of TGF-β receptor signaling in osteoblasts leads to decreased bone remodeling and increased trabecular bone mass. Development 126:4267–4279.

82. Grabstein KH, Eisenman J, Shanebeck K, Rauch C, Srinivasan S, Fung V, Beers C, Richardson J, Schoenborn MA, Ahdieh M, Johnson L, Alderson MR, Watson JD, Anderson DM, Giri JG 1994 Cloning of a T cell growth factor that interacts with the β chain of the interleukin-2 receptor. Science 264:965–968.

83. Ogata Y, Kukita A, Kukita T, Komine M, Miyahara A, Miyazaki A, Kohashi O 1999 A novel role of IL-15 in the development of osteoclasts: Inability to replace its activity with IL-2. J Immunol 162:2754–2760.

84. van Bezooijen RL, Farih-Sips HCM, Papapoulos SE, Lowik CWGM 1999 Interleukin 17: A new bone acting cytokine in vitro. J Bone Miner Res 14:1513–1521.

85. Kotake S, Udagawa N, Takahashi N, Matzuzaki K, Itoh K, Iyama S, Saito S, Inoue K, Kamatani N, Gillespie MT, Martin TJ, Suda T 1999 IL-17 in synovial fluids from patients with rheumatoid arthritis is a potent stimulator of osteoclastogenesis. J Clin Invest 103:1345–1352.

86. Udagawa N, Horwood NJ, Elliot J, Mackay A, Owens J, Okamura H, Kurimoto M, Chambers TJ, Martin TJ, Gillespie MT 1997 Interleukin 18 (interferon-γ inducing factor) is produced by osteoblasts and acts via granulocyte-macrophage colony stimulating factor and not via interferon-γ to inhibit osteoclast formation. J Exp Med 185:1005–1017.

87. Horwood NJ, Udagawa N, Elliott J, Grail D, Okamura H, Kurimoto M, Dunn AR, Martin T, Gillespie MT 1998 Interleukin 18 inhibits osteoclast formation via T cell production of granulocyte macrophage colony-stimulating factor. J Clin Invest 101:595–603.

88. Thomassen E, Bird TA, Renshaw BR, Kennedy MK, Sims JE 1998 Binding of interleukin-18 to the interleukin-1 receptor homological receptor IL-1RP1 leads to activation of signaling pathways similar to those used by interleukin-1. J Interferon Cytokine Res 18:1077–1088.

89. Oreffo RO, Teti A, Triffitt JT, Francis MJ, Carano A, Zallone AZ 1988 Effect of vitamin A on bone resorption: Evidence for direct stimulation of isolated chicken osteoclasts by retinol and retinoic acid. J Bone Miner Res 3:203–210.

90. Tashjian AH Jr, Voelkel EF, Lloyd W, Derynck R, Winkler ME, Levine L 1986 Actions of growth factors on plasma calcium: Epidermal growth factor and human transforming growth factor-α cause elevation of plasma calcium in mice. J Clin Invest 78:1405–1409.

91. Ibbotson KJ, Harrod J, Gowen M, D'Souza S, Smith DD, Winkler ME, Derynck R, Mundy GR 1986 Human recombinant transforming growth factor alpha stimulates bone resorption and inhibits formation in vitro. Proc Natl Acad Sci USA 83:2228–2232.

92. Stern PH, Krieger NS, Nissenson RA, Williams RD, Winkler ME, Derynck R, Strewler GL 1985 Human transforming growth factor alpha stimulates bone resorption in vitro. J Clin Invest 76:2016–2020.

93. Takahashi N, MacDonald BR, Hon J, Winkler ME, Derynck R, Mundy GR, Roodman GD 1986 Recombinant human transforming growth factor alpha stimulates the formation of osteoclast-like cells in long term human marrow cultures. J Clin Invest 78:894–898.

94. Kanatani M, Sugimoto T, Kano J, Kanzawa M, Chihara K 2003 Effect of high phosphate concentration on osteoclast differentiation as well as bone-resorbing activity. J Cell Physiol 196:180–189.

95. Kaji H, Sugimoto T, Kanatani M, Chihara K 1996 High extracellular calcium stimulates osteoclast-like cell formation and bone-resorbing activity in the presence of osteoblastic cells. J Bone Miner Res 11:912–920.

96. Tashjian AH, Voelkel EF, Levine L, Goldhaber P 1972 Evidence that the bone resorption-stimulating factor produced by mouse fibrosarcoma cells is prostaglandin E2: A new model for the hypercalcemia of cancer. J Exp Med 136:1329–1343.

97. Gallwitz WE, Mundy GR, Lee CH, Qiao M, Roodman GD, Raftery M, Gaskell SJ, Bonewald LF 1993 5-Lipoxygenase metabolites of arachidonic acid stimulate isolated osteoclasts to resorb calcified matrices. J Biol Chem 268:10087–10094.

98. Flynn MA, Qiao M, Garcia C, Dallas M, Bonewald LF 1999 Avian osteoclast cells are stimulated to resorb calcified matrices by and possess receptors for leukotriene B4. Calcif Tissue Int 64:154–159.

99. Bonewald LF, Flynn M, Qiao M, Dallas MR, Mundy GR, Boyce BF

100. Mundy GR, Shapiro JL, Bandelin JG, Canalis EM, Raisz LG 1976 Direct stimulation of bone resorption by thyroid hormones. J Clin Invest 58:529–534.

101. Mundy GR, Rick ME, Turcotte R, Kowalski MA 1978 Pathogenesis of hypercalcemia in lymphosarcoma cell leukemia: Role of an osteoclast activating factor-like substance and mechanism of action for glucocorticoid therapy. Am J Med 65:600–606.

102. Lindsay R, Hart DM, Forrest C, Baird C 1980 Prevention of spinal osteoporosis in oophorectomised women. Lancet 12:1151–1153.

103. Oursler MJ, Osdoby P, Pyfferoen J, Riggs BL, Spelsberg TC 1991 Avian osteoclasts as estrogen target cells. Proc Natl Acad Sci USA 88:6613–6617.

104. Girasole G, Jilka RL, Passeri G, Boswell S, Boder G, Williams DC, Manolagas SC 1992 17 beta-estradiol inhibits interleukin-6 production by bone marrow-derived stromal cells and osteoblasts in vitro: A potential mechanism for the anti-osteoporotic effect of estrogens. J Clin Invest 89:883–891.

105. Parfitt AM, Mundy GR, Roodman GD, Hughes DE, Boyce BF 1996 A new model for the regulation of bone resorption, with particular reference to the effects of bisphosphonates. J Bone Miner Res 11:150–159.

106. Reszka AA, Rodan GA 2003 Bisphosphonates: Mechanism of action. Curr Rheumatol Rep 5:65–74.

107. Mundy GR, Garret IR, Harris SE, Chan J, Chen D, Rossini G, Boyce BF, Zhao M, Gutierrez G 1999 Stimulation of bone formation in vitro and in rodents by statins. Science 286:1946–1949.

108. Black LJ, Sato M, Rowley ER, Magee DE, Bekele A, Williams DC, Cullinan GJ, Bendele R, Kauffman RF, Bensch WR, Frolik CA, Terminer JD, Bryant HU 1994 Raloxifene (LY139481 HCl) prevents bone loss and reduces serum cholesterol without causing uterine hypertrophy in ovariectomized rats. J Clin Invest 93:63–69.

109. Kousteni S, Chen JR, Bellido T, Han L, Ali AA, O'Brien CA, Plotkin L, Fu Q, Mancino AT, Wen Y, Vertino AM, Powers CC, Stewart SA, Ebert R, Parfitt AM, Weinstein RS, Jilka RL, Manolagas SC 2002 Reversal of bone loss in mice by nongenotropic signaling of sex steroids. Science 298:843–846.

110. Mundy GR, Rodan SB, Majeska RJ, DeMartino S, Trimmier C, Martin TJ, Rodan GA 1982 Unidirectional migration of osteosarcoma cells with osteoblast characteristics in response to products of bone resorption. Calcif Tissue Int 34:542–546.

111. Mundy GR, Poser JW 1985 Chemotactic activity of the gamma-carboxyglutamic acid containing protein in bone. Calcif Tis Int 35:164–168.

112. Pfeilschifter J, Bonewald L, Mundy GR 1990 Characterization of the latent transforming growth factor β complex in bone. J Bone Miner Res 5:49–58.

113. Dallas SL, Rosser JL, Mundy GR, Bonewald LF 2002 Proteolysis of latent transforming growth factor-beta (TGF-β)-binding protein by osteoclasts: A mechanism for release of TGF-β from bone matrix. J Biol Chem 277:21352–21360.

114. Pfeilschifter J, Wolf O, Naumann A, Minne HW, Mundy GR 1990 Chemotactic response of osteoblast-like cells to transforming growth factor β. J Bone Miner Res 5:825–830.

115. Grotendorst GR, Seppa HEJ, Kleinman HK, Martin GR 1981 Attachment of smooth muscle cells to collagen and their migration toward platelet-derived growth factor. Proc Natl Acad Sci USA 78:3669–3672.

116. Seppa H, Grotendorst G, Seppa S, Schiffmann E, Martin GR 1982 Platelet-derived growth factor is chemotactic for fibroblasts. J Cell Biol 92:584–588.

117. Senior RM, Griffin GL, Huang JS, Walz DA, Deuel TF 1983 Chemotactic activity of platelet alpha granule proteins for fibroblasts. J Cell Biol 96:382–385.

118. Canalis E, Pash J, Varghese S 1993 Skeletal growth factors. Crit Rev Eukaryot Gene Expr 3:155–166.

119. Manolagas SC 2000 Birth and death of bone cells: Regulatory mechanisms and implications for the pathogenesis and treatment of osteoporosis. Endocr Rev 21:15–37.

120. Canalis E, McCarthy T, Centrella M 1989 Growth factors and the regulation of bone remodeling. J Clin Invest 81:277–281.

121. Huelsken J, Birchmeier W 2001 New aspects of Wnt signaling pathways in higher vertebrates. Curr Opin Genet Dev 11:547–553.

122. Little RD, Carulli JP, Del Mastro RG, Dupuis J, Osborne M, Folz C, Manning SP, Swain PM, Zhao SC, Eustace B, Lappe MM, Spitzer L, Zweier S, Braunschweiger K, Benchekroun Y, Hu X, Adair R, Chee L, FitzGerald MG, Tulig C, Caruso A, Tzellas N, Bawa A, Franklin

B, McGuire S, Nogues X, Gong G, Allen KM, Anisowicz A, Morales AJ, Lomedico PT, Recker SM, Van Eerdewegh P, Recker RR, Johnson ML 2002 A mutation in the LDL Receptor related protein 5 gene results in the autosomal dominant high bone mass trait. Am J Hum Genet **70**:11–19.

123. Gong Y, Slee RB, Fukai N, Rawadi G, Roman-Roman S, Reginato AM, Wang H, Cundy T, Glorieux FH, Lev D, Zacharin M, Oexle K, Marcelino J, Suwairi W, Heeger S, Sabatakos G, Apte S, Adkins WN, Allgrove J, Arslan-Kirchner M, Batch JA, Beighton P, Black GC, Boles RG, Boon LM, Borrone C, Brunner HG, Carle GF, Dallapiccola B, De Paepe A, Floege B, Halfhide ML, Hall B, Hennekam RC, Hirose T, Jans A, Juppner H, Kim CA, Keppler-Noreuil K, Kohlschuetter A, LaCombe D, Lambert M, Lemyre E, Letteboer T, Peltonen L, Ramesar RS, Romanengo M, Somer H, Steichen-Gersdorf E, Steinmann B, Sullivan B, Superti-Furga A, Swoboda W, van den Boogaard MJ, Van Hul W, Vikkula M, Votruba M, Zabel B, Garcia T, Baron R, Olsen BR, Warman ML, the Osteoporosis-Pseudoglioma

Syndrome Collaborative Group 2001 LDL Receptor-Related Protein 5 (LRP5) affects bone accrual and eye development. Cell **107**:513–523.

124. Kato M, Patel MS, Levasseur R, Lobov I, Chang BH, Glass DA II, Hartmann C, Li L, Hwang TH, Brayton CF, Lang RA, Karsenty G, Chan L 2002 Cbfa1-independent decrease in osteoblast proliferation, osteopenia, and persistent embryonic eye vascularization in mice deficient in Lrp5, a Wnt coreceptor. J Cell Biol **157**:303–314.

125. Ducy P, Amling M, Takeda S, Priemel M, Schilling AF, Beil FT, Shen J, Vinson C, Rueger JM, Karsenty G 2000 Leptin inhibits bone formation through a hypothalamic relay: A central control of bone mass. Cell **100**:197–207.

126. Takeda S, Elefteriou F, Levasseur R, Liu X, Zhao L, Parker KL, Armstrong D, Ducy P, Karsenty G 2002 Leptin regulates bone formation via the sympathetic nervous system. Cell **111**:305–317.

127. Gordeladze JO, Roseland JE 2003 A unified model for the action of leptin on bone turnover. J Cell Biochem **88**:706–712.

Chapter 8.   Biomechanics of Bone

David B. Burr[1] and Charles H. Turner[2]

[1]Department of Anatomy and Cell Biology and [2]Department of Orthopedic Surgery, Indiana University School of Medicine, Indianapolis, Indiana

BIOMECHANICAL ROLES OF THE SKELETON

The skeleton serves several functions, but at least two key biomechanical roles. First, bones shield vital organs from trauma. Many protective bones have a sandwich structure, similar to corrugated cardboard, in which a compliant core separates two stiff plates. The porous spongy bone acts as a soft interface between the two bony plates. In the skull, mechanical energy resulting from blunt trauma concentrates mainly in the spongy bone separating the bony plates. Consequently, very little energy is transferred to the innermost bony plate, and the cranial vault is preserved. In addition, bones serve as levers against which muscles contract. To better distribute joint forces, the ends of long bones are broadened to reduce stress (force per unit area), and that stress is transmitted by trabecular bone in the metaphysis into the long bone cortex.

MATERIAL PROPERTIES OF BONE

To understand bone tissue as a structural material, it is necessary to introduce some terminology from materials science. Stress is the load per unit area and strain is the fractional or percentage change in length. Strain is a dimensionless ratio, but it is common to measure it in microstrain ($\mu\epsilon$). For example, if bone is deformed by 0.1%, its strain is 0.001, or 1000 $\mu\epsilon$. In humans, strains are generally less than 1000 $\mu\epsilon$ in tension and less than 2000 $\mu\epsilon$ in compression even during vigorous activities.[1] However, strains in the range of 3000–5000 $\mu\epsilon$ can be generated during activities that involve jumping or other types of impact loading.[2]

Materials can be characterized as weak or strong, ductile or brittle, stiff or compliant, based on the results of a mechanical stress-strain test (Fig. 1). The stress-strain curve is obtained by increasing stress to a bone specimen until it breaks. Before failure, the specimen deforms (strains). Strain is calculated as the amount of deformation divided by the original length of the specimen. The slope of the linear region of the stress-strain curve is called the Young's modulus of the material. This represents material stiffness; the greater the slope, the stiffer the material. A more gentle slope indicates a more compliant material. The height of the curve is the ultimate stress, one measure of strength. The point at which the stress-strain curve begins to bend is the yield point; that can be used as yet another measure of

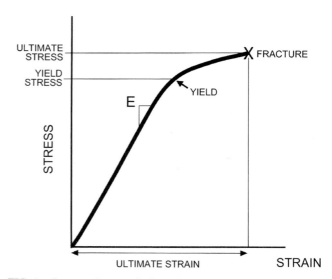

FIG. 1. Stress-strain curve for bone tissue. The stress at the peak of the curve, or ultimate stress, is one measure of strength. Another measure of strength is the stress at the yield point. Young's modulus (E) is defined by the slope of the linear portion of the curve. The strain from the yield point to failure (postyield strain) is a measure of brittleness. Bone is more brittle if it sustains less postyield strain.

Dr. Turner has served as a consultant for Novartis.

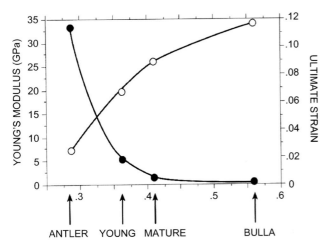

FIG. 2. Biomechanical properties of mineralized tissues. As mineral volume fraction (*x* axis) increases, Young's modulus (open circles) is improved, but ultimate strain (closed circles) decreases. Deer antler is less stiff (lower Young's modulus) and less brittle (higher ultimate strain), whereas the tympanic bulla from a fin whale is very brittle and stiff. Bone tissue from young cows is less stiff and brittle than tissue taken from mature (9 years old) cows. (Based on data from Currey[3].)

strength (yield strength). The area under the stress-strain curve is the amount of energy the tissue can withstand before failure. This tissue property is called modulus of toughness, or simply toughness. Toughness is important in bone biomechanics because a tough bone will be more resistant to fracture. Toughness is increased more by increasing the amount of strain that occurs after the yield point than by increasing either its strength or stiffness. A bone that can sustain little strain after yield is considered brittle. Interestingly, osteoporosis is commonly called the "brittle bone disease," although there is little or no evidence that osteoporotic bone is actually more brittle than normal, although it may be weaker and less rigid.

The degree of mineralization greatly affects material properties. Deer antler, which is not highly mineralized, sustains large ultimate strain but has a low Young's modulus (Fig. 2). This combination of properties makes an antler exceedingly difficult to break.[3] On the other hand, the tympanic bulla of a fin whale has high mineral content and a high Young's modulus, but a low ultimate strain, making it very brittle. The bulla is not as strong as antler or bone because of its brittleness. However, it is not designed for strength, but for acoustic properties. Long bone tissue has intermediate mechanical properties. Bone tissue becomes more mineralized and subsequently more brittle as it matures.

The design of long bones is a fortunate combination of the proper stiffness and toughness. Had bones been built like antlers, they would be too compliant to sustain the loads imposed on the skeleton. The disease condition osteomalacia results in compliant bones, which undergo creep (a slow deformation of a material under loading), resulting in bowing deformities. Had bones been more highly mineralized than they are, their stiffness would be greater but at the price of increased brittleness. Brittle bones would be more susceptible to fracture with mild trauma because they absorb

very little strain energy before they fail, that is, the area under the stress-strain curve is small.

Importance of Bone Size

Bone fragility could be largely eradicated if bones were massively overstructured. Large, dense bones last a lifetime without developing osteoporosis. A clinical example of skeletal overstructuring is the high bone mass (HBM) mutation in the *LRP5* gene, which results in bone mass that is about 5 SDs above normal.[4] Individuals with this mutation are effectively osteoporosis-free. However, for most people, bones are not designed for extreme longevity, as evidenced by the incidence of age-related bone fractures.

Long bones are, for the most part, thick-walled tubes. This geometry allows bones to carry loads effectively but remain relatively light. To understand the principle behind this, first consider that long bones are loaded mainly in bending.[5] The deflection of a beam in bending is given by $ML^2/8EI$, where M is the bending moment, L is length, E is Young's modulus, and I is the second moment of area. For a given value of M, beam deflection can be reduced by shortening the beam (decrease L), stiffening the beam material (increase E), or increasing I. The latter option applies best to bones; bone typically increases its bending strength by increasing I. For a tubular bone, the second moment of area I equals $\pi/4\,(r_o^4 - r_i^4)$, where r_o is the outer radius and r_i is the inner radius (Fig. 3). For mammalian long bones, r_o is about 1.8 times r_i giving $I = 0.71 r_o^4$. If the marrow cavity were filled completely, I would be $0.78 r_o^4$. Therefore, the

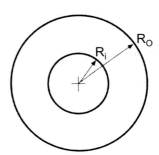

SECOND MOMENT OF AREA = $\pi/4\,(R_o^4 - R_i^4)$

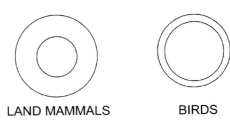

LAND MAMMALS   BIRDS

FIG. 3. The resistance to bending stresses for a long bone is represented by the second moment of area (*I*). Bones with larger values of *I* but less bone mass are more structurally efficient. The ratio of the diameter (*D*) to cortical thickness (*t*) is a measure of structural efficiency. Land mammals have *D/t* ratios of 4–5; for birds, *D/t* ratios can be 10 or greater.

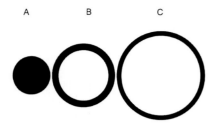

1.77	1.77	1.77	AREA (CM²)
0.25	0.64	1.13	SECOND MOMENT OF AREA (CM⁴)

FIG. 4. Tubular structures resist bending loads well because of efficient distribution of material. Bone area reflects BMD, but the second moment of the area is an indication of resistance to bending. The tubular structure in B has 2.5-fold greater second moment of area than a solid structure (A), although both have the same bone area. Increasing the diameter and decreasing the cortical thickness, as in C, increases the second moment of area further to 4.5-fold greater than A.

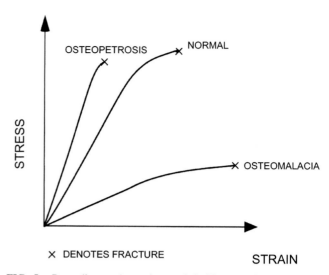

FIG. 5. Bone diseases have characteristic biomechanical profiles that require measurement of several mechanical parameters to properly resolve. Osteopetrotic bone is stiff but brittle, while osteomalacic bone is weak, compliant, and has little brittleness. Each of these diseases reduce energy to failure and thus increase bone fragility.

presence of a marrow cavity reduces the bending rigidity of the bone by less than 10%, but reduces its weight by over 15% (if we consider the weight of the marrow). The converse is also true; bone added to the periosteal surface increases bone bending strength many times more than the increase in bone area. Thus, addition of bone periosteally can increase bone strength, even when the absolute bone volume and bone mineral density (BMD) have not changed (Fig. 4).

What Measures Are Related to Fracture?

Strength and stiffness are typically used to define the "health" of a bone, but they are not so clearly, or physiologically, related to risk of fracture as the amount of energy required to cause fracture. A bone that is strong and stiff may require much less energy to fracture (the area under the curve) than a bone that is weaker and more compliant (Fig. 5). BMD is highly correlated with strength or stiffness,[6] but there is a more complex relationship between BMD and the energy required to cause fracture. For instance, a bone from an osteopetrotic patient will be very stiff, but also very brittle, resulting in reduced energy to failure and increased risk of fracture (Fig. 5). On the other hand, a bone with osteomalacia will tend to be poorly mineralized and weak, but very ductile (large ultimate displacement), resulting in increased energy to failure. Because of these properties, the bone may undergo large deformation without breaking.

The positive proportionality between mineral content and strength/stiffness causes some to equate the BMD with bone's risk of fracture. This is overly simplistic, because decreased BMD in some cases can be associated with maintained or increased strength, through compensatory structural and geometric adaptations such as the addition of a small amount of bone to the periosteal surface (Fig. 6).

Fatigue of Bone

Cyclic loading, even at low strains, causes a gradual reduction of strength and stiffness over time. This degradation of strength and modulus is called fatigue. In bone, the

reduction in mechanical properties is attributed to the formation of microcracks, which grow and coalesce with continued repetitive loading. Fatigue occurs more rapidly with intense exercise compared with normal activities. If left unchecked, fatigue of bone can lead to a stress fracture. The resistance to stress fracture in vivo is a function of the balance between crack initiation, crack growth, and crack repair through normal remodeling processes. However, bone is a fairly tough, fatigue-resistant material, and like other such composite materials, derives its fatigue properties from its resistance to crack growth rather than its resistance to crack initiation. Crack initiation is relatively easy, but the lamellar interfaces stop cracks from growing, redirect them longitudinally, and delay crack coalescence.

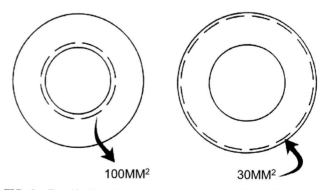

100MM²   30MM²

FIG. 6. Two idealized long bone cross-sections are shown. The one on the left represents a younger person's bone; the one on the right represents an older man's bone in which there is resorption of the endocortical surface but a small addition of bone to the periosteal surface. Despite the fact that 100 U of area were removed from the endocortical surface, and only 30 U were added to the periosteal surface, the sections have an identical bending strength. (Reprinted with permission from Martin RB, Burr, DB 1989 Structure, Function, and Adaptation of Compact Bone. Raven Press, New York, NY, USA, p. 231.)

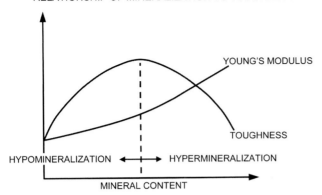

RELATIONSHIP OF MINERALIZATION TO TOUGHNESS

YOUNG'S MODULUS

TOUGHNESS

HYPOMINERALIZATION ←——→ HYPERMINERALIZATION

MINERAL CONTENT

FIG. 7. The stiffness of bone (Young's modulus) increases nonlinearly with increased mineralization, but bone's toughness is reduced at either high or low levels of mineralization. Bone toughness is maximized when 64–66% (by dry weight) of the matrix is composed of mineral. (Reprinted with permission from Wainwright, SA, Biggs WD, Currey, JD, Gosline JM 1976 Mechanical Design in Organisms. Halsted Press, New York, NY, USA.)

EFFECTS OF MATRIX COMPOSITION

Bone tissue is a two-phase porous composite material composed mostly of collagen and mineral, with mechanical properties determined primarily by the amounts, arrangement, and molecular structure of these primary constituents. The mineral component confers strength and stiffness to the tissue. The collagen phase is less brittle. Its important role may be to improve the overall toughness of the bone tissue.

Contribution of Bone Mineral

The ratio of mineral to collagen in bone affects both bone's strength and brittleness.[6,7] A moderate increase in bone mineral increases strength, thus improving resistance to fracture. Excessive mineral content increases brittleness and can be detrimental (Fig. 7).[8] The maturity and perfection of the mineral crystal undoubtedly has an effect on biomechanical properties, apart from the amount of mineral, but the specific effect is unknown. Reports using infrared spectrometry[9] suggest that larger crystals are present in bone from older osteoporotic women and that increased crystallinity itself or changes in the morphology of the mineral crystal may decrease the amount of postyield deformation that occurs before ultimate failure.

Bone strength and stiffness increase disproportionately to increases in bone mineral content (BMC).[6] Density is also strongly related to fatigue life. A 6% increase in density can result in a 3-fold longer fatigue life, whereas a 5% decrease in density is associated with a 50% decrease in fatigue life.[10]

Contribution of Collagen

Collagen has a small influence on the strength and stiffness of bone, but improves bone's toughness.[11] The most obvious clinical example of the mechanical effects of a collagen defect is osteogenesis imperfecta (OI). OI is a family of heritable disorders that involve mutations in the *type I procollagen* genes. People with OI have a markedly increased risk of fracture and often present with multiple fractures at a young age. This is likely caused by a combination of poor bone tissue properties, together with low bone volume and thin long bone cortices.

Variation in collagen content and structure can also improve the mechanical properties of bone. The *COL1A1* gene polymorphism, which encodes the $\alpha1(I)$ protein chain of type I collagen and alters the ratio of the α-1 and α-2 chains, is associated with a 5.9-fold increase in fracture risk in postmenopausal women and a 4.8-fold increase when prevalence is adjusted for age, body mass index (BMI), and BMD.[12,13] There is a stronger association between the COL1A1 Sp1 binding site polymorphism and osteoporotic fracture than between these and BMD or BMI at both the lumbar spine and the femoral neck.[14]

It has been speculated that intramolecular cross-links enhance bone toughness, whereas intermolecular bonds are less important.[15] The maturity of the cross-links may not be very important to bone's mechanical properties.[15,16]

The orientation of collagen fibers may be critically important to strength. Linear regression analyses have demonstrated that collagen fiber orientation explains 71% of the variation in bone tensile strength,[17] whereas the combination of mineralization and collagen fiber orientation explains up to 88% of the variation in elastic modulus.[18] The orientation of collagen fibers tends to be tightly regulated by the nature of the applied stress on bone.[19,20]

INFLUENCE OF AGE AND OSTEOPOROSIS ON BIOMECHANICAL PROPERTIES

The strength of cortical bone declines 2–5% per decade, while the amount of energy absorbed before failure of cortical bone declines 7–12% per decade. The decline in cancellous bone strength is between 8–10% per decade.

As one ages, there is an inherent fragility in the bone tissue that allows it to be damaged more easily from cyclic loading.[21] In addition, with age, bone is less able to sustain further deformation once it is damaged.[22] This decline in bone's ability to absorb energy is clinically important in making bones in elderly people more prone to failure from any impact load, such as one resulting from a fall. The reasons for these age-related changes are unclear but may be associated with slower bone turnover, increased tissue mineralization, and/or molecular changes in the mineral and/or collagen moieties.

Decreased fracture toughness in bones from older people is indicative of a change in the quality of bone tissue with age. Tough materials can sustain large amounts of damage without failure. Bone that is highly mineralized tends not to sustain much damage before failure and is not very tough, typical of a more brittle structure. Reduced toughness may partly explain the observation that fracture risk in older people is greater than predicted by the loss of bone mass alone.

Changes to the collagen content or molecular stability with age may contribute to either enhance bone strength or impair it. The age-related decline in collagen content is associated nonlinearly with a reduction in strength and stiffness, although cause and effect have not been established. In osteoporotic women, fewer reducible collagen cross-links with no change in collagen concentration[23] increase bone fragility.[24] The increased lysine hydroxylation found in newly synthesized bone matrix from osteoporotic patients is correlated to decreased strength in three-point bending.[25]

Periosteal apposition of bone with age serves a biomechanically important function by compensating for reduced tissue properties (or reduced bone volume) in men (Fig. 6), but this compensation is not sufficient to offset the larger losses of bone that occur in modern populations of women.[26] Before menopause, women lose bone at the rate of 4% per decade from the femoral neck, but maintain strength. Postmenopausally, however, the increased rate of loss (7% per decade) is not compensated and results in estimated femoral neck stresses that are 4–12% higher than in younger women.[27] Similar periosteal compensations have been shown for the vertebral body in men but not in women.[28]

INFLUENCE OF MICRODAMAGE ACCUMULATION ON BIOMECHANICAL PROPERTIES

By definition, accumulation of microdamage in any material reduces its elastic modulus. Stiffness loss occurs before the microscopic appearance of cracks,[29,30] so that histologically visible microdamage in bone presumes a loss of bone stiffness. Animal and postmortem human studies show that microdamage accumulation also reduces bone strength.[31] Importantly, microcrack accumulation has an effect on bone toughness. A 2- to 3-fold elevation of microdamage accumulation in the vertebrae or a 5- to 7-fold increase in the rib produced as a consequence of a suppression of remodeling was associated with a 20% reduction in bone toughness without a reduction in strength.[32,33] This is consistent with the prediction made by Currey et al.,[7] who proposed, based on ex vivo studies, that skeletal damage accumulation would have greater effects on bone's resistance to fracture than on its strength.

INFLUENCE OF DRUG THERAPIES ON BIOMECHANICAL PROPERTIES OF BONE

Therapeutic bone active agents have specific effects on matrix properties, mineralization, microdamage accumulation, and bone turnover. The effects on bone quality and fragility can be striking. Examples include high-dose fluoride or etidronate treatments, which impair bone mineralization and can cause severe bone fragility.[34,35]

Other osteoporosis drugs have more subtle effects on bone quality.[36] Each of these affects the mechanical properties of the bone. Often cortical and cancellous bone compartments are affected differently.

Effects of Antiresorptive Agents

Antiresorptive therapies prevent bone loss by suppressing bone turnover, which in turn increases the tissue age of the bone because old bone is not as readily replaced by new bone. Increased bone tissue age is associated with increased mineral content, increased mineral homogeneity, and increased microdamage accumulation. Also, suppressed bone turnover may decrease the porosity of cortical bone and the number of resorption pits in trabeculae.

Increased mineralization caused by antiresorptive drugs has both positive and negative effects on bone quality. There is an optimum range of mineralization to maximize bone toughness. The amount of energy that can be absorbed before failure (toughness) is reduced by either hypo- or hypermineralization (Fig. 7). Bisphosphonate treatment increases tissue mineralization above that found in osteopenic subjects.[37–39] This increased mineralization might account for much of the observed increase in BMD and reduced fracture risk found with risedronate, alendronate, or raloxifene.[40] If mineralization is increased further, past the optimum in Fig. 7, the bone tissue will become less resistant to fracture and consequently more fragile.

One effect of remodeling suppression is that it increases the homogeneity of the bone tissue as more of the tissue becomes mineralized to the same degree.[41,42] Because the effectiveness of bone in stopping cracks is positively proportional to the stiffness ratio across its internal interfaces, a homogeneous material will be less effective in slowing or stopping cracks initiated in the bone matrix. This would allow cracks to grow more quickly to critical size and ultimately increase fracture risk.

Rapid turnover accelerates osteoclastic resorption on trabecular surfaces that can reduce the resistance of trabecular struts to failure by buckling.[43] Ultimately, accelerated resorption will increase the probability for perforation and elimination of trabecular struts.[44,45] Reduced turnover by antiresorptive treatments may reduce fracture risk by more than expected given the magnitude of BMD increases by simply preventing this weakening of trabecular struts, although suppressed turnover will also reduce the bone's ability to repair microdamage.

Bisphosphonates alter three-dimensional trabecular architecture, independent of the change in BMD, making the cancellous bone more plate-like and denser, with thicker and more trabeculae compared with those of untreated controls.[46] Trabecular architecture becomes more isotropic with bisphosphonate treatment, perhaps providing better protection against fracture risk in falls that load the bone in unusual directions. The combination of architectural changes and reduced trabecular perforation may provide a rationale for the clinical observation that fracture risk decreased by 50–60% in the first year of bisphosphonate therapy despite only a 5% increase in BMD.[47]

The impressive fracture risk reduction seen in the first year of treatment with antiresorptive agents seems to be most prominent at trabecular bone sites. Antiresorptive agents have little effect on cortical bone geometry.[32,44,48] Consequently, increased strength of cortical bone, if it occurs, must occur through increased tissue mineralization and/or decreased cortical porosity rather than through geometric changes.

SUMMARY OF THE CHANGES OF CORTICAL BONE
AFTER hPTH TREATMENT

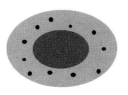
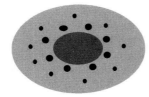

CONTROL

POROSITIES WERE
HOMOGENOUS

AFTER hPTH TREATMENT

BONE AREA INCREASED THROUGH:
• PERIOSTEAL EXPANSION
• MARROW AREA CONTRACTION
POROSITIES NEAR ENDOCORTICAL SURFACE
STRENGTH MAINTAINED OR INCREASED

FIG. 8. Treatment with human parathyroid hormone fragment, PTH(1-34), increases porosity of cortical bone, but because these porosities are mostly close to the marrow cavity, they have little effect on strength. The periosteal apposition that is associated with PTH(1-34) treatment completely compensates for the increased porosity so that bone strength is maintained or even increased.

Effects of Anabolic Agents

The current paradigm for anabolic therapy is intermittent treatment with parathyroid hormone (PTH) or a fragment of this peptide [PTH(1-34)]. The PTH fragment increases bone formation substantially, but also accelerates bone turnover. As a consequence, PTH decreases the mean tissue age of bone, which decreases BMC and microdamage accumulation while increasing porosity. PTH increases bone strength primarily through increased bone volume and improved cancellous architecture.

The acceleration of bone turnover increases the amount of bone that is hypomineralized and makes the tissue more compliant. It also increases the heterogeneity of the bone tissue, creating mixed populations of older bone and new bone. This creates stiffness variations that would slow crack growth, increase toughness, and delay or prevent fracture. These effects are likely to remain as long as PTH treatment is continued.

PTH has a beneficial effect on trabecular architecture through a different mechanism than the antiresorptive agents. Treatment with recombinant PTH(1-34) increases cancellous bone volume and improves trabecular architecture by increasing trabecular number. This occurs through longitudinal tunneling, converting thickened trabecular to multiple struts of normal thickness.[49] This change in architecture, in combination with increased net bone formation, is associated with increased bone strength. Clinically, the effect of these changes is to reduce fracture risk by more than 60% with 1 year of treatment.[50]

In cortical bone, PTH(1-34) increases turnover and cortical porosity, but this effect is most apparent close to the marrow cavity. The bone near the marrow cavity carries less stress than does the periosteal bone. Consequently, increased porosity near the endosteal surface has only a small negative effect on bone strength. The small loss of bone consequent to increased turnover is offset by increased periosteal apposition, which maintains or improves bone strength (Fig. 8).[51] This is likely the mechanism for the observed reduction in nonvertebral fractures.[50]

REFERENCES

1. Burr DB, Milgrom C, Fyhrie D, Forwood M, Nyska M, Finestone A, Hoshaw S, Saiag E, Simkin A 1996 In vivo measurement of human tibial strains during vigorous activity. Bone 18:405–410.
2. Milgrom C, Finestone A, Levi Y, Simkin A, Ekenman I, Mendelson S, Millgram M, Nyska M, Benjuya N, Burr DB 2000 Do high impact exercises produce higher tibial strains than running? Br J Sports Med 34:195–199.
3. Currey JD 1990 Physical characteristics affecting the tensile failure properties of compact bone. J Biomech 23:837–844.
4. Little RD, Carulli JP, Del Mastro RG, Dupuis J, Osborne M, Folz C, Manning SP, Swain PM, Zhao SC, Eustace B, Lappe MM, Spitzer L, Zweier S, Braunschweiger K, Benchekroun Y, Hu X, Adair R, Chee L, FitzGerald MG, Tulig C, Caruso A, Tzellas N, Bawa A, Franklin B, McGuire S, Nogues X, Gong G, Allen KM, Anisowicz A, Morales AJ, Lomedico PT, Recker SM, Van Eerdewegh P, Recker RR, Johnson ML 2002 A mutation in the LDL receptor-related protein 5 gene results in the autosomal dominant high-bone-mass trait. Am J Hum Gen 70:11–19.
5. Rubin CT, Lanyon LE 1982 Limb mechanics as a function of speed and gait: A study of functional strains in the radius and tibia of horse and dog. J Exp Biol 101:187–211.
6. Currey J 2002 Bones: Structure and Mechanics. University Press, Princeton, NJ, USA.
7. Currey JD, Brear K, Zioupos P 1996 The effects of aging and changes in mineral content in degrading the toughness of human femora. J Biomech 29:257–260.
8. Wainwright SA, Biggs WD, Currey JD, Gosline JM 1976 Mechanical Design in Organisms. Halsted Press, New York, NY, USA.
9. Paschalis EP, Betts F, diCarlo E, Mendelsohn R, Boskey A 1997 FTIR microspectroscopic analysis of human iliac crest biopsies from untreated osteoporotic bone. Calcif Tiss Int 61:487–492.
10. Carter DR, Hayes WC 1976 Bone compressive strength: The influence of density and strain rate. Science 194:1174–1176.
11. Wang X, Shen X, Li X, Agrawal CM 2002 Age-related changes in the collagen network and the toughness of bone. Bone 31:1–7.
12. Langdahl BL, Ralston SH, Grant SFA, Eriksen RF 1998 An Sp1 binding site polymorphism in the COL1A1 gene predicts osteoporotic fractures in both men and women. J Bone Miner Res 13:1384–1389.
13. Bernad M, Martinex MW, Escalona M, González ML, González C, Garcés MV, Del Campo MT, Martín Mola E, Maderò R, Carreñò L 2002 Polymorphism in the Type I collagen (COL1A1) gene and risk of fractures in postmenopausal women. Bone 30:223–228.
14. Mann V, Hobson EE, Li B, Stewart TL, Grant SFA, Robins SP, Aspden RM, Ralston SH 2001 A COL1A1 Sp1 binding site polymorphism predisposes to osteoporotic fracture by affecting bone density and quality. J Clin Invest 197:899–907.
15. Zioupos P, Currey JD, Hamer AJ 1999 The role of collagen in the declining mechanical properties of aging human cortical bone. J Biomed Mater Res 45:108–116.
16. Bailey AJ, Sims TJ, Ebbesen EN, Mansell JP, Thomsen JS, Mosekilde Li 1999 Age-related changes in the biochemical properties of human cancellous bone collagen: Relationship to bone strength. Calcif Tiss Int 65:203–210.
17. Martin RB, Ishida J 1989 The relative effects of collagen fiber orientation, porosity, density, and mineralization on bone strength. J Biomech 22:419–426.
18. Martin RB, Boardman DL 1993 The effects of collagen fiber orientation, porosity, density and mineralization on bovine cortical bone bending properties. J Biomech 26:1047–1054.
19. Riggs CM, Vaughan LC, Evans GP, Lanyon LE, Boyde A 1993 Mechanical implications of collagen fibre orientation in cortical bone of the equine radius. Anat Embryol (Berl) 187:239–248.
20. Takano Y, Turner CH, Owan I, Martin RB, Lau ST, Forwood MR, Burr DB 1999 Elastic anisotropy and collagen orientation of osteonal bone are dependent on the mechanical strain distribution. J Orthop Res 17:59–66.
21. Courtney AC, Hayes WC, Gibson LJ 1996 Age-related differences in post-yield damage in human cortical bone. Experiment and model. J Biomech 29:63–1471.
22. McCalden RW, McGeough JA, Barker MB, Court-Brown CM 1993 Age-related changes in the tensile properties of cortical bone. J Bone Joint Surg Am 75A:1193–1205.

23. Oxlund H, Mosekilde Li, Ørtoft G 1996 Reduced concentration of collagen reducible cross links in human trabecular bone with respect to age and osteoporosis. Bone **19:**479–484.
24. Bailey AJ, Wotton SF, Sims TJ, Thompson PW 1993 Biochemical changes in the collagen of human osteoporotic bone matrix. Connect Tiss Res **29:**119–132.
25. Knott L, Bailey AJ 1998 Collagen cross links in mineralizing tissues: A review of their chemistry, function and clinical relevance. Bone **22:**181–187.
26. Martin RB, Atkinson PJ 1977 Age and sex-related changes in the structure and strength of the human femoral shaft. J Biomech **10:**223–231.
27. Beck TJ, Oreskovic TL, Stone KL, Ruff CB, Ensrud K, Nevitt MC, Genant HK, Cummings SR 2001 Structural adaptation to changing skeletal load in the progression toward hip fragility: The study of osteoporotic fractures. J Bone Miner Res **16:**1108–1119.
28. Duan Y, Turner CH, Kim B-T, Seeman E 2001 Sexual dimorphism in bone fragility is more the result of gender differences in age-related bone gain than bone loss. J Bone Miner Res **16:**2267–2275.
29. Schaffler MB, Boyce TM, Fyhrie DP 1996 Tissue and matrix failure modes in human compact bone during tensile fatigue. Trans Orthop Res Soc **21:**57.
30. Burr DB, Turner CH, Naick P, Forwood MR, Ambrosius W, Hasan MS, Pidaparti R 1998 Does microdamage accumulation affect the mechanical properties of bone? J Biomech **31:**337–345.
31. Burr DB, Forwood MR, Fyhrie DP, Martin RB, Schaffler MB, Turner CH 1997 Bone microdamage and skeletal fragility in osteoporotic and stress fractures. J Bone Miner Res **12:**6–15.
32. Mashiba T, Hirano T, Turner CH, Forwood MR, Johnston CC, Burr DB 2000 Suppressed bone turnover by bisphosphonates increases microdamage accumulation and reduces some biomechanical properties in dog rib. J Bone Miner Res **15:**613–620.
33. Mashiba T, Turner CH, Hirano T, Forwood MR, Johnston CC, Burr DB 2001 Effects of suppressed bone turnover by bisphosphonates on microdamage accumulation and biomechanical properties in clinically relevant skeletal sites in beagles. Bone **28:**524–531.
34. Lundy MW, Stauffer M, Wergedal JE, Baylink DJ, Featherstone JD, Hodgson SF, Riggs BL 1995 Histomorphometric analysis of iliac crest bone biopsies in placebo-treated versus fluoride-treated subjects. Osteoporos Int **5:**115–129.
35. Hirano T, Turner CH, Forwood MR, Johnston CC Jr, Burr DB 2000 Does suppression of bone turnover impair mechanical properties by allowing microdamage accumulation? Bone **27:**13–20.
36. Turner CH 2002 Biomechanics of bone: Determinants of skeletal fragility and bone quality. Osteoporos Int **13:**97–104.
37. Meunier PJ, Boivin G 1997 Bone mineral density reflects bone mass but also the degree of mineralization of bone: Therapeutic implications. Bone **21:**373–377.
38. Boivin G, Chavassieux PM, Santora AC, Yates J, Meunier PJ 2000 Alendronate increases bone strength by increasing the mean degree of mineralization of bone tissue in osteoporotic women. Bone **27:**687–694.
39. Nuzzo S, Lafage-Proust MH, Martin-Badosa E, Boivin G, Thomas T, Alexandre C, Peyrin F 2002 Synchrotron radiation microtomography allows the analysis of three-dimensional microarchitecture and degree of mineralization of human iliac crest biopsy specimens: Effects of etidronate treatment. J Bone Miner Res **17:**1372–1382.
40. Cranney A, Guyatt G, Griffith L, Wells G, Tugwell P, Rosen C 2002 IX: Summary of meta-analyses of therapies for postmenopausal osteoporosis. Endocr Rev **23:**570–578.
41. Roschger P, Rinnerthaler S, Yates J, Rodan GA, Fratzl P, Klaushofer K 2001 Alendronate increases degree and uniformity of mineralization in cancellous bone and decreases the porosity in cortical bone of osteoporotic women. Bone **29:**185–191.
42. Boivin G, Meunier PJ 2002 The degree of mineralization of bone tissue measured by computerized quantitative contact microradiography. Calcif Tiss Int **70:**503–511.
43. Parfitt AM 2002 High bone turnover is intrinsically harmful: Two paths to a similar conclusion. J Bone Miner Res **17:**1558–1559.
44. Riggs BL, Melton LJ III 2002 Bone turnover matters: The raloxifene treatment paradox of dramatic decreases in vertebral fractures without commensurate increases in bone density. J Bone Miner Res **17:**11–14.
45. Riggs BL, Melton LJ III 2002 The Riggs/Melton view. J Bone Miner Res **17:**1560.
46. Borah B, Dufresne TE, Chmielewski PA, Gross GJ, Prenger MC, Phipps RJ 2002 Risedronate preserves trabecular architecture and increases bone strength in vertebra of ovariectomized minipigs as measured by three-dimensional microcomputed tomography. J Bone Miner Res **17:**1139–1147.
47. Cummings SR, Karpf DB, Harris F, Genant HK, Ensrud K, LaCroix AZ, Black DM 2002 Improvement in spine bone density and reduction in risk of vertebral fractures during treatment with antiresorptive drugs. Am J Med **112:**281–289.
48. Ott SM, Aleksik A, Lu Y, Harper K, Lips P 2002 Bone histomorphometric and biochemical marker results of a 2-year placebo-controlled trial of raloxifene in postmenopausal women. J Bone Miner Res **17:**341–348.
49. Jerome CP, Burr DB, Van Bibber T, Hock JM, Brommage R 2001 Treatment with human parathyroid hormone (1–34) for 18 months increases cancellous bone volume and improves trabecular architecture in ovariectomized cynomolgus monkeys (Macaca fascicularis). Bone **28:**150–159.
50. Neer RM, Arnaud CD, Zanchetta JR, Prince R, Gaich GA, Reginster JY, Hodsman AB, Eriksen EF, Ish-Shalom S, Genant HK, Wang O, Mitlak BH 2001 Effect of parathyroid hormone (1–34) on fractures and bone mineral density in postmenopausal women with osteoporosis. N Engl J Med **344:**1434–1441.
51. Burr DB, Hirano T, Turner CH, Hotchkiss C, Brommage R, Hock JM 2001 Intermittently administered human parathyroid hormone (1–34) treatment increases intracortical bone turnover and porosity without reducing bone strength in the humerus of ovariectomized cynomolgus monkeys. J Bone Miner Res **16:**157–165.

Chapter 9.   Skeletal Physiology: Fetus and Neonate

Christopher S. Kovacs

Faculty of Medicine, Endocrinology, Memorial University of Newfoundland, St. John's, Newfoundland, Canada

INTRODUCTION

Because of the obvious limitations in studying human fetuses and (to a lesser degree) neonates, human regulation of fetal and neonatal mineral homeostasis must be largely inferred from studies in animals. Some observations in animals may not apply to humans. This chapter briefly reviews existing human and animal data, including older studies of surgically manipulated animals and recent studies of mice engineered to lack calcitropic hormones or receptors. Detailed references are available in two recent, comprehensive reviews.[1,2]

FETUS

Much of normal mineral and bone homeostasis in the adult can be explained by the interactions of parathyroid hormone (PTH), 1,25-dihydroxyvitamin D or calcitriol (1,25-D), calcitonin, and the sex steroids. Many of our pharmacologic therapies for osteoporosis and other metabolic bone diseases are based on these hormones (or analogs of them) and the roles they play in the adult.

In contrast to the adult, comparatively little is known about how mineral and bone homeostasis is regulated in the fetus. It is evident that fetal mineral metabolism has been uniquely adapted to meet the specific needs of this developmental period, including the requirement to maintain an extracellular level of calcium (and other minerals) that is physiologically appropriate for fetal tissues, and to provide sufficient calcium (and other minerals) to fully mineralize the skeleton before birth. Mineralization occurs rapidly in late gestation, such that a human accretes 80% of the required 30 g of calcium in the third trimester, whereas a rat accretes 95% of the required 12.5 mg of calcium in the last 5 days of its 3-week gestation.

Minerals Ions and Calcitropic Hormones

A consistent finding among human and other mammalian fetuses is a total and ionized calcium concentration that is significantly higher than the maternal level during late gestation. Similarly, serum phosphate is significantly elevated, and serum magnesium is minimally elevated above the maternal concentration. The physiological importance of these elevated levels is not known. A calcium level equal to the maternal calcium concentration (and not above it) seems to be sufficient to ensure adequate mineralization of the fetal skeleton, and fetal survival to term is unaffected by extremes of hypocalcemia in several animal models. The increased calcium level is robustly maintained despite chronic, severe maternal hypocalcemia of a variety of causes. For example, adult humans and mice with nonfunctional vitamin D receptors have severe hypocalcemia, but murine fetuses with the same abnormality have normal serum calcium concentrations.[1]

Calcitropic hormone levels are also maintained at levels that differ from the adult. These differences seem to reflect the relatively different roles that these hormones play in the fetus and are not an artifact of altered metabolism or clearance of these hormones. Intact PTH levels are much lower than maternal PTH levels near the end of gestation, but it is unknown whether fetal PTH levels are low throughout gestation after the formation of the parathyroids, or only in late gestation. The low level of PTH is critically important, because fetal mice lacking parathyroids and PTH have marked hypocalcemia and undermineralized skeletons.[3] Circulating 1,25-D levels are also lower than the maternal level in late gestation and seem to be largely if not completely derived from fetal sources. The low circulating levels of 1,25-D in the fetus may be a response to high serum phosphate and suppressed PTH levels in late gestation. With respect to 1,25-D, the low levels of this hormone may reflect its relative unimportance for fetal mineral homeostasis, because both vitamin D deficiency and absence of vitamin D receptors do not impair serum mineral concentrations or the mineralization of the fetal skeleton. Fetal calcitonin levels are higher than maternal levels and are thought to reflect increased synthesis of the hormone. Apart from responding appropriately to changes in the serum calcium concentration, there is little evidence of an essential role for calcitonin in fetal mineral homeostasis.

Parathyroid hormone-related protein (PTHrP) is normally not present in the human adult circulation (outside of pregnancy and lactation), but in cord blood, PTHrP levels are up to 15-fold higher than that of PTH. PTHrP is produced in many tissues and plays multiple roles during embryonic and fetal development (see chapter on Parathyroid Hormone-

A

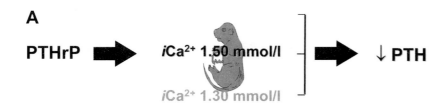

PTHrP ➡ iCa^{2+} 1.50 mmol/l

iCa^{2+} 1.30 mmol/l

➡ ↓ PTH

B

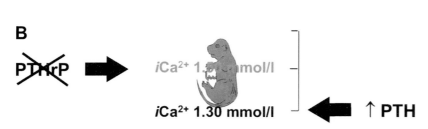

P̶T̶H̶r̶P̶ ➡ iCa^{2+} 1.~~~mol/l

iCa^{2+} 1.30 mmol/l

⬅ ↑ PTH

FIG. 1. Fetal blood calcium regulation. (A) Normal high fetal calcium level, which is dependent on PTHrP, activates the parathyroid CaSR, and PTH is suppressed. (B) In the absence of PTHrP, the fetal calcium level falls to a level that is now set by the parathyroid CaSR; PTH is stimulated to maintain the ionized calcium at the normal adult level (=maternal). (Reprinted from Pediatric Bone, Glorieux FH, Pettifor JM, Jüppner H, Fetal mineral homeostasis, pp. 271-302, 2003 with permission from Elsevier.)

Related Protein). The absence of PTHrP (in the *Pthrp*-null fetal mouse) leads to abnormalities of chondrocyte differentiation and skeletal development,[4] modest hypocalcemia,[5] and reduced placental calcium transfer (see below). Such *Pthrp*-null fetuses have increased PTH levels[6] but still remain modestly hypocalcemic, indicating that PTH does not make up for lack of PTHrP in maintaining a normal calcium concentration in the fetal circulation.

The role (if any) of the sex steroids in fetal skeletal development and mineral accretion is unknown, largely because the relevant analyses have not been performed in the relevant mouse models, and corresponding human data are absent. Estrogen receptor α and β knockout mice have been shown to have altered skeletal metabolism that develops postnatally, but the fetal skeleton has not been examined in detail. Similarly, postnatal skeletal roles of RANK, RANK ligand, and osteoprotegerin have been demonstrated in relevant knockout mice, but the role that this system plays in fetal mineral metabolism is not yet known.

Fetal Parathyroids

Intact parathyroid glands are required for maintenance of normal fetal calcium, magnesium, and phosphate levels; lack of parathyroids and PTH causes a greater fall in the fetal blood calcium than lack of PTHrP. Fetal parathyroids are also required for normal accretion of mineral by the skeleton and may be required for regulation of placental mineral transfer, as discussed below. Studies in fetal lambs have indicated that the fetal parathyroids may contribute to mineral homeostasis by producing both PTH and PTHrP, while detailed study of rats indicate that the fetal parathyroids produce only PTH. Whether human fetal parathyroids produce PTH alone, or PTH and PTHrP together, is unclear.

Calcium Sensing Receptor

The calcium sensing receptor (CaSR) sets the serum calcium level in adults by regulating PTH, but it does not seem to set the serum calcium level in fetuses. Instead, the fetal serum calcium is driven above the maternal level by the action of PTHrP, while in turn, the CaSR appropriately suppresses PTH in response to this elevated calcium level (Fig. 1A). In the absence of PTHrP (*Pthrp*-null mice), the fetal serum calcium falls to the normal adult level and the serum PTH is increased, consistent with the normal function of the CaSR to maintain the calcium concentration at the adult level (Fig. 1B). Inactivating mutations of the CaSR (*Casr*-null fetuses) lead to increases in serum calcium, PTH, 1-,25-D, and bone turnover of fetuses, resulting in a lower skeletal calcium content by term. The CaSR is also expressed within placenta as demonstrated in humans and mice, and this may indicate that the CaSR participates in the regulation of placental mineral transfer. *Casr*-null fetuses have a reduced rate of placental calcium transfer, but whether this is a direct consequence of the loss of placental CaSR is not known.[7]

Fetal Kidneys and Amniotic Fluid

Fetal kidneys partly regulate calcium homeostasis by adjusting the relative reabsorption and excretion of calcium, magnesium, and phosphate in response to the filtered load and other factors, such as PTHrP and PTH. The fetal kidneys also synthesize 1,25-D, but because absence of vitamin D receptors in fetal mice does not impair fetal calcium homeostasis or placental calcium transfer, it seems likely that renal production of 1,25-D is relatively unimportant.

Renal calcium handling in fetal life may be less important compared with the adult for the regulation of calcium homeostasis, because calcium excreted by the kidneys is not permanently lost. Fetal urine is the major source of fluid and solute in the amniotic fluid, and fetal swallowing of amniotic fluid is a pathway by which excreted calcium can be made available again to the fetus.

Placental Mineral Ion Transport

As noted above, the bulk of placental calcium and other mineral transfer occurs late in gestation at a rapid rate. Active transport of calcium, magnesium, and phosphate across the placenta is necessary for the fetal requirement to be met; only placental calcium transfer has been studied in detail. Analogous to calcium transfer across the intestinal mucosa, it has been theorized that calcium diffuses into calcium-transporting cells through maternal-facing basement membranes, is carried across these cells by calcium binding proteins, and is actively extruded at the fetal-facing basement membranes by Ca^{2+}-ATPase.

Data from animal models indicates that a normal rate of maternal-to-fetal calcium transfer can usually be maintained despite the presence of maternal hypocalcemia or maternal hormone deficiencies such as aparathyroidism, vitamin D deficiency, and absence of the vitamin D receptor. Whether the same is true for human pregnancies is less certain (see Fetal Response to Maternal Hypoparathyroidism section). A "normal" rate of maternal-fetal calcium transfer does not necessarily imply that the fetus is unaffected by maternal hypocalcemia. Instead, it is an indication of the resilience of the fetal-placental unit to be able to extract the required amount of calcium from a maternal circulation that has a severely lower calcium concentration than normal.

Fetal regulation of placental calcium transfer has been studied in a number of different animal models. Thyroparathyroidectomy in fetal lambs results in a reduced rate of placental calcium transfer, suggesting that the parathyroids are required for this process.[8] In contrast, studies in mice lacking parathyroids as a consequence of ablation of the *Hoxa3* gene have a normal rate of placental calcium transfer.[3] The discrepancy between these findings in lambs and mice may be caused by whether or not the parathyroids are an important source of PTHrP in the circulation, as discussed above. Studies in fetal lambs and in *Pthrp*-null fetal mice are in agreement that PTHrP, and in particular, midmolecular forms of PTHrP, stimulate placental calcium transfer.[5,9,10] PTH does not seem to be involved in this process, and there is little evidence that calcitonin or 1,25-D are required either.

Fetal Skeleton

A complete cartilaginous skeleton with digits and intact joints is present by the eighth week of gestation in humans. Primary ossification centers form in the vertebrae and long bones between the 8th and 12th weeks, but it is not until the third trimester that the bulk of mineralization occurs. At the 34th week of gestation, secondary ossification centers form in the femurs, but otherwise most epiphyses are cartilaginous at birth, with secondary ossification centers appearing in other bones in the neonate and child.[11]

The skeleton must undergo substantial growth and be sufficiently mineralized by the end of gestation to support the organism, but as in the adult, the fetal skeleton participates in the regulation of mineral homeostasis. Calcium accreted by the fetal skeleton can be subsequently resorbed to help maintain the concentration of calcium in the blood. Functioning fetal parathyroid glands are needed for normal skeletal mineral accretion, and both hypoparathyroidism (thyroparathyroidectomized fetal lambs and aparathyroid fetal mice) and hyperparathyroidism (including *Casr*-null fetal mice) reduce the net amount of skeletal mineral accreted by term.

Further comparative study of fetal mice lacking parathyroids or PTHrP has clarified the relative and interlocking roles of PTH and PTHrP in the regulation of the development and mineralization of the fetal skeleton. PTHrP produced locally in the growth plate directs the development of the cartilaginous scaffold that is later broken down and transformed into endochondral bone,[12] while PTH controls the mineralization of bone through its contribution to maintaining the fetal blood calcium and magnesium.[6] In the absence of PTHrP, a severe chondrodysplasia results,[4] but the fetal skeleton is fully mineralized.[6] In the absence of parathyroids and PTH, endochondral bone forms normally but is significantly undermineralized.[6] The blood calcium and magnesium were also significantly reduced in aparathyroid fetuses, and this may explain why lack of PTH impaired skeletal mineralization. That is, by reducing the amount of mineral presented to the skeletal surface and to osteoblasts, lack of PTH thereby impaired mineral accretion by the skeleton. When both parathyroids and PTHrP are deleted, the typical *Pthrp*-null chondrodysplasia results, but the skeleton is smaller and contains less mineral.[6] Therefore, normal mineralization of the fetal skeleton requires intact fetal parathyroid glands and adequate delivery of minerals to the fetal circulation. While both PTH and PTHrP are involved, PTH plays the more critical role in ensuring full mineralization of the skeleton before term.

Fetal Response to Maternal Hyperparathyroidism

In humans, maternal primary hyperparathyroidism has been associated with adverse fetal outcomes, including spontaneous abortion and stillbirth, which are thought to result from suppression of the fetal parathyroid glands. Because PTH cannot cross the placenta, fetal parathyroid suppression may result from increased calcium flux across the placenta to the fetus, facilitated by maternal hypercalcemia. Similar suppression of fetal parathyroids occurs when the mother has hypercalcemia caused by familial hypocalciuric hypercalcemia. Chronic elevation of the maternal serum calcium in mice results in suppression of the fetal PTH level,[7] but fetal outcome is not notably affected by this.

Fetal Response to Maternal Hypoparathyroidism

Maternal hypoparathyroidism during human pregnancy can cause fetal hyperparathyroidism. This is characterized by fetal parathyroid gland hyperplasia, generalized skeletal demineralization, subperiosteal bone resorption, bowing of the long bones, osteitis fibrosa cystica, rib and limb fractures, low birth weight, spontaneous abortion, stillbirth, and neonatal death. Similar skeletal findings have been reported in the fetuses and neonates of women with pseudohypoparathyroidism, renal tubular acidosis, and chronic renal failure. These changes in human skeletons differ from what has been found in animal models of maternal hypocalcemia, in which the fetal skeleton and the blood calcium is generally normal.

Integrated Fetal Calcium Homeostasis

The evidence discussed in the preceding sections suggests the following summary models.

© 2003 American Society for Bone and Mineral Research

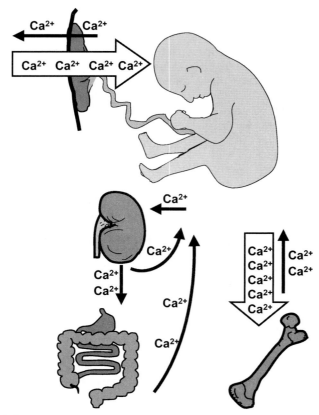

FIG. 2. Calcium sources in fetal life. (Reprinted from Pediatric Bone, Glorieux FH, Pettifor JM, Jüppner H, Fetal mineral homeostasis, pp. 271-302, 2003 with permission from Elsevier.)

Calcium Sources. The main flux of calcium and other minerals is across the placenta and into fetal bone, but calcium is also made available to the fetal circulation through several routes (Fig. 2). The kidneys reabsorb calcium; calcium excreted by the kidneys into the urine, and amniotic fluid may be swallowed and reabsorbed; calcium is also resorbed from the developing skeleton. Some calcium returns to the maternal circulation (backflux). The maternal skeleton is a potential source of mineral, and it may be compromised in mineral deficiency states to provide to the fetus.

Blood Calcium Regulation. The fetal blood calcium is set at a level higher than the maternal level through the actions of PTHrP and PTH acting in concert (among other potential factors; Fig. 3). The CaSR suppresses PTH in response to the high calcium level, but the low level of PTH is critically required for maintaining the blood calcium and facilitating mineral accretion by the skeleton. 1,25-D synthesis and secretion are, in turn, suppressed by low PTH and high blood calcium and phosphate. The parathyroids may play a central role by producing PTH and PTHrP or may produce PTH alone while PTHrP is produced by the placenta and other fetal tissues.

PTH and PTHrP, both present in the fetal circulation, independently and additively regulate the fetal blood calcium, with PTH having the greater effect. Neither hormone

can make up for absence of the other; if one is missing, the blood calcium is reduced, and if both are missing, the blood calcium is reduced even further. PTH may contribute to the blood calcium through actions on the PTH/PTHrP (PTH1) receptor in classic target tissues (kidney, bone), whereas PTHrP may contribute through placental calcium transfer and actions on the PTH1 receptor and other receptors.

The normal elevation of the fetal blood calcium above the maternal calcium concentration was historically taken as proof that placental calcium transfer is an active process. However, the fetal blood calcium level is not simply determined by the rate of placental calcium transfer because placental calcium transfer is normal in aparathyroid mice and increased in mice lacking the PTH1 receptor, but both phenotypes have significantly reduced blood calcium levels.[3,5] Also, *Casr*-null fetuses have reduced placental calcium transfer but markedly increased blood calcium levels.[7]

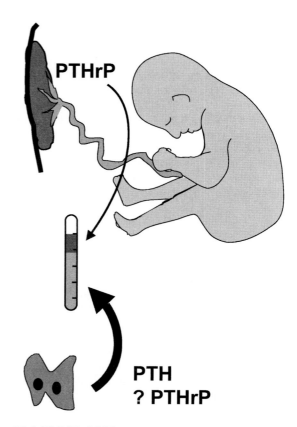

FIG. 3. Fetal blood calcium regulation. PTH has a more dominant effect on fetal blood calcium regulation than PTHrP, with blood calcium represented schematically as a thermometer (light gray = contribution of PTH; dark gray = contribution of PTHrP). In the absence of PTHrP, the blood calcium falls to the maternal level. In the absence of PTH (*Hoxa3*-null that has absent PTH but normal circulating PTHrP levels), the blood calcium falls well below the maternal calcium concentration. In the absence of both PTHrP and PTH (*Hoxa3/Pthrp* double mutant), the blood calcium falls even further than in the absence of PTH alone. (Reprinted from Pediatric Bone, Glorieux FH, Pettifor JM, Jüppner H, Fetal mineral homeostasis, pp. 271-302, 2003 with permission from Elsevier.)

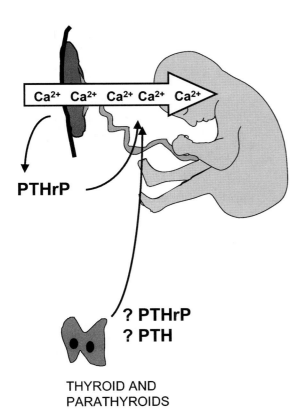

FIG. 4. Placental calcium transfer is regulated by PTHrP but not by PTH; whether the parathyroids produce PTHrP or not is uncertain. (Reprinted from Pediatric Bone, Glorieux FH, Pettifor JM, Jüppner H, Fetal mineral homeostasis, pp. 271-302, 2003 with permission from Elsevier.)

Placental Calcium Transfer. Placental calcium transfer is regulated by PTHrP but not by PTH (Fig. 4), and the placenta (and possibly the parathyroids) is likely an important source of PTHrP.

Skeletal Mineralization. PTH and PTHrP have separate roles with respect to skeletal development and mineralization (Fig. 5). PTH normally acts systemically to direct the mineralization of the bone matrix by maintaining the blood calcium at the adult level and possibly by direct actions on osteoblasts within the bone matrix. In contrast, PTHrP acts both locally within the growth plate to direct endochondral bone development and outside of bone to affect skeletal development and mineralization by contributing to the regulation of the blood calcium and placental calcium transfer. PTH has the more critical role in maintaining skeletal mineral accretion.

The rate of placental calcium transfer has been historically considered to be the rate-limiting step for skeletal mineral accretion. However, this is not correct because accretion of mineral was reduced in the presence of both normal and increased placental calcium transfer.[1] The rate limiting step seems to be the blood calcium level, which in turn, is largely determined by PTH. The level of blood calcium achieved in the *Pthrp*-null—that is, the normal adult level—is sufficient to allow normal accretion of mineral, while lower levels of blood calcium impair it.

NEONATE

After cutting the umbilical cord and abruptly losing the placental calcium infusion (and placental sources of PTHrP), a rapid adjustment in the regulation of mineral homeostasis occurs over hours to days. The neonate becomes dependent on intestinal calcium intake, skeletal calcium stores, and renal calcium reabsorption to maintain a normal blood calcium at a time of continued skeletal growth. PTH and 1,25-D become more important, whereas PTHrP becomes less involved in neonatal calcium homeostasis.

Mineral Ions and Calcitropic Hormones

Birth marks the onset of a fall in the total and ionized calcium concentration, likely provoked by loss of the placental calcium pump and placental-derived PTHrP, and a rise in pH induced by the onset of breathing. Studies in rodents indicate a fall in total and ionized calcium levels to 60% of the fetal value by 6–12 h after birth and a subsequent rise to the normal adult value over the succeeding week. Although data are less complete in humans, the progression in ionized and total calcium values seems to be similar. The ionized calcium in normal neonates falls from the umbilical cord level of 1.45 mM to a mean of 1.20 mM by 24 h after birth.[13] Babies delivered by elective C-section

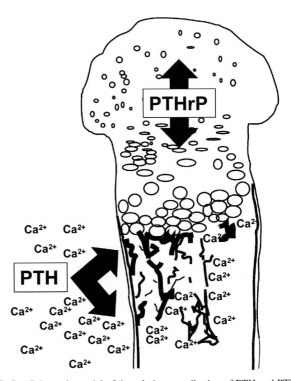

FIG. 5. Schematic model of the relative contribution of PTH and PTHrP to endochondral bone formation and skeletal mineralization. PTHrP is produced within the cartilaginous growth plate and directs the development of this scaffold that will later be broken down and replaced by bone. PTH reaches the skeleton systemically from the parathyroids and directs the accretion of mineral by the developing bone matrix. (Reprinted from Pediatric Bone, Glorieux FH, Pettifor JM, Jüppner H, Fetal mineral homeostasis, pp. 271-302, 2003 with permission from Elsevier.)

© 2003 American Society for Bone and Mineral Research

were found to have lower blood calcium and higher PTH levels at birth compared with babies delivered by spontaneous vaginal delivery,[14] indicating that the mode of delivery can affect early neonatal mineral homeostasis.

Phosphate initially rises over the first 24 h of postnatal life in humans and then gradually declines. The intact PTH level has been found to rise briskly to within or near the normal adult range by 24–48 h after birth.[2] The increase in PTH follows the early postnatal drop in the serum ionized calcium and precedes the subsequent rise in ionized calcium and 1,25-D and the fall in phosphate. During the first 48 h, the parathyroid glands have been found to respond sluggishly to more severe falls in the ionized calcium, such as that caused by exchange transfusion with citrated blood. The degree of responsiveness to acute hypocalcemia seems to increase with postnatal age.

In humans, 1,25-D rises to adult levels over the first 48 h of postnatal life, likely in response to the rise in PTH. Serum calcitonin rises 2- to 10-fold over cord blood levels over the same time interval and then gradually declines. Infants that are premature, asphyxiated, or hypocalcemic have the highest postnatal calcitonin levels; consequently, hypercalcitoninemia has been suggested to cause neonatal hypocalcemia. However, other studies indicate that the postnatal rise in calcitonin levels does not correlate to the fall in serum calcium.

PTHrP secretion from placenta, amnion, and umbilical cord is lost at birth; secretion from the parathyroid glands (if ever present) is also apparently lost sometime after birth, because PTHrP circulates at low to undetectable levels during normal adult life in humans and animals. Animal studies suggest that PTHrP may persist in the neonatal circulation for some time, whether secreted by the parathyroids or caused by absorption of PTHrP from milk (milk contains PTHrP at concentrations 10,000-fold higher than the level in the fetal circulation). Whether PTHrP present in milk contributes to the regulation of neonatal mineral homeostasis is unknown.

Intestinal Absorption of Calcium

In newborns, intestinal calcium absorption is a passive, nonsaturable process that is not dependent on vitamin D and 1,25-D. The high lactose content of milk has been shown to specifically increase the efficiency of intestinal calcium absorption and net bioavailability of dietary calcium, through effects on paracellular diffusion in the distal small bowel. With increasing postnatal age, the vitamin D receptor begins to appear in intestinal cells, and mucosal levels of the calcium binding protein calbindin$_{9K}$-D increase sharply. Around the same time, vitamin D–dependent active transport of calcium becomes noticeable, whereas passive transfer of calcium declines. By the time of weaning in rodents, the intestine is less permeable to passive absorption of calcium, and active transport has become the dominant means by which calcium is transferred into the intestinal mucosa. Data from newborn humans are less complete, but the onset of 1,25-D–dependent active transport of calcium follows a similar postnatal course. The normal postnatal maturation of the neonatal intestine may limit the ability of preterm humans to accrete sufficient calcium for skeletal mineralization and to regulate the blood calcium.

Renal Handling of Calcium

Although data are limited, urinary calcium excretion rises in humans over the first 2 weeks, consistent with a concurrent 2-fold rise in glomerular filtration rate. The neonatal kidney show a response to exogenously administered PTH that increases with postnatal age.

Skeletal Calcium Metabolism

In humans, the neonatal skeleton continues to accrete calcium at a rate of about 150 mg/kg/day, similar to the rate of the late-term fetus. Vitamin D deficiency or loss of the vitamin D receptor (which has no effect on mineral homeostasis of the fetus) becomes obvious during the neonatal period because of the onset of dependence on intestinal calcium transport for supply of calcium. In human vitamin D deficiency, hypocalcemia appears late in the first or second week, and rickets develops after 2 to 3 months.

Although parathyroidectomy and vitamin D deficiency in rats, and loss of vitamin D receptors in mice, will eventually result in hypocalcemia and hyperphosphatemia, by the time of weaning, neonatal rats and mice still have normal serum mineral concentrations and skeletal mineral content. These findings suggest that factors other than PTH and vitamin D (such as lactose, and perhaps, PTHrP in milk) may be required for normal accretion of calcium in the first several weeks when the pup is suckling and intestinal calcium absorption is not yet fully 1,25-D dependent.

Premature infants are prone to develop metabolic bone disease of prematurity, a form of rickets precipitated by loss of the placental calcium pump at a time when the skeleton is accreting calcium at a peak rate. It is not caused by vitamin D deficiency but seems to be the consequence of inadequate calcium and phosphate intake to meet the demands of the mineralizing neonatal skeleton. Special oral or parenteral formulas that are high in calcium and phosphorus content will correct the demineralization process and allow normal skeletal accretion of these minerals.

Neonatal Response to Maternal Hyper- or Hypoparathyroidism

Maternal hyperparathyroidism results in suppression of the neonatal parathyroid glands for some time after birth (the suppression can be permanent), and hypocalcemia, tetany, and even death may occur. The mechanism of the prolonged suppression is not known but may be caused by chronic exposure to increased flux of calcium across the placenta during fetal development. Suppression has been observed in infants of women with familial hypocalciuric hypercalcemia.

Maternal hypoparathyroidism in humans has resulted in neonatal parathyroid gland hyperplasia, as noted above in the fetal section. The serum calcium level of the neonate has usually been reported to be normal, whereas the PTH level (older assays) has been found to be elevated. The skeletal findings generally resolve over the first several months after birth, but acute interventions may be required to raise or lower the blood calcium in the neonate. In addition, subtotal parathyroidectomy may be required to control more severe, autonomous disease.

Maternal hypocalcemia of any cause may result in parathyroid gland hyperplasia and hyperparathyroidism in the fetus and neonate. In women with pseudohypoparathyroidism, children that do not inherit the genetic disorder are usually normal at birth, although transient neonatal hyperparathyroidism has been reported in some cases. Furthermore, children that did inherit the condition may also be normal at birth and gradually develop the full biochemical features of pseudohypoparathyroidism over the first several years of life.

Neonatal Hypocalcemia

Neonatal hypocalcemia typically presents as seizures that onset between 4 and 28 days of age. The preterm infant is particularly prone to hypocalcemia, having lost the placental calcium infusion at a time when the skeleton is rapidly accreting calcium and the intestinal calcium absorption is relatively inefficient. In addition to prematurity, other causes of neonatal hypocalcemia include congenital hypoparathyroidism, magnesium deficiency, maternal diabetes, vitamin D deficiency or resistance, and hyperphosphatemia.

Neonatal hypocalcemia can occur as a complication of maternal diabetes in pregnancy in up to 50% of cases, although tight control of the maternal glucose during pregnancy reduces the incidence. The cause of hypocalcemia is likely to be multifactorial but may include neonatal hypomagnesemia as a consequence of maternal glucosuria during pregnancy. Studies in rats have also suggested that maternal diabetes reduces placental mineral transport and skeletal mineral accretion, which in turn predisposes the neonate to develop hypocalcemia and hypomagnesemia.

REFERENCES

1. Kovacs CS 2003 Fetal mineral homeostasis. In: Glorieux FH, Pettifor JM, Jüppner H (eds.) Pediatric Bone: Biology and Diseases. Academic Press, San Diego, CA, USA, pp. 271–302.
2. Kovacs CS, Kronenberg HM 1997 Maternal-fetal calcium and bone metabolism during pregnancy, puerperium and lactation. Endocr Rev **18:**832–872.
3. Kovacs CS, Manley NR, Moseley JM, Martin TJ, Kronenberg HM 2001 Fetal parathyroids are not required to maintain placental calcium transport. J Clin Invest **107:**1007–1015.
4. Karaplis AC, Luz A, Glowacki J, Bronson RT, Tybulewicz VL, Kronenberg HM, Mulligan RC 1994 Lethal skeletal dysplasia from targeted disruption of the parathyroid hormone-related peptide gene. Genes Dev **8:**277–289.
5. Kovacs CS, Lanske B, Hunzelman JL, Guo J, Karaplis AC, Kronenberg HM 1996 Parathyroid hormone-related peptide (PTHrP) regulates fetal-placental calcium transport through a receptor distinct from the PTH/PTHrP receptor. Proc Natl Acad Sci USA **93:**15233–15238.
6. Kovacs CS, Chafe LL, Fudge NJ, Friel JK, Manley NR 2001 PTH regulates fetal blood calcium and skeletal mineralization independently of PTHrP. Endocrinology **142:**4983–4993.
7. Kovacs CS, Ho-Pao CL, Hunzelman JL, Lanske B, Fox J, Seidman JG, Seidman CE, Kronenberg HM 1998 Regulation of murine fetal-placental calcium metabolism by the calcium-sensing receptor. J Clin Invest **101:**2812–2820.
8. Care AD, Caple IW, Abbas SK, Pickard DW 1986 The effect of fetal thyroparathyroidectomy on the transport of calcium across the ovine placenta to the fetus. Placenta **7:**417–424.
9. Rodda CP, Kubota M, Heath JA, Ebeling PR, Moseley JM, Care AD, Caple IW, Martin TJ 1988 Evidence for a novel parathyroid hormone-related protein in fetal lamb parathyroid glands and sheep placenta: Comparisons with a similar protein implicated in humoral hypercalcaemia of malignancy. J Endocrinol **117:**261–271.
10. Care AD, Abbas SK, Pickard DW, Barri M, Drinkhill M, Findlay JB, White IR, Caple IW 1990 Stimulation of ovine placental transport of calcium and magnesium by mid-molecule fragments of human parathyroid hormone-related protein. Exp Physiol **75:**605–608.
11. Moore KL, Persaud TVN 1998 The Developing Human, 6th ed. W. B. Saunders, Philadelphia, PA, USA.
12. Karsenty G 2001 Chondrogenesis just ain't what it used to be. J Clin Invest **107:**405–407.
13. Loughead JL, Mimouni F, Tsang RC 1988 Serum ionized calcium concentrations in normal neonates. Am J Dis Child **142:**516–518.
14. Bagnoli F, Bruchi S, Garosi G, Pecciarini L, Bracci R 1990 Relationship between mode of delivery and neonatal calcium homeostasis. Eur J Pediatr **149:**800–803.

Chapter 10.   Childhood and Adolescence

Vicente Gilsanz[1] and Dorothy A. Nelson[2]

[1]Department of Radiology, Children's Hospital of Los Angeles, Los Angeles, California; and [2]Department of Internal Medicine, Wayne State University, Detroit, Michigan

INTRODUCTION

Childhood and adolescence are characterized by longitudinal growth as well as by changes in skeletal size and shape. Bone mass increases dramatically during growth, and it is becoming increasingly clear that the amount of bone accrued during these life periods may be an important determinant of future resistance to fractures. Thus, considerable interest is placed on defining the determinants that account for the physiological variations in skeletal growth, because they will provide the best means for identification of individuals and populations that are at greatest risk of osteoporosis and other disorders of bone and mineral metabolism.

The development of precise noninvasive methods for measuring bone mineral content (BMC) and bone mineral density (BMD) has significantly improved our ability to study the influence of genetic and environmental factors on the attainment of bone mass. Pediatric applications of the most commonly used methods, DXA and quantitative computed tomography (QCT), will be discussed below. Inherent differences in these measurement methods have sometimes led investigators to different conclusions about the timing

The authors have no conflict of interest.

and characteristics of bone growth and accumulation of bone mass.

ACCUMULATION OF BONE MASS AND PEAK BONE MASS

Skeletal mass increases from approximately 70–95 g at birth to 2400–3300 g in young women and men, respectively.[1] These gains are achieved through longitudinal growth, which results from a combination of bone modeling and remodeling. These processes occur at different rates and at different times at primary and secondary sites of bone formation.

Longitudinal studies of total body BMC measurements show that gains in bone mass are very rapid during adolescence and that up to 25% of peak bone mass (PBM) is acquired during the 2-year period across peak height velocity.[2] At peak height velocity, boys and girls have reached 90% of their adult stature, but only 57% of their adult BMC. At least 90% of PBM is acquired by age 18.[2]

The human skeleton contains approximately 85% cortical bone and 15% cancellous bone, and studies have shown that the patterns of gain during growth (like those of the rate of bone loss with aging) differ considerably between these two skeletal compartments.[3,4] The density of cancellous bone is strongly influenced by hormonal and/or metabolic factors associated with sexual development during late adolescence.[5] On average, cancellous bone density in the spine increases by 13% during puberty in white boys and girls. After controlling for puberty, vertebral bone density fails to correlate significantly with age, sex, weight, height, surface area, or body mass index (BMI).[5] The increase in the density of cancellous bone during the later stages of puberty is likely a reflection of a greater thickness of the trabeculae.

The factors that account for the increase in cancellous vertebral bone density during late puberty remain to be determined. It is reasonable to suspect that many of the physical changes undergone, such as the accelerated growth spurt and the increases in body and bone mass, are, at least in part, mediated by the actions of sex steroids.[6] Some of these effects may be caused by changes in protein and calcium metabolism induced by sex steroids, or alternatively, they may be secondary to the cascade of events triggered by the increase in growth hormone and insulin-like growth factor I (IGF-I) production observed after sex steroid exposure.

The exact age at which values for bone mass reach their peak at various skeletal sites has not yet been determined with certainty. It is likely that the timing of peak values differs between the axial and appendicular skeletons, and between men and women. Moreover, differences among studies are, in part, a reflection of the different modalities used for measuring bone mass.

In the axial skeleton, peak bone mass may be achieved by the end of the second decade of life. Studies in women using CT have demonstrated that the density and the size of vertebral bone reach their peak soon after the time of sexual and skeletal maturity,[5,7] corroborating anatomical data indicating trabecular bone loss as early as the third decade of life, and no change in the cross-sectional area of the verte-

bral body from 15 to 90 years of age.[8,9] The data regarding whether vertebral cross-sectional area in men continues to grow after cessation of longitudinal growth is controversial; whereas some authors find no change in the cross-sectional dimensions after skeletal maturity, others have suggested that vertebral size increases with age throughout adulthood.[9]

In the appendicular skeleton, the range of ages published in cross-sectional studies for the timing of peak bone mass has varied significantly, from 17–18 years of age to as late as 35 years of age.[10–13] Longitudinal DXA studies indicate that the rate of increase in skeletal mass slows markedly in late adolescence and that peak values in the femoral neck, like those in the spine, are achieved near the end of puberty in normal females.[7,14]

GENETIC INFLUENCE ON BONE ACCUMULATION DURING GROWTH

Heredity is an important determinant of bone mass. Convergent data from mother–daughter pairs, sib pairs, and twin studies have estimated the heritability of bone mass to account for 60–80% of its variance.[15–17] The magnitude of the genetic effect varies with age and between skeletal sites; it is higher in the young than in the elderly and in the spine than in the extremities.[18] Further support for this genetic influence comes from studies showing reduced bone mass in daughters of osteoporotic women compared with controls,[17] in men and women with first-degree relatives who have osteoporosis,[19] and more recently, in investigations reporting a link between several "candidate" genes and bone mass.

In a study of a large group of female subjects, polymorphisms of the vitamin D receptor (VDR) gene at a *Bsm*I restriction site were associated with BMD in prepubertal and adolescent girls.[20] Girls with BB genotype had significantly lower spinal BMD SD scores than girls with Bb and bb genotypes.[20] In contrast, polymorphisms at the start codon site of the *VDR* gene, detected with the *Fok*I restriction enzyme, were not associated with BMD at any skeletal site in prepubertal girls.[21] An association between femoral and spinal BMD and the VDR genotype at the *Apa*I and *Bsm*I restriction sites has been shown using CT in prepubertal American girls of Hispanic descent.[22] In this study, girls with aa and bb genotypes showed significantly higher volumetric BMD values than girls with the other genotypes, both at the spine and the femur. A polymorphism in the Sp1-binding site of the gene encoding for collagen type Iα1 was also found to explain some of the variability in vertebral BMD in this cohort of prepubertal girls.[23] In contrast, no relationship between the VDR genotype at *Bsm*I site and forearm BMD or rates of gain of BMD, was found in Norwegian boys and girls.[24]

Effect of Sex

Observations using CT indicate that, throughout life, females have smaller vertebral cross-sectional area compared with males, even after accounting for differences in body size. On average, the cross-sectional area of the vertebral bodies is 11% smaller in prepubertal girls than in prepubertal boys matched for age, height, and weight.[25] This disparity increases with growth and is greatest at skeletal maturity, when the cross-sectional dimensions of the vertebrae are about 25% smaller in women than in men, even after taking into consideration differences in body size.[26] Thus, the phenotypic basis for the 4- to 8-fold higher incidence of vertebral fractures in women compared with that in men may lie in the smaller size of the female vertebra.

In contrast, the cross-sectional dimensions of the femur do not differ between males and females matched for age, height, and weight.[27] The cross-sectional and cortical bone areas at the midshaft of the femur are primarily related to body weight, regardless of sex, a notion consistent with analytical models proposing that long bone cross-sectional growth is strongly driven by mechanical loads.[27,28]

Recent evidence also indicates that BMD is similar in boys and girls before puberty. Data obtained with DXA in two large samples of healthy subjects clearly indicated that there were no sex differences in BMC and BMD during the prepubertal period.[29,30] In the study by Nguyen et al.,[29] BMD values during puberty in girls were higher in the pelvis and spine, while measures in postpubertal boys were higher in the whole skeleton. Peak BMC and BMD was achieved between the ages of 20 and 25 years and occurred much earlier in girls than in boys.

Effect of Ethnicity

Most reports of ethnic differences in bone mass during childhood, based on absorptiometric methods, have indicated a higher bone mass among blacks compared with whites.[30-34] It is important to note that this generalization holds only for U.S. populations. For example "black" Gambian children have a smaller bone mass than British children,[35] and black children in South Africa have a similar appendicular bone mass to white children.[36] In one U.S. study based on DXA, spine bone density in 218 children was not affected by age, sex, race, or lifestyle when Tanner Stage and weight were taken into account.[37]

Pediatric studies using CT indicate that, regardless of sex, ethnicity has significant and differential effects on the density and the size of the bones in the axial and appendicular skeletons.[38] In the axial skeleton, the density of cancellous bone in the vertebral bodies is greater in black than in white adolescents. This difference first becomes apparent during late stages of puberty and persists throughout life.[39] Based on CT data, cancellous bone density is similar in black and white children before puberty, but during puberty it increases in all adolescents. The magnitude of the increase from prepubertal to postpubertal values is, however, substantially greater in black than in white subjects (34% versus 11%, respectively).[38] The cross-sectional areas of the vertebral bodies, however, do not differ between black and white children.[38] Thus, theoretically, the structural basis for the lower vertebral bone strength and the greater incidence of fractures in the axial skeleton of white subjects resides in their lower cancellous bone density. In contrast, in the appendicular skeleton, ethnicity influences the cross-sectional areas of the femurs but not the cortical bone area

nor the material density of cortical bone.[38] Although values for femoral cross-sectional area increase with height, weight, and other anthropometric parameters in all children, this measurement is substantially greater in black children.[38] As the same amount of cortical bone placed further from the center of the bone results in greater bone strength, the skeletal advantage for blacks in the appendicular skeleton is likely the consequence of the greater cross-sectional size of the bones.[28]

Limited data from Asian and Hispanic youth suggest that their bone mass is similar to that of white, but much lower than that of black children.[40,41] Differences in bone and body size account for much of the apparent observed ethnic differences in BMD among non-Hispanic, Hispanic, and Asian children.[40,41]

TRACKING OF BONE MASS

The amount of bone that is gained during adolescence is the main contributor to PBM, which in turn, is a major determinant of osteoporosis and fracture risk in older adulthood. Recent evidence seems to indicate that the morphological traits that contribute to the strength of the bone track throughout life, from childhood to adulthood; values remaining in the same position relative to population percentiles.[29,42,43] In one study, DXA bone mineral measurements of premenopausal mothers and prepubertal daughters showed considerable familial resemblance at all skeletal sites.[42] Moreover, DXA values in the daughters 2 years later correlated strongly with baseline values. Similarly, longitudinal CT measurements of cross-sectional areas of the vertebrae and femora and of cancellous bone density in healthy children indicated that measures at early puberty predicted values at sexual maturity.[43] When baseline values were divided into quartiles, a linear relation across pubertal stages was observed for each quartile (Fig. 1). The regression lines differed among quartiles, paralleled each other, and did not overlap. Therefore, individual volumetric BMD and bone size tracked through growth, maintaining the same position in the normal distribution at the end of puberty as was present in the prepubertal period. Thus, we are now in a position to identify those children who are genetically prone to develop low values for peak bone mass and toward whom osteoporosis prevention trials should be geared.

PEDIATRIC BONE MASS MEASUREMENT

DXA

The most commonly used quantitative radiologic method to assess bone mass in children, as in adults, is DXA. The standard software from most DXA manufacturers, however, was designed with adult patients in mind, so special software for pediatrics has been developed by some manufacturers. The software may require longer scanning time, which can make cooperation from children difficult, resulting in motion artifacts and other inaccuracies.[44]

The preferred anatomic sites for DXA measurements in adults (lumbar spine, proximal femur, and forearm) are problematic when measured in the growing skeleton where

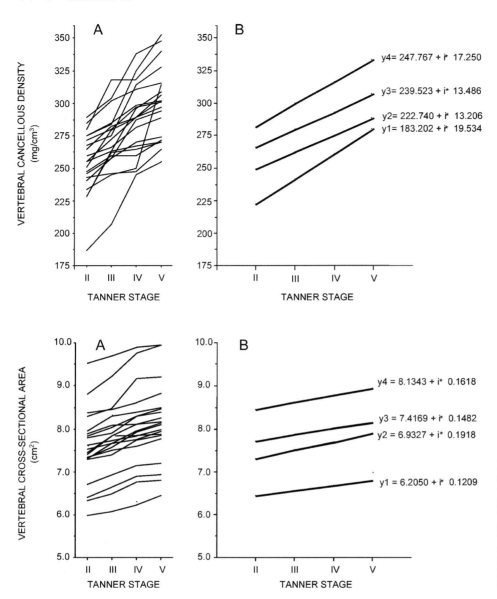

FIG. 1. Longitudinal measurements of vertebral cancellous bone density (upper) and vertebral cross-sectional area (lower) in 20 girls from Tanner stages 2–5 of sexual development. Values are shown for (A) each girl and (B) for each quartile. (Reproduced with permission of The Endocrine Society from Loro ML, et al., 2000 Early identification of children predisposed to low peak bone mass and osteoporosis later in life. J Clin Endocrinol Metab **85**:3908–3918.)

size and shape change with age. There is also tremendous variability in growth and body size at any given chronologic age. Because of these factors that affect regional BMD in children, whole body BMC has been recommended for pediatric studies.[45]

Normative data for DXA values in pediatrics is available in the literature and is included in some DXA software packages. It should, however, be noted that different DXA manufacturers display substantial variation in BMD values of the same bone. Therefore, caution is advised before using published normative data for clinical use, and institutional and device-specific norms are preferable to published references.

Bone mass determinations in children with DXA have been done at all ages, including newborns[46,47] and infants.[48,49] In general, values measured at different skeletal sites increase from infancy to adulthood (Fig. 2).[14,37,50–53] The relationship between age and BMC in the lumbar spine seems to be represented by a segmented polynomial curve[50–52,54]; a rapid increase during childhood is followed by an even greater increase during puberty that ends in the third decade of life.[7,14,50,52,54–56] Similar relationships may be seen in the femoral neck[14,51,54] and the entire skeleton.[51,54] However, radial DXA values in children have not been found to be influenced by puberty.[54]

Radiation exposure involved in DXA examinations is extremely low. The subject effective dose has been estimated to be about 1 μSv for lumbar spine measurements and about 4 μSv for whole skeleton scans.[57] In children, the precision of DXA measurements ranges from 0.8% to 2.5% in most studies.[46,48,50,56]

Several limitations of DXA must be stressed with reference to bone measurements during childhood, when major changes in body composition, body size, and skeletal mass occur. DXA is a projectional technique and its measurements are based on the two-dimensional projection of a three-dimensional structure. Thus, DXA values are a function of three skeletal parameters: the size of the bone being

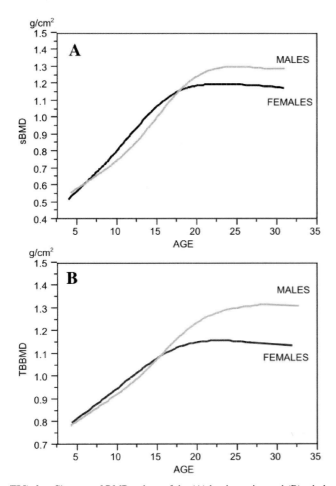

FIG. 2. Changes of BMD values of the (A) lumbar spine and (B) whole body with chronologic age. The acceleration during adolescence is followed by a plateau phase in early adulthood. DXA measurements performed in 319 healthy subjects (156 female, 163 male) from 4 to 32 years of age are shown. (Courtesy of Stefano Mora, MD, Milan, Italy.)

bone, changes in DXA measurements are observed if fat is distributed inhomogeneously around the bone measured. It has been calculated that inhomogeneous fat distribution in soft tissues, resulting in a difference of a 2-cm fat layer between soft tissue area and bone area, will influence DXA measurements by 10%.[64] While this is not of concern when studying subjects whose weight and body size remain constant, longitudinal DXA values in children are subject to considerable error, and measurements may reflect the changes in body size and composition that occur with growth more than true changes in bone density. This disadvantage especially limits the use of DXA in studies of children with eating disorders, such as obesity or anorexia nervosa.

QCT

QCT bone measurements can be obtained at any skeletal site with a standard clinical CT scanner using an external bone mineral reference phantom for calibration and specially developed software. The ability of QCT to assess both the volume and the density of bone in the axial and appendicular skeletons, without influence from body or skeletal size, is the major advantage of this modality when used in children. Unfortunately, CT scanners are expensive, large, nonportable machines that require costly maintenance and considerable technological expertise for proper function. Moreover, this equipment is usually located in the radiology department and is under constant clinical demand, creating a lack of accessibility. These disadvantages have partially been overcome by the recent development of smaller, mobile, less expensive peripheral QCT (pQCT) scanners designed exclusively for bone measurements. These smaller scanners, however, can only assess the bones of the appendicular skeleton.

The radiation exposure from QCT measurements is related to the technique used and can be as low as 150 mrem (1.5 mSv) localized to the region of interest in the appendicular or axial skeleton. The total body equivalent dose of radiation is approximately 4–9 mrems (40–90 μSv), and this figure includes the radiation associated with screening digital radiographs used to localize the site of measurement.[57,65] This amount of radiation is far lower than that associated with other CT imaging procedures, accounting for the wide range of published figures for the radiation dose associated with CT measurements. It is also less than many other commonly used radiographic diagnostic tests.

In the axial skeleton, QCT has principally been used to determine cancellous bone density (mg/cm^3) in the vertebral bodies, and less frequently, the dimensions of the vertebrae (Fig. 3). It should be noted that because the vertebrae of children contains proportionally more bone and less fat than that of elderly subjects, both the precision and accuracy of QCT cancellous bone density determinations in children are far better than that reported for adults. Coefficients of variation for determinations of cancellous bone density, vertebral body height, and vertebral cross-sectional area have been calculated as 1.5%, 1.3%, and 0.8%, respectively.[25] Unfortunately, the cortical bone in the vertebral body is not thick enough to avoid inaccuracies associated to bone averaging errors.

In the appendicular skeleton, three bone parameters can

examined, the volume of the bone, and its mineral density.[58] These values are frequently expressed as measurements of the bone content per surface area (g/cm^2), as determined by scan radiographs. However, scan radiographs only provide an approximation of the size of the bone and any correction based on these radiographs is only a very rough estimate of the "density." Attempts to overcome this disadvantage with the use of correction factors, that is, the squared root of the projected area, the height of the subject, the width of the bone, assuming the cross-sectional area of the vertebrae is a cube,[55,58,59] a cylinder with a circular base,[53,60] or a cylinder with an elliptic base area,[61] are subject to error, because there is no closed formula that defines the shape of the vertebrae. Similarly, although correction formulas have been proposed for the femur and the mid-radius,[53,56,62,63] they are also prone to error, because they cannot account for the marked changes in the size, as well as the shape, of the bone during growth.

Inaccuracies in DXA values can also result from the unknown composition of the soft tissues adjacent to the bone being analyzed. Because corrections for soft tissues are based on a homogenous distribution of fat around the

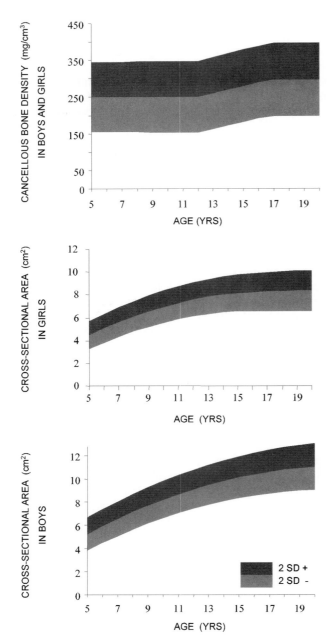

FIG. 3. Normative data for vertebral cancellous bone density and cross-sectional area in children and adolescents. Values for bone density are similar for boys and girls, while those for cross-sectional area differ.

be measured by QCT, the cross-sectional area (cm²) of the bone, the cortical bone area (cm²), and the cortical bone density.[66,67] To this effect, the outer and inner boundaries of the cortex are identified by specially developed software at the place of the maximum slope of the profile through the bone. The area within the outer cortical shell represents the cross-sectional area, while the area between the outer and inner shells represents the cortical bone area. The mean CT numbers of the pixels within the inner and outer cortical shells provide the average density of the bone. The coefficients of variation for repeated QCT measurements of cortical bone density, cortical bone area, and cross-sectional area of the femur range between 0.6% and 1.5%.[27,66,67]

Unfortunately, the reproducibility of measurements of cancellous bone density is poor because of the large anatomical variability of the metaphysis of the long bone.

ENVIRONMENTAL AND HORMONAL INFLUENCE ON BONE ACCUMULATION DURING GROWTH

Physical Activity

The beneficial effects of exercise on bone mass are well documented through multiple observational and retrospective studies indicating that weight bearing activities increase bone mass. Studies of prepubertal female gymnasts showed a larger cross-sectional area of the forearm, despite a shorter stature,[68] and areal BMD values expressed as SD scores were significantly greater than zero (the predicted mean of the controls) in the arms, legs, and spine, all weight-bearing sites.[68] In other studies, children and adolescents who were physically active accrued more bone mineral than their sedentary peers,[2,69] and a more recent study demonstrated that physical activity levels measured by accelerometry and parental report were positively associated with total body BMC and BMD measurements in preschool children.[70]

Studies comparing the effects of different physical exercises on bone indicated that high-impact exercises resulted in the greatest increases in bone mass in adolescents.[71] Similarly, gymnasts had higher spine and femur BMD than swimmers or sedentary girls.[72] Amateur athletes involved in weight-bearing sports (rugby, soccer, endurance running, fighting sports, bodybuilding) had higher values for total body and legs BMD than amateur sportsmen involved in active loading activities (swimming, rowing).[73]

Several randomized trials involving weight-bearing activity interventions for bone mass gains have been conducted in children and adolescents.[74–79] Exercise session attendance ranged from 50% to 97%; exercise adherence is therefore a potentially serious threat to the internal validity of the results. However, the most recent studies showed very high rates of adherence. With one exception at 36+ months,[74] the duration of the interventions was 6–12 months. All studies reported significant changes in femoral BMD, and four studies indicated increases in lumbar spine BMD and BMC in the intervention groups.

Whether the beneficial effect of physical activity on the growing skeleton is maintained in adulthood is unknown, because no prospective study has been designed to address this question. However, the results of most, but not all, retrospective analyses indicate that, indeed, the enhancement of bone acquisition during growth caused by exercise interventions may be long lasting. Lifetime tennis players, playing at a lower level of intensity then during youth, have remarkably higher forearm mineral content than control subjects.[80] Retired soccer players have high BMD during the first 10–20 years after cessation of sport, but their BMD is lower compared with active players.[81] Other studies suggest that BMD values are maintained at about 0.5–1.0 SD above the age-predicted mean in athletes who have been retired for 10–20 years.[68,82–84] Peri- and postmenopausal women who participated in sport activities during adolescence showed BMD measurements at the lumbar spine and femur that were remarkably higher than those of women who did not participate in physical activities during youth.[85] In a recent follow-up study of 27 years, lifetime physical activity was related to adult BMD, indicating the importance of continuing exercise after growth.[86] In contrast, a decrease in spinal BMD has been reported in runners who ceased exercising.[87] Similarly, cessation of exercise led to the return of BMD values to pretraining levels in 12 women who performed unilateral leg press for 1 year.[88]

Calcium Intake

The earliest data suggesting an influence of dietary calcium on PBM come from a study of two Croatian populations with substantially different calcium intakes.[89] The differences seen in bone mass were present at 30 years of age, suggesting that the effects of dietary calcium probably occurred during growth rather than in adulthood. Moreover, some epidemiological studies have shown an increased prevalence of osteoporosis in regions where dietary calcium intake is extremely low.[90]

The most convincing evidence that calcium consumption influences rates of bone mineral accrual rates comes from controlled supplementation trials in young healthy subjects. These studies showed that subjects given additional calcium for 1–3 years had greater gains than did controls.[91–96] Although bone size increased as a result of added dietary calcium in two studies,[91,95] the response to calcium varied with skeletal site, pretreatment calcium consumption, and pubertal stage. Greater bone mineral gains have been generally reported at cortical skeletal sites in prepubertal subjects and in girls whose habitual dietary intake was less than 850 mg per day.[95]

Whether short-term increases in bone mineral observed in these trials will translate into a clinically relevant reduction in osteoporosis risk is yet unknown. The magnitude of gains in BMC or BMD in most studies was modest; less than 5%. Moreover, the beneficial effect of calcium supplementation does not seem to last and most studies reported that the benefits of intervention disappeared once the treatment was stopped. However, in other studies the benefits persisted 12 months after discontinuation of supplement.

Hormonal Status

The presence of low bone mass in patients with abnormal pubertal development show the critical role that pubertal hormone changes have on mineral acquisition. Adult patients with hypogonadotropic hypogonadism commonly have low BMD values, resulting from inadequate bone mineral accrual during puberty.[97] Androgen receptors mediate the effects of testosterone in bone but their function is generally exerted after conversion to estrogen by a specific aromatase present in osteoblastic cells.[98] Thus, the more important sex steroid involved in skeletal maturation is estrogen.[99] Amenorrheic teens have lower lumbar bone density than girls with normal menses.[100] In addition, male patients with aromatase deficiency, or estrogen receptor defects resulting in complete resistance, have a phenotype that includes tall stature, normal secondary sexual characteristics, severe osteoporosis, and skeletal immaturity (delayed physeal closure), despite normal serum levels of tes-

tosterone.[101,102] Idiopathic delayed puberty has also been implicated as a cause of reduced peak bone mass.[103]

The effect that pregnancy and lactation have on bone acquisition in teenagers is yet to be fully defined. Normal pregnancy places a demand on calcium homeostasis, because the fetus and the placenta draw calcium from the maternal circulation to mineralize the fetal skeleton, and low BMD has been reported during pregnancy. Whether pregnancy during adolescence negatively influences bone density and PBM is a subject of great importance and is yet to be elucidated.

Reduced bone density is commonly seen in growth hormone (GH)-deficient children who fail to acquire bone mineral at the expected rate.[104,105] Part of the bone mass deficit in these patients is because of reduced bone size. Much of the GH action on bone is mediated through IGF-I, which functions as a bone trophic hormone that positively affects osteoblasts, and stimulates collagen synthesis. In humans, IGF-I serum levels have been found to be positively correlated to bone size measured at the midshaft of the femur.[106]

SUMMARY

Skeletal mass is accrued throughout childhood and adolescence and is largely determined by genetic and/or familial factors. A child's sex affects bone mass after puberty, while many ethnic differences seem to be present throughout growth. The influence of gonadal steroids is of major importance during puberty, while many factors such as other hormonal influences, physical activity type and intensity, and dietary calcium intake affect bone acquisition throughout growth. Bone mass measurements such as DXA and CT, while limited in some respects for pediatric applications, can be very important in assessing a child's skeletal status and growth.

REFERENCES

1. Trotter M, Hixon BB 1974 Sequential changes in weight, density, and percentage ash weight of human skeletons from an early fetal period through old age. Anat Rec **179:**1–18.
2. Bailey DA, McKay HA, Mirwald RL, Crocker PR, Faulkner RA 1999 A six-year longitudinal study of the relationship of physical activity to bone mineral accrual in growing children: The University of Saskatchewan bone mineral accrual study. J Bone Miner Res **14:**1672–1679.
3. Riggs BL, Wahner HW, Dunn WL, Mazess RB, Offord KP, Mellon LJ 1981 Differential changes in bone mineral density of the appendicular skeleton with aging. J Clin Invest **67:**328–335.
4. Mora S, Goodman WG, Loro ML, Roe TF, Sayre J, Gilsanz V 1994 Age-related changes in cortical and cancellous vertebral bone density in girls: Assessment with quantitative CT. AJR Am J Roentgenol **162:**405–409.
5. Gilsanz V, Gibbens DT, Carlson M, Boechat MI, Cann CE, Schulz EE 1988 Peak trabecular vertebral density: A comparison of adolescent and adult females. Calcif Tissue Int **43:**260–262.
6. Mauras N, Haymond MW, Darmaun D, Vieira NE, Abrams SA, Yergey A 1994 Calcium and protein kinetics in prepubertal boys - positive effects of testosterone. J Clin Invest **93:**1014–1019.
7. Theintz G, Buchs B, Rizzoli R, Slosman D, Clavien H, Sizonenko PC, Bonjour JP 1992 Longitudinal monitoring of bone mass accumulation in healthy adolescents: Evidence for a marked reduction after 16 years of age at the levels of lumbar spine and femoral neck in female subjects. J Clin Endocrinol Metab **75:**1060–1065.
8. Marcus R, Kosen J, Pfefferbaum A, Horning A 1983 Age-related loss

of trabecular bone in premenopausal women: A biopsy study. Calcif Tiss Int **35**:406–409.

9. Mosekilde L 1989 Sex differences in age-related loss of vertebral trabecular bone mass and structure - biomechanical consequences. Bone **10**:425–432.

10. Halioua L, Anderson JJB 1990 Age and anthropometric determinants of radial bone mass in premenopausal Caucasian women: A cross-sectional study. Osteoporos Int **1**:50–55.

11. Gordon CL, Halton JM, Atkinson S, Webber CE 1991 The contributions of growth and puberty to peak bone mass. Growth Dev Aging **55**:257–262.

12. Recker RR, Davies KM, Hinders SM, Heaney RP, Stegman MR, Kimmel DB 1992 Bone gain in young adult women. JAMA **268**:2403–2408.

13. Matkovic V, Jelic T, Wardlaw GM, Ilich JZ, Goel PK, Wright JK, Andon MB, Smith KT, Heaney RP 1994 Timing of peak bone mass in Caucasian females and its implication for the prevention of osteoporosis. J Clin Invest **93**:799–808.

14. Bonjour JP, Theintz G, Buchs B, Slosman B, Rizzoli R 1991 Critical years and stages of puberty for spinal and femoral bone mass accumulation during adolescence. J Clin Endocrinol Metab **73**:555–563.

15. Christian JC, Yu PL, Slemenda CW, Johnston CC 1989 Heritability of bone mass: A longitudinal study in ageing male twins. Am J Hum Genet **44**:429–433.

16. Pocock NA, Eisman JA, Hopper JL, Yeates MG, Sambrook PN, Ebert S 1991 Genetic determinants of bone mass in adults: A twin study. J Clin Invest **80**:706–710.

17. Seeman E, Hopper JL, Bach LA, Cooper ME, Parkinson E, McKay J, Jerums G 1989 Reduced bone mass in daughters of women with osteoporosis. N Engl J Med **320**:554–558.

18. Slemenda CW, Christian JC, Williams CJ, Norton JA, Johnston CC Jr 1991 Genetic determinants of bone mass in adult women: A reevaluation of the twin model and the potential importance of gene interaction on heritability estimates. J Bone Miner Res **6**:561–567.

19. Evans RA, Marel GH, Lancaster EK, Kos S, Evans M, Wong YP 1988 Bone mass is low in relatives of osteoporotic patients. Ann Intern Med **109**:870–873.

20. Ferrari SL, Rizzoli R, Slosman DO, Bonjour JP 1998 Do dietary calcium and age explain the controversy surrounding the relationship between bone mineral density and vitamin D receptor gene polymorphism? J Bone Miner Res **13**:363–370.

21. Ferrari SL, Rizzoli R, Manen D, Slosman DA, Bonjour JP 1998 Vitamin D receptor gene start codon polymorphisms (*Fok*I) and bone mineral density: Interaction with age, dietary calcium, and 3'-end region polymorphisms. J Bone Miner Res **13**:925–930.

22. Sainz J, Van Tornout JM, Loro ML, Sayre J, Roe TF, Gilsanz V 1997 Vitamin D receptor gene polymorphisms and bone density in prepubertal girls. N Engl J Med **337**:77–82.

23. Sainz J, Van Tornout JM, Sayre J, Kaufman F, Gilsanz V 1999 Association of collagen type 1 α1 gene polymorphism with bone density in early childhood. J Clin Endocrinol Metab **84**:853–855.

24. Gunnes M, Berg JP, Hasle J, Lehmann EH 1997 Lack of relationship between vitamin D receptor genotype and forearm bone gain in healthy children, adolescents, and young adults. J Clin Endocrinol Metab **82**:851–855.

25. Gilsanz V, Boechat MI, Roe TF, Loro ML, Sayre JW, Goodman WG 1994 Gender differences in vertebral body sizes in children and adolescents. Radiology **190**:673–677.

26. Gilsanz V, Boechat MI, Gilsanz R, Loro ML, Roe TF, Goodman WG 1994 Gender differences in vertebral sizes in adults: Biomechanical implications. Radiology **190**:678–682.

27. Gilsanz V, Kovanlikaya A, Costin G, Roe TF, Sayre J, Kaufman F 1997 Differential effect of gender on the size of the bones in the axial and appendicular skeletons. J Clin Endocrinol Metab **82**:1603–1607.

28. Van der Meulen MCH, Beaupre GS, Carter DR 1993 Mechanobiologic influences in long bone cross-sectional growth. Bone **14**:635–642.

29. Nguyen TV, Maynard LM, Towne B, Roche AF, Wisemandle W, Li J, Guo SS, Chumlea WC, Siervogel R 2001 Sex differences in bone mass acquisition during growth. J Clin Densitom **4**:147–157.

30. Nelson DA, Simpson PM, Johnson CC, Barondess DA, Kleerekoper M 1997 The accumulation of whole body skeletal mass in third- and fourth-grade children: Effects of age, gender, ethnicity and body composition. Bone Miner **20**:73–78.

31. Bell NH, Shary J, Stevens J, Garza M, Gordon L, Edwards J 1991 Demonstration that bone mass is greater in black than in white children. J Bone Miner Res **6**:719–723.

32. Laraque D, Arena I, Karp J, Gruskay D 1990 Bone mineral content in black pre-schoolers: Normative data using single photon absorptiometry. Pediatr Radiol **20**:461–463.

33. Li JY, Specker BL, Ho ML, Tsang RC 1989 Bone mineral content in black and white children 1 to 6 years of age. Early appearance of race and sex differences. Am J Dis Child **143**:1346–1349.

34. Thomas KA, Cook SD, Bennett JT, Whitecloud TSHI, Rice JC 1991 Femoral neck and lumbar spine mineral densities in a normal population 3–20 years of age. J Pediatr Orthop **11**:48–58.

35. Prentice A, Laskey MA, Shaw J, Cole TJ, Fraser DR 1990 Bone mineral content of Gambian and British children aged 0–36 months. Bone Miner **10**:211–224.

36. Patel DN, Pettifor JM, Becker PJ, Grieve C, Leschner K 1992 The effect of ethnic group on appendicular bone mass in children. J Bone Miner Res **7**:263–272.

37. Southard RN, Morris JD, Mahan JD, Hayes JR, Torch MA, Sommer A, Zipf WB 1991 Bone mass in healthy children: Measurements with quantitative DXA. Radiology **179**:735–738.

38. Gilsanz V, Skaggs DL, Kovanlikaya A, Sayre J, Loro ML, Kaufman F, Korenman SG 1998 Differential effect of race on the axial and appendicular skeletons of children. J Clin Endocrinol Metab **83**:1420–1427.

39. Kleerekoper M, Nelson DA, Flynn MJ, Pawluszka AS, Jacobsen G, Peterson EL 1994 Comparison of radiographic absorptiometry with dual energy x-ray absorptiometry and quantitative computed tomography in normal older white and black women. J Bone Miner Res **9**:1745–1750.

40. Bachrach LK, Hastie T, Wang MC, Balasubramanian N, Marcus R 1999 Bone mineral acquisition in healthy asian, hispanic, black, and caucasian youth: A longitudinal study. J Clin Endocrinol Metab **84**:4702–4712.

41. Horlick MB, Rosenbaum M, Nicolson M, Levine LS, Fedun B, Wang J, Pierson RN Jr, Leibel RL 2000 Effect of puberty on the relationship between circulating leptin and body composition. J Clin Endocrinol Metab **85**:2509–2518.

42. Ferrari S, Rizzoli R, Slosman D, Bonjour JP 1998 Familial resemblance for bone mineral mass is expressed before puberty. J Clin Endocrinol Metab **83**:358–361.

43. Loro ML, Sayre J, Roe TF, Goran MI, Kaufman FR, Gilsanz V 2000 Early identification of children predisposed to low peak bone mass and osteoporosis later in life. J Clin Endocrinol Metab **85**:3908–3918.

44. Koo WWK, Massom LR, Walters J 1995 Validation of accuracy and precision of dual energy x-ray absorptiometry for infants. J Bone Miner Res **10**:1111–1115.

45. Nelson DA, Koo WK 1995 Interpretation of bone mass measurements in the growing skeleton. Calcif Tissue Int **65**:1–3.

46. Braillon PM, Salle BL, Brunet J, Glorieux FH, Delmas PD, Meunier PJ 1992 Dual energy x-ray absorptiometry measurement of bone mineral content in newborns: Validation of the technique. Pediatr Res **32**:77–80.

47. Lapillonne AA, Glorieux FH, Salle BL, Braillon PM, Chambon M, Rigo J, Putet G, Senterre J 1994 Mineral balance and whole body bone mineral content in very low-birth-weight infants. Acta Paediatr Suppl **405**:117–122.

48. Koo WW, Walters J, Bush AJ 1995 Technical considerations of dual-energy x-ray absorptiometry-based bone mineral measurements for pediatric subjects. J Bone Miner Res **10**:1998–2004.

49. Rupich RC, Specker BL, Lieuw-A-Fa M, Ho M 1996 Gender and race differences in bone mass during infancy. Calcif Tissue Int **58**:395–397.

50. del Rio L, Carrascosa A, Pons F, Gusinyé M, Yeste D, Domenech F 1994 Bone mineral density of the lumbar spine in white Mediterranean Spanish children and adolescents: Changes related to age, sex, and puberty. Pediatr Res **35**:362–366.

51. Faulkner RA, Bailey DA, Drinkwater DT, McKay HA, Arnold C, Wilkinson AA 1996 Bone densitometry in Canadian children. Calcif Tissue Int **59**:344–351.

52. Glastre C, Braillon P, David L, Cochat P, Meunier PJ, Delmas PD 1990 Measurement of bone mineral content of the lumbar spine by dual energy x-ray absorptiometry in normal children: Correlations with growth parameters. J Clin Endocrinol Metab **70**:1330–1333.

53. Kröger H, Kotaniemi A, Vainio P, Alhava E 1992 Bone densitometry of the spine and femur in children by dual-energy x-ray absorptiometry. Bone Miner **17**:75–85.

54. Zanchetta JR, Plotkin H, Alvarez-Filgueira ML 1995 Bone mass in children: Normative values for the 2–20-year-old population. Bone **14**:3S–39S.

55. Katzman DK, Bachrach LK, Carter DR, Marcus R 1991 Clinical and

anthropometric correlates of bone mineral acquisition in healthy adolescent girls. J Clin Endocrinol (Oxf) Metab **73**:1332–1339.

56. Kröger H, Kotaniemi A, Kröger L, Alhava E 1993 Development of bone mass and bone density of the spine and femoral neck - a prospective study of 65 children and adolescents. Bone **23**:171–182.

57. Kalender WA 1992 Effective dose values in bone mineral measurements by photon absorptiometry and computed tomography. Osteoporos Int **2**:82–87.

58. Carter DR, Bouxsein ML, Marcus R 1992 New approaches for interpreting projected bone densitometry data. J Bone Miner Res **7**:137–145.

59. Jergas M, Breitenseher M, Gluer CC, Genant HK 1995 Estimates of volumetric bone density from projectional measurements improve the discriminatory capability of dual x-ray absorptiometry. J Bone Miner Res **10**:1101–1110.

60. Salle BL, Braillon P, Glorieux FG, Brunet J, Cavero E, Meunier PJ 1992 Lumbar bone mineral content measured by dual energy X-ray absorptiometry in newborns and infants. Acta Paediatr **81**:953–958.

61. Peel NFA, Eastell R 1994 Diagnostic value of estimated volumetric bone mineral density of the lumbar spine in osteoporosis. J Bone Miner Res **9**:317–320.

62. Lu PW, Cowell CT, Lloyd-Jones SA, Briody JN, Howman-Giles R 1996 Volumetric bone mineral density in normal subjects, aged 5–27 years. J Clin Endocrinol Metab **81**:1586–1590.

63. Moro M, van der Meulen MCH, Kiratli BJ, Marcus R, Bachrach LK, Carter DR 1996 Body mass is the primary determinant of midfemoral bone acquisition during adolescent growth. Bone Miner **19**:519–526.

64. Hangartner TN 1990 Influence of fat on bone measurements with dual-energy absorptiometry. Bone Miner **9**:71–78.

65. Cann CE 1991 Why, when and how to measure bone mass: A guide for the beginning user. In: Frey GD, Yester MV (ed.) Expanding the Role of Medical Physics in Nuclear Medicine. American Physics Institute, Washington, DC, USA, pp. 250–279.

66. Hangartner TN, Gilsanz V 1996 Evaluation of cortical bone by computed tomography. J Bone Miner Res **11**:1518–1525.

67. Kovanlikaya A, Loro ML, Hangartner TN, Reynolds RA, Roe TF, Gilsanz V 1996 Osteopenia in children: CT assessment. Radiology **198**:781–784.

68. Bass S, Pearce G, Bradney M, Hendrich E, Delmas PD, Harding A, Seeman E 1998 Exercise before puberty may confer residual benefits in bone density in adulthood: Studies in active prepubertal and retired female gymnasts. J Bone Miner Res **13**:500–507.

69. Cooper C, Cawley M, Bhalla A, Egger P, Ring F, Morton L, Barker D 1995 Childhood growth, physical activity, and peak bone mass in women. J Bone Miner Res **10**:940–947.

70. Janz KF, Burns TL, Torner JC, Levy SM, Paulos R, Willing MC, Warren JJ 2001 Physical activity and bone measures in young children: The Iowa bone development study. Pediatrics **107**:1387–1393.

71. Lima F, DeFalco V, Baima J, Carazzato JG, Pereira RM 2001 Effect of impact load and active load on bone metabolism and body composition of adolescent athletes. Med Sci Sports Exerc **33**:1318–1323.

72. Courteix D, Lespessailles E, Peres SL, Obert P, Germain P, Benhamou CL 1998 Effect of physical training on bone mineral density in prepubertal girls: A comparative study between impact-loading and non-impact-loading sports. Osteoporos Int **8**:152–158.

73. Morel J, Combe B, Francisco J, Bernard J 2001 Bone mineral density of 704 amateur sportsmen involved in different physical activities. Osteoporos Int **12**:152–157.

74. Sundberg M, Gardsell P, Johnell O, Karlsson MK, Ornstein E, Sandstedt B, Sernbo I 2001 Peripubertal moderate exercise increases bone mass in boys but not in girls: A population-based intervention study. Osteoporos Int **12**:230–238.

75. Petit MA, McKay HA, MacKelvie KJ, Heinonen A, Khan KM, Beck TJ 2002 A randomized school-based jumping intervention confers site and maturity specific benefits on bone structural properties in girls: A hip structural analysis study. J Bone Miner Res **17**:363–372.

76. Heinonen H, Sievanen H, Kannus P, Oja P, Pasanen M, Vuori I 2000 High-impact exercise and bones in growing girls: A 9-month controlled trial. Osteoporos Int **11**:1010–1017.

77. Fuchs RK, Buauer JJ, Snow CM 2001 Jumping improves hip and lumbar spine bone mass in prepubescent children: A randomized controlled trial. J Bone Miner Res **16**:148–156.

78. Bradney M, Pearce G, Naughton G, Sullivan C, Bass S, Beck T, Carlson J, Seeman E 1998 Moderate exercise during growth in prepubertal boys: Changes in bone mass, size, volumetric density, and bone strength. A controlled prospective study. J Bone Miner Res **13**:1814–1821.

79. Morris FL, Naughton GA, Gibbs JL, Carlson JS, Wark JD 1997 Prospective ten-month exercise intervention in premenarcheal girls: Positive effects on bone and lean mass. J Bone Miner Res **12**:1453–1462.

80. Huddleston AL, Rockwell D, Kulund DN, Harrison RB 1980 Bone mass in lifetime tennis athletes. JAMA **244**:1107–1109.

81. Karlsson MK, Linden C, Karlsson C, Johnell O, Obrant K, Seeman E 2000 Exercise during growth and bone mineral density and fractures in old age. Lancet **355**:469–470.

82. Khan KM, Grren RM, Saul A, Bennell KL, Crichton KJ, Hopper JL 1996 Retired elite female ballet dancers and nonathletic controls have similar bone mineral density at weight bearing sites. J Bone Miner Res **11**:1566–1574.

83. Karlsson MK, Hasserius R, Obrant KJ 1996 Bone mineral density in athletes during and after career: A comparison between loaded and unloaded skeletal regions. Calcif Tissue Int **59**:245–248.

84. Etherington J, Harris PA, Nandra D, Hart DJ, Wolman RL, Doyle DV, Spector TD 1996 The effect of weight-bearing exercise on bone mineral density: A study of female ex-elite athletes and the general population. J Bone Miner Res **11**:1333–1338.

85. Puntila E, Kroger H, Lakke T, Honkanen R, Tupperainen M 1997 Physical activity in adolescence and bone density in peri- and postmenopausal women: A population based study. Bone **21**:363–367.

86. Delvaux K, Lefevre J, Philippaerts R, Dequeker J, Thomis M, Vanreusel B, Claessens A, Eynde BV, Beunen G, Lysens R 2001 Bone mass and lifetime physical activity in Flemish males: A 27 year follow-up study. Med Sci Sports Exerc **33**:1868–1875.

87. Michel BA, Lane NE, Bjorkengren A, Bloch DA, Fries JF 1992 Impact of running on lumbar bone density: A 5-year longitudinal study. J Rheumatol **19**:1759–1763.

88. Vuori I, Heinonen A, Sievanan H, Kannus P, Pasanen M, Oja P 1994 Effect of unilateral strength training and detraining on bone mineral density and content in young women: A study of mechanical loading and deloading on human bones. Calcif Tissue Int **55**:59–67.

89. Matkovic V, Kostial K, Simonovic I, Buzinz R, Brodarec A, Nordin BE 1979 Bone status and fracture rates in two regions of Yugoslavia. Am J Clin Nutr **32**:540–549.

90. Heaney RP 1992 Calcium in the prevention and treatment of osteoporosis. J Intern Med **231**:169–180.

91. Lee WTK, Leung SSF, Leung DM, Cheng JC 1996 A follow-up study on the effects of calcium-supplement withdrawal and puberty on bone acquisition in children. Am J Clin Nutr **64**:71–77.

92. Lloyd T, Andon MB, Rollings N, Martel JK, Landis JR, Demers LM, Eggli DF, Kieselhorst K, Kulin HE 1993 Calcium supplementation and bone mineral density in adolescent girls. JAMA **270**:841–844.

93. Johnston CC Jr, Miller JZ, Slemenda CW, Reister TK, Hui S, Christian JC, Peacock M 1992 Calcium supplementation and increases in bone mineral density in children. N Engl J Med **327**:82–87.

94. Chan GM, Hoffman K, McMurry M 1995 Effects of dairy products on bone and body composition in pubertal girls. J Pediatr **126**:551–556.

95. Bonjour JP, Carrie AL, Ferrari S, Clavien H, Slosman D, Theintz G, Rizzoli 1997 Calcium-enriched foods and bone mass growth in prepubertal girls: A randomized double blind, placebo-controlled trial. J Clin Invest **99**:1287–1294.

96. Nowson CA, Green RM, Hopper JL, Sherwin AJ, Young D, Kaymakci B, Guest CS, Smid M, Larkins RG, Wark J 1997 A co-twin study of the effect of calcium supplementation on bone density during adolescence. Osetoporos Int **7**:219–225.

97. Finkelstein JS, Klibanski A, Neer RM, Greenspan SL, Rosenthal DI, Crowley WF Jr 1987 Osteoporosis in men with idiopathic hypogonadotropic hypogonadism. Ann Intern Med **106**:354–361.

98. Abu EO, Horner A, Kusec V, Triffitt JT, Compston JE 1997 The localization of androgen receptors in human bone. J Clin Endocrinol Metab **82**:3493–3497.

99. Frank GR 1995 The role of estrogen in pubertal skeletal physiology: Epiphyseal maturation and mineralization of the skeleton. Acta Paediatr **84**:627–630.

100. Hergenroeder AC 1995 Bone mineralization, hypothalamic amenorrhea, and sex steroid therapy in female adolescents and young adults. J Pediatr **126**:683–689.

101. Carani C, Qin K, Simoni M, Faustini-Fustini M, Serpente S, Boyd J, Korach KS, Simpson ER 1997 Effect of testosterone and estradiol in a man with aromatase deficiency. N Engl J Med **337**:91–95.

102. Smith EP, Boyd J, Frank GR, Takahashi H, Cohen RM, Specker B 1994 Estrogen resistance caused by a mutation in the estrogen-receptor gene in a man. N Engl J Med **331**:1056–1061.

103. Finkelstein JS, Klibanski A, Neer RM 1996 A longitudinal evaluation of bone mineral density in adult men with histories of delayed puberty. J Clin Endocrinol Metab **81:**1152–1155.
104. Boot AM, Engels MA, Boerma GJ, Krenning EP, DeMuinck Keizer-Schrama SM 1997 Changes in bone mineral density, body composition and lipid metabolism during growth hormone (GH) treatment in children with GH deficiency. J Clin Endocrinol Metab **82:**2423–2428.
105. Baroncelli GI, Bertelloni S, Ceccarelli C, Saggese G 1998 Measurement of volumetric bone mineral density accurately determines degree of lumbar undermineralization in children with growth hormone deficiency. J Clin Endocrinol Metab **83:**3150–3154.
106. Mora S, Pitukcheewanont P, Nelson JC, Gilsanz V 1999 Serum levels of insulin-like growth factor-I and the density, volume and cross-sectional area of bone in children. J Clin Endocrinol Metab **84:**2780–2783.

Chapter 11.   Skeletal Physiology: Pregnancy and Lactation

Christopher S. Kovacs[1] and Henry M. Kronenberg[2]

[1]*Faculty of Medicine, Endocrinology, Health Sciences Centre, Memorial University of Newfoundland, St. John's, Newfoundland, Canada; and* [2]*Endocrine Unit, Massachusetts General Hospital and Harvard Medical School, Boston, Massachusetts*

INTRODUCTION

Normal pregnancy places a demand on the calcium homeostatic mechanisms of the human female as the fetus and placenta draw calcium from the maternal circulation to mineralize the fetal skeleton. Similar demands are placed on the lactating woman, to supply sufficient calcium to the breast milk and enable continued skeletal growth in a nursing infant. Despite a similar magnitude of calcium demand presented to pregnant and lactating women, the adjustments made in each of these reproductive periods differ significantly (Fig. 1). These hormone-mediated adjustments normally satisfy the daily calcium needs of the fetus and infant without long-term consequences to the maternal skeleton. Detailed references on this subject are available in two comprehensive reviews.[1,2]

PREGNANCY

In total, the developing fetal skeleton gains up to 33 g of calcium, and about 80% of the accretion occurs during the third trimester, when the fetal skeleton is rapidly mineralizing. This calcium demand seems to be largely met by a doubling of maternal intestinal calcium absorption, mediated by 1,25-dihydroxyvitamin D and other factors.

Mineral Ions and Calcitropic Hormones

Normal pregnancy results in altered levels of calcium and the calcitropic hormones as schematically depicted in Fig. 2.[1] The total serum calcium falls early in pregnancy because of a fall in the serum albumin. This decrease should not be mistaken for true hypocalcemia, because the ionized calcium (the physiologically important fraction) remains constant. Serum phosphate levels are also normal during pregnancy.

The serum parathyroid hormone (PTH) level, when measured with a two-site immunoradiometric assay (IRMA), falls to the low-normal range (i.e., 10–30% of the mean nonpregnant value) during the first trimester, but increases

steadily to the mid-normal range by term. Total 1,25-dihydroxyvitamin D levels double early in pregnancy and maintain this increase until term; free 1,25-dihydroxyvitamin D levels are increased from the third trimester and possibly earlier. The rise in 1,25-dihydroxyvitamin D may be largely independent of changes in PTH, because PTH levels are typically decreasing at the time of the increase in 1,25-dihydroxyvitamin D. The maternal kidneys likely account for most, if not all, of the rise in 1,25-dihydroxyvitamin D during pregnancy, although the decidua, placenta, and fetal kidneys may contribute a small amount. The relative contribution of the maternal kidneys is based on several lines of evidence,[1] including the report of an anephric woman on hemodialysis who had low 1,25-dihydroxyvitamin D levels before and during a pregnancy. The renal 1α-hydroxylase is upregulated in response to factors such as PTH-related protein (PTHrP), estradiol, prolactin, and placental lactogen.

Serum calcitonin levels are also increased during pregnancy. It has been speculated that this increased level of calcitonin reflects its postulated role in protecting the ma-

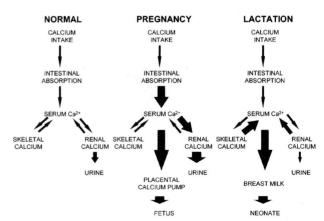

FIG. 1. Schematic illustration contrasting calcium homeostasis in human pregnancy and lactation compared with normal. The thickness of arrows indicates a relative increase or decrease with respect to the normal and nonpregnant state. (Reprinted with permission of The Endocrine Society from Kovacs CS, Kronenberg HM 1997 Maternal-fetal calcium and bone metabolism during pregnancy, puerperium and lactation. Endocr Rev **18:** 832–872.)

The authors have no conflict of interest.

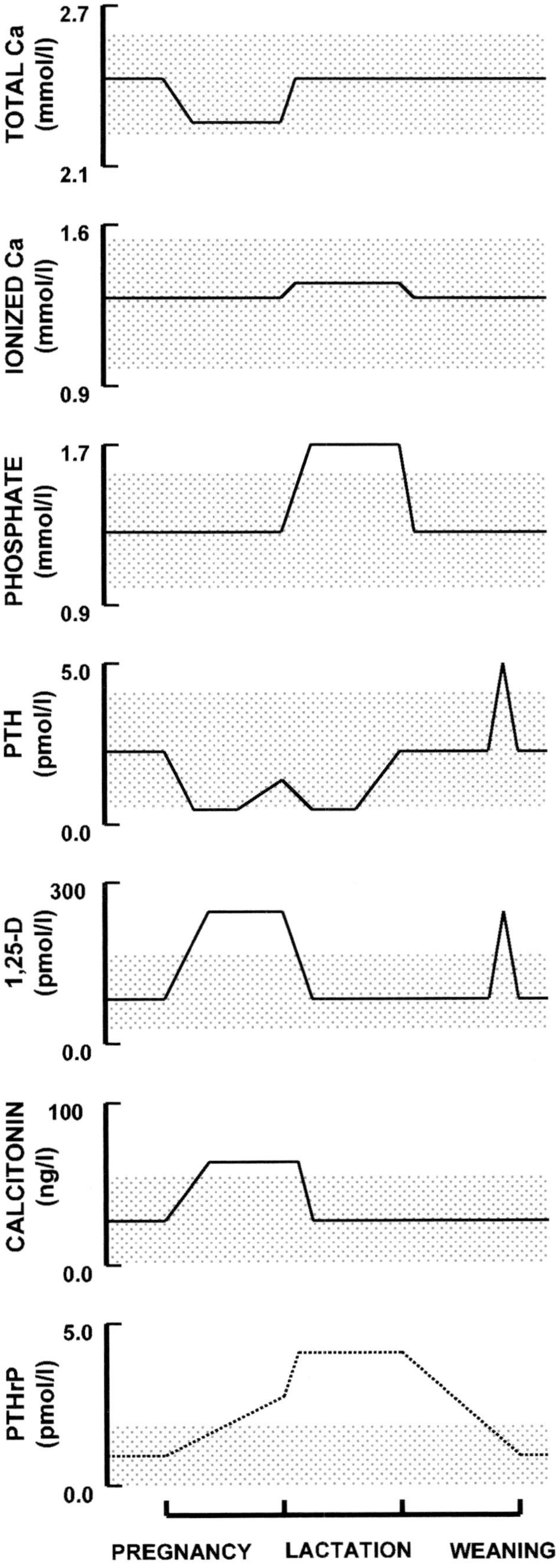

ternal skeleton from excessive resorption of calcium, but this hypothesis remains unproved.

PTHrP levels are increased during pregnancy, as determined by assays that detect PTHrP fragments encompassing amino acids 1–86. Because PTHrP is produced by many tissues in the fetus and mother (including the placenta, amnion, decidua, umbilical cord, fetal parathyroids, and breast), it is not clear which source(s) contribute to the rise detected in the maternal circulation. PTHrP may contribute to the elevations in 1,25-dihydroxyvitamin D and suppression of PTH that are noted during pregnancy. PTHrP may have other roles during pregnancy, such as regulating placental calcium transport in the fetus.[1,3] Also, PTHrP may have a role in protecting the maternal skeleton during pregnancy, because the carboxy-terminal portion of PTHrP ("osteostatin") has been shown to inhibit osteoclastic bone resorption.[4]

Pregnancy induces significant changes in the levels of other hormones, including the sex steroids, prolactin, placental lactogen, and insulin-like growth factor (IGF)-1. Each of these may have direct or indirect effects on calcium and bone metabolism during pregnancy, but these issues have been largely unexplored.

Intestinal Absorption of Calcium

Intestinal absorption of calcium is doubled during pregnancy from as early as 12 weeks of gestation (the earliest time-point studied); this seems to be a major maternal adaptation to meet the fetal need for calcium. This increase may be largely the result of a 1,25-dihydroxyvitamin D–mediated increase in intestinal calbindin$_{9K}$-D and other proteins; prolactin and placental lactogen (and possibly other factors) may also mediate part of the increase in intestinal calcium absorption. The increased absorption of calcium early in pregnancy may allow the maternal skeleton to store calcium in advance of the peak fetal demands that occur later in pregnancy.

Renal Handling of Calcium

The 24-h urine calcium excretion is increased as early as the 12th week of gestation (the earliest time-point studied), and the amounted excreted may exceed the normal range. The elevated calcitonin levels of pregnancy might also promote renal calcium excretion. Because fasting urine calcium values are normal or low, the increase in 24-h urine calcium likely reflects the increased intestinal absorption of calcium (absorptive hypercalciuria).

FIG. 2. Schematic illustration of the longitudinal changes in calcium, phosphate, and calcitropic hormone levels that occur during pregnancy and lactation. Normal adult ranges are indicated by the shaded areas. The progression in PTHrP levels has been depicted by a dashed line to reflect that the data are less complete; the implied comparison of PTHrP levels in late pregnancy and lactation are uncertain extrapolations because no reports followed patients serially. In both situations, PTHrP levels are elevated. (Adapted with permission of The Endocrine Society from Kovacs CS, Kronenberg HM 1997 Maternal-fetal calcium and bone metabolism during pregnancy, puerperium and lactation. Endocr Rev **18**:832–872.)

© 2003 American Society for Bone and Mineral Research

Skeletal Calcium Metabolism

Animal models indicate that histomorphometric parameters of bone turnover are increased during pregnancy, but comparable histomorphometric data are not available for human pregnancy. In one study,[5] 15 women who electively terminated a pregnancy in the first trimester (8–10 weeks) had bone biopsy evidence of increased bone resorption, including increased resorption surface, increased numbers of resorption cavities, and decreased osteoid. These findings were not present in biopsy specimens obtained from non-pregnant controls or in biopsy specimens obtained at term from 13 women who had elective C-sections.

Most human studies of skeletal calcium metabolism in pregnancy have examined changes in serum markers of bone formation and urine markers of bone resorption. These studies are fraught with a number of confounding variables, including lack of prepregnancy baseline values; effects of hemodilution in pregnancy on serum markers; increased glomerular filtration rate (GFR) and renal clearance; altered creatinine excretion; placental, uterine, and fetal contribution to the markers; degradation and clearance by the placenta; and lack of diurnally timed or fasted specimens. Given these limitations, many studies have reported that urinary markers of bone resorption (24-h collection) are increased from early to mid-pregnancy (including deoxy-pyridinoline, pyridinoline, and hydroxyproline). Conversely, serum markers of bone formation (generally not corrected for hemodilution or increased GFR) are often decreased from prepregnancy or nonpregnant values in early or mid-pregnancy, rising to normal or above before term (including osteocalcin, procollagen I carboxypeptides, and bone specific alkaline phosphatase). It is conceivable that the bone formation markers are artifactually lowered by normal hemodilution and increased renal clearance of pregnancy, obscuring any real increase in the level of the markers. Total alkaline phosphatase rises early in pregnancy largely because of contributions from the placental fraction; it is not a useful marker of bone formation in pregnancy.

Based on the scant bone biopsy data and the measurements of bone markers (with aforementioned confounding factors), one may cautiously conclude that bone turnover is increased in pregnancy, from as early as the 10th week of gestation. There is comparatively little maternal-fetal calcium transfer occurring at this stage of pregnancy compared with the peak rate of calcium transfer in the third trimester. One might have anticipated that markers of bone turnover would increase particularly in the third trimester, but in fact, no marked increase is seen at that time.

Changes in skeletal calcium content have been assessed through the use of sequential bone density studies during pregnancy. Because of concerns about fetal radiation exposure, few such studies have been done. Such studies are confounded by the changes in body composition and weight during normal pregnancy that can lead to artifactual changes in the bone density reading obtained. Using single and/or dual-photon absorptiometry, several prospective studies did not find a significant change in cortical or trabecular bone density during pregnancy.[1] Three recent studies have used DXA before conception and after delivery.[6–8] In two of the studies,

maternal lumbar spine bone density had dropped 4.5% and 3.5%, respectively, when preconception readings were compared with readings obtained an average of 2 [6] and 6 weeks postpartum.[7] The third study found no change in lumbar spine bone density measurements obtained preconception and within 1–2 weeks postdelivery.[8] Each study involved 16 or fewer subjects. Because the puerperium is associated with bone density losses of 1–3% per month (see LACTATION), it is possible that obtaining the second measurement 2–6 weeks after delivery contributed to the bone loss documented in the first two studies. Other longitudinal studies have found a progressive decrease during pregnancy in indices thought to correlate with bone mineral density (BMD), as determined by ultrasonographic measurements at another peripheral site, the os calcis. None of all the aforementioned studies can address the question as to whether skeletal calcium content is increased early in pregnancy in advance of the third trimester. Further studies, with larger numbers of patients, will be needed to clarify the extent of bone loss during pregnancy.

It seems certain that any acute changes in bone metabolism during pregnancy do not cause long-term changes in skeletal calcium content or strength. Numerous studies of osteoporotic or osteopenic women have failed to find a significant association of parity with bone density or fracture risk.[1,9] Although many of these studies could not separate out the effects of parity from those of lactation, it may be reasonable to conclude that if parity has any effect on bone density or fracture risk, it must be only a very modest effect.

Osteoporosis in Pregnancy

Occasionally, a woman may present with fragility fractures and low BMD during or shortly after pregnancy; the possibility that the woman had low bone density before pregnancy cannot be excluded. Some women may experience excessive resorption of calcium from the skeleton because of changes in mineral metabolism induced by pregnancy and other factors such as low dietary calcium intake and vitamin D insufficiency. The apparently increased rate of bone turnover in pregnancy may contribute to fracture risk, because a high rate of bone turnover is an independent risk factor for fragility fractures outside of pregnancy. Therefore, fragility fractures in pregnancy or the puerperium may be a consequence of pre-existing low bone density and increased bone turnover, among other possible factors. Additional changes in mineral metabolism occur during lactation that may further increase fracture risk in some women (see below).

Focal, transient osteoporosis of the hip is a rare, self-limited form of pregnancy-associated osteoporosis. It is probably not a manifestation of altered calcitropic hormone levels or mineral balance during pregnancy, but rather might be a consequence of local factors. The theories proposed to explain the condition include femoral venous stasis because of the gravid uterus, reflex sympathetic dystrophy, ischemia, trauma, viral infections, marrow hypertrophy, immobilization, and fetal pressure on the obturator nerve. These patients present with unilateral or bilateral hip pain, limp, and/or hip fracture in the third trimester. There is objective evidence of reduced bone density of the symptomatic femoral head and neck that has been shown by magnetic resonance imaging (MRI) to be the consequence of increased water content of the femoral head and the marrow cavity; a joint effusion may also be present. The symptoms and the radiological appearance usually resolve within 2–6 months postpartum.

Primary Hyperparathyroidism

Although probably a rare condition (there are no data available on its prevalence), primary hyperparathyroidism in pregnancy has been associated in the literature with an alarming rate of adverse outcomes in the fetus and neonate, including a 30% rate of spontaneous abortion or stillbirth. The adverse postnatal outcomes are thought to result from suppression of the fetal and neonatal parathyroid glands; this suppression may occasionally be prolonged after birth for months. To prevent these adverse outcomes, surgical correction of primary hyperparathyroidism during the second trimester has been almost universally recommended. Several case series have found elective surgery to be well tolerated and to dramatically reduce the rate of adverse events compared with the earlier cases reported in the literature. However, many of the women in those early cases had a relatively severe form of primary hyperparathyroidism that is not often seen today (symptomatic, with nephrocalcinosis and renal insufficiency). Whether the milder, asymptomatic form of primary hyperparathyroidism commonly seen today has the same risk of adverse fetal or neonatal outcomes has not been determined.

Familial Hypocalciuric Hypercalcemia

Although familial hypocalciuric hypercalcemia (FHH) has not been reported to adversely affect the mother during pregnancy, the maternal hypercalcemia can cause fetal and neonatal parathyroid suppression with subsequent tetany.

Hypoparathyroidism and Pseudohypoparathyroidism

Early in pregnancy, hypoparathyroid women may have fewer hypocalcemic symptoms and require less supplemental calcium. This is consistent with a limited role for PTH in the pregnant woman and suggests that an increase in 1,25-dihydroxyvitamin D and/or increased intestinal calcium absorption will occur in the absence of PTH. However, it is clear from other case reports that some pregnant hypoparathyroid women may require increased calcitriol replacement to avoid worsening hypocalcemia. It is important to maintain a normal ionized calcium level in pregnant women because maternal hypocalcemia has been associated with the development of intrauterine fetal hyperparathyroidism and fetal death. Late in pregnancy, hypercalcemia may occur in hypoparathyroid women unless the calcitriol dosage is substantially reduced or discontinued. This effect may be mediated by the increasing levels of PTHrP in the maternal circulation in late pregnancy.

In limited case reports of pseudohypoparathyroidism, pregnancy has been noted to normalize the serum calcium level, reduce the PTH level by one-half, and increase the 1,25-dihydroxyvitamin D level 2- to 3-fold.[10] The mechanism by which pseudohypoparathyroidism is improved in pregnancy remains unclear.

LACTATION

The typical daily loss of calcium in breast milk has been estimated to range from 280 to 400 mg, although daily losses as great as 1000 mg calcium have been reported. A temporary demineralization of the skeleton seems to be the main mechanism by which lactating humans meet these calcium requirements. This demineralization does not seem to be mediated by PTH or 1,25-dihydroxyvitamin D, but may be mediated by PTHrP in the setting of a fall in estrogen levels.

Mineral Ions and Calcitropic Hormones

The normal lactational changes in maternal calcium, phosphate, and calcitropic hormone levels are schematically depicted in Fig. 2.[1] The mean ionized calcium level of exclusively lactating women is increased, although it remains within the normal range. Serum phosphate levels are also higher during lactation, and the level may exceed the normal range. Because reabsorption of phosphate by the kidneys seems to be increased, the increased serum phosphate levels may, therefore, reflect the combined effects of increased flux of phosphate into the blood from diet and from skeletal resorption in the setting of decreased renal phosphate excretion.

Intact PTH, as determined by a two-site IRMA assay, has been found to be reduced 50% or more in lactating women during the first several months. It rises to normal at weaning, but may rise above normal after weaning. In contrast to the high 1,25-dihydroxyvitamin D levels of pregnancy, maternal free and bound 1,25-dihydroxyvitamin D levels fall to normal within days of parturition and remain there throughout lactation. Calcitonin levels fall to normal after the first 6 weeks postpartum.

PTHrP levels, as measured by two-site IRMA assays, are significantly higher in lactating women than in nonpregnant controls. The source of PTHrP may be the breast, because PTHrP has been detected in breast milk at concentrations exceeding 10,000 times the level found in the blood of patients with hypercalcemia of malignancy or normal human controls. Furthermore, lactating mice with the PTHrP gene ablated only from breast tissue have lower blood levels of PTHrP than control lactating mice.[11] A small rise in the maternal level of PTHrP can be demonstrated after suckling.[12] The primary role of PTHrP in the breast or breast milk is not clear. Studies in animals suggest that PTHrP may regulate mammary development and blood flow and the calcium content of milk. In addition, PTHrP reaching the maternal circulation from the lactating breast may cause resorption of calcium from the maternal skeleton, renal tubular reabsorption of calcium, and (indirectly) suppression of PTH. In support of this hypothesis, PTHrP levels have been found to correlate negatively with PTH levels and positively with the ionized calcium levels of lactating women.[12,13] Also, PTHrP levels correlate with the loss of BMD during lactation in humans.[14] Furthermore, observations in aparathyroid women provide evidence of the impact of PTHrP in calcium homeostasis during lactation (see below).

Intestinal Absorption of Calcium

Intestinal calcium absorption decreases to the nonpregnant rate from the increased rate of pregnancy. This corresponds to the fall in 1,25-dihydroxyvitamin D levels to normal.

Renal Handling of Calcium

In humans, the glomerular filtration rate falls during lactation, and the renal excretion of calcium is typically reduced to levels as low as 50 mg/24 h. This suggests that the tubular reabsorption of calcium must be increased to account for reduced calcium excretion in the setting of increased serum calcium.

Skeletal Calcium Metabolism

Histomorphometric data from animals consistently show increased bone turnover during lactation, and losses of 35% or more of bone mineral are achieved during 2–3 weeks of normal lactation in the rat.[1] Comparative histomorphometric data are lacking for humans, and in place of that, serum markers of bone formation and urinary markers of bone resorption have been assessed in numerous cross-sectional and prospective studies of lactation. Some of the confounding factors discussed with respect to pregnancy apply to the use of these markers in lactating women. In this instance, the glomerular filtration rate is reduced, and the intravascular volume is more contracted. Urinary markers of bone resorption (24-h collection) have been reported to be elevated 2- to 3-fold during lactation and are higher than the levels attained in the third trimester. Serum markers of bone formation (not adjusted for hemoconcentration or reduced GFR) are generally high during lactation and increased over the levels attained during the third trimester. Total alkaline phosphatase falls immediately postpartum because of loss of the placental fraction, but may still remain above normal because of the elevation in the bone-specific fraction. Despite the confounding variables, these findings suggest that bone turnover is significantly increased during lactation.

Serial measurements of bone density during lactation (by SPA, DPA, or DXA) have shown a fall of 3.0–10.0% in bone mineral content (BMC) after 2–6 months of lactation at trabecular sites (lumbar spine, hip, femur, and distal radius), with smaller losses at cortical sites.[1,9] The loss occurs at a peak rate of 1–3% per month, far exceeding the rate of 1–3% per year that can occur in women with postmenopausal osteoporosis who are considered to be losing bone rapidly. Loss of bone mineral from the maternal skeleton seems to be a normal consequence of lactation and may not be preventable by raising the calcium intake above the recommended dietary allowance. Several recent studies have demonstrated that calcium supplementation does not significantly reduce the amount of bone lost during

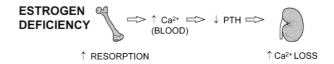

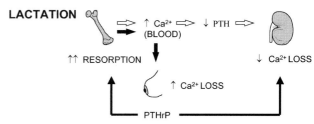

FIG. 3. Acute estrogen deficiency (e.g., GnRH analog therapy) increases skeletal resorption and raises the blood calcium; in turn, PTH is suppressed and renal calcium losses are increased. During lactation, the combined effects of PTHrP (secreted by the breast) and estrogen deficiency increase skeletal resorption, reduce renal calcium losses, and raise the blood calcium, but calcium is directed into breast milk. (Reprinted with permission of The Endocrine Society from Kovacs CS, Kronenberg HM 1997 Maternal-fetal calcium and bone metabolism during pregnancy, puerperium and lactation. Endocr Rev **18:**832–872.)

lactation.[15–18] Not surprisingly, the lactational decrease in BMD correlates with the amount of calcium lost in the breast milk.[19]

The mechanisms controlling the rapid loss of skeletal calcium content are not well understood. The reduced estrogen levels of lactation are clearly important but are unlikely to be the sole explanation. To estimate the effects of estrogen deficiency during lactation, it is worth noting the alterations in calcium and bone metabolism that occur in reproductive-age women who have estrogen deficiency induced by gonadotropin releasing hormone (GnRH) agonist therapy for endometriosis and other conditions. Six months of acute estrogen deficiency induced by GnRH agonist therapy leads to 1–4% losses in trabecular (but not cortical) bone density, increased urinary calcium excretion, and suppression of 1,25-dihydroxyvitamin D and PTH levels.[1] In lactation, women are not as estrogen deficient but lose more BMD (at both trabecular and cortical sites), have normal (as opposed to low) 1,25-dihydroxyvitamin D levels, and have reduced (as opposed to increased) urinary calcium excretion. The difference between isolated estrogen deficiency and lactation may be caused by the effects of other factors (such as PTHrP) that add to the effects of estrogen withdrawal in lactation (Fig. 3).

The bone density losses of lactation seem to be substantially reversed during weaning.[1,9,17] This corresponds to a gain in bone density of 0.5–2% per month in the woman who has weaned her infant. The mechanism for this restoration of bone density is uncertain and largely unexplored. In the long-term, the consequences of lactation-induced depletion of bone mineral seem clinically unimportant. The vast majority of epidemiologic studies of pre- and postmenopausal women have found no adverse effect of a history of lactation on peak bone mass, bone density, or hip fracture risk.

Osteoporosis of Lactation

Rarely, a woman will suffer a fragility fracture during lactation, and osteoporotic readings will be confirmed by DXA. Like osteoporosis in pregnancy, this may represent a coincidental, unrelated disease; the woman may have had low bone density before conception. Alternatively, some cases might represent an exacerbation of the normal degree of skeletal demineralization that occurs during lactation and a continuum from changes in bone density and bone turnover that may have occurred during pregnancy. For example, excessive PTHrP release from the lactating breast into the maternal circulation could cause excessive bone resorption, osteoporosis, and fractures in some of these cases. PTHrP levels were high in one case of lactational osteoporosis and were found to remain elevated for months after weaning.[20] However, the extent to which PTHrP contributes to the reduction of bone density during lactation has yet to be established.

Hypoparathyroidism and Pseudohypoparathyroidism

Calcitriol requirements of hypoparathyroid women fall early in the postpartum period, especially if the woman breastfeeds, and hypercalcemia may occur if the calcitriol dosage is not substantially reduced.[21] As observed in one recent case, this is consistent with PTHrP reaching the maternal circulation in amounts sufficient to allow stimulation of 1,25-dihydroxyvitamin D synthesis and maintenance of normal (or slightly increased) maternal serum calcium.[22]

The management of pseudohypoparathyroidism has been less well documented. Because these patients are likely resistant to the renal actions of PTHrP and the placental sources of 1,25-dihydroxyvitamin D are lost at parturition, the calcitriol requirements might well increase and may require further adjustments during lactation.

IMPLICATIONS

The studies of pregnant women suggest that the fetal calcium demand is met in large part by intestinal calcium absorption, which more than doubles from early in pregnancy. The studies of biochemical markers of bone turnover, DXA, and ultrasound are not conclusive, but are compatible with the possibility that the maternal skeleton does contribute calcium to the developing fetus. In comparison, the studies in lactating women suggest that skeletal calcium resorption is a dominant mechanism by which calcium is supplied to the breast milk, while renal calcium conservation is also apparent. These observations indicate that the maternal adaptations to pregnancy and lactation have evolved differently over time, such that dietary calcium absorption dominates in pregnancy, whereas the temporary borrowing of calcium from the skeleton seems to dominate during lactation. Lactation seems to program an obligatory skeletal calcium loss irrespective of maternal calcium intake, but the calcium is completely restored to the skeleton after weaning. The rapidity of calcium loss and regain by the skeleton of the lactating woman are through mechanisms that are at best, only partly understood. A full elucidation of the mechanisms of bone loss and restoration in the lactating woman might lead to the development of novel approaches to the treatment of osteoporosis and other metabolic bone diseases. Finally, while it is apparent that some women will experience fragility fractures as a consequence of pregnancy or lactation, the vast majority of women can be assured that the changes in calcium and bone metabolism during pregnancy and lactation are normal, healthy, and without adverse consequences in the long-term.

REFERENCES

1. Kovacs CS, Kronenberg HM 1997 Maternal-fetal calcium and bone metabolism during pregnancy, puerperium and lactation. Endocr Rev **18**:832–872.
2. Kovacs CS 2003 Fetal mineral homeostasis. In: Glorieux FH, Pettifor JM, Jüppner H (eds.) Pediatric Bone: Biology and Diseases. Academic Press, San Diego, CA, USA, pp. 271–302.
3. Kovacs CS, Lanske B, Hunzelman JL, Guo J, Karaplis AC, Kronenberg HM 1996 Parathyroid hormone-related peptide (PTHrP) regulates fetal-placental calcium transport through a receptor distinct from the PTH/PTHrP receptor. Proc Natl Acad Sci USA **93**:15233–15238.
4. Cornish J, Callon KE, Nicholson GC, Reid IR 1997 Parathyroid hormone-related protein-(107–139) inhibits bone resorption in vivo. Endocrinology **138**:1299–1304.
5. Purdie DW, Aaron JE, Selby PL 1988 Bone histology and mineral homeostasis in human pregnancy. Br J Obstet Gynaecol **95**:849–854.
6. Naylor KE, Iqbal P, Fledelius C, Fraser RB, Eastell R 2000 The effect of pregnancy on bone density and bone turnover. J Bone Miner Res **15**:129–137.
7. Black AJ, Topping J, Durham B, Farquharson RG, Fraser WD 2000 A detailed assessment of alterations in bone turnover, calcium homeostasis, and bone density in normal pregnancy. J Bone Miner Res **15**:557–563.
8. Ritchie LD, Fung EB, Halloran BP, Turnlund JR, Van Loan MD, Cann CE, King JC 1998 A longitudinal study of calcium homeostasis during human pregnancy and lactation and after resumption of menses. Am J Clin Nutr **67**:693–701.
9. Sowers M 1996 Pregnancy and lactation as risk factors for subsequent bone loss and osteoporosis. J Bone Miner Res **11**:1052–1060.
10. Breslau NA, Zerwekh JE 1986 Relationship of estrogen and pregnancy to calcium homeostasis in pseudohypoparathyroidism. J Clin Endocrinol Metab **62**:45–51.
11. VanHouten J, Dann P, Stewart A, Watson C, Karaplis A, Wysolmerski J 2001 Mammary-specific deletion of PTHrP reduces bone turnover and preserves bone mass during lactation. J Bone Miner Res **16**:S1; S137.
12. Dobnig H, Kainer F, Stepan V, Winter R, Lipp R, Schaffer M, Kahr A, Nocnik S, Patterer G, Leb G 1995 Elevated parathyroid hormone-related peptide levels after human gestation: Relationship to changes in bone and mineral metabolism. J Clin Endocrinol Metab **80**:3699–3707.
13. Kovacs CS, Chik CL 1995 Hyperprolactinemia caused by lactation and pituitary adenomas is associated with altered serum calcium, phosphate, parathyroid hormone (PTH), and PTH-related peptide levels. J Clin Endocrinol Metab **80**:3036–3042.
14. Sowers MF, Hollis BW, Shapiro B, Randolph J, Janney CA, Zhang D, Schork A, Crutchfield M, Stanczyk F, Russell-Aulet M 1996 Elevated parathyroid hormone-related peptide associated with lactation and bone density loss. J Am Med Assoc **276**:549–554.
15. Cross NA, Hillman LS, Allen SH, Krause GF 1995 Changes in bone mineral density and markers of bone remodeling during lactation and postweaning in women consuming high amounts of calcium. J Bone Miner Res **10**:1312–1320.
16. Kalkwarf HJ, Specker BL, Bianchi DC, Ranz J, Ho M 1997 The effect of calcium supplementation on bone density during lactation and after weaning. N Engl J Med **337**:523–528.
17. Polatti F, Capuzzo E, Viazzo F, Colleoni R, Klersy C 1999 Bone mineral changes during and after lactation. Obstet Gynecol **94**:52–56.
18. Kolthoff N, Eiken P, Kristensen B, Nielsen SP 1998 Bone mineral changes during pregnancy and lactation: A longitudinal cohort study. Clin Sci (Colch) **94**:405–412.

19. Laskey MA, Prentice A, Hanratty LA, Jarjou LM, Dibba B, Beavan SR, Cole TJ 1998 Bone changes after 3 mo of lactation: Influence of calcium intake, breast-milk output, and vitamin D-receptor genotype. Am J Clin Nutr 67:685–692.
20. Reid IR, Wattie DJ, Evans MC, Budayr AA 1992 Post-pregnancy osteoporosis associated with hypercalcaemia. Clin Endocrinol (Oxf) 37:298–303.
21. Caplan RH, Beguin EA 1990 Hypercalcemia in a calcitriol-treated hypoparathyroid woman during lactation. Obstet Gynecol 76:485–489.
22. Mather KJ, Chik CL, Corenblum B 1999 Maintenance of serum calcium by parathyroid hormone-related peptide during lactation in a hypoparathyroid patient. J Clin Endocrinol Metab 84:424–427.

Chapter 12.   Menopause

Ian R. Reid

Department of Medicine, University of Auckland, Auckland, New Zealand

INTRODUCTION

Menopause refers to the cessation of menstruation, which occurs at about 48–50 years of age in healthy women. The decline in ovarian hormone production is gradual and starts several years before the last period. Changes in bone mass and calcium metabolism are evident during this perimenopausal transition.[1] Estrogen is the ovarian product that has the greatest impact on mineral metabolism, although both progesterone and ovarian androgens may have some influence. Menopause ushers in a period of bone loss that extends until the end of life and is the central contributor to the development of osteoporotic fractures in older women.

EFFECTS ON BONE

Before menopause, there is virtually no bone loss in most regions of the skeleton, and fracture rates are stable. The most obvious effect of menopause on bone is an increase in the incidence of fractures—in the forearms and vertebrae, this is clearly apparent within the first postmenopausal decade. This is attributable to the rapid decline in bone mass that occurs in the perimenopausal years. Bone loss is more marked in trabecular than in cortical bone because the former has a far greater surface area over which bone resorption can take place. Thus, the fractures that occur early in the menopause are in trabecular-rich regions of the skeleton such as the distal forearm and vertebrae. The loss of bone and increase in fracture rates are preventable with estrogen replacement, and these benefits must be weighed against well-documented side effects.[2,3]

The perimenopausal increase in bone loss is associated with increased bone resorption.[4] Bone biopsy specimens in normal postmenopausal women show an increase in the fraction of bone surfaces at which resorption is taking place and an increase in the depth of resorption pits. These changes follow from an increase in the activation frequency of remodeling units and a prolongation of their resorptive phase, and result in the perforation and loss of trabeculae. In cortical bone, there is an increase in its porosity. After menopause, indices of bone resorption are twice the levels found in premenopausal women.[5] There is also an increase in markers of bone formation, but these are only about 50%

above premenopausal levels,[5] leading to negative bone balance. The changes in histomorphometric indices and biochemical markers can be returned to premenopausal levels with estrogen replacement therapy.

The changes in bone turnover that accompany menopause are in part accounted for by the direct actions of estrogen on bone cells. Estrogen receptors are present in both osteoblasts[6,7] and osteoclasts.[8] Estrogen promotes the development of osteoblasts, in preference to adipocytes, from their common precursor cell,[9] increases osteoblast proliferation,[10] and increases production of a number of osteoblast proteins (e.g., insulin-like growth factor-1,[11] type I procollagen,[11] transforming growth factor-β [TGF-β],[12,13] and bone morphogenetic protein-6).[14] Thus, estrogen tends to have an anabolic effect on the isolated osteoblast, and it may also be important in maintaining osteocyte function.[15] In vivo, however, the initiation of estrogen replacement therapy is usually associated with a reduction in osteoblast numbers and activity.[16] This is accounted for by the tight coupling of osteoblast activity to that of osteoclasts and the overriding effect of estrogen to reduce osteoclastic bone resorption.[8,17] However, there is now evidence that high concentrations of estrogen increase some histomorphometric indices of osteoblast activity (e.g., mean wall thickness) in humans, possibly by increasing osteoblast synthesis of growth factors.[18] Estrogen may also reduce osteoblast apoptosis.[19] Estrogen's suppression of osteoclast activity is in part mediated by increased osteoclast apoptosis.[20]

Many studies now indicate that bone marrow stromal and mononuclear cells are also important target cells for sex hormones in bone. These cells produce cytokines such as interleukin-1 (IL-1), interleukin-6 (IL-6), and tumor necrosis factor-α (TNFα), which are potent stimulators of osteoclast recruitment and/or activity.[21] Estrogen decreases production of each of these cytokines in vitro[22–24] and in vivo,[25] and may also modulate levels of receptors for IL-1.[26] The increase in osteoclast numbers and bone loss after ovariectomy is reduced by blockers of IL-6,[22] IL-1, or TNFβ.[27] Mice not expressing the *IL-6* gene do not lose bone after ovariectomy.[28] IL-1 and TNFα may act in part by regulating stromal cell production of IL-6 and macrophage colony-stimulating factor.[29] These cells also produce osteoprotegerin and RANKL, which stimulate and inhibit osteoclast development, respectively. Estrogen increases levels of the former[30] and reduces the effects of the

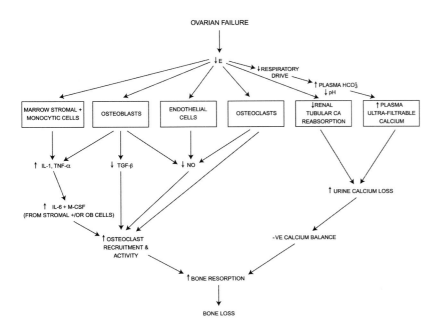

FIG. 1. The potential pathways by which menopause leads to bone loss. For simplicity, the figure does not show a contribution from loss of the anabolic effect of estrogen on the osteoblast. The fall in ovarian production of androgens and progesterone also contributes to some of these changes.

latter.[31] Estrogen's reduction in bone resorption may also be contributed to by its increasing levels of nitric oxide and TGFβ, both of which are potent inhibitors of osteoclast differentiation and bone resorption.[12,32] Thus, estrogen effects on production of cytokines and growth factors within the bone marrow micro-environment may act together with its direct effects on bone cells to modulate both bone resorption and bone formation. There may also be a contribution from estrogen's regulation of the release of systemic factors, such as growth hormone.[33]

EFFECTS ON CALCIUM METABOLISM

The bone loss that follows menopause is accompanied by negative changes in external calcium balance, which are approximately equally contributed to by decreases in intestinal calcium absorption and by increases in urinary calcium loss.[34] The reduction in intestinal calcium absorption is accompanied by reduced circulating concentrations of total but not free 1,25-dihydroxyvitamin D [1,25(OH)$_2$D], suggesting that the principal effect of estrogen on vitamin D metabolism is on synthesis of the protein that carries 1,25(OH)$_2$D in plasma.[35] Thus, oral administration of estrogen to postmenopausal women increases total 1,25(OH)$_2$D concentrations,[36] but use of transdermal estrogen, which bypasses the liver where vitamin D–binding globulin is synthesized, does not.[37] However, estrogen may directly regulate intestinal calcium absorption independently of vitamin D.[38]

In the kidney, it is clear that tubular reabsorption of calcium is higher in the presence of estrogen.[39–41] One study[39] found higher parathyroid hormone (PTH) concentrations in the presence of estrogen and inferred that this was the mechanism of the renal calcium conservation. However, higher PTH levels have not been the finding in a number of other studies.[42] Thus, it is likely that estrogen directly modulates renal tubular calcium absorption through its own receptor, which is present in the kidney.[43,44]

The changes in the handling of calcium by the gut and

kidney could each be a *cause* of postmenopausal bone loss, or they could represent homeostatic *responses* to it. If the former were the case, then PTH concentrations would be elevated in postmenopausal women to maintain plasma calcium concentrations in the face of intestinal and renal losses. This, in turn, would cause bone loss. If, on the other hand, bone loss were the primary event, then suppression of PTH would be expected, leading to secondary declines in intestinal and renal calcium absorption. The effect of menopause on PTH concentrations has been addressed many times without any consistent pattern emerging. This suggests that the situation is more complicated than this simple formulation suggests. Possibly, estrogen has direct effects on bone, kidney, and gut, and the opposing effects on PTH secretion of these actions lead to inconsistent changes in PTH concentrations. Furthermore, estrogen may directly modulate PTH secretion.[45,46]

There are small but consistently demonstrable effects of menopause on circulating concentrations of calcium. Total calcium is 0.05 mM higher after menopause.[47] This is partly attributable to a contraction of the plasma volume and resulting increase in albumin concentrations that occurs in the absence of estrogen,[48,49] and partly to an increase in plasma bicarbonate, which leads to an increase in the complexed fraction of plasma calcium.[35,40,41] The higher bicarbonate levels of postmenopausal women are attributable to a respiratory acidosis, which results from the loss of the respiratory stimulatory effects of progesterone on the central nervous system, an action that is potentiated by estrogen.[50,51] Despite changes in protein-bound and complexed calcium fractions, ionized calcium concentrations are usually found to be the same in pre- and postmenopausal women.

SUMMARY

The effects of menopause on skeletal physiology are summarized in Fig 1. The major effect is an increase in bone turnover, which is dominantly an increase in bone resorption. This results in bone loss that may be contributed to by reductions in both intestinal and renal tubular absorption of calcium. Bone loss persists throughout the entire postmenopausal period and results in a high risk of fractures in those women whose peak bone mass was in the lower part of the normal range.

REFERENCES

1. Okano H, Mizunuma H, Soda M, Kagami I, Miyamoto S, Ohsawa M, Ibuki Y, Shiraki M, Suzuki T, Shibata H 1998 The long-term effect of menopause on postmenopausal bone loss in Japanese women - results from a prospective study. J Bone Miner Res 13:303–309.
2. Lindsay R, Hart DM, Forrest C, Baird C 1980 Prevention of spinal osteoporosis in oophorectomised women. Lancet 2:1151–1153.
3. Rossouw JE, Anderson GL, Prentice RL, LaCroix AZ, Kooperberg C, Stefanick ML, Jackson RD, Beresford SAA, Howard BV, Johnson KC, Kotchen M, Ockene J 2002 Risks and benefits of estrogen plus progestin in healthy postmenopausal women - Principal results from the Women's Health Initiative randomized controlled trial. JAMA 288:321–333.
4. Heaney RP, Recker RR, Saville PD 1978 Menopausal changes in bone remodeling. J Lab Clin Med 92:964–970.
5. Garnero P, Sornayrendu E, Chapuy MC, Delmas PD 1996 Increased bone turnover in late postmenopausal women is a major determinant of osteoporosis. J Bone Miner Res 11:337–349.
6. Komm BS, Terpening CM, Benz DJ, Graeme KA, O'Malley BW, Haussler MR 1988 Estrogen binding receptor mRNA, and biologic response in osteoblast-like osteosarcoma cells. Science 241:81–84.
7. Eriksen EF, Colvard DS, Berg NJ, Graham ML, Mann KG, Spelsberg TC, Riggs BL 1988 Evidence of estrogen receptors in normal human osteoblast-like cells. Science 241:84–86.
8. Oursler M, Osdoby P, Pyfferoen J, Riggs BL, Spelsberg TC 1991 Avian osteoclasts as estrogen target cells. Proc Natl Acad Sci USA 88:6613–6617.
9. Okazaki R, Inoue D, Shibata M, Saika M, Kido S, Ooka H, Tomiyama H, Sakamoto Y, Matsumoto T 2002 Estrogen promotes early osteoblast differentiation and inhibits adipocyte differentiation in mouse bone marrow stromal cell lines that express estrogen receptor (ER) alpha or beta. Endocrinology 143:2349–2356.
10. Fujita M, Urano T, Horie K, Ikeda K, Tsukui T, Fukuoka H, Tsutsumi O, Ouchi Y, Inoue S 2002 Estrogen activates cyclin-dependent kinases 4 and 6 through induction of cyclin D in rat primary osteoblasts. Biochem Biophys Res Commun 299:222–228.
11. Ernst M, Heath JK, Rodan GA 1989 Estradiol effects on proliferation, messenger ribonucleic acid for collagen and insulin-like growth factor-I, and parathyroid hormone-stimulated adenylate cyclase activity in osteoblastic cells from calvariae and long bones. Endocrinology 125:825–833.
12. Yang NN, Bryant HU, Hardikar S, Sato M, Galvin RJS, Glasebrook AL, Termine JD 1996 Estrogen and raloxifene stimulate transforming growth factor-beta-3 gene expression in rat bone - a potential mechanism for estrogen- or raloxifene-mediated bone maintenance. Endocrinology 137:2075–2084.
13. Oursler MJ, Cortese C, Keeting PE, Anderson MA, Bonde SK, Riggs BL, Spelsberg TC 1991 Modulation of transforming growth factor-β production in normal human osteoblast-like cells by 17β-estradiol and parathyroid hormone. Endocrinology 129:3313–3320.
14. Rickard DJ, Hofbauer LC, Bonde SK, Gori F, Spelsberg TC, Lawrence B 1998 Bone morphogenetic protein-6-production in human osteoblastic cell lines - selective regulation by estrogen. J Clin Invest 101:413–422.
15. Tomkinson A, Reeve J, Shaw RW, Noble BS 1997 The death of osteocytes via apoptosis accompanies estrogen withdrawal in human bone. J Clin Endocrinol Metab 82:3128–3135.
16. Vedi S, Compston JE 1996 The effects of long-term hormone replacement therapy on bone remodeling in postmenopausal women. Bone 19:535–539.
17. Oursler MJ, Pederson L, Fitzpatrick L, Riggs BL, Spelsberg T 1994 Human giant cell tumors of the bone (osteoclastomas) are estrogen target cells. Proc Natl Acad Sci USA 91:5227–5231.
18. Bord S, Beavan S, Ireland D, Horner A, Compston JE 2001 Mechanisms by which high-dose estrogen therapy produces anabolic skeletal effects in postmenopausal women: Role of locally produced growth factors. Bone 29:216–222.
19. Gohel A, McCarthy MB, Gronowicz G 1999 Estrogen prevents glucocorticoid-induced apoptosis in osteoblasts in vivo and in vitro. Endocrinology 140:5339–5347.
20. Kameda T, Mano H, Yuasa T, Mori Y, Miyazawa K, Shiokawa M, Nakamaru Y, Hiroi E, Hiura K, Kameda A, Yang NN, Hakeda Y, Kumegawa M 1997 Estrogen inhibits bone resorption by directly inducing apoptosis of the bone-resorbing osteoclasts. J Exp Med 186:489–495.
21. Manolagas SC, Jilka RL 1995 Mechanisms of disease: Bone marrow, cytokines, and bone remodeling - Emerging insights into the pathophysiology of osteoporosis. N Engl J Med 332:305–311.
22. Jilka RL, Hangoc G, Girasole G, Passeri G, Williams DC, Abrams JS, Boyce B, Broxmeyer H, Manolagas SC 1992 Increased osteoclast development after estrogen loss: Mediation by interleukin-6. Science 257:88–91.
23. Girasole G, Jilka RL, Passeri G, Boswell S, Boder G, Williams DC, Manolagas SC 1992 Marrow-derived stromal cells and osteoblasts in vitro: A potential mechanism for the antiosteoporotic effects of estrogens. J Clin Invest 89:883–891.
24. Pacifici R, Rifas L, McCracken R, Vered I, McMurtry C, Avioli LV, Peck WA 1989 Ovarian steroid treatment blocks a postmenopausal increase in blood monocyte interleukin 1 release. Proc Natl Acad Sci USA 86:2398–2402.
25. Rogers A, Eastell R 1998 Effects of estrogen therapy of postmenopausal women on cytokines measured in peripheral blood. J Bone Miner Res 13:1577–1586.
26. Sunyer T, Lewis J, Collin-Osdoby P, Osdoby P 1999 Estrogen's bone-protective effects may involve differential IL-1 receptor regulation in human osteoclast-like cells. J Clin Invest 103:1409–1418.
27. Kimble RB, Matayoshi AB, Vannice JL, Kung VT, Williams C, Pacifici R 1995 Simultaneous block of interleukin-1 and tumor necrosis factor is required to completely prevent bone loss in the early postovariectomy period. Endocrinology 136:3054–3061.
28. Poli V, Balena R, Fattori E, Markatos A, Yamamoto M, Tanaka H, Ciliberto G, Rodan GA, Costantini F 1994 Interleukin-6 deficient mice are protected from bone loss caused by estrogen depletion. EMBO J 13:1189–1196.
29. Kimble RB, Srivastava S, Ross FP, Matayoshi A, Pacifici R 1996 Estrogen deficiency increases the ability of stromal cells to support murine osteoclastogenesis via an interleukin-1-and tumor necrosis factor-mediated stimulation of macrophage colony-stimulating factor production. J Biol Chem 271:28890–28897.
30. Hofbauer LC, Khosla S, Dunstan CR, Lacey DL, Spelsberg TC, Riggs BL 1999 Estrogen stimulates gene expression and protein production of osteoprotegerin in human osteoblastic cells. Endocrinology 140:4367–4370.
31. Srivastava S, Toraldo G, Weitzmann MN, Cenci S, Ross FP, Pacifici R 2001 Estrogen decreases osteoclast formation by down-regulating receptor activator of NF-kappa B ligand (RANKL)-induced JNK activation. J Biol Chem 276:8836–8840.
32. Ralston SH 1997 The Michael-Mason-Prize essay 1997 - nitric oxide and bone - what a gas. Br J Rheumatol 36:831–838.
33. Friend KE, Hartman ML, Pezzoli SS, Clasey JL, Thorner MO 1996 Both oral and transdermal estrogen increase growth hormone release in postmenopausal women - a clinical research center study. J Clin Endocrinol Metab 81:2250–2256.
34. Heaney RP, Recker RR, Saville PD 1978 Menopausal changes in calcium balance performance. J Lab Clin Med 92:953–963.
35. Prince RL, Dick I, Garcia-Webb P, Retallack RW 1990 The effects of the menopause on calcitriol and parathyroid hormone: Responses to a low dietary calcium stress test. J Clin Endocrinol Metab 70:1119–1123.
36. Civitelli R, Agnusdei D, Nardi P, Zacchei F, Avioli LV, Gennari C 1988 Effects of one-year treatment with estrogens on bone mass, intestinal calcium absorption, and 25-hydroxyvitamin D-1-alpha-hydroxylase reserve in postmenopausal osteoporosis. Calcif Tissue Int 42:77–86.
37. Selby PL, Peacock M 1986 The effect of transdermal oestrogen on bone, calcium-regulating hormones and liver in postmenopausal women. Clin Endocrinol (Oxf) 25:543–547.
38. Arjandi BH, Salih MA, Herbert DC, Sims SH, Kalu DN 1993 Evidence for estrogen receptor-linked calcium transport in the intestine. Bone Miner 21:63–74.
39. McKane WR, Khosla S, Burritt MF, Kao PC, Wilson DM, Ory SJ, Riggs BL 1995 Mechanism of renal calcium conservation with estrogen replacement therapy in women in early postmenopause - A clinical research center study. J Clin Endocrinol Metab 80:3458–3464.
40. Nordin BEC, Need AG, Morris HA, Horowitz M, Robertson WG 1991 Evidence for a renal calcium leak in postmenopausal women. J Clin Endocrinol Metab 72:401–407.
41. Adami S, Gatti D, Bertoldo F, Rossini M, FrattaPasini A, Zamberlan N, Facci E, LoCascio V 1992 The effects of menopause and estrogen

replacement therapy on the renal handling of calcium. Osteoporos Int **2:**180–185.

42. Prince RL 1994 Counterpoint: Estrogen effects on calcitropic hormones and calcium homeostasis. Endocr Rev **15:**301–309.

43. Hagenfeldt Y, Eriksson HA 1988 The estrogen receptor in the rat kidney. J Steroid Biochem Mol Biol **31:**49–56.

44. Criddle RA, Zheng MH, Dick IM, Callus B, Prince RL 1997 Estrogen responsiveness of renal calbindin-d-28k gene expression in rat kidney. J Cell Biochem **65:**340–348.

45. Greenberg C, Kukreja SC, Bowser EN, Hargis GK, Henderson WJ, Williams GA 1987 Parathyroid hormone secretion: Effect of estradiol and progesterone. Metabolism **36:**151–154.

46. Duarte B, Hargis GK, Kukreja SC 1988 Effects of estradiol and progesterone on parathyroid hormone secretion from human parathyroid tissue. J Clin Endocrinol Metab **66:**584–587.

47. Sokoll LJ, Dawson-Hughes B 1989 Effect of menopause and aging on serum total and ionized calcium and protein concentrations. Calcif Tissue Int **44:**181–185.

48. Minkoff JR, Young G, Grant B, Marcus R 1986 Interactions of medroxyprogesterone acetate with estrogen on the calcium-parathyroid axis in post-menopausal women. Maturitas **8:**35–45.

49. Aitken JM, Lindsay R, Hart DM 1974 The redistribution of body sodium in women on long-term estrogen therapy. Clin Sci Mol Med **47:**179–187.

50. Bayliss DA, Millhorn DE 1992 Central neural mechanisms of progesterone action: Application to the respiratory system. J Appl Physiol **73:**393–404.

51. Orr-Walker BJ, Horne AM, Evans MC, Grey AB, Murray MAF, McNeil AR, Reid IR 1999 Hormone replacement therapy causes a respiratory alkalosis in normal postmenopausal women. J Clin Endocrinol Metab **84:**1997–2001.

Chapter 13. Age-Related Osteoporosis

Clifford J. Rosen[1] and Douglas P. Kiel[2]

[1]*St. Joseph Hospital, Maine Center for Osteoporosis Research and Education, Bangor, Maine; and *[2]*HRCA Research and Training Institute, Boston, Massachusetts*

INTRODUCTION

Age-related fractures are the most common manifestation of osteoporosis and are responsible for the greatest proportion of the morbidity and mortality from this disease. Biochemical, biomechanical, and nonskeletal factors contribute to fragility fractures in the elderly. In this overview, we will focus on the skeletal and nonskeletal pathways that contribute to osteoporotic fractures in the older individual.

BONE REMODELING IN THE ELDERLY

Over a lifespan, women lose approximately 42% of their spinal and 58% of their femoral bone mass.[1] Surprisingly, rates of bone loss in the eight and ninth decades of life may be comparable with or even exceed those found in the immediate peri- and postmenopausal period of some women.[2,3] This is because of uncoupling in the bone remodeling cycle of older individuals, resulting in a marked increase in bone resorption but no change or a decrease in bone formation.[4,5] These alterations in bone turnover can be detected by biochemical markers of bone remodeling that include bone resorption indices (e.g., urinary and serum N-telopeptide, C-telopeptide, and urinary free and total deoxypyridinoline) and bone formation markers (e.g., osteocalcin, procollagen peptide, bone specific alkaline phosphatase). In general, bone turnover markers are significantly higher in older than younger postmenopausal women, and these indices are inversely related to bone mineral density (BMD).[6] For example, in the EPIDOS trial of elderly European females, the highest levels of osteocalcin, N-telopeptide, C-telopeptide, and bone-specific alkaline phosphatase were noted for those in the lowest tertile of femoral bone density.[7] Also, increased bone resorption indices were associated with a greater fracture risk independent of BMD.[7] For those women in EPIDOS with low bone density and a high bone resorption rate, there was a nearly 5-fold greater risk of a hip fracture.

In contrast to a consistent pattern of high bone resorption indices, bone formation markers in the elderly are more variable. Serum osteocalcin levels are high in elderly individuals, but this may be indicative of an increase in bone turnover rather than reflecting a true rise in bone formation.[7] On the other hand, bone-specific alkaline phosphatase and procollagen peptide levels have been reported to be high, normal, or low in elderly men and women.[8] Bone histomorphometric indices in elders are also quite variable. Thus, although there is strong evidence for an age-associated rise in bone resorption, changes in bone formation are inconsistent. Still there is uncoupling of the remodeling unit that leads to bone loss, altered skeletal architecture, and an increased propensity to fractures.

FACTORS THAT CONTRIBUTE TO AGE-RELATED BONE LOSS

Nutritional Factors

By far the most common cause of increased bone resorption in older individuals is calcium deficiency. Very low calcium intake (i.e., less than 800 mg per day) and vitamin D insufficiency are very common in the elderly and are caused by a number of factors, including dietary changes, lack of sunlight exposure, malabsorption, and anorexia. The end result of low calcium intake is persistent secondary hyperparathyroidism, which in turn, leads to increased bone resorption, often accentuated by occult vitamin D deficiency, especially in women living in northern latitudes.[9] Longitudinal trials of elderly men and women supplemented with calcium and vitamin D have demonstrated preservation of BMD and a reduction in osteoporotic fractures.[10,11] These studies led the National Academy of Science to recommend an increase in the minimal daily requirement for calcium intake in people over 65 years of age to 1500 mg/day.[12]

The authors have no conflict of interest.

© 2003 American Society for Bone and Mineral Research

Besides calcium and vitamin D, other nutritional factors may also play a role in age-related osteoporosis, including total protein intake, and even overall patterns of dietary intakes.[13-15] Protein/calorie malnutrition stimulates bone resorption and impairs bone formation both directly and through other mechanisms such as reduced serum insulin-like growth factor-I.[16] Vitamin K deficiency may contribute to an increased risk of osteoporotic fractures, possibly through effects on the carboxylation of bone proteins such as osteocalcin.[17] At least one observational study suggested that vitamin A intake might be associated with low BMD.[18] Recently, a case control study demonstrated a significant relationship between excessive intake of vitamin A and age-related fractures.[19]

Hormonal Factors

Estrogen deficiency has long been recognized as a major cause of bone loss in the first decade after menopause. More recently, investigators have identified a strong relationship between endogenous estrogen and bone mass in elderly men and women. In one prospective study, Slemenda et al. noted that both estrogens and androgens were independent predictors of bone loss in older postmenopausal women.[20] In both the Rancho Bernardo cohort and the Framingham Cohort, estradiol levels were very strongly related to BMD at the spine, hip, and forearm.[21,22]

Males also suffer from age-related bone loss, and evidence suggests that absolute estrogen levels, rather than testosterone concentrations, are essential for maintenance of BMD. In the Rancho Bernardo cohort, serum estradiol levels in elderly men correlated closely with bone mass at several sites.[21] Recently, Falahati-Nini et al. demonstrated that small amounts of estradiol were essential for preventing bone resorption in men, in part by upregulating osteoprotogerin (OPG).[23,24] Endogenous testosterone also plays a role in regulating bone turnover possibly more on the formation side than in respect to resorption. Serum testosterone levels decline with age at a rate of approximately 1.2% per year, whereas sex hormone binding globulin (SHBG) levels rise. Males treated with androgen antagonists or gonadotropin agonists for prostate cancer metastases rapidly lose bone mass and may be at high risk for subsequent osteoporotic fractures.[25] Overall, it seems likely that both androgens and estrogens are important in the elderly male. However, whether changes in male hormone levels are causally related to age related bone loss in men will have to await large-scale prospective studies.

Changes in the growth hormone(GH)/insulin-like growth factor I (IGF-I) axis may contribute to age-related bone loss. GH secretion declines 14% per decade and is the principle cause for low serum IGF-I concentrations in both elderly men and women.[26] However, it is likely that part of the impairment in bone formation noted in elderly individuals is more closely related to alterations in several insulin-like growth factor binding proteins than IGF-I itself.[26] Similarly, the adrenal androgens, DHEA and DHEA-S, also decline precipitously with age and are 10–20% of young adult serum levels.[27] Some studies have shown a positive correlation between DHEA levels and bone mass in the elderly, whereas others have failed to show any relationship.

Heritable and Environmental Factors

Age-related bone loss can be dramatic in some individuals, and this decline cannot be attributed solely to hormonal or nutritional factors. Several investigators have hypothesized that there is genetic programming that, when triggered by environmental factors, may lead to bone loss, especially in the elderly. Some animal models, but not others, have demonstrated a heritable component to age-related bone loss.[28] In humans, the multiplicity of environmental factors makes the determination of fracture heritability complicated, although recent publications suggest a genetic component.[29] On the other hand, environmental agents such as smoking, alcohol, and medications such as glucocorticoids and anticonvulsants, may contribute to an excessive rate of bone loss in some elders.

FRACTURES AND FALLS IN THE ELDERLY

In elderly individuals, decreased bone strength, as reflected by BMD, is only one of many important contributors to overall hip fracture risk. Other factors include propensity to fall, inability to correct a postural imbalance, characteristics of the faller such as height and muscle activity, the orientation of the fall, adequacy of local tissue shock absorbers, and characteristics of the impact surface. For its part, the resistance of a skeletal structure to failure (i.e., fracture) depends on the geometry of the bone, the material properties of the calcified tissue, and the location and direction of the loads to which the bone is subjected (i.e., during a fall or other activities). Estimations of the forces generated within the bone in response to a given load can be estimated using basic engineering principles. Those forces can then be compared with the strengths of the tissue. The ratio of the impact force expected during a fall to the force required to cause the bone to fail incorporates the two major determinants of fracture risk. When this ratio is close to or more than 1, the structure is at great risk of failure.

In the elderly, this ratio is 0.3 at the femoral neck for simple stance and normal ambulation. For stair climbing, it is about 0.6. In falls, the ratio ranges from 1 to greater than 70.[30] These calculations are complicated by considerable uncertainty about the loads to which hips are actually subjected during falls. For example, skeletal structures at high risk for age-related fracture, such as the hip, change their geometry with aging and bone remodeling, making it difficult to ascertain the true force of failure in vivo. Most of the energy from a fall dissipates before actual injury, and yet the residual force at impact remains two orders of magnitude greater than the energy required to fracture elderly femurs. This would suggest that a simple fall is easily capable of fracturing the proximal femur.

Falls in older people are rarely because of a single cause (Fig. 1). Falls usually occur when a threat to the normal homeostatic mechanisms that maintain postural stability is superimposed on underlying age-related declines in balance, ambulation, and cardiovascular function. In some cases, this may involve an acute illness such as a fever or infection, an environmental stress such as a newly initiated drug, or an unsafe walking surface. Regardless of the nature of the stress, an elderly person may not be able to compensate because of either age-related declines in function or

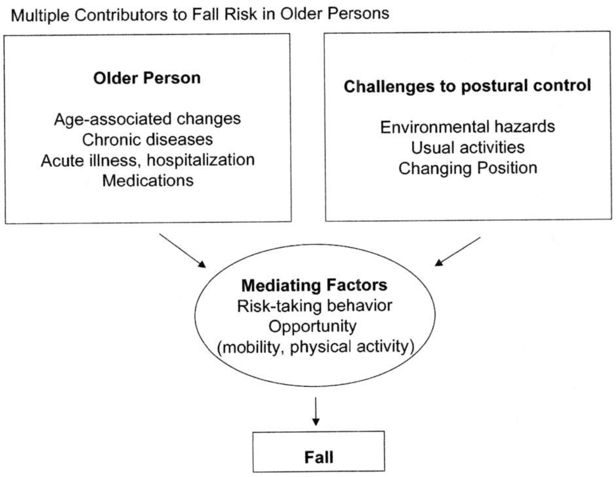

Older Person

Age-associated changes
Chronic diseases
Acute illness, hospitalization
Medications

Challenges to postural control

Environmental hazards
Usual activities
Changing Position

Mediating Factors
Risk-taking behavior
Opportunity
(mobility, physical activity)

Fall

FIG. 1. Falls are rarely because of a single cause. Characteristics of older persons (including age-related changes as well as acute illnesses), combined with everyday challenges to postural stability and mediating factors such as risk-taking behaviors, all contribute to the increased risk of falls with age. (Reproduced with permission from King MB, Tinetti ME 1995 Falls in community-dwelling older persons. J Am Geriatr Soc **43:**1146–1154.)

severe chronic disease. It is unlikely for an extrinsic stress to completely explain the circumstances of a fall. Older persons, by virtue of their age alone, experience declines in physiologic function, have greater numbers of chronic diseases, acute illnesses, and hospitalizations, and use multiple medications. Superimposed on these age-related characteristics, challenges to postural control may have a greater impact in aged persons according to their risk-taking behavior and opportunity to fall. Thus, those individuals who are completely immobile may not be at risk of falling despite multiple predisposing factors. On the other hand, persons who are either vigorous or only slightly frail may be at higher risk compared with individuals in between those extremes, due in part to more risk taking and inability to compensate for postural changes. Despite the importance of falls, bone density still remains a major predictor of fracture risk,[31] regardless of age.[32]

In one large study for hip fracture risk in elderly women, the subjects were grouped into three categories according to number of risk factors, for fracture other than bone density. Across all three risk groups, bone density remained an important predictor for fracture.[31]

APPROACH TO FRACTURE PREVENTION IN THE ELDERLY PATIENT

Because older persons have lower bone density to start, are continuing to lose bone, and are in the age group most likely to fracture, interventions would be expected to be most cost-effective when initiated in these individuals. The interventions can be divided into two groups: (1) those that reduce the applied load to the skeleton (fall prevention, passive protective systems), and (2) those that preserve or increase bone density.

Interventions That Reduce the Applied Load

Interventions to prevent falls must be predicated on an assessment of fall risk. This should include a history of falls,

because a history of falls is the single most important risk factor for a subsequent fall. If that history is positive, additional information can be obtained surrounding the events of the fall, because this information may identify important factors for targeting risk-factor modification strategies. The physical assessment of fall risk should include orthostatic vital sign measurement, a test of visual acuity, hearing, cardiac exam, extremity exam, and a test of the postural stability system as a whole using any of several recently developed assessment tools such as the "Get Up and Go" test.[33,34] Because some of the unfavorable outcomes of major fractures such as hip fractures are highly dependent on the premorbid status of an older patient, fracture prevention efforts should include a thorough assessment of underlying disability and frailty of the older person, because these factors influence long-term outcomes.[35]

For fall prevention interventions, the pooled results from several studies suggest that an intervention in which older people are assessed by a health professional trained to identify intrinsic and environmental risk factors is likely to reduce the fall rate (odds ratio = 0.79; 95% CI, 0.65–0.96).[36] Because falls to the side that impact on the hip are the primary determinant of hip fracture,[37] protective trochanteric padding devices have been developed.[38] Over the past 5 years, randomized, controlled trials have largely confirmed that hip protectors can reduce hip fracture, but subject compliance has been low.[39] Another way to reduce the energy delivered to the hip during a fall is to design flooring materials that will absorb energy rather than deliver the energy of a fall directly to the trochanter. Such flooring materials are currently being tested with the goal of using them in high-risk environments such as nursing homes.

Interventions That Preserve or Increase Bone Density

In addition to the attention to adequate basic nutritional factors, the use of therapeutic agents in the treatment of osteoporosis in the elderly person may be useful. Because older persons are at the greatest risk of fracture and fracture reduction has been demonstrated for estrogen therapy,[40] nasal calcitonin,[41] alendronate,[42] risedronate,[43] and parathyroid hormone,[44] potentially fewer elderly persons would have to be treated for less duration to prevent fractures than a younger population at lower risk of fracture.[45–48]

REFERENCES

1. Riggs BL, Wahner W, Seeman E, Offord KP, Dunn WL, Mazess RB, Johnson KA, Melton LJ III 1982 Changes in bone mineral density of the proximal femur and spine with aging: Differences between the postmenopausal and senile osteoporosis syndromes. J Clin Invest **70:**716–723.
2. Ensrud KE, Palermo L, Black DM, Cauley J, Jergas M, Orwoll ES, Nevitt MC, Fox KM, Cummings SR 1995 Hip and calcaneal bone loss increase with advancing age: Longitudinal results from the study of osteoporotic fractures. J Bone Miner Res **10:**1778–1787.
3. Hannan MT, Felson DT, Dawson-Hughes B, Tucker KL, Cupples LA, Wilson PW, Kiel DP 2000 Risk factors for longitudinal bone loss in elderly men and women: The Framingham Osteoporosis Study. J Bone Miner Res **15:**710–720.
4. Ensrud KE, Palmero L, Black MD, Cauley J, Jergas M, Orwoll ES, Nevitt MC, Fox KM, Cummings SR 1995 Hip and calcaneal bone loss increase with advancing age. J Bone Miner Res **10:**1778–1787.
5. Ross PD, Knowlton W 1998 Rapid bone loss is associated with

increased levels of biochemical markers. J Bone Miner Res **13:**297–302.

6. Dresner-Pollak R, Parker RA, Poku M, Thompson J, Seibel MJ, Greenspan SL 1996 Biochemical markers of bone turnover reflect femoral bone loss in elderly women. Calcif Tiss Int **59:**328–333.

7. Garnero P, Hausherr E, Chapuy MC, Marcelli C, Grandjean H, Muller C, Cormier C, Breart G, Meunier PJ, Delmas PD 1996 Markers of bone resorption predict hip fracture in elderly women: The EPIDOS prospective study. J Bone Miner Res **11:**1531–1538.

8. Bollen AM, Kiyak HA, Eyre DR 1997 Longitudinal evaluation of a bone resorption marker in elderly subjects. Osteoporos Int **7:**544–549.

9. Chapuy MC, Schott AM, Garnero P, Hans D, Delmas PD, Meunier PJ 1996 Healthy elderly French women living at home have secondary hyperparathyroidism and high bone turnover in winter. J Clin Endocrinol Metab **81:**1129–1133.

10. Dawson-Hughes B, Harris SS, Krall EA, Dallal GE 1997 Effect of calcium and vitamin D on bone density in men and women 65 years of age and older. N Engl J Med **337:**670–676.

11. Recker RR, Hinders S, Davies M, Heaney RP, Stegman MR, Lappe JM, Kimmel DB 1996 Correcting calcium deficiency prevents spine fractures in elderly women. J Bone Miner Res **11:**1961–1966.

12. NIH Consensus Conference 1995 Optimal calcium intake. JAMA **272:**1942–1948.

13. Dawson-Hughes B, Harris SS 2002 Calcium intake influences the association of protein intake with rates of bone loss in elderly men and women. Am J Clin Nutr **75:**773–779.

14. Hannan MT, Tucker KL, Dawson-Hughes B, Cupples LA, Felson DT, Kiel DP 2000 Effect of dietary protein on bone loss in elderly men and women: The Framingham Osteoporosis Study. J Bone Miner Res **15:**2504–2512.

15. Tucker KL, Chen H, Hannan MT, Cupples LA, Wilson PW, Felson D, Kiel DP 2002 Bone mineral density and dietary patterns in older adults: The Framingham Osteoporosis Study. Am J Clin Nutr **76:**245–252.

16. Schurch MA, Rizzoli R, Slosman D, Vadas L, Vergnaud P, Bonjour JP 1998 Protein supplements increase serum insulin-like growth factor-I levels and attenuate proximal femur bone loss in patients with recent hip fracture. A randomized, double-blind, placebo-controlled trial. Ann Intern Med **128:**801–890.

17. McKeown NM, Jacques PF, Gundberg CM, Peterson JW, Tucker KL, Kiel DP, Wilson PW, Booth SL 2002 Dietary and nondietary determinants of vitamin K biochemical measures in men and women. J Nutr **132:**1329–1334.

18. Promislow JH, Goodman-Gruen D, Slymen DJ, Barrett-Connor E 2002 Retinol intake and bone mineral density in the elderly: The Rancho Bernardo Study. J Bone Miner Res **17:**1349–1358.

19. Michaelsson K, Lithell H, Vessby B, Melhus H 2003 Serum retinol levels and the risk of fracture. N Engl J Med **348:**287–294.

20. Slemenda CW, Longcope C, Zhou L, Hui S, Peacock M, Johnston CC 1997 Sex steroids and bone mass in older men: Positive associations with serum estrogens and negative associations with androgens. J Clin Invest **100:**1755–1759.

21. Greendale GA, Edelstein S, Barrett-Connor E 1997 Endogenous sex steroids and bone mineral density in older women and men: The Rancho Bernardo Study. J Bone Miner Res **12:**1833–1843.

22. Amin S, Zhang Y, Sawin CT, Evans SR, Hannan MT, Kiel DP, Wilson PW, Felson DT 2000 Association of hypogonadism and estradiol levels with bone mineral density in elderly men from the Framingham study. Ann Intern Med **133:**951–963.

23. Khosla S, Atkinson EJ, Dunstan CR, O'Fallon WM 2002 Effect of estrogen versus testosterone on circulating osteoprotegerin and other cytokine levels in normal elderly men. J Clin Endocrinol Metab **87:**1550–1554.

24. Falahati-Nini A, Riggs BL, Atkinson EJ, O'Fallon WM, Eastell R, Khosla S 2000 Relative contribution of testosterone and estrogen in regulating bone resorption and formation in normal elderly men. J Clin Invest **106:**1553–1560.

25. Smith MR, Finkelstein JS, McGovern FJ, Zietman AL, Fallon MA, Schoenfeld DA, Kantoff PW 2002 Changes in body composition during androgen deprivation therapy for prostate cancer. J Clin Endocrinol Metab **87:**599–603.

26. Rosen CJ, Donahue LR, Hunter SJ 1994 IGFs and bone: The osteoporosis connection. Proc Soc Exp Biol Med **206:**83–102.

27. Barrett-Connor E, Kritz-Silverstein D, Edelstein SL 1993 A prospective study of DHEAS and bone mineral density in older men and women. Am J Epidemiol **137:**201–206.

28. Halloran BP, Ferguson VL, Simske SJ, Burghardt A, Venton LL,

29. Majumdar S 2002 Changes in bone structure and mass with advancing age in the male C57BL/6J mouse. J Bone Miner Res **17:**1044–1050.

29. Deng HW, Mahaney MC, Williams JT, Li J, Conway T, Davies KM, Li JL, Deng H, Recker RR 2002 Relevance of the genes for bone mass variation to susceptibility to osteoporotic fractures and its implications to gene search for complex human disease. Genet Epidemiol **22:**12–25.

30. Hayes WC 1991 Biomechanics of cortical and trabecular bone: Implications for assessment of fracture risk. In: Mow VC, Hayes WC (eds.) Basic Orthopaedic Biomechanics. Raven Press, New York, NY, USA, pp. 93–142.

31. Cummings SR, Nevitt MC, Browner WS, Stone K, Fox KM, Ensrud KE, Cauley J, Black D, Vogt TM 1995 Risk factors for hip fracture in white women. N Engl J Med **332:**767–773.

32. Nevitt MC, Johnell O, Black DM, Ensrud K, Genant HK, Cummings SR 1994 Bone mineral density predicts non-spine fractures in very elderly women. Osteoporos Int **4:**325–331.

33. Mathias A, Nayak USL, Isaacs B 1986 Balance in elderly patients: The "get-up and go" test. Arch Phys Med Rehabil **67:**387–389.

34. Tinetti ME 1986 Performance-oriented assessment of mobility problems in elderly patients. J Am Geriatr Soc **34:**119–126.

35. Leibson CL, Tosteson ANA, Gabriel SE, Ransom JE, Melton LJ 2002 Mortality, disability, and nursing home use for persons with and without hip fracture: A population-based study. J Am Geriatr Soc **50:**1644–1650.

36. Gillespie LD, Gillespie WJ, Robertson MC, Lamb SE, Cumming RG, Rowe BH 2001 Interventions for preventing falls in elderly people. Cochrane Database Syst Rev 2001(3):CD000340.

37. Greenspan SL, Myers ER, Kiel DP, Parker RA, Hayes WC, Resnick NM 1998 Fall direction, bone mineral density, and function: Risk factors for hip fracture in frail nursing home elderly. Am J Med **104:**539–545.

38. Nevitt MC, Cummings SR, the Study of Osteoporotic Fractures Research Group 1993 Type of fall and risk of hip and wrist fractures: The study of osteoporotic fractures. J Am Geriatr Soc **41:**1226–1234.

39. Parker MJ, Gillespie LD, Gillespie WJ 2001 Hip protectors for preventing hip fractures in the elderly. Cochrane Database Sys Rev 2001(2):CD001255.

40. Writing Group for the Women's Health Initiative Investigators 2002 Risks and benefits of estrogen plus progestin in healthy postmenopausal women. JAMA **288:**321–333.

41. Chesnut CH, Silverman SL, Andriano K, Ettinger B, Genant HK, Gimona A, Harris S, Kiel DP, LeBoff M, Maricic MJ, Miller P, Moniz C, Peacock M, Richardson P, Watts N, Baylink DJ for the PROOF Study Group 2000 A randomized trial of nasal spray salmon calcitonin in postmenopausal women with established osteoporosis: The Prevent Recurrence of Osteoporotic Fractures Study. Am J Med **109:**267–276.

42. Black DM, Cummings SR, Karpf DB, Cauley JA, Thompson DE, Nevitt MC, Bauer DC, Genant HK, Haskell WL, Marcus R, Ott SM, Torner JC, Quandt SA, Reiss TF, Ensrud KE 1996 Randomised trial of effect of alendronate on risk of fracture in women with existing vertebral fractures. Lancet **348:**1535–1541.

43. McClung MR, Geusens P, Miller PD, Zippel H, Bensen WG, Roux C, Adami S, Fogelman I, Diamond T, Eastell R, Meunier PJ, Reginster JY 2001 Effect of risedronate on the risk of hip fracture in elderly women. Hip Intervention Program Study Group. NEJ Medicine **344:**333–340.

44. Neer RM, Arnaud CD, Zanchetta JR, Prince R, Gaich GA, Reginster JY, Hodsman AB, Eriksen EF, Ish-Shalom S, Genant HK, Wang O, Mitlak BH 2001 Effect of parathyroid hormone (1–34) on fractures and bone mineral density in postmenopausal women with osteoporosis. NEJ Medicine **344:**1434–1441.

45. Lufkin EG, Wahner HW, O'Fallon WM, Hodgson SF, Kotowicz MA, Lane AW, Judd HL, Caplan RH, Riggs BL 1992 Treatment of postmenopausal osteoporosis with transdermal estrogen. Ann Intern Med **117:**1–9.

46. Overgaard K, Hansen MA, Jensen SB, Christiansen C 1992 Effect of salcatonin given intranasally on bone mass and fracture rates in established osteoporosis: A dose-response study. BMJ **305:**556–561.

47. Black DM, Cummings SR, Karpf DB, Cauley JA, Thompson DE, Nevitt MC, Bauer DC, Genant HK, Haskell WL, Marcus R, Ott SM, Torner JC, Quandt SA, Reiss TF, Ensrud KE 1996 Randomised trial of effect of alendronate on risk of fracture in women with existing vertebral fractures. Lancet **348:**1535–1541.

48. Liberman UA, Weiss SR, Broll J, Minne HW, Quan H, Bell NH, Rodriguez-Portales J, Downs RW Jr, Dequeker J, Favus M 1995 Effect of oral alendronate on bone mineral density and the incidence of fractures in postmenopausal osteoporosis. N Engl J Med **333:**1437–1443.

Chapter 14. Intestinal Absorption of Calcium, Magnesium, and Phosphate

Jacob Lemann, Jr.[1] and Murray J. Favus[2]

[1]*Nephrology Section, Tulane University School of Medicine, New Orleans, Louisiana; and* [2]*Department of Medicine, University of Chicago, Chicago, Illinois*

INTRODUCTION

Intestinal absorption of Ca, Mg, and PO_4 determines the supply of these minerals to meet the needs of increasing body mass, especially bone mineralization, during growth and the ongoing needs related to tissue turnover and bone remodeling in adults. The quantities of Ca, Mg, and PO_4 that are absorbed by the intestine are determined by the availability of these minerals in the diet and by the capacity of the intestine to absorb them. In general, intestinal mineral absorption represents the sum of two transport processes: saturable transcellular absorption that is physiologically regulated and nonsaturable paracellular absorption that is dependent on mineral concentration within the lumen of the gut.

Serum concentrations, urinary concentrations, and urinary excretion rates of Ca, Mg, or PO_4 are easily and routinely measured in the evaluation and care of patients with disorders of mineral metabolism and bone. However, quantitation of intestinal absorption of Ca, Mg, and PO_4 is difficult and has generally been assessed only in a research setting. Several techniques are available:

1. Metabolic balance. Subjects are fed constant diets, and the diets are analyzed for Ca, Mg, and PO_4. The subjects must be adapted to the diet for 7–10 days, especially if the quantity of Ca, Mg, or PO_4 in the diet differs significantly from a given subject's customary intake. In addition, because defecation occurs at irregular intervals, the subjects are continuously fed a measured quantity of a nonabsorbable marker that can be easily and reliably quantitated in the feces to verify achievement of the steady state and to assign a time interval to the stool collections. Polyethylene glycol (PEG), chromium sesquioxide, or small segments of radio-opaque tubing are often used as markers. After the adaptation period, feces are collected during a balance period of at least 6 days duration and analyzed for Ca, Mg, and PO_4. Dietary intake minus average daily fecal excretion during the balance period provides an estimate of net intestinal absorption of Ca, Mg, or PO_4.

2. Absorption from a single meal after intestinal washout. After overnight fasting, subjects undergo intestinal lavage over a period of 4 h with a solution that does not cause either net intestinal absorption or secretion of water and electrolytes. Four hours after completion of lavage, they are fed a meal together with a known amount of the nonabsorbable marker PEG. A duplicate meal is analyzed for Ca, Mg, and PO_4. Twelve hours after the meal, intestinal lavage is repeated for 4 h. The rectal effluent is collected, and together with any stool passed after ingestion of the meal, analyzed for Ca, Mg, PO_4, and PEG. Intake in the meal minus effluent excretion, corrected for the recovery of PEG, provides an estimate of net intestinal absorption of Ca, Mg, or PO_4. The study can also be repeated on a separate day when the subjects ingest only PEG without food to measure the quantities of Ca, Mg, or PO_4 secreted into the intestine. Total intestinal Ca, Mg, or PO_4 absorption (true absorption) can then be calculated as the sum of net absorption from the meal minus the quantity appearing in the effluent during fasting.

Both the balance method and the intestinal washout method provide estimates of actual net mineral input to the body from the intestine.

3. Absorption of isotopic minerals. A measured quantity of ^{47}Ca is administered orally. The fraction of the dose absorbed can be estimated either by external counting of radioisotope in the arm at a fixed time after dosing, by counting of isotope in serial blood samples and expressing fractional absorption as percent of dose/liter plasma when counts peak or by collecting and counting isotope excreted in the feces over 4–6 days after dosing and subtracting isotope excreted from the dose. Alternatively and more precisely, a measured quantity of ^{45}Ca can be administered intravenously together with the oral dose of ^{47}Ca. Ca absorption can then be estimated from the ratio of isotope concentrations, or specific activities in serum or urine or absorption rate can be estimated by compartmental kinetic analysis using multiple serum samples collected over 4–6 h after dosing. The stable isotopes ^{42}Ca and ^{44}Ca have also been used with measurement by mass spectrometry.

The authors have no conflict of interest.

Absorption of isotopic Mg and of isotopic PO_4 have not been studied because ^{28}Mg has a half-life of only 21 h and because of the unacceptably intense β-emission of ^{32}P.

4. Segmental intestinal absorption. After an overnight fast, a triple-lumen tube is passed to the duodenum, jejunum, ileum, or colon. Perfusate, containing Ca, Mg, or PO_4, together with a nonabsorbable marker, is instilled through the proximal lumen and aspirated at a constant rate from both the middle lumen, where mixing of the perfusate with intestinal contents has been completed, and from the distal lumen, which is the end of the intestinal study segment between the middle and distal lumens, usually 30 cm in length. Absorption of Ca, Mg, or PO_4 can then be estimated by the change in mineral concentration in the fluid aspirated distally relative to that aspirated at the end of the mixing segment, taking into account the simultaneous change in PEG concentration as a measure of perfusate absorption.

5. Indirect assessment of intestinal mineral absorption. After overnight fasting and collection of control urine and blood specimens, subjects are given 25 mmol Ca (1000 mg) orally, usually as calcium gluconate. Two subsequent 2-h urines are collected together with blood samples 1 and 3 h after the load. Fasting $U_{Ca}V$/ glomerular filtration rate (GFR), calculated as $([Ca]_{urine} \times [Creatinine]_{plasma})/[Creatinine]_{urine}$, is normally <0.035 mM GFR (<0.13 mg/100 ml GFR). Among subjects exhibiting normal rate of intestinal Ca absorption, the increment in $U_{Ca}V$/GFR after the load is <0.05 mM GFR (<0.20 mg/100 ml GFR). Greater increases in $U_{Ca}V$/GFR after the oral Ca load provide evidence for increased intestinal Ca absorption.

CALCIUM

The relationship between net intestinal Ca absorption/day (dietary Ca intake/day minus fecal Ca excretion/day) and dietary Ca intake/day, derived from metabolic balance studies of healthy adults, is illustrated in Fig. 1. On average, net intestinal Ca absorption is less than zero (e.g., fecal Ca excretion/day exceeds dietary Ca intake/day) when dietary Ca intake/ day is <5 mmol/day (<200 mg/day). Thus, on average, healthy adults require daily Ca intakes >10 mmol/ day (>400 mg/day) to maintain Ca balance, taking into account both the inability of the normal kidney to excrete urine that is essentially free of Ca (unlike Na, Mg, or PO_4) as well as ongoing minor skin losses of Ca. As dietary Ca intake/day rises from minimal intakes of 3–5 mmol/day (120–200 mg/day), net intestinal Ca absorption/day increases, but in progressively decreasing quantity, such that when Ca intake exceeds about 25 mmol/day (1000 mg/day), net intestinal Ca absorption tends to plateau at an average value of about 7.5 mmol/day (300 mg/day). The curvilinear relationship between net intestinal Ca absorption and dietary Ca intake reflects the sum of two absorptive mechanisms: active, saturable absorption and passive absorption, dependent on the concentration gradient between intestinal lumen and blood. The wide variation of net intestinal Ca absorption among healthy adults at any given level of di-

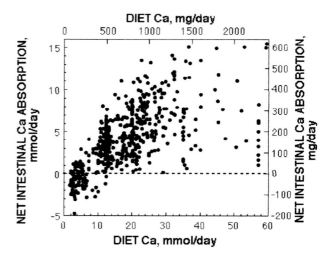

FIG. 1. Net intestinal Ca absorption in humans as measured by the metabolic balance method in relation to dietary Ca intake. Adapted from data in references 20–63.

etary intake that is seen in Fig. 1, especially when dietary Ca intake exceeds 15–20 mmol/day (600–800 mg/day), is presumed to primarily reflect variation in active Ca absorption between subjects.

Currently, 1,25-dihydroxyvitamin D [1,25(OH)$_2$D; calcitriol] is the only recognized hormonal stimulus of active intestinal Ca absorption, which occurs principally in the duodenum and jejunum. Whether absorption is measured by the balance technique, intestinal washout after a meal, or by isotopic methods, or whether absorption is expressed as a percentage of dietary or meal intake or isotope administered, Ca absorption increases as plasma calcitriol increases by an average of about 0.2% Ca absorbed/pmol 1,25(OH)$_2$D vitamin D/liter or about 0.5% Ca absorbed/pg 1,25(OH)$_2$D/ ml.

The interaction of dietary Ca intake and serum 1,25(OH)$_2$D concentrations as determinants of net intestinal Ca absorption is depicted in Fig. 2. When dietary Ca intake is very low, in the range of 4 mmol/day (160 mg/day), net intestinal Ca absorption reaches a maximum of about 3 mmol/day (120 mg/day), even when serum 1,25(OH)$_2$D levels are higher than the upper limit of the normal range (>135 pM or >56 pg/ml). In contrast, when dietary Ca intake is normal, 20 mmol/day (800 mg/day), net intestinal Ca absorption may exceed 10 mmol/day (400 mg/day), a value in the upper range of the wide normal variation shown in Fig. 1, when serum 1,25(OH)$_2$D levels average 120 pM (50 pg/ml), a concentration that is within the upper limit of the normal range.

This effect of the amount of Ca available to limit absorption has also been directly documented during perfusion studies of jejunal Ca absorption, as shown in Fig. 3. Ca absorption rises progressively as the jejunum is perfused with solutions containing 1, 2.5, 5, or 10 mM Ca, tending to plateau at the highest Ca concentration. Those studies also showed that Ca absorption is higher at any given perfusate Ca concentration among subjects who had been eating a low Ca diet (7.5 mmol/day; 300 mg/day) for 1 month than among subjects eating diets providing large amounts of Ca

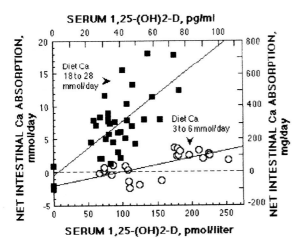

FIG. 2. Net intestinal Ca absorption in relation to serum 1,25(OH)$_2$D concentrations among subjects fed normal Ca diets alone [including anephric subjects with undetectable 1,25(OH)$_2$D levels] or also given calcitriol [solid symbols: Net intestinal Ca absorption (mmol/day) = −0.4 + 0.082 × Serum 1,25(OH)$_2$D (pM); r = 0.71) and among healthy subjects fed low Ca diets alone or also given calcitriol [open symbols: Net intestinal Ca absorption (mmol/day) = −2.0 + 0.021 × Serum 1,25(OH)$_2$D (pM); r = 0.56]. Adapted from data in references 55, 57, 58, 59, 60, and 62.

(50 mmol/day; 2000 mg/day). The increase in Ca absorption is caused by dietary Ca deprivation stimulation of parathyroid hormone (PTH) secretion and the resultant increase in renal 1,25(OH)$_2$D synthesis. The converse is also true, because high dietary Ca reduces PTH secretion and inhibits 1,25(OH)$_2$D synthesis. Thus, reduced net intestinal Ca absorption occurs when dietary Ca intake is limited, when serum 1,25(OH)$_2$D concentrations are low, or when the intestine is unresponsive to this hormone. Increased intestinal Ca absorption occurs when serum 1,25(OH)$_2$D concentrations are high or high-normal due to upregulation by 1,25(OH)$_2$D of it's own receptor. There are possible mechanisms that are independent of 1,25(OH)$_2$D. Very high Ca

TABLE 1. CAUSES OF REDUCED AND INCREASED INTESTINAL Ca ABSORPTION

Increased Ca absorption	Decreased Ca absorption
Increased renal 1,25(OH)$_2$D production	Very low dietary Ca intake
Growth	Decreased 1,25(OH)$_2$D
Pregnancy	Vitamin D deficiency
Lactation	Vitamin D–dependent rickets, type 1
Primary hyperparathyroidism	Chronic renal insufficiency
Idiopathic hypercalciuria (some types)	Hypoparathyroidism
Increased extrarenal 1,25(OH)$_2$D production	Aging
Sarcoidosis and other granulomas	With normal 1,25(OH)$_2$D production
B-cell lymphoma	Glucocorticoid excess
With normal plasma 1,25(OH)$_2$D	Thyroid hormone excess
Idiopathic hypercalciuria (some types)	Intestinal malabsorption including short-bowel syndrome

intakes also increase absorption, but such an increase in passive Ca absorption is accompanied by suppression of serum 1,25(OH)$_2$D. As a result, the increase in absorption would be blunted. The major conditions that reduce or enhance intestinal Ca absorption are listed in Table 1.

MAGNESIUM

The relationship between net intestinal Mg absorption/day (dietary Mg intake/day minus fecal Mg excretion/day) and dietary Mg intake/day, derived from metabolic balance studies, is illustrated in Fig. 4. Net intestinal Mg absorption is directly related to dietary Mg intake, on the average about 35–40% being absorbed when dietary Mg intake is in the normal range for adults of 7–30 mmol/day (168–720 mg/day). Because Mg is a constituent of all cells, and normal

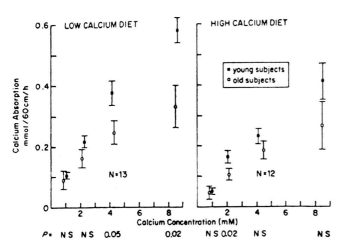

FIG. 3. Interaction of age and prior dietary Ca intake on jejunal Ca absorption from perfusate containing 1, 2.5, 5, or 10 mM Ca. Seven young and six old subjects were studied on a low Ca diet, and six old and six young subjects were studied on a high Ca diet. p values are by grouped t-test. Reproduced with permission from Am J Clin Nutr **32:**2052–2060.

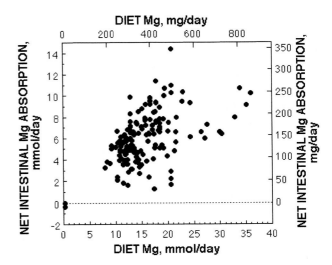

FIG. 4. Net intestinal Mg absorption in relation to dietary Mg intake. Adapted from data in references 22, 29, 31, 33, 35, 43, 52, 54, 58, 60, 61, 62, 65, and 69.

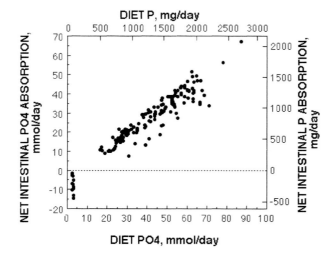

FIG. 5. Net intestinal PO_4 absorption in relation to dietary PO_4 intake. Net intestinal PO_4 (mmol/day) $= -5.4 + 0.77 \times$ Dietary PO_4 (mmol/day); $r = 0.95$. Adapted from data in references 20, 21, 22, 25, 26, 28, 29, 31, 33, 35, 37, 39, 40, 41, 42, 43, 46, 47, 52, 54, 56, 58, 60, 61, 62, and 63.

diets contain foods of cellular origin, dietary Mg intake is generally proportional to total caloric intake, thus assuring adequate intake and intestinal Mg absorption. The data in Fig. 3 also include observations from studies of Mg balances using synthetic diets that are nearly Mg-free. Net intestinal Mg absorption is less than zero (e.g., fecal Mg excretion/day exceeds dietary Mg intake/day) only when dietary Mg intake is <2 mmol/day (48 mg/day). The variation in net intestinal Mg absorption among healthy subjects at any given normal level of dietary Mg intake seems to be related to other constituents of the diet, such as PO_4 content, which complex Mg within the intestinal lumen and limit absorption. In contrast to Ca absorption, Mg absorption is not increased by serum $1,25(OH)_2D$, as plasma concentrations vary from undetectable to high among adults with no correlation with Mg absorption. Dietary Mg intakes exceeding 35 mmol/day (840 mg/day) seldom occur spontaneously. Only a small fraction of oral Mg supplementation taken as a cathartic [$Mg(OH)_2$, Mg-citrate] may be absorbed. Such high intake of Mg is apt to lead to hypermagnesemia only in the presence of significant reductions in kidney function. Thus, Mg-containing laxatives and antacids should not be given to patients with kidney disease. Reduced intestinal Mg absorption occurs with diffuse intestinal diseases causing malabsorption or as a consequence of laxative abuse.

PHOSPHATE

Intestinal PO_4 absorption, like the absorption of Ca, is dependent on both passive PO_4 transport related to the lumenal [PO_4] prevailing after a meal, and on active PO_4 transport that is stimulated by $1,25(OH)_2D$. The relationship between net intestinal PO_4 absorption/day (dietary PO_4 intake/day minus fecal PO_4 excretion/day) and dietary PO_4 intake/day, derived from metabolic balance studies, is shown in Fig. 5. As for Mg absorption in relation to dietary Mg intake, PO_4 absorption is directly related to dietary PO_4

intake. Because PO_4 is a major constituent of all cells, dietary PO_4 intake seldom is <20 mmol/day (<620 mg P/day). Based on studies using synthetic diets providing only 2–3 mmol PO_4/day (62–93 mg P/day), there is net intestinal secretion of PO_4 when dietary PO_4 intake is <10 mmol/day (<310 mg P/day); fecal PO_4 excretion exceeds dietary PO_4 intake. When dietary PO_4 intake varies over the usual normal range of 25–60 mmol/day (775–1860 mg P/day), 60–80% of dietary PO_4 is absorbed. Higher oral PO_4 intakes seldom occur spontaneously.

Intestinal PO_4 absorption is reduced in vitamin D deficiency. The administration of $1,25(OH)_2D$ to patients with chronic renal failure stimulates jejunal PO_4 absorption. However, experimental elevations of serum $1,25(OH)_2D$ in healthy, vitamin D–replete subjects does not further stimulate jejunal PO_4 absorption significantly. As shown in Fig. 6, fractional PO_4 absorption estimated by the balance technique increases only slightly, although significantly, as serum $1,25(OH)_2D$ concentrations vary from normal to experimentally elevated in adults fed diets adequate in PO_4. Even in the presence of undetectable serum $1,25(OH)_2D$ levels, patients with chronic renal failure exhibit significant concentration-dependent jejunal PO_4 absorption (Fig. 6). Thus, the availability of PO_4 in the diet seems to be the major determinant of net PO_4 input to the body from the intestine. Continuing absorption of dietary PO_4 is a major factor in the pathogenesis of secondary hyperparathyroidism occurring among patients with progressive kidney disease. Net intestinal PO_4 absorption among patients with chronic kidney disease is nearly identical to that among normal subjects, as dietary PO_4 intake varies over the range of 10–50 mmol/day (310–1550 mg P/day). As a consequence, cathartics, as well as enemas that contain large amounts of NaH_2PO_4/Na_2HPO_4, should not be given to

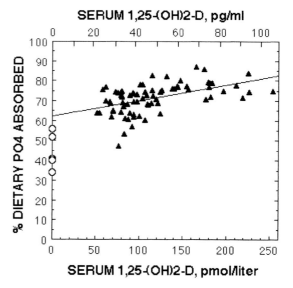

FIG. 6. Relationship between percent dietary PO_4 absorbed ([Net intestinal PO_4 absorption $\times$ 100]/[Dietary PO_4 intake]) and serum $1,25(OH)_2D$ concentrations in vitamin D–replete adults eating diets containing normal amounts of PO_4 alone or also given calcitriol. Data from five anephric patients [three of five also taking $Al(OH)_3$] with undetectable serum $1,25(OH)_2D$ concentrations are also shown.

patients with renal failure. Intestinal PO_4 absorption is also not apparently significantly reduced among patients with other disorders associated with chronic hyperphosphatemia such as hypoparathyroidism and tumoral calcinosis. Because of the ability of Al^{3+} and of Ca^{2+} to form insoluble PO_4 salts and thus limit intestinal PO_4 absorption, aluminum hydroxide gel, aluminum carbonate, and more recently in an attempt prevent the potential toxicity of aluminum, calcium carbonate, calcium acetate, or calcium citrate are routinely used in the care of patients with advanced renal failure. Chronic abuse of aluminum-containing antacids, by inhibiting absorption of dietary PO_4 and reabsorption of PO_4 entering the lumen of the gut in intestinal secretions, can rarely result in PO_4 depletion. PO_4 malabsorption can also occur with diffuse disease of the small intestine.

SUGGESTED READINGS

1. Favus MJ 2002 Intestinal absorption of calcium, magnesium, and phosphorus. In: Coe FL, Favus MJ (eds.) Disorders of Bone and Mineral Metabolism, 2nd ed. Lippincott Williams Wilkins, Philadelphia, PA, USA, pp. 48–73.
2. Lemann J Jr 2002 Idiopathic hypercalciuria. In: Coe FL, Favus MJ (eds.) Disorders of Bone and Mineral Metabolism, 2nd ed. Lippincott Williams Wilkins, Philadelphia, PA, USA, pp. 673–697.
3. Wasserman RH 1997 Vitamin D and the intestinal absorption of calcium and phosphorus. In: Feldman D, Glorieux FH, Pike JW (eds.) Vitamin D. Academic Press, San Diego, CA, USA, pp. 259–273.
4. Sheikh MS, Ramirez A, Emmett M, Santa Ana C, Schiller LR, Fordtran JS 1988 Role of vitamin D-dependent and vitamin D-independent mechanisms in absorption of food calcium. J Clin Invest 81:126–132.
5. Sheikh MS, Santa Ana CA, Nicar MJ, Schiller LR, Fordtran JS 1987 Gastrointestinal absorption from milk and calcium salts. N Engl J Med 317:532–536.
6. Favus MJ 1985 Factors that influence absorption and secretion of calcium in the small intestine and colon. Am J Physiol 248:G147–G157.
7. Portale AA, Booth BE, Halloran BE, Morris RC Jr 1984 Effect of diet phosphorus on circulating concentration of 1,25-dihydroxyvitamin D and immunoreactive parathyroid hormone in children with moderate renal insufficiency. J Clin Invest 73:1580–1589.
8. Maierhofer WJ, Lemann J, Gray RW, Cheung HS 1984 Dietary calcium and serum $1,25(OH)_2$-vitamin D as determinants of calcium balance in healthy men. Kidney Int 26:752–759.
9. Wilz DR, Gray RW, Dominguez JH, Lemann J 1979 Plasma $1,25(OH)_2$-vitamin D concentrations and net intestinal absorption of calcium, phosphate and magnesium in humans. Am J Clin Nutr 32:2052–2060.
10. Ireland P, Fordtran JS 1973 Effect of dietary calcium and age on jejunal calcium absorption in humans studied by intestinal perfusion. J Clin Invest 52:2672–2680.
11. Malm OJ 1958 Calcium requirement and adaptation in adult men. Scand J Clin Lab Invest Suppl 35:1–289.
12. Albright F, Reifenstein EC Jr 1948 The Parathyroid Glands and Metabolic Bone Disease. The Williams & Wilkins Company, Baltimore, MD, USA.

Chapter 15.   Calcium, Magnesium, and Phosphorus: Renal Handling and Urinary Excretion

David A. Bushinsky

Departments of Medicine and of Pharmacology and Physiology, University of Rochester School of Medicine and Dentistry, Nephrology Unit, Strong Memorial Hospital, Rochester, New York

INTRODUCTION

Adult, nonpregnant, humans have no appreciable daily net gain or loss of body calcium, magnesium, or phosphorus. This remarkable homeostasis is achieved by the coordinated interaction of the intestine, the site of net absorption; the kidney, the site of net excretion; and the bone, the largest repository of these ions in the body.[1,2] This neutral body ionic balance requires that net intestinal mineral absorption must equal renal mineral excretion. In this chapter we will discuss renal filtration, reabsorption, and the factors that influence urinary excretion of these ions.

CALCIUM

Filtration

The concentration of serum calcium is maintained at between 9.0 and 10.4 mg/dl or between 2.25 and 2.6 mM.[1,2] Approximately 40% of serum calcium is protein bound, especially to albumin and to lesser extent globulins and other proteins, and is not filtered by the glomerulous. Approximately 10% of calcium is complexed to phosphate, citrate, carbonate, and other anions, and the remaining 50% exists in the ionized form. The complexed and ionized calcium, which together are termed the ultrafiltrable calcium, are freely filtered by the glomerulous, and this ultrafiltrate has a calcium concentration of approximately 1.5 mM.

A typical 70-kg male with a normal glomerular filtration rate of 180 liters/day will filter approximately 270 mmol of calcium per day (180 liters/day $\times$ 1.5 mM).[2] This quantity of calcium, over 10 g, is far more than the calcium content of the entire extracellular fluid compartment and far more than the quantity of net intestinal calcium absorption, which is approximately 4 mmol/day. To maintain neutral calcium balance, approximately 98% of the filtered calcium must be reabsorbed along the renal tubule.

Intuitively, the process of massive filtration coupled to almost complete reabsorption of the filtrate seems energetically wasteful; however, one must consider that calcium is but one component of this ultrafiltrate. There are many other

The author has no conflict of interest.

PROXIMAL TUBULE

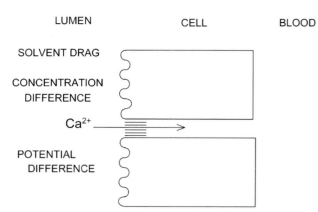

FIG. 1. Predominant mode of calcium transport in the proximal tubule: paracellular calcium transport.

THICK ASCENDING LIMB

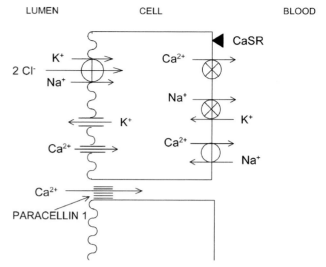

FIG. 2. Paracellular and transcellular calcium transport in the thick ascending limb of the loop of Henle.

substances, for example, creatinine and urea, which undergo filtration and virtually no reabsorption, resulting in complete excretion. Thus, substantial filtration followed by selective reabsorption allows precise control of excretion.

Reabsorption

Approximately 70% of filtered calcium is reabsorbed in the proximal tubule (Fig. 1). Proximal reabsorption is thought to be predominantly passive for two principle reasons: sodium and calcium are reabsorbed in parallel, and the proximal tubule epithelium is very "leaky" in that there is a large calcium flux from the bath to the lumen observed in micropuncture experiments.[3] The mechanism of proximal calcium reabsorption seems to be predominantly paracellular, with salt and water carrying calcium from the lumen to the interstitium through the transport mechanism of solvent drag. However, there is clear evidence for active transport of calcium in the latter portions of the proximal tubule.

Approximately 20% of filtered calcium is reabsorbed in the loop of Henle (Fig. 2). There appears to be little calcium transport in the thin descending or thin ascending limbs of Henle's loop. However, in the thick ascending limb of the loop of Henle (TALH), the lumen-positive voltage, generated by the Na-K-2Cl transporter with subsequent back leak of potassium, provides a strong driving force for paracellular calcium reabsorption. The loop diuretics, such as furosemide, impair calcium reabsorption in this segment by decreasing lumen-positive voltage.

The calcium sensing receptor (CaSR) is a G-protein–coupled receptor with abundant expression in the kidney; in the loop of Henle, the receptor is present along the basolateral surface.[4,5] An increase in peritubular calcium decreases tubular calcium reabsorption also by decreasing the lumen positive voltage. In addition there appears to be active calcium transport especially near the kidney cortex.

The protein, paracellin 1, is expressed in the thick ascending limb tight junctions. Mutations in this protein result in a selective defect in paracellular calcium (and magnesium) reabsorption.[6] Alterations in basolateral calcium

(and magnesium) may directly regulate divalent ion permeability at this site.

The distal convoluted tubule is responsible for approximately 8% of calcium reabsorption and is the major site of regulation of urine calcium excretion (Fig. 3). In this segment, active calcium transport occurs against both electrical and chemical gradients. Here calcium enters the cytosol down an electrical and chemical gradient through a recently identified renal epithelial calcium channel (ECaC), which is a member of the transient receptor potential (TRP) superfamily of channels.[7,8] ECaC is significantly more permeable to calcium than to sodium and has a principle role in the regulation of cellular calcium entry especially by $1,25(OH)_2D_3$ and perhaps by calcium itself.

The calcium is shuttled across the cell through a vitamin D–dependent calcium binding protein, calbindin-D_{28K}, which has been localized to the distal convoluted tubule and the more distal tubule segments.[9] This binding protein allows large amounts of calcium to be ferried across the cytosol without altering the free intracellular calcium con-

DISTAL CONVOLUTED TUBULE

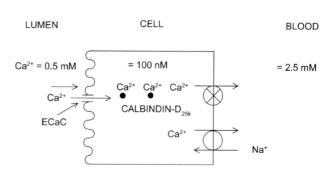

FIG. 3. Calcium transport in the distal convoluted tubule.

TABLE 1. FACTORS INFLUENCING CALCIUM EXCRETION

Glomerular filtration
  Increased
    Hypercalcemia
  Decreased
    Hypocalcemia
    Renal insufficiency
Tubular reabsorption
  Increased
    Extracellular fluid volume depletion
    Hypocalcemia
    Phosphate administration
    Metabolic alkalosis
    Parathyroid hormone
    Parathyroid hormone related protein
    Thiazide diuretics
    Familial hypocalciuric hypercalcemia and other genetic disorders
  Decreased
    Extracellular fluid volume expansion
    Hypercalcemia
    Phosphate depletion
    Metabolic acidosis
    Loop diuretics
    Cyclosporin A
    Autosomal dominant hypocalcemia
    Dent's disease
    Bartter's syndrome
    Other genetic disorders

centration. Calbindin-D$_{28K}$ co-localizes and may interact with ECaC to regulate calcium transport.[10]

At the basolateral membrane, calcium is transported against a large chemical gradient to the interstium. Active calcium transport is mediated principally through sodium for calcium exchange and also through a magnesium-dependent calcium ATPase. While transport of calcium generally follows sodium in this segment, reabsorption and subsequent excretion of the two ions can be dissociated providing further evidence for the regulation of calcium reabsorption in the distal convoluted tubule.

There appears to be reabsorption of less than 5% of filtered calcium in the collecting duct.

Factors Affecting Reabsorption

Ions

Sodium. Extracellular fluid volume expansion with saline infusion increases urinary sodium and calcium excretion, whereas extracellular fluid volume contraction decreases urinary sodium and calcium excretion (Table 1). Volume expansion principally causes a decrease in proximal tubule sodium and calcium reabsorption, which is independent of alterations in parathyroid hormone (PTH), although a decrease in distal calcium reabsorption may also occur.

Calcium. Increases in dietary calcium result in an increase in urinary calcium; approximately 6–8% of an increase in dietary calcium appears in the urine. Hypercalcemia will increase both ionized and complexed calcium, resulting in an increase in the ultrafiltrable calcium. However, this in-

crease in serum calcium will be opposed by a decrease in the glomerular filtration rate mediated through a decrease in the glomerular capillary ultrafiltration coefficient. Hypercalcemia results in a decline in reabsorption in the proximal tubule, in the loop of Henle, and in the distal tubule segments resulting in greater urinary excretion of calcium than sodium. Hypocalcemia will result in a decrease in ultrafiltrable calcium and an increase in the glomerular filtration rate. The hypocalcemia-induced decline in PTH will result in enhanced tubular calcium reabsorption and a fall in urinary calcium excretion.

The CaSR is on the basolateral membrane of TALH.[4,5] In this segment, calcium reabsorption is driven primarily by the lumen-positive voltage, which is generated by the Na-K-2Cl transporter. Activation of the CaSR by calcium decreases the activity of the potassium channel and limits the lumen positive voltage leading to a decrease in tubular calcium reabsorption.[11] Calcium may also alter the permeability of paracellin 1, leading to a decrease in calcium reabsorption. In the inner medullary collecting duct of the rat, CaSR co-localizes with the water channel aquaphorin-2,[12] perhaps helping to explain the polyuria observed in patients with hypercalcemia.

Phosphate. Phosphate administration, whether by the oral or intravenous route, reduces urine calcium excretion; micropuncture studies implicate an increase in distal calcium reabsorption. There are several extrarenal mechanisms that can contribute to the hypocalciuria of phosphate administration. An increase in phosphate will directly stimulate PTH secretion[13] and can lower ionized calcium also enhancing PTH secretion; the increased PTH will enhance calcium reabsorption. Phosphate will complex with calcium in the intestine, decreasing the amount of calcium available for absorption and can complex with calcium in the bone and soft tissues resulting in a decrease in the filtered load of calcium.

Phosphate depletion will result in hypercalciuria. While a defect in proximal tubule calcium reabsorption is controversial, there seems to be a direct effect of phosphate to decrease calcium reabsorption in the distal nephron.

Proton (H$^+$). Acute and chronic metabolic acidosis leads to an increase in urine calcium excretion, whereas metabolic alkalosis leads to a decrease in calcium excretion. Micropuncture studies show that during acute metabolic acidosis proximal tubule calcium reabsorption declines in parallel with a decrease in tubule bicarbonate concentration. During chronic metabolic acidosis, proximal tubule calcium reabsorption is unchanged, whereas there is a decrease in distal calcium reabsorption. The decreased calcium reabsorption is not mediated through changes in PTH or filtered load, but appears to be mediated by a direct effect of protons on the tubule. Bone seems to be the source of the additional urinary calcium because intestinal calcium absorption is not increased.[14,15] Respiratory acidosis seems to cause a minimal increase in calcium excretion compared with a similar decrement in pH caused by metabolic acidosis.

On a daily basis, humans generate approximately 1 mEq/

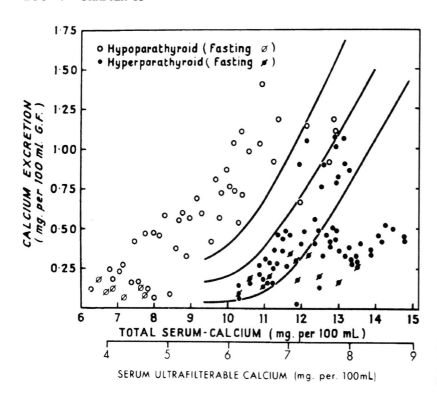

FIG. 4. Urinary excretion of calcium as a function of serum calcium concentration in normal subjects (solid line) and in patients with hypoparathyroidism (triangles) and hyperparathyroidism (circles). Dashed lines, ±SD; shaded area, the normal physiologic range. (Reprinted with permission from Nordin BEC, Peacock M 1969 Role of kidney in regulation of plasma-calcium. Lancet **2:**1280–1283.)

kg/24 h of protons.[15] This endogenous acid production is related to the metabolism of sulfur-containing amino acids (especially cysteine and methionine), which are found in animal protein. A very mild, almost undetectable, metabolic acidosis results before excretion of these acids.[16] Any impairment of renal function, as occurs as part of the aging process, results in a greater degree of metabolic acidosis.[17] When elderly patients are given potassium bicarbonate to neutralize their endogenous acid production, there is a decrease in urine calcium excretion.[16] Compared with sodium bicarbonate, potassium bicarbonate results in a greater decrement in calcium excretion perhaps because potassium administration does not result in extracellular fluid volume expansion.

Hormones

PTH and PTH Related Peptide. PTH is a principle regulator of renal tubule calcium reabsorption, with increasing levels of PTH increasing renal tubule calcium reabsorption[1,18] (Fig. 4). PTH will reduce glomerular filtration, and thus the filtered load of calcium, by reducing the glomerular ultrafiltration coefficient. The effects of PTH on proximal renal tubule calcium reabsorption remain controversial. PTH seems to increase active calcium transport in the TALH. However, PTH clearly increases calcium reabsorption in the distal convoluted tubule apparently through facilitating the opening of ECaC. The actions of PTH are mimicked by cyclic adenosine monophosphate (cAMP).

Although PTH clearly increases net renal tubule calcium reabsorption, patients with hyperparathyroidism are often hypercalciuric.[19] The PTH-induced increased tubule calcium reabsorption leads to hypercalcemia and an increased filtered load of calcium, which leads to increased urinary

calcium excretion. PTH also stimulates the conversion of $25(OH)D_3$ to $1,25(OH)_2D_3$ in the renal proximal tubule, resulting in enhanced intestinal calcium absorption and bone resorption; both lead to a further increase in the filtered load of calcium.

PTHrp is secreted by malignant cells and shares significant amino acid homology with PTH.[1,4] While not detected on standard PTH assays, this hormone mimics the actions of PTH on renal calcium reabsorption.

$1,25(OH)_2D_3$. The direct effects of $1,25(OH)_2D_3$ on renal tubule calcium reabsorption are complex, difficult to study, and not well understood. Vitamin D depletion will reduce renal tubule calcium reabsorption irrespective of the presence of PTH, and repletion of vitamin D will increase calcium reabsorption. However, administration of $1,25(OH)_2D_3$ to parathyroidectomized rats does not alter calcium reabsorption. Administration of vitamin D to humans results in hypercalciuria, although this effect may be mediated by the actions of vitamin D on the intestine and/or the bone. In mouse distal tubule cell culture, $1,25(OH)_2D_3$ did not alter calcium reabsorption but enhanced the effects of PTH on calcium transport,[20] while active calcium transport in primary cultures of cortical collecting duct cells was enhanced by $1,25(OH)_2D_3$. Vitamin D will increase renal calbindin-D_{28K}, which could augment renal tubular calcium reabsorption.

Calcitonin and Others. While calcitonin will increase calcium reabsorption in cultured distal convoluted cells, the in vivo effects of calcitonin are not straightforward. Physiologic doses of calcitonin are hypocalciuric, whereas supraphysiologic doses are hypercalciuric. Glucocorticoids, insulin, and glucagon have been reported to decrease tubular calcium reabsorption.

Diuretics

Thiazide. The acute administration of thiazide diuretics, including hydrochlorothiazide, chlorthalidone, or indapamide, results in an increase in urine sodium excretion with a small but variable change in urine calcium excretion. With chronic thiazide administration the increased sodium excretion continues; however, there is a marked increase in tubular calcium reabsorption and hypocalciuria. The dissociation of sodium and calcium excretion occurs in the distal convoluted tubule. Here, thiazides inhibit sodium chloride transport, leading to a hyperpolarization of the cell membrane. Because cellular calcium entry is mediated by calcium channels in the luminal cell membrane, hyperpolarization of this membrane enhances calcium entry and leads to increased calcium reabsorption. Administration of sodium can reverse the hypocalciuria, suggesting that thiazides also increase proximal renal tubule calcium reabsorption, in part, through inducing volume depletion. Thiazide administration is integral in the treatment of calcium nephrolithiasis because a reduction in urinary calcium excretion will reduce urinary supersaturation and stone formation.[12,21]

Loop. The acute administration of the loop diuretics, including furosemide, torosemide, or ethacrynic acid, results in a marked increase in urine calcium and sodium excretion. The loop diuretics inhibit the Na-K-2Cl transporter in the TALH, leading to a decrease in the positive lumen potential and a decline in calcium reabsorption at this site. As opposed to thiazide diuretics, which decrease sodium and increase calcium reabsorption, the loop diuretics cause a decrease in the reabsorption of both ions. As long as the lost urinary sodium is replaced, the hypercalciuria continues. Loop diuretic administration is useful in acute treatment of hypercalcemia.[22]

Cyclosporin A. Administration of cyclosporin A decreases renal tubular calcium reabsorption, perhaps because of a cyclosporin-induced decrease in calbindin-D_{28K}.[23]

Renal Function. During renal insufficiency, renal calcium filtration falls in direct proportion to the decline in the glomerular filtration rate. In addition, there is enhanced calcium reabsorption secondary to the usual increase in PTH. The increase in PTH is multifactorial.[2,24] It appears secondary to the decrease in renal $1,25(OH)_2D_3$ synthesis, resulting from a decrease in renal mass and from an increase in serum phosphorus caused by a decrease in renal phosphorus excretion. The fall in $1,25(OH)_2D_3$ not only decreases intestinal calcium absorption resulting in hypocalcemia and subsequent increased PTH secretion, but the decreased $1,25(OH)_2D_3$ leads to a direct increase in PTH secretion. The increase in phosphorus directly increases serum PTH.

Genetic Abnormalities. An inactivating mutation of CaSR, as seen in patients with familial hypocalciuric hypercalce-mia, will lead to an elevation of PTH, increased renal calcium reabsorption, and hypercalcemia.[11] Conversely an activating mutation of CaSR, as seen in patients with autosomal dominant hypocalcemia, will lead to inappropriately normal or low levels of PTH, decreased renal tubule calcium reabsorption, and hypocalcemia. Dent's disease is a rare, familiar proximal tubular defect leading to decreased renal tubular calcium reabsorption apparently associated with a defect in the chloride channel. The relationship between the chloride channel defect in Dent's disease and the decrease in renal tubular calcium reabsorption is not clear. Bartter's syndrome is associated with a decrease in renal tubular calcium reabsorption caused by any of several mutations affecting the thick ascending limb. Some patients with Bartter's syndrome have a defect in the gene encoding for the Na-K-2Cl transporter, some have abnormalities in the potassium channel, and others in the chloride channel. Any of these defects lead to a decrease in the lumen positive voltage driving the paracellular calcium reabsorption. A number of other genetic disorders, such as renal tubular acidosis, have been associated with alterations in renal tubular calcium transport.[11]

MAGNESIUM

Filtration

In humans, the concentration of serum magnesium is maintained at a constant level between 1.8 and 2.2 mg/dl or 1.5 and 1.9 mEq/liter.[22] Of the total serum magnesium, approximately 30% is protein bound, 55% is ionized, and 15% is complexed; the ionized and complexed magnesium constitute the ultrafiltrable magnesium. The concentration of free magnesium is influenced by pH, with a fall in pH increasing the proportion of ionized magnesium.

A 70-kg male with a glomerular filtration rate of 180 liters/day and a mean serum magnesium concentration of 1.8 mEq/liter filters approximately 227 mEq of magnesium per day because approximately 70% of serum magnesium is ultrafiltrable (180 liters/day $\times$ 1.8 mEq/liter $\times$ 0.7). Urine magnesium excretion averages about 12 mEq per day, indicating that approximately 95% of the glomerular filtrate is reabsorbed before excretion.

Reabsorption

Approximately 15% of filtered magnesium is reabsorbed in the proximal convoluted and straight tubule.[25] Magnesium reabsorption follows that of sodium and water and seems to be a passive paracellular process, including solvent drag, dependent on sodium and water reabsorption and the luminal concentration of magnesium. This is in contrast to calcium, where there is reabsorption of approximately 70% of the filtered load in this segment.

About 70% of magnesium is reabsorbed in the cortical TALH, with no reabsorption in the medullary TALH, through a paracellular route driven, as with calcium, by the positive lumen potential generated by the Na-K-2Cl transporter.[26] The CaSR also is sensitive to magnesium, and an elevated magnesium concentration will decrease potassium movement into the lumen of the TALH, leading to a de-

TABLE 2. FACTORS INFLUENCING MAGNESIUM REABSORPTION

Glomerular filtration
    Increased
        Hypermagnesemia
    Decreased
        Hypomagnesemia
        Renal insufficiency
Tubular reabsorption
    Increased
        Extracellular fluid volume expansion
        Hypomagnesemia
        Hypocalcemia
        Metabolic alkalosis
        Parathyroid hormone
    Decreased
        Extracellular fluid volume depletion
        Hypermagnesemia
        Phosphate depletion
        Hypercalcemia
        Loop diuretics
        Aminoglycoside antibiotics
        Cisplantin
        Cyclosporine
        Ethanol
        Gitelman's syndrome
        Other genetic disorders

creased lumen positive voltage and a decrease in magnesium reabsorption. Paracellin-1 is present in the tight junction and seems to have a regulatory role in magnesium reabsorption.[26]

Approximately 10% of magnesium is reabsorbed in the distal convoluted tubule through a transcellular, active transport process. Magnesium transport into the cytosol is through selective channels and extrusion into the interstitium is apparently mediated by a sodium for magnesium cotransporter.

Factors Affecting Reabsorption

Ions

Sodium. Extracellular fluid volume expansion with sodium chloride decreases tubular magnesium reabsorption and increases urinary magnesium excretion (Table 2). There is decreased proximal magnesium reabsorption, which parallels the decline in sodium reabsorption. Because the distal portions of the nephron are normally incapable of increased magnesium reabsorption, the increased delivery to the distal portions of the nephron appears in the urine.

Magnesium. Hypermagnesemia increases urine magnesium excretion. There is an increased filtered load of magnesium, which, despite some increased proximal tubular magnesium reabsorption, results in increased delivery to the loop of Henle. Magnesium reabsorption in the TALH seems to decline, apparently because of activation of the CaSR by magnesium, resulting in increased distal delivery and excretion of magnesium. Hypomagnesemia results in a prompt fall in urine magnesium excretion. There is little change in

proximal reabsorption and an increase in magnesium reabsorption in the TALH.

Phosphate. Phosphate depletion results in an increase in magnesium excretion because of a defect in reabsorption in the TALH, which can result in significant hypomagnesemia.

Calcium. Hypercalcemia leads to a prompt decline in overall magnesium reabsorption.[3] There is decreased magnesium reabsorption in both the proximal tubule and the TALH, the latter caused by activation of the CaSR, and perhaps, alteration in the tight junction permeability caused by effects on paracellin-1. Hypocalcemia leads to an increase in overall tubule magnesium reabsorption.

Proton. Metabolic alkalosis consistently increases renal tubular magnesium reabsorption, and metabolic acidosis seems to inhibit reabsorption. Magnesium reabsorption in the distal nephron seems to be directly correlated with the level of luminal bicarbonate concentration.

Hormones. To date, no specific hormone has been identified that regulates renal magnesium reabsorption. PTH increases magnesium reabsorption; however, the PTH-induced hypercalcemia opposes this increase in reabsorption.

Diuretics. The loop diuretics lead to a marked increase in magnesium excretion.[22] In contrast to their effects on calcium excretion, the thiazide diuretics cause a minimal increase in magnesium excretion.

Other Medications. The aminoglycoside antibiotics, cisplatin and cyclosporine, have been shown to inhibit magnesium reabsorption in the TALH, leading to increased urinary magnesium excretion.

Ethanol. Chronic, but not acute, administration of ethanol has been shown to decrease renal tubular magnesium reabsorption.

Renal Function. Any impairment of renal function will lead to a parallel decline in magnesium excretion. Continued dietary magnesium intake will result in marked hypermagnesemia. Patients with renal insufficiency must limit magnesium intake, which is often found in high concentrations in oral antacids and cathartics, to avoid hypermagnesemia.[22]

Genetic Disorders. There are a number of primary inherited disorders of magnesium reabsorption, which are generally associated with disorders in calcium transport.[26,27] Gitelman's syndrome presents with renal magnesium wasting and is associated with mutations in the chlorothiazide-sensitive NaCl co-transporter expressed in the distal convoluted tubule. Bartter's syndrome is not often associated with significant disturbances in the serum magnesium concentra-

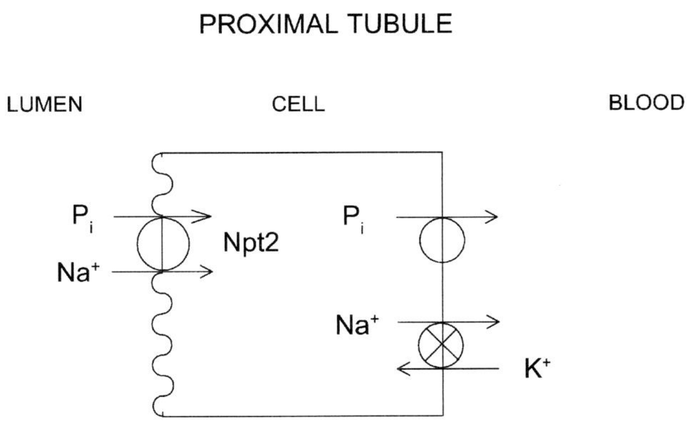

PROXIMAL TUBULE

FIG. 5. Phosphorus transport in the proximal tubule.

tion. Because the CaSR also senses magnesium, alterations in this receptor affect renal magnesium transport.

PHOSPHORUS

Filtration

The concentration of serum phosphorus in adults ranges between 2.5 and 4.5 mg/dl or 0.81 and 1.45 mM.[2,22] Serum phosphorus levels are highest in infants and decrease in childhood, reaching the normal adult levels in late adolescence. Approximately 70% of blood phosphorus is organic and contained within phospholipids, and 30% of the blood phosphorus is inorganic. Of the inorganic phosphorus, the majority, 85%, is free and circulates as monohydrogen or dihydrogen phosphate or complexed with sodium, magnesium, or calcium, whereas the minority, 15%, is protein bound.

A 70-kg male with a glomerular filtration rate of 180 liters/day and a mean serum phosphorus concentration of 1.25 mM filters approximately 200 mmol of phosphorus per day because approximately 85% of serum phosphorus is ultrafiltrable (180 liters/day $\times$ 1.25 mmol/liter $\times$ 0.85).[22] Urine phosphorus excretion averages about 25 mmol/day so that approximately 12.5% of the glomerular filtrate is excreted in the urine.

Reabsorption

The bulk of phosphorus reabsorption, 85%, occurs in the proximal tubule (Fig. 5). Proximal phosphorus transport occurs against an electrochemical gradient.[3] Reabsorption seems to be transcellular, absorptive, and dependent on the low concentration of intracellular sodium maintained by the basolateral Na-K-ATPase. The majority of phosphorus absorption occurs in the initial 25% of the proximal tubule. Transport seems more robust in the deeper juxtamedullary nephrons compared with the more cortical nephrons.

Three sodium gradient-dependent phosphate cotransporters (Npt1-Npt3) have been identified, of which Npt2 is responsible for approximately 85% of proximal tubule renal phosphate transport, is highly regulated, and is present on the apical brush border membrane.[28] Npt1 seems responsible for approximately 15% of the proximal phosphate and does not seem to be regulated.[29] Fibroblast

growth factor 23 (FGF-23) has been recently identified as a regulator of Npt2.[30] Elevated levels of FGF-23 have been detected in patients with renal phosphate wasting and hypophosphatemia. FGF-23 is metabolized by the *PHEX* gene (phosphate-regulating gene with homologies to the endopeptidases on the X chromosome), and mutations in *PHEX* can also cause hypophosphatemia because of the inability to metabolize FGF-23.[30]

Once inside the cell, the absorbed phosphorus equilibrates with cytosolic phosphorus; elimination of luminal phosphorus leads to a marked decline in intracellular phosphorus. Phosphorus transport across the basolateral membrane occurs down a favorable electrochemical gradient using an anion exchanger. It is tightly regulated to avoid depletion of intracellular phosphate.

There seems to be little phosphorus transport in the loop of Henle. A small quantity of phosphorus is reabsorbed in the distal convoluted tubule, especially in the absence of PTH. Whether there is phosphorus reabsorption more distally is not clear.

The overall tubular maximum for the reabsorption of phosphorus is approximately equal to the normal amount of phosphorus filtered by the glomerulous. Thus, any appreciable increase in the filtered load of phosphorus leads to an increase in urinary phosphorus excretion.

Factors Affecting Reabsorption

Ions

Phosphorus. A low phosphorus intake will stimulate tubular phosphorus reabsorption, whereas a high phosphorus

TABLE 3. FACTORS INFLUENCING PHOSPHORUS REABSORPTION

Filtration
  Increased
    Hyperphosphatemia
    Mild hypercalcemia
  Decreased
    Hypophosphatemia
    Renal insufficiency
    Moderate hypercalcemia
Tubular reabsorption
  Increased
    Phosphorus depletion
    Hypercalcemia
    Extracellular fluid volume depletion
    Chronic metabolic alkalosis
  Decreased
    Phosphorus excess
    Hypocalcemia
    Extracellular fluid volume expansion
    Acute metabolic alkalosis
    Chronic metabolic acidosis
    Parathyroid hormone
    Parathyroid hormone related protein
    FGF-23
    $1,25(OH)_2D_3$
    Thiazide diuretics
    X-linked hypophosphatemic rickets
    Autosomal dominant hypophosphatemic rickets
    Other metabolic and genetic disorders

intake will inhibit phosphorus reabsorption (Table 3). Alterations in phosphorus intake alter renal phosphorus reabsorption independent of changes in PTH, extracellular fluid volume, or the level of serum calcium. Variations in phosphorus intake lead to an inverse modulation in the maximum rate of transport of the proximal tubule Npt2 cotransporter within hours and alter the level of phosphorus reabsorption. The precise role of FGF-23 in regulating daily renal phosphorus excretion remains to be determined.

Calcium. Chronic hypercalcemia decreases, while chronic hypocalcemia increases, renal reabsorption of phosphorus. Acute changes in calcium have numerous effects on phosphorus filtration and reabsorption. An acute increase in serum calcium will decrease the glomerular filtration rate because of a decrease in the ultrafiltration coefficient and the renal blood flow. Increases in calcium lead to a release in red blood cell phosphorus and an increase in serum phosphorus; however, the phosphorus may bind to calcium and protein forming an unfilterable complex. Calcium is a principle regulator of PTH, which is phosphaturic. In general, filtered phosphorus seems to increase with mild increases in serum calcium and decrease as the level of calcium rises.

Sodium. Extracellular fluid volume expansion decreases renal tubular phosphorus reabsorption and volume concentration increases reabsorption. Volume expansion leads to a decrease in proximal sodium and phosphorus reabsorption.

Proton. Whereas acute metabolic acidosis does not significantly alter renal tubular phosphorus reabsorption, acute metabolic alkalosis leads to a decline in phosphorus reabsorption. Chronic metabolic acidosis decreases tubular phosphorus reabsorption through modulation of the Npt2 cotransporter independent of changes in PTH, whereas chronic alkalosis increases reabsorption.

Hormones

PTH and PTHrP. PTH is a principle regulator of renal phosphorus reabsorption and excretion; the hormone is phosphaturic. PTH regulates phosphorus reabsorption principally through regulation of the proximal Npt2 cotransporter. PTH also seems to decrease distal tubular reabsorption. PTHrP mimics the action of PTH on renal tubular phosphorus reabsorption. The hypophosphaturia of phosphorus depletion overrides the hyperphosphaturia induced by PTH.

FGF-23. FGF-23 is detectable in normal individuals and is elevated in many patients with renal phosphate wasting and hypophosphatemia, suggesting that FGF-23 is a principle regulator either directly or through another factor, of renal phosphate excretion.

$1,25(OH)_2D_3$. Chronic excess of $1,25(OH)_2D_3$ results in a decrease in renal phosphorus reabsorption and causes phos-

phaturia. Vitamin D increases intestinal phosphorus absorption resulting hyperphosphatemia and an increased filtered load of phosphorus.

Others. Insulin increases, whereas glucocorticoids and glucagon decrease, renal phosphorus reabsorption. The effect of calcitonin on phosphorus reabsorption is unclear.

Diuretics. Both the loop and thiazide diuretics are phosphaturic.

Renal Function. During renal insufficiency, urine phosphorus excretion remains relatively constant until the glomerular filtration rate falls to about 25% of normal.[15,31] Phosphorus excretion is maintained in the presence of a fall in glomerular filtration rate and the subsequent decline in the filtered load of phosphorus by the phosphaturic effect of elevated PTH levels. Renal insufficiency and failure are principle causes of hyperphosphatemia, which has an integral role in the pathogenesis of renal osteodystrophy.[31]

Acquired Metabolic and Genetic Abnormalities. X-linked hypophosphatemic rickets appears to be caused by the inability of *PHEX* to metabolize the phosphaturic factor FGF-23.[30] Autosomal dominant hypophosphatemic rickets may be caused by mutations in FGF-23 that prevent its metabolism. Tumors, especially of the mesenchyme, produce excessive amounts of FGF-23, resulting in hyperphosphaturia.

REFERENCES

1. Bushinsky DA, Monk RD 1998 Calcium. Lancet **352:**306–311.
2. Bushinsky DA 2001 Disorders of calcium and phosphorus homeostasis. In: Greenberg A (ed.) Primer on Kidney Diseases. Academic Press, San Diego, CA, USA, pp. 107–115.
3. Suki WN, Rouse D 1996 Renal transport of calcium, magnesium, and phosphate. In: Brenner BM (ed.) The Kidney. W. B. Saunders, Philadelphia, PA, USA, pp. 472–515.
4. Brown EM, Pollock M, Hebert SC 1998 The extracellular calcium-sensing receptor: Its role in health and disease. Annu Rev Med **49:** 15–29.
5. Motoyama HI, Friedman PA 2002 Calcium-sensing receptor regulation of PTH-dependent calcium absorption by mouse cortical ascending limbs. Am J Physiol Renal Physiol **283:**F399–F406.
6. Blanchard A, Jeunemaitre X, Coudol P, Dechaux M, Froissart M, May A, Demontis R, Fournier A, Paillard M, Houillier P 2001 Paracellin-1 is critical for magnesium and calcium reabsorption in the human thick ascending limb of Henle. Kidney Int **59:**2206–2215.
7. Hoenderop JG, Nilius B, Bindels RJ 2002 ECaC: The gatekeeper of transepithelial Ca^{2+} transport. Biochim Biophys Acta **1600:**6–11.
8. Hoenderop JG, Nilius B, Bindels RJ 2002 Molecular mechanism of active Ca^{2+} reabsorption in the distal nephron. Annu Rev Physiol **64:**529–549.
9. Sooy K, Kohut J, Christakos S 2000 The role of calbindin and 1,25 dihydroxyvitamin D_3 in the kidney. Curr Opin Nephrol Hypertens **9:**341–347.
10. Hoenderop JG, Dardenne O, Van Abel M, Van Der Kemp A, Van Os CH, St. Arnaud R, Bindels RJ 2002 Modulation of renal Ca^{2+} transport protein genes by dietary Ca^{2+} and 1,25-dihydroxyvitamin D_3 in 25-hydroxyvitamin D3–1α-hydroxylase knockout mice. FASEB **16:** 1398–1406.
11. Scheinman SJ, Guay-Woodford LM, Thakker RV, Warnock DG 1999 Genetic disorders of renal electrolyte transport. N Engl J Med **340:** 1177–1187.

12. Reilly RF, Ellison DH 2000 Mammalian distal tubule: Physiology, pathophysiology, and molecular anatomy. Physiol Rev 80:277–313.
13. Slatopolsky E, Finch J, Denda M, Ritter C, Zhong M, Dusso A, MacDonald PN, Brown AJ 1996 Phosphorus restriction prevents parathyroid gland growth. High phosphorus directly stimulates PTH secretion in vitro. J Clin Invest 97:2534–2540.
14. Bushinsky DA, Frick KK 2000 The effects of acid on bone. Curr Opin Nephrol Hypertens 9:369–379.
15. Bushinsky DA 1995 The contribution of acidosis to renal osteodystrophy. Kidney Int 47:1816–1832.
16. Sebastian A, Harris ST, Ottaway JH, Todd KM, Morris RC Jr 1994 Improved mineral balance and skeletal metabolism in postmenopausal women treated with potassium bicarbonate. N Engl J Med 330:1776–1781.
17. Bushinsky DA 1998 Acid-base imbalance and the skeleton. In: Burckhardt P, Dawson-Hughes B, Heaney RP (eds.) Nutritional Aspects of Osteoporosis. Serono Symposia USA, Norwell, MA, USA, pp. 208–217.
18. Nordin BEC, Peacock M 1969 Role of kidney in regulation of plasma-calcium. Lancet 2:1280–1283.
19. Monk RD, Bushinsky DA 1996 Pathogenesis of idiopathic hypercalciuria. In: Coe F, Favus M, Pak C, Parks J, Preminger G (eds.) Kidney Stones: Medical and Surgical Management. Lippincott-Raven, Philadelphia, PA, USA, pp. 759–772.
20. Friedman PA, Gesek FA 1995 Cellular calcium transport in renal epithelia: Measurement, mechanisms and regulation. Physiol Rev 75:429–471.
21. Bushinsky DA 2000 Renal lithiasis. In: Humes HD (ed.) Kelly's Textbook of Medicine. Lippincott Williams & Wilkins, New York, NY, USA, pp. 1243–1248.
22. Monk RD, Bushinsky DA 1999 Treatment of calcium, phosphorus, and magnesium disorders. In: Halperin M (ed.) Therapy in Nephrology and Hypertension: A Companion to Brenner and Rector's The Kidney. W. B. Saunders Co., Philadelphia, PA, USA, pp. 303–315.
23. Yang C, Kim J, Kim Y, Cha JH, Mim SY, Kim YO, Shin YS, Kim YS Bang BK 1998 Inhibition of calbindin D28K expression by cyclosporin A in rat kidney: The possible pathogenesis of cyclosporin A-induced hypercalciuria. J Am Soc Nephrol 9:1416–1426.
24. Bushinsky DA 1997 Bone disease in moderate renal failure: Cause, nature and prevention. Annu Rev Med 48:167–176.
25. Yu AS 2001 Evolving concepts in epithelial magnesium transport. Curr Opin Nephrol Hypertens 10:649–653.
26. Cole DE, Quamme GA 2000 Inherited disorders of renal magnesium handling. J Am Soc Nephol 11:1937–1947.
27. Warnock DG 2002 Renal genetic disorders related to K^+ and Mg^{2+}. Annu Rev Physiol 64:845–876.
28. Kumar R 2002 New insights into phosphate homeostasis: Fibroblast growth factor 23 and frizzled-related protein-4 are phosphaturic factors derived from tumors associated with osteomalacia. Curr Opin Nephrol Hypertens 11:547–553.
29. Magagnin S, Werner A, Markovich D, Sorribas V, Stange G, Biber J, Murer H 1993 Expression cloning of human and rat renal cortex Na/Pi cotransport. Proc Natl Acad Sci USA 90:5979–5983.
30. Strewler GJ 2001 FGF23, hypophosphatemia, and rickets: Has phosphatonin been found? Proc Natl Acad Sci USA 98:5945–5946.
31. Bushinsky DA 1997 Renal osteodystrophy. In: Jamison R, Wilkinson B (eds.) Nephrology. Chapman and Hall, London, UK, pp. 369–382.

Chapter 16. Mineral Balance and Homeostasis

Arthur E. Broadus

Department of Internal Medicine, Yale University School of Medicine, New Haven, Connecticut

INTRODUCTION

Life began in the primordial sea, rich in potassium and magnesium and poor in sodium, and it is felt that the present composition of the cytosol reflects this ancient heritage. With time, geologic changes altered the composition of the seas to one rich in sodium and calcium, and primitive organisms adapted to this altered milieu by developing ion pumps to maintain cytosolic homeostasis and the asymmetry of the concentrations of monovalent and divalent cations across their plasma membranes. The evolution of these pumps and channels can be viewed as one of the most fundamental developments in cell biology.

The progression to terrestrial life carried with it a complete dependence on minerals from the environment. With this came the evolution of the mineral exchange mechanisms in intestine, kidney, and bone, as well as the key systemic hormones, parathyroid hormone (PTH) and 1,25-dihydroxyvitamin D [1,25(OH)$_2$D], which regulate these exchange mechanisms. This integrated regulatory system has many checks and balances and serves as an elegant example of biological control.

Calcium

An adult human contains approximately 1000 g of calcium.[1] About 99% of this calcium is in the skeleton in the form of hydroxyapatite, and 1% is contained in the extracellular fluids and soft tissues. The extracellular concentration of calcium ions (Ca^{2+}) is in the range of 10^{-3} M, whereas the concentration of Ca^{2+} in the cytosol is about 10^{-6} M.

Calcium plays two predominant physiologic roles in the organism. In bone, calcium salts provide the structural integrity of the skeleton. In extracellular fluids and in the cytosol, the concentration of Ca^{2+} is critically important to the maintenance and control of a number of biochemical processes. The concentrations of Ca^{2+} in both compartments are maintained with great constancy.

Phosphorus

An adult human contains approximately 600 g of phosphorus. About 85% of this is present in crystalline form in the skeleton and plays a structural role. About 15% is present in the extracellular fluids, largely in the form of inorganic phosphate ions, and in soft tissues, almost totally in the form of phosphate esters. Intracellular phosphate esters and phosphorylated intermediates are involved in a

The author has no conflict of interest.

number of important biochemical processes, including the generation and transfer of cellular energy. Intracellular and extracellular concentrations of phosphorus (in the form of the phosphate divalent anion) are approximately 1×10^{-4} and 2×10^{-4} M, respectively, and these concentrations are less rigidly maintained than are those of calcium and magnesium.

Magnesium

An adult human contains approximately 25 g or 2000 mEq of magnesium. About two-thirds is present in the skeleton and one-third is in soft tissues. The magnesium in bone is not an integral part of the hydroxyapatite lattice structure but appears to be located on the crystal surface. Only a minor fraction of the magnesium in bone is freely exchangeable with extracellular magnesium. Magnesium is the most abundant intracellular divalent cation, and cellular magnesium is important as a cofactor for a number of enzymatic reactions and in the regulation of neuromuscular excitability. Approximately 1% of the total body magnesium is contained in the extracellular compartment, but its concentration in plasma does not provide a reliable index of either total body or soft tissue magnesium content. The concentration of magnesium ions (Mg^{2+}) is about 5×10^{-4} M in the cytosol as well as in the extracellular fluids, and its concentration in both compartments is rigidly maintained.

EXTRACELLULAR MINERAL METABOLISM

Calcium

There are three definable fractions of calcium in serum: ionized calcium (about 50%), protein-bound calcium (about 40%), and calcium that is complexed, mostly to citrate and phosphate ions (about 10%).[1] Both the complexed and ionized fractions are ultrafiltrable, so that about 60% of the total calcium in serum crosses semipermeable membranes (e.g., the glomerulus). About 90% of the protein-bound calcium is bound to albumin and the remainder to globulins. Alterations in the serum albumin concentration have a major influence on the measured total serum calcium concentration. At pH 7.4, each g/dl of albumin binds 0.8 mg/dl of calcium, and this simple relationship can be used to "correct" the total serum calcium concentration when circulating albumin is abnormal (e.g., given measured albumin and calcium concentrations of 2.0 g/dl and 7.4 mg/dl, respectively, the corrected serum calcium concentration is 9.0 mg/dl, assuming a normal mean serum albumin concentration of 4.0 g/dl). Calcium is bound largely to the carboxyl groups in albumin, and this binding is highly pH-dependent. Acute acidosis decreases binding and increases ionized calcium, and acute alkalosis increases binding with a consequent decrease in ionized calcium. For example, the pH dependency of calcium binding to carboxyl groups is the explanation for the reduction in ionized calcium that is responsible for the neuromuscular symptoms that characterize the hyperventilation syndrome (which produces a respiratory alkalosis). Such changes are not reflected in the total serum calcium concentration and can only be appreciated by actual measurement of ionized calcium at the ambient serum pH. Calcium concentrations are typically recorded in mg/dl (mg %); these concentrations can be converted to molar units simply by dividing by 4 (e.g., 10 mg/dl converts to 2.5 mM).

It is the ionized fraction of calcium (Ca^{2+}) that is physiologically important and that is rigidly maintained by the combined effects of PTH and $1,25(OH)_2D$.[2] Examples of the physiological functions of extracellular Ca^{2+} include (1) serving as a cofactor in the coagulation cascade (e.g., for factors VII, IX, X, and prothrombin), (2) maintenance of normal mineral ion product required for skeletal mineralization, and (3) contributing stability to plasma membranes by binding to phospholipids in the lipid bilayer and also regulating the permeability of plasma membranes to sodium ions. A reduction in ionized calcium increases sodium permeability and enhances the excitability of all excitable tissues; an increase in ionized calcium has the opposite effect.

Phosphorus

The inorganic phosphate in serum also exists as three fractions: ionized, protein-bound, and complexed. Protein binding is relatively insignificant for phosphate, representing some 10% of the total, but about 35% is complexed to sodium, calcium, and magnesium. Approximately 90% of the inorganic phosphate in serum is ultrafiltrable. The major ionic species of phosphate in serum at pH 7.4 is the divalent anion (HPO_4^{2-}).

In contrast to the rigid regulation of the concentration of calcium in serum, the serum phosphorus concentration varies quite widely throughout the day and is influenced by age, sex, diet, pH, and a wide variety of hormones. An adequate serum phosphate concentration is required to maintain an ion product sufficient for normal mineralization.

Magnesium

About 55% of serum magnesium is ionized, with 30% being protein bound and about 15% complexed. The protein-bound fractions interact with the carboxyl groups of albumin and is influenced by pH in a fashion analogous to that of calcium. It is the ionized fraction of magnesium that is physiologically important (e.g., to plasma membrane excitability). The extracellular concentration of ionized magnesium is tightly controlled by the tubular maximum or threshold for magnesium in the nephron.[3]

Only fasting measurements of serum calcium and phosphorus should be considered reliable.

CELLULAR MINERAL METABOLISM

A detailed summary of the numerous metabolic functions of calcium, magnesium, and phosphorus within cell is beyond the scope of this syllabus. The section attempts simply to highlight some of the important roles of these ions in cellular physiology.

Calcium

The control of cellular calcium homeostasis is complex, and the regulation of the concentration of the calcium ion in the cytosol is as rigidly maintained as is its concentration in the extracellular fluids.[4] Cells are bathed with approximately 10^{-3} M Ca^{2+}. The concentration of Ca^{2+} in the cytoplasm is approximately 10^{-6} M, or one-thousandth that in extracellular fluids. Cytosolic calcium is to some extent buffered by binding to other cytoplasmic constituents, and certain cells contain specific calcium-binding proteins that may serve as buffers and/or calcium transport proteins within the cytosol. The mitochondria and microsomes contain 90–99% of the intracellular calcium, bound largely to organic and inorganic phosphates. The calcium content of these organelles is sufficient to replenish cytosolic calcium some 500 times.

The low Ca^{2+} concentration in the cytosol is maintained by three groups of channel/pump/exchanger systems: an external system located in the plasma membrane and two internal systems located in the microsomal membrane and the inner mitochondrial membrane. Calcium diffuses into the cytosol across these three membranes. Each of the three systems is oriented in a direction of calcium egress from the cytosol; each requires energy, and each shares a high affinity for calcium (K_m approximately 10^{-6} M).

The importance of the three calcium transport systems in regulating cellular calcium metabolism varies considerably from cell to cell depending on the function of a particular cell type. Several examples serve to illustrate how the details of cellular calcium homeostasis have been adapted to subserve the specific physiologic function of a given cell type.

Calcium ions constitute the coupling factor that links excitation and contraction in all forms of skeletal and cardiac muscle. In striated muscle, the microsomes are extensively developed as the sarcoplasmic reticulum, which serves as the principal storehouse of intracellular calcium in muscle and is the most highly developed calcium transport structure known. Depolarization of the plasma membrane is accompanied by a small amount of voltage-gated calcium entry into the cell, and this acts as a trigger to release large quantities of calcium stored in the sarcoplasmic reticulum. The abrupt increase in cytosolic calcium interacts with troponin, a specific calcium-binding protein, leading to a conformational change and the actin-myosin interaction that constitutes muscle contraction. The reticulum vesicles are capable of reaccumulating the large quantity of cytosolic calcium with the extreme speed required by the relaxation process.

In most mammalian cells other than muscle, the principal internal calcium transport system is that of the inner mitochondrial membrane. In most cells, calcium serves as a second messenger, mediating the effects of membrane signals on the release of secretory products (e.g., neurotransmitters and endocrine secretions such as insulin and aldosterone).[4] The calcium messenger system involves a flow of information along several pathways such as the calmodulin and protein kinase C pathways. It is now recognized that in many such cells the several branches of the calcium messenger system and the cyclic adenosine monophosphate (cAMP) messenger system are intimately related, and that such systems are integrated in such a way that the net cellular response to a given stimulus is determined by a complex interplay ("cross-talk") between these systems.

The EF hand proteins comprise a large protein family that can act as "calcium sensors" as well as "calcium effectors" within the cell.[4] Calcium binding to these proteins alters their confirmation in such a way as to enhance their hydrophobicity, markedly changing the way in which they bind to protein targets.

Phosphorus

The transport of phosphate ions across the plasma membrane and the membranes of intracellular organelles proceeds passively but is determined by the movement of cations, mostly calcium. The phosphate content in mitochondria is high, where it exists largely in the form of calcium salts. The cytoplasmic concentration of free phosphate ions is quite low, and the remaining portion of intracellular phosphate is either bound or in the form of organic phosphate esters. These phosphate esters play a wide variety of critically important roles in cellular metabolism: purine nucleotides provide the cell with stored energy; phosphorylated intermediates are concerned with energy conservation and transfer; phospholipids are major constituents of cell membranes; and the phosphorylation of proteins is a critically important means of regulating their function.

Magnesium

Magnesium is the most abundant intracellular divalent cation and the second most abundant intracellular cation after potassium. Approximately 60% of cellular magnesium is contained in the mitochondria, and it is estimated that only 5–10% of intracellular magnesium ions exist free in the cytoplasm. The transport mechanism responsible for maintaining the asymmetric distribution of magnesium in intracellular compartments are far less well studied that the corresponding calcium transport systems, but it is clear that the cellular metabolism of calcium and of magnesium are regulated independently. Magnesium is an essential cofactor for a wide variety of key enzymes, including essentially all enzymes concerned with the transfer of phosphate groups, all reactions that require ATP, and each of the steps concerned with replication, transcription, and translation of genetic information.

MINERAL ION BALANCE AND MECHANISMS FOR MAINTAINING SYSTEMIC MINERAL HOMEOSTASIS

Mineral ion influx in the intestine, bone, and kidney, and the regulation of these processes by PTH and $1,25(OH)_2D$ are described in detail in other chapters in this primer (see also reference 2). The information in the sections that follow attempts to integrate these processes at the level of the intact organism, and it describes briefly the fine set of checks and balances that regulate mineral homeostasis in vivo.

The term *mineral ion balance* refers to the state of mineral homeostasis in the organism vis-à-vis the environment. In zero balance, mineral intake and accretion exactly match mineral losses. In positive balance, mineral intake and accretion exceed mineral losses. In negative balance, mineral

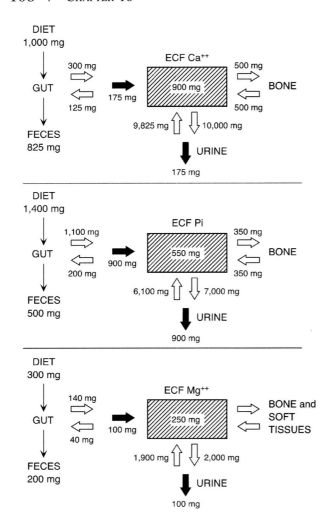

FIG. 1. Schematic representations of calcium, phosphorus, and magnesium fluxes in a normal adult in zero mineral ion balance. Open arrows denote unidirectional mineral fluxes, and solid arrows denote net fluxes; all values are given in mg/dl. (Endocrinology and Metabolism 1987:1358–1361 with permission from The McGraw-Hill Companies, Inc., New York, NY)

losses exceed mineral intake and accretion. A growing child is in positive mineral balance, whereas an immobilized patient or a weightless astronaut is in negative mineral balance. Formal balance studies are a relic of the past, but the concept of balance is central to even a cursory understanding of systemic mineral ion homeostasis. Figure 1 is a schematic representation of calcium, phosphorous, and magnesium metabolism in a normal adult on an average diet who is in zero mineral ion balance.

Calcium

The total extracellular pool of calcium is approximately 900 mg. This pool is in dynamic equilibrium with calcium entering and existing through the intestine, bone, and renal tubule. In zero balance, bone resorption and formation are equivalent at about 500 mg/day, and the net quantity of calcium absorbed by the intestine, approximately 175 mg per day, is quantitatively excreted into the urine. Thus,

under normal circumstances, net calcium absorption provides a surplus of calcium that considerably exceeds systemic requirements.

Several points illustrated in this schema merit some emphasis. The first is the quantitative importance of the kidney in the regulation of calcium homeostasis. The filtered load of calcium is a whopping 10,000 mg/day, and 10% of this, or 1000 mg/day, is under the control of PTH-regulated reabsorption in the distal nephron. The second is the elegance of biological control that must underlie a system in which calcium absorption and excretion are matched on essentially a milligram-for-milligram basis.

Phosphorus

The extracellular pool of orthophosphate is approximately 550 mg (Fig. 1). The pool is in dynamic equilibrium with phosphate entry and exit through the intestine, bone, kidney, and soft tissues (not depicted in the Fig. 1). In zero balance, fractional net phosphorus is about two-thirds of phosphorus intake; this amount represents a vast excess over systemic requirements and is quantitatively excreted into the urine.

Again, several points merit emphasis. The first is that the absorption of phosphate in the intestine is far less rigidly regulated than is the absorption of calcium. The second is the dominant role of the kidney; in this case, it is the threshold for phosphate reabsorption in the proximal tubule (tubular maximum for phosphate/glomerular filtration rate [TmP/GFR]) that serves as the setpoint that defines the fasting serum phosphorus concentration, and it is the setpoint that is regulated by PTH.[5] The term "phosphotonin" is used in connection with a protein (e.g., F6F-23) or a protein family that can also modulate TmP/GFR, possibly as a consequence of phosphate sensing somewhere in the organism. This is a rapidly evolving area that is treated in more detail elsewhere in this primer.

Magnesium

The extracellular pool of magnesium is approximately 250 mg and is in bidirectional equilibrium with magnesium fluxes across the intestine, kidney, bone, and soft tissues (Fig. 1). In zero balance, the magnesium derived from net intestinal absorption, approximately 100 mg per day, represents a systemic surplus and is quantitatively excreted. The kidney is responsible for regulating the serum magnesium concentration by a Tm-limited process that is reminiscent of the setpoint for phosphorus, except that the TmMg is not hormonally regulated.[3]

In summary, two key points are made in the preceding paragraphs: (1) normally, hormonal and/or intrinsic mechanisms of mineral ion absorption in the intestine provide the organism with a mineral supply that exceeds systemic mineral needs by a considerable measure, and (2) the renal tubule plays the dominant quantitative role in maintaining normal mineral homeostasis. Within the framework, minor fluctuations in systemic requirements are easily met by the surfeit of normal mineral absorption and do not require hormonal adjustments.

SYSTEMIC CALCIUM HOMEOSTASIS AND MAINTENANCE OF A NORMAL SERUM CALCIUM CONCENTRATION

The parathyroid chief cell is exquisitely sensitive to the ionized serum calcium concentration and is capable of responding to changes in this concentration so small that they are immeasurable by human hands.[2] The calcium receptor is the sensing device that is the core of the chief cell's sensitivity.[6] The integrated actions of PTH on distal tubular calcium reabsorption, bone resorption, and $1,25(OH)_2D$-mediated intestinal calcium absorption are responsible for the fine regulation of the serum ionized calcium concentration. The precision of this integrated control is such that, in a normal individual, serum ionized calcium probably fluctuates by no more than 0.1 mg/dl in either direction from its normal setpoint value throughout the day.

Distal tubular calcium reabsorption and osteoclastic bone resorption are the major control points in minute-to-minute serum calcium homeostasis; of these two processes, the effect of PTH on the distal tubule is quantitatively the more important. Indeed, the 1000 mg/dl of calcium that is under PTH control as it passes through the distal nephron is the centerpiece of the organism's ability to fine tune the serum calcium concentration. The effects of PTH on the acute phase of bone resorption and calcium reclamation in the distal tubule together constitute a classic "short-loop" feedback system, in that the calcium so provided feeds back directly on the parathyroid chief cell.

The parathyroid-renal [PTH-$1,25(OH)_2D$] axis is reminiscent of the pituitary-adrenal (ACTH-cortisol) axis, and use of the axis concept and terminology is encouraged. Whereas $1,25(OH)_2D$ can influence PTH secretion directly as a short-loop feedback, the essence of the PTH-$1,25(OH)_2D$ axis in practice is a long-loop feedback system in which $1,25(OH)_2D$-mediated calcium absorption provides the ultimate feedback on the parathyroid chief cell. This "long-loop" system is the only means by which the organism can regulate its capacity to obtain calcium from the environment, and it is therefore a crucial component of the organism's response to either a prolonged or a major hypocalcemic challenge. Maximal adjustments to the rate of calcium absorption in the intestine through the PTH-$1,25(OH)_2D$ axis require 24–48 h to become fully operative, so that this system has little to do with minute-to-minute regulation.

A 12- to 15-h fast in a normal individual represents a minor hypocalcemic challenge that requires only subtle hormonal readjustments for correction. The total quantity of calcium lost into the urine during this time is in the range of 50–75 mg. An immeasurable decrease in serum calcium occurs, leading to a slight increase in PTH secretion. The dip in serum calcium is corrected by an increased efficiency of calcium reclamation in the distal tubule and by the rapid resorptive response to PTH in bone; by 12 h, only minor increases in $1,25(OH)_2D$ synthesis will have occurred.

An abrupt reduction in dietary calcium intake to less that 100 mg per day or the administration of 80 mg of furosemide represent moderate hypocalcemic challenges; in each case, the initial deficit of calcium is in the range of 100–150 mg per day. A series of adjustments occurs, lead-

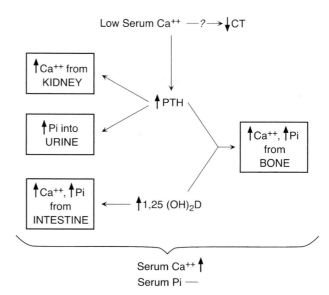

FIG. 2. The sequence of adjustments that are called into play in response to a moderate hypocalcemic challenge. (Endocrinology and Metabolism 1987:1358–1361 with permission from The McGraw-Hill Companies, Inc., New York, NY)

ing to a new steady state by 48 h (Fig. 2). A moderate increase in the secretion rate of PTH results in (1) increased calcium reabsorption from the distal tubule, (2) increased mobilization of calcium and phosphorus from bone, and (3) increased synthesis of $1,25(OH)_2D$, which participates with PTH in bone resorption and increases the efficiency of calcium and phosphorus absorption in the intestine. The increased circulating concentration of PTH resets the renal tubular phosphate threshold (TmP/GFR) at a lower level so that the increased amount of phosphorus mobilized from bone and absorbed from the intestine is quantitatively excreted into the urine. In the new steady state, serum calcium has returned to normal, serum phosphorus is unchanged or very slightly reduced, and a state of mild secondary hyperparathyroidism and efficient intestinal mineral absorption exists. At this point, the initial requirement for calcium mobilization from the skeleton is largely replaced by the enhanced absorption of calcium in the intestine.

The systemic mechanisms for the prevention of hypercalcemia consist of a reversal of the sequence just described, namely, an inhibition of PTH and $1,25(OH)_2D$ synthesis, with a reduction in calcium mobilization from bone, resorption from the intestine, and reclamation from the distal tubule. Whether the putative effects of calcitonin are of pathophysiologic importance in humans remains unclear. The bottleneck in the system's defense against hypercalcemia is the limited capacity of the kidneys to excrete calcium. In theory, normal kidneys can excrete a calcium load of 1000 mg or more per day. In practice, calcium excretion rates in this range are not often seen. Limitations in the theoretical ability of the kidney to combat hypercalcemia include (1) the fact that abnormalities in distal tubular reabsorption are actually involved in the genesis of hypercalcemia in a number of conditions (e.g., primary hyperparathyroidism), (2) the fact that a degree of renal impairment frequently accompanies many hypercalcemic conditions (e.g., the nephrocalcinosis that is associated with sarcoidosis or with the milk-alkali syndrome), and (3) the fact that an increased calcium concentration inhibits the ability of the renal tubule to conserve water, which may lead to a vicious cycle of dehydration and worsening hypercemia. One or more of these limitations can usually be demonstrated in any given patient with hypercalcemia.

A patient with advanced breast carcinoma metastatic to bone represents a severe hypercalcemic challenge. In such a patient, calcium is mobilized from bone, usually by local osteolytic mechanisms. Parathyroid function and 1,25(OH)$_2$D synthesis are appropriately suppressed, and the normal mechanisms of bone resorption, intestinal calcium absorption, and distal tubular calcium reabsorption are virtually eliminated. Initially, these adjustments may lead to a compensated steady state in which approximately 800-1000 mg per day of mobilized calcium is excreted, with a serum calcium that is high-normal or only slightly elevated. With advancing disease or, as often occurs, with immobilization resulting form the basic disease process or an intercurrent illness, the quantity of mobilized calcium overwhelms the renal capacity for calcium excretion, and the spiral of hypercalcemia, dehydration, and worsening hypercalcemia begins. In this circumstance, the serum calcium may climb from 10 to 15 mg/dl within 48 h.

SYSTEMIC PHOSPHORUS HOMEOSTASIS AND MAINTENANCE OF A NORMAL SERUM PHOSPHORUS CONCENTRATION

The kidney plays the dominant role in systemic phosphorus homeostasis and maintains the serum phosphorus concentration at a value that is very close to the tubular phosphorus threshold or TmP/GFR.[5] Because of the normal efficiency and lack of fine regulation of phosphorus absorption in the intestine, only in unusual circumstances (e.g., prolonged use of phosphate-binding antacids) is the systemic supply of phosphorus a limiting factor in phosphorus homeostasis. Thus, most disorders associated with chronic hypophosphatemia and/or phosphorus depletion in humans result from alterations in TmP/GRF (e.g., familial hypophosphatemic rickets or primary hyperparathyroidism). Similarly, most conditions of chronic hyperphosphatemia result from either intrinsic (e.g., renal impairment) or extrinsic (e.g., hypoparathyroidism) abnormalities in the renal threshold for phosphorus. In contrast, acute hypophosphatemia most commonly results from the flux of extracellular phosphate ions into soft tissues.

The PTH receptors in proximal tubule that mediate regulation of TmP/GFR and those in the distal nephron that regulate Ca^{2+} resorption are coupled to different intracellular signal transduction systems. This results in the use of Ca^{2+} as a second messenger associated with phosphate reabsorption in the case of proximal tubular cell, whereas, in the distal tubular cell, PTH regulates the reversible insertion of calcium channels into the luminal membrane, this being the means by which distal tubular calcium reabsorption is controlled. This is a particularly interesting example of specialized Ca^{2+} deployment/handling in the different cell types of the same organ.[7]

The sequence of events initiated in the face of a hy-

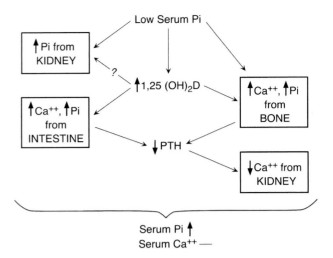

FIG. 3. The sequence of adjustments initiated in response to hypophosphatemia. (Endocrinology and Metabolism 1987:1358–1361 with permission from The McGraw-Hill Companies, Inc., New York, NY)

pophosphatemic challenge (Fig. 3) includes (1) stimulation of 1,25(OH)$_2$D synthesis in the kidney, (2) enhanced mobilization of phosphorus and calcium from bone, and (3) a hypophosphatemia-induced increase in TmP/GFR (possibly mediated by phosphotonin). The increased circulating concentration of 1,25(OH)$_2$D leads to increases in phosphorus and calcium absorption in the intestine and provides an additional stimulus for phosphorus and calcium mobilization from bone. The increased flow of calcium from bone and the intestine results in an inhibition of PTH secretion, which diverts the systemic flow of calcium into the urine and further increases TmP/GFR. The net result of this sequence of adjustments is a return of the serum phosphorus concentration to normal without change in the serum calcium concentration.

The defense against hyperphosphatemia consists largely of a reversal of the sequence of adjustments just described. The principal humoral factor that combats hyperphosphatemia is PTH, but the sequence of events is indirect. The product of the concentrations of calcium and phosphorus in serum is referred to as the mineral ion (Ca × P) product. This product tends to be a biological constant, in the sense that an increase in the concentration of one member leads to a reciprocal change in the concentration of the other. Thus, an acute rise in the serum phosphorus concentration produces a transient fall in the concentration of serum ionized calcium and a stimulation of PTH secretion, which reduces TmP/GFR and leads to a readjustment in serum phosphorus and calcium concentration. A prolonged rise in the serum phosphorus concentration results in (1) an intrinsic downward adjustment in TmP/GFR that is independent of PTH (possibly mediated via phosphotonin), (2) a reduction in circulating 1,25(OH)$_2$D with a concomitant reduction in the fractional absorption of phosphorus in the intestine, and (3) a persistent increase in PTH secretion (that can ultimately lead to chief cell hyperplasia). If hyperphosphatemia is prolonged and severe (e.g., as occurs in chronic renal insufficiency), the degree of secondary hyperparathyroidism is sufficient to lead to parathyroid bone disease.

SYSTEMIC MAGNESIUM HOMEOSTASIS AND MAINTENANCE OF A NORMAL SERUM MAGNESIUM CONCENTRATION

The understanding of systemic magnesium homeostasis remains at a relatively primitive state. Unlike calcium and phosphorus, there seems to be no important systemic or hormonal regulation of the magnesium concentration in the extracellular fluids. Instead, maintenance of the serum magnesium concentration seems to result from the combined fluxes of magnesium at the levels of the intestine, kidney, intracellular fluids, and perhaps the skeleton. The kidney is primarily responsible for the regulation of the serum magnesium concentration.[3]

The fractional absorption of magnesium is approximately 30%. In conditions of dietary magnesium excess, a smaller proportion may be absorbed, and in conditions of dietary magnesium deficiency, a higher proportion may be absorbed. The cellular mechanisms mediating magnesium in the small intestine are poorly defined but would seem to consist of both passive and facilitated (but not active) elements. These elements do not seem to be sensitive to PTH, calcitonin, or $1.25(OH)_2D$. Thus, the net quantity of magnesium absorbed seems to be primarily a function of magnesium intake.

Of the approximately 2000 mg of magnesium filtered per day, 96% is reabsorbed along the nephron, and about 4% is excreted in the urine (fractional magnesium excretion). The mechanisms of magnesium reabsorption along the nephron at a cellular level are poorly understood, but as is the case for calcium and phosphorus, it is possible to define a renal magnesium threshold or tubular maximum for magnesium (TmMg). The TmMg represents the net effects of magnesium reabsorption of different sites along the nephron. The TmMg is approximately 1.4 mg/dl when expressed as a function of the ultrafiltrable serum magnesium concentration or 2.0 mg/dl when expressed as a function of the total serum magnesium concentration.[3] The tubular maximum functions essentially as a setpoint for reabsorption, such that magnesium filtered at a concentration above the TmMg is excreted and that filtered at a concentration beneath the TmMg is retained. As in the intestine, renal tubular magnesium handling does not seem to be regulated by systemic of hormonal mechanisms in any important way.

In summary, systemic magnesium homeostasis does not seem to be hormonally regulated and therefore reflects largely the quantitative interplay of net magnesium absorption in the intestine and the fractional excretion of magnesium by the kidney. The fractional excretion of magnesium as a Tm-limited process and is primarily responsible for maintaining the serum magnesium concentration within rather narrow limits. The fine regulation of the serum magnesium concentration in the absence of hormonal controls provides an excellent example of the biological power of a Tm-limited transport process.

REFERENCES

1. Bringhurst FR 2001 Regulation of calcium and phosphate homeostasis. In: DeGroot LJ, Jameson JL (eds.) Endocrinology, 4th ed. Saunders, Philadelphia, PA, USA, pp. 1029–1052.
2. 2001 Bilezikian JP, Marcus R, Levine MA (eds.) The Parathyroids, 2nd ed. Raven Press, New York, NY, USA.
3. Rude RK 1993 Magnesium metabolism and deficiency. Endocrinol Metab Clin North Am 22:377–390.
4. Carafoli E 2002 Calcium signaling: A tale for all seasons. Proc Natl Acad Sci USA 99:1115–1112.
5. Bijvoet OLM 1969 Relation of plasma phosphate concentration to renal tubular reabsorption of phosphate. Clin Sci 37:230–236.
6. Brown EM, Conigrave A, Chattopadhyay N 2001 Receptors and signaling for calcium ions. In: Bilezikian JP, Marcus R, Levine MA (eds.) The Parathyroids, 2nd ed. Raven Press, New York, NY, USA, pp. 127–142.
7. Friedman PA, Tenenhouse HS 2002 Renal handling of calcium and phosphorus. In: Coe FL, Favus MJ (eds.) Disorders of Bone and Mineral Metabolism, 2nd ed. Lippincott Williams and Wilkins, Philadelphia, PA, USA, pp. 3–33.

Chapter 17. Calcium-Sensing Receptor

Edward M. Brown

Division of Endocrinology, Diabetes and Hypertension, Brigham and Women's Hospital, Harvard Medical School, Boston, Massachusetts

INTRODUCTION

In any given individual, the extracellular ionized calcium concentration (Ca_o^{2+}) is maintained within a remarkably narrow range, varying by only a few percent over the course of a day, a week, or for that manner, much of a lifetime. Calcium plays numerous critical roles both intra- and extracellularly; therefore, it is not surprising that the availability of this ion within the extracellular fluids is regulated so closely. The extracellular calcium-sensing receptor (CaR or CaSR) acts as the body's thermostat for calcium or "calciostat." It is a cell surface, G-protein–coupled receptor capable of detecting perturbations in the serum ionized calcium concentration of only a few percent. It does so principally through its presence in the chief cells of the parathyroid gland, the thyroidal C-cells, and cells along the kidney tubules involved in mineral ion homeostasis. Even minute changes in Ca_o^{2+} modulate the functions of these cells so as to restore normocalcemia. The CaR enables extracellular calcium ions, acting through their own cell

Dr. Brown has received research funding from NPS Pharmaceuticals.

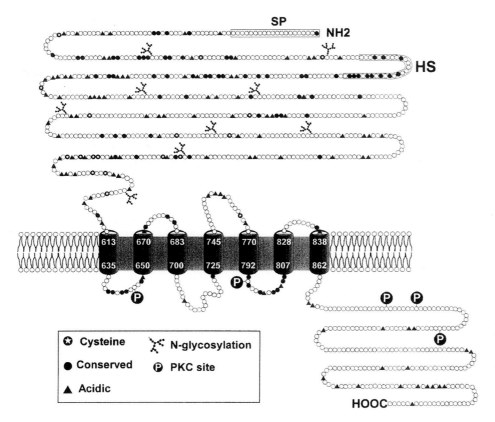

FIG. 1. Predicted structure of the human CaR. SP, signal peptide; HS, hydrophobic segment. (Modified from Metabolic Bone Diseases, Krane SM, Avioli LV, Familial benign hypocalciuric hypercalcemia and other syndromes of altered responsiveness to extracellular calcium, pp. 479–499, 1997 with permission from Elsevier.)

surface receptor, to act in effect, in a hormone-like role as an extracellular first messenger. This chapter will discuss the structure, function, and biological roles of the CaR, particularly with regard to its central role in mineral ion homeostasis.

CaR: ISOLATION, STRUCTURE, AND INTRACELLULAR SIGNALING

The CaR was the first receptor isolated whose principal physiological ligand is an inorganic ion. Studies carried out over two decades, examining the effects of extracellular calcium ions on intracellular second messengers in parathyroid cells, had suggested that calcium exerts its action through a cell surface, G-protein–coupled receptor (GPCR). This prediction was confirmed when the receptor was cloned using expression cloning in *Xenopus laevis*.[1] The CaR has three structural domains, a large extracellular domain (ECD), the seven membrane-spanning "serpentine" motif characteristic of the GPCRs, and a long intracellular, carboxyterminal (C)-tail (Fig. 1). The ECD of the CaR is heavily glycosylated, which is important for its efficient cell surface expression. The biologically active form of the receptor is a dimer, linked together by two disulfide bonds (at cys129 and cys131) between the ECDs of two monomers. The CaR's ECD has important determinants for binding extracellular calcium ions, although the locations of these sites are currently unknown. After the binding of calcium to the ECD, the receptor modulates the functions of the G-proteins that couple it to intracellular signaling pathways (see below). This initiation of signaling involves the

binding of G-proteins to the receptor's intracellular loops—especially the second and third loops—and the proximal portion of the C-tail.

The CaR belongs to a subfamily (family C) of the large superfamily of GPCRs—which also includes receptors for glutamate, gamma aminobutyric acid (GABA), pheromones, and odorants—that share very large extracellular domains (ECDs) of ~600 amino acid residues.[2] The recently solved three-dimensional structure of one of the eight G-protein–coupled receptors for glutamate (mGluR1) revealed that its ECD (and probably those of other family C receptors as well) has a bilobed, "venus flytrap" structure. Glutamate binding occurs within a crevice between the two lobes of each monomer and likely stabilizes the active conformations of the receptor. Elegant studies using molecular modeling and mutagenesis have extended this model to predict the three-dimensional structure of the CaR and to identify portions of the receptor important for dimerization and activation.[3,4] It will be of great interest to eventually determine the precise locations of the CaR's binding sites for calcium using the same approach combined with X-ray crystallography, because the receptor exhibits marked positive cooperativity. This cooperativity is largely responsible for the steepness of the inverse sigmoidal relationship between parathyroid hormone (PTH) release and Ca_o^{2+} that maintains the level of blood calcium within a very narrow range (see Fig. 2 and discussion below).

There are several lines of evidence documenting that the CaR actually serves as the "calciostat" for calcium homeostasis, including experiments-in-nature causing muta-

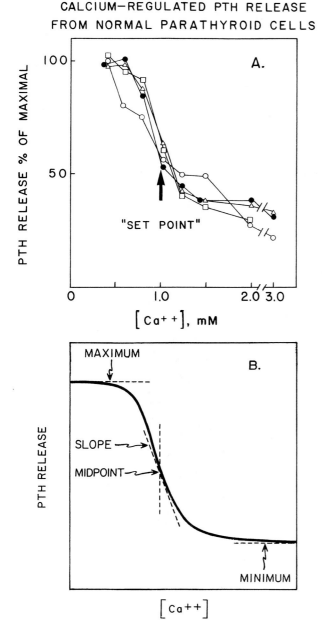

CALCIUM—REGULATED PTH RELEASE
FROM NORMAL PARATHYROID CELLS

A.

"SET POINT"

B.

MAXIMUM

SLOPE

MIDPOINT

MINIMUM

FIG. 2. (A) Relationship between PTH secretion and extracellular calcium in normal human parathyroid cells. Dispersed parathyroid cells were incubated with the indicated levels of calcium and PTH was determined by radioimmunoassay. (B) The four parameters describing the inverse sigmoidal relationship between the extracellular calcium concentration and PTH release in vivo and in vitro: A, maximal secretory rate; B, slope of the curve at the midpoint; C, midpoint or set-point of the curve (the level of calcium producing half of the maximal decrease in secretory rate; D, minimal secretory rate. (Reproduced from Contemporary Issues in Nephrology, vol. 2, Brenner BM, Stein H, Divalent ion homeostasis, pp. 479–499, 1997 with permission from Elsevier.)

tions in the human receptor as well as mouse models in which the receptor has been "knocked-out."[5] Persons heterozygous or homozygous for inactivating mutations exhibit mild to moderate or moderate to severe hypercalcemia, respectively, owing to "resistance" of the CaR to Ca_o^{2+}. The heterozygous state produces a condition known as familial

hypocalciuric hypercalcemia (FHH) or familial benign hypocalciuric hypercalcemia (FBHH).[6] Homozygous mutations, in contrast, usually cause neonatal severe hyperparathyroidism (NSHPT), which can be fatal if parathyroidectomy is not performed urgently within the immediate postnatal period.[7] Not surprisingly, mice heterozygous or homozygous for targeted inactivation of the receptor display biochemical and phenotypic findings similar to those of FHH and NSHPT, respectively. Persons with activating mutations of the CaR display varying degrees of hypocalcemia because of "oversensitivity" of the receptor to Ca_o^{2+}.[7,8] Thus, the calcium-sensing receptor plays a central, nonredundant role in maintaining normalcy of Ca_o^{2+}.

While Ca_o^{2+} is undoubtedly the CaR's principal physiological ligand in vivo, the receptor is activated by a number of other ligands, at least two of which—magnesium and certain amino acids[9]—are likely to be physiologically relevant. Although magnesium is about 2-fold less potent than calcium in its actions on the CaR and the level of Mg_o^{2+} is lower than that of Ca_o^{2+}, persons with inactivating or activating mutations of the receptor tend to have increases or decreases in their serum magnesium concentrations, respectively. These alterations in serum magnesium encompass changes within the normal range to frank hyper- or hypomagnesemia. Thus, it is likely that the CaR contributes to "setting" the normal level of extracellular magnesium.

More recent studies have shown that certain amino acids, especially aromatic amino acids, allosterically activate the CaR,[9] effectively sensitizing the receptor to any given level of Ca_o^{2+}. It is possible, therefore, that the CaR serves a more generalized role as a "nutrient" receptor, recognizing not only divalent cations but also amino acids. For instance, both calcium and aromatic amino acids increase gastrin release and acid production in the stomach—actions that may well be mediated by the CaR. There are additional circumstances in which calcium and protein metabolism appear to be linked in ways that could be mediated by the CaR. A high protein intake promotes hypercalciuria, an action traditionally ascribed to the acid load generated by metabolism of the protein; however, stimulation of renal CaRs by high circulating levels of amino acids could also contribute to the hypercalciuria. Furthermore, a low protein intake in normal subjects, as well as in patients with renal impairment, is associated with elevated levels of PTH. This association could be mediated, in part, by the parathyroid glands sensing a reduction in "nutrient" availability (e.g., the sum of divalent cation and amino acids, and responding with enhanced PTH secretion).

In addition to these endogenous ligands, allosteric activators of the CaR, so-called "calcimimetics,"[10] have been developed, as have CaR antagonists, termed "calcilytics."[11] Calcimimetics are currently in clinical trials for the treatment of primary and uremic secondary hyperparathyroidism and may eventually provide an effective medical treatment for these conditions. Calcilytics provide a means of stimulating endogenous PTH secretion by "tricking" the parathyroid glands into sensing hypocalcemia. They may provide an alternative to the injection of PTH and its analogs as an anabolic treatment of osteoporosis.[11]

The CaR modulates several intracellular signaling systems. It activates phospholipases C (PLC), D (PLD), and A_2

(PLA$_2$) by coupling to the G-protein, G$_{q/11}$. Stimulation of PLC generates diacylglycerol, which activates protein kinase C (PKC), and inositol trisphosphate, which raises the cytosolic calcium concentration by releasing calcium from intracellular stores. PLA$_2$ and PLD are activated in a PKC-dependent manner; the former generates arachidonic acid, which can be further metabolized to generate a host of messenger molecules (e.g., through the cyclo-oxygenase and lipoxygenase pathways). The CaR also stimulates influx of extracellular calcium by activating Ca^{2+}-permeable ion channels by mechanisms that remain to be elucidated. The receptor also activates three mitogen-activated protein kinases (MAPKs)—ERK1/2, p38 MAPK, and JNK. All three of these MAPKs phosphorylate cytosolic as well as nuclear proteins—the latter modulating the expression of genes controlling processes such as cell proliferation, differentiation, and apoptosis, processes that are all regulated by the CaR. Finally, the CaR inhibits adenylate cyclase, in some but not all cases, through the inhibitory G-protein, G$_i$.

ROLE OF THE CaR IN THE PARATHYROID

Raising Ca$_o^{2+}$ exerts three key actions on the parathyroid—inhibiting PTH secretion, PTH gene expression, and parathyroid cellular proliferation.[2] There is a steep inverse sigmoidal relationship between the circulating level of PTH in vivo or PTH secretion in vitro and Ca$_o^{2+}$ (Fig. 2). Key parameters describing this relationship are the midpoint or set-point, which contributes to "setting" the level of Ca$_o^{2+}$, and the slope at the set-point, the steepness of which participates importantly in ensuring that Ca$_o^{2+}$ fluctuates over a narrow range in vivo. The deranged Ca$_o^{2+}$-regulated PTH secretion in patients with inactivating or activating mutations of the CaR, as well as in mice with knockout of the *CaR* gene, prove the CaR's central role in controlling this aspect of parathyroid function. Furthermore, the marked parathyroid cellular hyperplasia in infants with NSHPT and mice homozygous for knockout of the *CaR* gene indicate that the receptor, directly or indirectly, tonically suppresses parathyroid cellular proliferation.[5] Preliminary evidence also supports a role for the CaR in mediating the known inhibitory action of Ca$_o^{2+}$ on PTH gene expression. High Ca$_o^{2+}$ also increases the intracellular degradation of PTH, leading to a reduction in the ratio of intact hormone to carboxyterminal fragments of PTH that are secreted. This action of high Ca$_o^{2+}$ could be mediated through the CaR, although this possibility has not been formally tested. These actions of high Ca$_o^{2+}$ provide for a highly orchestrated, temporal, and hierarchical control of PTH secretion that permits a graded series of responses depending on the nature of the hyper- or hypocalcemic stimulus. The most rapid response to hypocalcemia, for example, is increased secretion of this Ca$_o^{2+}$-elevating hormone, which occurs within seconds. A reduced rate of intracellular degradation of PTH then increases the amount of intact, bioactive PTH available for secretion within about 30 minutes. Increased transcription of the *PTH* gene and greater stability of pre-proPTH mRNA augments the amount of PTH synthesized by each parathyroid cell within hours to a day or so. Finally, enhanced parathyroid cellular proliferation occurs within days to weeks or longer and can increase the functional mass of parathyroid tissue enormously. Therefore, depending on the severity and duration of the hypocalcemic stimulus, the parathyroid glands can mount one, several, or all of these responses for ensuring that sufficient PTH is secreted to normalize Ca$_o^{2+}$.

While considerable progress has been made in documenting the effects of the CaR on parathyroid function, much remains to be learned about the cellular mechanisms through which it exerts these actions.[12] Despite several decades of study, the principal intracellular signal transduction pathway(s) through which the CaR regulates PTH secretion and other aspects of parathyroid function remains to be firmly established.

In addition to the CaR regulating parathyroid function, several factors regulate CaR gene expression in ways that may have physiological or pathophysiological relevance. In chicken but not in rat parathyroid, elevating Ca$_o^{2+}$ upregulates the expression of the CaR gene, thereby potentiating the actions of a given level of Ca$_o^{2+}$. Elevated levels of 1,25 dihydroxyvitamin D in vivo in the rat increase CaR mRNA in parathyroid, which sensitize the parathyroid to Ca$_o^{2+}$ under circumstances when vitamin D levels are high and less PTH may be needed to maintain Ca$_o^{2+}$ homeostasis. Interestingly, high Ca$_o^{2+}$ in the rat upregulates the expression of the vitamin D receptor (VDR), while vitamin D upregulates its own receptor. Therefore, Ca$_o^{2+}$ and 1,25-dihydroxyvitamin D can potentiate their own as well as one another's actions. Interleukin (IL)-1β is another factor upregulating CaR expression in the parathyroid, in association with inhibition of PTH release. This IL-1β–mediated increase in CaR expression could contribute to the mild hypocalcemia and inappropriately normal circulating PTH levels in patients with burn injury or other inflammatory states.

Conditions associated with reduced CaR expression include primary and uremic secondary hyperparathyroidism in humans. This reduction in receptor expression may contribute to the deranged Ca$_o^{2+}$-regulated PTH secretion in these conditions, both of which can show an increase in set-point for PTH release that would reset the level of Ca$_o^{2+}$ upward. Furthermore, high phosphorus intake in the setting of experimental renal insufficiency in the rat downregulates CaR expression.[13] This change in CaR expression is of unknown functional significance, however, because the restoration of normal parathyroid function after reinstitution of a low phosphorus diet precedes the associated increase in CaR expression in this animal model.

ROLE OF THE CaR IN THE C-CELL

In contrast to the inhibitory effect of high Ca$_o^{2+}$ on PTH secretion, elevated Ca$_o^{2+}$ stimulates secretion of the Ca$_o^{2+}$-lowering hormone, calcitonin (CT), by the thyroidal C-cells. Calcitonin has been reported to inhibit bone resorption and at supraphysiological concentrations to stimulate urinary calcium excretion—actions that cause significant hypocalcemia in rodents, but not in adult humans, in whom the hormone contributes little to normal Ca$_o^{2+}$ homeostasis. However, this hormone can be useful in treating states with increased bone resorption (e.g., Paget's disease of bone).

Before the cloning of the CaR, the mechanism by which Ca_o^{2+} modulates CT secretion was thought to differ fundamentally from that in the parathyroid. The availability of DNA and antibody probes for the CaR, however, made it clear that the receptor is expressed in C-cells. Subsequent studies have clarified how the receptor regulates CT secretion. By activating calcium- and sodium-permeable ion channels, the CaR produces cellular depolarization, which then activates voltage-dependent calcium channels, thereby stimulating CT secretion by classical, calcium-dependent, stimulus-secretion coupling.

ROLE OF THE CaR IN THE KIDNEY

Calcium exerts numerous actions on the kidney, several of which are relevant to the physiology and pathophysiology of mineral ion metabolism.[2] For example, high Ca_o^{2+} inhibits the 1-hydroxylation of 25-hydroxyvitamin D, reduces renin secretion, promotes hypercalciuria, and reduces urinary concentrating ability. Studies over the past decade have supported the CaR's roles in mediating several of these actions.

The CaR is expressed in several segments of the nephron.[14] It resides on the basolateral surface of the medullary (MTAL) and cortical thick ascending limbs (CTAL) of Henle's loop of as well as the macula densa. It is present predominantly on the basolateral membrane of the distal convoluted tubule (DCT). In the most distal nephron, it resides on the apical surface of the inner medullary collecting duct (IMCD), where vasopressin increases renal tubular reabsorption of water during dehydration. In several of these locations, available data strongly implicate the CaR in mediating known actions of Ca_o^{2+} on these segments of the nephron.

In the MTAL, the CaR inhibits NaCl reabsorption, thereby impairing generation of the hypertonic interstitium required for vasopressin to maximally stimulate water reabsorption in the IMCD.[15] As will be discussed below, the CaR also inhibits the action of vasopressin in the IMCD,[16] further limiting the capacity of the kidney to concentrate the urine. These two actions of the CaR on the renal concentrating mechanism very likely account for the known inhibitory effect of hypercalcemia on urinary concentrating ability (Fig. 3).

In the CTAL, the CaR inhibits the overall activity of the mechanism that drives the paracellular reabsorption of NaCl, Ca^{2+} and Mg^{2+}.[15] Hormones (e.g., PTH) that stimulate Ca^{2+} and Mg^{2+} reabsorption in CTAL do so by cyclic adenosine monophosphate (cAMP)-dependent stimulation of the $Na^+/K^+/2Cl^-$ cotransporter and the apical recycling K^+ channel (Fig. 4). This augments the lumen positive transepithelial potential, thereby promoting reabsorption of NaCl and divalent cations through the paracellular route. The CaR likely inhibits this process by reducing the activities of the $Na^+/K^+/2Cl^-$ cotransporter and the apical K^+ channel by a PLA_2-dependent mechanism as well as by reducing cAMP generation (Fig. 4). Thus, in addition to decreasing renal calcium reabsorption by CaR-mediated inhibition of PTH secretion, the CaR also blocks the action of PTH on this nephron segment to further reduce renal

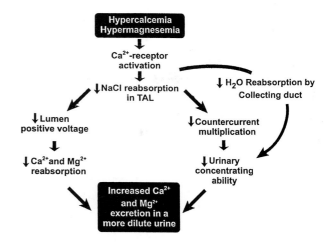

FIG. 3. Renal mechanisms through which the CaR decreases maximal urinary concentrating capacity in the face of CaR-mediated hypercalciuria (or hypermagnesuria). (Reproduced with permission from MedPub, Inc. Regul Peptide Lett **7**:43–47.)

calcium and magnesium reabsorption by a direct renal action of Ca_o^{2+}. The role of the CaR in directly regulating renal tubular reabsorption of Ca^{2+} is strongly supported by the fact that persons with FHH exhibit a marked reduction in their capacity to upregulate Ca_o^{2+} excretion in the CTAL in the face of hypercalcemia—even after parathyroidectomy.

In the DCT, reabsorption of calcium and magnesium take place through the transcellular route. Calcium initially enters the cells through a recently cloned, calcium-permeable channel in the luminal membrane called ECaC or CaT2[17,18] and then exits the basolateral membrane through the Na^+/Ca^{2+}-exchanger and/or Ca^{2+}-ATPase. Calcium, presumably acting through the CaR, can inhibit its own transcellular absorption in MDCK cells—a model of the DCT—by inhibiting the Ca^{2+}-ATPase.[19] Thus, as in the CTAL, the CaR may directly inhibit tubular reabsorption of calcium in the DCT in addition to doing so indirectly by inhibiting PTH release.

In the IMCD, available data strongly implicate the CaR in modulating vasopressin-stimulated water reabsorption in a physiologically important manner.[16] Consistent with the CaR's presence on the apical but not the basolateral surface of the IMCD, perfusion of the luminal (but not the basolateral side) of isolated IMCD segments with elevated levels of Ca_o^{2+} inhibits vasopressin-stimulated water flow by about 40%.[16] The role of the CaR in this process is supported by the fact that persons with FHH can concentrate their urine to a greater extent than subjects with primary hyperparathyroidism and an equivalent degree of hypercalcemia.[20] That is, similar to the resistance of PTH secretion and renal calcium reabsorption (most likely in the CTAL) to Ca_o^{2+} in FHH, there also appears to be resistance of the IMCD to the normal inhibitory action of Ca_o^{2+} on vasopressin-stimulated water flow.

Vasopressin stimulates water reabsorption in this nephron segment by causing the insertion of aquaporin-2-containing vesicles resident below the apical membrane of the cells into the luminal plasma membrane. The hypertonic interstitium surrounding the IMCD then enables passive reabsorp-

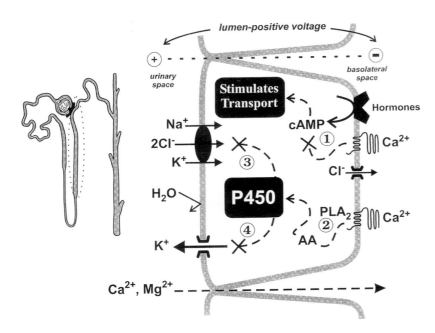

FIG. 4. Mechanisms through which the CaR controls reabsorption of calcium and magnesium in the CTAL. PTH acts on the CTAL through its basolateral receptor to increase cAMP levels, thereby increasing the overall activity of the $Na^+/K^+/2Cl^-$ cotransporter and recycling K^+ channel, which in turn, increases the lumen positive potential that drives paracellular reabsorption of Ca^{2+} and Mg^{2+}. Activation of the CaR inhibits this process by inhibiting adenylate cyclase and generating arachidonic acid (AA), which is metabolized to products of the p450 pathway that inhibit the K^+ channel and $Na^+/K^+/2Cl^-$ cotransporter. Both of these processes diminish the lumen positive potential and pari passu reabsorption of the divalent cations. (Reproduced from Bone, 20, Brown EM, Hebert SC, Calcium-receptor regulated parathyroid and renal function, pp. 303–309, 1997 with permission from Elsevier.)

tion of water. Because vasopressin exerts its effect on aquaporin-2 trafficking by activating adenylate cyclase, the CaR could inhibit this process, at least in part, by inhibiting vasopressin-stimulated cAMP accumulation. By inhibiting vasopressin-stimulated water flow, the CaR would, in effect, set an upper limit to the level of Ca^{2+} that could be reached within the distal nephron, which could potentially reduce the risk of renal stone formation. Furthermore, if there were habitual intake of excess calcium (e.g., in the milk-alkali syndrome), an elevated level of Ca_o^{2+}, through CaR-mediated inhibition of NaCl reabsorption in the MTAL, would "wash out" the medullary interstitium and further limit the concentration of Ca_o^{2+} that could be achieved in the IMCD under the influence of vasopressin (Fig. 3).

CaR IN BONE AND INTESTINE

Is the CaR also present in the other two major Ca_o^{2+}-translocating tissues, bone and intestine, that contribute to maintaining Ca^{2+} homeostasis? High Ca_o^{2+} stimulates bone formation and inhibits bone resorption in vitro. These actions of Ca^{2+} could contribute to calcium homeostasis by allowing bone to serve as a "sink" and reservoir for calcium ions to buffer changes in Ca_o^{2+} when the latter is high and low, respectively. The role of the CaR, however, if any, in mediating these actions of Ca_o^{2+} remains uncertain. Some authors,[21] but not others,[22] have identified the CaR in osteoblast and osteoclast precursors as well as in mature osteoblasts and osteoclasts. Moreover, the pharmacology for the effects of various divalent and trivalent cations on the functions of cells of both the osteoclast and osteoblast lineages differ in some cases from those expected of the CaR.[23,24] Thus, while there is general agreement that Ca_o^{2+} modulates several functions of osteoblasts and osteoclasts and their precursors that are important for bone turnover, the

identification of the relevant Ca_o^{2+}-sensing mechanism(s) has been elusive.

The CaR is known to be expressed in epithelial cells along the gastrointestinal tract that are involved in the absorption of dietary calcium (e.g., in the proximal small and large intestines).[25] It is also expressed in the enteric nervous system, where it could potentially mediate the known inhibitory and stimulatory actions of high and low levels of Ca_o^{2+}, respectively, on gastrointestinal motility. Further studies are needed, however, to determine whether the receptor has any physiologically relevant actions on the absorption of mineral ions from the intestine or other aspects of the gastrointestinal function relevant to mineral ion metabolism.

SUMMARY

The CaR serves as the crucial Ca_o^{2+} sensor in the parathyroid chief cells, C-cells, and cells along the nephron that participate in the control of renal calcium reabsorption. In response to small changes in Ca_o^{2+}, the CaR modulates the secretion of the Ca_o^{2+}-elevating hormone, PTH, and the Ca_o^{2+}-lowering hormone, CT, in ways that will restore normocalcemia. In addition to regulating the production of these calciotropic hormones, it exerts direct actions on the kidney (i.e., in the CTAL). Thus, by inhibiting PTH production and stimulating CT secretion as well as by promoting urinary calcium excretion, indirectly through PTH and directly through its actions in CTAL, the CaR enables Ca_o^{2+} to serve as the body's most effective Ca_o^{2+}-lowering hormone.

REFERENCES

1. Brown EM, Gamba G, Riccardi D, Lombardi M, Butters R, Kifor O, Sun A, Hediger MA, Lytton J, Hebert SC 1993 Cloning and charac-

terization of an extracellular Ca$^{(2+)}$-sensing receptor from bovine parathyroid. Nature **366**:575–580.

2. Brown EM, MacLeod RJ 2001 Extracellular calcium sensing and extracellular calcium signaling. Physiol Rev **81**:239–297.

3. Reyez-Cruz G, Hu J, Goldsmith PK, Steinbach PJ, Spiegel AM 2001 Human Ca^{2+} receptor extracellular domain. Analysis of function of lobe I deletion mutants. J Biol Chem **276**:32145–32151.

4. Hu J, Reyes-Cruz G, Chen W, Jacobson KA, Spiegel AM 2002 Identification of acidic residues in the extracellular loops of the seven transmembrane domain of the human Ca^{2+} receptor critical for response to Ca^{2+} and a positive allosteric modulator. J Biol Chem **277**:46622–46631.

5. Ho C, Conner DA, Pollak MR, Ladd DJ, Kifor O, Warren HB, Brown EM, Seidman JG, Seidman CE 1995 A mouse model of human familial hypocalciuric hypercalcemia and neonatal severe hyperparathyroidism. Nat Genet **11**:389–394.

6. Pollak MR, Brown EM, Chou YH, Hebert SC, Marx SJ, Steinmann B, Levi T, Seidman CE, Seidman JG 1993 Mutations in the human Ca$^{(2+)}$-sensing receptor gene cause familial hypocalciuric hypercalcemia and neonatal severe hyperparathyroidism. Cell **75**:1297–1303.

7. Brown EM 1999 Physiology and pathophysiology of the extracellular calcium-sensing receptor. Am J Med **106**:238–253.

8. Pollak MR, Brown EM, Estep HL, McLaine PN, Kifor O, Park J, Hebert SC, Seidman CE, Seidman JG 1994 Autosomal dominant hypocalcaemia caused by a Ca$^{(2+)}$-sensing receptor gene mutation. Nat Genet **8**:303–307.

9. Conigrave AD, Quinn SJ, Brown EM 2000 L-amino acid sensing by the extracellular Ca^{2+}-sensing receptor. Proc Natl Acad Sci USA **97**:4814–4819.

10. Nemeth EF, Steffey ME, Hammerland LG, Hung BC, Van Wagenen BC, DelMar EG, Balandrin MF 1998 Calcimimetics with potent and selective activity on the parathyroid calcium receptor. Proc Natl Acad Sci USA **95**:4040–4045.

11. Gowen M, Stroup GB, Dodds RA, James IE, Votta BJ, Smith BR, Bhatnagar PK, Lago AM, Callahan JF, DelMar EG, Miller MA, Nemeth EF, Fox J 2000 Antagonizing the parathyroid calcium receptor stimulates parathyroid hormone secretion and bone formation in osteopenic rats. J Clin Invest **105**:1595–1604.

12. Diaz R, El-Hajj Fuleihan G, Brown EM 1998 Regulation of parathyroid function. In: Fray J (ed.) Handbook of Physiology, vol. 3. Oxford University Press, New York, NY, USA, pp. 607–662.

13. Brown AJ, Ritter CS, Finch JL, Slatopolsky EA 1999 Decreased calcium-sensing receptor expression in hyperplastic parathyroid glands of uremic rats: Role of dietary phosphate. Kidney Int **55**:1284–1292.

14. Riccardi D, Lee WS, Lee K, Segre GV, Brown EM, Hebert SC 1996 Localization of the extracellular Ca$^{(2+)}$-sensing receptor and PTH/PTHrP receptor in rat kidney. Am J Physiol **271**:F951–F956.

15. Hebert SC, Brown EM, Harris HW 1997 Role of the Ca^{2+}-sensing Receptor in divalent mineral ion homeostasis. J Exp Biol **200**:295–302.

16. Sands JM, Naruse M, Baum M, Jo I, Hebert SC, Brown EM, Harris HW 1997 Apical extracellular calcium/polyvalent cation-sensing receptor regulates vasopressin-elicited water permeability in rat kidney inner medullary collecting duct. J Clin Invest **99**:1399–1405.

17. Hoenderop JGJ, Van de Graaf AWCM, Hartog A, van de Graaf SFJ, van Os CH, Willems PHGM, Bindels RJM 1999 Molecular identification of the apical Ca^{2+} channel in 1, 25-dihydroxyvitamin D3-responsive epithelia. J Biol Chem **274**:8375–8378.

18. Peng JB, Chen XZ, Berger UV, Vassilev PM, Brown EM, Hediger MA 2000 A rat kidney-specific calcium transporter in the distal nephron. J Biol Chem **275**:28186–28194.

19. Blankenship KA, Williams JJ, Lawrence MS, McLeish KR, Dean WL, Arthur JM 2001 The calcium-sensing receptor regulates calcium absorption in MDCK cells by inhibition of PMCA. Am J Physiol Renal Physiol **280**:F815–F822.

20. Marx SJ, Attie MF, Stock JL, Spiegel AM, Levine MA 1981 Maximal urine-concentrating ability: Familial hypocalciuric hypercalcemia versus typical primary hyperparathyroidism. J Clin Endocrinol Metab **52**:736–740.

21. Chang W, Tu C, Chen T-H, Komuves L, Oda Y, Pratt S, Miller S, Shoback D 1999 Expression and signal transduction of calcium-sensing receptors in cartilage and bone. Endocrinology **140**:5883–5893.

22. Pi M, Hinson TK, Quarles L 1999 Failure to detect the extracellular calcium-sensing receptor (CasR) in human osteoblast cell lines. J Bone Miner Res **14**:1310–1319.

23. Zaidi M, Adebanjo OA, Moonga BS, Sun L, Huang CL 1999 Emerging insights into the role of calcium ions in osteoclast regulation. J Bone Miner Res **14**:669–674.

24. Quarles DL, Hartle JE II, Siddhanti SR, Guo R, Hinson TK 1997 A distinct cation-sensing mechanism in MC3T3–E1 osteoblasts functionally related to the calcium receptor. J Bone Miner Res **12**:393–402.

25. Chattopadhyay N, Cheng I, Rogers K, Riccardi D, Hall A, Diaz R, Hebert SC, Soybel DI, Brown EM 1998 Identification and localization of extracellular Ca$^{(2+)}$-sensing receptor in rat intestine. Am J Physiol **274**:G122–G130.

Chapter 18. Parathyroid Hormone

Harald Jüppner and Henry M. Kronenberg

Endocrine Unit, Departments of Pediatrics and Medicine, Harvard Medical School, Massachusetts General Hospital, Boston, Massachusetts

INTRODUCTION

Parathyroid hormone (PTH) and the active form of vitamin D, 1,25-dihydroxy-vitamin D_3 [1,25(OH)$_2$D$_3$], are the principle regulators of calcium homeostasis for humans and most likely all terrestrial vertebrates.[1,2] In bone, PTH stimulates the release of calcium and phosphate, and in the kidney, it stimulates the reabsorption of calcium and inhibits the reabsorption of phosphate. Furthermore, PTH stimulates the activity of the renal 1-α-hydroxylase, thereby enhancing the synthesis of 1,25(OH)$_2$D$_3$, which in turn increases the intestinal absorption of calcium and phosphate. As a result of these PTH-dependent actions, blood calcium concentration rises and blood phosphate concentration declines. The extracellular calcium concentration is the most important physiological regulator of the minute-to-minute secretion of PTH. A rise in blood calcium concentration decreases PTH secretion, while a decrease in blood calcium increases PTH secretion. 1,25(OH)$_2$D$_3$ and low phosphate, as well as an increase in calcium, all act to decrease the synthesis of PTH. The mutual regulatory interactions of PTH, calcium, 1,25(OH)$_2$D$_3$, and phosphate can thus maintain the blood calcium level constant, even in the presence of significant fluctuations in dietary calcium, bone metabolism, or renal function. In this chapter, we review the structure and biosynthesis of PTH, the regulation of its secretion, and the physiologic actions of PTH, and

The authors have no conflict of interest.

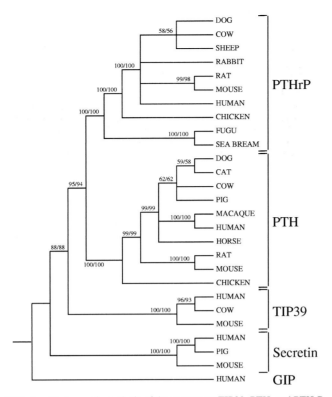

FIG. 1. Phylogenetic analysis of the precursors TIP39, PTH, and PTHrP, and the some peptides of the secretin family. (Reproduced with permission of The Endocrine Society from John M, Arai M, Rubin D, Jonsson K, Jüppner H, 2002 Identification and characterization of the murine and human gene encoding the tuberoinfundibular peptide of 39 residues (TIP39). Endocrinology **143**:1047–1057.)

examine the cellular and subcellular mechanisms responsible for those actions.

PTH

During evolution, the parathyroid glands first appear as discrete organs in amphibians, that is, with the migration of vertebrates from an aquatic to a terrestrial existence. In mammals, PTH is produced by the parathyroid glands, although small amounts of its mRNA have also been detected in the rat hypothalamus.[1] PTH is a single chain polypeptide that comprises in all investigated mammalian species 84 amino acids; chicken PTH, the only non-mammalian homolog isolated thus far, contains 88 residues (Fig. 1). The amino-terminal region of PTH, which is associated with most of its known biological actions, shows high homology among the different vertebrate species. The middle and carboxy-terminal regions show greater sequence variation, and these portions of the PTH molecule seem to have distinct biological properties that are probably mediated through distinct receptors.[3] However, the physiological importance of these actions needs further clarification.

Within the first 34 residues, PTH shares significant amino acid sequence conservation with the PTH-related peptide (PTHrP), which was initially discovered as the cause of the humoral hypercalcemia of malignancy syndrome.[4] Both peptides are derived from genes that presumably evolved through an ancient gene duplication event from a common precursor and thus share similarities in their intron-exon organization. PTH and PTHrP are furthermore distantly related to the tuberoinfundibular peptide of 39 residues (TIP39),[5] and the *TIP39* gene has an organization similar to those encoding PTH and PTHrP[6] (Fig. 2).

THE PARATHYROID CELL

Regulation of PTH Synthesis and Secretion and Parathyroid Cell Proliferation

Although a large number of factors modulate parathyroid function in vitro, only a few regulators are known to be of physiological relevance in vivo.[7] The extracellular concentration of calcium (Ca^{2+}_o) is the most important determinant of the minute-to-minute secretory rate of the parathyroid gland; low Ca^{2+}_o stimulates, whereas increased Ca^{2+}_o inhibits PTH secretion and suppresses PTH gene expression and parathyroid cellular proliferation. $1,25(OH)_2D_3$ inhibits

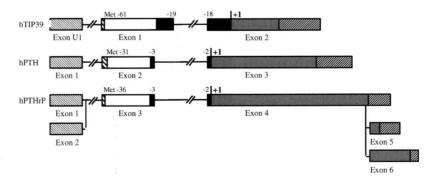

FIG. 2. Structures of the genes encoding human TIP39, human PTH, and human PTHrP. Boxed areas are exons and their names are shown underneath (because the start of exon U1 of the TIP39 gene is unknown, the box is open on the left site), white boxes denote presequences, black boxes denote prosequences (for TIP39 presumed), gray stippled boxes denote the mature sequences; noncoding regions are shown as striped boxes. The small striped boxes preceding the white boxes denote untranslated exonic sequences (4 bp for TIP39; 5 bp for PTH; 22 bp for PTHrP). The positions of the initiator methionine based on the secreted peptide are noted above the graphs; the positions where pro-sequences are interrupted by an intron are noted above the graph. +1 denotes the relative position of the beginning of the secreted peptide. (Reproduced with permission of The Endocrine Society from John M, Arai M, Rubin D, Jonsson K, Jüppner H, 2002 Identification and characterization of the murine and human gene encoding the tuberoinfundibular peptide of 39 residues (TIP39). Endocrinology **143**:1047–1057.)

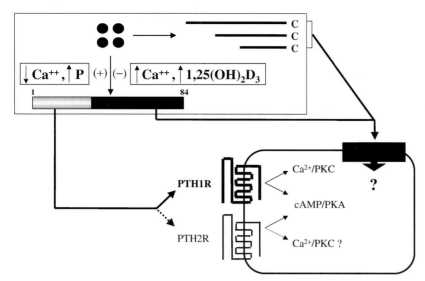

FIG. 3. PTH production and activation of different receptors. Intact PTH and different fragments are secreted from the parathyroid glands. Low ionized calcium and elevated phosphate increase PTH synthesis and secretion, while increased ionized calcium and 1,25(OH)$_2$D$_3$ led to a decrease; note that the regulatory actions of calcium are mediated through the calcium-sensing receptor. Different receptors interact with the amino- or carboxy-terminal portion of intact PTH. Through its amino-terminal portion, PTH activates the PTH/PTHrP receptor (PTH1R), a G-protein–coupled receptor that mediates its actions through at least two different signaling pathways, cAMP/KPA and Ca^{2+}/PKC. The closely related PTH2-receptor (PTH2R) is most likely the primary receptor for the tuberoinfundibular peptide of 39 residues (TIP39); however, at least the human PTH2R is also activated by amino-terminal PTH. Another receptor, which has not yet been cloned, interacts only with the carboxy-terminal portion of PTH.

expression of the *PTH* gene and may also directly reduce PTH secretion and parathyroid cellular proliferation. Phosphate, the most recently recognized direct modulator of parathyroid function, stimulates PTH gene expression, and probably indirectly, PTH secretion, as well as parathyroid cellular proliferation[8,9] (Fig. 3).

The parathyroid cell has a temporal hierarchy of responses to changes in Ca$^{2+}_o$, which can mount a progressively larger increase in PTH secretion in response to prolonged hypocalcemia.[7] To meet acute hypocalcemic challenges, PTH, stored in secretory vesicles, is rapidly secreted by exocytosis (e.g., over seconds to a few minutes). For the correction of prolonged hypocalcemia, parathyroid cells reduce the intracellular degradation of PTH (over minutes to about an hour), increase PTH gene expression (over several hours to a few days), and enhance the proliferative activity of parathyroid cells (over days to weeks or longer). Many, if not all, of these processes are controlled by a G-protein–coupled receptor that recognizes extracellular calcium ions as its principal physiological ligand. This calcium-sensing receptor (CaR) is expressed on the surface of parathyroid cells and several other cell types that are involved in regulating mineral ion homeostasis.[10]

Physiological Regulation of PTH Secretion

There is a steep inverse sigmoidal relationship between PTH levels and Ca$^{2+}_o$ in vivo and in vitro.[7] The steepness of this curve ensures large changes in PTH for small alterations in Ca$^{2+}_o$ and contributes importantly to the near constancy with which Ca$^{2+}_o$ is maintained in vivo. Parathyroid cells readily detect alterations in Ca$^{2+}_o$ of only a few percent. The mid-point or set-point of this parathyroid function curve is a key determinant of the level at which Ca$^{2+}_o$ is "set" in vivo. The parathyroid cell responds to changes in Ca$^{2+}_o$ within a matter of seconds, and it has sufficient stored PTH to sustain a maximal secretory response for 60–90 minutes. 1,25(OH)$_2$D$_3$ reduces PTH secretion in vitro,[11] while elevations in the

extracellular phosphate concentration stimulate PTH secretion.[8,9] These changes in PTH secretion caused by 1,25(OH)$_2$D$_3$ phosphate are, however, not immediate and may reflect primary actions on PTH synthesis.

Regulation of Intracellular Degradation of PTH

The pool of stored, intracellular PTH in the parathyroid cell is finite, being sufficient to sustain PTH secretion at maximal rates for only 60–90 minutes. The cell must therefore have mechanisms to increase hormone synthesis and release in response to more sustained hypocalcemia. One such adaptive mechanism is to reduce the intracellular degradation of the hormone, thereby increasing the net amount of intact, biologically active PTH that is available for secretion. During hypocalcemia, the bulk of the hormone that is released from the parathyroid cell is intact PTH(1-84). As the level of Ca$^{2+}_o$ increases, a greater fraction of intracellular PTH is degraded, and with overt hypercalcemia, the majority of the secreted immunoreactive PTH consists of carboxy-terminal fragments.[1]

Physiological Control of PTH Gene Expression

The second adaptive mechanism of the parathyroid cell to sustained reductions in Ca$^{2+}_o$ is to increase the cellular levels of PTH mRNA, which takes several hours. Reductions in Ca$^{2+}_o$ increase, while elevations reduce, the cellular levels of PTH mRNA by affecting the transcription rate of the PTH gene as well as through additional, post-transcriptional mechanisms.[2] Available data suggest that phosphate ions also directly regulate PTH gene expression. Hypo- and hyperphosphatemia in the rat lower and raise, respectively, the levels of the mRNA for PTH through a mechanism of action that is independent of changes in Ca$^{2+}_o$ or 1,25(OH)$_2$D$_3$.[2] This action of an elevated extracellular phosphate concentration could potentially contribute importantly to the secondary hyperparathyroidism frequently encountered in states with a chronically high serum phosphate, such as the secondary hyperparathyroidism in end-stage renal failure. It will be of interest to determine whether phosphate-sensing involves a receptor-mediated mechanism similar to that through which Ca^{2+}_o regulates parathyroid and kidney function.

Metabolites of vitamin D, principally $1,25(OH)_2D_3$, play an important role in the long-term regulation of parathyroid function and may act at several levels, including the control of PTH secretion,[11] as noted before, and control of expression the *PTH* gene, the *CaR* gene,[7] and the vitamin D receptor (*VDR*) gene, as well as the regulation of parathyroid cellular proliferation.[2] By far, the most important metabolite of vitamin D modulating parathyroid function is $1,25(OH)_2D_3$, which acts principally through an intracellular receptor that functions as a nuclear transcription factor, often in concert with other such transcription factors (i.e., those for retinoic acid or glucocorticoids). $1,25(OH)_2D_3$ reduces the levels of the mRNA encoding PTH through an action mediated by DNA sequences upstream from the *PTH* gene. $1,25(OH)_2D_3$-induced upregulation of the level of VDR expression in parathyroid could act as a feed-forward mechanism to potentiate its own inhibitory action(s) on parathyroid function.[2] High Ca^{2+}_o and $1,25(OH)_2D_3$ coordinately increase the mRNA for the VDR.[7] Some of the "noncalcemic" analogs of $1,25(OH)_2D_3$ (e.g., 22-oxacalcitriol, calcipotriol, and 19-nor-1,25-dihydroxyvitamin D2) inhibit PTH secretion while producing relatively little stimulation of intestinal calcium absorption and of bone resorption, the biological actions that underlie the hypercalcemic effects of $1,25(OH)_2D_3$.[12] Therefore, these synthetic vitamin D analogs may represent attractive candidates for treating the hyperparathyroidism of chronic renal insufficiency, because hypercalcemia resulting from the gastrointestinal and skeletal actions of $1,25(OH)_2D_3$ often becomes a factor limiting the treatment of such patients.

Physiological Regulation of Parathyroid Cellular Proliferation

The final adaptive mechanism contributing to changes in the overall level of parathyroid gland secretory activity is the adjustment of the rate of parathyroid cellular proliferation. Under normal conditions, there is little or no proliferative activity of parathyroid cells. The parathyroid glands, however, can enlarge greatly during states of chronic hypocalcemia, particularly in the setting of renal failure [probably because of a combination of hypocalcemia, hyperphosphatemia and low levels of $1,25(OH)_2D_3$ in the latter condition].[7] This enlargement cannot be accounted for solely by cellular hypertrophy, although the latter does contribute to the overall increase in glandular mass. The ability of calcium administration to prevent parathyroid hyperplasia in mice with deleted vitamin D receptors illustrates the importance of calcium in regulating parathyroid cell number.[13] Calcium acts to prevent hyperplasia through activation of the CaSR, because mutational inactivation of the CaSR in humans and mice leads to parathyroid hyperplasia at birth and because calcimimetic compounds that activate the CaSR can prevent parathyroid hyperplasia in experimental uremia.[14]

PARATHYROID HORMONE ACTION

Receptors for PTH

PTH-dependent regulation of mineral ion homeostasis is largely mediated through the PTH/PTHrP receptor (PTHIR), which is coupled to adenylate cyclase through $G_s\alpha$ and to phospholipase C through the G_q family of signaling proteins[1,3] (see Fig. 3). While most PTH/PTHrP receptor-dependent actions involve activation of adenylyl cyclase, some actions seem to require phospholipase C-mediated events. These dual signaling properties are particularly relevant because the PTH/PTHrP receptor was recently shown to interact in vitro, through a PDZ-domain, with Na^+/H^+ exchange regulatory factors NHERF1 and NHERF2. In the presence of NHERF2 (and probably also NHERF1), the activated PTH/PTHrP receptor preferentially activated phospholipase C and inhibited adenylyl cyclase through stimulation of inhibitory G proteins ($G_{i/o}$ proteins).[15] NHERF-dependent changes in PTH/PTHrP receptor signaling may thus account for some of different tissue- and cell-specific actions induced by PTH or PTHrP.

The PTH/PTHrP receptor belongs to a distinct family of G-protein–coupled receptors and mediates with similar or indistinguishable efficacy biological actions of both PTH and PTHrP.[3] The PTH/PTHrP receptor is most abundantly expressed in the target tissues for PTH's actions, that is, kidney and bone, but it is also found in a large variety of other fetal and adult tissues and at particularly high concentrations in growth plate chondrocytes.[1,3] In tissues other than kidney and bone, the PTH/PTHrP receptor most likely mediates the para-/autocrine actions of PTHrP, rather than the endocrine actions of PTH. Of considerable importance is the receptor's role in cartilage and bone development, because it mediates in this tissue the PTHrP-dependent regulation of chondrocyte proliferation and differentiation; thus, it has a major role in bone development and growth.[16,17]

The PTH/PTHrP receptor seems to be the most important receptor mediating the actions of PTH and PTHrP. There is considerable pharmacologic evidence, however, for the existence of other receptors that are activated by either PTH and/or PTHrP, including a receptor/binding protein that interacts with the carboxy-terminal portion of PTH and may be involved in mediating the hypocalcemic actions of this portion of the molecule.[3,18,19] However, most of these putative receptors have not yet been cloned, and their biological functions, some of which may be unrelated to the control of calcium and phosphorus homeostasis, remain poorly characterized. Only cDNAs encoding the PTH2-receptor have been isolated thus far.[3,20,21] The human PTH2 receptor, but not the homolog of this receptor from other species, is activated by PTH; PTHrP does not activate any the different PTH2 receptor species unless residues 5 and 23 are replaced with the corresponding PTH-specific amino acids.[1,3] However, the natural ligand for the PTH2-receptor seems to be TIP39, a recently identified hypothalamic peptide.[22,23] Expression of the PTH-2 receptor is restricted to relatively few tissues, that is, placenta, pancreas, blood vessels, testis, and brain, and although most biological function(s) mediated through this receptor remain

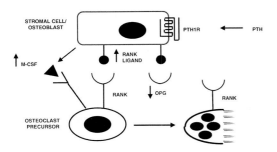

FIG. 4. PTH actions on bone. The PTH/PTHrP receptor (PTH1R) is expressed on stromal cells/osteoblasts. On receptor activation by PTH, expression of M-CSF and RANK ligand are increased, which then enhances the formation of osteoclasts from precursors and the activity of already existing mature osteoclasts. In response to PTH, expression of OPG, a decoy receptor for RANK ligand, is decreased thus reducing the activity of existing osteoclasts and the formation of mature osteoclasts from precursor cells.

to be determined, it may have a role in the regulation of renal blood flow.[20,24,25]

Actions of PTH on Bone

PTH has complex and only partially understood actions on bone that require the presence of and often direct contact between several different specialized cell types, including osteoblasts, bone marrow stromal cells, hematopoetic precursors of osteoclasts, and mature osteoclasts.[26] Administration of PTH leads to the release of calcium from a rapidly turning-over pool of calcium near the surface of bone; after several hours, calcium is also released from an additional pool that turns over more slowly.[27] Chronic administration of PTH (or increased secretion of PTH associated with primary hyperparathyroidism) leads to an increase in osteoclast cell number and activity.[28] The release of calcium is accompanied by the release of phosphate and matrix components, such as degradation products of collagen. Paradoxically, particularly when given intermittently, PTH administration leads to the formation of increased amounts of trabecular bone[29,30]; these anabolic actions of PTH are currently being explored for the prevention and treatment of osteoporosis.[31]

The osteoblast and its precursor, the marrow stromal cell, have central roles in directing both the catabolic (bone resorption) and anabolic (bone formation) actions of PTH (Fig. 4). Only a subset of stromal cells and osteoblasts synthesize mRNA encoding the PTH/PTHrP receptor.[32] Although cell lines capable of differentiating into osteoclasts have been shown to have PTH/PTHrP receptors,[33–38] these receptors are not needed or sufficient for the stimulation of osteoclastic development by PTH.[39] Elegant studies of co-cultures of osteoblasts/stromal cells and osteoclast precursors had shown that PTH affects osteoclast maturation and functions only indirectly through its actions on cells of the osteoblast lineage, which express abundant amounts of the PTH/PTHrP receptor.[26] A key osteoblastic protein that activates osteoclast development and activity of mature osteoclasts is RANK ligand (also termed osteoclast-differentiating factor [ODF], TRANCE, or osteoprotegerin-ligand), a member of the tumor necrosis factor (TNF) family

of proteins, which is anchored by a single hydrophobic membrane-spanning domain to the cell surface of osteoblasts.[40–42] On interaction with RANK, a member of the TNF receptor family, expressed on preosteoclasts, these precursors differentiate into mature osteoclasts, if macrophage colony-stimulating factor (M-CSF) is also present.[41,42] RANKL also increases the bone-resorbing properties of mature osteoclasts. PTH stimulates the expression of RANKL on the cell surface of osteoblasts,[41] and the same response is stimulated by other molecules, that is, interleukin 11 (IL-11), prostaglandin E_2, and 1,25-dihydroxyvitamin D_3, which were previously noted to stimulate the formation of osteoclasts. PTH also stimulates the synthesis of M-CSF.[42]

The interactions of osteoblastic RANKL and its osteoclastic receptor RANK are further controlled by a secreted protein, osteoprotegerin (OPG), a soluble "decoy" receptor with homology to the RANK and other members of the TNF receptor family. The effects of overexpression of OPG in transgenic mice,[43] as well as the ablation the OPG gene,[44] suggest that this binding protein importantly modulates the communication between osteoblasts and osteoclasts.[44] PTH inhibits the expression of OPG in osteoblast cells.[45] Thus, by increasing M-CSF and RANKL and inhibiting OPG expressed locally by cells of the osteoblast lineage, PTH stimulates osteoclastogenesis and the activity of mature osteoclasts.

The mechanisms whereby PTH increases bone formation are complicated and less well understood (see Fig. 4). PTH increases the number of osteoblasts by increasing the number of osteoprogenitors cells,[46] by decreasing apoptosis of preosteoblasts and osteoblasts,[47,48] by increasing osteoblast proliferation,[49] and perhaps by converting inactive bone lining cells to active osteoblasts.[50] On the other hand, when added to cells in culture, PTH stops preosteoblastic cells from becoming mature osteoblasts. It also changes the activity of mature osteoblasts. In cell culture systems, PTH inhibits the production of collagen and other matrix proteins, perhaps partly by steering the key osteoblast transcription factor, RUNX2 (also called CBFA-1), to proteosome-mediated destruction.[51] The prominent action of PTH in vivo to increase bone formation may result from the production by osteoblasts of growth factors such as IGF-1 and fibroblast growth factor (FGF)-2, as well as from the release of growth factors from matrix after PTH-induced osteoclast action.

With complicated actions both on bone formation and bone resorption, it is perhaps not surprising that the net effects of PTH on bone can be either anabolic (net increase in bone mass) or catabolic (net decrease in bone mass). Depending on the dose of PTH, the mode of administration (intermittent versus continuous), the animal species, and the specific site (trabecular bone versus cortical bone), PTH can be either anabolic or catabolic.

Actions of PTH in Kidney

In kidney, PTH has three major biological functions that are essential for the regulation of mineral ion homeostasis: stimulating the reabsorption of calcium, inhibiting the reabsorption of phosphate, and enhancing the synthesis of

$1,25(OH)_2D_3$. Each of these actions of PTH contributes to the maintenance of blood calcium concentrations, and to a lesser extent, phosphate concentrations, within narrow limits.

Phosphate is normally reabsorbed from the glomerular filtrate both in the proximal and distal tubules, and at both these sites, reabsorption is inhibited by PTH.[52] Best studied is its effect on proximal tubular cells where phosphate is transported into the cell against an electrochemical gradient. To accomplish this task, an ATP-dependent sodium pump, Na^+/K^+ ATPase, drives sodium from the cell. Because of the concentration gradient for sodium established by this pump and through the actions of a membrane-anchored co-transporter, Npt2a (previously termed NaPi2), sodium re-enters the cell along with phosphate.[53] PTH blocks this sodium-dependent phosphate co-transport by reducing the amount of the Npt2a protein on the cell surface, primarily by increasing its internalization and subsequent lysosomal degradation,[54,55] but also by decreasing its synthesis.[56] PTH is only one of several determinants of Npt2a expression, as dietary phosphate restriction leads, independent of changes in blood concentrations of PTH, to a markedly enhanced renal phosphate reabsorption, and thus a virtual elimination of urinary phosphate losses.[57] The complete lack of Npt2a expression through ablation of its gene, leads to severe renal phosphate wasting, and other abnormalities that are similar to those observed in hereditary hypophosphatemic rickets with hypercalciuria (HHRH).[58] Interestingly, heterozygous NPT2a mutations were recently identified in two patients with nephrolithiasis and osteoporosis associated with hypophosphatemia caused by impaired renal tubular reabsorption.[59]

In the distal tubule, PTH also inhibits phosphate reabsorption; the transporter(s) that are involved in this process have not yet been identified. Teleologically, the PTH-stimulated phosphaturia can be viewed as a way of handling the release of phosphate from bone that accompanies the PTH-stimulated release of calcium from bone. Furthermore, because of the quantitative dominance of the phosphaturia, blood phosphate falls in response to PTH. This hypophosphatemia reinforces the effect of PTH on bone, because low levels of blood phosphate stimulate bone resorption.

Most calcium reabsorption occurs in the proximal tubule,[60–62] but only the calcium reabsorption in the distal nephron is PTH dependent.[57] Although the kidneys reabsorb calcium more efficiently when stimulated by PTH, the absolute amount of calcium in the urine usually increases when the circulating concentrations of PTH are chronically elevated to levels sufficient to produce hypercalcemia, as in patients with primary hyperparathyroidism. However, this increase in urinary calcium excretion is caused by the substantial increase in the filtered load of calcium, which is caused by hypercalcemia as a result of increased bone resorption and increased intestinal absorption of calcium, rather than by impaired renal tubular handling of calcium.

PTH also activates the mitochondrial 25-hydroxyvitamin D-1-α-hydroxylase in proximal tubular cells; this leads to an elevation of the blood $1,25(OH)_2D_3$ concentration,[63,64] which in turn is a potent inducer of intestinal calcium absorption (as well as of bone resorption). This effect of PTH is not immediate, because the stimulation of

$1,25(OH)_2D_3$ synthesis occurs over several hours and requires the synthesis of new mRNA and protein.[65–67] Along with its action on the 1-α-hydroxylase, PTH decreases the activity of the renal 25-hydroxyvitamin D-24-hydroxylase, thus enhancing the effect on $1,25(OH)_2D_3$ synthesis. Other factors, particularly low blood phosphate concentration, also markedly increase the synthesis of this biologically active vitamin D metabolite, while hypercalcemia, as would be generated by sustained increases in PTH, directly suppresses, independent of blood levels of PTH or phosphate, the 1-α-hydroxylase activity and thus limits in a homeostatic manner the production of $1,25(OH)_2D_3$.[68,69]

Because of its effectiveness in raising blood calcium concentration, $1,25(OH)_2D_3$ is widely used, along with oral calcium supplementation, in the treatment of hypoparathyroidism (and pseudohypoparathyroidism). However, because $1,25(OH)_2D_3$ cannot mimic the renal, calcium-sparing effects of PTH, urine calcium excretion can rise quickly as serum calcium approaches the normal range, particularly when the underlying hypoparathyroidism is caused by activating mutations in the calcium-sensing receptor, as in autosomal dominant hypocalcemia with hypercalciuria.[7] In both groups of patients, but particularly the latter, the blood calcium is best kept at or below the normal range, with periodic monitoring of 24-h urinary calcium excretion to avoid the long-term consequences of hypercalciuria.

Molecular Defects in the PTH/PTHrP Receptor

The endocrine actions of PTH, and the autocrine/paracrine actions of PTHrP, are mediated through the PTH/PTHrP receptor. A single G-protein–coupled receptor is thus essential for the biological roles of two distinct ligands, which are important for regulation of calcium homeostasis and for the regulation of chondrocyte proliferation and differentiation, respectively. The ablation of one allele encoding the PTH/PTHrP receptor gene in mice revealed no discernible abnormality, while the ablation of both alleles resulted, depending on the mouse strain, in fetal death during mid- or late gestation and severe skeletal abnormalities.[16] Based on the functional properties of the PTH/PTHrP receptor and based on the findings in gene-ablated mice, it seems likely that receptor mutations in humans would most likely affect mineral ion homeostasis and bone development.

Mutations in the PTH/PTHrP receptor were initially suspected as a cause of pseudohypoparathyroidism type Ib (PHP-Ib), in which patients exhibit PTH-resistant hypocalcemia and hyperphosphatemia.[70,71] However, these patients lack discernible growth plate abnormalities, indicating that the actions of PTHrP are appropriately mediated. It was therefore not surprising, at least in retrospect, that PTH/PTHrP receptor mutations could not be identified in PHP-Ib patients[70,71]; in fact, PHP-Ib is now known to be a paternally imprinted disorder that is caused by an yet unknown molecular mutation that appears to reside more than 50 kb upstream of the *GNAS1* gene.[72,73]

PTH/PTHrP receptor mutations have, however, been identified in two rare genetic disorders: Jansen's metaphyseal chondrodysplasia and Blomstrand's lethal chondrodysplasia. Activating mutations that lead to ligand-independent accumulation of cyclic adenosine monophosphate (cAMP) were identified as the cause of the autosomal dominant Jansen's disease, which is characterized by short-limbed dwarfism, severe hypercalcemia, and hypophosphatemia, despite normal or undetectable levels of PTH and PTHrP in the circulation.[17] Inactivating PTH/PTHrP receptor mutations (homozygous or compound heterozygous) were identified in patients with Blomstrand's disease, who are typically born prematurely and die at birth or shortly thereafter. These patients present with advanced bone maturation, accelerated chondrocyte differentiation, and, most likely, severe abnormalities in mineral ion homeostasis.[17] Two rare genetic human disorders thus provide important new insights concerning the biological importance of the PTH/PTHrP receptor in mediating actions of both PTH and PTHrP.

REFERENCES

1. Jüppner H, Gardella T, Brown E, Kronenberg H, Potts J Jr 2000 Parathyroid hormone and parathyroid hormone-related peptide in the regulation of calcium homeostasis and bone development. In: DeGroot L, Jameson J (eds.) Endocrinology. W. B. Saunders Company, Philadelphia, PA, USA, pp. 969–998.
2. Silver J, Naveh-Many T, Kronenberg HM 2002 Parathyroid hormone. In: Bilezikian JP, Raisz LG, Rodan GA (eds.) Principles of Bone Biology, vol. 1. Academic Press, New York, NY, USA, pp. 407–422.
3. Gardella TJ, Jüppner H, Bringhurst FR, Potts JT Jr 2002 Receptors for parathyroid hormone (PTH) and PTH-related peptide. In: Bilezikian J, Raisz L, Rodan G (eds.) Principles of Bone Biology. Academic Press, San Diego, CA, USA, pp. 389–405.
4. Yang KH, Stewart AF 1996 Parathyroid hormone-related protein: The gene, its mRNA species, and protein products. In: Bilezikian JP, Raisz LG, Rodan RA (eds.) Principles of Bone Biology. Academic Press, New York, NY, USA, pp. 347–362.
5. Usdin TB, Hoare SRJ, Wang T, Mezey E, Kowalak JA 1999 Tip39: A new neuropeptide and PTH2-receptor agonist from hypothalamus. Nature Neurosci 2:941–943.
6. John M, Arai M, Rubin D, Jonsson K, Jüppner H 2002 Identification and characterization of the murine and human gene encoding the tuberoinfundibular peptide of 39 residues (TIP39). Endocrinology 143:1047–1057.
7. Diaz R, El-Hajj GF, Brown E 1998 Regulation of parathyroid function. In: Fray JGS (ed.) Handbook of Physiology, vol. 3. Oxford University Press, New York, NY, USA, pp. 607–662.
8. Almaden Y, Canalejo A, Hernandez A, Ballesteros E, Garcia-Navarro S, Torres A, Rodriguez M 1996 Direct effect of phosphorus on PTH secretion from whole rat parathyroid glands in vitro. J Bone Miner Res 11:970–976.
9. Slatopolsky E, Finch J, Denda M, Ritter C, Zhong M, Dusso A, MacDonald P, Brown A 1996 Phosphorus restriction prevents parathyroid gland growth. High phosphorus directly stimulates PTH secretion in vitro. J Clin Invest 97:2534–2540.
10. Brown EM, Gamba G, Riccardi D, Lombardi M, Butters R, Kifor O, Sun A, Hediger MA, Lytton J, Hebert SC 1993 Cloning and characterization of an extracellular Ca^{2+}-sensing receptor from bovine parathyroid. Nature 366:575–580.
11. Au W 1984 Inhibition by 1,25 dihydroxycholecalciferol of parathyroid gland in organ culture. Calcif Tiss Int 36:384–391.
12. Slatopolsky E, Finch J, Ritter C, Denda M, Morrissey J, Brown A, DeLuca H 1995 A new analog of calcitrol, 19-nor-1, 25-$(OH)_2D_2$, suppress parathyroid hormone secretion in uremic rats in the absence of hypercalcemia. Am J Kidney Dis 26:852–860.
13. Li YC, Amling M, Pirro AE, Priemel M, Meuse J, Baron R, Delling G, Demay MB 1998 Normalization of mineral ion homeostasis by dietary means prevents hyperparathyroidism, rickets, and osteomalacia, but not alopecia in vitamin D receptor-ablated mice. Endocrinology 139:4391–4396.
14. Wada M, Nagano N, Furuya Y, Chin J, Nemeth EF, Fox J 2000 Calcimimetic NPS R-568 prevents parathyroid hyperplasia in rats with severe secondary hyperparathyroidism. Kidney Int 57:50–58.
15. Mahon M, Donowitz M, Yun C, Segre G 2002 Na(+)/H(+) exchanger regulatory factor 2 directs parathyroid hormone 1 receptor signalling. Nature 417:858–861.
16. Lanske B, Kronenberg H 1998 Parathyroid hormone-related peptide (PTHrP) and parathyroid hormone (PTH)/PTHrP receptor. Crit Rev Eukaryot Gene Expr 8:297–320.
17. Jüppner H, Schipani E, Silve C 2002 Jansen's metaphyseal chondrodysplasia and Blomstrand's lethal chondrodysplasia: Two genetic disorders caused by PTH/PTHrP receptor mutations. In: Bilezikian J, Raisz L, Rodan G (eds.) Principles of Bone Biology. Academic Press, San Diego, CA, USA, pp. 1117–1135.
18. Slatopolsky E, Finch J, Clay P, Martin D, Sicard G, Singer G, Gao P, Cantor T, Dusso A 2000 A novel mechanism for skeletal resistance in uremia. Kidney Int 58:753–761.
19. Nguyen-Yamamoto L, Rousseau L, Brossard JH, Lepage R, D'Amour P 2001 Synthetic carboxyl-terminal fragments of parathyroid hormone (PTH) decrease ionized calcium concentration in rats by acting on a receptor different from the PTH/PTH-related peptide receptor. Endocrinology 142:1386–1392.
20. Usdin TB, Gruber C, Bonner TI 1995 Identification and functional expression of a receptor selectively recognizing parathyroid hormone, the PTH2 receptor. J Biol Chem 270:15455–15458.
21. Rubin DA, Hellman P, Zon LI, Lobb CJ, Bergwitz C, Jüppner H 1999 A G protein-coupled receptor from zebrafish is activated by human parathyroid hormone and not by human or teleost parathyroid hormone-related peptide: Implications for the evolutionary conservation of calcium-regulating peptide hormones. J Biol Chem 274:23035–23042.
22. Usdin TB 1997 Evidence for a parathyroid hormone-2 receptor selective ligand in the hypothalamus. Endocrinology 138:831–834.
23. Hoare SRJ, Rubin DA, Jüppner H, Usdin TB 2000 Evaluating the ligand specificity of zebrafish parathyroid hormone (PTH) receptors: Comparison of PTH, PTH-related protein and tuberoinfundibular peptide of 39 residues. Endocrinology 141:3080–3086.
24. Usdin TB, Bonner TI, Harta G, Mezey E 1996 Distribution of PTH-2 receptor messenger RNA in rat. Endocrinology 137:4285–4297.
25. Eichinger A, Fiaschi-Taesch N, Massfelder T, Fritsch S, Barthelmebs M, Helwig J 2002 Transcript expression of the tuberoinfundibular peptide (TIP)39/PTH2 receptor system and non-PTH1 receptor-mediated tonic effects of TIP39 and other PTH2 receptor ligands in renal vessels. Endocrinology 143:3036–3043.
26. Suda T, Udagawa N, Takahashi N 1996 Cells of bone: Osteoclast generation. In: Bilezikian JP, Raisz LG, Rodan GA (eds.) Principles of Bone Biology. Academic Press, New York, NY, USA, pp. 87–102.
27. Talmage RV, Elliott JR 1958 Removal of calcium from bone as influenced by the parathyroids. Endocrinology 62:717–722.
28. Mundy GR, Roodman GD 1987 Osteoclast ontogeny and function. In: Peck WA (ed.) Bone and Mineral Research, vol. 5. Elsevier, Amsterdam, The Netherlands, pp. 209–280.
29. Finkelstein JS 1996 Pharmacological mechanisms of therapeutics: Parathyroid hormone. In: Bilezikian JP, Raisz LG, Rodan GA (eds.) Principles of Bone Biology. Academic Press, New York, NY, USA, pp. 993–1005.
30. Dempster DW, Cosman F, Parisien M, Shen V, Lindsay R 1993 Anabolic actions of parathyroid hormone on bone [published erratum appears in Endocr Rev 1994 Apr;15(2):261. Endocr Rev 14:690–709.
31. Neer R, Arnaud C, Zanchetta J, Prince R, Gaich G, Reginster J, Hodsman A, Eriksen E, Ish-Shalom S, Genant H, Wang O, Mitlak B 2001 Effect of parathyroid hormone (1–34) on fractures and bone mineral density in postmenopausal women with osteoporosis. N Engl J Med 344:1434–1441.
32. Lee K, Deeds JD, Chiba S, Un-no M, Bond AT, Segre GV 1994 Parathyroid hormone induces sequential c-fos expression in bone cells in vivo: In situ localization of its receptor and c-fos messenger ribonucleic acids. Endocrinology 134:441–450.
33. Mears DC 1971 Effects of parathyroid hormone and thyrocalcitonin on the membrane potential of osteoclasts. Endocrinology 88:1021–1028.
34. Ferrier J, Ward A, Kanehisa J, Heersche JN 1986 Electrophysiological responses of osteoclasts to hormones. J Cell Physiol 128:23–26.
35. Teti A, Rizzoli R, Zallone AZ 1991 Parathyroid hormone binding to cultured avian osteoclasts. Biochem Biophys Res Commun 174:1217–1222.
36. Hakeda Y, Hiura K, Sato T, Okazaki R, Matsumoto T, Ogata E, Ishitani R, Kumegawa M 1989 Existence of parathyroid hormone binding sites on murine hemopoietic blast cells. Biochem Biophys Res Commun 163:1481–1486.
37. Rouleau MF, Mitchell L, Goltzman D 1988 In vivo distribution of parathyroid hormone receptors in bone: Evidence that a predominant

osseous target cell is not the mature osteoblast. Endocrinology **123:** 187–191.

38. Silve CM, Hradek GT, Jones AL, Arnaud CD 1982 Parathyroid hormone receptor in intact embryonic chicken bone: Characterization and cellular localization. J Cell Biol **94:**379–386.

39. Liu BY, Guo J, Lanske B, Divieti P, Kronenberg HM, Bringhurst FR 1998 Conditionally immortalized murine bone marrow stromal cells mediate parathyroid hormone-dependent osteoclastogenesis in vitro. Endocrinology **139:**1952–1964.

40. Lacey DL, Timms E, Tan HL, Kelley MJ, Dunstan CR, Burgess T, Elliott R, Colombero A, Elliott G, Scully S, Hsu H, Sullivan J, Hawkins N, Davy E, Capparelli C, Eli A, Qian YX, Kaufman S, Sarosi I, Shalhoub V, Senaldi G, Guo J, Delaney J, Boyle WJ 1998 Osteoprotegerin ligand is a cytokine that regulates osteoclast differentiation and activation. Cell **93:**165–176.

41. Yasuda H, Shima N, Nakagawa N, Yamaguchi K, Kinosaki M, Mochizuki SI, Tomoyasu A, Yano K, Goto M, Murakami A, Tsuda E, Morinaga T, Higashio K, Udagawa N, Takahashi N, Suda T 1998 Osteoclast differentiation factor is a ligand for osteoprotegerin/osteoclastogenesis-inhibitory factor and is identical to TRANCE/RANKL. Proc Natl Acad Sci USA **95:**3597–3602.

42. Suda T, Takahashi N, Udagawa N, Jimi E, Gillespie MT, Martin TJ 1999 Modulation of osteoclast differentiation and function by the new members of the tumor necrosis factor receptor and ligand families. Endocr Rev **20:**345–357.

43. Simonet SW, Lacey DL, Dunstan CR, Kelley M, Chang MS, Luthy R, Nyugen HQ, Wooden S, Bennett L, Boone T, Shimamoto G, DeRose M, Elliott R, Colombero A, Tan HL, Trail G, Sullivan J, Davy E, Bucay N, Renshaw-Gegg L, Huges TM, Hill D, Pattison W, Campbell P, Sander S, Van G, Tarpley J, Derby P, Lee R 1997 Osteoprotegerin: A novel secreted protein involved in the regulation of bone density. Cell **89:**309–319.

44. Bucay N, Sarosi I, Dunstan DR, Morony S, Tarpley J, Capparelli C, Scully S, Tan HL, Xu W, Lacey DL, Boyle WJ, Simonet WS 1998 Osteoprotegerin-deficient mice develop early onset osteoporosis and arterial calcification. Genes Dev **12:**1260–1268.

45. Horwood NJ, Elliott J, Martin TJ, Gillespie MT 1998 Osteotropic agents regulate the expression of osteoclast differentiation factor and osteoprotegerin in osteoblastic stromal cells. Endocrinology **139:** 4743–4746.

46. Aubin JE, Heersche JNM 2001 Cellular actions of parathyroid hormone on osteoblast and osteoclast differentiation. In: Bilezikian JP, Marcus R, Levine MA (eds.) The Parathyroids, Basic and Clinical Concepts, 2nd ed. Academic Press, San Diego, CA, USA, pp. 199–211.

47. Jilka RL, Weinstein RS, Bellido T, Roberson P, Parfitt AM, Manolagas SC 1999 Increased bone formation by prevention of osteoblast apoptosis with parathyroid hormone. J Clin Invest **104:**439–446.

48. Manolagas SC 2000 Birth and death of bone cells: Basic regulatory mechanisms and implications for the pathogenesis and treatment of osteoporosis. Endocr Rev **21:**115–137.

49. Canalis E, Centrella M, Burch W, McCarthy TL 1989 Insulin-like growth factor I mediates selective anabolic effects of parathyroid hormone in bone cultures. J Clin Invest **83:**60–65.

50. Dobnig H, Turner RT 1995 Evidence that intermittent treatment with parathyroid hormone increases bone formation in adult rats by activation of bone lining cells. Endocrinology **136:**3632–3638.

51. Tintut Y, Parhami F, Le V, Karsenty G, Demer LL 1999 Inhibition of osteoblast-specific transcription factor Cbfa1 by the cAMP pathway in osteoblastic cells.Ubiquitin/proteasome-dependent regulation. J Bioln Chem **274:**28875–28879.

52. Bringhurst FR 1989 Calcium and phosphate distribution, turnover, and metabolic actions. In: DeGroot LJ (ed.) Endocrinology, 2nd ed., vol. 2. W. B. Saunders Co., Philadelphia, PA, USA, pp. 805–843.

53. Cheng L, Sacktor B 1981 Sodium gradient-dependent phosphate transport in renal brush border vesicles. J Biol Chem **256:**1556–1564.

54. Pfister MF, Ruf I, Stange G, Ziegler U, Lederer E, Biber J, Murer H 1998 Parathyroid hormone leads to the lysomal degradation of the renal type II Na/P$_i$ cotransporter. Proc Natl Acad Sci USA **95:**1909–1914.

55. Murer H, Hernando N, Forster I, Biber J 2000 Proximal tubular phosphate reabsorption: Molecular mechanisms. Physiol Rev **80:** 1373–1409.

56. Malmström K, Murer H 1987 Parathyroid hormone regulates phosphate transport in OK cells via an irreversible inactivation of a membrane protein. FEBS Lett **216:**257–260.

57. Drezner MK 1996 Phosphorus homeostasis and related disorders. In: Bilezikian JP, Raisz LG, Rodan GA (eds.) Principles in Bone Biology. Academic Press, New York, NY, USA, pp. 263–276.

58. Beck L, Karaplis AC, Amizuka N, Hewson AS, Ozawa H, Tenenhouse HS 1998 Targeted inactivation of *Ntp2* in mice leads to severe renal phosphate wasting, hypercalciuria, and skeletal abnormalities. Proc Natl Acad Sci USA **95:**5372–5377.

59. Prie D, Huart V, Bakouh N, Planelles G, Dellis O, Gerard B, Hulin P, Benque-Blanchet F, Silve C, Grandchamp B, Friedlander G 2002 Nephrolithiasis and osteoporosis associated with hypophosphatemia caused by mutations in the type 2a sodium-phosphate cotransporter. N Engl J Med **347:**983–991.

60. Suki WN 1979 Calcium transport in the nephron. Am J Physiol **237:**F1–F6.

61. Torikai S, Wang M-S, Klein KL, Kurokawa K 1981 Adenylate cyclase and cell cyclic AMP of rat cortical thick ascending limb of Henle. Kidney Int **20:**649–654.

62. Morel F, Imbert-Teboul M, Chabardes D 1981 Distribution of hormone-dependent adenylate cyclase in the nephron and its physiological significance. Annu Rev Physiol **43:**569–581.

63. Garabedian M, Holick MF, Deluca HF, Boyle IT 1972 Control of 25-hydrocholecalciferol metabolism by parathyroid glands. Proc Natl Acad Sci USA **69:**1673–1676.

64. Fraser DR, Kodicek E 1973 Regulation of 25-hydroxycholecalciferol-1-hydroxylase activity in kidney by parathyroid hormone. Nature **241:**163–166.

65. Fox J, Mathew MB 1991 Heterogeneous response to PTH in aging rates: Evidence for skeletal PTH resistance. Am J Physiol **260:**E933–E937.

66. Norman AW, Roth J, Orci L 1982 The vitamin D endocrine system: Steroid metabolisms, hormone receptors and biological response. Endocr Rev **3:**331–366.

67. Murayama A, Takeyama K, Kitanaka S, Kodera Y, Kawaguchi Y, Hosoya T, Kato S 1999 Positive and negative regulations of the renal 25-hydroxyvitamin D3 1alpha-hydroxylase gene by parathyroid hormone, calcitonin, and 1alpha, 25(OH)2D3 in intact animals. Endocrinology **140:**2224–2231.

68. Shigematsu T, Horiuchi N, Ogura Y 1986 Human parathyroid hormone inhibits renal 24-hydroxylase activity of 25-hydroxyvitamin D3 by a mechanism involving adenosine 3′, 5′-monophosphate in rats. Endocrinology **118:**1583–1589.

69. Tanaka Y, Lorenc RS, Deluca HF 1975 The role of 1,25-dihydroxyvitamin D3 and parathyroid hormone in the regulation of chick renal 25-hydroxy-vitamin D3–24-hydroxylase. Arch Biochem Biophys **171:**521–526.

70. Bastep M, Jüppner H 2000 Pseudohypoparathyroidism: New insights into an old disease. In: Strewler GJ (ed.) Endocrinology and Metabolism Clinics of North America: Hormones and Disorders of Mineral Metabolism, vol. 29. W. B. Saunders, Philadelphia, PA, USA, pp. 569–589.

71. Jan de Boer SM, Levine MA 2001 Pseudohypoparathyroidism: Clinical, Biochemical, and Molecular Features. In: Bilezikian JP, Markus R, Levine NA (eds.) The Parathyroids: Basic and Clinical Concepts. Academic Press, New York, NY, USA, pp. 807–825.

72. Jüppner H, Schipani E, Bastepe M, Cole DEC, Lawson ML, Mannstadt M, Hendy GN, Plotkin H, Koshiyama H, Koh T, Crawford JD, Olsen BR, Vikkula M 1998 The gene responsible for pseudohypoparathyroidism type Ib is paternally imprinted and maps in four unrelated kindreds to chromosome 20q13.3. Proc Natl Acad Sci USA **95:**11798–11803.

73. Bastepe M, Pincus JE, Sugimoto T, Tojo K, Kanatani M, Azuma Y, Kruse K, Rosenbloom AL, Koshiyama H, Jüppner H 2001 Positional dissociation between the genetic mutation responsible for pseudohypoparathyroidism type Ib and the associated methylation defect at exon A/B: Evidence for a long-range regulatory element within the imprinted *GNAS1* locus. Hum Mol Genet **10:**1231–1241.

Chapter 19.   Parathyroid Hormone-Related Protein

Gordon J. Strewler[1] and Robert A. Nissenson[2]

[1]*Department of Medicine, Beth Israel-Deaconess Medical Center and Harvard Medical School, Boston, Massachusetts; and*
[2]*Departments of Medicine and Physiology, University of California, and Veterans Affairs Medical Center, San Francisco, California*

INTRODUCTION

The parathyroid hormone-related protein (PTHrP) is a second member of the PTH family. Originally discovered as the cause of hypercalcemia in malignancy,[1] PTHrP has proven to act in many tissues to regulate both development and function, and its recognition has expanded our concept of the role of the PTH/PTHrP family beyond the horizons of calcium homeostasis to include developmental and regulatory functions in a variety of tissues.[2–4]

The characteristics of the clinical syndrome of humoral hypercalcemia are discussed elsewhere. As in primary hyperparathyroidism, hypercalcemia in malignancy is characterized by a decreased renal threshold for phosphate, leading to hypophosphatemia, and by increased urinary excretion of cyclic adenosine monophosphate (cAMP).[5] However, PTH is suppressed in malignancy-associated hypercalcemia. The finding that PTH was suppressed in a syndrome that so resembled primary hyperparathyroidism biochemically suggested that a distinct molecule secreted by tumors could mimic PTH, and this led to the development of bioassay techniques to search for a PTH-like factor in tumors that produced hypercalcemia. These assays guided the isolation and ultimate identification of what proved to be a PTH-related protein (also called PTH-like protein). As predicted, the tumor-derived protein proved to be an able mimic of PTH, for reasons that became clear when its structure could be determined.

Human PTHrP is encoded by a single-copy gene located on chromosome 12.[3] The human *PTHrP* gene, with three promoters, nine exons, and complex patterns of alternative exon splicing, is much more complicated than the *PTH* gene. However, it is clear from the protein structure and from similarities in gene organization that both arose from a common ancestral gene. The amino acid sequence of PTHrP is homologous with the sequence of PTH only at the amino terminus, where 8 of the first 13 amino acids in PTH and PTHrP are identical (Fig. 1). This homologous domain, limited as it is, involves a crucial region of the molecule that is known to be required for activation of the shared PTH/PTHrP receptor, and thus explains the ability of PTHrP to mimic PTH as an inducer of bone resorption, renal phosphate wasting, and hypercalcemia in malignancy. Beyond this region, the sequences of PTH and PTHrP have little in common. Even in the primary receptor-binding domain (amino acids 18–34), PTH and PTHrP do not have recognizable primary sequence similarities, although the binding domain has a common α-helical secondary structure in both peptides. Compared with the 84-amino acid peptide PTH, PTHrP is considerably longer, with three isoforms of 139, 141, and 173 amino acids, whose sequences are identical through amino acid 139.[3] These isoforms arise from alternative RNA splicing. Although the protein isoforms are expressed differentially in individual tissues and tumors, their relative importance in normal physiology and humoral hypercalcemia are unknown.

The isoforms of PTHrP are cleaved by prohormone convertases within cells that secrete them to produce a variety of secreted peptides (Fig. 2). These include an amino-terminal fragment that possesses the ability to bind to the classic PTH/PTHrP receptor and a midregion fragment that has biological actions that are distinct from those of amino-terminal PTHrP (e.g., stimulation of placental calcium transport). Carboxy-terminal fragments are also predicted to be secretory fragments, and they can be detected in the blood. Carboxy-terminal PTHrP peptides that induce calcium transients in hippocampal neurons[6] also appear to be capable of inhibiting bone resorption in some systems,[7,8] and one peptide, PTHrP(107-139), has been named osteostatin. Thus, PTHrP is a polyhormone, the precursor of multiple biologically active peptides. In this regard, PTHrP resembles proopiomelanocortin, the pituitary precursor of adrenocorticotrophin (ACTH), melanocyte-stimulating hormone (MSH), β-lipotropin, and the endorphins and enkephalins.

PTHrP and PTH bind with equivalent affinities to a common receptor, the PTH/PTHrP receptor,[9,10] and consequently they have very similar ranges of biological activities. Both produce hypercalcemia, hypophosphatemia as a consequence of reduced renal reabsorption of phosphate, and accelerated production of 1,25-dihydroxyvitamin D by the kidney.[2,9] However, each of the hormones also has its own receptors: in the case of PTH, the PTH-2 receptor does not recognize PTHrP. In the case of PTHrP, receptors in brain[11] and skin[12] recognize the amino-terminal domain of PTHrP exclusively. There must be additional PTHrP receptors to mediate the effects of midregion and carboxy-terminal PTHrP peptides, but these have yet to be identified.

There is little doubt that PTHrP is the major cause of hypercalcemia in malignancy.[1] Infusion of PTHrP can reproduce most aspects of the clinical syndrome of hypercalcemia, serum levels of PTHrP are increased in hypercalcemia,[13] and neutralizing antibodies to PTHrP can reverse hypercalcemia induced in animals by human tumor cells.[14] This indicates that secretion of PTHrP is not merely associated with hypercalcemia but necessary for its develop-

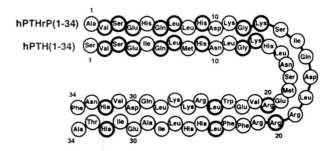

FIG. 1. Amino-terminal amino acid sequence of hPTHrP is compared with that of hPTH.

The authors have no conflict of interest.

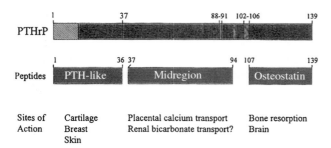

Sites of   Cartilage   Placental calcium transport   Bone resorption
Action   Breast   Renal bicarbonate transport?   Brain
                Skin

FIG. 2. (Top) Structural features of PTHrP. The PTH-homologous domain PTHrP(1-13) is delineated by slashed lines, and potential cleavage sites are shown as lines or cross-hatched regions. (Middle) Peptides known or postulated to be derived from PTHrP. (Bottom) Proven or postulated sites of action of individual PTHrP peptides are shown beneath each peptide.

ment. The specific tumors that characteristically produce humoral hypercalcemia by secreting PTHrP include squamous, renal, and breast carcinoma. PTHrP also plays a causative role in the hypercalcemia that is associated with islet cell tumors, pheochromocytoma, and the adult T-cell leukemia syndrome, where PTHrP is produced by malignant T-lymphocytes infected with the etiologic agent of this disorder, the human T-cell lymphotrophic virus.[15] It has recently been suggested that PTHrP also has a role in some cases of multiple myeloma[16] and in sarcoidosis.[17]

The normal circulating level of PTHrP is considerably lower than the level of PTH, and it is doubtful that PTHrP has a major role in the day-to-day maintenance of calcium homeostasis. It is clear, however, that PTHrP has vital functions in development and in normal physiology, primarily local ones at the cell or tissue level. PTHrP is widely present in fetal tissues, including cartilage, many epithelial surfaces, skeletal and heart muscle, distal renal tubules, hair follicles, brain, and placenta.

As an approach to understanding the physiological roles of PTHrP, both copies of the *PTHrP* gene in the mouse have been disrupted by targeted mutations introduced by homologous recombination.[18] Although mice heterozygous for the loss of PTHrP have a subtle phenotype,[19] in the homozygous state, loss of the *PTHrP* gene is an embryonic lethal mutation. Homozygotes survive until near the time of parturition but have multiple anomalies in the development of cartilage and bone. Their limbs are short and their rib cages are small because of defective proliferation of chondrocytes during endochondral bone formation, as well as premature maturation and apoptosis of chondrocytes.[18,20] A similar phenotype occurs in humans with Blomstrand chondrodysplasia,[21] and in Jansen's metaphyseal chondrodysplasia, a constitutively active PTH/PTHrP receptor produces a converse phenotype in cartilage (mimicking PTHrP action) as well as hypercalcemia (mimicking PTH action).[22] In the regulation of endochondral bone formation, PTHrP is under the control of the secreted morphogen Indian hedgehog, one of a family of developmental patterning genes, the vertebrate orthologs of the *Drosophila* segmentation gene *Hedgehog*.[23] The system seems to be designed to provide a feedback loop from early hypertrophic chondrocytes to coordinate the exit of proliferating chondro-

cytes from the cell cycle and their subsequent transformation into the hypertrophic layer.[24]

PTHrP is widely expressed in developing and adult tissues and has a number of physiologic functions. Genetic models to elucidate these functions are now available, because it has been possible to rescue PTHrP knockout mice from lethality by expressing either PTHrP or a constitutively active receptor in cartilage,[25,26] allowing other phenotypes to be expressed. To date, these models have disclosed important roles of PTHrP in mammary glands, which is virtually absent in rescued PTHrP knockout mice, the teeth, which fail to erupt, and the skin and hair. In all cases, PTHrP is a signaling molecule in epithelial-mesenchymal interactions in which PTHrP is secreted by epithelial cells and signals for a mesenchymal response.

Secretion of PTHrP from the ingrowing epithelial sprouts in developing breast tissue permits branching morphogenesis of mammary glands by activating receptors in the underlying mesenchyme.[25] Presumably this interaction induces a mesenchymal signal that is sent back to the epithelium of the ducts to induce their proliferation. When overexpressed, PTHrP induces a mesenchymal signal that leads to ectopic nipple formation.[27] PTHrP appears to have additional roles to play in lactating mammary tissue. There, expression of PTHrP is under the control of prolactin,[28]

TABLE 1. SITES OF EXPRESSION AND PROPOSED ACTIONS OF PTHrP

Sites of expression	Proposed actions
Mesenchymal tissues	
Cartilage	Promotes proliferation of chondrocytes; inhibits terminal differentiation and apoptosis of chondrocytes
Bone	Inhibits bone resorption
Smooth muscle	Released in response to stretch; relaxes smooth muscle
Vascular	
Myometrium	
Urinary bladder	
Cardiac muscle	Required for development; positive chronotropic stimulus; indirect positive inotropic stimulus
Skeletal muscle	Unknown
Epithelial tissues	
Mammary	Induces branching morphogenesis; secreted into milk, blood, regulates bone loss during lactation?
Epidermis	Unknown
Hair follicle	Inhibits anagen
Intestine	Unknown
Tooth enamel	Induces osteoclastic resorption of overlying bone
Endocrine tissues	
Parathyroid	Unknown
Pancreatic islets	Stimulates insulin secretion and somatic growth
Pituitary	Unknown
Placenta	Stimulates placental calcium transport
Central nervous system	Released from cerebellar granular neurons in response to L-type calcium channels; receptors in cerebellum, hippocampus, hypothalamus

and PTHrP is secreted into milk at concentrations 10,000-fold higher than its serum concentration.[29] There is growing evidence in the mouse that PTHrP released into the circulation from lactating mammary tissue signals for bone resorption and thus regulates the response of maternal calcium metabolism to the stress of lactation. Whether this is physiologically important in humans is uncertain.[30]

The failure of tooth eruption in rescued PTHrP knockout mice can be attributed to another epithelial-mesenchymal interaction. The formation of the teeth appears normal, but PTHrP is absent from the enamel epithelium, which caps the tooth rudiment as it pushes its way through the overlying alveolar bone to erupt. Restoration of PTHrP expression to enamel epithelium restores tooth eruption.[31] This implies that PTHrP secreted by the epithelial layer is targeted to receptors in the overlying bone, where it activates resorption of alveolar bone by osteoclasts to allow passage of the tooth.[32] The signaling circuit in alveolar bone is distinctive, because there is no general defect in osteoclast function in transgenic mice to produce an osteopetrotic phenotype.

It has long been known that to supply calcium to the mineralizing skeleton of the fetus, calcium is transported across the placenta by a placental pump, maintaining a serum calcium level that is higher in the fetus than in the mother. This maternal-fetal gradient is abolished in PTHrP knockout mice,[33] indicating that PTHrP is the principal regulator of placental calcium transport. The source of PTHrP may be liver or placenta itself.[34] The transport of calcium can be restored by infusion of midregional fragments or PTHrP, but not by amino-terminal PTHrP or by PTH.[33,35,36] Thus, for the regulation of systemic calcium economy, the fetus uses a midregion peptide from PTHrP, perhaps secreted from the parathyroid gland, in much the same way that PTH is used in the postnatal state.

PTHrP is secreted by a variety of smooth muscle beds,[37] where it is released in response to stretch,[38,39] and it acts as a smooth muscle dilator through binding to the PTH/PTHrP receptor.[40] This sets up the circuitry for a short loop feedback system in which PTHrP would respond to stretch by relaxing smooth muscle locally. This circuitry could be operative in uterine smooth muscle at the time of parturition or in the urinary bladder. Targeted expression of PTHrP in vascular smooth muscle causes a fall in blood pressure, suggesting possible short loop feedback regulation of vascular tone.[41] In the heart, PTHrP is required for normal cardiomyocyte development.[42] PTHrP is released by atrial and ventricular myocytes[43] and has a positive chronotropic effect, as well as a positive inotropic effect that probably results from coronary vasodilation.[44,45] PTHrP is also released from stromal cells of the spleen and other organs in response to endotoxic shock,[46] and neutralization of PTHrP effects with antibodies prolongs survival after administration of lethal doses of endotoxin.[47]

In the arterial wall, PTHrP is expressed in proliferating vascular smooth muscle cells in culture and after balloon angioplasty in vivo.[48] The level of PTHrP is increased in atherosclerotic coronary arteries.[49] Exposure of rat vascular smooth muscle cells to PTHrP has an antimitotic effect, suggesting that locally released PTHrP would act to throttle the response to a proliferative stimulus.[50] In contrast, when transfected into A10 rat vascular smooth muscle cells,

PTHrP induces marked proliferation.[51] The proliferative response does not occur with transfection of mutant forms of PTHrP from which polybasic amino acid sequences between residues 88 and 106 had been deleted. These sequences have been shown to function as a nuclear localization sequence in other cells,[52] and wild-type PTHrP, but not the deletion mutants, is targeted to the nucleus of A10 cells. It thus appears possible that in addition to binding to cell surface receptors, PTHrP can have direct nuclear actions, termed *intracrine* actions. Because secreted fragments of PTHrP and its intracrine actions seem to have opposing effects on proliferation, PTHrP could interplay in a complex fashion with other proliferative factors in determining the response of the vascular wall to injury or atherosclerosis.

Potential intracrine actions of PTHrP have recently been shown to extend beyond vascular smooth muscle cells.[53] It is possible that this represents a major alternate signaling pathway for PTHrP in addition to G-protein signaling through the PTH/PTHrP receptor, although this has yet to be definitively established. Intracrine signaling by PTHrP can occur through multiple mechanisms.[54] In some cases, secreted PTHrP may be taken up by cells through endocytosis, with subsequent trafficking of the protein to the nucleus.[55,56] It is not clear whether this endocytosis requires the binding of PTHrP to the PTH/PTHrP receptor. A second possibility is that initiation of translation of PTHrP mRNA may occur through an alternative start site, resulting in the synthesis of a cytoplasmic form of the peptide capable of entering the nucleus.[57] Finally, PTHrP may be transported in retrograde fashion from the endoplasmic reticulum to the cytoplasm.[58] The nuclear localization of PTHrP seems to be regulated by phosphorylation of the protein, with PTHrP appearing either in the nuclear matrix or in the nucleolus, depending on the system.[55] In some cases, nuclear localization of PTHrP varies markedly as a function of the progression of cells through the cell cycle, suggesting a functional role of PTHrP in cell proliferation and/or survival.[59] Indeed, there is evidence that the intracrine actions of PTHrP can promote cell proliferation or survival, depending on the cell type.[52,60,61] Nuclear PTHrP may also function as a regulator of gene expression, as has recently been suggested in prostate cancer cells.[62] Additional studies are needed to determine how intracrine signaling cooperates with classical PTH/PTHrP receptor signaling in mediating the pleiotropic biological effects of PTHrP.

REFERENCES

1. Wysolmerski JJ, Broadus AE 1994 Hypercalcemia of malignancy-the central role of parathyroid hormone-related protein. Annu Rev Med **45:**189–200.
2. Halloran BP, Nissenson RA 1992 Parathyroid Hormone-Related Protein: Normal Physiology and Its Role in Cancer. CRC Press, Boca Raton, FL, USA.
3. Broadus A, Stewart A 1994 Parathyroid hormone-related protein: Structure, processing, and physiological actions. In: Bilezikian J, Levine M, Marcus R (eds.) The Parathyroids. Raven Press, New York, NY, USA, pp. 259–339.
4. Wysolmerski JJ, Stewart AF 1998 The physiology of parathyroid hormone-related protein-an emerging role as a developmental factor. Annu Rev Physiol **60:**431–460.
5. Stewart AF, Horst R, Deftos LJ, Cadman EC, Lang R, Broadus AE 1980 Biochemical evaluation of patients with cancer-associated hypercalcemia. N Engl J Med **303:**1377–1383.
6. Fukayama S, Tashjian AH Jr, Davis JN, Chisholm JC 1995 Signaling by

N- and C-terminal sequences of parathyroid hormone-related protein in hippocampal neurons. Proc Natl Acad Sci USA **92**:10182–10186.

7. Fenton AJ, Kemp BE, Kent GN, Moseley JM, Zheng MH, Rowe DJ, Britto JM, Martin TJ, Nicholson GC 1991 A carboxyl-terminal peptide from the parathyroid hormone-related protein inhibits bone resorption by osteoclasts. Endocrinology **129**:1762–1768.

8. Cornish J, Callon KE, Nicholson GC, Reid IR 1997 Parathyroid hormone-related protein-(107–139) inhibits bone resorption in vivo. Endocrinology **138**:1299–1304.

9. Orloff JJ, Wu TL, Stewart AF 1989 Parathyroid hormone-like proteins: Biochemical responses and receptor interactions. Endocr Rev **10**:476–495.

10. Orloff JJ, Reddy D, de Papp AE, Yang KH, Soifer NE, Stewart AF 1994 Parathyroid hormone-related protein as a prohormone: Posttranslational processing and receptor interactions. Endocr Rev **15**:40–60.

11. Yamamoto S, Morimoto I, Yanagihara N, Zeki K, Fujihira T, Izumi F, Yamashita H, Eto S 1997 Parathyroid hormone-related peptide-(1–34) [PTHrP-(1–34)] induces vasopressin release from the rat supraoptic nucleus in vitro through a novel receptor distinct from a Type I or Type II PTH/PTHrP receptor. Endocrinology **138**:2066–2072.

12. Orloff JJ, Ganz MB, Ribaudo AE, Burtis WJ, Reiss M, Milstone LMS, Stewart AF 1992 Analysis of PTHrP binding and signal transduction mechanisms in benign and malignant squamous cells. Am J Physiol **262**:E599–E607.

13. Burtis WJ, Brady TG, Orloff JJ, Ersbak JB, Warrell RP Jr, Olson BR, Wu TL, Mitnick ME, Broadus AE, Stewart AF 1990 Immunochemical characterization of circulating parathyroid hormone-related protein in patients with humoral hypercalcemia of cancer. N Engl J Med **322**:1106–1112.

14. Kukreja SC, Shevrin DH, Wimbiscus SA, Ebeling PR, Danks JA, Rodda CP, Wood WI, Martin TJ 1988 Antibodies to parathyroid hormone-related protein lower serum calcium in athymic mouse models. J Clin Invest **82**:1798–1802.

15. Ikeda K, Ohno H, Hane M, Yokoi H, Okada M, Honma T, Yamada A, Tatsumi Y, Tanaka T, Saitoh T, Hirose S, Mori S, Takeuchi Y, Fukumoto S, Terukina S, Iguchi H, Kiriyama T, Ogata E, Matsumoto T 1994 Development of a sensitive two-site immunoradiometric assay for parathyroid hormone-related peptide: Evidence for elevated levels in plasma from patients with adult T-cell leukemia/lymphoma and B-cell lymphoma. J Clin Endocrinol Metab **79**:1322–1327.

16. Firkin F, Seymour JF, Watson AM, Grill V, Martin TJ 1996 Parathyroid hormone-related protein in hypercalcaemia associated with haematological malignancy. Br J Haematol **94**:486–492.

17. Zeimer HJ, Greenaway TM, Slavin J, Hards DK, Zhou H, Doery JCG, Hunter AN, Duffield A, Martin TJ, Grill V 1998 Parathyroid-hormone-related protein in sarcoidosis. Am J Pathol **152**:17–21.

18. Karaplis AC, Luz A, Glowacki J, Bronson RT, Tybulewicz VLJ, Kronenberg HM, Mulligan RC 1994 Lethal skeletal dysplasia from targeted disruption of the parathyroid hormone-related peptide gene. Genes Dev **8**:277–289.

19. Amizuka N, Karaplis AC, Henderson JE, Warshawsky H, Lipman ML, Matsuki, Y, Ejiri S, Tanaka M, Izumi N, Ozawa H, Goltzman D 1996 Haploinsufficiency of parathyroid hormone-related peptide (PTHrP) results in abnormal postnatal bone development. Dev Biol **175**:166–176.

20. Amling M, Neff L, Tanaka S, Inoue D, Kuida K, Weir E, Philbrick WM, Broadus AE, Baron R 1997 BCL-2 lies downstream of parathyroid hormone-related peptide in a signaling pathway that regulates chondrocyte maturation during skeletal development. J Cell Biol **136**:205–213.

21. Jobert AS, Zhang P, Couvineau A, Bonaventure J, Roume J, Le Merrer M, Silve C 1988 Absence of functional receptors for parathyroid hormone and parathyroid hormone-related peptide in Blomstrand chondrodysplasia. J Clin Invest **102**:34–40.

22. Schipani E, Langman CB, Parfitt AM, Jensen GS, Kikuchi S, Kooh SW, Cole WG, Juppner H 1996 Constitutively activated receptors for parathyroid hormone and parathyroidhormone-related peptide in Jansen's metaphyseal chondrodysplasia. N Engl J Med **335**:708–714.

23. Vortkamp A, Lee K, Lanske B, Segre GV, Kronenberg HM, Tabin CJ 1996 Regulation of rate of cartilage differentiation by Indian hedgehog and PTH-related protein. Science **273**:613–622.

24. Kronenberg HM 2003 Developmental regulation of the growth plate. Nature **423**:332–336.

25. Wysolmerski JJ, Philbrick WM, Dunbar ME, Lanske B, Kronenberg H, Karaplis A, Broadus AE 1998 Rescue of the parathyroid hormone-related protein knockout mouse demonstrates that parathyroid hormone-related protein is essential for mammary gland development. Development **125**:1285–1294.

26. Schipani E, Lanske B, Hunzelman J, Luz A, Kovacs CS, Lee K, Pirro A, Kronenberg HM, Juppner H 1997 Targeted expression of constitutively active receptors for parathyroid hormone and parathyroid hormone-related peptide delays endochondral bone formation and rescues mice that lack parathyroid hormone-related peptide. Proc Natl Acad Sci USA **94**:13689–13694.

27. Foley J, Dann P, Hong J, Cosgrove J, Dreyer B, Rimm D, Dunbar M, Philbrick W, Wysolmerski J 2001 Parathyroid hormone-related protein maintains mammary epithelial fate and triggers nipple skin differentiation during embryonic breast development. Development **128**:513–525.

28. Thiede MA, Rodan GA 1988 Expression of a calcium-mobilizing parathyroid hormone-like peptide in lactating mammary tissue. Science **242**:278–280.

29. Budayr AA, Halloran BP, King JC, Diep D, Nissenson RA, Strewler GJ 1989 High levels of a parathyroid hormone-like protein in milk. Proc Natl Acad Sci USA **86**:7183–7185.

30. Kovacs CS, Kronenberg HM 1997 Maternal-fetal calcium and bone metabolism during pregnancy, puerperium, and lactation. Endocr Rev **18**:832–872.

31. Philbrick WM, Dreyer BE, Nakchbandi IA, Karaplis AC 1998 Parathyroid hormone-related protein is required for tooth eruption. Proc Natl Acad Sci USA **95**:11846–11851.

32. Nakchbandi IA, Weir EE, Insogna KL, Philbrick WM, Broadus AE 2000 Parathyroid hormone-related protein induces spontaneous osteoclast formation via a paracrine cascade. Proc Natl Acad Sci USA **97**:7296–7300.

33. Kovacs CS, Lanske B, Hunzelman JL, Guo J, Karaplis AC, Kronenberg HM 1996 Parathyroid hormone-related peptide (PTHrP) regulates fetal-placental calcium transport through a receptor distinct from the PTH/PTHrP receptor. Proc Natl Acad Sci USA **93**:15233–15238.

34. Kovacs CS, Manley NR, Moseley JM, Martin TJ, Kronenberg HM 2001 Fetal parathyroids are not required to maintain placental calcium transport. J Clin Invest **107**:1007–1015.

35. Abbas SK, Pickard DW, Rodda CP, Heath JA, Hammonds RG, Wood WI, Caple IW, Martin TJ, Care AD 1989 Stimulation of ovine placental calcium transport by purified natural and recombinant parathyroid hormone-related protein (PTHrP) preparations. Q J Exp Physiol **74**:549–552.

36. Care AD, Abbas SK, Pickard DW, Barri M, Drinkhill M, Findlay JB, White IR, Caple IW 1990 Stimulation of ovine placental transport of calcium and magnesium by mid-molecule fragments of human parathyroid hormone-related protein. Exp Physiol **75**:605–608.

37. Massfelder T, Helwig JJ, Stewart AF 1996 Parathyroid hormone-related protein as a cardiovascular regulatory peptide. Endocrinology **137**:3151–3153.

38. Yamamoto M, Harm SC, Grasser WA, Thiede MA 1992 Parathyroid hormone-related protein in the rat urinary bladder: A smooth muscle relaxant produced locally in response to mechanical stretch. Proc Natl Acad Sci USA **89**:5326–5330.

39. Thiede MA, Daifotis AG, Weir EC, Brines ML, Burtis WJ, Ikeda K, Dreyer BE, Garfield RE, Broadus AE 1990 Intrauterine occupancy controls expression of the parathyroid hormone-related peptide gene in preterm rat myometrium. Proc Natl Acad Sci USA **87**:6969–6973.

40. Nickols GA, Nana AD, Nickols MA, DiPette DJ, Asimakis GK 1989 Hypotension and cardiac stimulation due to the parathyroid hormone-related protein, humoral hypercalcemia of malignancy factor. Endocrinology **125**:834–841.

41. Maeda S, Sutliff RL, Qian J, Lorenz JN, Wang J, Tang H, Nakayama T, Weber C, Witte D, Strauch AR, Paul RJ, Fagin JA, Clemens TL 1999 Targeted overexpression of parathyroid hormone-related protein (PTHrP) to vascular smooth muscle in transgenic mice lowers blood pressure and alters vascular contractility. Endocrinology **140**:1815–1825.

42. Qian J, Colbert MC, Witte D, Kuan CY, Gruenstein E, Osinska H, Lanske B, Kronenberg HM, Clemens TL 2003 Midgestational lethality in mice lacking the parathyroid hormone(PTH)/PTH-related peptide receptor is associated with abrupt cardiomyocyte death. Endocrinology **144**:1053–1061.

43. Deftos LJ, Burton DW, Brandt DW 1993 Parathyroid hormone-like protein is a secretory product of atrial myocytes. J Clin Invest **92**:727–735.

44. Ogino K, Burkhoff D, Bilezikian JP 1995 The hemodynamic basis for the cardiac effects of parathyroid hormone (PTH) and PTH-related protein. Endocrinology **136**:3024–3030.

45. Hara M, Liu YM, Zhen LC, Cohen IS, Yu HG, Danilo P, Ogino K, Bilezikian JP, Rosen MR 1997 Positive chronotropic actions of parathyroid hormone and parathyroid hormone-related peptide are associ-

ated with increases in the current, I-F, and the slope of the pacemaker potential. Circulation **96:**3704–3709.

46. Funk JL, Krul EJ, Moser AH, Shigenaga JK, Strewler GJ, Grunfeld C, Feingold KR 1993 Endotoxin increases parathyroid hormone-related protein mRNA levels in mouse spleen. Mediation by tumor necrosis factor. J Clin Invest **92:**2546–2552.

47. Funk JL, Moser AH, Strewler GJ, Feingold KR, Grunfeld C 1996 Parathyroid hormone-related protein is induced during lethal endotoxemia and contributes to endotoxin-induced mortality in rodents. Mol Med **2:**204–210.

48. Ozeki S, Ohtsuru A, Seto S, Takeshita S, Yano H, Nakayama T, Ito M, Yokota T, Nobuyoshi M, Segre GV, Yamashita S, Yano K 1996 Evidence that implicates the parathyroid hormone-related peptide in vascular stenosis -increased gene expression in the intima of injured rat carotid arteries and human restenotic coronary lesions. Arterioscler Thromb Vasc Biol **16:**565–575.

49. Nakayama T, Ohtsuru A, Enomoto H, Namba H, Ozeki S, Shibata Y, Yokota T, Nobuyoshi M, Ito M, Sekine I, Yamashita S 1994 Coronary atherosclerotic smooth muscle cells overexpress human parathyroid hormone-related peptides. Biochem Biophys Res Commun **200:**1028–1035.

50. Pirola CJ, Wang HM, Kamyar A, Wu S, Enomoto H, Sharifi B, Forrester JS, Clemens TL, Fagin JA 1993 Angiotensin II regulates parathyroid hormone-related protein expression in cultured rat aortic smooth muscle cells through transcriptional and post-transcriptional mechanisms. J Biol Chem **268:**1987–1994.

51. Massfelder T, Dann P, Wu TL, Vasavada R, Helwig JJ, Stewart AF 1997 Opposing mitogenic and anti-mitogenic actions of parathyroid hormone-related protein in vascular smooth muscle cells—a critical role for nuclear targeting. Proc Natl Acad Sci USA **94:**13630–13635.

52. Henderson JE, Amizuka N, Warshawsky H, Biasotto D, Lanske BM, Goltzman D, Karaplis AC 1995 Nucleolar localization of parathyroid hormone-related peptide enhances survival of chondrocytes under conditions that promote apoptotic cell death. Mol Cell Biol **15:**4064–4075.

53. Amizuka N, Oda K, Shimomura J, Maeda T 2002 Biological action of parathyroid hormone (PTH)-related peptide (PTHrP) mediated either

54. by the PTH/PTHrP receptor or the nucleolar translocation in chondrocytes. Anatom Sci Int **77:**225–236.

54. Fiaschi-Taesch NM, Stewart AF 2003 Minireview: Parathyroid hormone-related protein as an intracrine factor–trafficking mechanisms and functional consequences. Endocrinology **144:**407–411.

55. Lam MH, House CM, Tiganis T, Mitchelhill KI, Sarcevic B, Cures A, Ramsay R, Kemp BE, Martin TJ, Gillespie MT 1999 Phosphorylation at the cyclin-dependent kinases site (Thr85) of parathyroid hormone-related protein negatively regulates its nuclear localization. J Biol Chem **274:**18559–18566.

56. Aarts MM, Rix A, Guo J, Bringhurst R, Henderson JE 1999 The nucleolar targeting signal (NTS) of parathyroid hormone related protein mediates endocytosis and nucleolar translocation. J Bone Miner Res **14:**1493–1503.

57. Nguyen M, He B, Karaplis A 2001 Nuclear forms of parathyroid hormone-related peptide are translated from non-AUG start sites downstream from the initiator methionine. Endocrinology **142:**694–703.

58. Nguyen MT, Karaplis AC 1998 The nucleus: A target site for parathyroid hormone-related peptide (PTHrP) action. J Cell Biochem **70:**193–199.

59. Lam MH, Olsen SL, Rankin WA, Ho PW, Martin TJ, Gillespie MT, Moseley JM 1997 PTHrP and cell division: Expression and localization of PTHrP in a keratinocyte cell line (HaCaT) during the cell cycle. J Cell Physiol **173:**433–446.

60. de Miguel F, Fiaschi-Taesch N, Lopez-Talavera JC, Takane KK, Massfelder T, Helwig JJ, Stewart AF 2001 The C-terminal region of PTHrP, in addition to the nuclear localization signal, is essential for the intracrine stimulation of proliferation in vascular smooth muscle cells. Endocrinology **142:**4096–4105.

61. Falzon M, Du P 2000 Enhanced growth of MCF-7 breast cancer cells overexpressing parathyroid hormone-related peptide. Endocrinology **141:**1882–1892.

62. Gujral A, Burton DW, Terkeltaub R, Deftos LJ 2001 Parathyroid hormone-related protein induces interleukin 8 production by prostate cancer cells via a novel intracrine mechanism not mediated by its classical nuclear localization sequence. Cancer Res **61:**2282–2288.

Chapter 20.   Vitamin D: Photobiology, Metabolism, Mechanism of Action, and Clinical Applications

Michael F. Holick

Section of Endocrinology, Diabetes and Metabolism, Department of Medicine, Boston University Medical Center, Boston, Massachusetts

INTRODUCTION

Vitamin D is a secosteroid that is made in the skin by the action of sunlight.[1] Vitamin D (D represents either or both D_2 and D_3) is biologically inert and must undergo two successive hydroxylations in the liver and kidney to become the biologically active 1,25-dihydroxyvitamin D [$1,25(OH)_2D$].[1–5] $1,25(OH)_2D$'s main biological effect is to maintain the serum calcium within the normal range. It accomplishes this by increasing the efficiency of intestinal absorption of dietary calcium and by recruiting stem cells in the bone to become mature osteoclasts, which in turn, mobilize calcium stores from the bone into the circulation.[1–5] The renal production of $1,25(OH)_2D$ is tightly regulated by serum calcium levels through the action of parathyroid hormone (PTH) and phosphorus (Fig. 1). There are a wide variety

of inborn and acquired disorders in the metabolism of vitamin D that can lead to both hypo- and hypercalcemic conditions. $1,25(OH)_2D$ not only regulates calcium metabolism but also is capable of inhibiting the proliferation and inducing terminal differentiation of a variety of normal and cancer cells, modulating the immune system, enhancing insulin secretion, and downregulating the renin/angiotension system. Active vitamin D compounds are used for the treatment of the hyperproliferative skin disease psoriasis and are being developed to treat some cancers and type 1 diabetes.

PHOTOBIOLOGY OF VITAMIN D_3

During exposure to sunlight, cutaneous 7-dehydrocholesterol (7-DHC, provitamin D_3), the immediate precursor of cholesterol, absorbs solar radiation with energies between 290 and 315 nm (ultraviolet B [UVB]), which in turn, causes the transformation of 7-DHC to previtamin D_3

The author has no conflict of interest.

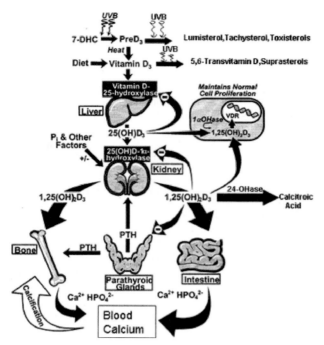

FIG. 1. The photochemical, thermal, and metabolic pathways for vitamin D. During exposure to sunlight (UVB), 7-DHC is converted to previtamin D₃ (preD₃). PreD₃ undergoes thermal isomerization to vitamin D₃, and vitamin D from the diet, along with the skin's vitamin D, enters the circulation and is metabolized sequentially in the liver and kidney to 25(OH)D and 1,25(OH)₂D. Serum phosphorus (Pi) and PTH levels are major regulators of renal 1,25(OH)₂D production. 24-OHase is responsible for the degradation of 1,25(OH)₂D to calcitroic acid. 25(OH)D can also enter other nonrenal tissues including colon, prostate, and breast, where it undergoes transformation to 1,25(OH)₂D. It then interacts with its VDR to induce genes that regulate cell growth.

(Fig. 1).[1–4] Once formed, previtamin D₃ undergoes a membrane-enhanced temperature-dependent isomerization over a period of a few hours to vitamin D₃ (Fig. 1). Vitamin D₃ is translocated from the skin into the circulation, where it is bound to the vitamin D–binding protein.[1–4]

There are no documented cases of vitamin intoxication caused by excessive exposure to sunlight. The likely mechanism for this is that once previtamin D₃ and vitamin D₃ are formed, they absorb solar UVB radiation and are transformed into several biologically inert photoproducts (Fig. 1).[1–3]

A variety of factors can alter the cutaneous production of vitamin D₃. Melanin, an excellent natural sunscreen, competes with 7-DHC for UVB photons, thereby reducing the production of vitamin D₃.[1–3] People of skin color require longer exposure (5- to 10-fold) to sunlight to make the same amount of vitamin D₃ as their white counterparts.[1–3] Aging diminishes the concentration of 7-DHC in the epidermis. Compared with a young adult, a person over the age of 70 years produced less than 30% of the amount of vitamin D₃ when exposed to the same amount of simulated sunlight.[1–3] Latitude, time of day, and season of the year dramatically affect the production of vitamin D₃ in the skin (Fig. 2). At a latitude of 42°N (Boston), sunlight is incapable of producing vitamin D₃ in the skin between the months of November through February. At 52°N (Edmonton, Canada), this period is extended to October through March.[1–3] Casual exposure to sunlight provides most (80–100%) of our vitamin D requirement. The inability of the sun to produce vitamin D₃ in the far northern and southern latitudes during the winter requires both children and adults to take a vitamin D supplement to prevent vitamin D deficiency. For children and young adults, the cutaneous production of vitamin D₃ during the spring, summer, and fall is often in excess and is stored in the fat so that it can be used during the winter months. However, both children and adults who always wear sun protection may not make enough vitamin D₃, and therefore, do not have sufficient vitamin D stores for winter use and will become vitamin D deficient unless a

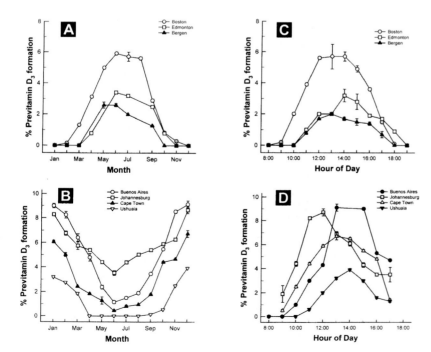

FIG. 2. Influence of season, time of day, and latitude on the synthesis of previtamin D₃ in the (A and C) Northern and (B and D) Southern Hemispheres. The hour indicated in C and D is the end of the 1-h exposure time. The data for hour of the day were collected in July. The data represent the means ± SE of triplicate determinations.

vitamin D supplement is taken. Exposure to sunlight at lower latitudes such as Los Angeles (34°N), Puerto Rico (18°N), and Buenos Aires (34°S) results in the cutaneous production of vitamin D_3 during the entire year (Fig. 2).[1–3] During the summer months in Boston, exposure to sunlight from the hours of 9:00 a.m. to 5:00 p.m. Eastern Daylight Savings Time (EDST) contains sufficient UVB radiation to produce previtamin D_3 in the skin. In the spring and fall months, vitamin D_3 production commences at 10:00 a.m. and ceases after 3:00 p.m. EDT (Fig. 2). Topical use of a sunscreen with a sun protection factor of 8 (SPF 8) will substantially reduce, by greater than 97%, the cutaneous production of vitamin D_3.[1–3] Chronic use of sunscreens can result in vitamin D insufficiency.[3] Although sunscreen use is extremely valuable for the prevention of skin cancer and the damaging effects caused by excessive exposure to the sun, both children and adults who depend on sunlight for their vitamin D_3 should consider exposure of hands, face, and arms or arms and legs to suberythemal amounts of sunlight (25% of the amount that would cause a mild pinkness to the skin) two to three times a week before topically applying a sunscreen with an SPF of 15. Thus, they can take advantage of the beneficial effect of sunlight while preventing the damaging effects of chronic excessive exposure to sunlight.

FOOD SOURCES OF VITAMIN D AND THE RECOMMENDED ADEQUATE INTAKE

Vitamin D is rare in foods. The major natural sources of vitamin D are oily fish such as salmon and mackerel as well as fish liver oils including cod liver oil.[1–3] Vitamin D can also be obtained from foods fortified with vitamin D including some cereals, bread products, and milk. Other dairy products including ice cream, yogurt, and cheese are not fortified with vitamin D. An evaluation of the vitamin D content in milk throughout the United States and Canada, however, revealed that almost 50% of the milk samples did not contain within 50% of the amount of vitamin D stated on the label and approximately 15% of skim milk samples contained no detectable vitamin D.[6] Multivitamin and pharmaceutical preparations containing vitamin D are reliable sources of vitamin D. The new recommended adequate intake (AI) for vitamin D for infants, all children, and adults up to the age of 50 years is 200 IU(5 μg)/day. For adults 51–70 and 71+ years, the AIs are 400 IU and 600 IU/day, respectively. Because there is no evidence that increasing vitamin D intake had any benefit during pregnancy and lactation, the AI for these women is also 200 IU/day.[7] There is mounting evidence that in the absence of sunlight, the AI for vitamin D in adults is between 600 and 1000 IU/day. [1–3,8–10]

METABOLISM OF VITAMIN D

Vitamin D_2, which comes from yeasts and plants, and vitamin D_3, which is found in oily fish and cod liver oil and is made in the skin, have essentially the same biological potency in humans.[1–4] The differences between vitamin D_2 and vitamin D_3 are a double bond between C_{22} and C_{23} and a methyl group on C_{24} for vitamin D_2.[1–3] Once vitamin D_2 or vitamin D_3 enters the circulation, they are bound to the vitamin D–binding protein and transported to the liver where the cytochrome P_{450}-vitamin D-25-hydroxylase (CYP27A1) introduces an OH on carbon 25 to produce 25-hydroxyvitamin D [25(OH)D] (Fig. 1).[1–4] 25(OH)D enters the circulation and is the major circulating form of vitamin D. Because the hepatic vitamin D-25-hydroxylase is not tightly regulated, an increase in the cutaneous production of vitamin D_3 or ingestion of vitamin D will result in an increase in circulating levels of 25(OH)D.[1–5,8] Therefore, its measurement is used to determine whether a patient is vitamin D deficient, vitamin D sufficient, or vitamin D intoxicated.[1–4]

25(OH)D is biologically inert. It is transported to the kidney where the cytochrome P_{450}-mono-oxygenase, 25(OH)D-1α-hydroxylase (1-OHase; CYP27B1), metabolizes 25(OH)D to 1,25(OH)$_2$D (Fig. 1).[1–4] Although the kidney is the major source of circulating 1,25(OH)$_2$D, there is strong evidence that a wide variety of tissues and cells, including activated macrophages, osteoblasts, keratinocytes, prostate, colon, and breast, express the 1-OHase and have the ability to produce 1,25(OH)$_2$D.[1–4] In addition, during pregnancy, the placenta produces 1,25(OH)$_2$D.[4] However, because anephric patients have very low or undetectable levels of 1,25(OH)$_2$D in their blood, the extrarenal sites of 1,25(OH)$_2$D production do not appear to play a role in calcium homeostasis. The local production of 1,25(OH)$_2$D in tissues not associated with calcium homeostasis may be for the purpose of regulating cell growth.[1–3]

When serum ionized calcium declines, there is an increase in the production and secretion of PTH. PTH has a variety of biological functions on calcium metabolism. It also regulates calcium homeostasis by enhancing the renal conversion of 25(OH)D to 1,25(OH)$_2$D (Fig. 1).[1–5] It does this indirectly through its renal wasting of phosphorus resulting in decreased intracellular and blood levels of phosphorus. Hypophosphatemia and hyperphosphatemia are associated with increased and decreased circulating concentrations of 1,25(OH)$_2$D, respectively.[11] A variety of other hormones associated with growth and development of the skeleton or calcium regulation, including growth hormone and prolactin, indirectly increase the renal production of 1,25(OH)$_2$D. Aged osteoporotic patients may lose their ability to upregulate the renal production of 1,25(OH)$_2$D by PTH.[12,13] This, along with a decrease in the amount of vitamin D receptor in elders' small intestine,[14] may help explain the age-related decrease in the efficiency of intestinal calcium absorption.

Both 25(OH)D and 1,25(OH)$_2$D undergo a 24-hydroxylation by the 25(OH)D-24-hydroxylase (CYP24) to form 24,25-dihydroxyvitamin D [24,25(OH)$_2$D] and 1,24,25-trihydroxyvitamin D, respectively. 1,25(OH)$_2$D is metabolized in all of its target tissues, as well as in the liver and kidney. [1–5,15–17] It undergoes several hydroxylations in the side-chain by the 25(OH)D-24-hydroxylase, causing the cleavage of the side-chain between carbons 23 and 24 and resulting in the biologically inert water soluble acid, calcitroic acid (Fig. 1).[1–5,15–17] These metabolites are considered to be biologically inert and are the first step in

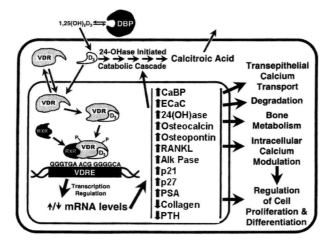

FIG. 3. A schematic representation of the mechanism of action of 1,25(OH)$_2$D in various target cells resulting in a variety of biological responses. The free form of 1,25(OH)$_2$D$_3$ enters the target cell and interacts with its nuclear VDR, which is phosphorylated (Pi). The 1,25(OH)$_2$D–VDR complex combines with the retinoic acid X receptor (RXR) to form a heterodimer, which in turn interacts with the VDRE, causing an enhancement or inhibition of transcription of vitamin D–responsive genes including calcium binding protein (CaBP), ECaC, 24-OHase, RANKL, alkaline phosphatase (alk Pase), prostate specific antigen (PSA), and PTH.

their biodegradation. Although more than 50 different metabolites of vitamin D have been identified, only 1,25(OH)$_2$D is believed to be important for most, if not all, of the biological actions of vitamin D on calcium and bone metabolism.[1–5,15–17]

MOLECULAR BIOLOGY OF VITAMIN D

The mechanism of action of 1,25(OH)$_2$D is similar to that of estrogen and other steroids. All target tissues for vitamin D contain a nuclear vitamin D receptor for 1,25(OH)$_2$D (VDR). This vitamin D receptor has a 1000-fold higher affinity for 1,25(OH)$_2$D compared with 25(OH)D and other dihydroxylated metabolites of vitamin D.[1–5,15] Analogous to other steroid hormones, the free 1,25(OH)$_2$D in the circulation enters its target cell, where it is recognized by its nuclear receptor (Fig. 3). The exact sequence by which 1,25(OH)$_2$D interacts with its receptor and causes activation of transcription of specific genes whose products are involved in the stimulation of biological responses caused by vitamin D is not completely clarified (Fig. 3). However, it is known that the VDR must complex with a retinoic acid X receptor (RXR) to form a heterodimeric complex with 1,25(OH)$_2$D$_3$.[15] Once formed, it interacts with several transcriptional factors, and this complex binds to a specific vitamin D–responsive element (VDRE) within the DNA. The DNA binding motif for VDR, which is present in the N terminus of the molecule containing the zinc fingers, interacts with the VDRE, which is composed of two tandem repeated hexa-nucleotide sequences separated by three base pairs (Fig. 3).[18,19] This interaction leads to the transcription of the gene and the synthesis of new mRNAs for a variety of proteins.[1–4,18–20]

The *VDR* gene has nine exons that give rise to the VDR,

which contains a DNA-binding domain in the N-terminal region and a hormone-binding domain in the C-terminal region (Fig. 4). Specific exon mutations have been identified that cause resistance to 1,25(OH)$_2$D, causing vitamin D–resistant rickets (also known as vitamin D–dependent rickets type II).[4,21] There are also mutations in the exons and introns that can lead to polymorphisms of the *VDR* gene that do not cause any biologically significant alteration in the amino acid composition of the VDR. These polymorphisms are thought to be important in the transcription of the *VDR* gene and/or stabilization of the resultant VDR mRNA. There is some evidence that these polymorphisms may lead to a differential responsiveness to 1,25(OH)$_2$D$_3$ in the intestine and bone, thereby playing a role in peak bone mass and the development of osteoporosis and other diseases.[22]

BIOLOGICAL FUNCTIONS OF VITAMIN D IN THE INTESTINE AND BONE

The major physiologic function of vitamin D is to maintain serum calcium at a physiologically acceptable level to maximize a wide variety of metabolic functions, signal transduction, and neuromuscular activity.[1–4] It accomplishes this by interacting with its receptor in the small intestine. Recent evidence suggests that 1,25(OH)$_2$D enhances calcium entry through an epithelial calcium channel (ECaC). This calcium channel is induced by 1,25(OH)$_2$D. 1,25(OH)$_2$D also induces several proteins in the small intestine, including calcium binding protein calbindin 9K, alkaline phosphatase, low affinity Ca ATPase, brush border actin, calmodulin, and several brush border proteins of 80–90 kDa. These facilitate the movement of calcium through the cytoplasm and transfer the calcium across the basal lateral membrane into the circulation.[4,20,23] 1,25(OH)$_2$D causes a biphasic response on intestinal calcium absorption in vitamin D–deficient animals. A rapid response occurs within 2 h and peaks by 6 h and another that begins after 12 h and peaks at 24 h, suggesting that there is

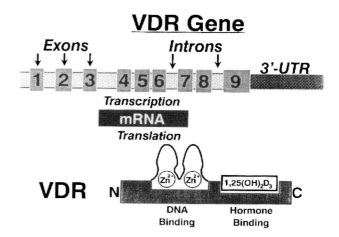

FIG. 4. Structure of the *VDR* gene, showing the nine exons and intervening introns and the 3'-untranslated region. The nine exons are transcribed into the VDR mRNA, which in turn is translated into the VDRs that contain a DNA and hormone-binding domains.

a rapid action of $1,25(OH)_2D$ on intestinal calcium absorption and a more prolonged nuclear mediated response.[23,24] $1,25(OH)_2D$ also enhances the absorption of dietary phosphorus. Although calcium and phosphorus absorption occur along the entire length of the small intestine, most of the phosphorus transport occurs in the jejunum and ileum, unlike calcium absorption, which principally occurs in the duodenum. The net result is that there is an increase in the efficiency of intestinal calcium and phosphorus absorption. In the vitamin D–deficient state, no more than 10–15% of dietary calcium and 60% of dietary phosphorus is absorbed in the gastrointestinal tract. However, with adequate vitamin D, adults absorb approximately 30% of dietary calcium and 70–80% of dietary phosphorus by the $1,25(OH)_2D$-mediated processes. During pregnancy, lactation, and growth spurts, circulating concentrations of $1,25(OH)_2D$ increase, thereby increasing the efficiency of intestinal calcium absorption by as much as 50–80%.[1–4]

When there is inadequate dietary calcium to satisfy the body's calcium requirement, $1,25(OH)_2D$ interacts with the VDR in osteoblasts, resulting in signal transduction to produce RANKL on their surface. The pre-osteoclasts have the RANK receptor for RANKL.[1–4,25] The direct contact of the pre-osteoclast's RANK with the osteoblast's RANKL results in signal transduction to induce pre-osteoclasts to become mature osteoclasts. The mature osteoclasts release hydrochloric acid and proteolytic enzymes to dissolve bone and matrix releasing calcium into the extracellular space. $1,25(OH)_2D$ also increases the expression of alkaline phosphatase, osteocalcin, osteopontin, and a variety of cytokines in osteoblasts.[4,25]

The major function of $1,25(OH)_2D$ for the bone mineralization process is to maintain a calcium $\times$ phosphorus product in the circulation that is in a supersaturated state, thereby resulting in the passive mineralization of the collagen matrix (osteoid) laid down by osteoblasts. $1,25(OH)_2D$ does not have a direct active role in the mineralization process; its responsibility is to maintain blood levels of calcium and phosphorus in the normal range for proper mineralization to occur.[1–4] There are some vitamin D analogs that have increased activity in osteoblasts, which stimulates them to produce more matrix and enhances bone formation.

NONCALCEMIC ACTIVITIES OF $1,25(OH)_2D_3$

Most tissues and cells in the body have a VDR, including brain, prostate, breast, gonads, colon, pancreas, monocytes, and activated T- and B-lymphocytes. Although the exact physiologic function of $1,25(OH)_2D$ in these tissues is not fully understood, $1,25(OH)_2D$ has varied biological activities that have important physiologic implications and pharmacologic applications. Most normal cell types and many tumor cells have a VDR. $1,25(OH)_2D_3$ and its analogs will often inhibit proliferation and induce terminal differentiation of normal cells, such as keratinocytes and cancer cells of the prostate, colon, breast, lymphoproliferative system, and lung.[1–4] The antiproliferative property of $1,25(OH)_2D_3$, and its analogs have been successfully developed to treat the hyperproliferative skin disorder psoriasis

and are in development to treat prostate, breast, and colon cancer.[26,27]

It is recognized that the kidney has a VDR. It has been assumed that its only functions were to downregulate its own synthesis and to enhance the $25(OH)D$-24-OHase expression to increase $1,25(OH)_2D_3$ degradation. However, $1,25(OH)_2D$ has been reported to also downregulate renin production in the kidney, suggesting that $1,25(OH)_2D$ may influence blood pressure control.[28] β-islet cells have a VDR and $1,25(OH)_2D_3$ has been reported to be a stimulator of insulin production and secretion[1–4] either directly through its interaction with the β-islet cell's VDR or indirectly by raising the serum concentration of calcium.

Activated T- and B-lymphocytes, monocytes, and macrophages all respond to $1,25(OH)_2D$, resulting in the modulation of their immune functions.[1,2,4] Thus, it has been suggested that vitamin D sufficiency may be important in decreasing risk of common autoimmune diseases such as multiple sclerosis and diabetes type 1[1,2,4,29] (Fig. 5).

NONRENAL SYNTHESIS OF $1,25(OH)_2D_3$

The 1-OHase was cloned and various point mutations have been identified for pseudovitamin D–deficient rickets (vitamin D–dependent rickets type 1).[21,30] In 1-OHase knockout mice, reproductive and immune dysfunction has been reported. The cloning of the 1-OHase has provided the impetus to explore the expression of this mitochondrial enzyme in nonrenal tissues, including prostate, colon, skin, breast, and osteoblast.[1,2,4] Although the physiologic function of the extrarenal 1-OHase is not well understood, there is mounting evidence that the local cellular production of $1,25(OH)_2D$ may be important for regulation of cell growth and other cellular activities. It is believed that once $1,25(OH)_2D$ is made and carries out its physiologic function, it is rapidly catabolized to calcitroic acid and therefore does not enter into the circulation to increase circulating concentrations of $1,25(OH)_2D$[1,2] (Fig. 5). Clearly, further studies are needed to help clarify the importance of the nonrenal 1-OHase in normal and cancer tissues.

REGULATION OF PTH SECRETION BY $1,25(OH)_2D$

The parathyroid chief cell has a VDR, and it responds to $1,25(OH)_2D_3$ by decreasing the expression of the *PTH* gene and decreasing PTH synthesis and secretion. Patients with long-standing secondary and tertiary hyperparathyroidism can develop within the parathyroid gland islands of PTH-secreting cells that have little or no VDR and therefore are no longer responsive to the PTH-lowering effect of $1,25(OH)_2D$.[31] Thus, the goal in patients with mild to moderate renal failure is to suppress secondary hyperparathyroidism. This can be accomplished by maintaining normal serum calcium concentrations first by controlling for hyperphosphatemia, which is one of the most potent downregulators of renal production of $1,25(OH)_2D_3$. However, when the serum phosphorus levels are maintained in the normal range and there continues to be an increase in PTH levels in the circulation, the use of oral or intravenous $1,25(OH)_2D_3$ and its less calcemic analogs 19-nor-1,25-

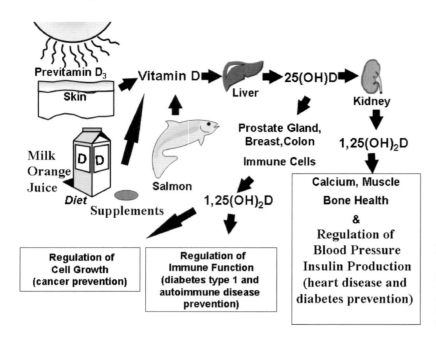

FIG. 5. Sources of vitamin D and its metabolism to $1,25(OH)_2D$ in the kidney and extra renal tissues, including prostate gland, breast, colon, and immune cells. Once produced, $1,25(OH)_2D$ has a multitude of biological actions on calcium, muscle, and bone health, regulation of blood pressure and insulin production, regulation of immune function, and regulation of cell growth.

dihydroxyvitamin D_2, 1α-hydroxyvitamin D_3 or 1,24-epi-dihydroxyvitamin D_2 to maintain serum calcium levels and directly suppress PTH expression is warranted.[32]

CLINICAL APPLICATIONS

Hypocalcemic Disorders

There are a variety of hypocalcemic disorders that are directly associated with acquired and inherited disorders in the acquisition of vitamin D, its metabolism to $1,25(OH)_2D$, and the cellular recognition of $1,25(OH)_2D$.[1–5,21,33–35] Vitamin D deficiency can be caused by a decreased synthesis of vitamin D_3 in the skin because of (1) excessive sunscreen use, (2) clothing of all sun exposed areas, (3) aging, (4) changes in season of the year, and (5) increased latitude.[1–3] Intestinal malabsorption of vitamin D associated with fat malabsorption syndromes, including Crohn's disease, sprue, Whipple's disease, and hepatic dysfunction, is recognizable by low or undetectable circulating concentrations of $25(OH)D$.[4,33] Increased vitamin D deposition in body fat is the cause of vitamin D deficiency in obesity.[1,2] Dilantin and phenobarbital can alter the kinetics for the metabolism of vitamin D to $25(OH)D$ requiring that these patients receive two to five times the AI for vitamin D to correct this abnormality.[33] Because the liver has such a large capacity to produce $25(OH)D$, usually greater than 90% of the liver has to be dysfunctional before it is incapable of making an adequate quantity of $25(OH)D$. Often the fat malabsorption associated with the liver failure is the cause for vitamin D deficiency.[4,33] Patients with nephrotic syndrome excreting greater than 4 g of protein/24 h can have lower $25(OH)D$ because of the coexcretion of the vitamin D binding protein (DBP) with its $25(OH)D$.[33]

Acquired disorders in the metabolism of $25(OH)D$ to $1,25(OH)_2D$ can cause hypocalcemia. Patients with chronic renal failure with a glomelular filtration rate (GFR) of less than 30% of normal have decreased reserved capacity to produce $1,25(OH)_2D$.[1,4,33] Hyperphosphatemia and hypoparathyroidism will result in the decreased production of $1,25(OH)_2D$.[4,11,33] Oncogenic osteomalacia, a rare acquired disorder, which produces fibroblast growth factor 23 (FGF-23), and X-linked hypophosphatemic rickets caused by a defect in the catabolism of FGF-23 are associated with hypocalcemia, hypophosphatemia, and very inappropriately low levels of $1,25(OH)_2D$.[4,33,34]

There are two rare inherited hypocalcemic disorders that are caused by either a deficiency in the renal production of $1,25(OH)_2D$ (vitamin D–dependent rickets type I) or a defect or deficiency in the VDR [$1,25(OH)_2D$–resistant syndrome].[4,21,33]

Hypercalcemic Disorders

Excessive ingestion of vitamin D (usually greater than that 5000–10,000 IU/day) for many months can cause vitamin D intoxication that is recognized by markedly elevated levels of $25(OH)D$ (usually >125 ng/ml) and usually normal levels of $1,25(OH)_2D$, hypercalcemia, and hyperphosphatemia.[8,33,35,36] Ingestion of excessive quantities of $25(OH)D_3$, 1α-OH-D_3, $1,25(OH)_2D_3$, dihydrotachysterol, or exuberant use of topical calcipotriene (Dovonex) for psoriasis can cause vitamin D intoxication.[4,26,33] Because activated macrophages convert in an unregulated fashion $25(OH)D$ to $1,25(OH)_2D$, chronic granulomatous diseases such as sarcoidosis and tuberculosis are often associated with increased serum levels of $1,25(OH)_2D$ that results in hypercalciuria and hypercalcemia.[4,33,37] Rarely, lymphomas associated with hypercalcemia are caused by increased production of $1,25(OH)_2D$ by macrophages associated with the lymphomatous tissue. Primary hyperparathyroidism and hypophosphatemia are also associated with increase renal production of $1,25(OH)_2D$.[4,11,33]

CONSEQUENCES AND TREATMENT OF VITAMIN D DEFICIENCY

Vitamin D plays a critical role in the mineralization of the skeleton at all ages. As the body depletes its stores of vitamin D because of lack of exposure to sunlight or a deficiency of vitamin D in the diet, the efficiency of intestinal calcium absorption decreases from approximately 30–40% to no more than 10–15%. This causes a decrease in the ionized calcium concentration in the blood, which signals the calcium sensor in the parathyroid glands, resulting in an increase in the synthesis and secretion of PTH.[1,24,33] PTH not only tries to conserve calcium by increasing renal tubular reabsorption of calcium but also plays an active role in mobilizing stem cells to become active bone calcium resorbing osteoclasts. PTH also increases tubular excretion of phosphorus, causing hypophosphatemia. The net effect of vitamin D insufficiency and vitamin D deficiency is a normal serum calcium, elevated PTH, and alkaline phosphatase, and a low or low normal fasting serum phosphorus. The hallmark of vitamin D deficiency is a low (<20 ng/ml) or undetectable level of 25(OH)D in the blood.[1,2,4,33] The secondary hyperparathyroidism and low calcium × phosphorus product is thought to be responsible for the increase in unmineralized osteoid, which is the hallmark of rickets/osteomalacia.[2] In addition, the secondary hyperparathyroidism causes increased osteoclastic activity, resulting in calcium wasting from the bone, which in turn can precipitate or exacerbate osteoporosis.

Vitamin D deficiency is a major cause of metabolic bone disease in older adults. Rickets is, once again, becoming a major health problem for infants of mothers of color who exclusively breastfeed their children and do not supplement them with vitamin D.[1,2,33,38] Vitamin D deficiency is underappreciated in the population at large. The NHANES III survey revealed that 42% of black women ages 15–49 years were vitamin D deficient throughout the United States at the end of the winter.[39] Vitamin D deficiency is common in the elderly, especially those who are infirm and in nursing homes.[1–3,9,33] Approximately 50% of free-living elders were found to be vitamin D deficient throughout the year. Even healthy young adults are at risk. A study in students and young medical doctors aged 18–29 years in Boston at the end of the winter revealed 32% were vitamin D deficient and a significant number had secondary hyperparathyroidism.[40] Vitamin D deficiency not only robs the skeleton of precious calcium stores, but causes osteomalacia. This disease, unlike osteoporosis, causes vague symptoms of bone pain, bone achiness, muscle aches, and pains and muscle weakness. These symptoms are often dismissed by physicians, or the patient is given the diagnosis of fibromyalgia. A recent study revealed that 88% of women with muscle pain, weakness, and bone pain were caused by vitamin D deficiency.[41]

Casual exposure to sunlight is the best source of vitamin D. Because the skin has such a large capacity to produce vitamin D3, children and adults of all ages can obtain their vitamin D requirement from exposure to sunlight. For young adults a whole body exposure to one minimum erythemal dose (a slight pinkness to the skin) of simulated

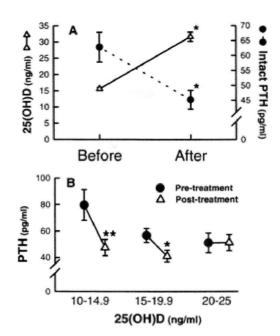

FIG. 6. (Top) Healthy adults aged 49–83 received 50,000 IU of vitamin D₂ once a week for 8 weeks. Serum levels of 25(OH)D and intact PTH are shown before and after receiving vitamin D₂. (Bottom) These same patients with serum 25(OH)D above 10 ng/ml (considered to be the lowest limit of the normal range by many laboratories) and below 25 ng/ml were stratified regarding their PTH levels before and immediately after therapy. The data clearly show significant declines in PTH when the initial serum 25(OH)D levels were between 11 and 19 ng/ml, suggesting that patients were deficient in vitamin D until the 25(OH)D was above 20 ng/ml. Based on this and other data, the new recommendation is that patients should have a blood level of at least 20 ng/ml and preferably 30 ng/ml of 25(OH)D to maximize bone and cellular health.

sunlight was found to be equivalent to taking a single oral dose of between 10,000 and 25,000 IU of vitamin D.[1–3] Therefore, children and adults only need minimum exposure of unprotected skin to sunlight followed by the application of a sunscreen or use of other sun protective measures, including clothing. In Boston, we recommend that white men and women expose face and arms or arms and legs to sunlight three times a week for about 25% of time that it would cause a mild sunburn in the spring, summer, and fall.[1–3,5]

Patients with vitamin D deficiency require immediate attention with aggressive therapy. Trying to replete vitamin D deficiency with a multivitamin or with a few multivitamins containing 400 IU of vitamin D is not only not effective but can be potentially dangerous because these multivitamins often contain the safe upper limit of vitamin A. The vitamin D tank is empty and requires rapid filling. This can be accomplished by giving a pharmacologic dose of vitamin D orally of 50,000 IU of vitamin D once a week for 8 weeks; this will often correct vitamin D deficiency as measured by an increase in 25(OH)D above 20 ng/ml[42] (Fig. 6). If this is not achieved, an additional 8-week course is reasonable. Alternatively, intramuscular injections of between 50,000 and 500,000 IU of vitamin D will help correct vitamin D deficiency. However, this method can often be painful, and the vitamin D is variably absorbed into the body. Patients who are chronically vitamin D deficient are often given 50,000 IU of vitamin D once or twice a month after correction of their vitamin D deficiency. The fortification of some orange juice and other juice products with vitamin D[43] offers an additional source of vitamin D to those who do not drink milk.[43] The goal is to have blood levels of 25(OH)D of at least 30 ng/ml to achieve the maximum benefit for skeletal and cellular health.[1,2]

CONCLUSION

When evaluating patients for hypo- and hypercalcemic conditions, it is appropriate to consider the patient's vitamin D status as well as whether they suffer from either an acquired or inherited disorder in the acquisition and/or metabolism of vitamin D. Because the assay for vitamin D is not available to clinicians, the best assay to determine vitamin D status is 25(OH)D. The $1,25(OH)_2D$ assay is not only useless in determining vitamin D status, but it can also be misleading because $1,25(OH)_2D$ levels can be normal or elevated in a vitamin D–deficient patient. Only when there is a suspicion that there is an acquired or inherited disorder in the metabolism of 25(OH)D is it reasonable to measure circulating $1,25(OH)_2D$ concentrations. Although there are a variety of other metabolites of vitamin D in the circulation, the measurement of other vitamin D metabolites has not proved to be of any significant value. It has been suggested that there may be a correlation with the development of metabolic bone disease with polymorphism for the vitamin D receptor gene.[22] Although these data are intriguing, the information is, at this time, of limited clinical value but may someday provide an insight as to a person's potential maximum bone density. The noncalcemic actions of $1,25(OH)_2D_3$ have great promise for clinical applications in the future (Fig. 5). The activated vitamin D compounds $1,25(OH)_2D_3$, $1,24(OH)_2D_3$, and calcipotriene herald a new pharmacologic approach for treating psoriasis.[26] The recent report of a 2MD analog that markedly increased bone density in rodents offers a novel approach of developing vitamin D analogs as anabolic drugs to treat osteoporosis.[44] Combination therapy of $1,25(OH)_2D_3$ and its analogs with other cancer drugs offers promise in treating many lethal cancers.[45] In addition, vitamin D analogs are being developed to treat or mitigate common autoimmune disorders including multiple sclerosis and diabetes type 1. Clearly the vitamin D field of research remains robust.

REFERENCES

1. Holick MF 2002 Vitamin D: The underappreciated D-lightful hormone that is important for skeletal and cellular health. Curr Opin Endocrinol Diabetes 9:87–98.
2. Holick MF 2003 Calciotropic hormones and the skin: A millennium perspective. J Cell Biochem 88:296–307.
3. Holick MF 1994 Vitamin D: New horizons for the 21st century. Am J Clin Nutr 60:619–630.
4. Bouillon R 2001 Vitamin D: From photosynthesis, metabolism and action to clinical applications. In: Degroot LL and Jameson JL (eds.) Endocrinology, 4th ed., vol. 2. W. B. Saunders Co., Philadelphia, PA, USA, pp. 1009–1028.
5. DeLuca H 1988 The vitamin D story: A collaborative effort of basic science and clinical medicine. FASEB J 2:224–236.
6. Holick MF, Shao Q, Liu WW, Chen TC 1992 The vitamin D content of fortified milk and infant formula. N Engl J Med 326:1178–1181.
7. Standing Committee on the Scientific Evaluation Dietary Reference Intakes (ed.) 1999 Calcium. Dietary Reference Intakes for Calcium, Phosphorus, Magnesium, Vitamin D, and Fluoride. Institute of Medicine, National Academy Press, Washington, DC, USA, pp. 71–145.
8. Barger-Lux MJ, Heaney RP, Dowell S, Chen TC, Holick MF 1998 Vitamin D and its major metabolites: Serum levels after graded oral dosing in healthy men. Osteoporos Int 8:222–230.
9. Dawson-Hughes B, Dallal GE, Krall EA, Harris S, Sokoll LJ, Falconer G 1991 Effect of vitamin D supplementation on wintertime and overall bone loss in healthy postmenopausal women. Ann Intern Med 115:505–512.
10. Vieth R 1999 Vitamin D supplementation, 25-hydroxyvitamin D concentrations, and safety. Am J Clin Nutr 69:842–856.
11. Portale AA, Halloran BP, Morris RC Jr 1989 Physiologic regulation of the serum concentration of 1,25-dihydroxyvitamin D by phosphorus in normal men. J Clin Invest 83:1494–1499.
12. Slovik DM, Adams JS, Neer RM, Holick MF, Potts JT 1981 Deficient production of 1,25-dihydroxyvitamin D in elderly osteoporotic patients. N Engl J Med 305:372–374.
13. Riggs BL, Hamstra A, DeLuca HF 1981 Assessment of 25-hydroxyvitamin D 1α-hydroxylase reserve in postmenopausal osteoporosis by administration of parathyroid extract. J Clin Endocrinol Metab 53:833–835.
14. Ebeling PR, Sandgren ME, DiMagno EP, Lane AW, DeLuca HF, Riggs BL 1992 Evidence of an age-related decrease in intestinal responsiveness to vitamin D: Relationship between serum 1,25-dihydroxyvitamin D3 and intestinal vitamin D receptor concentration in normal women. J Clin Endocrinol Metab 75:176–182.
15. McCary LC, DeLuca HF 1999 Functional metabolism and molecular biology of vitamin D action. In: Holick MF (ed.) Vitamin D: Physiology, Molecular Biology, and Clinical Applications. Humana Press, Totowa, NJ, USA, pp. 39–56.
16. Reddy GS, Tserng KY, Thomas BR, Dayal R, Norman AW 1987 Isolation and identification of 1,23-dihydroxy-25, 25, 26, 27-tetranorvitamin D3, a new metabolite of 1,25-dihydroxyvitamin D3 produced in rat kidney. Biochemistry 26:324–331.
17. Jones G 1999 Metabolism and catabolism of vitamin D, its metabolites, and clinically relevant analogs. In: Holick MF (ed.) Vitamin D: Physiology, Molecular Biology, and Clinical Applications. Humana Press, Totowa, NJ, USA, pp. 57–84.
18. Freedman LP 1999 Multimeric coactivator complexes for steroid/nuclear receptors. Trends Endocrinol Metab 10:403–407.
19. MacDonald PN 1999 Molecular biology of the vitamin D receptor. In: Holick MF (ed.) Vitamin D: Physiology, Molecular Biology, and Clinical Applications. Humana Press, Totowa, NJ, USA, pp. 39–56.
20. Raval-Pandya M, Porta AR, Christakos S 1999 Mechanism of action of 1,25-dihydroxyvitamin D3 on intestinal calcium absorption and renal calcium transport. In: Holick MF (ed.) Vitamin D: Physiology, Molecular Biology, and Clinical Applications. Humana Press, Totowa, NJ, USA, pp. 163–173.
21. Demay MB 1995 Hereditary defects in vitamin D metabolism and vitamin D receptor defects. In: Degroot LJ (ed.) Endocrinology, 13th ed., vol. 2. Saunders Co., Philadelphia, PA, USA, pp. 1173–1178.
22. Cooper GS, Umbach DM 1996 Are vitamin D receptor polymorphisms associated with bone mineral density? A meta-analysis. J Bone Miner Res 11:1841–1849.
23. Bouillon R, Van Cromphaut S, Carmeliet G 2003 Intestinal calcium absorption: Molecular vitamin D mediated mechanisms. J Cell Biochem 88:332–339.
24. Baran DT 1999 Nongenomic rapid effects of vitamin D. In: Holick MF (ed.) Vitamin D: Physiology, Molecular Biology, and Clinical Applications. Humana Press, Totowa, NJ, USA, pp. 195–205.
25. Khosla S 2001 The OPG/RANKL/RANK system. Endocrinology 142:5050–5055.
26. Holick MF 1998 Clinical efficacy of 1,25-dihydroxyvitamin D3 and its analogues in the treatment of psoriasis. Retinoids 14:12–17.
27. Guyton KZ, Kensler TW, Posner GH 2001 Cancer chemoprevention using natural vitamin D and synthetic analogs. Annu Rev Pharmacol Toxicol 41:421–442.
28. Li Y, Kong J, Wei M, Chen ZF, Liu S, Cao LP 2002 1,25-dihydroxyvitamin D3 is a negative endocrine regulator of the renin-angiotensin system. J Clin Invest 110:229–238.
29. Hypponen E, Laara E, Jarvelin M-R, Virtanen SM 2001 Intake of

vitamin D and risk of type 1 diabetes: A birth-cohort study. Lancet **358:**1500–1503.

30. Kitanaka S, Takeyama KI, Murayama A, Sato T, Okumura K, Nogami M, Hasegawa Y, Nimi H, Yanagisawa J, Tanaka T, Kato S 1988 Inactivating mutations in the human 25-hydroxyvitamin D$_3$ 1α-hydroxylase gene in patients with pseudovitamin D-deficient rickets. N Engl J Med **338:**653–661.

31. Fukuda N, Tanaka H, Tominaga R, Fukagawa M, Kurokawa K, Seino Y 1993 Decreased 1,25-dihydroxyvitamin D$_3$ receptor density is associated with a more severe form of parathyroid hyperplasia in chronic uremic patients. J Clin Invest **92:**1436–1443.

32. Delmez JA, Tindira C, Grooms P, Dusso A, Windus DW, Slatopolsky E 1989 Parathyroid hormone suppression by intravenous 1,25-dihydroxyvitamin D: A role for increased sensitivity to calcium. J Clin Invest **83:**1349–1355.

33. Holick MF 2001 Evaluation and treatment of disorders in calcium, phosphorus, and magnesium metabolism. In: Noble J (ed.) Textbook of Primary Care Medicine, 3rd ed. Mosby, Inc., St. Louis, MO, USA, pp. 886–898.

34. Christie PT, Harding B, Nesbit MA, Whyte MP, Thakker RV 2001 X-linked hypophosphatemia attributable to pseudoexons of the PHEX gene. J Clin Endocrinol Metab **86:**3840–3844.

35. Vieth R 1999 The mechanisms of vitamin D toxicity. Bone Miner **11:**267–272.

36. Jacobus CH, Holick MF, Shao Q, Chen TC, Holm IA, Kolodny JM, El-Hajj Fuleihan G, Seely E 1992 Hypervitaminosis D associated with drinking milk. N Engl J Med **326:**1173–1177.

37. Adams JS, Gacad MA, Anders A, Endres DB, Sharma OP 1986 Biochemical indicators of disordered vitamin D and calcium homeostasis in sarcoidosis. Sarcoidosis Vasc Diffuse Lung Dis **3:**1–6.

38. Kreiter SR, Schwartz RP, Kirkman HN, Charlton PA, Calikoglu AS, Davenport M 2000 Nutritional rickets in African American breast-fed infants. J Pediatr **137:**2–6.

39. Nesby-O'Dell S, Scanlon KS, Cogswell ME, Gillespie C, Hollis BW, Looker AC 2002 Hypovitaminosis D prevalence and determinants among African American and white women of reproductive age: Third national health and nutrition examination survey, 1988–1994. Am J Clin Nutr **76:**187–192.

40. Tangpricha V, Pearce EN, Chen TC, Holick MF 2002 Vitamin D insufficiency among free-living healthy young adults. Am J Med **112:**659–662.

41. Glerup H, Mikkelsen K, Poulsen L, Hass E, Overbeck S, Thomesen J, Charles P, Eriksen EF 2000 Commonly recommended daily intake of vitamin D is not sufficient if sunlight exposure is limited. J Intern Med **247:**260–268.

42. Malabanan A, Veronikis IE, Holick MF 1998 Redefining vitamin D insufficiency. Lancet **351:**805–806.

43. Tangpricha V, Koutkia P, Rieke SM, Chen TC, Perez AA, Holick MF 2003 Fortification of orange juice with vitamin D: A novel approach to enhance vitamin D nutritional health. Am J Clin Nutr. **77:**1478–1483.

44. Shevde NK, Plum LA, Clagett-Dame M, Yamamoto H, Pike JW, DeLuca HF 2002 A potent analog of 1α-25-dihydroxyvitamin D$_3$ selectively induces bone formation. Proc Natl Acad Sci USA **99:** 13487–13491.

45. Beer TM, Eilers KM, Garzotto M, Egorin MJ, Lowe BA, Henner WD 2003 Weekly high-dose calcitriol and docetaxel in metastatic androgen-independent prostate cancer. J Clin Oncol **21:**123–128.

Chapter 21. Calcitonin

Leonard J. Deftos

Department of Medicine, University of California and San Diego Veterans Affairs Medical Center, San Diego, California

INTRODUCTION

Calcitonin (CT) is a 32 amino acid peptide secreted primarily by thyroidal C-cells but also by cells of the diffuse neuroendocrine system. Its main skeletal effect is to inhibit osteoclastic bone resorption. This property has led to its use for disorders characterized by increased bone resorption. Parenteral and nasal formulations of the peptide are used for the treatment of Paget's disease, osteoporosis, and the hypercalcemia of malignancy. The secretion of CT is regulated acutely by blood calcium and chronically by gender and perhaps age. CT is metabolized by the kidney and the liver. The *CT* gene encodes other neuropeptides. CT is also a tumor marker for medullary thyroid carcinoma, the signal tumor of multiple endocrine neoplasia (MEN) type II.[1]

BIOCHEMISTRY

Over a dozen species of CT, including human, have been sequenced. Common features include a 1–7 amino-terminal disulfide bridge, a glycine at residue 28, and a carboxy-terminal proline amide residue. Five of the nine amino-terminal residues are identical in all CT species. The greatest divergence resides in the interior 27 amino acids. Basic amino acid substitutions enhance potency. Thus, the non-mammalian CTs have the most potency, even in mammalian systems. In contrast to parathyroid hormone (PTH), a biologically active fragment of CT has not been discovered. However, an amphipathic backbone seems to enhance potency.[1,2]

MOLECULAR BIOLOGY

The *CT* gene consists of six exons separated by introns (Fig. 1). Two distinct mature mRNAs are generated from differential splicing of the exon regions in the initial gene transcript. One translates as a 141-residue CT precursor, the other as a 128-residue precursor for *CT* gene–related peptide (CGRP). CT is the major post-translationally processed peptide in C-cells, whereas CGRP, a 37-amino acid peptide, is the major processed peptide in neurons. The main biological effect of CGRP is vasodilation, but it also functions as a neurotransmitter and does react with the CT receptor. The relevance of CGRP to skeletal metabolism is unknown, but it may be produced in skeletal tissue and exert a local regulatory effect. An alternative splicing pathway for the *CT* gene has been recently described. It produces a carboxy-terminal C-pro CT with eight different terminal amino acids. The *CT* gene predicts the presence of other processed peptides, and there is more than one copy of this gene.[1–3]

This author has no conflict of interest.

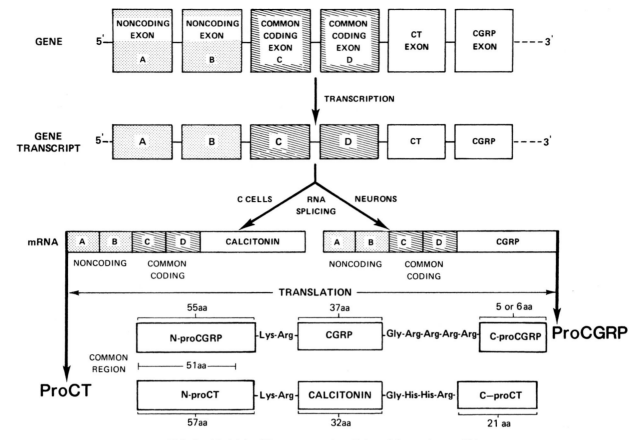

FIG. 1. Model for CT gene expression. (Adapted from reference 23.)

BIOSYNTHESIS

Thyroidal C-cells are the primary source of CT in mammals, and the ultimobranchial gland is the primary source in submammals.[1,3] C-cells are neural crest derivatives, and they also produce CGRP, the second CT gene product. Other tissue sources of CT have been described, notably the pituitary cells and widely distributed neuroendocrine cells.[4] Although CT may have paracrine effects at these sites, the nonthyroidal sources of CT are not likely to contribute to its peripheral concentration. However, malignant transformation can occur in both ectopic and eutopic cells that produce CT, and the peptide then becomes a tumor marker.[1] The best example of the latter is medullary thyroid carcinoma, and of the former, small-cell lung cancer. Many of the tumors associated with ectopic CT production probably derive this potential from their common neural crest origin with thyroidal C-cells.[1–3]

BIOLOGICAL EFFECTS

CT's main biological effect is to inhibit osteoclastic bone resorption.[1] Within minutes of its administration, CT causes the osteoclast to shrink in size and to decrease its bone-resorbing activity.[2] This dramatic and complex event is accompanied by the production of cyclic adenosine monophosphate (cAMP) and by increased cytosolic calcium in the osteoclast.[1–3,5] In a situation where bone turnover is sufficiently high, CT will produce hypocalcemia and hypophosphatemia. CT has also been reported to inhibit osteocytes and stimulate osteoblasts, but these effects are controversial.[6] Analgesia is a commonly reported effect of CT treatment.[7] Calciuria, phosphaturia, and gastrointestinal effects on calcium flux have been reported for CT, but they occur at concentrations of the hormone that are supraphysiologic.[1–3] It should be noted, however, that the concentration of the peptide at its several sites of biosynthesis may be sufficiently high to explain some extraskeletal effects of CT by a paracrine mechanism.[1] Thus, CT may exert physiologic effects on the pituitary and central nervous system.[1,4] Furthermore, the demonstration of CT and CT receptors at intracranial sites may qualify CT as a neurotransmitter.[1,2] Other effects of CT have been reported. It has been observed to act as an anti-inflammatory agent, to promote fracture and wound healing, to be uricosuric, to be antihypertensive, and to impair glucose tolerance. The importance of these latter effects is yet to be determined.[1–3]

CT AS A DRUG

CT's main biological action of inhibiting osteoclastic bone resorption has resulted in its successful use in disease states characterized by increased bone resorption and the consequent hypercalcemia.[1–3] CT can be used in Paget's disease, in which osteoclastic bone resorption is dramatically increased; in osteoporosis, in which the increase of bone resorption may be more subtle; and in the treatment of hypercalcemia of malignancy.[3] Newer pharmacologic preparations of CT may have improved therapeutic effects.[7] The nasal preparation of CT has superseded the original parental preparation in clinical use.[3,7]

Secretion

Ambient calcium concentration is the most important regulator of CT secretion.[1] When blood calcium rises acutely, there is a proportional increase in CT secretion, and an acute decrease in blood calcium produces a corresponding decrease in plasma CT. However, the effects of chronic hypercalcemia and chronic hypocalcemia are not fully defined, and conflicting results have been reported.[8,9] It seems likely that the C-cells can respond to mild hypercalcemia by increasing CT secretion, but, if the hypercalcemia is severe and/or prolonged, the C-cells probably exhaust their secretory reserve. The inhibitory effect on CT secretion by hypocalcemia is difficult to show. Chronic hypocalcemia seems to decrease the secretory challenge to C-cells, and they increase their stores of CT; these stores can be released on appropriate stimulation.[10]

Metabolism

The metabolism of CT is a complex process that involves many organ systems. Evidence has been reported for degradation of the hormone by kidney, liver, bone, and even the thyroid gland.[1–3] Like many other peptide hormones, CT disappears from plasma in a multiexponential manner that includes an early half-life measured in minutes. In most studies, the kidney seems to be the most important organ of clearance for CT. Inactivation of the hormone seems more important than renal excretion, because relatively little CT can be detected in urine. Metabolism of the peptide during inflammatory disease may result in the production of specific forms of CT that can be identified by selective immunoassays.[11]

Gastrointestinal Factors

Gastrointestinal peptides, especially those of the gastrin-cholecystokinin family, are potent CT secretagogues when administered parenterally in supraphysiologic concentrations.[1,2] This observation has led to the postulate that there is an entero-C-cell regulatory pathway for CT secretion. However, only meals that contain sufficient calcium to raise the blood calcium have been demonstrated to increase CT secretion in humans.[8] Thus, the secretory relationship between the gastrointestinal tract and C-cells in human needs further exploration to determine its physiologic significance. Nevertheless, pentagastrin as well as glucagon can be used as stimulatory test for CT secretion.

PROVOCATIVE TESTING FOR CT-PRODUCING TUMORS

The stimulatory effect of calcium and gastrointestinal (GI) peptides, especially pentagastrin, on CT secretion has led to their use as provocative tests for the secretion of CT in patients suspected of having medullary thyroid carcinoma (MTC), a neoplastic disorder of thyroidal C-cells that can occur in a familial pattern as part of MEN type II.[1] Most tumors respond with increased CT secretion to the administration of either calcium or pentagastrin or their combination, but either agent can sometimes give misleading results. Therefore, in clinically compelling situations, both agents should be considered for diagnostic testing. CT measurements can also be used to monitor the effectiveness of therapy, usually thyroidectomy, in patients with MTC.[1–3]

GENDER AND AGE

Most investigators find that women have lower CT levels than men.[5,12] The mechanism of this difference is unclear but may be accounted for in part by a stimulating effect of gonadal steroids on CT secretion.[13,14] The effect of age on CT secretion is more controversial[5,12–15]: newborns seem to have a higher serum level of the hormone, and in adults, a progressive decline with age has been reported by several laboratories.[5,15] However, stable adult levels have also been observed.[12] It is likely that the different assay procedures used in different studies account for the conflicting results. Thus, the serum concentration of some forms of CT may decline with age, whereas others do not.[5,12] The physiologic significance of the various circulating forms of CT measured by different assay procedures has not been defined. Nonmonomeric, as well as monomeric, forms of circulating CT species are biologically active,[1–3] and some procedures may not accurately reflect biologically active CT in blood.

CLINICAL ABNORMALITIES OF CT SECRETION

MTC

MTC is a tumor of the CT-producing C-cells of the thyroid gland.[1] Although a rare tumor, it can occur in a familial pattern as part of MEN type II. MTC is generally regarded as intermediate between the aggressive behavior of anaplastic thyroid carcinoma and the more indolent behavior of papillary and follicular thyroid carcinoma. The most common presentation is a thyroid nodule, and the most common symptom is diarrhea. These tumors usually produce diagnostically elevated serum concentrations of CT. Therefore, immunoassay for CT in serum can be used to diagnose the presence of MTC with an exceptional degree of accuracy and specificity. In a small but increasing percentage of patients, however, basal hormone levels are indistinguishable from normal. Many of these subjects represent the early stages of C-cell neoplasia or hyperplasia, most amenable to surgical cure. To identify these patients with early disease, provocative tests for CT secretion, previously discussed, have been developed that can identify MTC in a patient whose diagnosis could have been missed if basal CT determinations only had been performed. Abnormalities of the RET oncogene are the genetic basis for inherited MTC and provide the basis for genetic testing.[1]

Other CT-Producing Neoplasms

Neoplastic disorders of other neuroendocrine cells can also produce abnormally elevated amounts of CT. The best known example is small-cell lung cancer. However, other tumors, such as carcinoids and islet cell tumors of the pancreas, can also overexpress CT.[1,2]

Renal Disease

There are increases in immunoassayable CT with both acute and chronic renal failure, but considerable disagreement exists regarding the mechanism and significance of these increases.[1–3] Because the secretion and/or metabolism of CT is abnormal in renal disease and because renal osteodystrophy is characterized by increased bone resorption, CT, which acts to inhibit bone resorption, has been implicated, but not conclusively, in the pathogenesis of uremic osteodystrophy.[1,2]

Hypercalciuria

Elevated levels of CT have been demonstrated in patients with hypercalciuria.[16] The physiologic significance of enhanced CT secretion is unknown, but it may represent a compensatory response to intestinal hyperabsorption of calcium. Although CT in high concentrations has both phosphaturic and calciuric actions in humans, it is not likely that a primary alteration in CT secretion contributes to the development of hypercalciuria.[1]

Bone Disease

No skeletal disease has been conclusively attributed to CT abnormalities.[1–3] Although women have lower CT levels than men, there is conflicting evidence as to whether endogenous secretion of the hormone contributes to the pathogenesis of osteoporosis.[14,17,18] Nevertheless, CT has been of therapeutic benefit in osteoporosis.[7] Reduced CT reserve in women may contribute to the greater severity of osteitis fibrosa cystica in women with primary hyperparathyroidism.[9] Skeletal abnormalities have not been identified in patients following thyroidectomy.[1,2] However, the recent demonstration in pyknodysostosis of dysfunctional mutations of the gene for cathepsin K,[19] responsible for collagen degradation by osteoclasts, and the high levels of serum calcitonin reported in this disease,[20] suggest an intriguing link between skeletal dysplasia and calcitonin secretion. For example, the increased calcitonin may be compensatory for the impaired osteoclastic resorption.

Hypercalcemia and Hypocalcemia

Calcium challenge is a well-documented stimulus for CT secretion. Although increased CT secretion has only inconsistently been associated with chronic hypercalcemia,[8,9] an exaggerated response of CT to secretagogues has been convincingly observed in several hypocalcemic states.[10]

Calcitonin Receptor

CT mediates its biological effects through the CT receptor (CRT).[21] CTRs have been cloned from the pig, human, rat, mouse, and rabbit, but a nonmammalian CTR has yet to be cloned. CTRs are most robustly expressed in osteoclasts but also are expressed in several other sites, including the central nervous system. The mammalian CTRs share common structural and functional motifs, signal through several pathways, and can exist in several isoforms with insert sequences or deletions or both in their intracellular and extracellular domains. These isoforms arise from alternative splicing of receptor mRNA transcribed from a single gene. Some of the isoforms of the CTR seem to have differential ligand specificity, perhaps accounting for the pleiotropic effects of the hormone.[21]

Salmon calcitonin (SCT) apparently conforms best to the structural requirements for binding and signaling of mammalian CTRs, perhaps explaining its greater potency in humans and mammals and its sustained receptor binding and activation of cAMP.[7,21] An isoform of the CTR that is expressed in rat brain seems to preferentially recognize SCT, and binding sites for SCT are present at several sites in the central nervous system (CNS). It is thus speculated that an SCT-like ligand is produced by mammals. There is some evidence for this in both humans and murine. Finally, it is also notable that another nonmammalian CT, chicken CT (CCT), also seems more potent in humans than human CT, and that a CCT-like ligand may be expressed in humans.[21]

Ligand Families for CT

Long known to be related to CGRP1 and 2, CT recently was recognized to be related in sequence to two other peptides, adrenomedullin and amylin.[22] Although all of these peptides share the feature of being neuromodulators, they also appear to have unique hormone actions. The effects of CT were described earlier. CGRP1 and CGRP2 are potent vasodilators an immunomodulators, with actions in the CNS and at may other targets. Adrenomedullin also is a potent vasodilator with some CNS actions. The actions of amylin are related to carbohydrate metabolism, to gastric emptying, and to CNS function.[23]

Receptor Modulation

Despite their distinct bioactivities, the family of CT-related ligands shows some cross-reactivity at each other's receptors, although they generally bear only partial homology.[23] The interaction of ligands among these receptors is influenced by newly discovered receptor-modulating proteins.[22,23] This modulation expands the repertoire of biological actions that can be mediated by receptors and their ligands. One modulator, termed CGRP-receptor component protein (CGRP-RCP), consists of a hydrophilic protein that is highly conserved across species and found in virtually all tissues. The second group of receptor modulators is a family of proteins termed receptor activity–modifying proteins (RAMPs) and comprises three members, RAMPs1 to 3.[23] RAMPs interact with a distinct calcitonin receptor-like receptor (CRLR) and transports it to the cell-membrane surface.[24] RAMP1 transport of CRLR results in a terminally glycosylated receptor that recognizes CGRP, whereas RAMP2 and 3 expression produces a core glycosylated receptor that recognizes adrenomedullin. Receptor modulation is another molecular mechanism of genetic economy whereby specific ligands can acquire functions beyond those allowed by a simple lock-and-key model of receptor specificity.[23,25]

ROLE OF CT IN MINERAL METABOLISM

The exact physiologic role of CT in calcium homeostasis and skeletal metabolism has not been established in humans, and many questions remain unanswered about the significance of this hormone in humans. Does CT secretion decline with age? Do gonadal steroids regulate the secretion of CT? Do the lower levels of serum CT in women contribute to the pathogenesis of age-related loss of bone mass and osteoporosis? Do extrathyroidal sources of CT participate in the regulation of skeletal metabolism? Are there primary and secondary abnormalities of CT secretion in diseases of skeletal and calcium homeostasis? The conclusive answers to these questions await clinical studies with an assay procedure that directly measures the biological activity of CT in blood. Furthermore, accurate local measurements of CT and its effects may be necessary to elucidate the emerging role of CT as a paracrine and autocrine agent.

REFERENCES

1. Deftos LJ, Sherman SI, Gagel RF 2001 Multiglandular endocrine disorders. In: Felig P, Frohman LA (eds.) Endocrinology and Metabolism, 4th ed. McGraw Hill, New York, NY, USA, pp. 1355–1382.
2. Inzerillo AM, Zaidi M, Huang CL 2002 Calcitonin: The other thyroid hormone. Thyroid 12:791–798.
3. Zaidi M, Inzerillo AM, Moonga BS, Bevis JR, Huang CL-H 2002 Forty years of calcitonin-where are we now? A tribute to the work of Iain MacIntyre, FRS. Bone 30:655–663.
4. Deftos LJ 1987 Pituitary cells secrete calcitonin in the reverse hemolytic plaque assay. Biochem Biophys Res Commun 146:1350–1356.
5. Deftos LJ, Weisman MH, Williams GH, Karpf DB, Frumar AM, Davidson BH, Parthemore JG, Judd HL 1980 Influence of age and sex on plasma calcitonin in human beings. N Engl J Med 302:1351–1353.
6. Wallach S, Farley JR, Baylink DJ, Brenne-Gati L 1993 Effects of calcitonin on bone quality and osteoblastic function. Calcif Tissue Int 52:335–339.
7. Silverman SL, Azria M 2002 The analgesic role of calcitonin following osteoporotic fracture. Osteoporos Int 13:858–867.
8. Austin LA, Heath H III 1981 Calcitonin-physiology and pathophysiology. N Engl J Med 304:269–278.
9. Parthemore JG, Deftos LJ 1979 Secretion of calcitonin in primary hyperparathyroidism. J Clin Endocrinol Metab 49:223–226.
10. Deftos LJ, Powell D, Parthemore JG, Potts JT Jr 1973 Secretion of calcitonin in hypocalcemic states in man. J Clin Invest 52:3109–3114.
11. Muller B, White JC, Nylen ES, Snider RH, Becker KL, Habene JF 2001 Ubiquitous expression of the calcitonin-i gene in multiple tissues in response to sepsis. J Clin Endocrinol Metab 86:396–404.
12. Tiegs RD, Body JJ, Barta JM, Health H III 1986 Secretion and metabolism of monomeric human calcitonin: Effects of age, sex, and thyroid damage. J Bone Miner Res 1:339–343.
13. Foresta C, Scanelli G, Zanatta GP, Busnardo B, Scandellari C 1987 Reduced calcitonin reserve in young hypogonadic osteoporotic men. Horm Metab Res 19:275–277.
14. Stevenson JC, White MC, Joplin GF, MacIntyre I 1982 Osteoporosis and calcitonin deficiency. BMJ 285:1010–1011.
15. Klein GL, Wadlington EL, Collins ED, Catherwood BD, Deftos LJ 1984 Calcitonin levels in sera of infants and children: Relations to age and periods of bone growth. Calcif Tissue Int 36:635–638.
16. Ivey JJ, Roos BA, Shen FH, Baylink DJ 1981 Increased immunoreactive calcitonin in idiopathic hypercalciuria. Metab Bone Dis Relat Res 3:29–32.
17. Taggart HM, Ivey JJ, Sisom K, Chestnut CH III, Baylink DJ, Huber MB 1982 Deficient calcitonin response to calcium stimulation in postmenopausal osteoporosis. Lancet 1:475–478.
18. Tiegs RD, Body JJ, Wahner HW, Barta J, Riggs BL, Heath H III 1985 Calcitonin secretion in postmenopausal osteoporosis. N Engl J Med 312:1097–2000.
19. Motyckova G, Fisher DE 2002 Pycnodysostosis: Role and regulation of cathepsis K in osteoclast function and human disease. Curr Mol Med 2:407–421.
20. Baker RK, Wallach S, Tashjian AH Jr 1973 Plasma calcitonin in pycnodysostosis: Intermittently high basal levels and exaggerated responses to calcium and glucagons infusions. J Clin Endocrinol Metab 37:46–55.
21. Deftos LJ 1997 There's something fishy and perhaps even fowl about the mammalian calcitonin receptor and its ligand. Endocrinology 138:519–520.
22. Cornish J, Naot D 2002 Amylin and adrenomedullin: Novel regulators of bone growth. Curr Pharm 8:2009–2021.
23. Deftos LJ, Roos BA, Oates EL 1999 Calcitonin. In: Favus MJ (ed.) Primer on the Metabolic Bone Diseases and Disorders of Mineral Metabolism, 4th ed. Lippincott Williams & Wilkins, Philadelphia, PA, USA, pp. 99–104.
24. Muff R, Born W, Fishcer JA 2001 Adrenomedullin and related peptides: Receptors and accessory proteins. Peptides 22:1765–1772.
25. Purdue BW, Tilakaratne N, Sexton PM 2002 Molecular pharmacology of the calcitonin receptor. Receptors Channels 8:243–255.

Clinical Evaluation of Bone and Mineral Disorders

Chapter 22.   History and Physical Examination

Peter M. Sklarin,[1] Dolores M. Shoback,[2] and Craig B. Langman[3]

[1]Menlo Medical Clinic, Menlo Park, California; [2]Departments of Medicine and Endocrine, Veterans Affairs Medical Center, and Department of Medicine, University of California, San Francisco, California; and [3]Department of Pediatrics, Northwestern University Medical School, and Department of Nephrology and Mineral Metabolism, Children's Memorial Hospital, Chicago, Illinois

INTRODUCTION

With the availability of treatments that can prevent, control, or cure most metabolic bone diseases, early recognition is essential. An experienced clinician can accurately diagnose many bone disorders by history and physical examination alone. Many of these diseases have a subtle and insidious onset and are not often recognized until they have reached a severe stage. The clinician's challenge, therefore, is not only early diagnosis of existing disease, but also the identification of patients at risk. A careful history and thorough physical examination are the physician's most powerful tools in choosing whom to screen with diagnostic tests and deciding which patients will benefit most from preventive intervention or therapy.[1,2]

MEDICAL HISTORY

For the adult, an initial assessment should include the patient's age, gender, race, menopausal status, and a complete medical, pharmacologic, nutritional, and family history. For the child, a careful maternal gestational history with an emphasis on perinatal or neonatal mortality, birth history, feeding history, and level of usual activity is warranted. In some situations, the chief complaint leads directly to the diagnosis: for example, a hip fracture from osteoporosis, bowing deformity of the legs from rickets, numbness and tingling around the mouth and in the tips of the fingers in a patient with hypocalcemia, or polyuria with hypercalcemia. Other factors may provide strong evidence that an unspecified bone disease is present and prompt the physician to explore further. For example, severe back or bone pain, history of fracture with minimal trauma, prolonged immobilization, loss of height in elderly people, and sunlight deprivation all raise the index of suspicion for the presence of skeletal disease. In children, additional features of growth retardation or short stature, bone pain, muscle weakness, skeletal deformities, extraskeletal calcifications,

and waddling gait are suggestive of the presence of metabolic bone disease.

The duration of symptoms also is important: are they lifelong or new? Does the diet contain adequate calcium, phosphorus, and vitamin D? If the diet is insufficient, is there adequate sunlight exposure? Does the patient engage in regular weight-bearing exercise? Does an adult or child with osteopenia engage in activities at play or work that involve a high risk of trauma? A drug history is of vital importance, because many medicines, including over-the-counter preparations, can adversely affect the skeleton. Glucocorticoids, whether inhaled, taken orally, or administered systematically, thyroid hormone, anticonvulsants, and heparin may cause or worsen osteoporosis. Current use of long-acting benzodiazepines and high caffeine intake may increase the risk of osteoporotic hip fracture. Excessive alcohol intake is associated with hypomagnesemia, nutritional deficiencies of calcium, vitamin D, and protein, reduced sunlight exposure, and tendency to fall. Alcohol ingestion also may directly impair osteoblast function. Antacids containing aluminum may lead to aluminum-induced bone disease, typically in the setting of renal insufficiency. Cancer chemotherapy, even years previously, may affect bone. Long-term lithium therapy is associated with hypercalcemia and parathyroid hormone (PTH) hypersecretion.[1] Prolonged use of sodium fluoride or the bisphosphonate etidronate can result in osteomalacia. Hypervitaminosis A is associated with excessive bone resorption and bone pain, and vitamin D excess can result in hypercalcemia. Gonadotropin-releasing hormone agonists induce an estrogen-deficient state when given in a continuous manner and may result in reduced bone mass. Diuretics can confound test interpretation by increasing or decreasing urine calcium or by increasing serum alkaline phosphatase activity.[2]

The patient should be asked about any history of endocrine, renal, or gastrointestinal disease. Hyper- and hypoparathyroidism, hyperthyroidism, Cushing's syndrome, and sex hormone deficiency all may affect bone remodeling. Gastrectomy or gastric stapling, intestinal-malabsorption syndromes, chronic obstructive biliary disease, and pancre-

---

Dr. Shoback has served as a consultant for Eli Lilly & Co., Merck, and Procter & Gamble.

atic insufficiency all can result in osteopenia. Children with cystic fibrosis or chronic cholestatic liver disease are prone to osteopenia.

Data from the Study of Osteoporotic Fractures (SOF), a multicenter cohort of 9709 white women aged 65 years or older, identified historical factors that help to predict hip fracture in older women.[3] This study suggested that the risk of hip fracture is higher among women who have had previous fractures of any type after age 50 years, women who rate their own health as fair or poor, and women who spend ≤4 h a day on their feet. Among the SOF cohort, investigators found that the more weight a woman had gained since age 25 years, the lower her risk of hip fracture. However, if a woman weighed less than she had at the age of 25 years, this doubled her risk of hip fractures. Women who were tall at the age of 25 years also had a greater risk.

Because many of the metabolic bone disorders are heritable, a careful family history is important for purposes of screening and educating those at risk, or for recommending genetic counseling. In the SOF cohort, women with a maternal history of hip fracture had a 2-fold increased risk of hip fracture, independent of bone mass, height, and weight.[3] In certain conditions, the diagnosis is firmly established when other family members are tested. For example, in X-linked hypophosphatemic rickets (also called vitamin D–resistant rickets), the presence of isolated hypophosphatemia in a heterozygous woman confirms the presence of the trait and its hereditary pattern.

PHYSICAL EXAMINATION

Height and weight should be measured in all patients, and head circumference in children younger than 3 years. A Tanner sexual-maturity rating should be given to all children and adolescents. The clinician should look specifically for any bony deformities or masses, leg-length inequality, vertebral tenderness, a surgical scar on the neck (suggesting previous thyroid or parathyroid surgery), and abnormal gait. Often a single physical finding leads to a specific diagnosis. Blue or gray sclerae suggest osteogenesis imperfecta. These patients also may have deafness, ligamentous laxity with joint hypermobility, diaphoresis, dental defects, and they may bruise easily. Café au lait spots are present in the McCune-Albright syndrome, soft-tissue or mesenchymal tumors in oncogenic rickets/osteomalacia, and premature loss of deciduous teeth in hypophosphatasia. Alopecia, ranging from sparse hair to total alopecia without eyelashes, occurs in two-thirds of kindreds with vitamin D–dependent rickets type II.

In rickets, a constellation of physical findings provides the diagnosis. The patient may have short stature, bony tenderness, softened skull (craniotabes), parietal flattening, and frontal bossing. There is often palpable enlargement of the costochondral junctions (the "rachitic rosary"), thickening of the wrists and ankles, flared wrists from metaphyseal widening, Harrison's groove (a horizontal depression along the lower border of the chest, corresponding to the costal insertions of the diaphragm), bowing deformity of the long bones from weight bearing, and waddling gait. The patient also may have reduced muscle strength and tone, lax liga-

ments, an indentation of the sternum in response to the force exerted by the diaphragm and intercostal muscles, delayed eruption of permanent teeth, and enamel defects. Rickets affect the most rapidly growing bone. Because the skull is growing rapidly at birth, craniotabes is found in congenital rickets. A rachitic rosary is prominent during the first year of life, when the rib cage grows rapidly. Late rickets, which occurs at the time of adolescent growth spurt, results in a knock-knee deformity. In infants and young children, listlessness and irritability are common. In infants, floppiness and hypotonia are characteristic. Associated syndromic features in children should be evaluated as well during the examination, including ocular and otic abnormalities.

Hypocalcemia is characterized by neuromuscular irritability. This may include varying degrees of tetany, which usually begins with numbness and tingling around the mouth and in the tips of the fingers, followed by muscle spasms in the extremities and face. There may be thumb adduction, metacarpophalangeal joint flexion, and interphalangeal joint extension. Latent tetany can be demonstrated by eliciting Chvostek's sign or Trousseau's sign. Chvostek's sign is spasm of facial muscles elicited by tapping the facial nerve in the region of the parotid gland, just anterior to the ear lobe, below the zygomatic arch, or between the zygomatic arch and the corner of the mouth. The response ranges from a twitching of the lip at the corner of the mouth to a twitching of all the facial muscles on the stimulated side. Slightly positive reactions may occur in up to 10–15% of normal adults; it is commonly present in neonates without evidence of pathology. To elicit Trousseau's sign, a sphygmomanometer is inflated on the arm to 20 mm above the systolic blood pressure for 2–5 minutes. A positive response consists of carpal spasm with relaxation occurring 5–10 s after the cuff is deflated. Relaxation should not be immediate. Both Chvostek's and Trousseau's signs can be absent, however, even in severe hypocalcemia.

In patients with idiopathic hypoparathyroidism, the physician should look for signs of the polyglandular failure syndromes: chronic mucocutaneous candidiasis, Addison's disease, alopecia, vitiligo, premature ovarian failure, diabetes mellitus, autoimmune thyroid disease, and pernicious anemia. Pseudohypoparathyroidism presents a constellation of signs, including those of long-standing hypocalcemia and hyperphosphatemia. Symptoms of tetany are common and include carpopedal spasm, tetanic convulsions, paresthesias, muscle cramps, and stridor. There may be soft-tissue calcifications, and posterior subcapsular cataracts develop frequently. Albright's hereditary osteodystrophy refers to a constellation of findings seen in pseudohypoparathyroidism or pseudo-pseudohypoparathyroidism. It includes round facies, short stature, obesity, shortening of the digits (brachydactyly), subcutaneous ossification, and dental hypoplasia. Many patients are mentally retarded. A characteristic shortening of the fourth and fifth digits can be recognized as dimpling over the knuckles of a clenched fist (Archibald's sign).

Most patients with primary hyperparathyroidism usually have no abnormal physical findings. Enlarged parathyroid glands are usually palpable only when parathyroid carcinoma is present, and band keratopathy (calcium-phosphate deposition in the medial and lateral limbic margins of the cornea) is seen rarely and usually only by slit-lamp examination. Extreme elevations of serum calcium may produce an altered sensorium, hypertension, and nonspecific abdominal pain.

Patients with renal osteodystrophy often have characteristic physical findings. Spontaneous tendon rupture may occur in patients with advanced renal failure, almost always in association with marked secondary hyperparathyroidism. Bone deformities are common, especially in patients with severe aluminum toxicity. A funnel-chest abnormality may be produced by rib deformities and kyphoscoliosis. Pseudo-clubbing may result from enlargement of the distal tufts of the fingers as a result of osteitis fibrosa. Bowing of long bones, genu valgum, and ulnar deviation of the wrist may be seen in children before epiphyseal closure has occurred, and slipped epiphyses may occur in the periadolescent period.

Patients with Paget's disease usually have no signs of the disease. Over many years, however, progressive cranial involvement can produce increased head size, whereas bowing and enlargement of the long bones may occur with disease of the femur and tibia. Slowly progressive hearing loss, vertigo, tinnitus, or a combination of these can occur in up to 25% of patients with skull involvement. Commonly, there is redness with increased skin temperature over an affected bone. Defects in Bruch's membrane of the retina, termed angioid streaks, may be observed in about 10% of patients. Deformity of the facial bones (leontiasis ossea) may be seen in Paget's disease but is more common in fibrous dysplasia.

Patients with established osteoporosis often exhibit dorsal kyphosis or a gibbus (dowager's hump) and loss of height. They may have a protuberant abdomen (that the patient may confuse with obesity), ribs within the pelvic rim that may be bruised, paravertebral muscle spasm, and thin skin (McConkey's sign). The clinician should look for signs of secondary causes of osteoporosis (e.g., hypogonadism, Cushing's syndrome). In the SOF, four physical findings indicated an increased risk of hip fracture: the inability to rise from a chair without using one's arms, a resting pulse rate of >80 beats/min, poor depth perception, and poorer low-frequency contrast sensitivity.[3] By combining these clinical findings with a careful history, assessment of risk factors, and bone density measurement, it may be possible to make a good assessment of hip fracture risk.

With the availability of sophisticated diagnostic techniques to assess bone density and remodeling, the clinician is faced with new and difficult decisions about test interpretation and resource allocation. A complete history and physical examination continue to be the clinician's most important guides, often providing crucial clues to the origin of skeletal disorders in children and adults.

REFERENCES

1. Bilezikian JP, Marcus R, Levine MA (eds.) 2001 The Parathyroids: Basic and Clinical Concepts. Academic Press, San Diego, CA, USA.
2. DeGroot LJ, Jameson JL (eds.) 2001 Endocrinology, 4th ed. WB Saunders, Philadelphia, PA, USA.
3. Cummings SR, Nevitt MC, Browner WS, Stone K, Fox KM, Ensrud KE, Cauley J, Black D, Vogt TM 1995 Risk factors for hip fracture in white women: Study of Osteoporotic Fractures Research Group. N Engl J Med 322:767–773.

Chapter 23.   Fractures: Evaluation and Clinical Implications

Julie T. Lin,[1] Marjolein C. H. van der Meulen,[1,2] Elizabeth R. Myers,[1] and Joseph M. Lane[1]

[1]Hospital for Special Surgery, Metabolic Bone Disease Service, New York, New York; and [2]Mechanical and Aerospace Engineering, Cornell University, Ithaca, New York

INTRODUCTION

Osteoporotic fractures are a serious problem with many adverse consequences. Of the 1.5 million osteoporotic fractures that occur each year, 700,000 are vertebral fractures and 300,000 are hip fractures. Vertebral fractures can result in substantial skeletal deformity, pain, and functional limitations. Hip fractures are one of the most significant osteoporotic fractures because of their high morbidity and mortality. While medical management with anti-osteoporotic therapy such as bisphosphonates and parathyroid hormone can improve bone strength, medication management does not address the other contributing factors and only provides partial protection. Therapies that include fall prevention and the use of hip protectors show potential to effectively minimize the risk of falling and the risk of sustaining hip fracture after the fall, respectively. This chapter will address osteoporotic fracture etiology, fracture prevention strategies, and principles of fracture management.

FRACTURE ETIOLOGY: FACTOR OF RISK

Fractures of load-bearing structures, such as the skeleton, occur under two different circumstances: after repetitive loading and the accumulation of damage and after a single traumatic overload that exceeds the failure capacity of the structure. To understand the etiology of bone fracture, information is needed on the interplay between the load-bearing capacity of a bone at risk and the loads imposed onto that same bone. This idea can be captured in the *factor of risk*,[1] which is the ratio of the load applied to the bone over the load necessary to cause fracture. The factor of risk

The authors have no conflict of interest.

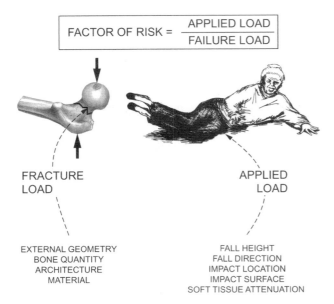

$$\text{FACTOR OF RISK} = \frac{\text{APPLIED LOAD}}{\text{FAILURE LOAD}}$$

FRACTURE LOAD

EXTERNAL GEOMETRY
BONE QUANTITY
ARCHITECTURE
MATERIAL

APPLIED LOAD

FALL HEIGHT
FALL DIRECTION
IMPACT LOCATION
IMPACT SURFACE
SOFT TISSUE ATTENUATION

FIG. 1. Example of determinants of factor of risk for the proximal femur under side impact.

can be conceptualized for either repetitive loading (fatigue) or single loading events. Most research to date has focused on the factor of risk for single loading events such as falls (see example in Fig. 1). For single events, if the applied load is much greater than the load necessary to cause fracture (factor of risk is much greater than one), bony failure will most likely occur. The applied loads are a function of activity at the time of fracture and conditions that transfer loads to the skeleton. The load necessary to cause fracture, which is the bone *failure load*, is determined by characteristics related to bone structure and content.

Determinants of Bone Failure Load

Osteoporotic fractures occur most commonly at anatomic sites with substantial volumes of cancellous bone, including the spine, hip, and forearm. To understand why fracture occurs after a single traumatic event, we need to consider the features of whole bones and the properties of cortical and cancellous bone that contribute to the load-bearing capacity of the hip and spine.

The ability of any load-bearing object to carry applied loads without failure is a function of several contributing factors.[2] At the whole bone level, the ability of a vertebra or femur to bear loads depends on the properties of the constituent material and how and where this material is located (bone geometry). At sites of osteoporotic fractures, the constituent material is generally cancellous bone, a complex structure in its own right.

If one removes a small cube of cancellous bone and applies forces to the surface, failure will be determined by how much material is present (bone quantity), where this material is distributed (architecture), and what the properties of the material are (tissue composition) (Fig. 2). The role of bone quantity in load-bearing has been studied extensively, as has architecture to a lesser degree; the rela-

tionship of tissue material properties to failure is the least well understood.

The volume of tissue contained within a region of cancellous bone is the bone volume fraction; similarly, the mass of bone tissue within the region is the apparent density. Cancellous apparent density is strongly related to load-bearing capacity and failure; the ultimate stress (failure load per cross-sectional area) is approximately proportional to the square of apparent density[3] (see review by ref. 4). However, two regions of similar apparent density can differ substantially in ultimate stress as a result of material architecture. The ultimate stress is generally greater when loading occurs along the direction of preferential trabecular orientation. In the lumbar vertebrae, the primary orientation is superior-inferior, and the ultimate stress along the superior-inferior direction is double the ultimate stress in the medial-lateral or anterior-posterior directions.[5] Correlations between trabecular architecture and failure properties are difficult to establish in sites with locally variable architecture, and many different measures are necessary to adequately characterize trabecular morphology. As our ability to image cancellous tissue in three-dimensions improves, so will our understanding of the architectural parameters relevant to fracture.

The final consideration in cancellous failure is the material properties of the tissue. Compositional changes in mineral content (such as osteomalacia) and matrix collagen cross-linking (such as osteogenesis imperfecta) are known to impact mechanical properties in well-controlled circumstances. However, precise relationships to failure load are not known at this time.

In the clinic, current in vivo imaging techniques cannot capture cancellous bone volume fraction and architecture. Therefore, assessment of failure properties must occur at the whole bone level and incorporate the above considerations

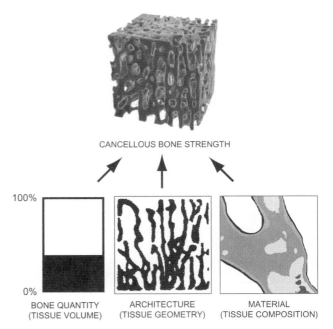

CANCELLOUS BONE STRENGTH

100%

0%

BONE QUANTITY
(TISSUE VOLUME)

ARCHITECTURE
(TISSUE GEOMETRY)

MATERIAL
(TISSUE COMPOSITION)

FIG. 2. Contributors to cancellous loading bearing ability include bone quantity, architecture, and material.

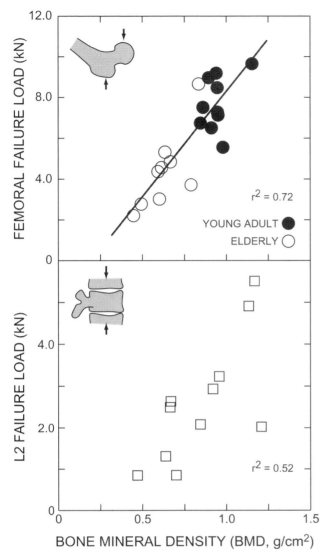

FIG. 3. Relationships between BMD and fracture load of the proximal femur and L2 vertebra. (Adapted from Courtney et al.[7] and Moro et al.[8])

of cancellous load-bearing capacity. Areal bone mineral density (BMD; g/cm^2), measured by DXA, is a single measure that captures both mineral content and bone size.[6] Because both material and geometric considerations impact failure, this integral measure does predict bone failure load. Laboratory tests of the proximal femur and lumbar vertebra show good correlation between failure load and DXA-measured BMD[7,8] (Fig. 3). As demonstrated in Fig. 3, the denominator of the factor of risk decreases as BMD decreases. This results in a higher factor of risk for a given set of loading conditions. In prospective clinical studies, there is considerable evidence that low BMD is associated with increased fracture rates for the hip and spine.[9,10]

Determinants of Applied Loads

Characterizing applied loads is difficult and depends on many factors. For hip fractures, which are most often associated with falls,[11] the magnitude and direction of the applied loads depend on the type of fall. Falls from standing height or higher have an increased risk of hip fracture compared with falls from lower heights.[12,13] In case-control studies, falls to the side with impact on or near the hip are strongly associated with hip fracture in both nursing home and community-dwelling elderly.[13–15]

Predictions of femoral peak impact forces for falls to the side from standing height have been extrapolated from experiments using human subjects in a pelvis-release configuration (a drop onto the side from a very small height).[16] Predictions of impact force range from 5000 to 12,500 N, which can be compared with values for femoral failure load of 2000–8000 N (Fig. 3). Thus, the factor of risk could easily be greater than one for this potentially harmful type of fall. Consequently, for elderly fallers, in whom femoral BMD is often low, falling from standing height, to the side, and impacting the hip are important contributing factors to hip fracture (Fig. 1).

Loads transmitted to the femur during impact depend on the impact surface and on attenuating properties of overlying soft tissues. Falling onto a hard surface is significantly

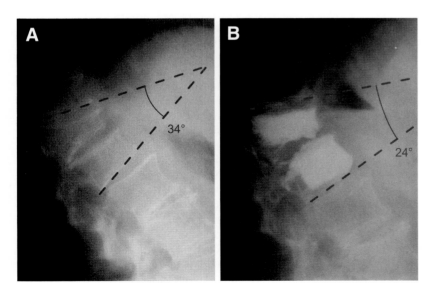

FIG. 4. Radiographs of lumbar spine before and after kyphoplasty. (A) Fractured vertebral bodies with 34° kyphotic angle indicated. (B) Vertebral bodies after restoration of height by kyphoplasty with 24° kyphotic angle indicated.

associated with hip fractures.[12] Low body mass index (BMI), which correlates with decreased soft tissue thickness over the greater trochanter and therefore decreased attenuation,[17,18] is positively associated with hip fracture rates.[11,15,19] As a result, for fallers with low levels of femoral BMD, hard impact surfaces and thin overlying soft tissues pose additional risk for hip fracture (Fig. 1).

FRACTURE PREVENTION STRATEGIES

There are several basic approaches to preventing fractures that are associated with falls: averting the fall, decreasing the severity of a fall if one does occur, or maintaining or even increasing bone strength and failure load. Tactics to reduce the impact of harmful falls include exercise to strengthen critical muscles, energy-absorbing flooring, and trochanteric padding. Interventions such as fall prevention or hip protectors are the focus of this section. Pharmacologic agents, exercise, and nutrition are all interventions that show potential for increasing bone mass and load-bearing capacity. Medical and exercise interventions that affect bone properties are discussed elsewhere; a brief review is given below.

Fall Prevention

More than 90% of hip fractures occur as a result of falls.[11,20] Falls represent an increasingly prevalent problem, both in nursing homes and in the community. In nursing homes, there are 1.5 falls/person/year and 0.29 falls/person/year onto the hip, with 20% of the latter group resulting in hip fracture.[21] In the community, 30% of those over 65 years of age fall each year.[22–24]

There are multiple risk factors for falls, including being elderly (65 years or older); having muscle weakness, gait and balance problems, functional limitations, visual impairment, and cognitive impairment; side effects of medications; environmental factors; and history of previous falls. In addition, poor performance on neuromuscular function tests, including body sway and gait speed, is correlated with falls.[25,26]

Screening for fall risk in elderly patients may be performed in the office or in any motion analysis center/ physical therapy gym if available. A history of falls and predisposing factors to falls can provide important information about appropriate interventions. A targeted neurologic exam, such as decreased vibration, may indicate proprioceptive impairments.[27] Assessing gait can help to identify specific muscle group deficiencies, unsafe gait patterns, and the need for assistive devices such as walkers and canes. Screening tests can be performed to evaluate the risk of falls: timed single limb stance for balance,[28,29] timed get up and go for functional gait performance,[30] and functional reach to assess flexibility and balance.[31,32]

Specific interventions to identify predisposing factors and reduce falls include physical therapy, Tai Chi, home hazard assessment and modification, withdrawal of psychotropic medications, and a multidisciplinary, multifactorial, health/ environmental risk factor screening and intervention program.[33] Exercise programs, such as Tai Chi and physical therapy, can improve balance and muscle strength in the elderly, decreasing falls by 46%.[34,35] Evaluation of the home with surveillance for risks such as cluttered obstacles or throw rugs can help to reduce fall risk. Occupational therapist home visits targeted at environmental hazards and facilitation of necessary home modifications resulted in reduced fall risk.[36] Decreased falls may be a consequence of home modifications and behavior changes such as increased awareness of the environment. Medications, particularly psychotropic drugs, have been implicated in falls,[27,37] and withdrawal of medicine reduces the number of falls and fall risk.[38]

A multiple risk factor intervention strategy, combining many of the single interventions discussed above, has been shown to result in a significant reduction in risk of falling among elderly persons in the community with risk factors for falls. Elder community dwellers treated by a combination of medication, behavioral adjustment, and exercise had fewer falls after 1 year.[39] The Prevention of Falls in the Elderly Trial (PROFET) demonstrated the benefit of a detailed medical and occupational therapy assessment with referral to relevant services in elderly community dwellers with history of falls.[40] After 12 months, the intervention group had a reduced risk of falling, reduced risk of recurrent falls, and lower odds of admission to the hospital.

Strategies to Decrease Applied Loads

In addition to fall prevention, applied loads can be reduced by several strategies, including strengthening critical muscles and absorbing the energy of a fall with flooring or padding.

Hip protectors are designed to pad the hip and are a simple approach to prevent hip fractures if falls do occur. There have been several randomized, controlled trials that have demonstrated them to be cost-efficient and efficacious in certain high risk groups. The primary obstacle in their use remains compliance, which is typically less than 50%.

These orthoses, usually made of polypropylene or polyethylene, are most commonly sewn or placed in undergarments. They may be worn as undergarments or may be worn on top of underwear. There are several types of hip protectors available for use, few of which have been specifically subjected to randomized controlled trials. The most widely used hip protector in the United States is Safehip (Tytex Inc., Woonsocket, RI, USA), which has an outer shield of polypropylene with an inner Plastazote lining. The KPH hip protector (Respecta, Helsinki, Finland) is an undergarment with a pocket in each side into which a removable hip protector is placed. The KPH2, a variant, was used in the largest randomized controlled trial to date.[41] The High Impact Protection System (HIPS) hip protector (Quertrop Medical, Gentofte, Finland), similar in design to the KPH, consists of a removable inner and outer shell placed into an undergarment with specially designed pockets. The Hip-Guard is a hip protector belt worn over clothing.

The largest randomized controlled trial to date involving hip protectors was performed by Kannus et al.[41] Subjects in the hip protector group had significantly fewer fractures, with respective rates of hip fracture of 21.3 and 46.0 per 1000 person-years in the hip protector and control groups, respectively. Hip fracture risk was reduced 60% with the use of hip protectors and more than 80% when the protector was worn at the time of fall. However, a meta-analysis of seven trials using hip protectors did not find a statistically significant difference in fracture occurrence between those allocated to wear hip protectors and controls.[42] Therefore, the efficacy of hip protectors under controlled, intention-to-treat circumstances is still to be determined.

Hip protectors are cost-effective because of associated economic savings and gains in quality-adjusted life years.[43,44] They can also improve self-confidence. Hip protector users have less fear of falling (43% versus 57%, respectively, in hip protector wearers versus controls) and have greater improvements in falls self-efficacy (one's belief in his/her ability to avoid falling).[45] In addition, hip protector wearers are more confident about going out and are three times more likely to believe they are offered protection from hip fractures.[46]

Hip protector acceptance and compliance are important and potentially limiting factors to successful implementation. Acceptance rates of subjects asked to use hip protectors in clinical trials can be as low as 69%.[47] Compliance rates are even lower, such as the 48% compliance rate reported by Kannus et al.[41] and the median rate of 57% reported by van Schoor et al.[47] in a review of previous studies. Patient noncompliance is attributed to complaints about the physical aspects of the hip protectors,[47] including their bulkiness, heat, tightness of waistband, and plastic cover[46]; the extra effort needed to wear them[48]; and difficulties in putting them on and taking them off.[46]

Appropriate candidates for hip protectors include those patients at risk for fall, osteoporotic patients, patients with fear of falling, and especially patients with prior hip fracture. Compliance remains the main obstacle to the successful use of hip protectors. Strategies to improve compliance include patient education, emphasizing the risks of fall, emphasizing greater freedom and quality of life, and providing constant reinforcement and positive feedback.

Strategies to Increase Bone Failure Load

Bone failure strength relates to bone quantity, architecture, and tissue composition. Calcium, vitamin D, estrogens, selective estrogen receptor modulators (SERMs), calcitonin, bisphosphonates, and parathyroid hormone (PTH) all alter bone failure strength in a positive fashion. With medical therapeutics, osteoporotic fracture risk is diminished and mechanical properties are enhanced. Before peak bone mass is achieved, appropriate nutrition and exercise can maximize peak bone strength. Compared with young adults, menopause and aging lead to less skeletal capacity to withstand loads and adversely affects factor of risk even in the presence of anti-osteoporotic therapy. The rationale and efficacy of drug treatments to prevent and manage osteoporotic patients is discussed elsewhere in this Primer.

FRACTURE MANAGEMENT AND TREATMENT

If the above measures are not successful, osteoporotic fractures can result. Orthopedic surgical management for the repair of osteoporotic fractures commonly results in failure of internal fixation. Mineral density of the involved bone directly relates to the holding strength of the internal fixation. Consequently, osteoporotic bone often lacks the strength to maintain the devices. The plate and screw fixation, when applied to fractures of the proximal and distal femur, have failure rates ranging from 10% to 25%, resulting from screw loosening and cut outs. The traditional technique of internal fixation must be altered to achieve success in osteoporotic bone by load sharing.

In most cases, osteoporotic patients are healthiest on the day of injury and are usually in the best condition to undergo surgery within the first 48 h after injury.[49,50] However, the judicious preoperative management to reverse medical decompensation causing or resulting from injury benefits survival.[50] The aim of the operative intervention is to achieve stable fracture fixation to permit early return to function and weight bearing. Although anatomic restoration is important for intra-articular fractures, metaphyseal and diaphyseal fractures are best managed by efforts to primarily achieve stability rather than anatomic reduction.

The primary mode of failure in internal fixation in osteoporotic bone is bone failure rather than implant breakage. Because BMD correlates linearly with the holding power of screws, osteoporotic bone often lacks the strength to hold plates and screws securely.[51–53] Traditionally, surgeons have resorted to cancellous bone grafting to augment or ensure rapid and complete healing of fractures. In osteoporotic bone, bone grafting plays several important roles including providing osteoinductive, osteoconductive, and osteogenic properties[54] and will stimulate new bone formation periosteally as well as in fracture gaps created by comminution.

The donor source for autogenous bone graft is usually the iliac crest. There is significant morbidity[55] and often the quantity and quality is not available or is insufficient. Thus, bone graft substitutes can provide an attractive alternative for autogenous graft in osteoporotic patients.[56] Bone graft substitutes include allograft bone, demineralized allograft bone products, and synthetic osteoconductive materials that can be used as bone void fillers. Several of these products have been demonstrated to be useful as alternatives to autogenous graft in treating acute fractures.[57,58] A comprehensive discussion of the orthopedic treatment of common osteoporotic appendicular fractures is provided elsewhere.

Vertebral fractures account for almost 50% of osteoporotic fractures. Only 250,000 of 700,000 are clinically symptomatic.[59,60] Of these fractures, falls account for 50%, lifting objects for 20%, and no recognized event in 30%.[61] Patients with multiple vertebral fractures have a 23–37% increased mortality rate depending on fracture severity and number of levels involved.[59,60] Traditional treatment consists of analgesics, osteoporotic medicine, bedrest, hyperextension braces, and physical therapy. In patients with persistent pain or evidence of ongoing collapse, the minimally invasive spine procedures vertebroplasty and kyphoplasty may be appropriate.[62,63]

Vertebroplasty uses direct bone cement injection into the vertebral body through a pedicular or extrapedicular approach under fluoroscopic control.[64–68] Eighty percent of patients show significant pain relief, and there is no further collapse of the vertebral body. No attempt is made to correct the kyphotic deformity or restoration of vertebral height and this high-pressure procedure may be associated with increased cement leakage[69] and possible acute respiratory distress syndrome (ARDS).

Kyphoplasty uses a balloon tamp to create a cavity and reduce the fracture. Once the cavity has been achieved, the low-pressure cementation may occur, which maintains the fracture reduction and the enhanced vertebral height. Again, pain relief is reported in 80–90% of patients, with a significant improvement in SF-36, some restoration of height in 80% of patients, and partial correction of the kyphosis.[62,69,70] There is a lower risk of cement leakage, and major complications occur very rarely.[71] The low complication rate is in part caused by the low-pressure fill of the bone void.

To date, vertebroplasty and kyphoplasty clearly lead to pain relief in cohort studies.[69] However, there have been no published randomized, controlled trials comparing cement reconstruction with standard palliative care or comparing vertebroplasty with kyphoplasty. With the lack of control groups, there is no definitive illustration of efficacy, and complete understanding of risk and benefit awaits additional studies. Therefore, the relative value of the two procedures remains to be determined by prospective randomized trials.[62] In addition, it is uncertain whether methylmethacrylate or hydroxyapatite-based ceramics should be used.[72] Nevertheless, these modes of therapy offer marked pain relief for the osteoporotic patient with vertebral fracture.[62,63]

While the acute fracture is addressed, often the underlying osteoporosis is neither diagnosed nor treated. However, a fragility fracture has a high correlation with the presence of underlying osteoporosis. Numerous studies of patients with Colles and hip fractures have documented the disconnect between surgical treatment of an osteoporotic fracture and therapeutic treatment of the underlying osteoporosis.

REFERENCES

1. Hayes WC, Myers ER, Robinovitch SN, van den Kroonenberg A, Courtney AC, McMahon TA 1996 Etiology and prevention of age-related hip fractures. Bone 18:77S–86S.
2. van der Meulen MC, Jepsen KJ, Mikic B 2001 Understanding bone strength: Size isn't everything. Bone 29:101–104.
3. Carter DR, Hayes WC 1977 The compressive behavior of bone as a two-phase porous structure. J Bone Jt Surg Am 59:954–962.
4. Keaveny TM 2001 Strength of trabecular bone. In: Cowin SC (ed.) Bone Mechanics Handbook, 2nd ed. CRC Press, Boca Raton, FL, USA, pp. 16-1–16-42.
5. Galante J, Rostoker W, Ray RD 1970 Physical properties of trabecular bone. Calcif Tissue Res 5:236–246.
6. Carter DR, Bouxsein ML, Marcus R 1992 New approaches for interpreting projected bone densitometry data. J Bone Miner Res 7:137–145.
7. Courtney AC, Wachtel EF, Myers ER, Hayes WC 1995 Age-related reductions in the strength of the femur tested in a fall-loading configuration. J Bone Joint Surg Am 77:387–395.
8. Moro M, Hecker AT, Bouxsein ML, Myers ER 1995 Failure load of thoracic vertebrae correlates with lumbar bone mineral density measured by DXA. Calcif Tissue Int 56:206–209.
9. Cummings SR, Bates D, Black DM 2002 Clinical use of bone densitometry: Scientific review. JAMA 288:1889–1897.
10. Marshall D, Johnell O, Wedel H 1996 Meta-analysis of how well measures of bone mineral density predicts occurrence of osteoporotic fractures. BMJ 312:1254–1259.
11. Grisso JA, Kelsey JL, Strom BL, Chiu GY, Maislin G, O'Brien LA, Hoffman S, Kaplan F 1991 Risk factors for falls as a cause of hip fracture in women. The Northeast Hip Fracture Study Group. N Engl J Med 324:1326–1331.
12. Grisso JA, Capezuti A, Schwartz A 1996 Falls as risk factors for fractures. In: Marcus R, Feldman D, Kelsey J (eds.) Osteoporosis. Academic Press, San Diego, CA, USA, pp. 599–611.
13. Hayes WC, Myers ER, Morris JM, Gerhart TN, Yett HS, Lipsitz LA 1993 Impact near the hip dominates fracture risk in elderly nursing home residents who fall. Calcif Tissue Int 52:192–198.
14. Nevitt MC, Cummings SR 1993 Type of fall and risk of hip and wrist fractures: The study of osteoporotic fractures. The Study of Osteoporotic Fractures Research Group. J Am Geriatr Soc 41:1226–1234.
15. Greenspan SL, Myers ER, Maitland LA, Resnick NM, Hayes WC 1994 Fall severity and bone mineral density as risk factors for hip fracture in ambulatory elderly. JAMA 271:128–133.
16. Robinovitch SN, Hayes WC, McMahon TA 1991 Prediction of femoral impact forces in falls on the hip. J Biomech Eng 113:366–374.
17. Maitland LA, Myers ER, Hipp JA, Hayes WC, Greenspan SL 1993 Read my hips: Measuring trochanteric soft tissue thickness. Calcif Tissue Int 52:85–89.
18. Robinovitch SN, McMahon TA, Hayes WC 1995 Force attenuation in trochanteric soft tissues during impact from a fall. J Orthop Res 13:956–962.
19. Pruzansky ME, Turano M, Luckey M, Senie R 1989 Low body weight as a risk factor for hip fractures in both black and white women. J Orthop Res 7:192–197.
20. Hedlund R, Lindgren U 1987 Trauma type, age, and gender as determinants of hip fracture. J Orthop Res 5:242–246.
21. Lauritzen JB 1996 Hip fractures: Incidence, risk factors, energy absorption, and prevention. Bone 18:65S–75S.
22. Blake AJ, Morgan K, Bendall MJ, Dallosso H, Ebrahim SB, Arie TH, Fentem PH, Bassey EJ 1988 Falls by elderly people at home: Prevalence and associated factors. Age Ageing 17:365–372.
23. Campbell AJ, Borrie MJ, Spears GF 1989 Risk factors for falls in a community-based prospective study of people 70 years and older. J Gerontol 44:M112–M117.
24. Tinetti ME, Speechley M, Ginter SF 1988 Risk factors for falls among elderly persons living in the community. N Engl J Med 319:1701–1707.
25. Lord SR, Clark RD, Webster IW 1991 Postural stability and associated physiological factors in a population of aged persons. J Gerontol 46:M69–M76.
26. Lord SR, Sambrook PN, Gilbert C, Kelly PJ, Nguyen T, Webster IW, Eisman JA 1994 Postural stability, falls and fractures in the elderly: Results from the Dubbo Osteoporosis Epidemiology Study. Med J Aust 160:688–691.
27. Tinetti ME 2003 Clinical practice. Preventing falls in elderly persons. N Engl J Med 348:42–49.
28. Birmingham TB 2000 Test-retest reliability of lower extremity functional instability measures. Clin J Sport Med 10:264–268.
29. Franchignoni F, Tesio L, Martino MT, Ricupero C 1998 Reliability of four simple, quantitative tests of balance and mobility in healthy elderly females. Aging (Milano) 10:26–31.
30. Podsiadlo D, Richardson S 1991 The timed "Up & Go": A test of basic functional mobility for frail elderly persons. J Am Geriatr Soc 39:142–148.
31. Duncan PW, Weiner DK, Chandler J, Studenski S 1990 Functional reach: A new clinical measure of balance. J Gerontol 45:M192–M197.
32. Weiner DK, Duncan PW, Chandler J, Studenski SA 1992 Functional reach: A marker of physical frailty. J Am Geriatr Soc 40:203–207.
33. Gillespie LD, Gillespie WJ, Robertson MC, Lamb SE, Cumming RG, Rowe BH 2001 Interventions for preventing falls in elderly people. Cochrane Database Syst Rev 3:CD000340.
34. Wolf SL, Barnhart HX, Kutner NG, McNeely E, Coogler C, Xu T 1996 Reducing frailty and falls in older persons: An investigation of Tai Chi and computerized balance training. Atlanta FICSIT Group. Frailty and Injuries: Cooperative Studies of Intervention Techniques. J Am Geriatr Soc 44:489–497.
35. Robertson MC, Gardner MM, Devlin N, McGee R, Campbell AJ 2001 Effectiveness and economic evaluation of a nurse delivered home exercise programme to prevent falls. 2: Controlled trial in multiple centres. BMJ 322:701–704.
36. Cumming RG, Thomas M, Szonyi G, Salkeld G, O'Neill E, Westbury C, Frampton G 1999 Home visits by an occupational therapist for assessment and modification of environmental hazards: A randomized trial of falls prevention. J Am Geriatr Soc 47:1397–1402.

37. Cumming R 1998 Epidemiology of medication-related falls and fractures in the elderly. Drugs Aging **12:**43–53.

38. Campbell AJ, Robertson MC, Gardner MM, Norton RN, Buchner DM 1999 Psychotropic medication withdrawal and a home-based exercise program to prevent falls: A randomized, controlled trial. J Am Geriatr Soc **47:**850–853.

39. Tinetti ME, Baker DI, McAvay G, Claus EB, Garrett P, Gottschalk M, Koch ML, Trainor K, Horwitz RI 1994 A multifactorial intervention to reduce the risk of falling among elderly people living in the community. N Engl J Med **331:**821–827.

40. Close J, Ellis M, Hooper R, Glucksman E, Jackson S, Swift C 1999 Prevention of falls in the elderly trial (PROFET): A randomised controlled trial. Lancet **353:**93–97.

41. Kannus P, Parkkari J, Niemi S, Pasanen M, Palvanen M, Jarvinen M, Vuori I 2000 Prevention of hip fracture in elderly people with use of a hip protector. N Engl J Med **343:**1506–1513.

42. Parker MJ, Gillespie LD, Gillespie WJ 2001 Hip protectors for preventing hip fractures in the elderly. Cochrane Database Syst Rev **2:**CD001255.

43. Colon-Emeric CS, Datta SK, Matchar DB 2003 An economic analysis of external hip protector use in ambulatory nursing facility residents. Age Ageing **32:**47–52.

44. Segui-Gomez M, Keuffel E, Frick KD 2002 Cost and effectiveness of hip protectors among the elderly. Int J Technol Assess Health Care **18:**55–66.

45. Cameron ID, Stafford B, Cumming RG, Birks C, Kurrle SE, Lockwood K, Quine S, Finnegan T, Salkeld G 2000 Hip protectors improve falls self-efficacy. Age Ageing **29:**57–62.

46. McAughey JM, McAdoo M 2002 Hip protectors. Acceptability of hip protectors was 35% at six months in the community. BMJ **324:**1454.

47. van Schoor NM, Devillé WL, Bouter LM, Lips P 2002 Acceptance and compliance with external hip protectors: A systematic review of the literature. Osteoporos Int **13:**917–924.

48. Cameron ID, Quine S 1994 Likely noncompliance with external hip protectors: Findings from focus groups. Arch Gerontol Geriatr Suppl **19:**273–281.

49. Aharonoff GB, Koval KJ, Skovron ML, Zuckerman JD 1997 Hip fractures in the elderly: Predictors of one year mortality. J Orthop Trauma **11:**162–165.

50. Kenzora JE, McCarthy RE, Lowell JD, Sledge CB 1984 Hip fracture mortality. Relation to age, treatment, preoperative illness, time of surgery, and complications. Clin Orthop **186:**45–56.

51. Sjostedt A, Zetterberg C, Hansson T, Hult E, Ekstrom L 1994 Bone mineral content and fixation strength of femoral neck fractures. A cadaver study. Acta Orthop Scand **65:**161–165.

52. Stromsoe KW, Hoiseth A, Alho A 1993 Holding power of the 4.5 mm AO/ASIF cortex screw in cortical bone in relation to bone mineral. Injury **24:**656–659.

53. Alho A 1993 Mineral and mechanics of bone fragility fractures. A review of fixation methods. Acta Orthop Scand **64:**227–232.

54. Aronson J, Cornell CH 1999 Bone healing and grafting. In: Beaty SH (ed.) Orthopaedic Knowledge Update 6. American Academy of Orthopaedic Surgeons, Rosemont, IL, USA, pp. 25–36.

55. Younger EM, Chapman MW 1989 Morbidity at bone graft donor sites. J Orthop Trauma **3:**192–194.

56. Gazdag AR, Lane JM, Glaser D, Forster RA 1995 Alternatives to autogenous bone graft: Efficacy and indications. J Am Acad Orthop Surg **3:**1–8.

57. Bucholz RW, Carlton A, Holmes R 1989 Interporous hydroxyapatite as a bone graft substitute in tibial plateau fractures. Clin Orthop **240:**53–62.

58. Chapman MW, Bucholz R, Cornell C 1997 Treatment of acute fractures with a collagen-calcium phosphate graft material. A randomized clinical trial. J Bone Joint Surg Am **79:**495–502.

59. Cooper C, Melton L Jr 1992 Vertebral fractures. BMJ **304:**1634–1635.

60. Kado DM, Browner WS, Palermo L, Nevitt MC, Genant HK, Cummings SR 1999 Vertebral fractures and mortality in older women: A prospective study. Study of Osteoporotic Fractures Research Group. Arch Intern Med **159:**1215–1220.

61. Myers ER, Wilson SE 1997 Biomechanics of osteoporosis and vertebral fracture. Spine **22:**25S–31S.

62. Watts NB, Harris ST, Genant HK 2001 Treatment of painful osteoporotic vertebral fractures with percutaneous vertebroplasty or kyphoplasty. Osteoporos Int **12:**429–437.

63. Garfin SR, Yuan HA, Reiley MA 2001 New technologies in spine: Kyphoplasty and vertebroplasty for the treatment of painful osteoporotic compression fractures. Spine **26:**1511–1515.

64. Deramond H, Depriester C, Galibert P, Le Gars D 1998 Percutaneous vertebroplasty with polymethylmethacrylate. Technique, indications, and results. Radiol Clin North Am **36:**533–546.

65. Gangi A, Kastler BA, Dietemann JL 1994 Percutaneous vertebroplasty guided by a combination of CT and fluoroscopy. Am J Neuroradiol **15:**83–86.

66. Grados F, Depriester C, Cayrolle G, Hardy N, Deramond H, Fardellone P 2000 Long-term observations of vertebral osteoporotic fractures treated by percutaneous vertebroplasty. Rheumatology (Oxford) **39:**1410–1414.

67. Jensen ME, Evans AJ, Mathis JM, Kallmes DF, Cloft HJ, Dion JE 1997 Percutaneous polymethylmethacrylate vertebroplasty in the treatment of osteoporotic vertebral body compression fractures: Technical aspects. Am J Neuroradiol **18:**1897–1904.

68. Cortet B, Cotten A, Boutry N, Flipo RM, Duquesnoy B, Chastanet P, Delcambre B 1999 Percutaneous vertebroplasty in the treatment of osteoporotic vertebral compression fractures: An open prospective study. J Rheumatol **26:**2222–2228.

69. Lieberman IH, Dudeney S, Reinhardt MK, Bell G 2001 Initial outcome and efficacy of "kyphoplasty" in the treatment of painful osteoporotic vertebral compression fractures. Spine **6:**1631–1638.

70. Lane JM, Johnson DE, Khan SN, Girardi FP, Cammisa FP 2002 Minimally invasive options for the treatment of osteoporotic vertebral compression fractures. Orthop Clin North Am **33:**431–438.

71. Phillips FM, Todd Wetzel F, Campbell-Hupp M 2002 An in vivo comparison of the potential for extravertebral cement leak after vertebroplasty and kyphoplasty. Spine **27:**2173–2178.

72. Bostrom MP, Lane JM 1997 Future directions. Augmentation of osteoporotic vertebral bodies. Spine **22:**38S–42S.

Chapter 24. Blood Calcium, Phosphorus, and Magnesium

Anthony A. Portale

Department of Pediatrics, University of California at San Francisco, San Francisco, California

SERUM CALCIUM CONCENTRATION

Calcium exists in serum in one of three forms: protein-bound calcium (40%), which is not filtered by the renal glomerulus, and ionized (48%) and complexed calcium (12%), which are filtered.[1] Complexed calcium is that bound to various anions such as phosphate, citrate, and bicarbonate. For clinical purposes, the total serum calcium concentration is the most commonly evaluated index of calcium status; however, the blood ionized calcium concentration provides a more precise estimate of an individual's calcium status, particularly in critically ill patients.

Total Calcium Concentration

Albumin accounts for 90% of the protein binding of calcium in serum; globulins account for the remainder.

The author has no conflict of interest.

TABLE 1. CHARACTERISTICS OF THE CIRCADIAN RHYTHMS IN BLOOD MINERAL CONCENTRATION IN HUMANS

	Concentration (mg/dl)		Amplitude (mg/dl)	Phase (h)	
	Fasting	24-h mean	(Nadir to peak)	Nadir	Peak
Total serum calcium	9.6	9.4	0.5	0300	1300
Blood ionized calcium	4.67	4.52	0.3	1900	1000
Serum phosphorus	3.6	4.0	1.2	1100	0200

Data are from references 4 and 17.

Calcium binds to anionic carboxylate groups on the albumin molecule, and fewer than 20% of the binding sites are occupied in normal serum. Conditions that change the serum concentration of albumin will affect the measured total calcium concentration, and under such circumstances, the total calcium concentration might not accurately reflect the calcium status of the patient. For example, in patients with nephrotic syndrome or hepatic cirrhosis, in whom the serum albumin concentration is decreased, the total calcium concentration will decrease, whereas the ionized calcium concentration may not change. Several algorithms or nomograms have been developed to correct the total calcium concentration for abnormal values of total protein or albumin or to estimate the "free" calcium concentration.[2] However, such algorithms do not precisely estimate the free calcium concentration and incorrectly predict the calcium status in 20–30% of subjects, as judged from measurement of ionized calcium concentration.[2] For routine clinical interpretation of serum calcium levels, the simplest formula to "correct" the total serum calcium concentration for changes in albumin concentration is the following[3]: for each 1 g/dl decrease in serum albumin concentration below 4.0 g/dl, add 0.8 mg/dl to the measured total calcium concentration; conversely, for each 1 g/dl increase in serum albumin concentration above 4.0 g/dl, subtract 0.8 mg/dl from the measured total calcium concentration. Because measurement of blood ionized calcium concentration is now widely available in clinical laboratories, the use of "corrected" values for total calcium or estimated values for "free" calcium should be abandoned.

The total serum calcium concentration exhibits a circadian rhythm characterized by a single nadir and peak, with amplitude (nadir to peak) of approximately 0.5 mg/dl (Table 1).[4,5] This rhythm is thought to reflect hemodynamic changes in serum albumin concentration that result from changes in body posture.[6] Prolonged upright posture or venostasis can result in hemoconcentration and thus show potentially misleading increases of about 0.5 mg/dl in serum calcium concentration. There is little difference between values taken in fasting and nonfasting states.

Normal values for serum total calcium concentration vary somewhat among clinical laboratories and range from 9.0 to 10.6 mg/dl. In men, the calcium concentration decreases with advancing age from a mean of ~9.6 mg/dl at the age of 20 to ~9.2 mg/dl at the age of 80 years, and the decrease can be accounted for by a decrease in serum albumin concentration.[7] In women, no change is observed with age. In children, the serum calcium concentration is higher than in adult subjects, being highest at 6–24 months of age, the mean ~10.2 mg/dl, decreasing to ~9.8 mg/dl at 6–8 years and decreasing further to adult values at 16–20 years[8,9] (Table 2).

For routine determination of total serum calcium concentration, most clinical laboratories use automated spectrophotometric techniques such as the o-cresolphthalein complexone method; the reference method is atomic absorption spectrophotometry.[10] Calcium concentrations expressed in mg/dl can be converted to mM by dividing by 4, and to mEq/liter by dividing by 2. The atomic weight of calcium is 40.08, and its valence is 2.

Ionized Calcium

Ionized calcium is the fraction of plasma calcium that is important for physiologic processes, such as muscle con-

TABLE 2. REPRESENTATIVE NORMAL VALUES FOR CONCENTRATIONS OF BLOOD IONIZED CALCIUM, SERUM TOTAL CALCIUM, PHOSPHORUS, AND MAGNESIUM

	Age (yr)	Blood ionized calcium		Serum total calcium	Phosphorus	Magnesium
		(mg/dl)	(mM)	(mg/dl)	(mg/dl)	(mg/dl)
Infants	0–0.25	4.9–5.6	(1.22–1.40)	8.8–11.3	4.8–7.4	1.6–2.5
	1–5	4.9–5.3	(1.22–1.32)	9.4–10.8	4.5–6.2	1.6–2.5
Children	6–12	4.6–5.3	(1.15–1.32)	9.4–10.3	3.6–5.8	1.7–2.3
Men	20	4.5–5.2	(1.12–1.30)	9.1–10.2	2.5–4.5	1.7–2.6
	50	4.5–5.2	(1.12–1.30)	8.9–10.0	2.3–4.1	1.7–2.6
	70	4.5–5.2	(1.12–1.30)	8.8–9.9	2.2–4.0	1.7–2.6
Women	20	4.5–5.2	(1.12–1.30)	8.8–10.0	2.5–4.5	1.7–2.6
	50	4.5–5.2	(1.12–1.30)	8.8–10.0	2.7–4.4	1.7–2.6
	70	4.5–5.2	(1.12–1.30)	8.8–10.0	2.9–4.8	1.7–2.6

Data are from references 7, 8, 9, 11, 12, 13, 14, 21, 22, and 26.

traction, blood coagulation, nerve conduction, hormone secretion (parathyroid hormone and 1,25-dihydroxyvitamin D) and action, ion transport, and bone mineralization. In the past, measurement of blood ionized calcium concentration was technically difficult and not widely available in clinical settings. Now readily and accurately measured in most hospital laboratories,[11] this measurement is most useful in critically ill patients, particularly those in whom serum protein levels are decreased, acid-base disturbances are present, or to whom large amounts of citrated blood products are given, such as with cardiac surgery or liver transplantation.

The range of values of ionized calcium for normal individuals must be established for each laboratory and will vary depending on which technique is used and whether the measurement is made in serum, plasma, or heparinized whole blood. Measured with currently available, ion-selective electrodes, serum ionized calcium concentrations in healthy adult men and women range from approximately 4.5 to 5.2 mg/dl (1.12–1.30 mM), without significant sex differences.[10,11] In healthy infants, ionized calcium levels decrease from ~5.8 mg/dl (1.45 mM) at birth to a nadir of 4.9 mg/dl (1.22 mM) at 24 h of life,[12] and increase slightly during the first week of life to 5.4 mg/dl (1.35 mM).[13] Values in young children are slightly higher (by about 0.1 mg/dl) than those in adults until after puberty.[10,14]

Calcium binding to albumin is strongly pH-dependent between pH 7 and 8; an acute increase or decrease in pH of 0.1 pH units will increase or decrease, respectively, the protein-bound fraction of calcium by about 0.12 mg/dl. Thus, in hypocalcemic patients with metabolic acidosis, rapid correction of acidemia with sodium bicarbonate can precipitate tetany, because of increased binding of calcium to albumin, and thereby a decrease in ionized calcium concentration. Blood ionized calcium concentrations exhibit a low-amplitude circadian rhythm characterized by a peak at 10:00 a.m. and a nadir at 6:00–8:00 p.m., with amplitude (nadir to peak) of 0.3 mg/dl.[4] Thus, specimens for analysis drawn after the morning give slightly lower values. Specimens must be obtained anaerobically to avoid spurious results caused by ex vivo changes in pH. Measurements made in heparinized whole blood tend to be slightly lower than those in serum, because of binding of calcium by heparin. Calcium binding to heparin can be minimized by using calcium-titrated heparin (Radiometer Corp., Copenhagen, Denmark) at a concentration of 50 IU/ml or lower or sodium or lithium heparin at a concentration of 15 U/ml or lower[15]; under these circumstances, values from serum, plasma, or whole blood are similar. For hospitalized patients, it is recommended that specimens be obtained in the morning fasting state to avoid possible effects of posture, diurnal variation, and food ingestion.

SERUM PHOSPHORUS CONCENTRATION

Phosphorus exists in plasma in two forms: an organic form principally consisting of phospholipids and an inorganic form.[16] Of the total plasma phosphorus of approximately 14 mg/dl, about 8 mg/dl is in the organic form and about 4 mg/dl in the inorganic form. In clinical settings,

only the inorganic orthophosphate form is routinely measured. About 15–20% of total plasma inorganic phosphorus is protein-bound. The remainder, which is filtered by the renal glomerulus, exists principally either as the undissociated or "free" phosphate ions, HPO_4^{2+} and $H_2PO_4^-$, which are present in serum in a ratio of 4:1 at pH 7.4, or as phosphate complexed with sodium, calcium, or magnesium.

The terms *phosphorus concentration* and *phosphate concentration* are often used interchangeably, and for clinical purposes, the choice matters little. Phosphorus in the form of the phosphate ion circulates in blood, is filtered by the renal glomerulus, and is transported across plasma membranes. However, the content of phosphate in plasma, urine, tissue, or foodstuffs is measured and expressed in terms of the amount of elemental phosphorus contained in the specimen, hence use of the term *phosphorus concentration*.

In healthy subjects ingesting typical diets, the serum phosphorus concentration exhibits a circadian rhythm, characterized by a decrease to a nadir just before noon, an increase to a plateau in late afternoon, and a small further increase to a peak shortly after midnight (Table 1).[4,17] The amplitude (nadir to peak) is approximately 1.2 mg/dl, or 30%, of the 24-h mean level. Increases or decreases in dietary intake of phosphorus induce substantial increases or decreases, respectively, in serum phosphorus levels during late morning, afternoon, and evening, but less or no change in morning fasting phosphorus levels.[17] To minimize the effect of dietary phosphorus on the serum phosphorus concentration, specimens for analysis should be obtained in the morning fasting state. Specimens obtained in the afternoon are more likely to be affected by diet and may be more useful in monitoring the effect of changes in dietary phosphorus on serum phosphorus concentrations, as in patients with renal insufficiency receiving phosphorus binding agents to suppress secondary hyperparathyroidism. With administration of the phosphorus binding agent aluminum hydroxide, the decrease in morning fasting phosphorus levels underestimated the severity of hypophosphatemia observed throughout much of the day.[17,18]

Factors other than time of day and diet can affect the serum phosphorus concentration. Presumably because of movement of phosphorus into the cell, intravenous infusion of glucose or insulin, ingestion of carbohydrate-rich meals, acute respiratory alkalosis, or infusion or endogenous release of epinephrine can decrease the serum phosphorus concentration acutely. The decrease in phosphorus concentration induced by acute respiratory alkalosis can be as great as 2.0 mg/dl.[19] Serum phosphorus concentration can be increased acutely by metabolic acidosis or by intravenous infusion of calcium, the latter presumably caused by efflux of inorganic phosphate from red blood cells.[20]

There are substantial effects of age on the fasting serum phosphorus concentration. Serum phosphorus levels are high in infants, ranging from 4.8 to 7.4 mg/dl (mean 6.2 mg/dl) in the first 3 months of life and decreasing to 4.5–5.8 mg/dl (mean 5.0 mg/dl) at the age of 1–2 years.[21] In mid-childhood, values range from 3.5 to 5.5 mg/dl (mean, 4.4 mg/dl) and decrease to adult values by late adolescence.[8,9,22] In adult males, serum phosphorus levels decrease with age from approximately 3.5 mg/dl at the age of 20 years to 3.0 mg/dl at the age of 70.[7,22] In women, the values are similar to those of men until after the menopause, when they increase slightly from ~3.4 mg/dl at the age of 50 to 3.7 mg/dl at the age of 70. Representative normal ranges for serum phosphorus concentration are depicted in Table 2.

The normal range for serum phosphorus concentration is laboratory-specific. Phosphorus concentration is most commonly determined using automated spectrophotometric techniques based on the reaction of phosphate ions with molybdate.[10] Phosphorus concentrations should be determined in serum or plasma that has been separated promptly from red blood cells. Prolonged standing or hemolysis of the specimen can lead to a spurious increase in phosphorus concentration. Concentrations of phosphorus expressed as mg/dl can be converted to mM by dividing by 3.1. The atomic weight of phosphorus is 30.98. Because plasma phosphate is a mixture of monovalent and divalent ions, the composite valence of phosphorus in serum (or intravenous solutions) at pH 7.4 is 1.8; at this pH, 1 mmol of phosphorus is equal to 1.8 mEq.

SERUM MAGNESIUM CONCENTRATION

As with calcium, magnesium exists in serum in three distinct forms: protein-bound magnesium (30%), which is not filtered by the renal glomerulus, and ionized (55%) and complexed (15%) magnesium, which are filtered.[16] Magnesium is bound principally to albumin in a pH-dependent manner similar to that of calcium. Ionized magnesium is the fraction that is important for physiologic processes, including neuromuscular transmission and cardiovascular tone. Measurement of ionized magnesium concentration using ion-selective electrodes is available in some laboratories; however, its clinical usefulness in evaluating body magnesium status remains to be determined.[23–25] For most clinical purposes, the total concentration of magnesium in serum is determined. Most laboratories use automated spectrophotometric techniques; the reference method is atomic absorption spectrophotometry.[10]

The serum total magnesium concentration is closely maintained within the narrow range of 1.7–2.6 mg/dl. There are no significant differences in magnesium concentration between men and women, nor with respect to age, and values in children are similar to those in adults (Table 2). The circadian variation in magnesium concentration is of low amplitude and not clinically significant. Prolonged standing or hemolysis of the specimen can lead to spurious increases in serum magnesium concentration. The whole blood ionized magnesium concentration in healthy volunteers ranges from 0.44 to 0.59 mM (mean, ~0.52 mM). Concentrations expressed as mg/dl can be converted to mM by dividing by 2.4, and to mEq/liter by dividing by 1.2. The atomic weight of magnesium is 24.31.

REFERENCES

1. Moore EW 1970 Ionized calcium in normal serum, ultrafiltrates, and whole blood determined by ion-exchange electrodes. J Clin Invest 49:318–334.
2. Ladenson JH, Lewis JW, Boyd JC 1978 Failure of total calcium corrected for protein, albumin, and ph to correctly assess free calcium status. J Clin Endocrinol Metab 46:986–993.
3. Editorial 1979 Serum calcium. Lancet 1:858–859.
4. Markowitz M, Rotkin L, Rosen JF 1981 Circadian rhythms of blood minerals in humans. Science 213:672–674.
5. Halloran BP, Portale AA, Castro M, Morris RCJ, Goldsmith RS 1985 Serum concentration of 1,25-dihydroxyvitamin D in the human: Diurnal variation. J Clin Endocrinol Metab 60:1104–1110.
6. Jubiz W, Canterbury JM, Reiss E, Tyler FH 1972 Circadian rhythm in serum parathyroid hormone concentration in human subjects: Correlation with serum calcium, phosphate, albumin, and growth hormone levels. J Clin Invest 51:2040–2046.
7. Keating FRJ, Jones JD, Elveback LR, Randall RV 1969 The relation of age and sex to distribution of values in healthy adults of serum, calcium inorganic phosphorus, magnesium, alkaline phosphatase, total proteins, albumin, and blood urea. J Lab Clin Med 73:825–834.
8. Arnaud SB, Goldsmith RS, Stickler GB, McCall JT, Arnaud CD 1973 Serum parathyroid hormone and blood minerals: Interrelationships in normal children. Pediatr Res 7:485–493
9. Burritt MF, Slockbower JM, Forsman RW, Offord KP, Bergstralh EJ, Smithson WA 1990 Pediatric reference intervals for 19 biologic variables in healthy children. Mayo Clin Proc 65:329–336.
10. Pesce AJ, Kaplan LA 1987 Methods in Clinical Chemistry. C. V. Mosby Company, St. Louis, MO, USA.
11. Bowers GN, Brassard C, Sena S 1986 Measurement of ionized calcium in serum with ion-selective electrodes: A mature technology that can meet the daily service needs. Clin Chem 32:1437–1447.
12. Loughead JL, Mimouni F, Tsang RC 1988 Serum ionized calcium concentrations in normal neonates. Am J Dis Child 142:516–518.
13. Nelson N, Finnstrom O, Larsson L 1987 Neonatal reference values for ionized calcium, phosphate and magnesium. Selection of reference population by optimality criteria. Scand J Clin Lab Invest 47:111–117.
14. Specker BL, Lichenstein P, Mimouni F, Gormley C, Tsang RC 1986 Calcium-regulating hormones and minerals from birth to 18 months of age: A cross-sectional study. II. Effects of sex, race, age, season, and diet on serum minerals, parathyroid hormone, and calcitonin. Pediatrics 77:891–896.
15. Boink ABTJ, Buckley BM, Christiansen TF, Covington AK, Maas AHJ, Müller-Plathe O, Sachs C, Siggaard-Andersen O and the International Federation of Clinical Chemistry 1991 Recommendation: Recommendation on sampling, transport and storage for the determination of the concentration of ionized calcium in whole blood, plasma and serum. Clin Chim Acta 202:S13–S22.
16. Marshall RW 1976 Plasma fractions. In: Nordin BEC (ed.) Calcium, Phosphate and Magnesium Metabolism. Churchill Livingston, London, UK, pp. 162–185.
17. Portale AA, Halloran BP, Morris RC Jr 1987 Dietary intake of phosphorus modulates the circadian rhythm in serum concentration of phosphorus: Implications for the renal production of 1,25-dihydroxyvitamin D. J Clin Invest 80:1147–1154.
18. Cam JM, Luck VA, Eastwood JB, De Wardener HE 1976 The effect of aluminum hydroxide orally on calcium, phosphorus and aluminum metabolism in normal subjects. Clin Sci Mol Med 51:407–414.
19. Mostellar ME, Tuttle EP 1964 Effects of alkalosis on plasma concentration and urinary excretion of inorganic phosphate in man. J Clin Invest 43:138–149.
20. Peraino RA, Suki WN 1980 Influence of calcium on renal handling of phosphate. In: Massry SG, Fleisch H (eds.) Renal Handling of Phosphate. Plenum, New York, NY, USA, pp. 287–306.
21. Brodehl J, Gellissen K, Weber HP 1982 Postnatal development of tubular phosphate reabsorption. Clin Nephrol 17:163–171.
22. Greenberg BG, Winters RW, Graham JB 1960 The normal range of serum inorganic phosphorus and its utility as discriminant in the diagnosis of congenital hypophosphatemia. J Clin Endocrinol Metab 20:364–379.
23. Saha H, Harmoinen A, Pietila K, Morsky P, Pasternack A 1996 Measurement of serum ionized versus total levels of magnesium and calcium in hemodialysis patients. Clin Nephrol 46:326–331.
24. Cook LA, Mimouni FB 1997 Whole blood ionized magnesium in the healthy neonate. J Am Coll Nutr 16:181–183.
25. Steinberger HA, Hanson CW 1998 Outcome-based justification for implementing new point-of-care tests: There is no difference between magnesium replacement based on ionized magnesium and total magnesium as a predictor of development of arrhythmias in the postoperative cardiac surgical patient. Clin Lab Manage Rev 12:87–90.
26. 1989 Meites S (ed.) Pediatric Clinical Chemistry. The American Association for Clinical Chemistry, Washington, DC, USA.

Chapter 25. Parathyroid Hormone, Parathyroid Hormone-Related Protein, and Vitamin D Metabolites

Lauren Golden, Karl Insogna, and John J. Wysolmerski

Section of Endocrinology and Metabolism, Department of Internal Medicine, Yale University School of Medicine, New Haven, Connecticut

INTRODUCTION

The ability to measure circulating levels of calciotropic hormones is a prerequisite for the accurate diagnosis and successful treatment of disorders of mineral metabolism and metabolic bone diseases. Although the current assays for parathyroid hormone (PTH), parathyroid hormone-related protein (PTHrP), and vitamin D metabolites are generally reliable and accurate, this was not the case as recently as the mid- to late 1980s. Even today, assays for these hormones are evolving as technology improves and as our knowledge of the physiology of calcium metabolism is advanced. In this chapter, we will review the current assays for each of these hormones and discuss how they are best used in clinical care. Before doing this, however, we will briefly describe the techniques used in the most common types of immunoassays.

RADIOIMMUNOASSAY

All hormone immunoassays rely on the ability of immunoglobulins to bind the molecule to be measured, and the specificity and affinity of the antibody–hormone interaction is the primary determinant of the sensitivity and specificity of the measurement. Historically, radioimmunoassays (RIAs) were the first type of immunoassays developed.[1,2] This format relies on the ability of unlabeled hormone in biological fluids to displace a trace amount of radioactively labeled hormone from its interaction with an antibody (Fig. 1). A fixed amount of antibody specific for the hormone of interest is incubated with a known small amount of a radiolabeled hormone or hormone fragment. Once the label has equilibrated with the antibody, a series of increasing known or standard quantities of unlabeled hormone are added and the amount of label remaining bound to the antibody at each standard dose is measured. This generates a curve that describes an inverse relationship between bound tracer and the concentration of unlabeled hormone, because increasing amounts of hormone in the sample displace more tracer. Patient samples are added to the antibody/radiolabel mix under identical conditions to the samples defining the standard curve. Comparing the amount of displacement of the radiotracer by the unknown sample to the standard curve allows the patient's hormone concentration to be calculated. This type of assay has also been adapted to the use of a hormone tracer conjugated to an enzyme that produces a specific color when provided with the correct substrate. This is called an ELISA.

IMMUNOMETRIC ASSAYS

Immunometric assays use the binding of a labeled antibody to the hormone being measured rather than the displacement of labeled hormone from an antibody[3,4] (Fig. 2). In the most common design, a first "capture" antibody bound to a solid phase such as a plastic bead or dish is used to remove the hormone of interest from a biological fluid. The capture antibody is present in great excess, so all the hormone present in the sample should be bound. Then a labeled, second "detection" antibody, which interacts with another portion of the hormone, is added and allowed to bind. After this reaction takes place, the hormone is sandwiched between two antibodies, one attached to a solid substrate and one that is labeled. Thus, these are often referred to as "sandwich" assays. The amount of label incorporated into these sandwiches is directly proportional to the amount of hormone in the sample. Similar to an RIA, the hormone concentration is extrapolated from a standard curve generated by a series of increasing amounts of purified hormone added to the assay. The type of label in these assays can vary. Most commonly, the detection antibody is radioactively labeled, so it is called an immunoradiometric assay (IRMA). However, the detection antibody can also be linked to enzymes that generate a colorimetric reaction to form an ELISA or that generate a chemiluminescent reaction to form an immunochemiluminometric assay.

MEASUREMENT OF PTH

Secretion and Metabolism of PTH

PTH is secreted by chief cells of the parathyroid gland in response to alterations in the concentration of extracellular

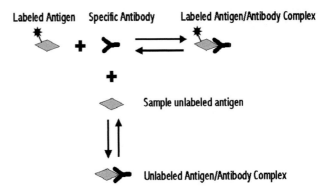

FIG. 1. Principles of the RIA. Labeled and unlabeled antigen compete for antibody binding. The unlabeled antigen (e.g., PTH) is present in the sample to be measured. In an RIA, the final step is to separate the antibody/antigen complexes and measure the amount of radioactivity bound by the antibody. The more radioactivity that is bound, the lower the amount of the antigen of interest in the sample. Conversely, a low level radioactivity bound to the antibody

---

The authors have no conflict of interest.

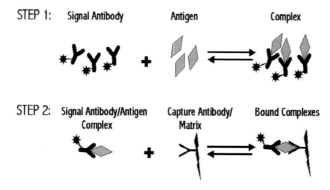

STEP 1:   Signal Antibody   Antigen   Complex

STEP 2:   Signal Antibody/Antigen   Capture Antibody/   Bound Complexes
          Complex   Matrix

FIG. 2. Principles of the immunoradiometric assay. Step 1: the signal antibody (radiolabeled monoclonal antibody) forms a complex with the antigen. Step 2: The signal antibody/antigen complex then reacts with the capture antibody, bound to solid matrix. Excess, unbound, radiolabeled signal

calcium. When calcium concentrations fall, PTH secretion is stimulated, and when calcium concentrations rise, it is suppressed.[5] The major secretory product and the biologically active form of the hormone is an 84 amino acid peptide [PTH(1-84)] that is derived from a pre-pro form of PTH initially translated within the parathyroid cells.[6,7] Although shorter amino-terminal fragments of PTH have biological activity, there is little convincing evidence that these forms actually circulate in detectable concentrations. PTH(1-84) has a short half-life, on the order of 2–3 minutes, and it circulates at low concentrations (7–36 pg/liter).[6,8] Once secreted, PTH(1-84) is rapidly metabolized, primarily in the liver but also to some extent in the kidney, to fragments containing the mid-region and carboxy-terminal portions of the molecule. These fragments of PTH have a much longer half-life in the circulation and are excreted by the kidney. Midregion and carboxy-terminal fragments have been estimated to represent between 50% and 90% of the total circulating PTH immunoreactivity, and they accumulate when renal function is impaired.[1,9–11] In addition to the liver and kidney, under conditions of hypercalcemia, parathyroid cells also metabolize PTH and secrete a portion in the form of midregion and C-terminal fragments.[12,13] To further complicate the issue, recently it has been shown that approximately 30% of what had previously been thought to represent intact, circulating PTH(1-84) is actually an N-terminally truncated fragment [PTH(7-84)] that may be secreted from the parathyroid gland itself.[14] The biological significance of the extensive metabolism of PTH remains uncertain. The fact that PTH(1-84) has a short half-life allows the circulating level of PTH to reflect closely the parathyroid secretory rate and thus provides a mechanism for the rapid adjustment of PTH levels in response to minute-to-minute changes in serum calcium. Beyond this, however, it has been shown that circulating PTH(7-84) can act as an antagonist of the PTH receptor (type I PTH/PTHrP receptor [PTH1R]), and it has been suggested that C-terminal fragments of PTH may exert biological effects through a novel receptor.[14–16] Whatever its physiologic role, the heterogeneity of circulating PTH has created obstacles for its accurate measurement in patients.

PTH Immunoassays

The oldest PTH assays are radioimmunoassays using antisera directed at the carboxy-terminal and midportion of the PTH molecule.[1,2,17] As a result, these assays detect not only PTH(1-84) but also the circulating midregion and/or carboxy-terminal fragments. Because these fragments accumulate in the circulation in renal failure, the RIAs are not useful in patients with significant degrees of renal insufficiency. However, in patients with normal renal function, they readily discriminate between baseline and elevated levels of PTH and can be used to diagnose patients with primary and secondary hyperparathyroidism. These assays continue to be used today, including at our institution. The assay we employ uses antisera directed at PTH(44-68), with PTH(37-84) as a trace.[2] In our experience and in that of others as well, this midregion assay is more sensitive than the intact PTH assay in detecting slight elevations in PTH levels in patients with mild primary hyperparathyroidism and in patients with secondary hyperparathyroidism not caused by renal disease.[2,18]

The standard PTH assays in use today are the so-called intact PTH(1-84) assays. There are now several commercially available versions, all of which are variations on the first immunoradiometric assay introduced in 1987.[3] These assays use antibodies to the C-terminal region of PTH(1-84) as the capture, and labeled antisera to the amino-terminal portion of PTH as the signal. For many years it was thought that these assays exclusively measured intact, biologically active PTH(1-84). However, in the past several years, it has become clear that the signal antibodies do not recognize the extreme amino-terminal portion of PTH and thus cross-react with the inactive PTH(7-84) fragment.[14] Immunometric assays with a similar format but using chemiluminescent or fluorimetric detection systems have been adapted to provide for rapid turnaround times in the operating room suite. These assays provide PTH measurements within 15 minutes and have allowed for near real-time monitoring of the response of circulating levels of PTH to parathyroid surgery.[19,20]

As alluded to in the previous paragraph, we now know that up to one-third of the immunoreactivity detected in the intact PTH IRMA is actually PTH(7-84), which is biologically inactive or perhaps even an antagonist of PTH(1-84).[14,16,21–25] This observation has prompted the development of a new generation of immunometric PTH assays that use signal antibodies recognizing the extreme amino terminus of PTH(1-84).[23,24] These assays, which have been termed "whole" or "bioactive" PTH assays, do not recognize PTH(7-84) and thus are truly specific for PTH(1-84). At the present, the terminology is somewhat confusing because the old immunometric assays are still referred to as intact PTH assays, which in retrospect, is a misnomer. These assays have provided us with several bits of new information. First, using the whole PTH assays, it is clear that the normal range of PTH concentration is lower than previously thought (7–36 pg/ml instead of 10–65 pg/ml). Second, different intact PTH assays vary in their crossreactivity with PTH(17-84). This likely explains the different normal ranges noted with intact PTH assays from different manufacturers. Finally, it has been reported that the relative proportion of PTH(7-84) to PTH(1-84) increases in patients with renal failure, leading to spurious elevations in the intact assays.[22,23] This might explain the observation that the degree of hyperparathyroidism in renal failure patients is often overestimated by the intact PTH assay compared with bone biopsy criteria.[26] Much of this extra PTH may be the PTH(7-84) fragment. However, most studies have demonstrated a tight correlation between the results from the whole PTH and intact PTH assays across a wide variety of clinical situations including renal failure and after renal transplantation.[14] The results from whole assays are always about 30% lower, but accounting for this difference, these assays do not appear to be able to discriminate better between hyperparathyroid and adynamic bone disease in patients with renal disease.[14,23–25] Therefore, the clinical use of the whole PTH and the intact PTH assays are probably similar. However, we anticipate that over time, the intact PTH assays will be supplanted by the newer whole PTH assays simply because it is logical to measure the bioactive PTH concentration as accurately as possible.

Measurement of PTH in Clinical Practice

The most common clinical use of PTH measurements is in the differential diagnosis of hypercalcemia. In this situation, the presence or absence of an elevated PTH level allows one to make the broad distinction between PTH-dependent and PTH-independent causes. For practical purposes, this reduces to making or excluding a diagnosis of primary hyperparathyroidism. In patients with normal renal function, all the currently available assays are able to do this. There exists a small group of patients with very mild primary hyperparathyroidism whose PTH levels are not frankly elevated. However, PTH levels need to be interpreted in the context of the serum calcium level. A PTH level at the upper end of the physiologic range is not normal when it occurs in a patient with an elevated serum calcium level, and this combination should suggest the diagnosis of primary hyperparathyroidism or familial hypocalciuric hypercalcemia (FHH). There is one preliminary report suggesting that the whole PTH assay format may more reliably show measurements above the normal range in this subgroup of patients with mild primary hyperparathyroidism.[27] If this observation is confirmed, this assay may be preferable for these patients. There is also a recent report of "normocalcemic" hyperparathyroidism.[28] Again, a high-normal serum calcium coupled with an elevated PTH level should arouse suspicion of primary hyperparathyroidism or FHH. Finally, the intact assay and presumably the whole PTH assay as well have the advantage over the PTH RIAs in being able to reliably document suppressed PTH levels. This is helpful in confirming a PTH-independent cause of hypercalcemia.

Primary hyperparathyroidism is usually caused by a parathyroid adenoma, and surgical removal of the adenomatous gland is curative. Parathyroidectomy traditionally has involved a bilateral neck exploration under general anesthesia to identify and remove the abnormal gland. In this approach, surgical success has been measured at the time of operation

by confirmation that parathyroid tissue was removed by frozen section and by the response of the calcium level postoperatively. However, the availability of rapid PTH immunometric assays with turn around times of 15 minutes or less has helped to revolutionize the approach to parathyroidectomy.[19,20] In what is rapidly becoming the standard approach, surgery can now be done in a directed fashion under local anesthesia, guided by the radiographic, preoperative localization of the adenoma.[29,30] Because the radiological studies are not perfect, using this approach, the surgeon requires confirmation that the proper gland has been resected. Given the rapid half-life of PTH and the suppression of normal parathyroid hormone secretion by hypercalcemia, a rapid decline in PTH levels provides this confirmation. In the series published to date, a 50% reduction in PTH levels within 5–10 minutes after resection of the suspected adenoma has been highly predictive of surgical cure.[19,20,29–31] This approach has also recently been used to monitor parathyroid function during thyroidectomy to help predict postoperative hypocalcemia.

The second most common setting in which PTH measurements are useful is in the diagnosis and monitoring of secondary hyperparathyroidism. This group of patients can be further divided into those with normal renal function and those with renal insufficiency. In the absence of renal insufficiency, secondary hyperparathyroidism occurs in response to calcium insufficiency. This can occur because of vitamin D deficiency, calcium malabsorption secondary to gastrointestinal disease, or renal calcium wasting. Depending on the severity and chronicity of these conditions, frank hypocalcemia may or may not be present. In addition to making the diagnosis, measuring PTH levels is useful to gauge the adequacy and/or response to therapy. In our experience, the midregion PTH RIA is more sensitive than the intact PTH assay in making the diagnosis of mild secondary hyperparathyroidism in patients with normal renal function.

Secondary hyperparathyroidism is a predictable consequence of progressive renal failure. The pathophysiology of parathyroid hyperfunction in renal disease is covered in depth elsewhere. The measurement of PTH levels is an important adjunct to the management of renal bone disease. Knowledge of the PTH level factors into the management of phosphate binder and vitamin D therapy. The measurement of PTH helps to identify patients at risk for adynamic bone disease or calciphylaxis. Finally, PTH levels are a factor in determining which patients are candidates for surgical treatment of parathyroid hyperplasia. The use of PTH RIAs is inappropriate in patients with renal insufficiency for reasons discussed previously. The use of the intact PTH assay has been very useful in following these patients. However, as discussed before, it is now known that the intact assays also measure fragments of PTH whose concentrations are elevated in renal failure.[14,21,22] For this reason, the whole PTH assay has been advertised to be superior in renal patients. However, it is still unclear if PTH(7-84) circulates in patients with renal failure in concentrations that are enough out of proportion to PTH(1-84) to make the whole PTH assay superior to the standard intact assay in this patient group.[25]

The last setting in which PTH levels may be useful is in

the management of metabolic bone disease and nephrolithiasis. Both primary and secondary hyperparathyroidism can contribute to bone loss in patients with osteoporosis. PTH levels do not need to be measured in all osteoporotic patients. However, the possibility of hyperparathyroidism should be considered, and if the serum calcium level or the urinary calcium excretion rate is abnormal, PTH levels should be obtained. Secondary hyperparathyroidism can complicate therapy for X-linked hypophosphatemic rickets, and PTH levels should be followed in these patients.[32] The population of patients with calcium-containing kidney stones is enriched for individuals with primary hyperparathyroidism, renal calcium wasting, and absorptive hypercalciuria.[33] In particular, stone patients with primary hyperparathyroidism can present with a phenotype consisting of minor elevations of serum calcium level, moderate elevations in $1,25(OH)_2$ vitamin D levels, and hypercalciuria.[34] Measuring PTH levels in patients with stones is helpful in recognizing these patients with mild hyperparathyroidism and in distinguishing between this disorder and the other possible etiologies for calcium stones.

MEASUREMENT OF PTHrP

Secretion and Metabolism of PTHrP

PTHrP is a growth factor or cytokine that was originally discovered as the cause of the clinical syndrome of humoral hypercalcemia of malignancy (HHM). The *PTH* and *PTHrP* genes are both derived from a common ancestor gene that most likely resembled the present day *PTHrP* gene. As a result, the two proteins share considerable amino-terminal homology that allows both PTHrP and PTH to bind and stimulate the same receptor-the type I PTH/PTHrP receptor (PTH1 receptor). Unlike PTH, which is expressed only in the parathyroids and hypothalamus, the *PTHrP* gene is widely expressed, and PTHrP is found in almost all tissues. However, normally PTHrP acts locally, in an autocrine or paracrine fashion, and appears to be excluded from the circulation. It is only in the setting of malignancy that significant amounts of PTHrP are found in the circulation and lead to the development of hypercalcemia by stimulating PTH1 receptors in bone and kidney that are meant to mediate the calciotropic actions of PTH.

The primary transcript of PTHrP is a prohormone much like proopiomelanocortin (POMC), and it is extensively processed within the cell to generate a series of PTHrP peptides. To date, several fragments of various sizes containing the amino-terminal portion of PTHrP have been described. These peptides have the ability to interact with the PTH1 receptor and exert PTH-like effects. In addition, midregion and C-terminal peptides have been described that may have their own receptors and exert biological effects. Most of the studies examining the production of various PTHrP peptides have been performed in cell culture systems. It is not clear exactly which peptides circulate in either normal people or in patients with HHM. The half-life of peptides containing the amino-terminal portion of PTHrP is short in human plasma, where they appear to be degraded by circulating proteases.[35–37] For this reason, the measure-

ment of PTHrP requires the immediate addition of protease inhibitors to collected samples. As discussed below, in most normal people, amino-terminal containing fragments of PTHrP either do not circulate, or do so at low concentrations, at or below the current threshold of sensitivity of the current assays (approximately 0.1 pM). One exception may be during lactation, when amino-terminal containing PTHrP has been measured in the circulation of nursing mothers.[38] In contrast, in normal people, midregion containing PTHrP peptides can be readily measured. C-terminal–containing fragments are undetectable in normal individuals, but they accumulate in patients with renal failure.[36,37]

Appreciable levels of amino-terminal containing PTHrP molecules are only found in the circulation of hypercalcemic patients with the HHM syndrome. Studies have suggested that the ability of a given tumor to cause this syndrome is likely related to that tumor's level of PTHrP gene expression.[39] It is likely also related to the tumor mass, because HHM tends to be a late complication in patients with large tumor burdens. One interesting unanswered issue is whether tumors somehow specifically counteract the barriers that normally exclude PTHrP from the circulation or whether they simply overwhelm them. Very little is known about the exact forms of PTHrP secreted by different tumors and if there is any peripheral organ-specific metabolism of these peptides.

PTHrP Immunoassays

Many immunoassays for PTHrP currently exist, although the majority are used primarily for research purposes. These include RIAs directed at the amino-terminal, midregion, and C-terminal portions of the molecule.[35,36] There are also immunometric assays directed at PTHrP(1-36) and PTHrP(1-74).[37] Although there have been reports of the use of several of these assays to measure PTHrP in different patient groups, it has been the immunometric assays that have shown the best discrimination between hypercalcemic patients with HHM and patients with hypercalcemia due to other causes.[37,40–42] These assays remain the standard for the measurement of PTHrP in clinical care. In an analogous fashion to the intact PTH assays, the original PTHrP IRMA used antisera to the midregion of PTHrP as the capture and antisera to the amino-terminus as the signal.[37] There are now commercial assays that employ this strategy but also ones that use amino-terminal antibodies as capture and midregion antibodies as signal.[40–42] Practically, what is important for the clinician to remember is that these assays all measure longer amino-terminal fragments of PTHrP containing at least the first 74–86 amino acids.

Measurement of PTHrP in Clinical Practice

The clinical use of measuring PTHrP is generally restricted to confirming the diagnosis of HHM. Most commonly, this syndrome occurs in patients with solid tumors without extensive bone metastases and represents approximately 80% of all cases of malignancy-associated hypercalcemia at our institution.[36,43] The most common types of tumors causing HHM include squamous tumors of the head and neck, squamous lung tumors, urothelial malignancies, and breast tumors. Breast tumors represent a gray area between hypercalcemia of the humoral variety and hypercalcemia mediated by bone metastases. Breast cancer cells make PTHrP, which may contribute in an important manner to the peritumoral bone resorption that leads to the establishment of osteolytic metastases.[44] If a given breast tumor makes enough PTHrP, it can also spill over into the circulation and cause hypercalcemia through the humoral route.[45] In addition to carcinomas, PTHrP can also be produced in sufficient quantities by some hematologic malignancies and by benign neoplasms, such as islet cell adenomas of the pancreas and pheochromocytomas, to cause hypercalcemia. In fact, the list of tumors documented to produce PTHrP and HHM at least once continues to grow.

In the vast majority of cases, the diagnosis of HHM is obvious because it occurs in patients with known tumors of one of the types enumerated above. However, hyperparathyroidism is a common disease and should always be ruled out even in this setting. The diagnosis of HHM is confirmed if the intact PTH level is suppressed and the PTHrP level is elevated. Given the lability of PTHrP in blood, if levels are to be checked, the blood sample should be drawn into a special collection vial containing protease inhibitors and should be placed on ice immediately. Plasma should be separated promptly and frozen until assayed. One issue in interpreting the results of PTHrP assays is the lack of a well-established reference range for human beings. In our experience, most normal, nonlactating individuals have undetectable circulating levels of PTHrP.[37] In the instructional guide to their commercial PTHrP(1-86) IRMA, the Nichols Institute reports that they detected PTHrP levels in 254 of 270 individuals using an assay with a sensitivity of 0.3 pM. The mean level was 0.5 pM, and they estimated a normal range of <1.3 pM. Obviously, these values are just at the threshold of the current assays. In studies of patients with HHM, the average level of PTHrP has been approximately 20 pM.[37,46] However, there is a broad range of values in these patients, and there is not good correlation between PTHrP levels and the degree of hypercalcemia. Thus, in hypercalcemic cancer patients with suppressed PTH levels, a measurable PTHrP level is likely significant. Certainly, any level over 5 pM should be considered abnormal. Routine therapy for malignancy-associated hypercalcemia does not alter PTHrP levels, so after the diagnosis of HHM is established, PTHrP levels do not need to be followed.

Apart from malignancy-associated hypercalcemia, PTHrP should not be measured in the routine evaluation of hypercalcemia. There have been rare case reports in which PTHrP has been implicated as the cause of hypercalcemia in inflammatory diseases and in benign breast disease.[47,48] In addition, as noted above, benign endocrine tumors have been noted to make PTHrP. Thus, measuring PTHrP levels may occasionally be helpful in unusual cases of hypercalcemia. However, these measurements should only be performed after other, more common causes of hypercalcemia are excluded.

MEASUREMENT OF VITAMIN D METABOLITES

Production and Metabolism of Vitamin D

Vitamin D (cholecalciferol, vitamin D_3) is a steroid hormone produced in the skin by exposure to solar or ultraviolet light.[49] Vitamin D enters the circulation and is transported bound to the vitamin D–binding protein. Hydroxylation of vitamin D_3 by the hepatic 25-hydroxylase produces 25-hydroxyvitamin D_3 [25(OH)D_3], the major circulating form of vitamin D.[50] At pharmacologic doses, 25(OH)D_3 has a biological effect on intestinal calcium absorption, as well as renal handling of calcium and phosphorus.[51,52] Subsequent hydroxylation of 25(OH)D_3 by the renal 1-α-hydroxylase converts 25(OH)D_3 to 1,25-dihydroxyvitamin D_3 [1,25(OH)$_2D_3$],[53] and it is this metabolite that has the greatest biological potency. 1,25(OH)$_2D_3$ circulates at concentrations that are approximately 1000-fold lower than 25(OH)D_3,[54] but on a molar basis is far more potent than the latter metabolite at enhancing intestinal calcium absorption and mobilizing calcium from bone. Metabolism of 1,25(OH)$_2D_3$ by the liver and kidney, as well as by target tissues (bone and intestine), results in the formation of 24,25-dihydroxyvitamin D_3 [24,25(OH)$_2D_3$] and 1,24,25 trihydroxy vitamin D_3 [1,24,25(OH)$_2D_3$].[3,55] Because these compounds are generally considered to be biologically inert, and only 25(OH)D_3 and 1,25(OH)$_2D_3$ have clinical relevance, the focus of this chapter will be on the measurement of 25(OH)D_3 and 1,25(OH)$_2D_3$.

Vitamin D Assays

Historically, assessment and quantitation of vitamin D metabolites presented significant methodologic challenges. Early assays were cumbersome and hampered by low specificity in distinguishing between various vitamin D metabolites. In addition, 1,25(OH)$_2D_3$ circulates at very low concentrations and is relatively unstable, necessitating the development of high sensitivity assays. Recent methodologic advances have dramatically improved our ability to quantitate vitamin D, with current RIAs optimized for rapid, accurate detection of 25(OH)D_3 and 1,25(OH)$_2D_3$.

25(OH)D_3

In the early 1970s, generation of tritiated vitamin D compounds ([^{3}H] vitamin D) with high specific activity[56] enabled the development of competitive protein-binding assays for vitamin D, and subsequently for 25(OH)D_3.[57,58] Early assays overestimated the amount of circulating vitamin D and were limited in their ability to distinguish between vitamin D metabolites. During the ensuing decade, these problems were overcome by the addition of extensive prepurification steps,[59] which greatly improved assay results but were quite cumbersome. In the interim, assays using ultraviolet quantitative high-performance liquid chromatography (HPLC) were described,[60,61] providing valid determinations of circulating 25(OH)D_3.

HPLC quantitation methods provided several advantages over early competitive protein-binding assays. HPLC allows individual quantitation of vitamin D metabolites, permitting distinction of $25(OH)D_2$ from $25(OH)D_3$ and thus overcoming this limitation of earlier assays. The steps of HPLC include sample extraction, solid-phase extraction chromatography, silica cartridge chromatography, and quantitative normal-phase high performance liquid chromatography. Given the high circulating concentrations of $25(OH)D_3$ (nanomole/liter range), $25(OH)D_3$ can be directly quantitated by ultraviolet detection after separation by normal-phase HPLC.[62] Although it produces superior results, HPLC quantitation methodology also uses tritiated tracers and liquid scintillation counting and requires the use of large sample sizes and expensive equipment.[62] Despite these relative disadvantages, HPLC quantitation assays emerged as the gold standard for measurements of $25(OH)D_3$.

The laborious nature of HPLC methodology and the increasing clinical demand for $25(OH)D_3$ analysis spurred the development of more rapid assay procedures for the measurement of $25(OH)D_3$. By the mid 1980s, RIAs were introduced to measure circulating $25(OH)D_3$. As described previously, RIAs rely on the ability of unlabeled hormone in biological fluids to displace a trace amount of radioactively labeled hormone from its interaction with an antibody (Fig. 1). Early assays continued to use tritiated vitamin D compounds ($[^3H]25(OH)D_3$) as tracers, but eliminated the need for sample prepurification, thus considerably simplifying the measurement process.[63] Subsequent modifications of RIA methodology introduced the use of an ^{125}I-labeled trace, obviating the use of tritiated compounds.[64]

The current method of choice for assessing $25(OH)D_3$ status is the ^{125}I-labeled $25(OH)D_3$ RIA. This was the first assay approved by the Food and Drug Administration (FDA) for use in clinical diagnosis and is available as a kit (DiaSorin Corp., Stillwater, MN, USA). The ^{125}I-based RIA involves four steps: extraction, incubation with primary antibody, precipitation with a secondary antibody, and quantitation. The primary antibody used in the ^{125}I-based RIA is raised against a synthetic vitamin D analog[23–27] (pentanorvitamin D-C22-carboxylic acid) and is coupled to bovine serum albumin (BSA).[63,64] The antibody cross-reacts equally with both vitamin $25(OH)D_2$ and $25(OH)D_3$ metabolites, although RIA measurements predominantly reflect levels of $25(OH)D_3$, which contributes the greatest percentage (93–94%) to the assessment of nutritional vitamin D status.[65] The ^{125}I-labeled $25(OH)D_3$ RIA accurately identifies vitamin D toxicity and deficiency in a variety of clinical situations.

FDA approval has now been granted to additional manufacturers (IDS Ltd., Tyne and Wear, UK; Nichols Institute, San Clemente, CA, USA) for ^{125}I-labeled $25(OH)D_3$ RIA kits. A recent study compared the performance of the new IDS Ltd. assay with that of the DiaSorin assay, as well as with ultraviolet quantitative HPLC, the gold standard for measurements of $25(OH)D_3$.[66] The IDS Ltd. kit underestimated total circulating $25(OH)D_3$ compared with the DiaSorin assay and HPLC. This was attributed to a lower recovery of $25(OH)D_2$ and differing affinity of the primary antibody for $25(OH)D_2$ and $25(OH)D_3$.

A chemiluminescence protein-binding assay for the detection of $25(OH)D_3$ has recently been approved by the FDA (Nichols Advantage Specialty Systems, Nichols Institute). This assay employs acridinium ester chemiluminescence detection technology and can be run using a fully automated random access immunoanalyzer. The steps involved include release of vitamin D metabolites from serum binding proteins (DBP), incubation with magnetic particles and acridinium ester-labeled anti-DBP polyclonal antibodies, and detection/quantitation. Preliminary studies suggest that this method yields excellent sample recovery, and values correlate well with those obtained using standard RIA and HPLC techniques.[67]

$1,25(OH)_2D_3$

Accurate quantitation of $1,25(OH)_2D_3$ presented even greater methodologic challenges than measurement of its 25-hydroxylated precursor. As noted earlier, $1,25(OH)_2D_3$ circulates at concentrations (picogram/milliliter range) that are approximately 1000-fold lower than $25(OH)D_3$, rendering it unsuitable for measurement by direct ultraviolet quantitation. In addition, $1,25(OH)_2D_3$ is relatively unstable and is extremely lipophilic, characteristics that presented additional hurdles to biochemists engaged in assay development. Nonetheless, an assay employing functional radioreceptor techniques was introduced in 1974.[68]

This radioreceptor assay (RRA) was based on isolation of the VDR from chick intestines, a process complicated by the lability of the isolated VDR protein. The RRA required sample isolation and purification using three laborious chromatographic steps and used tritiated vitamin D compounds as reporters. Although cumbersome, the RRA provided initial insights into vitamin D homeostasis. Subsequent modifications over the next 12 years refined the technique, reducing the volume of sample required and replacing early chromatographic systems with HPLC.[69–72] Ultimately, the need for HPLC prepurification steps was also eliminated with the introduction of a new assay in 1984 that relied on solid-phase extraction of $1,25(OH)_2D_3$.[73]

The new assay further advanced RRA techniques through the use of VDRs isolated from calf thymus; these receptors showed greater stability than those isolated from chick intestine. This procedure was developed into the first commercial kit for measurement of $1,25(OH)_2D_3$.[62] Additional improvements were introduced in 1986 that simplified the purification steps.[74] However, the specificity of the VDR for its ligand, $1,25(OH)_2D_3$, necessitated the use of $[^3H]1,25(OH)_2D_3$ and precluded the use of an ^{125}I-labeled tracer. Thus, despite all the improvements, the calf thymus RRA for $1,25(OH)_2D_3$ remains a labor-intensive endeavor. This prompted the development of new RIA techniques for the measurement of $1,25(OH)_2D_3$.

In 1996 Hollis et al.[75] developed and introduced a new RIA using an ^{125}I-labeled tracer to quantify circulating levels of $1,25(OH)_2D_3$. The ^{125}I-based RIA exhibits numerous advantages over previous methods. Importantly, it does not require the preparation or use of VDR receptors, greatly simplifying assay methodology. Use of an ^{125}I reporter allows rapid quantitation of $1,25(OH)_2D_3$. In addition, this technique involves generation of a standard curve at the time of sample processing, eliminating the need for individual sample recovery, dilution conversion, or recovery estimates.

TABLE 1. CONCENTRATIONS OF VITAMIN D METABOLITES, CALCIUM, AND PTH IN DISORDERS OF CALCIUM HOMEOSTASIS

	$25(OH)D_3$	$1,25(OH)_2D_3$	Calcium	PTH
Hypercalcemia				
Primary hyperparathyroidism	Normal	Normal/increased	Increased	Increased
Humoral hypercalcemia of malignancy	Normal	Decreased/normal	Increased	Decreased
Vitamin D toxicity				
Vitamin D	Increased	Decreased/normal	Increased	Decreased
$25(OH)D_3$	Increased	Decreased/normal	Increased	Decreased
$1,25(OH)_2D_3$	Normal	Increased	Increased	Decreased
Granulomatous diseases	Normal	Increased	Increased	Decreased/normal
Lymphoma	Normal	Decreased/increased	Increased	Decreased/normal
Familial hypocalciuric hypercalcemia	Normal	Normal/increased	Increased	Normal/increased
Idiopathic osteoporosis	Normal	Normal/increased	Increased	Decreased/normal
Milk alkali syndrome	Normal	Decreased	Increased	Decreased
Hypocalcemia				
Vitamin D deficiency				
Early	Decreased	Normal	Decreased/normal	Increased
Prolonged	Decreased	Decreased	Decreased	Increased
Renal dysfunction				
Renal failure	Normal	Decreased	Decreased	Increased
Nephrotic syndrome	Decreased	Decreased/normal	Ionized calcium decreased	Increased
Severe hepatocellular disease	Decreased	Normal/decreased	Ionized calcium decreased	Increased
Hypoparathyroidism	Normal	Decreased/normal	Decreased	Decreased
Pseudohypoparathyroidism	Normal	Decreased/normal	Decreased	Normal/increased
Vitamin D–dependent rickets	Normal/increased	Decreased	Decreased	Increased
Vitamin D–resistant rickets	Normal/increased	Increased	Decreased	Increased
Hyperphosphatemia	Normal	Decreased	Decreased	Increased
Hypomagnesemia	Normal	Decreased/normal	Decreased	Decreased

As noted in the above discussion of measurement of circulating $25(OH)D_3$, the success of an RIA depends on the ability of unlabeled hormone in biological fluids to displace trace amounts of radioactively labeled hormone from an antibody. Development of a valid RIA to measure $1,25(OH)_2D_3$ was hampered initially by the lack of specificity of available antibodies to $1,25(OH)_2D_3$. Early antibodies demonstrated approximately 1% cross-reactivity with more abundant metabolites of vitamin D [$24,25(OH)_2D_3$ and $25,26(OH)_2D_3$] and exhibited only 70% cross-reactivity with $1,25(OH)_2D_2$ and $1,25(OH)_2D_3$.[62] To circumvent this problem, early RIAs used dual-column chromatographic purification of serum samples before assay. Newer antibodies have been introduced that possess limited (0.1%) cross-reactivity with $24,25(OH)_2D_3$ and $25,26(OH)_2D_3$ and that cross-react equally with both $1,25(OH)_2D_2$ and $1,25(OH)_2D_3$. These newer antibodies have allowed simplification of the RIA to its current form: sample extraction using single-column solid-phase chromatography, incubation with primary antibody, precipitation with a secondary antibody, and quantitation. Recently, an ^{125}I-based RIA (DiaSorin) for $1,25(OH)_2D_3$ has been validated and approved for clinical use.[76]

Measurement of Vitamin D in Clinical Practice

The availability of sensitive, reliable assays for the quantitation of vitamin D metabolites is key to the diagnosis and management of a many disorders of skeletal and mineral homeostasis. Clinical entities in which concentrations of $25(OH)D_3$ and/or $1,25(OH)_2D_3$ are frequently altered are outlined in Table 1.

As discussed earlier, the clinically relevant vitamin D metabolites include $25(OH)D_3$, which reflects total body stores of vitamin D, and $1,25(OH)_2D_3$, the active or hormonal form of the vitamin. There are little data to support the routine measurement of vitamin D_3, as this precursor is rapidly cleared from the circulation after release from the skin. Similarly, there are no known biological functions for $24,25(OH)_2D_3$, the second most abundant vitamin D metabolite in serum,[77] although we have used it as a therapeutic in the treatment of X-linked hypophosphatemic rickets.[78] Recently, the ability of $1,25(OH)_2D_3$ analogs to inhibit cell proliferation has sparked renewed interest in their potential therapeutic applications in preventing neoplasias,[79] so measurement of these analogs may be of more clinical relevance in the future.

The remainder of this section will deal with specific applications of vitamin D measurements in clinical practice. Approaches to the patient with hypercalcemia, hypocalcemia, renal disease and osteoporosis are highlighted.

The Hypercalcemic Patient. The differential diagnosis of a patient presenting with hypercalcemia includes those syndromes manifesting both *hypercalcemia and hypercalciuria*

© 2003 American Society for Bone and Mineral Research

(most commonly primary hyperparathyroidism, humoral hypercalcemia of malignancy, local osteolytic hypercalcemia, vitamin D toxicity, granulomatous disorders) and those manifesting *hypercalcemia and hypocalciuria* (familial hypocalciuric hypercalcemia) (see Table 1).

Hypercalcemia and Hypercalciuria. The constellation of hypercalcemia, hypophosphatemia, hypercalciuria, and elevated levels of PTH establishes the diagnosis of primary hyperparathyroidism. Because circulating levels of $1,25(OH)_2D_3$ largely reflect PTH activity, elevations in circulating levels of $1,25(OH)_2D_3$ are often seen in patients with primary hyperparathyroidism (Fig. 3). However, this is not invariably the case, and elevations of serum $1,25(OH)_2D_3$ are not required to establish a diagnosis of primary hyperparathyroidism. As discussed elsewhere, a small cohort of hypercalcemic patients may present with PTH levels that are not frankly elevated but are inappropriate in the context of an elevated serum calcium. Elevations of $1,25(OH)_2D_3$ in this setting may help confirm the diagnosis of primary hyperparathyroidism. $1,25(OH)_2D_3$ ceases to be a reliable marker for PTH bioactivity in the setting of renal disease as discussed below.

Patients with non–PTH-mediated hypercalcemia may also present with hypercalcemia and hypercalciuria. In these syndromes, PTH levels are low because production of the hormone is suppressed by the hypercalcemia. Two common and serious causes of non–PTH-mediated hypercalcemia are humoral hypercalcemia of malignancy (HHM) and local osteolytic hypercalcemia (LOH). As discussed previously, HHM is mediated by tumor-derived PTHrP and shares many biochemical features with primary hyperparathyroidism. However, levels of $1,25(OH)_2D_3$ are inappropriately normal or frankly low in patients with HHM, while often elevated in patients with primary hyperparathyroidism (Fig. 3). LOH is a paracrine syndrome in which tumors metastatic to bone release local factors that stimulate osteoclastogenesis. It is commonly seen in patients with breast cancer, multiple myeloma, and other hematologic malignancies such as leukemia and lymphoma. Examples of molecules that may mediate LOH are interleukin-6 (IL-6) and locally produced PTHrP, which can act in a paracrine fashion when produced by breast tumors, as well as act systemically to produce HHM. $1,25(OH)_2D_3$ levels are low in patients with LOH.

Hypercalcemia as a result of vitamin D toxicity is most commonly caused by over-replacement with $1,25(OH)_2D_3$ and is associated with hypercalciuria.[80] It may also be seen after ingestion of large quantities of vitamin D or $25(OH)D_3$, because sufficiently high concentrations of $25(OH)D_3$ can bind the vitamin D receptor in intestine and bone. Thus, the biochemical profile of vitamin D metabolites in hypervitaminosis D is determined by the nature of the vitamin D metabolite ingested (Table 1). In the setting of intoxication with $1,25(OH)_2D_3$, levels of this metabolite are elevated, while levels of $25(OH)D_3$ are normal. Intoxication with vitamin D or $25(OH)D_3$ results in normal or reduced levels of $1,25(OH)_2D_3$ in the setting of elevated concentrations of vitamin D or $25(OH)D_3$.

The milk alkali syndrome is being seen with increasing frequency given the routine administration of calcium carbonate to prevent and treat osteoporosis. The milk alkali syndrome results from the excessive ingestion of calcium together with an absorbable alkali like bicarbonate. Patients present with hypercalcemia, hyperphosphatemia, and usually have some degree of renal insufficiency. In these patients, PTH and $1,25(OH)_2D$ levels are suppressed. $25(OH)D$ levels are usually normal.

Most granulomatous disorders, both noninfectious (e.g., sarcoidosis, berylliosis) and infectious (*Mycobacterium tuberculosis*, histoplasmosis), can be associated with hypercalcemia and hypercalciuria. This is most often seen in sarcoidosis, where up to 50% of patients may have hypercalciuria and 10% hypercalcemia at some point in the course of their disease. In nearly all cases the cause is unregulated overproduction of $1,25(OH)_2D_3$ by the granulomas.[81] This inflammatory tissue has the capacity to convert $25(OH)D_3$ to the active metabolite. Unlike the renal $1-\alpha$-hydroxylase, the enzyme in the granuloma is not regulated by PTH or phosphorous. Serum levels of $1,25(OH)_2D_3$ are usually frankly elevated in these individuals, but occasionally normal or high normal levels are seen. In these instances, granulomas may be located in particularly vitamin D–responsive tissues such as bone or intestine, resulting in local production of high levels of the metabolite that are not necessarily reflected in the serum values. Rarely, lymphomas can produce $1,25(OH)_2D_3$, leading to hypercalcemia.[82]

Hypercalcemia and Hypocalciuria. The combination of hypercalcemia and hypocalciuria, in the absence of exposure to thiazide diuretics, suggests the diagnosis of familial hypocalciuric hypercalcemia (FHH). In this disorder, $1,25(OH)_2D_3$ values are usually within the normal range, although they may be mildly elevated in some patients.[83,84]

The Hypocalcemic Patient. The differential diagnosis of hypocalcemia includes vitamin D deficiency, renal dysfunction, hepatic dysfunction, hypoparathyroidism, and vitamin D–dependent and vitamin D–resistant rickets. These disorders are discussed in detail in other chapters. Accurately distinguishing among the causes of hypocalcemia requires the measurement of vitamin D metabolites.

Total body stores of vitamin D are best assessed by measurement of $25(OH)D_3$. The long half-life of this metabolite allows it to serve as an accurate reflection of total vitamin D stores. Vitamin D deficiency occurs as a result of inadequate exposure to sunlight, poor dietary intake, and decreased intestinal absorption of vitamin D. With regard to intestinal absorption, there is extensive enterohepatic circulation of $25(OH)D_3$, which may be impaired in small bowel diseases leading to depletion of body stores.

Vitamin D deficiency causes rickets in childhood and osteomalacia in adults, two conditions discussed extensively elsewhere in this volume. Milder degrees of vitamin D deficiency, so called vitamin D_3 insufficiency, lead to subtle mineralization defects and/or osteopenia caused by secondary hyperparathyroidism. As vitamin D levels fall, PTH levels rise (secondary hyperparathyroidism; Fig. 4) in

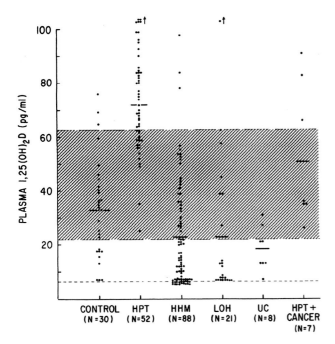

FIG. 3. Plasma 1,25(OH)$_2$D$_3$ values in six groups of patients. Control, patients with cancer and normal serum calcium values; HPT, primary hyperparathyroidism; HHM, humoral hypercalcemia of malignancy; LOH, local osteolytic hypercalcemia; UC, unclassified; HPT + Cancer, primary hyperparathyroidism and cancer. The numbers in parentheses indicate the numbers of patients on whom the measurement is available. (Reprinted with permission from Godsall JW, Burtis WJ, Insogna KL, Broadus AE, Stewart AF 1986 Nephrogenous cyclic AMP, adenylate cyclase-stimulating activity, and the humoral hypercalcemia of malignancy. Recent Prog Horm Res **42**:705–750. © 1986 The Endocrine Society.)

an effort to increase conversion of 25(OH)D to 1,25(OH)$_2$D$_3$ and increase calcium absorption. Thus, measurement of 1,25(OH)$_2$D$_3$ alone is misleading in this setting and does not accurately reflect vitamin D stores. As vitamin D deficiency progresses, 1,25(OH)$_2$D$_3$ levels may also become reduced.

Home-bound or institutionalized patients, particularly the elderly, are at risk for 25(OH)D$_3$ insufficiency and frank vitamin D deficiency caused by inadequate exposure to sunlight and poor nutritional intake. Vitamin D insufficiency and deficiency are associated with accelerated age-related bone loss[85] and an increased risk for hip fracture, and should be considered in the investigation of risk factors in the osteoporotic patient. Therapy with vitamin D (ergocalciferol, calciferol) is aimed at repletion of vitamin D stores, reflected by normalization of serum 25(OH)D$_3$ levels and a return of circulating PTH to the normal range. The lower limit of normal for serum 25(OH)D is an area of ongoing debate and controversy. Based on data like those shown in Fig. 4, as well as our own clinical experience, we consider serum 25(OH)D$_3$ values ≥20 ng/ml to be indicative of adequate vitamin D$_3$ stores. We consider values between 15 and 20 ng/ml to indicate vitamin D insufficiency, and values below 15 ng/ml to reflect vitamin D deficiency.

Patients with renal dysfunction manifest decreased levels of 1,25(OH)$_2$D$_3$ because of renal tubular damage that impairs the 1-α-hydroxylase enzyme that converts 25(OH)D$_3$

to 1,25(OH)$_2$D$_3$. The normal decline in renal function that attends aging may explain in part why intestinal calcium absorption falls with aging, [i.e., renal production of 1,25(OH)$_2$D$_3$ falls] and secondary hyperparathyroidism becomes more prevalent.[86] As renal function declines, hyperphosphatemia develops despite the actions of PTH, and this may also reduce conversion of 25(OH)D$_3$ to 1,25(OH)$_2$D$_3$, because phosphate suppresses the 1-α-hydroxylase enzyme. Thus, in patients with renal insufficiency, serum concentrations of phosphate and PTH may be elevated, whereas concentrations of calcium and 1,25(OH)$_2$D$_3$ are reduced, and concentrations of 25(OH)D$_3$ are normal.

Patients with severe nephrotic syndrome may present with low serum concentrations of calcium and 25(OH)D$_3$. These occur as a result of increased renal losses of both calcium and vitamin D–binding proteins, particularly albumin and DBP. Measurement of an ionized calcium and PTH level help distinguish true vitamin D deficiency from that caused by decreased protein binding in patients with the nephrotic syndrome. Patients with true vitamin D deficiency will manifest secondary hyperparathyroidism (i.e., elevated

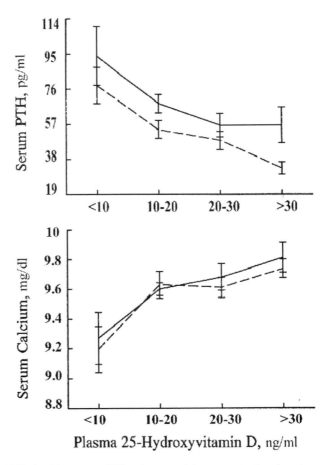

FIG. 4. Mean serum PTH and serum calcium concentrations by category of plasma 25(OH)D concentration in black (solid line) and white (dashed line) adults. Not the sharp increase in PTH when serum concentrations of 25(OH)D fall below 25 ng/ml. (Adapted with permission from Harris SS, Soteriades E, Coolidge JAS, Mudgal S, Dawson-Hughes B 2000 Vitamin D insufficiency and hyperparathyroidism in a low-income, multiracial elderly population. J Clin Endocrinol Metab **85**:4125–4130.)

levels of PTH in the context of low serum ionized calcium concentrations). Patients with nephrotic syndrome who are vitamin D sufficient should have normal serum ionized calcium concentrations and normal levels of PTH.

Chronic liver disease can lead to decreased hepatic synthesis of binding proteins (albumin, prealbumin, DBP), resulting in lowered total serum calcium and vitamin D levels, although free levels of both are normal. Hepatic 25-hydroxylase activity is usually preserved even in cases of severe hepatic insufficiency, so production of $25(OH)D_3$ from vitamin D is usually unaffected. However, these patients can experience vitamin D deficiency caused by poor nutritional intake, failure of enterohepatic circulation, or lack of sunlight exposure. Again, a low serum ionized calcium concentration in association with an elevated level of PTH suggests true vitamin D deficiency in these patients.[35] Treatment with $25(OH)D_3$, although ideal in this setting, is not practical in the United States, because this preparation of vitamin D is no longer available. Treatment with vitamin D is usually successful. Monitoring of serum calcium and PTH for resolution of secondary hyperparathyroidism guides dosing.

Patients presenting with either PTH deficiency (hypoparathyroidism) or PTH resistance (pseudohypoparathyroidism) have hypocalcemia and hyperphosphatemia. Concentrations of $1,25(OH)_2D_3$ are either reduced or inappropriately normal for the degree of associated hypocalcemia. This reflects a failure of PTH-induced activation of the renal 1-α-hydroxylase enzyme. As would be anticipated, concentrations of $25(OH)D_3$ are normal in these patients. This metabolic profile may also be seen in patients with severe magnesium deficiency, which is associated with reduced release of PTH from the parathyroid glands and perhaps a resistance to the action of PTH in target tissues.

Patients with vitamin D–dependent rickets type I have an inherited defect in the 1-α-hydroxylase enzyme leading to a failure of $1,25(OH)_2D_3$ synthesis. Those with vitamin D–dependent rickets type II exhibit target organ resistance to the action of $1,25(OH)_2D_3$ most often because of structural defects in the receptor. Both disorders manifest hypocalcemia and normal or increased levels of $25(OH)D_3$. Serum concentrations of $1,25(OH)_2D_3$ may be used to distinguish between the two disorders, because levels are predictably low in vitamin D–dependent rickets and markedly increased in patients with vitamin D–resistant rickets.

REFERENCES

1. Berson SA, Yalow RS 1968 Immunochemical heterogeneity of parathyroid hormone in plasma. J Clin Endocrinol Metab 28:1037–1047.
2. Mallette LE, Tuma SN, Berger RE, Kirkland J 1982 Radioimmunoassay for the middle region of human parathyroid hormone using an homologous antiserum with a carboxy-terminal fragment of bovine PTH as radioligand. J Clin Endocrinol Metab 54:1017–1024.
3. Nussbaum SR, Zahradnik RJ, Lavigne JR, Brennan GL, Nozawa-Ung K, Kim LV, Keutmann HT, Wang CA, Potts JT Jr, Segre GV 1987 Highly sensitive two-site immunoradiometric assay of parathyrin and its clinical utility in evaluating patients with hypercalcemia. Clin Chem 33:1364–1367.
4. Blind E, Schmidt-Gayk H, Scharla S, Flentje D, Fisher S, Gohring U, Hitzler W 1988 Two site assay of intact parathyroid hormone in the investigation of primary hyperparathyroidism and other disorders of calcium metabolism compared with a midregion assay. J Clin Endocrinol Metab 67:3543–3560.
5. Brown EM 2001 Physiology of calcium homeostasis. In: Bilezikian JP, Marcus R, Levine MA (eds.) The Parathyroids: Basic and Clinical Concepts, 2nd ed. Academic Press, San Diego, CA, USA, pp. 167–182.
6. Kronenberg HM, Bringhurst FR, Segre GV, Potts JT Jr 2001 Parathyroid hormone biosynthesis and metabolism. In: Bilezikian JP, Marcus R, Levine MA (eds.) The Parathyroids: Basic and Clinical Concepts, 2nd ed. Academic Press, San Diego, CA, USA, pp. 17–30.
7. Kemper B, Habener JF, Mulligan RC, Potts JT Jr, Rich A 1974 Pre-proparathyroid hormone: A direct translation product of parathyroid messenger RNA. Proc Natl Acad Sci USA 71:3731–3735.
8. Bringhurst FR, Stern AM, Yotts M, Mizrahi N, Segre GV, Potts JT Jr 1988 Peripheral metabolism of PTH: Fate of biologically active amino terminus in vivo. Am J Physiol 255:E886–E893.
9. Martin KJ, Hruska KA, Freitag JJ, Klahr S, Slatopolsky E 1979 The peripheral metabolism of parathyroid hormone. N Engl J Med 302:1092–1098.
10. Segre GV, D'Amour P, Hultman A, Potts J Jr 1981 Effects of hepatectomy, nephrectomy, and nephrectomy/uremia on the metabolism of parathyroid hormone in the rat. J Clin Invest 67:439–448.
11. Bringhurst FR, Segre GV, Lampman GW, Potts JT Jr 1982 Metabolism of parathyroid hormone by Kupffer cells: Analysis by reverse-phase high-performance liquid chromatography. Biochemistry 21:4252–4258.
12. D'Amour P, LaBelle F, LeCavalier L, Plourde V, Harvey D 1986 Influence of serum Ca concentration on circulating molecular forms of PTH in three species. Am J Physiol 251:E680–E687.
13. Hanley DA, Ayer LM 1986 Calcium-dependent release of carboxyl-terminal fragments of parathyroid hormone by hyperplastic human parathyroid tissue in vivo. J Clin Endocrinol Metab 63:1075–1079.
14. Blumsohn A, Hadari AA 2002 Parathyroid hormone: What are we measuring and does it matter? Ann Clin Biochem 39:169–172.
15. Slatopolsky E, Finch J, Clay P, Martin D, Sicard G, Singer G, Gao P, Cantor T, Dusso A 2000 A novel mechanism for skeletal resistance in uremia. Kidney Int 58:753–761.
16. Nguyen-Yamamoto L, Rousseau L, Brossard JH, Lepage R, D'Amour P 2001 Synthetic carboxyl-terminal fragments of parathyroid hormone (PTH) decrease ionized calcium concentration in rats by acting on a receptor different from the PTH/PTH-related peptide receptor. Endocrinology 142:1386–1392.
17. Segre GV, Habener JF, Powell D, Tregear GW, Potts JT Jr 1972 Parathyroid hormone in human plasma. Immunochemical characterization and biological implications. J Clin Invest 51:3163–3172.
18. Mallette LE, Wilson DP, Kirkland JL 1983 Evaluation of hypocalcemia with a highly sensitive, homologous radioimmunoassay for the midregion of parathyroid hormone. Pediatrics 71:64–69.
19. Nussbaum SR, Thompson AR, Hutcheson KA, Gaz RD, Wang CA 1988 Intraoperative measurement of parathyroid hormone in the surgical management of hyperparathyroidism. Surgery 104:1121–1127.
20. Irvin GL III, Deserio GT III 1994 A new, practical intraoperative parathyroid hormone assay. Am J Surg 168:466–468.
21. Brossard JH, Cloutier M, Roy L, Lepage R, Gascon-Barre M, D'Amour P 1996 Accumulation of a non-(1–84) molecular form of parathyroid hormone (PTH) detected by intact PTH assay in renal failure: Importance in the interpretation of PTH values. J Clin Endocrinol Metab 81:3923–3929.
22. Lepage R, D'Amour P, Boucher A, Hamel L, Demontigny C, Labelle F 1988 A non-(1–84) circulating parathyroid hormone (PTH) fragment interferes significantly with intact PTH commercial assay measurements in uremic samples. Clin Chem 44:805–809.
23. John MR, Goodman WG, Gao P, Cantor TL, Salusky IB, Jüppner H 1999 A novel immunoradiometric assay detects full-length human PTH but not amino-terminally truncated fragments: Implications for PTH measurements in renal failure. J Clin Endocrinol Metab 84:4287–4290.
24. Gao P, Scheibel S, D'Amour P, John MR, Rao SD, Schmidt-Gayk H, Cantor TL 2001 Development of a novel immunoradiometric assay exclusively for biologically active whole parathyroid hormone 1–84: Implications for improvement of accurate assessment of parathyroid function. J Bone Miner Res 16:605–614.
25. Godber IM, Parker CR, Lawson N, Hitch T, Porter CJ, Roe SD, Cassidy MJD, Hosking DJ 2002 Comparison of intact and 'whole molecule' parathyroid hormone assays in patients with histologically confirmed post-renal transplant osteodystrophy. Ann Clin Biochem 39:314–417.
26. Quarles LD, Lobough B, Murphy G 1992 Intact parathyroid hormone

over-estimates the presence and severity of parathyroid-mediated osseous abnormalities in uremia. J Clin Endocrinol Metab 75:145–150.

27. Silverberg SJ, Brown IN, Bilezikian JP, Deftos LJ 2000 A new highly sensitive assay for parathyroid hormone in primary hyperparathyroidism. J Bone Miner Res 15:S4;S167.

28. Bilezikian J, Potts J Jr 2002 Asymptomatic primary hyperparathyroidism: New issues and new questions-Bridging the past with the future. J Bone Miner Res 17:S2;N57–N67.

29. Sokoll LJ, Drew H, Udelsman R 2000 Intraoperative parathyroid hormone analysis: A study of 200 consecutive cases. Clin Chem 46:1662–1668.

30. Irvin GL, Stakianakis G, Yeung L, Deriso GT, Fishman LM, Molinari AS, Foss JN 1996 Ambulatory parathyroidectomy for primary hyperparathyroidism. Arch Surg 131:1074–1078.

31. Chen H, Sokoll LJ, Udelsman R 1999 Outpatient minimally invasive parathyroidectomy: A combination of sestamibi-SPECT localization, cervical block anesthesia, and intraoperative parathyroid hormone assay. Surgery 126:1016–1022.

32. Carpenter TO, Mitnick MA, Ellison A, Smith C, Insogna KL 1994 Nocturnal hyperparathyroidism: A frequent feature of X-linked hypophosphatemia. J Clin Endocrinol Metab 78:1378–1383.

33. Insogna KL, Broadus AE 1987 Nephrolithiasis. In: Felig P, Baxter JD, Broadus AE, Frohman LA (eds.) Endocrinology and Metabolism, 2nd ed. McGraw-Hill, New York, NY, USA, pp. 1500–1581.

34. Broadus AE, Horst RL, Lang R, Littledike ET, Rasumssen H 1980 The importance of 1,25 dihydroxyvitamin D in the pathogenesis of hypercalciuria and renal stone formation in primary hyperparathyroidism. N Engl J Med 302:421–426.

35. Strewler GJ 2000 The physiology of parathyroid hormone-related protein. N Engl J Med 342:177–185.

36. Philbrick WM, Wysolmerski JJ, Galbraith S, Holt E, Orloff JJ, Yang KH, Vasavada RC, Weir EC, Broadus AE, Stewart AF 1996 Defining the roles of parathyroid hormone-related protein in normal physiology. Physiol Rev 76:127–173.

37. Burtis WJ, Brady TG, Orloff JJ, Ersbak JB, Warrell RP, Olson BR, Wu TL, Mitnick MA, Broadus AE 1990 Immunochemical characterization of circulating parathyroid hormone-related protein in patients with humoral hypercalcemia of cancer. N Engl J Med 322:1106–1112.

38. Kovacs CS, Kronenberg HM 1997 Maternal-fetal calcium and bone metabolism during pregnancy, puerperium, and lactation. Endocr Rev 18:832–872.

39. Wysolmerski JJ, Vasavada R, Foley J, Weir EC, Burtis WJ, Kukrja SC, Guise TA, Broadus AE, Philbrick WM 1996 Transactivation of the PTHrP gene in squamous carcinomas predicts the occurrence of hypercalcemia in athymic mice. Cancer Res 56:1043–1049.

40. Pandian MR, Morgan CH, Carlton E, Segre GV 1992 Modified immunoradiometric assay of parathyroid hormone-related protein: Clinical application in the differential diagnosis of hypercalcemia. Clin Chem 38:282–288.

41. Ratcliffe WA, Norbury S, Heath DA, Ratcliffe JG 1991 Development and validation of an immunoradiometric assay of parathyrin-related protein in unextracted plasma. Clin Chem 37:678–685.

42. Wu T, Taylor R, Kao P 1997 Parathyroid-hormone-related peptide immunochemiluminometric assay. Ann Clin Lab Sci 27:384–389.

43. Stewart AF, Horst R, Deftos LJ, Cadman EC, Lang R, Broadus AE 1980 Biochemical evaluation of patients with cancer-associated hypercalcemia: Evidence for humoral and nonhumoral groups. N Engl J Med 303:1377–1383.

44. Yin JJ, Selander K, Chirgwin JM, Dallas M, Grubbs BG, Wieser R, Massagué J, Mundy GR, Guise TA 1999 TGF-β signaling blockade inhibits PTHrP secretion by breast cancer cells and bone metastases development. J Clin Invest 103:197–206.

45. Isales CM, Carcangiu ML, Stewart AF 1987 Hypercalcemia in breast cancer: Reassessment of the mechanism. Am J Med 82:1143–1147.

46. Budayr AA, Nissenson RA, Klein RF, Pun KK, Clark OH, Diep D, Arnaud CD, Strewler GJ 1989 Increased serum levels of a parathyroid hormone-like protein in malignancy-associated hypercalcemia. Ann Intern Med 111:807–812.

47. Khosla S, van Heerden JA, Gharib H, Jackson IT, Danks J, Hayman JA, Martin TJ 1990 Parathyroid hormone-related protein and hypercalcemia secondary to massive hyperplasia. N Engl J Med 322:1157.

48. Berar-Yanay N, Weiner P, Magadle R 2001 Hypercalcemia in systemic lupus erythematosus. Clin Rheumatol 20:147–149.

49. Fraser DR 1995 Fat-soluble vitamins: Vitamin D. Lancet 345:104–107.

50. Haussler MR, McCain TA 1977 Basic and clinical concepts relatied to vitamin d metabolism and action. N Engl J Med 297:974–983.

51. Kumar R 1997 Vitamin D and the kidney. In: Feldman D, Glorieux FH, Pike JW (eds.) Vitamin D. Academic Press, San Diego, CA, USA, pp. 275–292.

52. Breslau NA, Zerwekh JE 1997 Pharmacology of vitamin D preparations. In: Feldman D, Glorieux FH, Pike JW (eds.) Vitamin D. Academic Press, San Diego, CA, USA, pp. 607–618.

53. Holick MF 1995 Vitamin D: Photobiology, metabolism, and clinical applications. In: DeGroot L, Besser H, Burger HG, Jameson JL, Loriaux DC, Marshall JC, Odell WD, Potts JT Jr, Rubenstein AH (eds.) Endocrinology, 3rd ed. WB Saunders, Philadelphia, PA, USA, pp. 990–1013.

54. Broadus AE, Horst RL, Lang R, Littledike ET, Rasmussen H 1980 The importance of circulating 1,25-dihydroxyvitamin D in the pathogenesis of hypercalciuria and renal-stone formation in primary hyperparathyroidism. N Engl J Med 302:421–426.

55. Reichel H, Koeffler HP, Norman AW 1989 The role of the vitamin D endocrine system in health and disease. N Engl J Med 320:981–991.

56. Suda T, DeLuca HF, Hallick RB 1971 Synthesis of [26, 27–3H]-25-hydroxycholecalciferol. Ann Biochem 43:139–146.

57. Belsey R, DeLuca HF, Potts JT 1971 Competitive binding assay for vitamin D and 25-OH vitamin D. J Clin Endocrinol Metab 33:554–557.

58. Haddad JG, Chyu KJ 1971 Competitive protein-binding radioassay for 25-hydroxycholecalciferol. J Clin Endocrinol Metab 33:992–995.

59. Horst RL, Reinhardt TA, Beitz DC, Littledike ET 1981 A sensitive competitive protein binding assay for vitamin D in plasma. Steroids 37:581–591.

60. Jones G 1978 Assay of vitamins D2 and D3 in human plasma by high-performance liquid chromatography. Clin Chem 24:287–298.

61. Eisman JA, Sheperd RM, DeLuca HF 1977 Determination of 25-hydroxyvitamin D2 and 25-hydroxyvitamin D3 in human plasma using high-performance liquid chromatography. Ann Biochem 80:298–305.

62. Hollis BW 1997 Detection of vitamin D and its major metabolites. In: Feldman D, Glorieux FH, Pike JW (eds.) Vitamin D. Academic Press, San Diego, CA, USA, pp. 587–606.

63. Hollis BW, Napoli JL 1985 Improved radioimmunoassay for vitamin D and its use in assessing vitamin D status. Clin Chem 31:1815–1819.

64. Hollis BW, Kamerud JQ, Selvaag SR, Lorenz JD, Napoli JL 1993 Determination of vitamin D status by radioimmunoassay with an 125I-labeled tracer. Clin Chem 39:529–532.

65. Hollis BW, Pittard WB 1984 Evaluation of the total fetomaternal vitamin D relationships at term: Evidence for racial differences. J Clin Endocrinol Metab 1959:652–657.

66. Hollis BW 2000 Comparison of commercially available 125I-based RIA methods for the determination of circulating 25-hydroxyvitamin D. Clin Chem 46:1657–1661.

67. Roth H-J, Zahn I, Alkier R, Schmidt H 2001 Validation of the first automated chemiluminescence protein-binding assay for the detection of 25-hydroxycalciferol. Clin Lab 47:357–365.

68. Brumbaugh PF, Haussler DH, Bursac DM, Haussler MR 1974 Filter assay for 1,25-dihydroxyvitamin D3: Utilization of the hormone target tissue chromatin receptor. Biochemistry 13:4091–4097.

69. Haussler MR, McCain TA 1977 Basic and clinical concepts relatied to vitamin D metabolism and action. N Engl J Med 297:1041–1050.

70. Eisman JA, Hamsra AJ, Kream BE, DeLuca HF 1976 A sensitive, precise, and convenient method for determination of 1,25-dihydroxyvitamin Din human plasma. Arch Biochem Biophys 176:235–243.

71. Clemens TL, Hendy GN, Graham RF, Baggioline EG, Uskokovic MR, O'Riordan JLH 1978 A radioimmunoassay for 1,25-dihydroxyvitamin D3. Clin Sci Mol Med 54:329–332.

72. Hollis BW 1986 Assay of circulating 1,25-dihydroxyvitamin D involving a novel single-cartridge extraction and purification procedure. Clin Chem 32:2010–2063.

73. Reinhardt TA, Horst RL, Orf JW, Hollis BW 1984 A microassay for 1,25-dihydroxyvitamin D not requiring high performance liquid chromatography: Application to clinical studies. J Clin Endocrinol Metab 958:91–98.

74. Hollis BW 1986 Assay of circulating 1,25-dihydroxyvitamin D involving a novel single-cartridge extraction and purification procedure. Clin Chem 32:2060–2063.

75. Hollis BW, Kamerud JQ, Kurkowski A, Beaulieu J, Napoli JL 1996 Quantification of circulating 1,25-dihydroxyvitamin D by radioimmunoassay with an 125I-labeled tracer. Clin Chem 42:586–592.

76. Clive DR, Sudhaker D, Giacherio D, Gupta M, Schreiber MJ, Sackrison JL, MacFarlane GD 2002 Analytical and clinical validation of a radioimmunoassay for the measurement of 1,25 (OH)$_2$D$_3$. Clin Biochem **35**:517–521.
77. St-Arnaud R, Glorieux FH 1998 24, 25-Dihydroxyvitamin D: Active metabolite or inactive catabolite? Endocrinology **139**:3371–3374.
78. Carpenter TO, Keller M, Schwartz D, Mitnick MA, Smith C, Ellison A, Carey D, Comite F, Horst R, Travers R, Glorieux FH, Insogna KI 1996 24, 25-dihydroxyvitamin D supplementation corrects hyperparathyroidism and improves skeletal abnormalities in X-linked hypophosphatemic rickets–a clinical research center study. J Clin Endocrinol Metab **81**:2371–2388.
79. Brown AJ, Dusso A, Slatopolsky E 1994 Selective vitamin D analogs and their therapeutic applications. Semin Nephrol **14**:156–174.
80. Vieth R 1990 The mechanisms of vitamin D toxicity. Bone Miner 267–272.
81. Insogna KL, Dreyer BE, Mitnick MA, Ellison AF, Broadus AE 1988 Enhanced production rate of 1,25-dihydroxyvitamin D in sarcoidosis. J Clin Endocrinol Metab **66**:72–75.
82. Rosenthal N, Insogna K, Godsall W, Smaldone L, Waldron T, Stewart A 1985 1,25-Dihydroxyvitamin D as a humoral mediator of hypercalcemia in lymphoma. J Clin Endocrinol Metab **60**:29–33.
83. Firek AF, Kao PC, Heath H III 1991 Plasma intact parathyroid hormone (PTH) and PTH-related peptide in familial benign hypercalcemia: Greater responsiveness to endogenous PTH than in primary hyperparathyroidism. J Clin Endocrinol Metab **72**:541–546.
84. Kristiansen JH, Rodbro P, Christiansen C, Brochner MJ, Carl J 1985 Familial hypocalciuric hypercalcemia II: Intestinal calcium absorption and vitamin D metabolism. Clin Endocrinol (Oxf) **23**:511–515.
85. Fraser DR 1995 Vitamin D. Lancet **345**:104–107.
86. Slovik DM, Adams JS, Neer RM, Holick MF, Potts JT 1981 Deficient production of 1,25(oh)$_2$d$_3$ in elderly osteoporotic patients. N Engl J Med **305**:372–374.

Chapter 26.   Biochemical Markers of Bone Turnover

Sundeep Khosla[1] and Michael Kleerekoper[2]

[1]*Division of Endocrinology, Mayo Clinic, Rochester, Minnesota; and* [2]*Division of Endocrinology, Wayne State University, Detroit, Michigan*

INTRODUCTION

Throughout adult life, bone tissue is subject to a continuous process of turnover, whereby old bone is removed and replaced by new bone by the coupled processes of bone resorption and bone formation. Moreover, most states of increased bone turnover, such as postmenopausal osteoporosis, are associated with a net increase in bone resorption over formation, resulting in bone loss. Thus, while measurement of bone mineral density (BMD) is critical in the clinical evaluation of the patient at risk for osteoporosis, BMD represents a static parameter that provides no insight into the rate of bone turnover in a given patient. The ability to complement the static measurement of BMD with an assessment of the dynamic process of bone turnover could, in principle, enhance the ability of BMD to predict the risk of subsequent fracture. However, while it has been possible to measure BMD at various skeletal sites for almost 20 years, bone turnover could only be assessed in the past by combined calcium balance and isotope kinetic studies (which are time consuming and enormously expensive) or by tetracycline-based histomorphometry (which is invasive and expensive). Thus, the more recent availability of biochemical markers for bone turnover represent a major methodological advance. These measurements are noninvasive, relatively inexpensive, generally available, can measure changes in bone turnover over short intervals of time, and can be assessed repetitively. As with any new technology, however, where they fit into our clinical approach to patients with known or suspected osteoporosis is an evolving area. With this caveat in mind, this chapter reviews currently available biochemical markers for bone turnover and their potential clinical use in the evaluation and management of patients with osteoporosis.

CURRENTLY AVAILABLE BIOCHEMICAL MARKERS OF BONE TURNOVER

Table 1 lists currently available bone turnover markers. Each of the markers represents a product released into the circulation during the process of bone formation or resorption. Hence, it is useful to discuss the markers in the context of these processes.

The major synthetic product of osteoblasts is type I collagen; however, osteoblasts also synthesize and secrete a variety of noncollagenous proteins, two of which are clinically useful markers of osteoblastic activity, and by inference, bone formation. Bone specific alkaline phosphatase (BSAP) is an osteoblast product that is clearly essential for mineralization. Indeed, BSAP deficiency, as in the disease hypophosphatasia, results in defective mineralization of

TABLE 1. CURRENTLY AVAILABLE BONE BIOCHEMICAL MARKERS

Formation
Serum
Bone specific alkaline phosphatase (BSAP)
Osteocalcin (OC)
Carboxyterminal propeptide of type I collagen (PICP)
Aminoterminal propeptide of type I collagen (PINP)
Resorption
Urine
Hydroxyproline
Free and total pyridinolines (Pyd)
Free and total deoxypyridinolines (Dpd)
N-telopeptide of collagen cross-links (NTx)
C-telopeptide of collagen cross-links (CTx)
Serum
Cross-linked C-telopeptide of type I collagen (ICTP)
Tartrate-resistant acid phosphatase, TRACP
N-telopeptide of collagen cross-links (NTx)
C-telopeptide of collagen cross-links (CTx)

The authors have no conflict of interest.

bones and teeth.[1] The precise role of BSAP in the mineralization process, however, remains unclear. It may increase local concentrations of inorganic phosphate, destroy local inhibitors of mineral crystal growth, transport phosphate, or act as a calcium-binding protein or Ca^{2+}-ATPase.

Circulating AP activity is derived from several tissues, including intestine, spleen, kidney, placenta (in pregnancy), liver, bone, or from various tumors. Thus, measurement of total AP activity does not provide specific information on bone formation. However, because the two most common sources of elevated AP levels are liver and bone, a number of techniques, including heat denaturation, chemical inhibition of selective activity, gel electrophoresis, and precipitation by wheat germ lectin have been used to distinguish the liver versus bone isoforms of the enzyme. Recent assays, however, have used tissue specific monoclonal antibodies to measure the bone isoform which have 10–20% cross-reactivity with the liver isoform.

Osteocalcin (OC) is another noncollagenous protein secreted by osteoblasts and is widely accepted as a marker for osteoblastic activity, and hence, bone formation. However, it should be kept in mind that OC is incorporated into the matrix and is released into the circulation from the matrix during bone resorption, so the serum level at any one time has a component of both bone formation and resorption. Therefore, OC is more properly a marker of bone turnover rather than a specific marker of bone formation. It is a small protein of 49 amino acids, and in most species, contains three residues (at 17, 21, and 24) of γ-carboxyglutamic acid (Gla). The function of OC has not been identified, although its deposition in the bone matrix increases with hydroxyapatite deposition during skeletal growth. In vitro studies suggest that OC may function to limit the process of mineralization,[2] and in vivo studies using OC "knock-out" mice have found that these mice actually have increases in bone mass.[3]

In the circulation, OC is present as the intact molecule and as a fragment or fragments of the intact molecule. It is unclear whether fragmentation of the intact molecule occurs in the blood, occurs during bone resorption, or both. While older immunoassays that measured various OC fragments often gave widely discordant results even in the same individuals, newer assays measuring the major circulating forms of OC, which are either the intact molecule or a large N-terminal fragment spanning residues 1–43,[4] have shown much greater reliability as bone turnover markers.

As noted earlier, the major synthetic product of osteoblasts is type I collagen so, in principle, indices of type I collagen synthesis would appear to be ideal bone formation markers. Several such assays have been developed in recent years, directed against either the carboxy- or amino-extension peptides of the procollagen molecule. These extension peptides (carboxyterminal propeptide of type I collagen [PICP] and aminoterminal propeptide of type I procollagen [PINP]) guide assembly of the collagen triple helix and are cleaved from the newly formed molecule in a stoichiometric relationship with collagen biosynthesis. However, because type I collagen is not unique to bone, these peptides are also produced by other tissues that synthesize type I collagen, including skin.

Several immunoassays for PICP and PINP have been

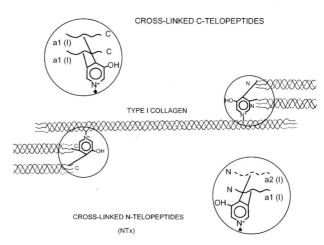

FIG. 1. Schematic showing the source of cross-linked N- and C-telopeptides of type I collagen from bone. The amino- and carboxy-terminals of the collagen chains are linked to adjacent collagen chains by these cross-links. The telopeptides are the regions of the collagen chains where this cross-linking occurs; during the process of collagen breakdown, these telopeptides are released into the circulation and cleared by the kidney. (Adapted from Endocrine Reviews **17**:333–368 with permission from The Endocrine Society.)

developed.[5,6] Clinically, however, neither of these seems to be as useful as either BSAP or OC in terms of distinguishing normal from disease states. This may, in part, be because of the inability of current assays to distinguish between bone and soft-tissue contributions to the circulating levels of these peptides.

In contrast to the bone formation markers, where the noncollagenous proteins produced by osteoblasts seem to be the most useful markers, it is the collagen degradation products, rather than specific osteoclast proteins, that are most useful as markers of bone resorption. As the skeleton is resorbed, the collagen breakdown products are released into the circulation and ultimately cleared by the kidney. The predominant amino acid of type I collagen is hydroxyproline, and assay of its level in the urine has been used for many years to assess bone resorption. However, hydroxyproline is not specific to bone collagen, and dietary protein sources can also contribute to urinary hydroxyproline excretion. Because of this, patients had to be on a collagen-free diet for 1–3 days before a 24-h collection for hydroxyproline measurement. It seems, however, that an overnight fast may be adequate to eliminate the effects of dietary collagen,[7] so this may be the preferred way to collect the specimen. Nonetheless, a major drawback of urinary hydroxyproline measurements is that they require high-pressure liquid chromatographic (HPLC) methods, which are relatively time-consuming and expensive.

The recent development of rapid and relatively inexpensive immunoassays for various collagen breakdown products represents perhaps the major advance in this area and one that is likely to greatly increase the clinical use of the bone resorption markers. Collagen molecules in the bone matrix are staggered to form fibrils that are joined by covalent cross-links (Fig. 1). These cross-links consist of hydroxylysyl-pyridinolines (Pyd) and lysyl-pyridinolines (deoxypyridinolines [Dpd]). Pyd is present in the skeleton more abundantly than Dpd, but Dpd has greater specificity because Pyd is present to some extent in type II collagen of cartilage and other connective tissues. The Pyd and Dpd cross-links occur at two intermolecular sites in the collagen molecule: at or near residue 930, where two aminotelopeptides are linked to a helical site (N-telopeptide of collagen cross-links [NTx]), and at residue 87, where two carboxytelopeptides are linked to a helical site (C-telopeptide of collagen cross-links [CTx]; Fig. 1).

When osteoclasts resorb bone, they release a variety of collagen degradation products into the circulation that are metabolized further by the liver and the kidney. Thus, urine contains both free Pyd and Dpd (approximately 40%) and peptide-bound Pyd and Dpd (approximately 60%). The initial assays for Pyd and Dpd measured both free and, following acid hydrolysis of urine, total Pyd and Dpd by fluorometry after HPLC.[8] While this likely remains the "gold standard" for measuring Pyd and Dpd in urine, it is relatively time-consuming and expensive, and there are now a number of immunoassays that can measure free Pyd and Dpd in urine.[9]

In addition to the free Pyd and Dpd assays, immunoassays are also now available to measure the amino- and carboxy-terminal telopeptides released during bone resorption (NTx and CTx, respectively).[10,11] There are, therefore, a number of rapid and relatively inexpensive methods for assessing urinary bone resorption markers, each with certain advantages and limitations (discussed below). Moreover, assays have also been developed to measure Dpd, NTx, and CTx in the circulation, which obviates the need for urine collections.

In addition to these assays, there has been another assay available for measuring serum cross-linked C-telopeptide of type I collagen (ICTP), which recognized an antigen in serum, but not in urine. While this assay has been available for several years, it has been relatively disappointing as a bone resorption marker,[12] and the peptides being recognized in serum have not been fully characterized.

Finally, the only osteoclast-specific product that has been evaluated to any extent as a bone resorption marker is TRACP. Acid phosphatase is a lysosomal enzyme that is present in a number of tissues, including bone, prostate, platelets, erythrocytes, and the spleen. Osteoclasts contain a TRACP that is released into the circulation. However, plasma TRACP is not entirely specific for the osteoclast, and the enzyme is relatively unstable in frozen samples. Because of these limitations, TRACP has not been used to any significant extent in the clinical assessment of patients, although the development of immunoassays using monoclonal antibodies specifically directed against the bone isoenzyme of TRACP may improve its clinical use.

GENERAL CONSIDERATIONS IN THE USE OF BONE BIOCHEMICAL MARKERS

Before discussing the specific clinical settings in which bone biochemical markers might be useful, it is helpful to review certain general issues regarding the use of these markers. First, urinary resorption markers are generally reported after normalizing to creatinine excretion. This has

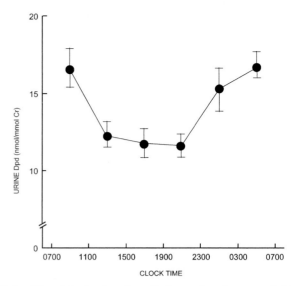

FIG. 2. Diurnal rhythm for urinary Dpd excretion of a group of elderly women (mean age, 71 $\pm$ 2 years). Note that urinary Dpd excretion increases by approximately 50% between 9:00 p.m. and 7:00 a.m. (Adapted from J Clin Endocrinol Metab **81:**1699–1703 with permission from The Endocrine Society.)

certain limitations, including variability in the creatinine measurement that contributes to the overall variability in the measurement of the urinary markers (see below), as well as potential artifactual changes in the urinary markers based on alterations in muscle mass. Thus, a more appropriate correction might be to express the urinary markers in terms of dl or liter of glomerular filtrate, although this is relatively cumbersome in the clinical setting. Nonetheless, this potential for artifact should be kept in mind when interpreting the urinary excretion markers. Serum assays for NTx and CTx are now available in several research and reference laboratories, and serum CTx is available in Europe on an automated platform. These advances, particularly automation, have substantially reduced the "noise" in the assays, although it is still seems best to obtain a fasting blood specimen.

A second issue is that many of the bone turnover markers have circadian rhythms, so the timing of sampling is of some importance. Thus, both serum OC and PICP levels peak in the early morning hours (between 4 and 8 a.m.), and have nadirs in the mid- to late afternoon.[13,14] BSAP, which has a long half-life in serum (1–2 days), however, does not show much circadian variability. All of the urinary and serum bone resorption markers also have significant circadian patterns, with peak levels occurring between 4 and 8 a.m.[15] (Fig. 2). For the urine markers, therefore, it is best to obtain either a 24-h urine collection or, if that is inconvenient for the patient, a second morning void sample can be used.

In adults, a third consideration is that most of the bone turnover markers tend to be positively associated with age,[16] except for a significant decline from adolescence to about age 25 years, as the phase of skeletal consolidation is completed.[13] This issue must be kept in mind when normative data for each of the markers are established. Moreover, unlike the current World Health Organization (WHO)

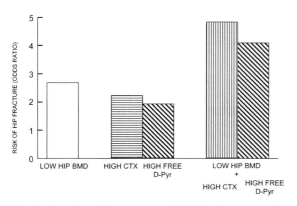

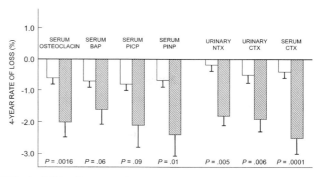

FIG. 3. Combination of the assessment of BMD and bone resorption rate to predict hip fracture risk in a cohort of elderly (mean age, 82.5 years) French women. Low BMD was defined by a value below 2.5 SD of the young adult mean and high bone resorption by urinary CTx or free Dpd values above 2.0 SD of the young adult mean. (Adapted from J Bone Miner Res 1996;**11**:1531–1538 with permission from the American Society for Bone and Mineral Research.)

FIG. 5. Mid-radius BMD change over 4 years in 305 healthy postmenopausal women with low (open bars) and high (shaded bars) bone turnover at baseline. High turnover was defined as bone marker levels above the upper limit of the premenopausal range. p values refer to the difference in the rate of bone loss between the two groups of bone turnover. (Adapted from J Bone Miner Res 1999;**14**:1614–1621 with permission from the American Society for Bone and Mineral Research.)

definitions for osteopenia and osteoporosis, there are currently no accepted criteria for defining "high" bone turnover. Thus, the clinician obtaining the bone turnover marker should be aware as to whether the reference range for that particular marker is based on young adult individuals (i.e., age 20 or 25–40 years) or age-matched individuals.

A fourth issue is the potential for differential changes in the various bone formation or resorption markers in different disease states or in response to different therapies. Thus, BSAP tends to show much larger increases in Paget's disease than OC; conversely, glucocorticoid therapy is associated with larger decrements in OC levels as opposed to BSAP levels.[17] Similarly, the urinary excretion of free and peptide-bound fractions of Pyd seems to be differently affected by bisphosphonate and estrogen therapy. Thus, bisphosphonate treatment has been reported to induce a specific decrease of cross-linked peptides without any change in the excretion of free cross-links, whereas estrogen

therapy decreases the urinary excretion of both forms of Pyd and Dpd.[11]

Finally, one has to be aware of the potential variability (technical and biological) of the various bone turnover markers. BMD can be measured by DXA with an accuracy of greater than 95% and a precision error for repeat measurements of between 0.5% and 2.5%. The technology needs to be this good because the rate of change in BMD is slow, and in many circumstances, the annual rate of change is less than the precision error of the measurement. In contrast, the biochemical markers of bone remodeling are subject to intra- and interassay variability (technical variability) as well as individual patient biological variability. As noted earlier, for the urine-based markers, this variability is compounded by the normalization to creatinine excretion, because there is considerable day-to-day variation of creatinine excretion in individual patients. In general, the long-term variability of the urine-based markers is on the order of 20–30%,[18,19] and the serum-based markers on the order of 10–15%,[20] but this is improved to 3–5% with automated assays. This issue will be considered further below, because it is critical to keep this in mind when these markers are used in the clinical setting.

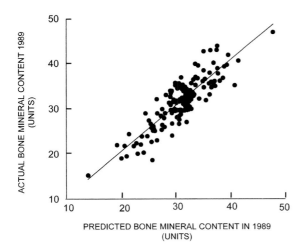

FIG. 4. Predicted vs. actual bone mineral content of the forearm in a group of early postmenopausal women studied 12 years apart. Bone mineral content was predicted using a combination of bone biochemical markers (see text for details). (Adapted from BMJ 1991;**303**:1548–1549 with permission from the BMJ Publishing Group.)

POTENTIAL CLINICAL USES OF BONE BIOCHEMICAL MARKERS

Prediction of Bone Mass

Bone biochemical markers assess balance between resorption and formation, and although bone turnover markers are generally inversely correlated with BMD,[21] these correlations are not strong enough to have any value in terms of predicting bone mass for a given individual. Thus, these markers cannot and should not be used to diagnose osteoporosis or to predict bone mass; direct measurement of BMD is extremely effective at accomplishing that.

Prediction of Fracture Risk

This represents perhaps the most intriguing use of bone biochemical markers, because in principle, assessment of

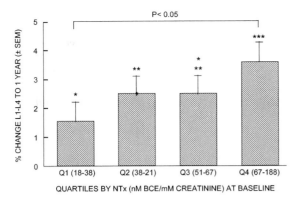

FIG. 6. Response to HT at the spine by quartiles of baseline NTx excretion in a group of early postmenopausal women (p values vs. baseline BMD: *p < 0.05; **p < 0.001; ***p < 0.0001). (Adapted from AM J Med **102**:29–37 with permission from Elsevier.)

bone turnover may provide additional information on fracture risk beyond that provided by BMD. Several studies now do suggest that bone turnover may be an independent predictor of fracture risk.[21–23] Thus, in a prospective cohort study of elderly (age >75 years) French women, urinary CTx and free Dpd excretion above the upper limit of the premenopausal range (i.e., mean +2 SD) was associated with an increased risk of hip fracture (Fig. 3), even after adjusting for femoral neck BMD.[23] In recent population-based studies in women, bone resorption markers were negatively correlated with BMD of the hip, spine, and forearm, and women with osteoporosis were more likely to have high bone turnover.[21] Moreover, a history of osteoporotic fractures of the hip, spine, or distal forearm was associated with reduced hip BMD and with elevated biochemical markers of bone resorption.[21] The mechanisms by which increased bone turnover adversely affects fracture risk include exacerbation of rates of bone loss[24] (see below), microarchitectural deterioration of the skeleton caused by perforation of trabeculae and loss of structural elements of bone,[25] or a reduction in bone strength caused by an enlarged remodeling space.[22,26] Thus, bone turnover, as assessed by biochemical markers, seems to have a significant impact on the risk of fracture independent of BMD. However, until more prospective data are available, particularly in younger women than those studied in the French cohort,[23] the routine use of bone biochemical markers to complement BMD measurements for prediction of fracture risk in an individual patient cannot be recommended at this time.

Prediction of Bone Loss

Estrogen deficiency at menopause increases the rate of bone remodeling, which results in high turnover bone loss. This is reflected by a significant increase in the mean value of markers of resorption and formation from before to after menopause. Moreover, the individual variability in the bone turnover markers also increases after menopause, reflecting a variable skeletal response among different individuals to estrogen deficiency. This is also reflected in the variable rates of bone loss observed among women after menopause. Several studies now indicate that, at least for groups of individuals, bone biochemical markers can be used to predict the rate of bone loss. Thus, Hansen et al.[24] measured the bone mineral content (BMC) of the forearm at baseline and 12 years later and attempted to predict the observed rate of bone loss by using a biochemical model that included fat mass, serum alkaline phosphatase activity, fasting urinary calcium to creatinine ratio, and fasting urinary hydroxyproline to creatinine ratio. Using these relative crude bone turnover markers, they were able to predict the observed bone mass 12 years later with a high degree of accuracy (Fig. 4). Thus, these and other data[27] do suggest that bone turnover markers, either individually or in combination,

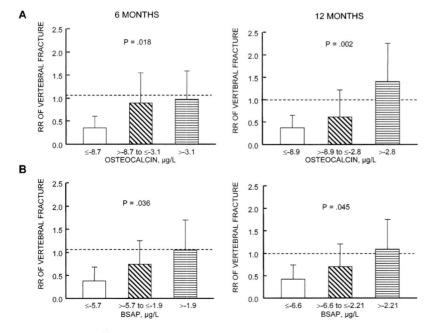

FIG. 7. The relative risk of new vertebral fractures (raloxifene vs. placebo) by tertiles of change in serum (A) OC and (B) BSAP after 6 and 12 months. The p values are for interaction and indicate the presence of a differential antifracture efficacy across tertiles for a model including tertile, therapy, and tertile × therapy. (Adapted from Osteoporos Int **12**:922–930 with permission from International Osteoporosis Foundation.)

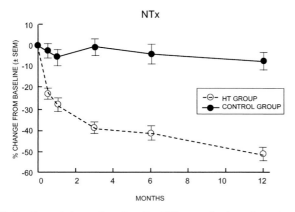

FIG. 8. Percent change from baseline NTx excretion in early postmenopausal women treated with HT or no therapy. (Adapted from Am J Med **102**:29–37 with permission from Elsevier.)

may be able to predict rates of bone loss, thereby complementing the static measurement of BMD. Recently, Garnero at al.[28] reported results of a 4-year prospective study of change in forearm BMD in early postmenopausal women as a function of bone turnover markers. Subjects were divided into those in whom the value for the marker being studied was within the reference interval for healthy premenopausal women (normal turnover group) or more than 2 SD above the mean value for premenopausal women (high turnover group). The study involved three markers of resorption and four formation markers. Women in the normal turnover group lost <1% of BMD over 4 years, whereas those in the high turnover group lost three to five times that amount of bone (Fig. 5).

Selection of Patients for Therapy

Several studies indicate that individuals with the highest levels of bone turnover seem to have the best response to antiresorptive therapy (i.e., with estrogen, calcitonin, or bisphosphonates). Thus, in a prospective 2-year study of hormone therapy (HT), Chesnut et al.[29] found that subjects in the highest quartiles for baseline urinary NTx excretion demonstrated the greatest gain in BMD in response to HT (Fig. 6). With the recent approval of the first formation-stimulation therapy (teriparatide), it is appropriate to speculate that this therapy would be more effective in patients with low bone turnover than in those with high turnover. As with the clinical trials using antiresorptive therapies, the clinical trials with teriparatide were not designed to specifically test this hypothesis, and no difference in baseline values for markers between responders and nonresponders was reported. This analysis only evaluated response in terms of change in BMD, not antifracture effectiveness. Such data may be forthcoming with further analysis of the data, as has recently been demonstrated with the antiresorptive drug raloxifene.[30] In that study, the changes in bone formation markers OC and BSAP were significant predictors of antifracture efficacy (Figs. 7A and 7B), whereas change in hip or spine BMD were not. Changes in urinary CTX were also not predictors of antifracture effectiveness, and it remains to

be seen whether this will change now that better assays for serum CTX, with less variability, are available.

It is likely that therapy for osteoporosis will evolve into combinations of antiresorptive and formation-stimulation drugs. The combinations and permutations of how this might occur are quite extensive. It would seem logical, particularly with the availability of more reliable serum assays for resorption as well as formation markers, that markers will play an increasing role in the selection and timing of therapies.

Monitoring Effectiveness of Therapy

This represents perhaps the best established clinical use of bone biochemical markers at present. Considerable data now indicate that after initiation of antiresorptive therapy, there is a significant reduction in markers of bone resorption within 4–6 weeks,[12,31] and in markers of bone formation, in 2–3 months.[12] Thus, bone turnover markers can be used to determine when therapy is ineffective. Antiresorptive agents should produce a reduction in the markers of resorption of between 20% and 80%, depending on the agent and the markers. Thus, despite the potential technical and biological variability of the markers, changes of this magnitude should be clinically meaningful. For most treatments, the nadir will be reached between 2 and 3 months after initiation and will remain constant as long as the patient is on therapy (Fig. 8).[29] Failure to show the expected reduction in resorption markers could indicate noncompliance with therapy or the possible need to change the dose or type of therapy. This use of bone biochemical markers offers a

TABLE 2. CURRENT AND POTENTIAL CLINICAL USE OF BIOCHEMICAL MARKERS OF BONE REMODELING

Clinical use	Quality of outcome
Diagnose osteoporosis	None
Predict bone mass	Very poor
Predict fracture occurrence	Strong, but unproven potential
Select patients for therapy	Possibly useful, when used in conjunction with bone mass measurement, at segregating fast from slow losers
	Without BMD, not until fracture prediction is better documented
Select specific therapy for patients	Will become more important as new classes of therapies, such as formation stimulation agents, are used (e.g., PTH)
Select specific dose for patients	Very useful when more than one dose is available (currently only estrogen and injectable calcitonin)
Monitor compliance with therapy	None, it is more cost-effective to ask patients
Monitor effectiveness of therapy	The most appropriate current use
Predict increases in bone mass on therapy	Yes, but not demonstrated in all studies with all therapies

Adapted with permission from Kleerekoper.[33]

© 2003 American Society for Bone and Mineral Research

marked advantage over using BMD to assess the effectiveness of therapy, because the interval between serial measurements of BMD must be at least 12 (and possibly 24) months before significant changes in BMD can be documented, or more importantly, the lack of change in BMD can be established with any certainty.

SUMMARY AND CONCLUSIONS

The availability of biochemical markers of bone formation and resorption that can be measured rapidly and relatively inexpensively represents a significant advance in the evaluation and treatment of patients at risk for or with osteoporosis. The markers provide a dynamic assessment of the skeleton that can potentially complement the static measurement of BMD. As with any new technology, however, one needs to understand their limitations and use them in the appropriate clinical setting. Table 2 summarizes the current and potential clinical use of these markers. Their use is likely to continue to increase with further clinical experience and technical refinements in the assays. This, in turn, has the potential for resulting in better selection of patients for therapy, tailoring specific therapies to different patients, and better monitoring of the effectiveness of therapy.

REFERENCES

1. Whyte MP 1994 Hypophosphatasia and the role of alkaline phosphatase in skeletal mineralization. Endocr Rev **15**:439–461.
2. Zhou H, Choong P, McCarthy R, Chou S, Martin T, Ng K 1994 In situ hybridization to show sequential expression of osteoblast gene markers during bone formation in vivo. J Bone Miner Res **9**:1489–1500.
3. Ducy P, Desbois C, Boyce B, Pinero G, Story B, Dunstan C, Smith E, Bonadio J, Goldstein S, Gundberg C, Bradley A, Karsenty G 1996 Increased bone formation in osteocalcin-deficient mice. Nature **382:**448–452.
4. Deftos LJ, Wolfert RL, Hill CS, Burton DW 1992 Two-site assays of bone Gla protein (osteocalcin) demonstrate immunochemical heterogeneity of the intact molecule. Clin Chem **38:**2318–2321.
5. Melkko J, Niemi S, Risteli L, Risteli J 1990 Radioimmunoassay of the carboxyterminal propeptide of human type I procollagen. Clin Chem **36:**1328–1332.
6. Melkko J, Kauppila S, Niemi S, Risteli L, Haukipuro K, Jukkola A, Risteli J 1996 Immunoassay for intact amino-terminal propeptide of human type I procollagen. Clin Chem **42:**947–954.
7. Wilson PS, Kleerekoper M, Bone H, Parfitt AM 1990 Urinary total hydroxyproline measured by HPLC: Comparison of spot and timed urine collections. Clin Chem **36:**388–389.
8. Black D, Duncan A, Robins SP 1988 Quantitative analysis of the pyridinium crosslinks of collagen in urine using ion-paired reversed-phase high-performance liquid chromatography. Anal Biochem **169:**197–203.
9. Robins SP, Woitge H, Hesley R, Ju J, Seyedin S, Seibel M 1994 Direct enzyme-linked immunoassay for urinary deoxypyridinoline as a specific marker for measuring bone resorption. J Bone Miner Res **9:**1643–1649.
10. Hanson DA, Weis MAE, Bollen A, Maslan SL, Singer FR, Eyre DR 1992 A specific immunoassay for monitoring human bone resorption: Quantitation of type I collagen cross-linked N-telopeptides in urine. J Bone Miner Res **7:**1251–1258.
11. Garnero P, Gineyts E, Arbault P, Christiansen C, Delmas PD 1995 Different effects of bisphosphonate and estrogen therapy on free and peptide-bound bone cross-links excretion. J Bone Miner Res **10:**641–649.
12. Garnero P, Shih WJ, Gineyts E, Karpf DB, Delmas PD 1994 Comparison of new biochemical markers of bone turnover in late postmenopausal osteoporotic women in response to alendronate treatment. J Clin Endocrinol Metab **79:**1693–1700.
13. Eastell R, Simmons PS, Colwell A, Assiri AM, Burritt MF, Russell RG, Riggs BL 1992 Nyctohemeral changes in bone turnover assessed by serum bone Gla-protein concentration and urinary deoxypyridinoline excretion: Effects of growth and ageing. Clin Sci **83:**375–382.
14. Hassager C, Risteli J, Risteli L, Jensen SB, Christiansen C 1992 Diurnal variation in serum markers of type I collagen synthesis and degradation in healthy premenopausal women. J Bone Miner Res **7:**1307–1311.
15. McKane WR, Khosla S, Egan KS, Robins SP, Burritt MF, Riggs BL 1996 Role of calcium intake in modulating age-related increases in parathyroid function and bone resorption. J Clin Endocrinol Metab **81:**1699–1703.
16. Khosla S, Melton LJI, Atkinson EJ, Klee GG, O'Fallon WM, Riggs BL 1998 Relationship of serum sex steroid levels with bone mineral density in aging women and men: A key role for bioavailable estrogen. J Clin Endocrinol Metab **83:**2266–2274.
17. Duda RJ Jr, O'Brien JF, Katzmann JA, Peterson JM, Mann KG, Riggs BL 1988 Concurrent assays of circulating bone Gla-protein and bone alkaline phosphatase: Effects of sex, age, and metabolic bone disease. J Clin Endocrinol Metab **66:**951–957.
18. Kleerekoper M, Wilson PS, Simpson P 1994 Within subject variability of biochemical markers of bone remodeling in normal older women. J Bone Miner Res **9:**1;S394.
19. Gertz BJ, Shao P, Hanson DA, Quan H, Harris ST, Genant HK 1994 Monitoring bone resorption in early postmenopausal women by an immunoassay for cross-linked collagen peptides in urine. J Bone Miner Res **9:**135–140.
20. Panteghini M, Pagani F 1995 Biological variation in bone-derived biochemical markers in serum. Scand J Clin Lab Invest **55:**609–616.
21. Melton LJI, Khosla S, Atkinson EJ, O'Fallon WM, Riggs BL 1997 Relationship of bone turnover to bone density and fractures. J Bone Miner Res **12:**1083–1091.
22. Riggs BL, Melton LJ III, O'Fallon WM 1996 Drug therapy for vertebral fractures in osteoporosis: Evidence that decreases in bone turnover and increases in bone mass both determine anti-fracture efficacy. Bone **18:**197S–201S.
23. Garnero P, Hausherr E, Chapuy MC, Marcelli C, Grandjean H, Muller C, Cormier C, Breart G, Meunier PJ, Delmas PD 1996 Markers of bone resorption predict hip fracture in elderly women: The EPIDOS Prospective Study. J Bone Miner Res **11:**1531–1538.
24. Hansen MA, Overgaard K, Riis BJ, Christiansen C 1991 Role of peak bone mass and bone loss in postmenopausal osteoporosis: 12 year study. BMJ **303:**1548–1549.
25. Parfitt AM 1984 Age-related structural changes in trabecular and cortical bone: Cellular mechanisms and biomechanical consequences. Calcif Tissue Int **36:**S123–S128.
26. Einhorn TA 1992 Bone strength: The bottom line. Calcif Tissue Int **51:**333–339.
27. Uebelhart D, Schlemmer A, Johansen JS, Gineyts E, Delmas PD 1991 Effect of menopause and hormone replacement therapy on the urinary excretion of pyridinium cross-links. J Clin Endocrinol Metab **72:**367–373.
28. Garnero P, Sornay-Rendu E, Duboeuf F, Delmas PD 1999 Markers of bone turnover predict postmenopausal forearm bone loss over 4 years: The OFELY study. J Bone Miner Res **14:**1614–1621.
29. Chesnut CH III, Bell NH, Clark GS, Drinkwater BL, English SC, Johnson CC Jr, Notelovitz M, Rosen C, Cain DF, Flessland KA, Mallinak NJ 1997 Hormone replacement therapy in postmenopausal women: Urinary N-telopeptide of type I collagen monitors therapeutic effect and predicts response of bone mineral density. Am J Med **102:**29–37.
30. Bjarnason NH, Sarkar S, Duong T, Mitlak B, Delmas PD, Christiansen C 2001 Six and twelve month changes in bone turnover are related to reduction in vertebral fracture risk during 3 years of raloxifene treatment in postmenopausal osteoporosis. Osteoporos Int **12:**922–930.
31. Prestwood KM, Pilbeam CC, Burleson JA, Woodiel FN, Delmas PD, Deftos LJ, Raisz LG 1994 The short term effects of conjugated estrogen on bone turnover in older women. J Clin Endocrinol Metab **79:**366–371.
32. Calvo MS, Eyre DR, Gundberg CM 1996 Molecular basis and clinical applications of biological markers of bone turnover. Endocr Rev **17:**333–368.
33. Kleerekoper M 1996 Biochemical markers of bone remodeling. Am J Med Sci **312:**270–277.

Chapter 27. Radiologic Evaluation of Bone Mineral in Children

Mary B. Leonard[1] and Richard M. Shore[2]

[1]Department of Pediatrics, Children's Hospital of Philadelphia, Philadelphia, Pennsylvania; and [2]Department of Radiology, Northwestern University Medical School, Chicago, Illinois

INTRODUCTION

Bone mineral evaluation in children is performed for different reasons than in adults, and the approaches used for this evaluation are consequently different. Recent years have seen a dramatic increase in interest in the effects of childhood diseases on bone mineralization. Bone mineralization has been examined across a broad spectrum of pediatric disorders, including cystic fibrosis, cerebral palsy, anorexia nervosa, renal failure, sickle cell disease, insulin-dependent diabetes, inborn errors of metabolism, and leukemia, with particular attention focused on many disorders requiring glucocorticoid therapy such as juvenile rheumatoid arthritis, inflammatory bowel disease, nephrotic syndrome, systemic lupus erythematosis, and organ transplantation.[1–22] These reports have led to recommendations for bone density screening protocols in children being considered for steroid therapy and ongoing monitoring of the response to therapy.[23–25] Treatment protocols with bisphosphonates, calcitonin, calcium, vitamin D, hormone replacement therapy, or growth hormone have been proposed for children and adolescents with decreased bone mass.[8,26–29] Nonetheless, there is significant controversy over the optimal measures of bone health in children, the unique limitations of existing technologies in children, and the availability of adequate reference data to characterize the impact of childhood diseases and their therapies.

Bone mineral evaluation in childhood must include both quantitative and qualitative assessment. Quantitative evaluation is essential because subjective assessment of bone density from skeletal radiographs is unreliable. In some cases, significant osteopenia may be present while skeletal radiographs still appear within normal limits. Even if osteopenia is demonstrated on radiographs, its appearance is highly dependent on technical factors such as beam energy, use of a grid, and the response characteristics of the film or computed radiography system. These factors prohibit meaningful serial evaluation of bone mineral status. Therefore, many excellent methods have been developed for determining the amount of bone mineral present.

However, quantitative evaluation alone is not sufficient because decreased bone mineral mass may be caused by several different processes. The quantitative methods should be used in conjunction with qualitative assessment of skeletal radiographs, as well as other clinical and laboratory data, to determine the mechanism and etiology of bone loss. Even children with known diagnoses, such as chronic renal failure, may have osteopenia from several different pathophysiological mechanisms, which may have different radiographic appearances. Rickets, other vitamin deficiencies or poisonings, osteoporosis, hyperparathyroidism, and osteogenesis imperfecta may have typical radiographic appearances. There are also qualitative findings that indicate that bone mineral deficiency is present, and these are important to recognize because they may be the first clinical indication of a bone mineral abnormality.

QUANTITATIVE MEASUREMENTS OF BONE LOSS IN CHILDREN

The techniques that are available for measuring bone mineral in children are similar to those used in adults, although their selection is influenced by the availability of normal values. Quantitative methods that have pediatric applications include radiogrammetry (measurement of cortical dimensions) and multiple methods of quantifying photon absorption by bone, with DXA being the most widely used method.

Radiogrammetry

Measurements of cortical dimensions are usually performed on hand films with measurement of the second metacarpal midshaft. At this site, standards have been established for different populations.[30,31] A high-detail film screen combination should be used, and the measurements of the outside and inside diameters of the cortex are made at midshaft. Based on these measurements, cortical thickness, cortical area, and percent cortical area can all be calculated. Cortical bone standards have also been developed for the humerus for neonates of varying gestational ages,[32] and this is a useful site because it is often included on neonatal chest radiographs. Premature infants can be followed longitudinally from birth to determine whether cortical bone mineral is growing along the normal growth curve as would have occurred in utero, or whether significant bone loss has occurred (Fig. 1). Standard have also been developed for a number of sites.[33]

Advantages of radiogrammetry include its simplicity, low cost, and availability of good standards that are age- and sex-specific and have been developed for several population groups in the United States, including whites, blacks, and Mexican Americans.[30] There are also many pediatric patients for whom radiogrammetry is the only quantitative method that may be used. For most neonates, cortical measurement of the humerus is usually the only available method.

Although some of the photon absorptiometry techniques have been adapted to neonates in research settings, this in not generally available. Beyond the neonatal period, DXA is often unsuccessful in children below 5 years of age because of the inability to adequately define bone margins and insufficient standards for those children. In addition to cal-

The authors have no conflict of interest.

culation of cortical thickness, these measurements can be used to determine if the bone loss is caused by endosteal resorption or lack of periosteal surface apposition. This is important because certain diseases affect these processes differently. In most causes of pediatric osteoporosis, other than renal osteodystrophy, the usual mechanism of bone loss is increased resorption along the endosteal surface, resulting in a larger medullary space.[34] However, in some

conditions, such as osteogenesis imperfecta and osteopenia associated with chronic illnesses such as juvenile rheumatoid arthritis or Crohn disease, there is lack of growth on the outer surface.[30,31,34] In most cases, a diminished outside diameter is indicative of lack of growth. An important exception is subperiosteal resorption caused by hyperparathyroidism, most often caused by chronic renal failure. Careful evaluation of the hand radiograph is needed to search for subperiosteal resorption, which is indicative of hyperparathyroidism, or intracortical resorption, which is seen with either hyperparathyroidism or other causes of rapid bone loss. A hand radiograph also permits the evaluation of skeletal maturation, allowing bone mineralization to be compared with either chronological age or skeletal age-matched control values.[34] The latter may be more realistic, particularly for disorders in which there is marked retardation of skeletal maturation or in delayed puberty.

The major disadvantage of radiogrammetry is that its precision is lower than that for the several forms of photon absorptiometry and hence it is not as useful for recognizing changes over serial examinations. Accuracy and precision are particularly decreased in circumstances where the endosteal cortical margin is not well defined. This occurs most often with conditions leading to rapid bone loss that produce a permeative pattern with a ragged margin. Furthermore, intracortical bone loss is not recognized by measurement of cortical thickness. Thus, if subperiosteal resorption or increased intracortical striations are seen on the hand radiograph, cortical measurements should not be used. Radiogrammetry also does not measure cancellous bone.

DXA

DXA was developed to provide rapid and precise measures of bone mineral at multiple sites with minimal radiation exposure. DXA machines use site-specific scans to measure the bone mass and bone density of the whole body and subregions of interest, namely the lumbar spine, hip, and forearm. DXA is, by far, the most commonly used method for the assessment of bone health in children. However, DXA has several limitations that are pronounced in the assessment of children. These can be broadly classified as (1) difficulties in scan acquisition because of limitations in the bone edge detection software in children with low bone mass and because of variation in the distance of the bone from the apex of the fan beam; (2) inadequacy of pediatric

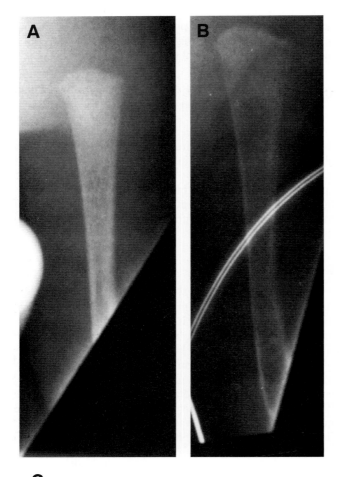

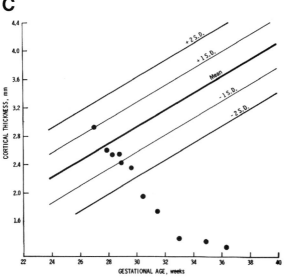

FIG. 1. Humerus of a premature infant (A) at birth and (B) 6 weeks later. Note the marked thinning of the cortex postnatally. Most of the loss has occurred by endosteal resorption. The outer diameter has shown little change, but the medullary diameter is considerably wider. (C) Longitudinal humeral cortical thickness measurements for this patient are shown against the in utero growth curve for humeral cortical thickness at birth. At birth, the cortical thickness was 1 SD above the mean, but it decreased rapidly thereafter. At 10 weeks after birth, equivalent to just above 36 weeks' gestational age, the bone mineral was very low, much lower than that of even a 22-week-old gestational age infant. (Poznanski AK, Kuhns LR, Guire KE 1980 New standards of cortical mass in the humerus of neonates: A means of evaluating loss in the premature infant. Radiology **134:**639–644 with permission from The Radiological Society of North America.)

reference data across varied maturation stages, ethnic groups, and gender groups in healthy children; and (3) difficulties in the interpretation of DXA results in children with impaired growth, altered body composition, or delayed maturation caused by childhood illness. Although varied techniques have been proposed to address these pitfalls, the third limitation remains the greatest challenge in the assessment of childhood osteopenia.

Scan Acquisition and Analysis. Pediatric DXA images often could not be analyzed with early-generation software because of failure of the bone edge detection algorithm to identify and measure completely all bones. In our experience, the DXA lumbar spine scan could not be analyzed using standard software (QDR 2000; Hologic, Inc., Waltham, MA, USA) in 40% of chronically ill children less than 12 years of age and in younger healthy children with lower bone mass, particularly those less than 6 years of age.[35] Although it was possible to use visual inspection to fill in the regions missed by standard software, this was an imprecise process. It resulted in loss of the systematic algorithm's threshold definition of bone edge and led to inaccuracies in measurements of bone mineralization. In an effort to address this limitation, software modifications were developed to improve detection of low density bone in children and severely osteopenic adults. While the new software performed well, this modification increased the detection of low density bone and resulted in a systematic decrease in the bone mineral density (BMD) measurement compared with the standard analysis.[35] Comparable effects were seen with whole body pediatric analyses.[36] The large magnitude of these differences demonstrated that different software options may not be used interchangeably in studies of BMD in children and use of older reference data requires attention to the analysis mode. More recently introduced is an automatic whole body measurement algorithm that dynamically adjusts bone detection thresholds and soft tissue determinations based on the subject's weight to provide improved bone mapping in all regions of the skeleton.[37] In addition, a new technique to improve the bone detection in the lumbar spine uses anatomical assumptions to refine the bone mapping process; the skeleton is assumed to be articulated, the center of mass of the vertebral bodies are assumed to lie near the center of the image, and adjacent vertebral bodies are assumed to lie within a certain distance of one another. Future studies are needed to evaluate the use of these new approaches in longitudinal studies and in children with altered body composition. These changes illustrate the rapidly evolving nature of the field.

Another limitation of DXA in children relates to the potential for projection error in the assessment of bone measures in subjects of differing body size and composition. This is especially relevant in children where bone mineral content (BMC) and bone area are considered separately, as discussed below. The earlier DXA scanners used a pencil beam design that used a pencil beam X-ray, obtaining a true projection of the scanned region.[38,39] Increasingly, pencil bean scanners have been replaced by a multiple detector array design coupled to a fan-shaped X-ray beam. These fan beam densitometers acquire scans by performing a single sweep of the patient with substantially shorter scanning times and improved geometric resolution. However, the fan beam technique causes an inherent magnification of scanned structures as the distance from the X-ray source, and hence from the apex of the fan beam, changes.[38,39] Pocock has shown that variations in soft tissue thickness between patients, by altering the distance of the skeleton from the fan beam X-ray source, are sufficiently large to cause significant errors in measures of bone geometry and BMC.[38,39] This effect may be even greater across the wide range of body sizes included in pediatric studies. While this error has minimal effect on areal bone mineral density (because BMC and area are affected to comparable degrees), magnification error may have dramatic effects on strategies in children where the BMC and bone area are considered separately. Again, changes in scan acquisition and analysis techniques dictate that investigators and clinicians consider hardware and software issues before adopting reference data or new analysis strategies.

Reference Data. Comparisons to appropriate pediatric bone mineral reference data are essential to describe accurately the clinical impact of childhood disease on bone development, to monitor changes in bone mineralization, and to identify patients for treatment protocols. Misclassification of a normal bone mineral result as representing osteopenia may result in undue parental anxiety, alterations in treatment of the underlying disease, or initiation of potentially harmful drugs to impact bone metabolism.

DXA is widely accepted as a quantitative measurement technique for assessing skeletal status in postmenopausal women. The diagnosis of osteoporosis in adults is based on the comparison of a measured BMD result with the average BMD of young adults at the time of peak bone mass, defined as a T-score.[40] A T-score ≤ -2.5 SDs below the mean peak bone mass is associated with increased fracture risk and is used for the diagnosis of osteoporosis. While the T-score is a standard component of DXA BMD results, it is clearly inappropriate to assess skeletal health in children through comparison with peak adult bone mass; T-scores should not be used in children. At present, there are no evidence-based guidelines for classification of bone health in children. Despite the growing body of normative data in children, there is little agreement on the quantitative definition of osteopenia and osteoporosis in children.

Earlier studies of bone mineralization in healthy children were conducted using single- or dual-photon absorptiometry,[41,42] or DXA in pencil beam mode.[43,44] Although these studies were instrumental in describing determinants of peak bone mass, they cannot be used as reference data for current research studies or clinical care because of the changes in bone density assessment technology. Changes in hardware and software technology, including fan-beam technology and low-density software analysis algorithms, result in significant alterations in the absolute levels of bone area, bone mass, and BMD, as discussed above.

A further shortcoming of some previous studies of bone health is their small sample size and the lack of more detailed information for children across various maturational stages, ethnic groups, and gender groups. Most pediatric BMD reference data sets used to calculate z-scores contain small numbers of subjects within each age category and may not accurately characterize normal variability in BMD. A systematic comparison of published pediatric DXA BMD normative data revealed differences in the age-specific means and SDs for BMD across five studies.[6,44–47] These differences had a significant impact on the diagnosis of osteopenia in children with chronic diseases.[48] For example, use of reference data that were not gender-specific resulted in significantly greater misclassification of males as osteopenic.[48]

Most BMD reference data sets in healthy children are based on chronologic age. There is considerable variability in bone mineralization according to body size and sexual maturation, especially during adolescence. Reference data should allow for assessment of bone mineralization in relation to body size and puberty stage, in addition to age. This is particularly important for the clinical care of children with chronic disease who frequently experience growth failure, malnutrition, and delayed sexual and skeletal maturation. Therefore, despite the widespread availability of data on normal children, the prevalence of osteopenia in many childhood diseases is not known. Furthermore, most studies have focused on trabecular BMD. Reference data that capture the bone structural changes that underpin cortical bone growth are needed.

Substantial effort is needed to develop adequate reference data and validate classification schemes of bone health in children. In 2002, the National Institutes of Health initiated a prospective longitudinal DXA study of BMD in a multiethnic sample of 1500 children and adolescents to be enrolled at five pediatric centers across the country.

Interpretation of DXA Results in Children. A significant limitation of DXA is the reliance on measurement of projected two-dimensional measures of BMD. DXA calculates an estimate of BMD expressed as grams per scanned region (e.g., individual vertebrae, whole body, or hip). Dividing the BMC (g) within the defined anatomical region by the projected area of the bone (cm^2) then generates "areal BMD" (g/cm^2). This BMD is not a measure of true volumetric density (g/cm^3) because it provides no information about the depth of bone. Bones of larger width and height also tend to be thicker. Because this third dimension is not factored into DXA estimates of areal BMD, DXA systematically underestimates the bone density of short people. Similarly, catch-up growth may result in the appearance of increasing areal bone mineral density when the volumetric BMD actually has not changed.

Recent pediatric studies have recognized the importance of short stature in the assessment of DXA-based measures of BMD in chronic childhood disease and have adjusted the DXA BMD result for height and/or weight.[5,49,50] Unfortunately, this too is an incomplete solution because healthy children of the same height or weight as a chronically ill child will be younger than the ill child. Skeletal maturity and Tanner stage are key determinants of bone mass and comparison with less mature controls is a flawed solution to the influence of bone size. Studies reporting BMD for age and BMD for height in chronically ill children have dem-

onstrated dramatic differences in the interpretation of these results.[51]

The confounding effect of skeletal geometry on DXA measures is now well recognized and multiple analytic strategies have been proposed to express DXA bone mass in a form that is less sensitive to differences in skeletal size. Carter et al. introduced an approach that uses the dimensions of the projected anterioposterior (AP) bone area to estimate the total vertebral volume.[52,53] Volume is estimated as Area$^{1.5}$. The AP BMC is then divided by this estimate of volume to generate "bone mineral apparent density" (BMAD). This approach assumes that bone depth increases proportionate to the square root of AP area. Kroger et al. developed an alternative mathematical approach for calculating apparent volumetric BMD using ancillary DXA-derived data, assuming that each vertebral body was approximated as a cylinder.[54] This technique was compared with magnetic resonance imaging (MRI) of lumbar vertebrae in adults.[55] The DXA-derived apparent volumetric BMD correlated moderately well with MRI-derived BMD and was not associated with body size ($R = 0.67–0.82$). Both of these approaches have been used to examine changes in bone density and size in growing children.[53,56]

In 1990, Beck et al. introduced an approach to derive femoral neck geometry from raw DXA bone mineral image data for an estimate of hip strength using single plane engineering stress analysis.[57] The program, Hip Strength Analysis (HSA) computed subperiosteal width, cross-sectional area cortical thickness, endosteal diameter, and section modulus at the femoral neck, intertrochanter, and femoral shaft regions. The HSA results showed better agreement with bone strength than routine DXA femoral neck BMD. This approach has yielded important insight into the structural basis of hip fragility in postmenopausal women and recently was applied in children.[58–61] Petit et al. used the HSA approach to determine the effects of a randomized school-based jumping intervention on hip structural properties in girls.[61] The early-pubertal girls in the intervention group showed significantly greater gains in femoral neck and intertrochanter BMD. Underpinning these changes were increased bone cross-sectional area and reduced endosteal expansion. Changes in subperiosteal dimensions did not differ. Structural changes improved bending strength at the femoral neck. These data show that innovative analysis techniques are needed to address site-specific effects of diseases and therapies in children.

Varied approaches have been advocated for the assessment of whole body bone mass. Investigators have proposed normalizing bone mass to body weight or lean mass.[44,62,63] Molgaard et al. proposed a multistaged approach to determine if differences in whole body BMC are caused by differences in bone size or bone density[50]: bone size is assessed relative to body size (bone area-for-height) and BMC is assessed relative to bone size (BMC-for-bone area). This approach has been used in studies of healthy children, as well as in children with chronic disease.[63–65] However, it is not known if this interpretation of the predominantly cortical whole body DXA scan accurately captures clinically significant differences in cortical bone health, that is, bone dimensions, density, and strength. Last, Taylor et al. reported that in children 2–9 years of age, subtotal BMD

Table 1. Bone Mineral Accretion During Childhood and Adolescence

	Changes with growth	Effect of ethnicity
Vertebral trabecular bone		
Density (mg/cm^3)	Constant through Tanner stages I–II; then increases during puberty	No differences until puberty, when the increase in blacks (34%) is greater than whites (11%)
Cross-sectional area (cm^2)	Increases during puberty	None
Appendicular cortical bone		
Density (mg/cm^3)	May be increased in females during puberty	None
Cross-sectional area (cm^2)	Cortical area increases proportionately greater than overall bone cross-sectional area. During puberty: greater periosteal apposition in males; greater endosteal apposition in females	Blacks have greater total cross-sectional area but similar cortical cross-sectional area (thinner cortex but greater strength)

(whole body BMD − head BMD) is predicted better by age than total whole body BMD, possibly because of an invalid adult algorithm for head BMD in adults.[66] They advocated excluding the head from analyses of whole body BMD in children.

Physical activity is a well-recognized determinant of bone mass.[67–69] The mechanostat theory proposes that bone dimensions expand in response to the magnitude and direction of the biomechanical forces to which it is subjected.[70] Mechanical forces on the skeleton arise from muscle contraction, and these forces generate signals that determine bone architecture. Furthermore, measures of lean tissue mass are generated by whole body DXA. Recent studies have demonstrated a strong correlation between muscle strength, muscle mass, and bone mass in healthy children.[71–73] These relationships are consistent with the theory that adaptation to changes in biomechanical usage during childhood results in changes in bone geometry, not density. Schoenau et al. advised that the evaluation of muscle strength should play a significant role in the assessment of skeletal disorders in childhood; the muscle and skeletal systems should be viewed as a functional unit.[72–74] This model proposes that the primary bone diseases have their cause in a direct disorder of the bone cells and/or synthesized matrix, resulting in an uncoupling of the normal bone-muscle relationship. The secondary bone diseases arise because of decreased muscle strength related to the underlying disease. Comparison of bone muscle relationships in children requires careful attention to height because the comparison of bone mass in two children with comparable muscle mass may result in the inappropriate comparison of two children of differing height.

Prediction of Fracture Risk. In adults, "current fracture risk" is defined as the risk potential 3–5 years after the bone mass has been measured. Multiple DXA studies have shown that the relative risk of fracture is increased 1.5–2.5 times for each SD reduction in BMD.[75–77] Until recently, data on fracture risk have been obtained predominantly on older white women. This is primarily because younger women fracture infrequently and are not included in studies designed to assess current fracture risk. These fracture risk data should not be applied to premenopausal women or to children.

The impact of skeletal properties on fracture risk in otherwise healthy children had not been addressed until recently. In the first prospective cohort study in children, Goulding et al. related baseline DXA measures of bone mass to subsequent fractures over a 4-year interval in otherwise healthy girls, ages 3–15 years.[78] Using multivariate models (adjusting for age, weight, and fracture history), each reduction of 1 SD of baseline total body DXA BMD, equivalent to a 6.4% difference, nearly doubled the risk of new fractures (hazard ratio [HR] per 1 SD decrease = 1.92; 95% CI, 1.31–2.81). Lumbar spine BMAD (an estimate of trabecular volumetric density) also predicted new fractures during the follow-up interval (HR per 1 SD decrease = 1.34; 95% CI, 1.02–1.75).

Although derived volumetric BMD measures are decreased in children with forearm fractures compared with healthy controls,[79] it is not known if BMAD or other adjusted DXA measures provide a better measure of fracture risk than routine DXA areal bone mineral density measures in children.[78]

A shortcoming of all of these techniques is that integrated measures of bone mass do not allow distinction between cortical and trabecular bone. DXA-based measures provide no information on bone architecture and are limited in their usefulness to differentiate the spectrum of bone accrual during growth. A three-dimensional structural analysis of trabecular architecture and cortical bone dimensions can be obtained by computed tomography. This technique offers an opportunity to overcome these limitations and advance our understanding of bone mineralization in children.

Quantitative Computed Tomography

Computed tomography (CT) provides an image unobscured by overlying structures.[80,81] The CT attenuation of different bone tissues provides quantitative information, referred to as quantitative CT (QCT). In contrast to DXA, this technique describes volumetric BMD, accurately measures bone dimensions, and distinguishes between cortical and trabecular bone.

The application of QCT techniques in children is illustrated by a series of important studies clarifying the distinction between increases in bone size and increases in bone density in the growing appendicular and axial skeleton,[82–85] as well as the nature of ethnic and gender differences in bone geometry and density. These studies are summarized

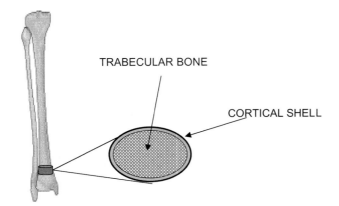

FIG. 2. Measurement of trabecular bone in the tibial diaphysis by pQCT. The trabecular measure is obtained in the distal metaphysis, providing measures of trabecular bone area and volumetric bone mineral density.

in Table 1. Trabecular bone density, measured in the lumbar spine, does not increase before puberty. During puberty, trabecular density increases, and the magnitude of the increase is greater in black than white subjects.[83] Gilsanz et al. reported that cortical bone density is constant across age, gender, and race.[82,83] However, a more recent study demonstrated greater cortical density in females after pubertal stage 3.[86] Black children have a greater total femoral cross-sectional area (cortical bone and bone marrow space combined) but similar cortical bone area, that is, the cortical bone is thinner. The greater distance of the cortical bone from the central axis increases the cross-sectional moment of inertia, and thereby, substantially increases bone strength. During puberty, males accrue bone predominantly on the periosteal surface, where the effect on bone strength is highest, whereas females gain bone on the endocortical surface, which has a lesser effect on bone stability.[85] In addition, the timing of menarche in females is associated with the endosteal dimensions in adulthood.[87]

To minimize radiation exposure, special high-resolution scanners were developed for the peripheral skeleton (pQCT), specifically, the radius or tibia. Figures 2 and 3 illustrate pQCT measurement sites in the tibia. The distal site is largely trabecular bone, while the mid-shaft is almost entirely cortical bone. The volume of each component is calculated from the scan thickness and cross-sectional area, and the density by attenuation of the X-ray beam. Bone strength can also be estimated by pQCT from the total bone area and cortical thickness and density.[88] For example, the studies of bone mineral accretion and bone strength reviewed above demonstrated that there are gender and ethnic differences in the development of bone strength during childhood and adolescence.[85] To date, most pQCT-based studies on bone mineral accrual in the distal radius have been conducted by Schoenau et al. at the Research Institute of Child Nutrition and the Children's Hospital, Cologne, Germany.[84,85,89–92] Reference data on 371 healthy children, adolescents, and young adults have been published.[89]

Technical Limitations of QCT Technologies. While DXA is ubiquitous, QCT and pQCT machines are less readily

available. QCT and pQCT are almost exclusively limited to research applications, and there is less experience with these techniques in children. The primary limitation in the assessment of cortical bone occurs in the event of thin cortical bone, when CT accuracy can be influenced by the small bone size.[81] The CT image is composed of many picture points (pixels) with definite edge lengths. If the cortical bone is thin, the partially filled in pixels at the cortical edges measure falsely low densities because of the significantly lower density of the surrounding soft tissues. The errors are the greatest in very thin bone where a greater proportion of pixels are only partially filled, referred to as "partial-volume effect." In general, if the voxel measure 0.40 mm and the cortical thickness is less than 2.5 mm, pQCT results for cortical volumetric BMD increase with cortical thickness, even if the actual mineral density of the cortical compartment is constant.[81,93] Disease states that cause cortical thinning may result in the false impression that there is also decreased cortical density. Cortical thickness in the midshaft of the radius is below 2.5 mm in most children under 14 years of age and in many adults.[90] Therefore, some investigators have moved to the tibia for pQCT assessments in children. QCT may be performed in the larger femur, which is less subject to partial volume effects.

The greatest difficulty in the pQCT assessment of trabecular bone is in the selection of the measurement site within the appendicular skeleton. Traditionally, trabecular bone is measured at the 4% site—the site whose distance to the distal endplate of the bone corresponds to 4% of the forearm length. The advantage of this location is that it contains metaphyseal trabecular bone. However, in children, this site may be immediately adjacent to, or superimposed on, the mineralized portion of the growth plate. Glancing this dense mineralized growth plate results in marked overestimation of trabecular BMD. On the other hand, trabecular density decreases dramatically proximal to the growth plate. There-

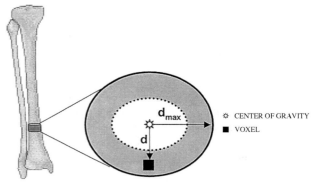

Total Cross-Sectional Area = area contained within the outer periosteal envelope

Cortical Cross-Sectional Area = area contained between the outer periosteal envelope and inner endosteal envelope

a = area of one voxel in the cortex (mm²)

d = distance of one voxel to the center of gravity (mm)

d_{max} = maximum distance (eccentricity) to the center of gravity (mm)

CD = volumetric cortical density in one voxel (mg/mm³)   ND = normal physiological density (1200 mg/mm³)

Stress Strain Index (SSI, mm³) = $\sum_{i} [(a_i \times d_i^2)(CD/ND)]/d_{max}$

FIG. 3. Measurement of cortical bone in the tibial diaphysis by pQCT. Cortical bone is assessed in the shaft of the tibia, where the bone is entirely cortical. Measures of cortical dimensions and density are used to calculate the parameters.

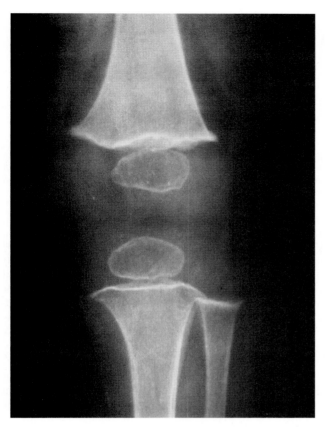

FIG. 4. Scurvy. The major radiographic manifestations of scurvy are those of osteopenia. The trabecular pattern is washed out with preservation of the cortex and zone of provisional calcification. In the epiphysis, this is manifest by maintenance of a white line (a zone of provisional equivalent region) around the epiphysis which is internally radiolucent. This produces the Wimberg ring of scurvy and is the equivalent of a picture frame vertebra of osteopenia in adults. In the metaphysis, the zone of provisional calcification is maintained (white line of Frankel) and this stands out compared with the lucent metaphyseal region beneath it (scurvy zone or Trummerfeld zone)

fore, investigators have used a different definition of the 4% site in children—the site whose distance to the most distal part of the growth plate corresponds to 4% of the forearm length. This technique will introduce difficulty in the longitudinal assessment of children as the growth plate moves distally. Other investigators have advocated measuring the trabecular bone a fixed distance from the endplate or growth plate to standardize measures as the bone grows. Studies comparing these difference strategies are ongoing in our laboratories and other pediatric centers.

QUALITATIVE EVALUATION OF RADIOGRAPHS

Overall Density

Subjective evaluation of radiographic density is a very inaccurate and inconsistent method for evaluation of bone loss.[94] In the spine, more than 50% of bone can be lost without any evidence on the radiograph because it is mostly cortical bone that is seen on plain radiographs, and much loss of cancellous bone can occur before it is visualized. Also, the apparent density is very dependent on the radio-

graphic technique. With higher kilovoltage, there is less of a difference between the absorption of calcium and soft tissue, making the bones appear more "washed out." Similarly, not using a high-ratio grid can make the bones look more osteopenic.

Appearance of the Cortex Compared With the Center of Bone

Although both cortical and trabecular bone are usually deficient in patients with osteopenia, there is often relative preservation of the thinned cortex, which stands out sharply against the very lucent trabecular region. This sign is sometimes useful in evaluation of the vertebrae,[95] producing a "picture-frame vertebra" with the well-defined vertebral margins surrounding the lucent trabecular center. Similarly, relative cortical preservation in the epiphyses characterizes Wimberger's ring of scurvy, which is simply a manifestation of severe osteopenia (Fig. 4).

Appearance of Trabecular Pattern

A coarse trabecular pattern may be useful in evaluating the presence and type of osteopenia; however, it can also be

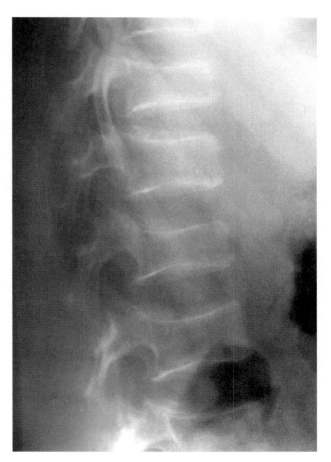

FIG. 5. Multiple compression fractures from osteoporosis in a boy with Crohn's disease. The vertebral bodies are flatter than normal, with indentations on the endplates. Compare with the vertebrae in Fig. 12, which show normal vertebral shape but are abnormally sclerotic.

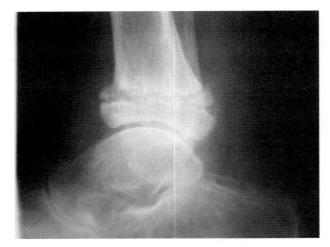

FIG. 6. Distal tibial metaphyseal fractures in patient with chronic renal failure and secondary hyperparathyroidism.

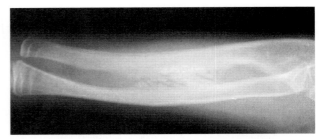

FIG. 8. Six-year-old girl with osteogenesis imperfecta type V showing characteristic ossification of the interosseous membrane. This form of osteogenesis imperfecta is also characterized by excessive callus formation with fracture healing.

quite inaccurate. Trabecular orientation is related to stress. With osteopenia there is relative preservation of those trabeculae that are aligned in the direction of maximum stress. In the spine, the vertically oriented trabeculae are preserved, and thus, prominent vertical striations are usually a sign of osteoporosis. Similarly, in the hip, coarse trabeculation may be an indication of osteopenia; in adults, the degree of osteopenia can be graded by the number of trabecular patterns present.[96] There is some difference in appearance between the coarse trabecular patterns in osteoporosis and hyperparathyroidism, but usually this is not a reliable differential sign.

Presence of Compression Fractures of the Spine or Fractures of Other Bones

The appearance of anterior wedging or concave endplate deformities in the spine, seen best in the lateral projections, is a good sign of bone loss[95] (Fig. 5). In children, vertebral compression fractures may occur without any history of

trauma in diseases associated with severe bone loss, such as osteogenesis imperfecta, rickets, juvenile rheumatoid arthritis, Crohn's disease, or corticosteroid therapy. Vertebral compressions may be the presenting sign of leukemia or neuroblastoma. Other disorders producing wedged vertebrae include Langerhans' cell histiocytosis, juvenile osteoporosis, Gaucher's disease, and Scheuermann's disease. A square impression on the endplate is seen characteristically in sickle cell disease.

Bone loss can be associated with a variety of fractures of the long bones as well as of the spine. Fracture location appearance may provide some clues regarding the underlying disorder. In hyperparathyroidism, fractures through the growth plates and metaphyses are not uncommon (Fig. 6). Metaphyseal fractures and vertebral compression fractures are also often seen with idiopathic juvenile osteoporosis. In contrast, most extremity fractures in osteogenesis imperfecta occur in the diaphysis. Recurrent olecranon avulsion fractures are also suggestive of osteogenesis imperfecta, and these may often be seen in patients with otherwise relatively normal appearing bones radiographically (Fig. 7). Overabundant callus with healing may be seen in children with neuromuscular abnormalities, particularly myelodysplasia, as well as those with osteogenesis type V, a disorder also

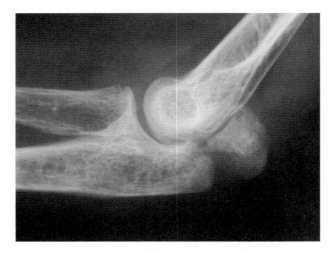

FIG. 7. Eight-year-old boy with osteogenesis imperfecta and recurrent olecranon avulsion fractures that occurred bilaterally.

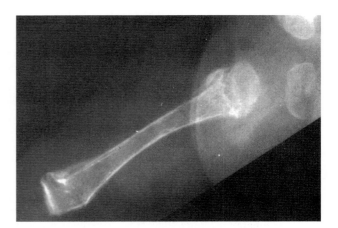

FIG. 9. Multiple femoral fractures in a premature neonate with bronchopulmonary dysplasia. There is callus around the upper femoral fracture. The lower fracture is angulated, with some callus on the lateral side. This is evidence of healing. The poorly mineralized bones in this infant fractured with no known trauma but from normal handling in the nursery.

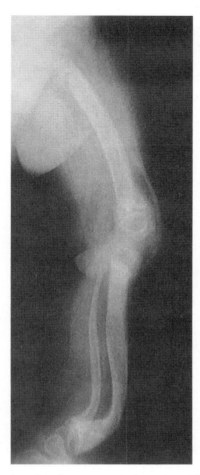

FIG. 10. Bowing of the lower extremity bones in a child with treated rickets. The legs may bend in any direction, depending on the stresses involved.

characterized by ossification of the interosseous membrane in the forearm (Fig. 8).[97] In premature neonates on total parenteral nutrition, most fractures occur without a history of trauma (Fig. 9).

Presence of Bowing of the Bones in Children

A number of conditions with osteopenia in children will result in bowing of the long bones, particularly rickets (Fig. 10), osteogenesis imperfecta, and fibrous dysplasia. In some cases, there may be associated small cortical breaks on the convex surface. In children with rickets, the bowing is a manifestation of osteomalacia. After treatment for rickets, the bones tend to straighten with growth over time.

Presence of Subperiosteal Resorption and Other Signs of Hyperparathyroidism

Subperiosteal resorption is a pathognomonic manifestation of hyperparathyroidism.[98,99] These resorptions are best seen on hand radiographs obtained with either industrial films or with mammography film screen combination, and they can be easily missed if ordinary screen exposures are obtained.[100] To identify the resorptions properly, the ra-

diographs may need to be examined with a magnifying glass. These findings are best seen along the radial aspect of the middle phalanges (Fig. 11A). The distal tufts may also be involved, but their involvement is not as specific as that of the phalanges because some irregularity of the tufts can occur normally. Thus, it is difficult to determine whether subtle tuft defects are caused by normal variation or by hyperparathyroidism. Subperiosteal resorption may also be seen in other areas of the body. Commonly involved areas, particularly in infants and young children, include the medial aspects of the femoral neck, proximal humerus (Fig. 11B), and proximal tibia (Fig. 11C), as well as near the metaphyseal areas of many other bones. The growth plate and metaphysis can have a rickets-like appearance, with somewhat greater widening at the lateral and medial ends than in the center. Some of the other radiographic findings of hyperparathyroidism in children are those that are often considered to be more characteristic of secondary hyperparathyroidism from renal disease than of primary hyperparathyroidism, although they can be seen in both conditions. These findings include bone sclerosis, which can produce a "rugger jersey" appearance in the spine (Fig. 12), a coarse trabecular pattern,[100,101] and arterial calcification.[102] The rugger jersey appearance is not specific for hyperparathyroidism and may also be seen in osteopetrosis. In children, slipping of various epiphyses, particularly the proximal femoral and the proximal humeral, may be seen (Fig. 13).[103] Less commonly, slips of other epiphyses may be seen, such as those for the ankle, which may lead to valgus deformity (Fig. 14). Signs of avascular necrosis may be seen, and metaphyseal fractures (Fig. 6) may be present and are often symmetrical. Well-circumscribed lucent areas from brown tumors may be seen in any part of the skeleton (Fig. 15) and are often considered more characteristic of primary than of secondary hyperparathyroidism. However, in children, they are seen more often with secondary hyperparathyroidism because it is much more common.

Presence of Linear Striations

Increased linear striations[104,105] in the cortex of the metacarpals as well as in other bones can be because of hyperparathyroidism, osteomalacia, and other causes of high bone turnover such as in hyperthyroidism. Some striation may be seen in normal children. Abnormal striations are usually not seen in slower forms of bone loss, such as that caused by chronic diseases or juvenile rheumatoid arthritis. When intracortical resorption is present, cortical thickness measurements do not accurately represent the amount of cortical bone and thus are not useful in determining bone loss.

Metaphyseal Changes in Rickets

Rickets is a condition of inadequate mineralization of osteoid and cartilage at the growing ends of bones in children. The radiologic hallmarks of this disorder are apparent widening of the physis from accumulation of nonmineralized osteoid and cartilage, irregularity of the metaphysis, and loss of definition of the zone of provisional calcification. The radiographic findings of rickets are best appreci-

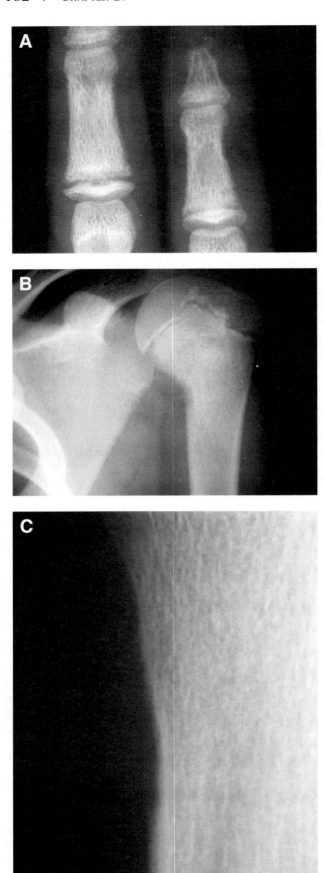

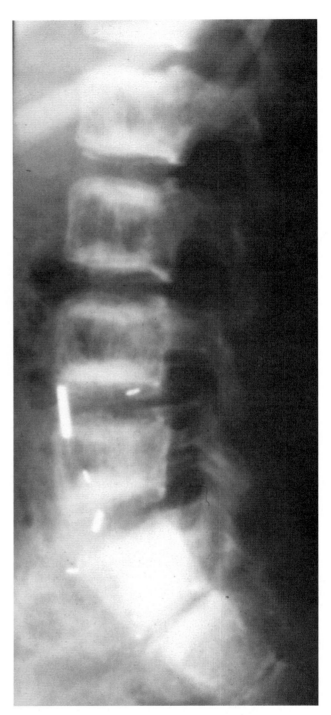

FIG. 12. "Rugger-jersey" spine in a child with renal osteodystrophy. The sclerotic bands on the upper and lower margins of each vertebra are characteristic of secondary hyperparathyroidism. Coarse trabeculae are seen in the vertebral bodies.

FIG. 11. Hyperparathyroidism. (A) Moderately severe findings. Subperiosteal resorption is present, more prominent along the radial than the ulnar aspects of the middle phalanges. (B) Erosion of the medial aspect of the proximal humerus. (C) Erosion of the medial aspect of the proximal tibia in hyperparathyroidism.

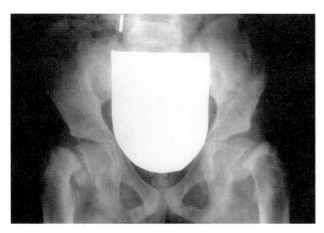

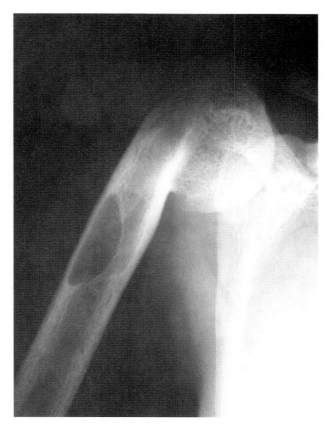

FIG. 13. Bilateral slipped capital femoral epiphyses in a child with renal osteodystrophy. Note the widened growth plates in the proximal femora and displacement of the femoral heads with respect to the neck. These are fractures through the growth plates. At the inferior margin of each growth plate, there is a small fragment of bone that probably broke from the metaphysis. The appearance is similar to that seen in developmental coxa vara. The lucency in the left femoral neck is a brown tumor, a manifestation of hyperparathyroidism.

ated by comparison of the acute phase with healing (Fig. 16). These changes are most severe in bones with the greatest growth, and thus are most pronounced in the distal

FIG. 15. Renal osteodystrophy. The varus deformity of proximal humerus is caused by a prior slipped epiphysis. The well defined lytic lesion of the proximal humeral diaphysis is a brown tumor of hyperparathyroidism.

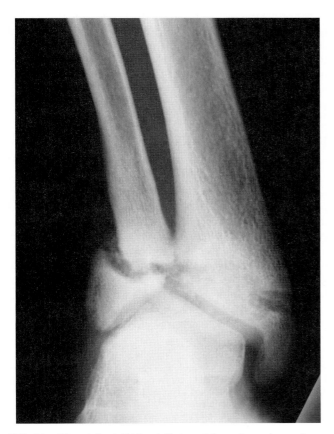

FIG. 14. Slipped distal tibial and fibular epiphyses in renal osteodystrophy. The slippage of the distal fibular epiphysis has led to valgus deformity.

femur and distal radius in most children. They are rarely seen in slow-growing bones, such as the tubular bones of the hand. Similarly, rachitic changes are greater during times of rapid growth, such as in infancy and adolescence, than during periods of slower growth. Conversely, growth failure may mask the radiographic manifestation of rickets, which then become apparent with improved growth (Fig. 17). Widening of the anterior ribs, the rachitic rosary, may be seen radiographically (Fig. 18). In osteitis fibrosa from hyperparathyroidism, accumulation of fibrous tissue in the metaphyses can produce lucencies that may appear similar to the nonmineralized osteoid of rickets. This may cause these disorders to be indistinguishable, although in some cases of hyperparathyroidism there is more erosion around the edge of the involved growth plate than is seen in rickets.[101]

All types of rickets have similar changes at the growth plate, and the radiological distinction among the various types of rickets may be difficult. Diagnosis is usually based on clinical and biochemical findings. Occasionally, differentiation by radiological appearance is possible. For example, the radiological appearance of X-linked hypophosphatemia (XLH, vitamin D–resistant rickets) differs from other causes of rickets by the relative infrequency of signs of secondary hyperparathyroidism in untreated cases. Furthermore, in older children with XLH, the long bones, particularly the femora, are usually thickened and bowed,

© 2003 American Society for Bone and Mineral Research

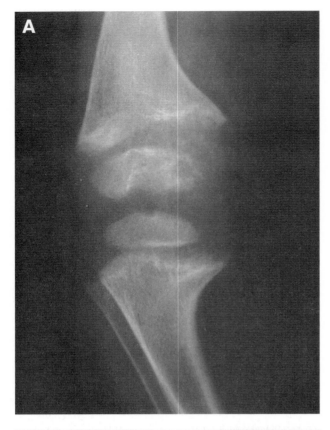

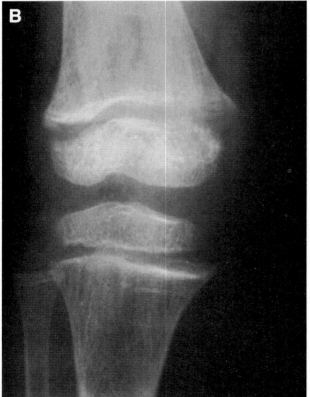

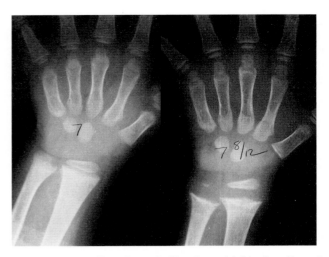

FIG. 17. Rickets, effect of growth. Chronic renal failure from Fanconi-Bickel syndrome. Hand radiograph (obtained for bone age determination) at 7 years of age (left image) show mild flaring of the distal ulnar metaphysis that can be seen as a normal finding and no other findings of rickets. Because of short stature, therapy with growth hormone was begun. A follow-up radiograph (right image) shows marked widening of the distal radial and ulnar growth plates, poor mineralization of the zone of provisional calcification, and flaring of the metaphyses.

and this is not seen in other forms of rickets. For comparison, in vitamin D–dependent rickets, usually caused by absence of renal 1α-hydroxylase, the rachitic changes may be seen in younger infants than in other forms of rickets, and they are also associated with more severe findings of hyperparathyroidism. During the healing of rickets, initial calcification is usually at the zone of provisional calcification, leaving a lucent band between it and the irregular metaphysis, and this lucent band may be confused with leukemia or metaphyseal stress changes. During healing, apparent periosteal elevation may be present.

Disorders Mimicking Rickets

There are a number of conditions that can mimic rickets,[106] including copper deficiency, diphosphonate therapy, fluorosis, hypophosphatasia, primary and secondary hyperparathyroidism, Menkes' syndrome, Schwachman syndrome, and various forms of metaphyseal chondrodysplasia, particularly Jansen syndrome in the neonate and McKusick and Schmidt forms in older children. Mucolipidosis II and osteopetrosis in infants may have manifestations similar to rickets. Among these conditions mimicking rickets, radiologic differentiation is often possible. For example, in Jansen syndrome, the epiphysis is markedly displaced from the metaphysis, much more so than in rickets (Fig. 19).

FIG. 16. Rickets before and after therapy. (A) Knee AP radiograph in 3.7-year-old girl with X-linked hypophosphatemia before therapy shows marked widening of the growth plates, loss of definition of the zone of provisional calcification, and cupping and fraying of the metaphysis. (B) Follow-up radiograph at 5.4 years of age shows substantial healing. The zones of provisional calcification are now well mineralized and the metaphyseal cupping and fraying have resolved. However, the physes are still wider than normal.

Later on, bizarre chondroid calcifications are seen in metaphyseal regions, which are even more characteristic. The serum calcium level may be elevated in Jansen syndrome, which also differentiates it from rickets. Hypophosphatasia can usually be distinguished from rickets, with the metaphyseal defects appearing more punched-out as opposed to the more uniform involvement of the growth plate in rickets. The rachitic-like changes of hyperparathyroidism can sometimes be differentiated by erosion along the edge of the growth plate. There are also a number of localized disorders that can mimic rickets. These include growth-plate fractures that have not been immobilized (Fig. 20), frostbite, radiation therapy, and chronic recurrent multifocal osteomyelitis.

Signs of Osteomalacia

Failure to mineralize osteoid seams adequately during the normal process of bone turnover defines osteomalacia. This process can occur in both children and adults, whereas rickets is limited to children before physeal closure. Radiologic differentiation of osteomalacia from other forms of osteopenia is difficult unless Looser zones, also called pseudofractures, are present. These are areas of cortical lucency with surrounding sclerosis that may not go completely through the cortex (Fig. 21). They are usually perpendicular to the cortex and are often seen along the medial side of the femoral neck and in the pubis or ischium, although they may also occur in other areas. The lucency represents nonmineralized osteoid, which accumulates at sites of increased bone turnover from stress. Although Looser zones are suggestive of osteomalacia, similar-appearing cortical lucencies may be seen in other disorders, including fibrous dysplasia and, in adults, Paget's disease.

Increased Bone Mineral with Sclerosis

Increased bone density on radiographs can be seen in a variety of bone dysplasias; the most classic of which is osteopetrosis. Although the bone appears dense and thick, it is very brittle and prone to fracture. Bands of density may also be seen and may mimic renal osteodystrophy in the spine.

Sclerosis may also be seen in the metaphyses (Fig. 22)

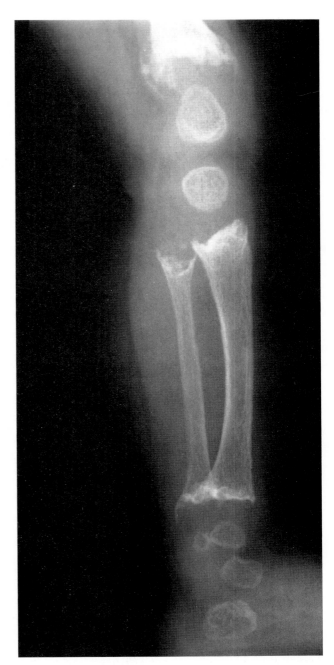

FIG. 19. Jansen metaphyseal chondrodysplasia. Note the irregular, somewhat sclerotic metaphyseal ends reminiscent of rickets. However, there is marked separation between the peculiar round epiphyses of the distal femur and proximal tibia and their respective metaphyses. With further maturation, this wide space fills in with irregular calcification, giving the characteristic appearance of Jansen syndrome, which is then not confused with rickets.

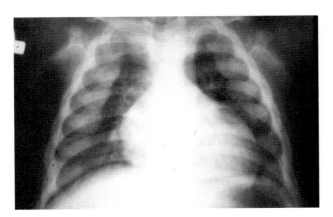

FIG. 18. Rachitic rosary. Chest X-ray shows widening of the anterior rib ends, a metaphyseal equivalent region, producing the rachitic rosary.

and vertebral end plates in response to bisphosphonate therapy for osteopenia.

APPROACH TO THE EVALUATION OF BONE MINERAL DISORDERS IN CHILDREN

The radiological evaluation of bone mineral disorders in children includes recognition that a bone mineral disorder is

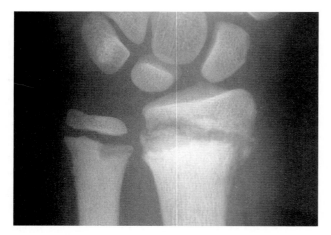

FIG. 20. Trauma mimicking rickets. Wrist radiograph in a young football player who continued to play with a sore wrist for a few weeks. Widening and irregularity of the growth plates are caused by unhealed growth-plate fractures of the radius and ulna. Because of continued athletic activity, motion between the fragments prevented healing. After casting, healing was complete.

present, determination of the disease process involved, and quantification of the severity of osteopenia. Thus, both qualitative and quantitative evaluation is essential. The

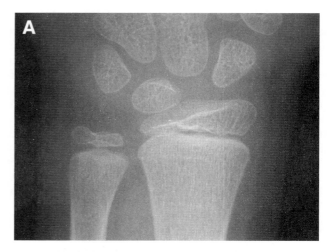

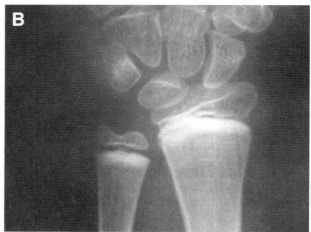

FIG. 22. Effect of bisphosphonate therapy. Wrist radiograph at (A) 9 years of age shows osteopenia, but no other abnormality. After bisphosphonate treatment for osteopenia, (B) a follow-up wrist radiograph shows marked sclerosis at the zone of provisional calcification.

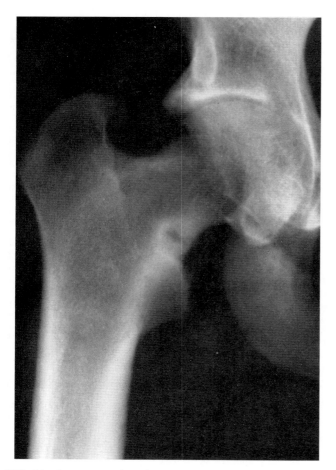

FIG. 21. Looser zone in a female with X-linked hypophosphatemic rickets and painful hips. The linear lucency in the medial portion of the femoral neck with sclerosis around it is a typical Looser zone (also called pseudofracture) and is indicative of osteomalacia.

steps involved are highly dependent on the clinical situation. In some cases, a radiographic diagnosis of rickets or hyperparathyroidism will be made on radiographs obtained for some other purpose. In these cases, further clinical and laboratory evaluation is needed to determine the underlying disease, and its effect on overall bone mineral status should be determined by quantitative techniques. In other cases, the suspicion of osteopenia is based strictly on the clinical situation, such as chronic corticosteroid therapy, and quantitative studies will determine whether osteopenia is present, and if so, how severe it is. In patients who have experienced multiple fractures, evaluation should be both qualitative to determine if signs of a metabolic bone disease is present as well as quantitative.

Quantitative bone mineral evaluation is dependent on patient age as well as available resources. In most cases, DXA will be the method of choice, and it has the versatility of being able to measure multiple sites including the lumbar spine, proximal femur, forearm bones, and whole body, However, pediatric age-specific standards are not available at all sites and at all ages. When DXA studies of the lumbar spine are compared with the pediatric standards that are built into the equipment by the manufacturer, they are adjusted for age, but not ethnicity, body size, or skeletal maturation. These considerations are important, but may conflict with one another (particularly when body size and maturation are discordant), and the mechanisms by which they can be used are not straightforward. QCT and pQCT offers considerable promise but are not generally available for pediatric use except in research settings.

Because of its lower accuracy and precision compared with photon absorptiometry methods, radiogrammetry is not as useful of a technique. However, it is still used in children below 5 years of age for whom DXA standards are not available. Despite its limitations, it is also useful to be able to use this technique to objectively determine whether osteopenia is present when interpreting hand radiographs (often obtained for bone age evaluation) or when observing the humeral diaphysis on neonatal chest radiographs.

REFERENCES

1. Boot AM, de Jongste JC, Verberne AA, Pols HA, de Muinck Keizer-Schrama SM 1997 Bone mineral density and bone metabolism of prepubertal children with asthma after long-term treatment with inhaled corticosteroids. Pediatr Pulmonol 24:379–384.

2. Boot AM, Engels MA, Boerma GJ, Krenning EP, De Muinck Keizer-Schrama SM 1997 Changes in bone mineral density, body composition, and lipid metabolism during growth hormone (GH) treatment in children with GH deficiency. J Clin Endocrinol Metab 82:2423–2428.

3. Boot AM, Nauta J, de Jong MC, Groothoff JW, Lilien MR, van Wijk JA, Kist-van Holthe JE, Hokken-Koelega AC, Pols HA, de Muinck Keizer-Schrama SM 1998 Bone mineral density, bone metabolism and body composition of children with chronic renal failure, with and without growth hormone treatment. Clin Endocrinol (Oxf) 49:665–672.

4. Boot AM, van den Heuvel-Eibrink MM, Hahlen K, Krenning EP, de Muinck Keizer-Schrama SM 1999 Bone mineral density in children with acute lymphoblastic leukaemia. Eur J Cancer 35:1693–1697.

5. Boot AM, Bouquet J, Krenning EP, de Muinck Keizer-Schrama SM 1998 Bone mineral density and nutritional status in children with chronic inflammatory bowel disease. Gut 42:188–194.

6. Henderson RC, Madsen CD 1996 Bone density in children and adolescents with cystic fibrosis. J Pediatr 128:28–34.

7. Klein GL, Herndon DN, Langman CB, Rutan TC, Young WE, Pembleton G, Nusynowitz M, Barnett JL, Broemeling LD, Sailer DE 1995 Long-term reduction in bone mass after severe burn injury in children. J Pediatr 126:252–256.

8. Nishioka T, Kurayama H, Yasuda T, Udagawa J, Matsumura C, Niimi H 1991 Nasal administration of salmon calcitonin for prevention of glucocorticoid-induced osteoporosis in children with nephrosis. J Pediatr 118:703–707.

9. Tenbrock K, Kruppa S, Mokov E, Querfeld U, Michalk D, Schonau E 2000 Analysis of muscle strength and bone structure in children with renal disease. Pediatr Nephrol 14:669–672.

10. Bunker MR, Thomas KA, Meyers ST, Texada T, Humbert JR, Cook SD, Gitter R 1998 Bone mineral density of the lumbar spine and proximal femur is decreased in children with sickle cell anemia. Am J Orthop 27:43–49.

11. Lettgen B, Jeken C, Reiners C 1994 Influence of steroid medication on bone mineral density in children with nephrotic syndrome. Pediatr Nephrol 8:667–670.

12. Sanchez CP, Salusky IB, Kuizon BD, Ramirez JA, Gales B, Ettenger RB, Goodman WG 1998 Bone disease in children and adolescents undergoing successful renal transplantation. Kidney Int 53:1358–1364.

13. Martinati LC, Bertoldo F, Gasperi E, Fortunati P, Lo Cascio V, Boner AL 1998 Longitudinal evaluation of bone mass in asthmatic children treated with inhaled beclomethasone dipropionate or cromolyn sodium. Allergy 53:705–708.

14. Lettgen B, Hauffa B, Mohlmann C, Jeken C, Reiners C 1995 Bone mineral density in children and adolescents with juvenile diabetes: Selective measurement of bone mineral density of trabecular and cortical bone using peripheral QCT. Horm Res 43:173–175.

15. Roe TF, Mora S, Costin G, Kaufman F, Carlson ME, Gilsanz V 1991 Vertebral bone density in insulin-dependent diabetic children. Metabolism 40:967–971.

16. Bhudhikanok GS, Wang MC, Marcus R, Harkins A, Moss RB, Bachrach LK 1998 Bone acquisition and loss in children and adults with cystic fibrosis: A longitudinal study. J Pediatr 133:18–27.

17. Humphries IR, Allen JR, Waters DL, Howman-Giles R, Gaskin KJ 1998 Volumetric bone mineral density in children with cystic fibrosis. Appl Radiat Isot 49:593–595.

18. Warner JT, Evans WD, Webb DK, Bell W, Gregory JW 1999 Relative osteopenia after treatment for acute lymphoblastic leukemia. Pediatr Res 45:544–551.

19. Schwahn B, Mokov E, Scheidhauer K, Lettgen B, Schonau E 1998 Decreased trabecular bone mineral density in patients with phenylketonuria measured by peripheral quantitative computed tomography. Acta Paediatr 87:61–63.

20. Dellert SF, Farrell MK, Specker BL, Heubi JE 1998 Bone mineral content in children with short bowel syndrome after discontinuation of parental nutrition. J Pediatr 132:516–519.

21. Atkinson SA, Halton JM, Bradley C, Wu B, Barr RD 1998 Bone and mineral abnormalities in childhood acute lymphoblastic leukemia: Influence of disease, drugs and nutrition. Int J Cancer 1:35–39.

22. Semeao EJ, Jawad AF, Stouffer NO, Zemel BS, Piccoli DA, Stallings VA 1999 Risk factors for low bone mineral density in children and young adults with Crohn's disease. J Pediatr 135:593–600.

23. Carpi J 1997 Do baseline bone scan before giving inhaled steroids for asthma. Pediatr News 31:5–6.

24. El-Desouki M, Al-Jurayyan N 1997 Bone mineral density and bone scintigraphy in children and adolescents with osteomalacia. Eur J Nucl Med Mol Imaging 24:202–205.

25. Ponder SW 1995 Clinical use of bone densitometry in children: Are we ready yet? Clin Pediatr 34:237–240.

26. Brumsen C, Hamdy NA, Papapoulos SE 1997 Long-term effects of bisphosphonates on the growing skeleton. Studies of young patients with severe osteoporosis. Medicine 76:266–283.

27. Saggese G, Baroncelli GI, Barsanti S 1996 Bone mineral density during growth hormone therapy. Paediatr Osteology 1105:109–114.

28. Langman CB, Thorson DK, Shaykin RA, Rock JA 1998 Alendronate therapy in osteopenic pediatric disorders. Bone 1:S457.

29. Robinson E, Bachrach LK, Katzman DK 2000 Use of hormone replacement therapy to reduce the risk of osteopenia in adolescent girls with anorexia nervosa. J Adolesc Health 26:343–348.

30. Poznanski AK 1974 The Hand in Radiologic Diagnosis. WB Saunders, Philadelphia, PA, USA.

31. Garn SM, Poznanski AK, Nagy JM 1971 Bone measurement in the differential diagnosis of osteopenia and osteoporosis. Radiology 100:509–518.

32. Poznanski AK, Kuhns LR, Guire KE 1980 New standards of cortical mass in the humerus of neonates: A means of evaluating bone loss in the premature infant. Radiology 134:639–644.

33. Virtama P, Helela T (eds.) 1969 Radiographic Measurements of Cortical Bone. Turku Auraprint Oy, Stockholm, The Netherlands.

34. Poznanski AK 1983 Radiologic evaluation of growth. In: Davidson M (ed.) Growth Retardation Among Children and Adolescents With Inflammatory Bowel Disease: Report of Workshop Conducted in Reston, Virginia, March 6–8, 1981. National Foundation for Ileitis and Colitis, New York, NY, USA, pp. 53–81.

35. Leonard MB, Feldman HI, Zemel BS, Berlin JA, Barden EM, Stallings VA 1998 Evaluation of low density spine software for the assessment of bone mineral density in children. J Bone Miner Res 13:1687–1690.

36. Zemel BS, Leonard MB, Stallings VA 2000 Evaluation of the Hologic experimental pediatric whole body analysis software in healthy children and children with chronic disease. J Bone Miner Res 15(Suppl 1):S400.

37. Kelly TL 2002 Pediatric whole body measurements. J Bone Miner Res 17(Suppl 1):S297.

38. Pocock NA 1997 Magnification error of femoral geometry using fan beam densitometers. Calcif Tissue Int 60:8–10.

39. Blake GM 1993 Dual X-ray absorptiometry: A comparison between fan beam and pencil beam scans. Br J Radiol 66:902–906.

40. The WHO Study Group 1994 Assessment of fracture risk and its application to screening for postmenopausal osteoporosis. Report of a WHO Study Group. World Health Organ Tech Rep Ser 843:1–129.

41. Hui SL, Johnston CC, Mazess RB 1985 Bone mass in normal children and young adults. Growth 49:34–43.

42. Bishop NJ, dePriester JA, Cole TJ, Lucas A 1992 Reference values for radial bone width and mineral content using single photon absorptiometry in healthy children aged 4 to 10 years. Acta Paediatr 81:463–468.

43. Bachrach LK, Hastie T, Wang MC, Narasimhan B, Marcus R 1999 Bone mineral acquisition in healthy Asian, Hispanic, black, and

Caucasian youth: A longitudinal study. J Clin Endocrinol Metab **84:**4702–4712.

44. Southard RN, Morris JD, Mahan JD, Hayes JR, Torch MA, Sommer A, Zipf WB 1991 Bone mass in healthy children: Measurement with quantitative DXA. Radiology **179:**735–738.

45. Bonjour JP, Theintz G, Buchs B, Slosman D, Rizzoli R 1991 Critical years and stages of puberty for spinal and femoral bone mass accumulation during adolescence. J Clin Endocrinol Metab **73:**555–563.

46. Faulkner RA, Bailey DA, Drinkwater DT, McKay HA, Arnold C, Wilkinson AA 1996 Bone densitometry in Canadian children 8–17 years of age. Calcif Tissue Int **59:**344–351.

47. Glastre C, Braillon P, David L, Cochat P, Meunier PJ, Delmas PD 1990 Measurement of bone mineral content of the lumbar spine by dual energy x-ray absorptiometry in normal children: Correlations with growth parameters. J Clin Endocrinol Metab **70:**1330–1333.

48. Leonard MB, Propert KJ, Zemel BS, Stallings VA, Feldman HI 1999 Discrepancies in pediatric bone mineral density reference data: Potential for misdiagnosis of osteopenia. J Pediatr **135:**182–188.

49. Klaus G, Paschen C, Wuster C, Kovacs GT, Barden J, Mehls O, Scharer K 1998 Weight-/height-related bone mineral density is not reduced after renal transplantation. Pediatr Nephrol **12:**343–348.

50. Molgaard C, Thomsen BL, Prentice A, Cole TJ, Michaelsen KF 1997 Whole body bone mineral content in healthy children and adolescents. Arch Dis Child **76:**9–15.

51. Leonard MB, Bachrach LK 2001 Assessment of bone mineralization following renal transplantation in children: Limitations of DXA and the confounding effects of delayed growth and development. Am J Transplant **1:**193–196.

52. Carter DR, Bouxsein ML, Marcus R 1992 New approaches for interpreting projected bone densitometry data. J Bone Miner Res **7:**137–145.

53. Katzman DK, Bachrach LK, Carter DR, Marcus R 1991 Clinical and anthropometric correlates of bone mineral acquisition in healthy adolescent girls. J Clin Endocrinol Metab **73:**1332–1339.

54. Kroger H, Kotaniemi A, Vainio P, Alhava E 1992 Bone densitometry of the spine and femur in children by dual-energy x-ray absorptiometry. Bone Miner **17:**75–85.

55. Kroger H, Vainio P, Nieminen J, Kotaniemi A 1995 Comparison of different models for interpreting bone mineral density measurements using DXA and MRI technology. Bone **17:**157–159.

56. Lu PW, Cowell CT, SA LL-J, Briody JN, Howman-Giles R 1996 Volumetric bone mineral density in normal subjects, aged 5–27 years. J Clin Endocrinol Metab **81:**1586–1590.

57. Beck TJ, Ruff CB, Warden KE, Scott WW, Rao GU 1990 Predicting femoral neck strength from bone mineral data. A structural approach. Invest Radiol **25:**6–18.

58. Beck TJ, Ruff CB, Scott WW Jr, Plato CC, Tobin JD, Quan CA 1992 Sex differences in geometry of the femoral neck with aging: A structural analysis of bone mineral data. Calcif Tissue Int **50:**24–29.

59. Beck TJ, Ruff CB, Bissessur K 1993 Age-related changes in female femoral neck geometry: Implications for bone strength. Calcif Tissue Int **1:**S41–S46.

60. Beck TJ, Stone KL, Oreskovic TL, Hochberg MC, Nevitt MC, Genant HK, Cummings SR 2001 Effects of current and discontinued estrogen replacement therapy on hip structural geometry: The study of osteoporotic fractures. J Bone Miner Res **16:**2103–2110.

61. Petit MA, McKay HA, MacKelvie KJ, Heinonen A, Khan KM, Beck TJ 2002 A randomized school-based jumping intervention confers site and maturity-specific benefits on bone structural properties in girls: A hip structural analysis study. J Bone Miner Res **17:**363–372.

62. Goulding A, Taylor RW, Jones IE, McAuley KA, Manning PJ, Williams SM 2000 Overweight and obese children have low bone mass and area for their weight. Int J Obes Relat Metab Disord **24:**627–632.

63. Weiler HA, Janzen L, Green K, Grabowski J, Seshia MM, Yuen KC 2000 Percent body fat and bone mass in healthy Canadian females 10 to 19 years of age. Bone **27:**203–207.

64. Laursen E, Molgaard C, Michaelsen K, Koch C, Muller J 1999 Bone mineral status in 134 patients with cystic fibrosis. Arch Dis Child **81:**235–240.

65. Nysom K, Molgaard C, Michaelsen KF 1998 Bone mineral density in the lumbar spine as determined by dual-energy X-ray absorptiometry. Comparison of whole-body scans and dedicated regional scans. Acta Radiol **39:**632–636.

66. Taylor A, Konrad PT, Norman ME, Harcke HT 1997 Total body bone mineral density in young children: Influence of head bone mineral density. J Bone Miner Res **12:**652–655.

67. Nordstrom P, Pettersson U, Lorentzon R 1998 Type of physical activity, muscle strength, and pubertal stage as determinants of bone

68. Slemenda CW, Miller JZ, Hui SL, Reister TK, Johnston CC 1991 Role of physical activity in the development of skeletal mass in children. J Bone Miner Res **6:**1227–1233.

69. Bailey DA, McKay HA, Mirwald RL, Crocker PR, Faulkner RA 1999 A six-year longitudinal study of the relationship of physical activity to bone mineral accrual in growing children: The University of Saskatchewan bone mineral accrual study. J Bone Miner Res **14:**1672–1679.

70. Frost HM 1997 Strain and other mechanical influences on bone strength and maintenance. Curr Opin Orthop **8:**60–70.

71. Ferretti JL, Capozza RF, Cointry GR, Garcia SL, Plotkin H, Alvarez Filgueira ML, Zanchetta JR 1998 Gender-related differences in the relationship between densitometric values of whole-body bone mineral content and lean body mass in humans between 2 and 87 years of age. Bone **22:**683–690.

72. Schonau E 1998 The development of the skeletal system in children and the influence of muscular strength. Horm Res **49:**27–31.

73. Schonau E, Westermann F, Mokow E, Scheidhauer K, Werhahn E, Stabrey A, Muller-Berghaus J 1998 The functional muscle-bone unit in health and disease. Paediatr Osteology **1154:**191–202.

74. Schonau E, Neu M, Mokov E, Wassmer G, Manz F 2000 Influence of puberty on muscle area and cortical bone area of the forearm in boys and girls. J Clin Endocrinol Metab **85:**1095–1098.

75. Cummings SR, Nevitt MC, Browner WS, Stone K, Fox KM, Ensrud KE, Cauley J, Black D, Vogt TM 1995 Risk factors for hip fracture in white women. Study of Osteoporotic Fractures Research Group. N Engl J Med **332:**767–773.

76. Cummings SR, Black DM, Nevitt MC, Browner W, Cauley J, Ensrud K, Genant HK, Palermo L, Scott J, Vogt TM 1993 Bone density at various sites for prediction of hip fractures. The Study of Osteoporotic Fractures Research Group. Lancet **341:**72–75.

77. Ross PD, Davis JW, Epstein RS, Wasnich RD 1991 Pre-existing fractures and bone mass predict vertebral fracture incidence in women. Ann Intern Med **114:**919–923.

78. Goulding A, Jones IE, Taylor RW, Manning PJ, Williams SM 2000 More broken bones: A 4-year double cohort study of young girls with and without distal forearm fractures. J Bone Miner Res **15:**2011–2018.

79. Goulding A, Cannan R, Williams SM, Gold EJ, Taylor RW, Lewis-Barned NJ 1998 Bone mineral density in girls with forearm fractures. J Bone Miner Res **13:**143–148.

80. Gilsanz V 1998 Bone density in children: A review of the available techniques and indications. Eur J Radiol **26:**177–182.

81. Hangartner TN, Gilsanz V 1996 Evaluation of cortical bone by computed tomography. J Bone Miner Res **11:**1518–1525.

82. Gilsanz V, Kovanlikaya A, Costin G, Roe TF, Sayre J, Kaufman F 1997 Differential effect of gender on the sizes of the bones in the axial and appendicular skeletons. J Clin Endocrinol Metab **82:**1603–1607.

83. Gilsanz V, Skaggs DL, Kovanlikaya A, Sayre J, Loro ML, Kaufman F, Korenman SG 1998 Differential effect of race on the axial and appendicular skeletons of children. J Clin Endocrinol Metab **83:**1420–1427.

84. Rauch F, Schoenau E 2001 Changes in bone density during childhood and adolescence: An approach based on bone's biological organization. J Bone Miner Res **16:**597–604.

85. Schoenau E, Neu CM, Rauch F, Manz F 2001 The development of bone strength at the proximal radius during childhood and adolescence. J Clin Endocrinol Metab **86:**613–618.

86. Schoenau E, Neu CM, Rauch F, Manz F 2002 Gender-specific pubertal changes in volumetric cortical bone mineral density at the proximal radius. Bone **31:**110–113.

87. Rauch F, Klein K, Allolio B, Schoenau E 1996 Age at menarche and cortical bone geometry in premenopausal women. Bone **25:** 69–73.

88. Ferretti JL 1995 Perspectives of pQCT technology associated to biomechanical studies in skeletal research employing rat models. Bone **17:**353S–364S.

89. Neu CM, Manz F, Rauch F, Merkel A, Schoenau E 2001 Bone densities and bone size at the distal radius in healthy children and adoloescents: A study using peripheral quantitative computed tomography. Bone **28:**227–232.

90. Rauch F, Tutlewski B, Fricke O, Rieger-Wettengl G, Schauseil-Zipf U, Herkenrath P, Neu CM, Schoenau E 2001 Analysis of cancellous bone turnover by multiple slice analysis at distal radius: A study using peripheral quantitative computed tomography. J Clin Densitom **4:**257–262.

91. Neu CM, Rauch F, Manz F, Schoenau E 2001 Modeling of cross-sectional bone size, mass and geometry at the proximal radius: A

study of normal bone development using peripheral quantitative computed tomography. Osteoporos Int **12**:538–547.

92. Rauch F, Neu C, Manz F, Schoenau E 2001 The development of metaphyseal cortex–implications for distal radius fractures during growth. J Bone Miner Res **16**:1547–1555.

93. Binkley TL, Specker BL 2000 pQCT measurement of bone parameters in young children: Validation of technique. J Clin Densitom **3**:9–14.

94. Epstein DM, Dalinka MK, Kaplan FS, Aronchick JM, Marinelli DL, Kundel HL 1986 Observer variation in the detection of osteopenia. Skeletal Radiol **15**:347–349.

95. Schneider R 1984 Radiologic methods of evaluating generalized osteopenia. Orthop Clin North Am **15**:631–651.

96. Singh M, Nagrath AR, Maini PS 1970 Changes in trabecular pattern of the upper end of the femur as an index of osteoporosis. J Bone Joint Surg Am **52**:457–467.

97. Glorieux FH, Rauch F, Plotkin H, Ward L, Travers R, Roughley P, Lalic L, Glorieux DF, Fassier F, Bishop NJ 2000 Type V osteogenesis imperfecta: A new form of brittle bone disease. J Bone Miner Res **15**:1650–1658.

98. Meema HE, Oreopoulos DG 1983 The mode of progression of subperiosteal resorption in the hyperparathyroidism of chronic renal failure. Skeletal Radiol **10**:157–160.

99. Debnam JW, Bates ML, Kopelman RC, Teitelbaum SL 1977 Radio-

100. Weiss A 1974 Incidence of subperiosteal resorption in hyperparathyroidism studied by fine detail bone radiography. Clin Radiol **25**:273–276.

101. Parfitt AM 1977 Clinical and radiographic manifestations of renal osteodystrophy. In: Davis DS (ed.) Calcium Metabolism in Renal Failure and Nephrolithiasis. John Wiley & Sons, New York, NY, USA, pp. 145–195.

102. Meema HE, Oreopoulos DG, DeVeber GA 1976 Arterial calcifications in severe chronic renal disease and their relationship to dialysis treatment, renal transplant, and parathyroidectomy. Radiology **121**:315–321.

103. Mehls O, Ritz E, Krempien B, Gilli G, Link K, Willich E, Scharer K 1975 Slipped epiphyses in renal osteodystrophy. Arch Dis Child **50**:545–554.

104. Meema HE, Meema S 1972 Comparison of microradioscopic and morphometric findings in the hand bones with densitometric findings in the proximal radius in thyrotoxicosis and in renal osteodystrophy. Invest Radiol **7**:88–96.

105. Meema HE, Oreopoulos DG, Meema S 1978 A roentgenologic study of cortical bone resorption in chronic renal failure. Radiology **126**:67–74.

106. Frame B, Poznanski AK 1980 Conditions that may be confused with rickets. In: DeLuca HJ (ed.) Pediatric Diseases Related to Calcium. Elsevier, New York, NY, USA, pp. 269–289.

logical pathological correlations in uremic bone disease. Radiology **125**:653–658.

Chapter 28.   Scintigraphy in Metabolic Bone Disease

Ignac Fogelman and Gary J.R. Cook

Department of Nuclear Medicine, Guys Hospital; and Department of Nuclear Medicine, Royal Marsden Hospital, London, United Kingdom

INTRODUCTION

Bone scintigraphy was first described by Fleming et al.[1] in 1961 by using strontium-85 as the radiopharmaceutical. Since then, both gamma cameras and radiopharmaceuticals have undergone substantial development. Gamma cameras are now able to perform high-resolution imaging in short scan times either as whole-body acquisitions or as a number of localized views of the skeleton. More recently, tomographic scintigraphic imaging has become more widely available, and its use has become routine in nuclear medicine, leading to improved sensitivity and specificity for lesion detection.

The most commonly used radiopharmaceuticals for bone imaging are labeled with technetium-99m (^{99m}Tc), a radionuclide available to all nuclear medicine departments and with physical properties that make it ideal for acquiring high resolution data on many physiologic and pathological processes. Diphosphonate compounds such as methylene diphosphonate (MDP), labeled with ^{99m}Tc, are the most commonly used radiopharmaceuticals for bone scintigraphy. These compounds have a basic structure that is discussed elsewhere in the primer.

The exact mechanism of localization of these compounds in bone is not fully understood, but it is probable that they bind to hydroxyapatite crystals. In a normal subject, approximately 30% of an injected dose of ^{99m}Tc-MDP remains in the skeleton, with the majority of uptake being within the first hour. Remaining tracer is cleared from extracellular fluid and blood by renal excretion, and imaging is usually performed at 3–4 h, before there has been significant physical decay of ^{99m}Tc and when the ratio between bone activity and background activity is maximal. The degree of accumulation in bone is dependent on local blood flow but is influenced more strongly by the degree of osteoblastic activity, and hence bone formation. Most pathological processes that involve bone result in increased local bone turnover, with both osteoblast and osteoclast activity being increased. A bone scan is therefore a functional map of bone turnover, which may be either focal or generalized throughout the skeleton.

Conventionally, bone scans are acquired and displayed as planar images, but in recent years, the use of tomography (single photon emission computed tomography [SPECT]) in nuclear medicine has become widely available and is increasingly used, particularly in the investigation of back pain. Although spatial resolution is not improved by tomography, there is heightened contrast between abnormalities and adjacent normal structures, increasing the sensitivity of lesion detection. In addition, tomography provides data in three dimensions, so anatomic localization of abnormalities is improved, allowing more specific diagnoses.

OSTEOPOROSIS

In clinical management of the metabolic bone diseases, the isotope bone scan is most useful in osteoporotic patients, in whom it has a valuable role in evaluation and manage-

The authors have no conflict of interest.

A

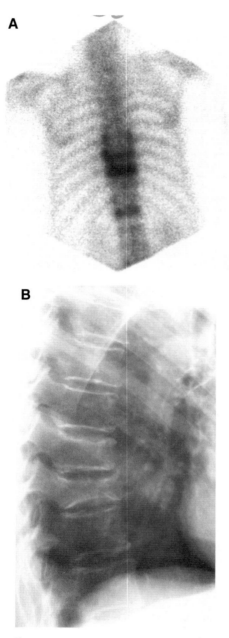

B

plains of back pain with multiple vertebral fractures on radiographs, and the bone scan is normal, then this essentially excludes recent fracture as a cause of symptoms. Other causes of pain should then be considered. Currently, a vertebral fracture is defined based on morphometry,[5] but morphometric abnormalities are not specific to fracture and, for example, may be caused by congenital vertebral anomalies. The bone scan may therefore have a role in deciding whether a morphometric abnormality is related to a fracture, provided that it is acquired within several months of the start of symptoms.

Ryan and Fogelman,[6] by comparing vertebral fractures identified with scintigraphy with morphometric radiographic changes, concluded that only in vertebrae with morphometric deformities >3 SDs below the normal mean can fractures be confidently diagnosed. To date, this approach has not been used in clinical practice, however.

Because of its great sensitivity, the bone scan also is useful in identifying unsuspected osteoporotic fractures at other sites such as ribs, pelvis, and hip. It also has an important role in assessing suspected fractures where radiography is unhelpful, either because of poor sensitivity related to the anatomic site of the fracture (e.g., sacrum; Fig. 2) or because adequate views are not obtainable because of the patient's discomfort.[2]

An isotope bone scan also may be valuable in patients in whom back pain persists for longer than one would expect

FIG. 1. A: 99mTc-methylene diphosphonate (MDP) bone scan showing typical linear uptake of vertebral fractures. (A) The different intensity suggests they occurred at different times. (B) The fractures are confirmed on the corresponding lateral radiograph.

ment.[2] The bone scan has no role in the diagnosis of osteoporosis per se but is most often used in established osteoporosis to diagnose vertebral fracture. The characteristic appearance of this type of fracture is of intense, linearly increased tracer uptake at the affected level. It should be noted that although the bone scan may become positive immediately after a fracture, it can take up to 2 weeks for the scan to become abnormal, especially in the elderly.[3] Subsequently, there is a gradual reduction in tracer uptake, with the scan normalizing between 3 and 18 months after the incident, the average being between 9 and 12 months[4] (Fig. 1). Because of this, the bone scan also is extremely useful in assessing the age of fractures. If a patient com-

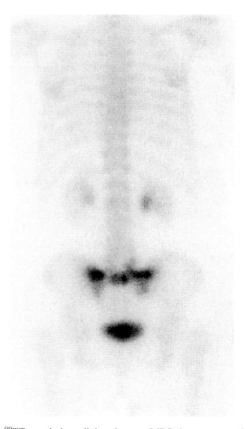

FIG. 2. 99mTc-methylene diphosphonate (MDP) bone scan performed in a woman with known osteoporosis and buttock pain, showing typical features of a sacral insufficiency fracture, which was not detected radiologically.

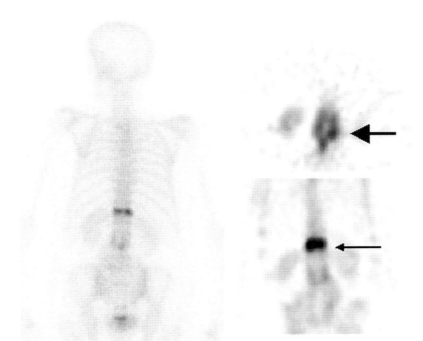

FIG. 3. ^{99m}Tc-methylene diphosphonate (MDP) planar (left) and single photon emission computed tomography (SPECT) transaxial (top) and coronal (bottom) images. Linear uptake typical of vertebral fracture is seen at T12 on the planar and coronal images (small arrow), but transaxial slices also show increased activity in the left sided facet joint at this level (large arrow).

after vertebral fracture. It is common to find that there has been additional unsuspected vertebral fracture. In addition, we are increasingly becoming aware that osteoporotic patients with chronic back pain may have unsuspected abnormalities affecting the facet joints.[2,7] It is not known whether this is related to physical disruption of the joint at the time of vertebral collapse or is caused by subsequent secondary degenerative or inflammatory changes. To identify abnormalities in the facet joints, SPECT imaging is essential (Fig. 3). On planar imaging alone, it is not possible to separate activity in the facet joints from associated activity in the vertebral body caused by fracture, and the three-dimensional properties of this technique allow confident anatomical placement of abnormal foci of increased activity. In the osteoporotic patient, it also is important to exclude secondary causes for pain, such as metastatic disease, infection, Paget's disease, and others.

PAGET'S DISEASE

The isotope bone scan is invaluable in the assessment of patients with suspected Paget's disease, both for diagnosis and to define the extent of skeletal involvement (Fig. 4). The majority of patients with Paget's disease have polyostotic disease (80–90%). The bone scan is a convenient way to evaluate the whole skeleton and has shown a greater sensitivity for detecting affected sites in symptomatic patients than have radiographic skeletal surveys.[8] Characteristically, affected bones show intensely increased activity, which starts at the end of a bone and spreads either proximally or distally, often showing a "V" or "flame-shaped" leading edge. Another clue that a scintigraphic abnormality is caused by Paget's disease rather than other focal skeletal pathology is that a whole bone is often involved, and this is most often evidenced in the pelvis, scapula, and vertebrae. In the vertebrae, the characteristic finding is of abnormal

tracer accumulation throughout the vertebra, affecting the body and posterior elements, including the spinous and transverse processes (Fig. 5).

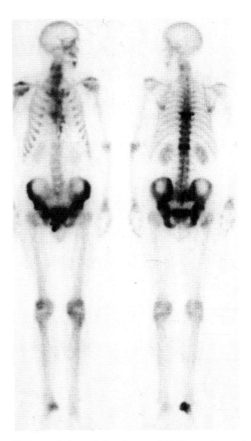

FIG. 4. ^{99m}Tc-methylene diphosphonate (MDP) anterior and posterior whole-body bone scan showing intense activity within a number of bones, with features typical of Paget's disease.

A

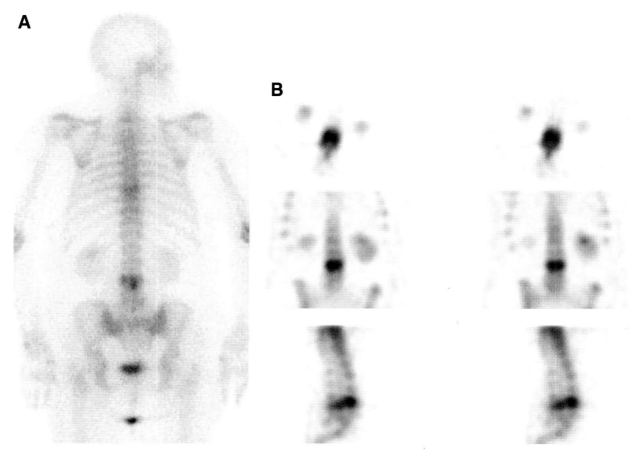

B

FIG. 5. (A) Whole-body bone scan and (B) single photon emission computed tomography (SPECT) slices (from top to bottom: transaxial, coronal, and sagittal) showing increased metabolic activity at L3. SPECT images show how the whole vertebra, including the body and posterior elements, are involved in a pattern typical of Paget's disease.

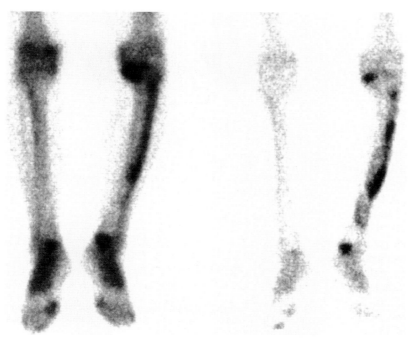

FIG. 6. ^{99m}Tc-methylene diphosphonate (MDP) bone scans of lower legs before (left) and 6 months after (right) treatment with intravenous bisphosphonates. The pretreatment scan shows the typical "flame-shaped" leading edge of Paget's disease in a bowed left tibia. After treatment, the tibial activity has become quite heterogeneous.

The skull may show a different pattern, with a ring of increased activity only in the margins of the lesion, representing what is recognized radiologically as osteoporosis circumscripta.

As powerful treatments for Paget's disease have become available in recent years, it is increasingly being recognized that preventive treatment with regard to possible complications is desirable, rather than simply treating symptomatic cases. Because of this, it is important to be able to accurately evaluate the extent of disease and response to treatment. However, the role of the bone scan with regard to treatment is not well defined.

A scan can be obtained approximately 3–6 months after therapy. It must be recognized that pagetic lesions may often respond in a heterogeneous manner, even in individual patients.[9] After intravenous bisphosphonate therapy, some bones may completely normalize, whereas the majority show some improvement, and a small proportion remain unchanged. Persistent active disease evident on bone scan may be an indication for more aggressive therapy in selected cases to achieve an optimal clinical result. Subsequently, the bone scan may also act as a sensitive measure of reactivation of disease, influencing decisions on further treatment. It is important to be aware that the bone scan appearances can be unusual after successful bisphosphonate treatment; resultant heterogeneous uptake sometimes mimicking metastatic disease and hence a complete clinical history is essential for correct interpretation (Fig. 6).

The radionuclide bone scan may occasionally identify complications of Paget's disease. An incremental fracture on the convex surface of a bowed long bone may be shown as a linear area of increased activity running perpendicular to the cortex. Although osteosarcoma complicating Paget's disease is very rare, clues that sarcomatous change may have occurred include a change to heterogeneous and irregular uptake within an area of bone, perhaps with some photon-deficient areas corresponding to bone destruction. However, the bone scan may be misleading in the event of fracture or sarcomatous change or both, as one attempts to identify focally increased tracer uptake against a high background of activity. It is important to perform radiographs of any symptomatic site in this situation.

HYPERPARATHYROIDISM

Most cases of primary hyperparathyroidism are asymptomatic and are unlikely to be associated with changes on bone scintigraphy. The diagnosis is a biochemical one, and the bone scan therefore has no routine role in diagnosis. Bone scans are often used to help differentiate the causes of hypercalcemia, in particular, hyperparathyroidism versus malignancy, and so typical features of metabolic bone disorders should be recognized. In hyperparathyroidism, there is increased skeletal turnover, and in the more severe cases, commonly seen as part of renal osteodystrophy, this will be evident scintigraphically. A bone scan may show a number of features in hyperparathyroidism, but the most important is the generalized increased uptake throughout the skeleton, which may be identified because of increased contrast between bone and soft tissues. Indeed, renal activity normally

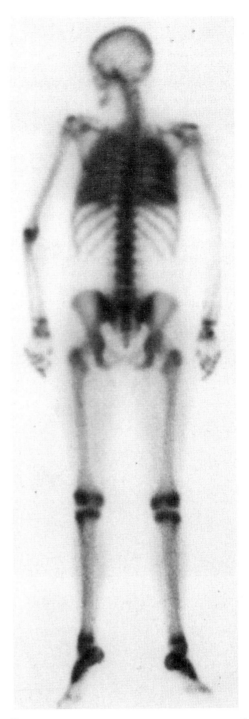

FIG. 7. ^{99m}Tc-methylene diphosphonate (MDP) bone scan of a patient with hyperparathyroidism resulting from chronic renal impairment, showing typical features of metabolic bone disease. In addition, diffuse lung activity is seen, indicating microcalcification.

clearly seen on a bone scan may not be evident. This appearance has been termed a "superscan" because of the apparent high-quality images caused by the high bone uptake (Fig. 7). Other typical features that have been described in bone scans in metabolic bone diseases include a prominent calvarium and mandible, beading of the costochondral junctions, and a "tie" sternum.

© 2003 American Society for Bone and Mineral Research

Severe forms of hyperparathyroidism may be associated with ectopic calcification, which may lead to uptake of bone radiopharmaceuticals into soft tissue, the most dramatic example being that of microcalcification in the lungs. Focal skeletal abnormalities may represent associated brown tumors, although these are rare.

Nuclear medicine is the most frequently used modality for imaging abnormal parathyroid glands before surgery. Experienced parathyroid surgeons do not usually require localization before surgery because all four parathyroid glands are examined preoperatively. However, even in experienced hands, it may be advantageous to localize a parathyroid adenoma preoperatively because this may reduce the time and complexity of surgery. If surgery fails, or if there is recurrent hyperparathyroidism, localization techniques are especially valuable because many of these cases have ectopic glands. Previously thallium 201/technetium 99m (^{201}Tl/^{99m}Tc) subtraction imaging was used. Here, the

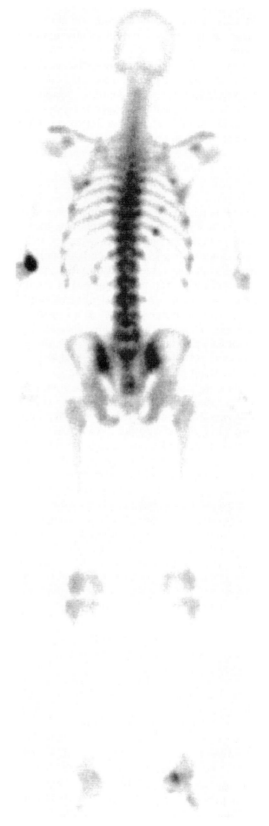

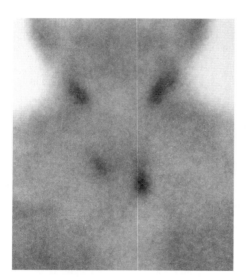

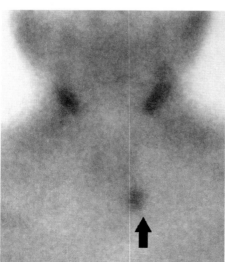

FIG. 8. ^{99m}Tc-sestamibi parathyroid scans taken at 20 minutes (top) and 3 h (bottom) after injection. The early image show uptake in the thyroid and parathyroid glands, but at 3 h, there is washout from the thyroid, leaving activity in a parathyroid adenoma (arrow).

FIG. 9. Whole-body bone scan showing enhanced uptake throughout the skeleton (increased bone / soft tissue ratio) together with multiple focal abnormalities in the ribs in a patient with chronic renal failure and biochemistry consistent with osteomalacia.

data from a thyroid ^{99m}Tc scan are digitally subtracted from a ^{201}T1 scan, which accumulates in both thyroid and parathyroid, leaving an image of parathyroid thallium activity. More recently, improved results were reported with the use of ^{99m}Tc sestamibi.[10] This agent accumulates in both thyroid and parathyroid tissue soon after injection, but after this, there is different washout, with the parathyroids retaining activity at 2–4 h compared with the thyroid (Fig. 8). Sensitivities of approximately 90% have been reported before surgery, although results are poorer in reoperative cases.[11]

RENAL OSTEODYSTROPHY

Renal osteodystrophy is caused by a combination of bone disorders as a consequence of chronic renal dysfunction and often show the most severe cases of metabolic bone disease. It may comprise osteoporosis, osteomalacia, adynamic bone, and secondary hyperparathyroidism in varying degrees. The commonest bone scan appearance is similar to a superscan from other metabolic bone disorders, and uptake of diphosphonate in areas of ectopic calcification also may be seen. A clue in differentiating this type of scintigraphic pattern from others is that there may be a lack of bladder activity in view of renal failure. Although rarely seen now, aluminum toxicity from hemodialysis causes a poor quality bone scan with reduced skeletal uptake and increased soft tissue activity, because aluminum blocks mineralization, and hence uptake of tracer. This pattern is applicable to other forms of adynamic bone disease.

OSTEOMALACIA

Patients with osteomalacia usually show similar features of a bone scan as described in hyperparathyroidism, although in the early stages of the disease, it may appear normal.[12] The reason that osteomalacia shows these features is not fully understood. Tracer avidity may reflect diffuse uptake in osteoid, although more probably it is

caused by the degree of secondary hyperparathyroidism that is present. In addition, the presence of focal lesions may represent pseudofractures or true fractures (Fig. 9). Pseudofractures are characteristically found in the ribs, the lateral border of the scapula, the pubic rami, and the medial femoral cortices. Although osteomalacia is usually a biochemical and/or histological diagnosis, the typical bone scan features can be helpful in suggesting the diagnosis. The detection of pseudofractures with this technique is more sensitive than that with radiography.[13]

REFERENCES

1. Fleming WH, McIlraith JD, King ER 1961 Photoscanning of bone lesions utilising strontium-85. Radiology **77**:635–636.
2. Cook GJR, Hannaford E, Lee M, Clarke SEM, Fogelman I 2002 The value of bone scintigraphy in the evaluation of osteoporotic patients with back pain. Scand J Rheumatol **31**:245–248.
3. Spitz J, Lauer I, Tittel K, Wiegand H 1993 Scintimetric evaluation of remodeling after bone fractures in man. J Nucl Med **34**:1403–1409.
4. Fogelman I, Carr D 1980 A comparison of bone scanning and radiology in the evaluation of patients with metabolic bone disease. Clin Radiol **31**:321–326.
5. Eastell R, Cedel SL, Wahner HW, Riggs BL, Melton LJ 1991 Classification of vertebral fractures. J Bone Miner Res **6**:207–215.
6. Ryan PJ, Fogelman I 1994 Osteoporotic vertebral fractures: Diagnosis with radiography and bone scintigraphy. Radiology **190**:669–672.
7. Ryan PJ, Evans P, Gibson T, Fogelman I 1992 Osteoporosis and chronic back pain: A study with single photon emission computed bone scintigraphy. J Bone Miner Res **7**:1455–1459.
8. Fogelman I, Carr D 1980 A comparison of bone scanning and radiology in the assessment of patients with symptomatic Paget's disease. Eur J Nucl Med **5**:417–421.
9. Ryan PJ, Gibson T, Fogelman I 1992 Bone scintigraphy following pamidronate therapy for Paget's disease of bone. J Nucl Med **33**:1589–1593.
10. McBiles M, Lambert AT, Cole MG, Kim SY 1995 Sestamibi parathyroid imaging. Semin Nucl Med **25**:221–234.
11. Chen CC, Skarulis MC, Fraker DL, Alexander HR, Marx SJ, Spiegel AM 1995 Technetium-99m-sestamibi imaging before reoperation for primary hyperparathyoidism. J Nucl Med **36**:2186–2191.
12. Fogelman I, McKillop JH, Bessent RG, Boyle IT, Turner JG, Greig WR 1978 The role of bone scanning in osteomalacia. J Nucl Med **19**:245–248.
13. Fogelman I, McKillop JH, Greig WR, Boyle IT 1977 Pseudofractures of the ribs detected by bone scanning. J Nucl Med **18**:1236–1237.

Chapter 29.   Radiology of Osteoporosis

Michael Jergas[1] and Harry K. Genant[2]

[1]Department of Radiology and Nuclear Medicine, St. Elisabeth-Krankenhaus, Teaching Hospital of the University of Cologne, Cologne, Germany; and [2]Department of Radiology, Medicine, Epidemiology and Orthopaedic Surgery, Osteoporosis and Arthritis Research Group, University of California San Francisco, San Francisco, California

INTRODUCTION

The term osteoporosis is widely used clinically to mean generalized loss of bone, or radiographic osteopenia, accompanied by relatively atraumatic fractures of the spine, wrist, hips, or ribs. Because of uncertainties of specific

radiologic interpretation, the term osteopenia ("poverty of bone") has been used as a generic designation for radiographic signs of decreased bone density of any cause. Radiographic findings suggestive of osteopenia and osteoporosis are frequently encountered in everyday medical practice and can result from a wide spectrum of diseases ranging from highly prevalent causes such as postmenopausal and involutional osteoporosis to rare endocrinologic and hereditary or acquired disorders (Table 1). Histologi-

The authors have no conflict of interest.

TABLE 1. DISORDERS ASSOCIATED WITH RADIOGRAPHIC
OSTEOPOROSIS (OSTEOPENIA)

I. Primary osteoporosis
   1. Involutional osteoporosis (postmenopausal and senile)
   2. Juvenile osteoporosis
II. Secondary osteoporosis
  A. Endocrine
    1. Adrenal cortex (Cushing's disease)
    2. Gonadal disorders (Hypogonadism)
    3. Pituitary (Hypopituitarism)
    4. Pancreas (Diabetes)
    5. Thyroid (Hyperthyroidism)
    6. Parathyroid (Hyperparathyroidism)
  B. Marrow replacement and expansion
    1. Myeloma
    2. Leukemia
    3. Metastatic disease
    4. Gaucher's disease
    5. Anemias (Sickle Cell Disease, Thalassemia)
  C. Drugs and substances
    1. Corticosteroids
    2. Heparin
    3. Anticonvulsants
    4. Immunosuppressants
    5. Alcohol (in combination with malnutrition)
  D. Chronic disease
    1. Chronic renal disease
    2. Hepatic insufficiency
    3. Gastrointestinal malabsorption
    4. Chronic inflammatory polyarthropathies
    5. Chronic immobilization
  E. Deficiency states
    1. Vitamin D
    2. Vitamin C (Scurvy)
    3. Calcium
    4. Malnutrition
  F. Inborn errors of metabolism
    1. Osteogenesis imperfecta
    2. Homocystinuria

cally, in each of these disorders, there is a deficient amount of osseous tissue, although different pathogenic mechanisms may be involved. Conventional radiography is widely available, and alone or in conjunction with other imaging techniques, is widely used for the detection of complications of osteopenia, for the differential diagnosis of osteopenia, or for subsequent follow-up examinations in specific clinical settings. Bone scintigraphy, computed tomography, and magnetic resonance imaging are additional diagnostic methods that are applied almost routinely to aid in the differential diagnosis of osteoporosis and its sequelae.

RADIOGRAPHIC FINDINGS IN OSTEOPENIA AND OSTEOPOROSIS

The absorption of X-rays by a tissue depends on the quality of the X-ray beam, the character of the atoms composing the tissue, the physical density of the tissue, and the thickness of the penetrated structure. The amount of X-ray absorption defines the density of X-ray shadow that a tissue casts on the film. Because the absorption rises with the third power of the atomic number, and because calcium

has a high atomic number, it is primarily the amount of calcium that affects the X-ray absorption of bone. The amount of calcium per unit mineralized bone volume in osteoporosis remains constant at about 35%.[1,2] Therefore, a decrease in the mineralized bone volume results in a decrease of the total bone calcium and consequently a decreased absorption of the X-ray beam. On the X-ray film, this phenomenon is referred to as increased radiolucency.

In addition to loss of bone mass, changes in bone structure occur, and these can be observed radiographically. Bone is composed of two compartments, cortical bone and trabecular bone. The structural changes seen in cortical bone loss represent bone resorption at different sites (e.g., the inner and outer surfaces of the cortex, or within the cortex in the Haversian and Volkmann channels). These three sites (endosteal, intracortical, and periosteal) may react differently to distinct metabolic stimuli, and careful investigation of the cortices may be of value in the differential diagnosis of metabolic disease affecting the skeleton (Fig. 1).

The normal process of cortical bone remodeling typically occurs in the endosteal "envelope," and the interpretation of subtle changes in this layer may be difficult at times. With increasing age, there is a widening of the marrow canal because of an imbalance of endosteal bone formation and resorption that leads to a "trabeculization" of the inner surface of the cortex (Fig. 2). Endosteal scalloping caused by resorption of the inner bone surface can be seen in high bone turnover states.

Intracortical bone resorption is pathological and may cause longitudinal striation or tunneling, predominantly in the subendosteal zone. These changes are seen in various high turnover metabolic diseases affecting the bone such as hyperparathyroidism, osteomalacia, renal osteodystrophy, acute osteoporosis from disuse or the reflex sympathetic dystrophy syndrome, but also may occur in postmenopausal osteoporosis. Intracortical tunneling is a hallmark of rapid bone turnover. It is usually not apparent in disease states with relatively low bone turnover such as senile osteoporosis. Accelerated endosteal and intracortical resorption with intracortical tunneling and an indistinct border of the inner cortical surface is best depicted with high-resolution radiographic techniques. Intracortical tunneling must be distinguished from nutritional foraminae, which are isolated and present with an oblique orientation. Intracortical resorption is also a sign of bone viability and is not seen in necrotic or allograft bone.

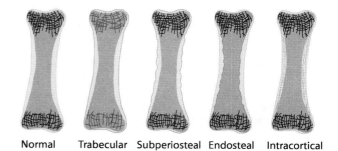

FIG. 1. Patterns of bone loss in the trabecular and cortical compartment of the long bones.

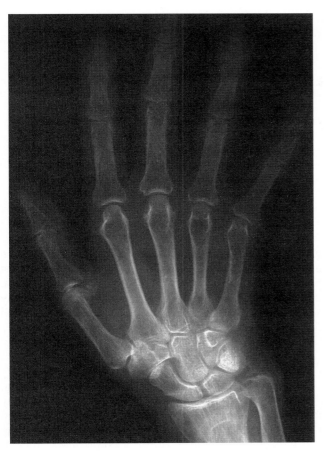

FIG. 2. Advanced involutional osteoporosis with cortical thinning and uniform trabecular resorption as depicted on this hand radiograph.

Subperiosteal bone resorption is associated with an irregular definition of the outer bone surface. This finding is pronounced in diseases with a high bone turnover, principally primary and secondary hyperparathyroidism. Rarely, it may also be present in other diseases. Cortical thinning with expansion of the medullary cavity occurs as endosteal bone resorption exceeds periosteal bone apposition in most adults. In the late stages of osteoporosis, the cortices appear paper thin, with the endosteal surface usually being smooth.

Trabecular bone responds faster to metabolic changes than does cortical bone.[3] Changes are most prominent in the axial skeleton and in the ends of the long and tubular bones of the appendicular skeleton (juxta-articular), for example, proximal femur, distal radius. These are sites with a relatively large amount of trabecular bone. Loss of trabecular bone (in cases with low rates of loss) occurs in a predictable pattern. Non–weight-bearing trabeculae are resorbed first. This leads to a relative prominence of the weight-bearing trabeculae. The remaining trabeculae may become thicker, which may result in a distinct radiographic pattern. For example, early changes of osteopenia in the lumbar spine include a rarefaction of the horizontal trabeculae accompanied by a relative accentuation of the vertical trabeculae, radiographically appearing as vertical striation of the bone. With decreasing density of the trabecular bone the cortical rim of the vertebrae is accentuated, and the vertebrae may have a "picture-frame" appearance. In addi-

tion to changes in the trabecular bone, thinning of the cortical bone occurs. Changes of the bone structure at distinct skeletal sites are assessed for the differential diagnosis of various skeletal conditions. For the evaluation of very subtle changes, such as different forms of bone resorption, high-resolution radiographic techniques with optical or geometric magnification may be required.[4]

The anatomic distribution of the osteopenia or osteoporosis depends on the underlying cause. Osteopenia can be generalized, affecting the whole skeleton, or regional, affecting only a part of the skeleton, usually in the appendicular skeleton. Typical examples of generalized osteopenias are involutional and postmenopausal osteoporosis and osteoporosis caused by endocrine disorders such as hyperparathyroidism, hyperthyroidism, osteomalacia, and hypogonadism. Regional forms of osteoporosis result from factors affecting only parts of the appendicular skeleton such as disuse, reflex sympathetic syndrome, and transient osteoporosis of large joints. The distribution of osteopenia may vary considerably between different diseases and may be suggestive of a specific diagnosis. Focal osteopenia primarily reflects an underlying cause such as inflammation, fracture, or tumor.

Thus, it seems that a number of characteristic features by conventional radiography make the diagnosis of osteopenia or osteoporosis possible. However, the detection of osteopenia by conventional radiography is inaccurate because it is influenced by many technical factors such as radiographic exposure factors, film development, soft tissue thickness of the patient, etc. It has been estimated that as much as 20–40% of bone mass must be lost before a decrease in bone density can be seen in lateral radiographs of the thoracic and lumbar spine.[5] Finally, the diagnosis of osteopenia from conventional radiographs is dependent on the experience of the reader and his/her subjective interpretation.[6]

In summary, a radiograph may reflect the amount of bone mass, histology, and gross morphology of the skeletal part examined. The principal findings of osteopenia are increased radiolucency; changes in bone microstructure, for example, rarefaction of trabeculae; thinning of the cortices, eventually resulting in changes of the gross bone morphology, that is, changes in the shape of the bone; and fractures.

DISEASES CHARACTERIZED BY GENERALIZED OSTEOPENIA

Involutional Osteoporosis

Involutional osteoporosis is the most common generalized skeletal disease. It has been classified as a type I or postmenopausal osteoporosis and a type II or senile osteoporosis.[7,8] Gallagher added a third type, meaning secondary osteoporosis (Table 2).[9] Although the importance of estrogen deficiency for postmenopausal osteoporosis has been established, the distinction between the first two types of osteoporosis is not generally accepted. Distinctions between postmenopausal and senile osteoporosis may sometimes be arbitrary, and the assignment of fracture sites to the different types of osteoporosis is uncertain. Postmenopausal osteoporosis is believed to represent that process occurring

TABLE 2. CLASSIFICATION OF OSTEOPOROSIS AFTER ALBRIGHT, RIGGS AND MELTON, AND GALLAGHER[7–9]

Type	I Postmenopausal	II Senile	III Secondary
Age	55–70	75–90	Any age
Years past menopause	5–15	25–40	
Sex ratio (female:male)		2:1	1:1
Fracture site	Spine	Hip, spine, pelvis, humerus	Spine, hip, peripheral skeleton
Bone loss			
Trabecular	+++	++	+++
Cortical	+	++	+++
Contributing factor			
Menopause	+++	++	++
Age	+	+++	++

in a subset of postmenopausal women, typically between the ages of 50 and 65 years. There is accelerated trabecular bone resorption related to estrogen deficiency, and the fracture pattern in this group of women primarily involves the spine and the wrist. In senile osteoporosis, there is a more proportionate loss of cortical and trabecular bone. The characteristic fractures of senile osteoporosis include fractures of the hip, the proximal humerus, the tibia, and the pelvis in elderly women and men, usually 75 years or older. Major factors in the etiology of senile osteoporosis include an age-related decrease in bone formation, diminished adrenal function, reduced intestinal calcium absorption, and the occurrence of secondary hyperparathyroidism.

The radiographic appearance of the skeleton in involutional osteoporosis may include all of the aforementioned characteristics for generalized osteoporosis. The high prevalence of involutional osteoporosis with its typical radiographic manifestations has lead to numerous attempts to diagnose and quantify osteoporosis based on its radiographic characteristics.

Osteopenia and Osteoporosis of the Axial Skeleton

The radiographic manifestation of osteopenia of the axial skeleton includes increased radiolucency of the vertebrae. The vertebral body's radiographic density may assume the density of the intervertebral disk space. Further findings include vertical striation of the vertebrae because of reinforcement of vertical trabeculae in the osteopenic vertebra, framed appearance of the vertebrae ("picture framing" or "empty box") caused by an accentuation of the cortical outline, and increased biconcavity of the vertebral endplates (Fig. 3). Biconcavity of the vertebrae results from protrusion of the intervertebral disk into the weakened vertebral body (Fig. 4). A classification of these characteristics can be found with the Saville index.[10] This index, however, has never gained widespread acceptance, because it is prone to great subjectivity and experience of the reader. Doyle et al. found that neither of aforementioned signs of osteopenia reflect the bone mineral status of an individual reliably and cannot be used for follow-up of osteopenic patients.[11] Thus, bone density measurements using dedicated densitometric methods have widely replaced the subjective analysis of bone density from conventional radiographs. Densitometric results may reveal osteopenia even if the bone loss is not detectable on a spine radiograph. Nevertheless, the aforementioned radiographic signs of osteoporosis have been found to be significantly related to measured bone density, and normal bone densitometry measurements may sometimes have to be considered false if the radiograph displays characteristic changes of osteopenia.[12,13]

Vertebral Fractures and Their Diagnosis

Vertebral fractures are the hallmarks of osteoporosis (Fig. 4), and although one may argue that osteopenia per se may not be diagnosed reliably from spinal radiographs, spinal radiography continues to be a substantial aid in diagnosing and following vertebral fractures.[14] Furthermore, in combination with a low bone density, a vertebral fracture has been recognized as a the strongest risk factor for future osteoporotic fractures.[15–17] Thus, the presence of vertebral fracture has become a key factor in patient evaluation as expressed in recent NOF guidelines.[18]

Changes in the gross morphology of the vertebral body have a wide range of appearances from increased concavity of the end plates to a complete destruction of the vertebral anatomy in vertebral crush fractures. In clinical practice, conventional radiographs of the thoracolumbar region in lateral projection are analyzed qualitatively by radiologists or experienced clinicians to identify vertebral deformities or fractures. For an experienced radiologist, this assessment generally is uncomplicated, and it can be aided by additional radiographic projections such as anteroposterior and oblique views, or by complimentary examinations such as bone scintigraphy, computed tomography, and magnetic resonance imaging.[19–21]

In the context of conducting epidemiologic studies or clinical drug trials in osteoporosis research, where vertebral fractures are an important endpoint(s), the requirements and expectations differ considerably from the clinical environment.[22] The examinations are frequently performed without specific clinical indications and without specific therapeutic ramifications. The evaluation for fractures is generally limited to lateral conventional thoracolumbar radiographs, and the number of subjects to be reviewed is often quite large, requiring high efficiency. The assessment may be performed by a variety of observers with different levels of experience. The detection of vertebral fractures certainly depends on the reader's expertise. Early experi-

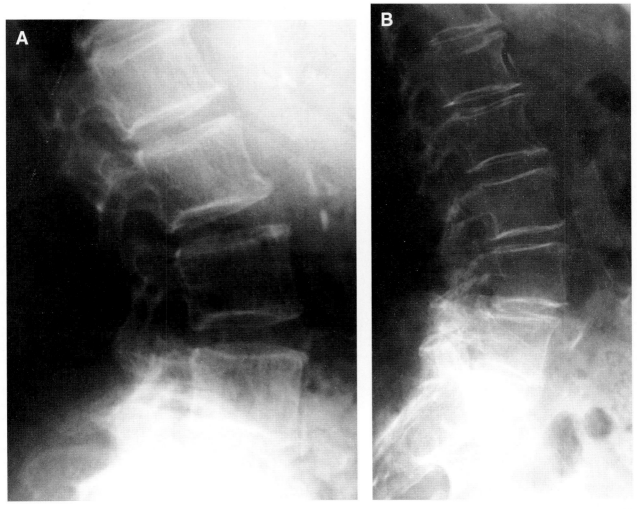

FIG. 3. Moderate postmenopausal osteoporosis of the thoracic spine with overall loss of bone density. (A) The cortices are thinned, and the vertebral bodies have a striated appearance because of loss of secondary trabeculae and reinforcement of sharply defined primary trabeculae. (B) As trabecular bone is lost, there is a relative accentuation of the cortex, resulting in the appearance of "picture framing."

ence with qualitative readings indicated that considerable variability in fracture identification exists when radiologists or clinicians interpreted radiographs without specific training, standardization, reference to an atlas, or prior consensus readings.[23–25]

Therefore, several approaches to standardizing visual qualitative readings have been proposed and applied in clinical studies. An early approach for a standardized description of vertebral fractures was made by Smith et al., who assigned one of three grades (normal, indeterminate, or osteoporotic) to a patient depending on the most severe deformity.[26] The spinal radiographs were evaluated on a per patient and not on a per vertebra basis, a serious limitation for the follow-up of vertebral fractures and also for the assessment of the severity of osteoporosis. Other standardized visual approaches allow for an assessment of vertebral deformities on a per vertebra rather than on a per patient basis and thus make a more accurate assessment of the fracture status of a person and the follow-up of individual fractures possible. Meunier et al. proposed an approach in which each vertebra is graded depending on its shape or deformity.[27] Grade 1 is assigned to a normal vertebra without any deformity, grade 2 is assigned to a biconcave vertebra, and grade 4 is assigned to an end plate fracture or a wedged or crushed vertebra. The sum of all grades of the vertebrae T7—L4 is the radiological vertebral index (RVI). This approach is limited because it considers only the type of the vertebral deformity, that is, biconcavity versus fracture, without assessing fracture severity. For prevalent fractures, each fracture, whether it is diminutive or severe, would have the same weight in the RVI, and for the application of this approach to follow-up examinations, this means that refractures of pre-existing fractures may not be detected at all. With the distinction between biconcavity and fracture in this approach, the concept of "vertebral deformity" versus vertebral fracture was introduced. However, it was not expressively attempted to distinguish nonfracture deformities such as degenerative remodeling from actual fracture appearances.

Nielsen et al. modified Meunier's radiological vertebral index and introduced the "vertebra deformity score" (VDS),[28] by which each vertebra from T4 to L5 is assigned

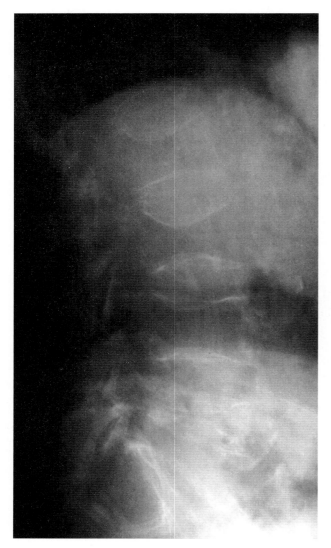

FIG. 4. Severe osteopenia. The transparency of the vertebral bodies matches that of the intervertebral disc space. There are multiple fractures of the vertebral endplates leading to biconcave deformities of the vertebrae as well as a severe fracture of L5.

an individual score from 0 to 3 depending on the type of vertebral deformity. This grading scheme is based on the reduction of the anterior, middle, and posterior vertebral heights, H_a, H_m, and H_p, respectively. A vertebral deformity (to be graded 1–3) is present when any vertebral height, H_a, H_m, or H_p, is reduced by at least 4 mm or 15%. A vertebral deformity score 0 is assigned to a normal vertebra without any vertebral height reduction. A VDS 1 deformity corresponds to a vertebral end plate deformity with the heights H_a and H_p being normal. A wedge deformity with a reduction of H_a and—to a lesser extent H_m—is assigned a VDS of 2. A compression deformity, which is assigned a VDS of 3, is characterized by a reduction of all vertebral heights H_a, H_m, and H_p. Grading all vertebrae T4–L5 using this score, the minimum VDS for the whole spine would thus be 0 with all vertebrae intact and the maximum score would be 42 with compression fractures of all vertebrae. The vertebral deformity score still relies on the type of deformity, that is,

the vertebral shape, and changes of the vertebral shape would be required to account for incident vertebral fractures on follow-up radiographs. A quantitative extension of the VDS with measurements of the vertebral heights has been proposed by Kleerekoper et al. to account for the continuous character of vertebral fractures.

The radiologist's perspective of vertebral fracture diagnosis, that is, considering the differential diagnosis as well as the severity of a fracture, is probably best reflected in the semiquantitative fracture assessment used in several studies.[14,29] The severity of a fracture is assessed solely by visual determination of the extent of vertebral height reduction and morphological change, and vertebral fractures are differentiated from other nonfracture deformities. With this approach, the type of the deformity (wedge, biconcavity, or compression) is no longer linked to the grading of a fracture as is done with the other standardized visual approaches. As depicted on Fig. 5, thoracic and lumbar vertebrae from T4 to L4 are graded on visual inspection and without direct vertebral measurement as normal (grade 0), mildly deformed (grade 1, approximately 20–25% reduction in anterior, middle, and/or posterior height and a reduction of 10–20% of the projected vertebral area), moderately deformed (grade 2, approximately 25–40% reduction in anterior, middle, and/or posterior height and a reduction of 20–40% of the projected vertebral area), and severely deformed (grade 3, approximately 40% or greater reduction in anterior, middle, and/or posterior height and in the projected vertebral area). In addition to height reductions, careful attention is given to alterations in the shape and configuration of the vertebrae relative to adjacent vertebrae and expected normal appearances. These features add a strong qualitative aspect to the interpretation and also render this method less readily definable. Several studies, however, have demonstrated that semiquantitative interpretation, after careful training and standardization, can produce results with excellent intra- and interobserver reproducibility within the same school of training.[14,30]

In a further effort to provide definable, reproducible, and objective methods to detect vertebral fractures and to accommodate the assessment of large numbers of radiographs by technicians (in the absence of radiologists or experienced clinicians), various quantitative morphometric approaches have been explored and used. Early studies using direct measurements of vertebral dimensions on lateral radiographs were described by Fletcher in 1946, Hurxthal in 1968, Jensen and Tougaard in 1981, and Kleerekoper et al. in 1984, with the rationale being a reduction in the subjectivity considered intrinsic to the qualitative assessment of spinal radiographs.[31–34]

Increasingly sophisticated morphometric approaches have been derived for the definition of vertebral dimensions, most of them making 4–10 points on a vertebral body to define vertebral heights (Fig. 6).[35–37] Typically, H_a, H_m, and H_p are measured, as is the projected vertebral area. Newer techniques are based on digitally captured conventional radiographs to assess the vertebral dimensions.[38–40] These techniques then rely on either marking points manually to define vertebral heights or finding those points and measuring in an automated or semiautomated fashion.

Hedlund and Gallagher used criteria such as percent

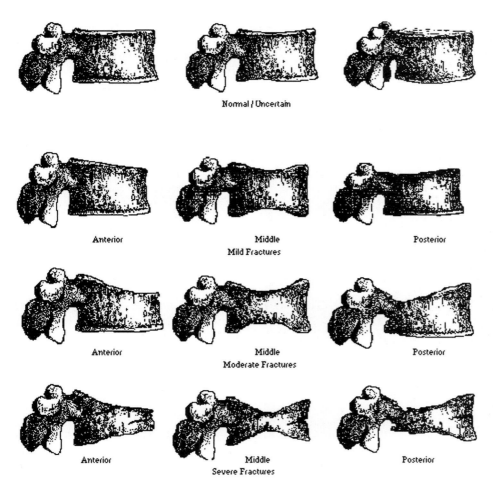

Normal / Uncertain

Anterior   Middle   Posterior
Mild Fractures

Anterior   Middle   Posterior
Moderate Fractures

Anterior   Middle   Posterior
Severe Fractures

FIG. 5. Grading scheme for a semiquantitative assessment of vertebral deformities after Genant. The drawing illustrates the reductions of vertebral height that correspond to the grade of deformity (Drawing courtesy of Dr. C.Y. Wu).

reduction of vertebral height, wedge angles, and areas in various combinations.[41] Davies et al. used two distinct morphometric cut-off thresholds for the detection of either vertebral compression or wedge fractures using vertebral height ratios that were defined by a radiologist's assessment of vertebral deformities.[42] Smith-Bindman et al. initially reported the use of vertebral level specific reductions in anterior, middle, or posterior height ratios expressed as a percentage relative to normal data.[43] Melton used this level-specific approach, and subsequently, Eastell et al. modified it by applying height ratio reductions in terms of standard deviations rather than percentage.[44] With this approach, each vertebral level has its own specific mean and SD. Minne et al. developed a method by which vertebral height measures are adjusted according to the height of T4 as a means of standardization, and the resulting values are compared with a normal population.[45] Black et al. derived a statistical method for establishing normative data from morphometric measures of vertebral heights based on deletion of the tails of the Gaussian distribution of an unselected population.[46] McCloskey et al. used vertebral height ratios and introduced an additional parameter defined as a predicted posterior height in addition to the measured posterior height.[47] Ross et al. further refined morphometric criteria for fracture by using height reductions in SDs based on the overall patient specific vertebral dimensions combined with population based level-specific vertebral dimensions.[48]

Several comprehensive studies have compared the various methods or cut-off criteria in the same populations to examine the impact of methodology on estimates of vertebral prevalence and on identification of individual patients or individual vertebrae as fractured. In these studies, the expected trade-offs between sensitivity and specificity were observed. Two- to 4-fold differences in estimates of fracture prevalence and generally poor or modest kappa scores between the different algorithms for defining fractures were reported.[43,49,50] Therefore, despite having developed sophisticated, describable, and objective methods, the application and interpretation of the results have been complicated by the large differences observed from one technique to the next. Unfortunately, no true gold standard for defining fractures exists, by which one can judge the methods or their variable cut-off criteria. However, as a first approximation, there is some rationale for comparing visual assessment and morphometric data on a per vertebra basis to develop a consensus interpretation based on the expertise of experienced radiologists and highly trained research assistants.[51] This may help to understand the reasons for concordant and discordant results and to use the strengths of the respective methods. When relying solely on quantitative morphometry, one has to consider that no real distinction between osteoporotic fractures and other nonfracture deformities can be made. Besides the uncertainties that are introduced by vertebral projection, differences in the applied technique and

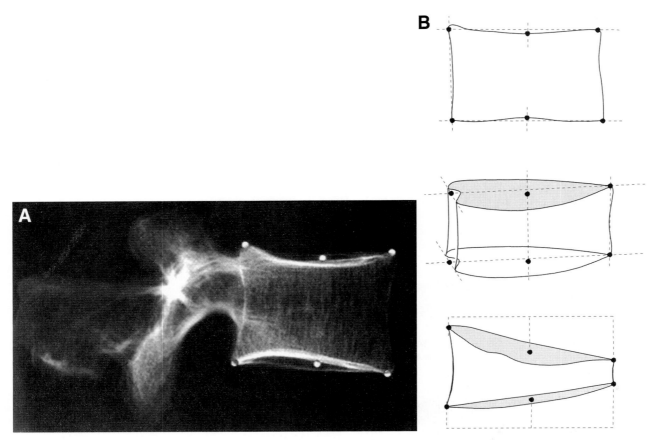

FIG. 6. (A) In six-point digitization, the endpoints of the vertebral heights are marked directly on the vertebra. Point placement is fairly easy when the vertebra is ideally projected with perfect superposition of the vertebral contours. (B) When the vertebra is rotated and oblique, point placement is more difficult.

intra- and interobserver precision of quantitative morphometry, this may have a substantial impact on the prevalence and to a lesser extent on the incidence of vertebral fractures in a population.

When comparing a standardized visual approach with quantitative morphometry, substantial differences between both techniques have been reported, while the agreement between different, centrally trained readers for the semiquantitative approach is reportedly very good.[14,30,50,52] This applies to the diagnosis of both prevalent and incident fractures. Drawing on the strength of each of the approaches both a quantitative approach as well as a standardized visual approach may be applied in combination to reliably diagnose vertebral fractures in clinical drug trials.[51,53,54]

It seems feasible that a more recently developed technique, the morphometric X-ray analysis (MXA; Fig. 7), which employs a DXA scanner for the depiction of the thoracolumbar spine, may overcome some of the drawbacks of conventional radiographs.[55,56] Especially, the effect of different projections and magnification effects between two films will be minimized because of the technical specifications of this technique. Furthermore, it is possible to assess bone density on the same scanner.[57] Other limitations like poorer image resolution and higher noise levels apply, however.[58] The restrictions that are inherent to quantitative morphometry also apply to MXA, potentially even more because image quality does not always warrant a thorough diagnostic evaluation of a vertebral deformity. While MXA may be helpful in the serial assessment of vertebral deformities, its diagnostic validity is still under investigation.[59–62]

Osteopenia and Osteoporosis at Other Skeletal Sites

The axial skeleton is not the only site where characteristic changes of osteopenia and osteoporosis can be depicted radiographically. Changes in the trabecular and cortical bone can also be seen in the appendicular skeleton. It is first apparent at the ends of long and tubular bones because of the predominance of cancellous bone in these regions. Endosteal resorption has a prominent role particularly in senile osteoporosis. The net result of this chronic process is widening of the medullary canal and thinning of the cortices. In late stages of senile osteoporosis, the cortices are paper-thin and the endosteal surfaces are smooth. In rapidly evolving postmenopausal osteoporosis, accelerated endosteal and intracortical bone resorption may be seen and can be directly assessed by high-resolution radiographic techniques. Methods to quantitate the changes at the peripheral skeleton have been proposed and also clinically applied (e.g., Singh index, radiogrammetry).[63–65] Conventional radiography is the basis for a number of recent studies exploring new aspects of assessing bone structure using sophisticated image analysis procedures such as fractal analysis or fast Fourier

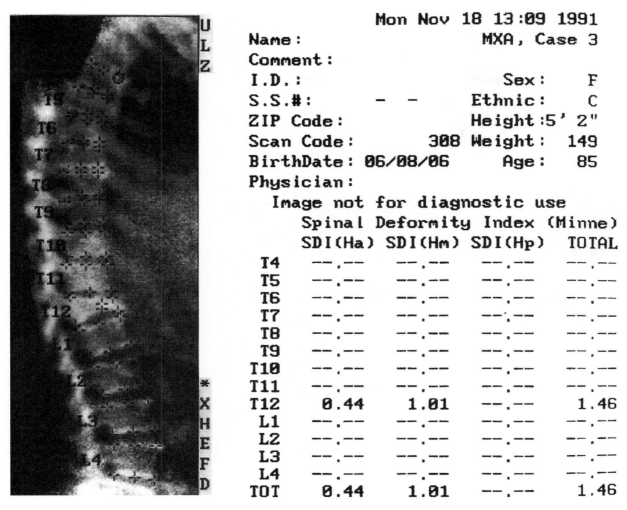

	Mon Nov 18 13:09 1991
Name :	MXA, Case 3

Comment :
I.D.:   Sex: F
S.S.#:   — —   Ethnic: C
ZIP Code: Height:5' 2"
Scan Code: 308 Weight: 149
BirthDate: 06/08/06   Age: 85
Physician :

Image not for diagnostic use
Spinal Deformity Index (Minne)

	SDI(Ha)	SDI(Hm)	SDI(Hp)	TOTAL
T4	--.--	--.--	--.--	--.--
T5	--.--	--.--	--.--	--.--
T6	--.--	--.--	--.--	--.--
T7	--.--	--.--	--.--	--.--
T8	--.--	--.--	--.--	--.--
T9	--.--	--.--	--.--	--.--
T10	--.--	--.--	--.--	--.--
T11	--.--	--.--	--.--	--.--
T12	0.44	1.01	--.--	1.46
L1	--.--	--.--	--.--	--.--
L2	--.--	--.--	--.--	--.--
L3	--.--	--.--	--.--	--.--
L4	--.--	--.--	--.--	--.--
TOT	0.44	1.01	--.--	1.46

FIG. 7. Morphometric X-ray absorptiometry (MXA) of the spine. In this example, a severe wedge fracture is detected at the T12 level using the spine deformity index.

transforms.[66–69] These techniques have also been applied to the study of bone structure using high-resolution images acquired with magnetic resonance imaging or computed tomography in a research setting.[70–75]

DIFFERENTIAL DIAGNOSIS OF REDUCED BONE MASS

Aside from senile and postmenopausal states, there are various other conditions that may be accompanied by generalized osteoporosis. While most of the previously mentioned radiographic characteristics are shared by a variety of conditions, there may be some apparent differences in the appearance of osteoporosis as compared with involutional osteoporosis.

Endocrine Disorders Associated With Osteoporosis

Hyperparathyroidism leads to both increased bone resorption and bone formation. Changes induced by hyperparathyroidism may affect all bone surfaces, resulting in subperiosteal, intracortical, endosteal, subchondral, subepiphyseal, subligamentous and subtendinous, and trabecular bone resorption.[76–78] Subperiosteal bone resorption is the most characteristic radiographic feature of hyperparathyroidism.[79] It is especially prominent in the hand, wrist, and foot, but may also be seen other sites (Fig. 8). Radiographically, the outer margin of the bone becomes indistinct. Scalloping and spiculation of the cortex may occur in later stages. Undermineralization of the tela ossea leads to the distinctive radiographic appearance of acro-osteolyses.[80] Intracortical resorption results in longitudinally oriented linear striations within the cortex, and endosteal bone resorption leads to scalloping of the inner cortex, cortical thinning, and widening of the medullary canal.[81]

Subchondral bone resorption frequently also affects the joints of the axial skeleton, causing undermineralization of the Tela ossea. For example, it may mimic widening of the sacroiliac joint space leading to "pseudo-widening" of the joint.[82] The osseous surface may collapse and thus may simulate subchondral lesions of inflammatory disease. Osteopenia occurs frequently in hyperparathyroidism and may be observed throughout the skeleton. Other radiographic signs of hyperparathyroidism include focal bone lesions ("brown tumors"), cartilage calcification, and bone sclerosis.[83] Increased amounts of trabecular bone leading to bone

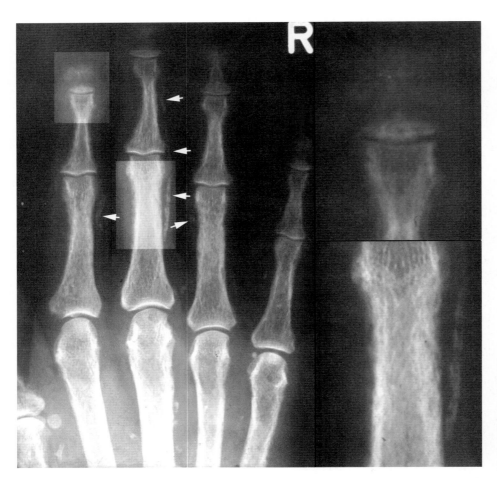

FIG. 8. Conventional radiograph of the hand in secondary hyperparathyroidism. The magnification illustrated periosteal bone resorption with indistinct delineation of the outer cortical border. There is also osteolytic appearance of the distal phalanges caused by undermineralization of the osseous substance. Calcification of the small vessels is present (arrows).

sclerosis may occur especially in patients with renal osteodystrophy and secondary hyperparathyroidism. Increased bone density may occur preferably in the axial skeleton, sometimes leading to deposition of bone in subchondral areas of the vertebral body, resulting in an appearance of radiodense bands across the superior and inferior border and normal or decreased density of the center ("rugger-jersey spine"; Fig. 9).[84]

While osteoporosis is defined by a reduction of regularly mineralized osteoid, findings in osteomalacia include an abnormally high amount of nonmineralized osteoid and a reduction in mineralized bone volume. Thus, radiographic abnormalities in osteomalacia include osteopenia (reduction of mineralized bone), coarsened, indistinct trabeculae, and unsharp delineation of cortical bone (excessive apposition of nonmineralized osteoid), deformities, insufficiency fractures, and true fractures (bone softening and weakening).[85] The deformations include bowing and bending of the long bones and biconcave deformities of the vertebrae.[86] Pseudofractures, or Looser's zones (focal accumulations of osteoid in compact bone at right angles of the long axis), are diagnostic of osteomalacia and are often bilateral and symmetrical. There are more than 50 different diseases that may cause osteomalacia, of which chronic renal insufficiency, hemodialysis, and renal transplantation are the most common causes.[87,88] Modern patient management has resulted in typical radiographic features of osteomalacia being present in only a minority of these patients.[89] A decrease of vitamin D in chronic renal insufficiency leads to osteomalacia (and rickets in the growing child). The additional secondary hyperparathyroidism leads to a superimposition of radiographic changes from both osteomalacia and secondary hyperparathyroidism.[90] This radiographic appearance is termed renal osteodystrophy. A common finding in secondary hyperparathyroidism associated with renal osteodystrophy is an osteosclerosis, resulting in typical appearance of the vertebral bodies as seen in the rugger-jersey spine.[87] Several other radiographic abnormalities may be frequently seen in renal osteodystrophy including amyloid deposits, destructive spondyloarthropathy, inflammatory changes, avascular necrosis, soft tissue calcifications, and arteriosclerosis.[91,92]

Hyperthyroidism is a high-turnover disease, and it is associated with an increase in both bone resorption and bone formation.[93] Because bone resorption exceeds bone formation, rapid bone loss may occur and result in generalized osteoporosis, with the largest effect on cortical bone.[94] This effect is especially pronounced in patients with thyrotoxicosis or with a history of thyrotoxicosis.[95] Suppressive doses of thyroid hormone have been reported to decrease or have no effect on bone density.[96] Radiological findings of hyperthyroidism-induced osteoporosis are those that are commonly seen in involutional or senile osteoporosis, including generalized osteopenia and cortical thinning and tunneling. The fractures associated with this condition affect the spine, the hip, and the distal radius.[97,98]

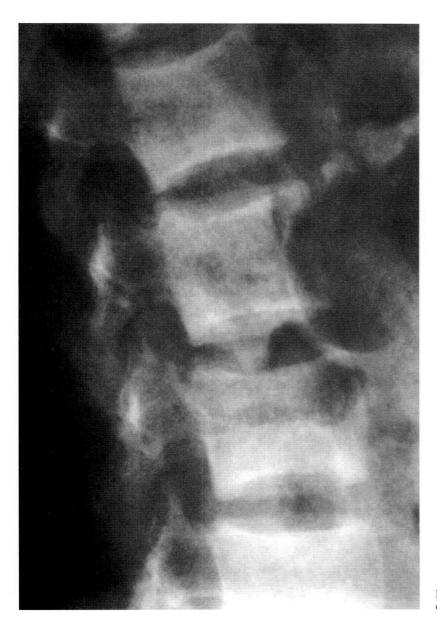

FIG. 9. Renal osteodystrophy presenting with subchondral bands of sclerosis, the "rugger-jersey" spine.

Medication-Induced Osteoporosis

Hypercortisolism from the use of corticosteroids is probably the most common cause of medication-induced generalized osteoporosis, whereas the endogenous form of hypercortisolism, Cushing's disease, is relatively rare.[99–101] Decreased bone formation and increased bone resorption have been observed in hypercortisolism. This has attributed to inhibition of osteoblast formation, either direct stimulation of osteoclast activity or increased secretion of parathyroid hormone. The typical radiographic appearance of steroid-induced osteoporosis comprises generalized osteoporosis, at predominantly trabecular sites, with decreased bone density and fractures of the axial but also of the appendicular skeleton. A characteristic finding in steroid-induced osteoporosis is the marginal condensation of the vertebral bodies resulting from exuberant callus formation. Osteonecrosis is another complication of hypercortisolism, most frequently involving the femoral head, and to a lesser extent the humeral head and the femoral condyles.[102,103]

Generalized osteoporosis has been observed in patients receiving high-dose heparin therapy.[104,105] The radiological features of heparin-induced osteoporosis include generalized osteopenia and vertebral compression fractures.[106] The pathophysiologic mechanism of heparin-induced osteoporosis is not completely clear, and there may be a prolonged effect on bone even after cessation of therapy.[107,108]

Other Causes of Generalized Osteoporosis

Malnutrition, chronic alcoholism (if associated with malnutrition), smoking and caffeine intake, and Marfan syndrome may cause generalized osteoporosis. Pregnancy-associated osteoporosis has been observed but is relatively uncommon.[109–113] Marrow abnormalities associated with osteoporosis include anemias (sickle cell anemia, thalassemia), plasma cell myeloma, leukemia, Gaucher's disease, and glycogen storage disease.[114,115] This list is certainly far from being complete, but it represents some of the major causes of osteoporosis. Additional imaging techniques such as computed tomography, magnetic resonance tomography, and bone scintigraphy, as well as clinical information, may be helpful in differential diagnosis of these various conditions associated with osteoporosis.[116–119]

There are some conditions of the growing skeleton that result in generalized osteoporosis. Rickets is characterized by inadequate mineralization of the bone matrix, and some of its radiographic appearance may resemble that of osteomalacia.[120] Widening of the growth plates, cupping of the metaphysis, and decreased density and irregularities of the metaphyseal margins may be present.[121] Epiphyseal ossification centers may show delayed ossification and unsharp borders.[122] Overgrowth of the hyaline cartilage may lead to prominence of costochondral junctions of the ribs (rachitic rosary). The child's age at the onset of the disease determines the pattern of bone deformity, with bowing of the long bone being more pronounced in infancy and early childhood and vertebral deformities and scoliosis in older children.[123] Further deformities that may be observed in rickets include pseudofractures, basilar invagination, and triradiate configuration of the pelvis.

Idiopathic juvenile osteoporosis is perhaps a self-limited disease of childhood with recovery occurring as puberty progresses.[124] A typical feature of this condition is the increased vulnerability of the metaphyses, often resulting in metaphyseal injuries of the knees and ankles. Idiopathic juvenile osteoporosis must be distinguished from osteogenesis imperfecta, another disease often presenting with radiographic signs of generalized osteoporosis.[125] The pathogenesis of osteogenesis imperfecta is quantitative or qualitative abnormalities of type I collagen. There are four major types of osteogenesis imperfecta, and the degree of osteoporosis in osteogenesis imperfecta depends strongly on the type of disease.[126] The clinical features of each type usually correspond to the type of mutation. The abnormal maturation of collagen seen in this disorder results in a primary defect in bone matrix. This, combined with a defective mineralization, results in overall loss of bone density involving both the axial and peripheral skeleton. Patients with type III disease have a significantly decreased bone density presenting with generalized osteopenia, thinned cortices, fractures of long bones and ribs, exuberant callus formation, and bone deformation.[127] The degree of osteopenia is highly variable, however, and at the mildest end of the spectrum some patients do not have any radiographic signs of osteopenia.[128]

REGIONAL OSTEOPOROSIS

Osteoporosis may also be confined to only a segment of the body. This type of osteoporosis is called regional osteoporosis, and it is commonly caused by some disorder of the appendicular skeleton. Osteoporosis caused by immobilization or disuse, characteristically occurs in the immobilized regions of patients with fractures, motor paralysis caused by central nervous system disease or trauma, and bone and joint inflammation.[129] Chronic and acute disease may vary in their radiographic appearance somewhat showing diffuse osteopenia, linear radiolucent bands, speckled radiolucent areas, and cortical bone resorption.

Reflex sympathetic dystrophy, sometimes also termed Sudeck's atrophy or algodystrophy, has the radiographic appearance of a high turnover process. It most often occurs in patients with trauma, such as Colles' fracture, but also in patients with any neurally related musculoskeletal, neurologic, or vascular condition such as hemiplegia or myocardial infarction.[130–132] This condition is probably related to overactivity of the sympathetic nervous system with increased blood flow and increased intravenous oxygen saturation in the affected extremity.[133,134] Its radiographic appearance includes soft tissue swelling as well as regional osteoporosis showing with bandlike, patchy, or periarticular osteoporosis. Additional radiographic features include subperiosteal bone resorption, intracortical tunneling, endosteal bone resorption with initial excavation, and scalloping of the endosteal surface and subsequent remodeling and widening of the medullary canal, as well as subchondral and juxtaarticular erosions.[135] Especially in the early stages of reflex sympathetic dystrophy, bone scintigraphy may be helpful to establish the diagnosis.[136,137]

Transient regional osteoporosis includes conditions that have in common the development of self-limited pain and radiographic osteopenia affecting one or several joints, most commonly the hip. Transient osteoporosis typically occurs in middle-aged men or women in the third trimester of pregnancy. At the onset of clinical symptoms, there may be normal radiographic findings, and within several weeks, patients develop variable osteopenia of the hip, sometimes involving the acetabulum. Some patients later develop similar changes in the opposite hip or in other joints, in which case the term regional migratory osteoporosis may be used. No specific therapy is required, because all patients recover. The cause of transient regional osteoporosis is not known, and it seems that it may be related to reflex sympathetic dystrophy. In some patients with clinically similar or identical manifestations, magnetic resonance imaging presents with transient regional bone marrow edema.[138,139] Because not all patients with identical clinical symptoms and transient bone marrow edema develop regional osteoporosis, the sensitivity as to the detection of regional osteoporosis has to be questioned as well as the interrelationship between transient regional osteoporosis and transient bone marrow edema. There also seems to be a relationship of transient bone marrow edema to ischemic necrosis of bone, and there is a need to define criteria for allowing differentiation of transient bone marrow edema and the edema pattern associated with osteonecrosis.[140–142]

QUANTIFYING BONE MINERAL IN CONVENTIONAL RADIOGRAPHY

Standardized Evaluation of Conventional Radiographs

The lack of methods to objectively assess bone density in the past made some researchers use the characteristic radiographic appearance of bone in osteoporosis to grade or classify osteoporosis, for example, Saville's score for clas-

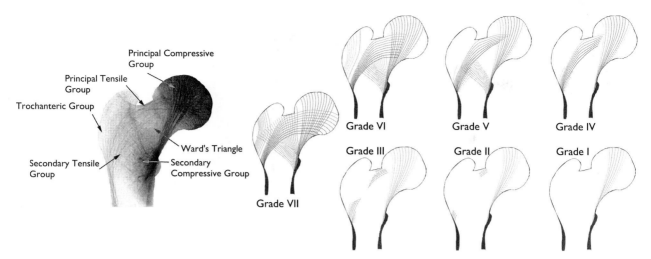

FIG. 10. The Singh index is based on the assumption that the trabeculae in the proximal femur disappear in a predictable sequence depending on their original thickness. The classification ranges from grade VII (normal, all trabecular groups visible) to grade I (marked reduction of even the principal compressive trabeculae), according to the degree of bone loss.

sifying vertebral osteoporosis.[10] Doyle et al. studied the single radiological criteria of osteoporosis. Except for biconcavity, the authors found none of the other criteria to be valid criteria for the diagnosis of osteoporosis.[11] *"Can Radiologists Detect Osteopenia on Plain Radiographs?"*, Garton et al. asked and concluded that, although the reproducibility of Saville's score was only moderate, bone density was significantly correlated with this score.[143] Aside from single criteria, the radiographic impression of the spine as a whole may hint to a reduced bone density.[13] Therefore, because it is essential for differential diagnosis of osteoporosis and for diagnosing and monitoring vertebral deformities, conventional radiography will remain an important diagnostic tool.

In an attempt to quantify the degree of osteoporosis, Barnett and Nordin, and in a similar form, Dent et al., proposed that the increased biconcavity of a vertebra could be used to diagnose and monitor osteoporosis.[144,145] The quotient of middle and anterior vertebral height today is associated with the names of Barnett and Nordin. However, the authors only used one vertebra to calculate their score (usually L3), which may not represent the bone mineral status of the whole spine.[6] Tracking the course of osteoporosis with reference to only one vertebra simply does not work.

The axial skeleton is not the only site where characteristic changes of osteopenia and osteoporosis can be depicted radiographically. Changes in the trabecular and cortical bone can also be seen in the appendicular skeleton, and methods for quantitating these changes have been proposed and also clinically applied.

Urist reported that, in women with hip fractures, the principal compressive trabeculae in the proximal femur become more prominent, while other groups of trabeculae are resorbed.[146] Based on this observation in women with advanced osteoporosis, Singh et al. in 1970 proposed a femoral index for the diagnosis of osteoporosis based on the assumption that the trabeculae in the proximal femur disappear in a predictable sequence depending on their original

thickness.[63] The authors considered that the thickness and spacing of trabeculae in the various trajectory groups (principal compressive, secondary compressive, greater trochanter, principal tensile, and secondary tensile group) depend on the intensity of stresses normally carried by these trabeculae, and with advancing bone loss, trabeculae that are thinner become invisible first on the radiograph. Singh and coworkers introduced a classification ranging from grade VII (normal, all trabecular groups visible) to grade I (marked reduction of even the principal compressive trabeculae) according to the degree of bone loss (Fig. 10). The authors reported a relatively good discrimination of individuals with and without vertebral fractures. A range of interobserver variation has been reported for the Singh index, with the variability being influenced strongly by the quality of the radiographs, the degree of osteoporosis, with moderate changes being harder to agree on than the extremes, and the experience of the observer.

Radiogrammetry

Radiogrammetry, a simple measurement of cortical thickness in virtually any tubular bone, is easy to perform with a caliper or with a graduated magnifying glass. Simple cortical measurements may be represented in several ways: one method involves summing the thickness of both cortices as an index of bone mass; another method uses the combined cortical thickness divided by the total bone width as a measure of density; finally, a circular cross-section of bone can be assumed with the measurements of bone width and cortical thickness converted to cortical areas that more closely parallel actual physical mass (Fig. 11). Radiogrammetry is applied most often to the metacarpal bones.[147] The correlation between radiogrammetric measurements and other methods of bone densitometry is generally regarded as only moderate.[148,149]

Simple cortical measurements, particularly when obtained at several anatomic sites, provide information that is more useful in clinical research than in individual patient

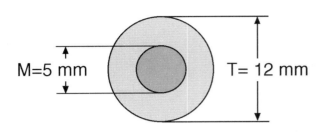

Combined Cortical Thickness (CCT)   T-M
Cortical Index   (T-M)/T
Cortical Area $0.785 * (T^2 - M^2)$

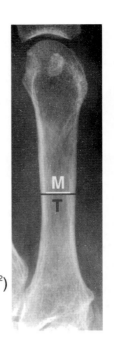

FIG. 11. For a long time, radiogrammetry represented the only quantitative method to evaluate changes of bone density by measuring the thickness of the cortical bone. The results may be expressed as combined cortical thickness, cortical index, or even an assumed cortical area. Typically, this measurement is performed on the second metacarpal bone. T, outer diameter (thickness); M, inner diameter (marrow canal).

management. Meema found radiogrammetry to be a good discriminator between postmenopausal women with and without vertebral fractures.[150,151] In the context of the large epidemiological Study of Osteoporotic Fractures, metacarpal radiogrammetry proved to be predictive of future incident hip fractures.[152] One major limitation of radiogrammetry is its failure to measure intracortical resorption or porosity and irregular endosteal scalloping or erosion. Because intracortical and trabecular bone resorptions are important indicators of high bone turnover states, the fact that they are not measured by this technique is significant. Despite its shortcomings when applied to individual patients, radiogrammetry remains an important research tool for studying changes in cortical bone.

A variation of radiogrammetry was introduced recently and is called Digital X-ray Radiogrammetry (DXR). Originally, in this technique, a radiogram of the forearm was scanned on a commercial high-resolution scanner, and the digital image of the forearm was analyzed using various regions of interest in three metacarpals and radius and ulna. In its most recent version, the analysis is restricted to the metacarpal bones II–IV. A bone mineral density (BMD) equivalent DXR bone density is calculated from cortical thickness of these bones, and image procession algorithms are applied to calculate additional parameters, striation, and porosity. Initial results showed the method provided adequate precision as well as a good association with age and with the history of fracture.[153,154]

Photodensitometry or Radiographic Absorptiometry

The photographic density on a film is roughly proportional to the mass of bone located in the X-ray beam. A relatively large change in bone mineral content (BMC; 25–50%) must occur, however, before it can be detected with visual observation of radiographs.[5,155] In an effort to quantitate bone mass, a number of investigators have measured the optical density of bone contained in radiographs, in which both the anatomic part to be studied and a reference wedge are included.[156–158] Simultaneous exposure of a reference system (usually an aluminum or hydroxyapatite wedge or step wedge) allows for reproducible determination of bone density with an appropriate exposure technique (Fig. 12). After film processing, bone and reference wedge are evaluated using a photo densitometer.

Photodensitometry is a low-dose and low-cost technique, which measures integral bone (trabecular and cortical). Multiple technical problems arise, however, such as nonuniformity of X-ray intensity beam hardening because of the polychromatic radiation source and variation in film sensitivity related to processing. Photodensitometry is limited to the peripheral skeleton because of soft tissue inhomogeneities. Various measurement sites in the upper and lower extremities are reported in the literature. Metacarpal or phalangeal bones are preferred sites. Several investigators confirmed the significant association with prevalent vertebral fractures as well as with future hip fractures.[159–162] However, there is still some controversial discussion on the diagnostic efficiency of radiographic absorptiometry.[163] As a plus, cost effectiveness, ease of use, and its theoretically ubiquitous availability make this technique an interesting option for the assessment of bone mass.

Even some of the methods used to study bone density at the axial skeleton are derived from radiographic absorptiometry. Photodensitometry cannot be applied to the axial skeleton because of the greater amount and inhomogeneity of the surrounding soft tissue. Krokowski and Schlungbaum reported on a photodensitometric method for determining the BMC at the lumbar spine already in 1959. The authors used two lateral radiographs of the lumbar spine taken at two distinct energies (62 and 250 kV) to calculate bone density in a region of interest.[164] This method described the basic principles of what was to become the most wide-

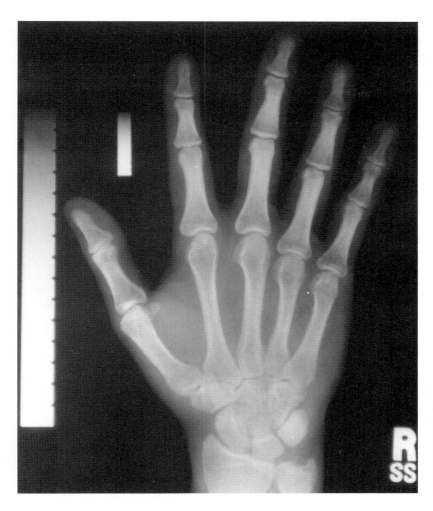

FIG. 12. In radiographic absorptiometry, the simultaneous exposure of a reference system (usually a wedge or step wedge consisting of aluminum or hydroxyapatite) allows for a reproducible determination of bone density with an appropriate exposure technique. By comparing the attenuation values of the reference with known density values, one determines corresponding density of a region of interest in the bone.

spread technique to assess bone density at the axial skeleton, dual-photon absorptiometry (DPA) or DXA.

REFERENCES

1. Albright F, Smith PH, Richardson AM 1941 Postmenopausal osteoporosis. Its clinical features. JAMA **116**:2465–2474.
2. LeGeros RZ 1994 Biological and synthetic apatites. In: Brown PW, Constantz B (eds.) Hydroxyapatite and Related Materials. CRC Press, Boca Raton, FL, USA, pp. 3–28.
3. Frost HM 1964 Dynamics of bone remodelling. In: Frost HM (ed.) Bone Biodynamics. Little Brown, Boston, MA, USA, pp. 315–334.
4. Genant HK, Doi K, Mall JC, Sickles EA 1977 Direct radiographic magnification for skeletal radiology. Radiology **123**:47–55.
5. Lachmann E, Whelan M 1936 The roentgen diagnosis of osteoporosis and its limitations. Radiology **26**:165–177.
6. Jergas M, Uffmann M, Escher H, Schaffstein J, Nitzschke E, Köster O 1994 Visuelle Beurteilung konventioneller Röntgenaufnahmen und duale Röntgenabsorptiometrie in der Diagnostik der Osteoporose. Z Orthop Ihre Grenzgeb **132**:91–98.
7. Albright F 1947 Osteoporosis. Ann Intern Med **27**:861–882.
8. Riggs BL, Melton LJ 1983 Evidence for two distinct syndromes of involutional osteoporosis. Am J Med **75**:899–901.
9. Gallagher JC 1990 The pathogenesis of osteoporosis. Bone Miner **9**:215–227.
10. Saville PD 1967 A quantitative approach to simple radiographic diagnosis of osteoporosis: Its application to the osteoporosis of rheumatoid arthritis. Arthritis Rheum **10**:416–422.
11. Doyle FH, Gutteridge DH, Joplin GF, Fraser R 1967 An assessment of radiological criteria used in the study of spinal osteoporosis. Br J Radiol **40**:241–250.
12. Jergas M, Uffmann M, Escher H, Glüer CC, Young KC, Grampp S, Köster O, Genant HK 1994 Interobserver variation in the detection of osteopenia by radiography and comparison with dual X-ray absorptiometry (DXA) of the lumbar spine. Skeletal Radiol **23**:195–199.
13. Ahmed AIH, Ilic D, Blake GM, Rymer JM, Fogelman I 1998 Review of 3530 referrals for bone density measurements of spine and femur: Evidence that radiographic osteopenia predicts low bone mass. Radiology **207**:619–624.
14. Genant HK, Wu CY, van Kuijk C, Nevitt M 1993 Vertebral fracture assessment using a semi-quantitative technique. J Bone Miner Res **8**:1137–1148.
15. Ross PD, Davis JW, Epstein RS, Wasnich RD 1991 Pre-existing fractures and bone mass predict vertebral fracture incidence in women. Ann Intern Med **114**:919–923.
16. Ross PD, Genant HK, Davis JW, Miller PD, Wasnich RD 1993 Predicting vertebral fracture incidence from prevalent fractures and bone density among non-black, osteoporotic women. Osteoporos Int **3**:120–126.
17. Kotowicz MA, Melton LJ III, Cooper C, Atkinson EJ, O'Fallon WM, Riggs LB 1994 Risk of hip fracture in women with vertebral fracture. J Bone Miner Res **9**:599–605.
18. National Osteoporosis Foundation 2000 Physician's Guide to Prevention and Treatment of Osteoporosis. National Osteoporosis Foundation, Washington, DC, USA.
19. McAfee PC, Yuan HA, Fredrickson BE, Lubicky JP 1983 The value of computed tomography in thoracolumbar fractures. An analysis of one hundred consecutive cases and a new classification. J Bone Joint Surg Am **65**:461–473.
20. Campbell SE, Phillips CD, Dubovsky E, Cail WS, Omary RA 1995 The value of CT in determining potential instability of simple wedge-compression fractures of the lumbar spine. AJNR Am J Neuroradiol **16**:1385–1392.

21. Ballock RT, Mackersie R, Abitbol JJ, Cervilla V, Resnick D, Garfin SR 1992 Can burst fractures be predicted from plain radiographs? J Bone Joint Surg Br **74:**147–150.
22. Kleerekoper M, Nelson DA, Peterson EL, Tilley BC 1992 Outcome variables in osteoporosis trials. Bone **13:**S29–S34.
23. Jensen GF, McNair P, Boesen J, Hegedüs V 1984 Validity in diagnosing osteoporosis. Euro J Radiol **4:**1–3.
24. Deyo RA, McNiesh LM, Cone RO III 1985 Observer variability in the interpretation of lumbar spine radiographs. Arthritis Rheum **28:**1066–1070.
25. Genant HK, Jergas M, van Kuijk C 1995 Vertebral Fracture in Osteoporosis. Radiology Research and Education Foundation, San Francisco, CA, USA.
26. Smith RW, Eyler WR, Mellinger RC 1960 On the incidence of senile osteoporosis. Ann Intern Med **52:**773–781.
27. Meunier PJ, Bressot C, Vignon E, Edouard C, Alexandre C, Courpron P, Laurent J 1978 Radiological and histological evolution of post-menopausal osteoporosis treated with sodium fluoride-vitamin D-calcium. Preliminary results. In: Courvoisier B, Donath A, Baud CA (eds.) Fluoride and Bone. Hans Huber Publishers, Bern, Germany, pp. 263–276.
28. Nielsen VAH, Pødenphant J, Martens S, Gotfredsen A, Riis BJ 1991 Precision in assessment of osteoporosis from spine radiographs. Euro J Radiol **13:**11–14.
29. Genant HK 1990 Radiographic assessment of the effects of intermittent cyclical treatment with etidronate. In: Christiansen C, Overgaard K (eds.) Third International Conference on Osteoporosis, vol. 3. Osteopress ApS, Copenhagen, Denmark, pp. 2047–2054.
30. Wu CY, Li J, Jergas M, Genant HK 1995 Comparison of semiquantitative and quantitative techniques for the assessment of prevalent and incident vertebral fractures. Osteoporos Int **5:**354–370.
31. Kleerekoper M, Parfitt AM, Ellis BI 1984 Measurement of vertebral fracture rates in osteoporosis. In: Christiansen C, Arnaud CD, Nordin BEC, Parfitt AM, Peck WA, Riggs BL (eds.) Copenhagen International Symposium on Osteoporosis June 3–8, 1984, vol. 1. Department of Clinical Chemistry, Glostrup Hospital, Copenhagen, Denmark, pp. 103–108.
32. Fletcher H 1947 Anterior vertebral wedging - Frequency and significance. Am J Roentgenol **57:**232–238.
33. Hurxthal L 1968 Measurement of anterior vertebral compressions and biconcave vertebrae. Am J Roentgenol **103:**635–644.
34. Jensen KK, Tougaard L 1981 A simple x-ray method for monitoring progress of osteoporosis. Lancet **2:**19–20.
35. Nelson D, Peterson E, Tilley B, O'Fallon W, Chao E, Riggs BL, Kleerekoper M 1990 Measurement of vertebral area on spine x-rays in osteoporosis: Reliability of digitizing techniques. J Bone Miner Res **5:**707–716.
36. Spencer NE, Steiger P, Cummings SR, Genant HK 1990 Placement for points for digitizing spine films. J Bone Miner Res **5:**S2;S247.
37. Jergas M, San Valentin R 1995 Techniques for the assessment of vertebral dimensions in quantitative morphometry. In: Genant HK, Jergas M, van Kuijk C (eds.) Vertebral Fracture in Osteoporosis. Radiology Research and Education Foundation, San Francisco, CA, USA, pp. 163–188.
38. Kalidis L, Felsenberg D, Kalender W, Eidloth H, Wieland E 1992 Morphometric analysis of digitized radiographs: Description of automatic evaluation. In: Ring EFG (ed.) Current research in osteoporosis and bone mineral measurement II: 1992. British Institute of Radiology, London, UK, pp. 14–16.
39. Evans SF, Nicholson PHF, Haddaway MJ, Davie MWJ 1993 Vertebral morphometry in women aged 50–81 years. Bone Miner **21:**29–40.
40. Wu C, van Kuijk C, Li J, Jiang Y, Chan M, Countryman P, Genant HK 2000 Comparison of digitized images with original radiography for semiquantitative assessment of osteoporotic fractures. Osteoporos Int **11:**25–30.
41. Hedlund LR, Gallagher JC 1988 Vertebral morphometry in diagnosis of spinal fractures. Bone Miner **5:**59–67.
42. Davies KM, Recker RR, Heaney RP 1993 Revisable criteria for vertebral deformity. Osteoporos Int **3:**265–270.
43. Smith-Bindman R, Cummings SR, Steiger P, Genant HK 1991 A comparison of morphometric definitions of vertebral fracture. J Bone Miner Res **6:**25–34.
44. Eastell R, Cedel SL, Wahner HW, Riggs BL, Melton LJ III 1991 Classification of vertebral fractures. J Bone Miner Res **6:**207–215.
45. Minne HW, Leidig G, Wüster C, Siromachkostov L, Baldauf G, Bickel R, Sauer P, Lojen M, Ziegler R 1988 A newly developed spine deformity index (SDI) to quantitate vertebral crush fractures in patients with osteoporosis. Bone Miner **3:**335–349.
46. Black DM, Cummings SR, Stone K, Hudes E, Palermo L, Steiger P 1991 A new approach to defining normal vertebral dimensions. J Bone Miner Res **6:**883–892.
47. McCloskey EV, Spector TD, Eyres KS, Fern ED, O'Rourke N, Vasikaran S, Kanis JA 1993 The assessment of vertebral deformity: A method for use in population studies and clinical trials. Osteoporos Int **3:**138–147.
48. Ross PD, Yhee YK, He Y-F, Davis JW, Kamimoto C, Epstein RS, Wasnich RD 1993 A new method for vertebral fracture diagnosis. J Bone Miner Res **8:**167–174.
49. Sauer P, Leidig G, Minne HW, Dudeck G, Schwarz W, Siromachkostov L, Ziegler R 1991 Spine deformity index (SDI) versus other objective procedures of vertebral fracture identification in patients with osteoporosis. J Bone Miner Res **6:**227–238.
50. Hansen M, Overgaard K, Nielsen V, Jensen G, Gotfredsen A, Christiansen C 1992 No secular increase in the prevalence of vertebral fractures due to postmenopausal osteoporosis. Osteoporos Int **2:**241–246.
51. Genant HK, Jergas M, Palermo L, Nevitt M, San Valentin R, Black D, Cummings SR 1996 Comparison of semiquantitative visual and quantitative morphometric assessment of prevalent and incident vertebral fractures in osteoporosis. J Bone Miner Res **11:**984–996.
52. Leidig-Bruckner G, Genant HK, Minne HW, Storm T, Thamsborg G, Bruckner T, Sauer P, Schilling T, Soerensen OH, Ziegler R 1994 Comparison of a semiquantitative and a quantitative method for assessing vertebral fractures in osteoporosis. Osteoporos Int **4:**154–161.
53. Cummings SR, Melton LJ III, Felsenberg D, National Osteoporosis Foundation Working Group on Vertebral Fracture 1995 Assessing vertebral fractures. J Bone Miner Res **10:**518–523.
54. Grados F, Roux C, de Vernejoul MC, Utard G, Sebert JL, Fardellone P 2001 Comparison of four morphometric definitions and a semiquantitative consensus reading for assessing prevalent vertebral fractures. Osteoporos Int **12:**716–722.
55. Steiger P, Weiss H, Stein JA 1993 Morphometric x-ray absorptiometry of the spine: A new method to assess vertebral osteoporosis. Proceedings of the 4th International Symposium on Osteoporosis and Consensus Development Conference. Hong Kong, p. 292.
56. Steiger P, Cummings SR, Genant HK, Weiss H 1994 Morphometric x-ray absorptiometry of the spine: Correlation in vivo with morphometric radiography. Osteoporos Int **4:**238–244.
57. Greenspan SL, von Stetten E, Emond SK, Jones L, Parker RA 2001 Instant vertebral assessment: A noninvasive dual X-ray absorptiometry technique to avoid misclassification and clinical mismanagement of osteoporosis. J Clin Densitom **4:**373–380.
58. Ferrar L, Jiang G, Eastell R 2001 Short-term precision for morphometric X-ray absorptiometry. Osteoporos Int **12:**710–715.
59. Chappard C, Kolta S, Fechtenbaum J, Dougados M, Roux C 1998 Clinical evaluation of spine morphometric X-ray absorptiometry. Br J Rheumatol **37:**496–501.
60. Ferrar L, Jiang G, Barrington NA, Eastell R 2000 Identification of vertebral deformities in women: Comparison of radiological assessment and quantitative morphometry using morphometric radiography and morphometric X-ray absorptiometry. J Bone Miner Res **15:**575–585.
61. Rea JA, Chen MB, Li J, Blake GM, Steiger P, Genant HK, Fogelman I 2000 Morphometric X-ray absorptiometry and morphometric radiography of the spine: A comparison of prevalent vertebral deformity identification. J Bone Miner Res **15:**564–574.
62. Guermazi A, Mohr A, Grigorian M, Taouli B, Genant HK 2002 Identification of vertebral fractures in osteoporosis. Semin Musculoskelet Radiol **6:**241–252.
63. Singh YM, Nagrath AR, Maini PS 1970 Changes in trabecular pattern of the upper end of the femur as an index of osteoporosis. J Bone Joint Surg Am **52:**457–467.
64. Barnett E, Nordin BEC 1961 Radiological assessment of bone density. I.-The clinical and radiological problem of thin bones. Br J Radiol **34:**683–692.
65. Meema HE, Meema S 1981 Radiogrammetry. In: Cohn SH (ed.) Non-invasive Measurements of Bone Mass. CRC Press, Boca Raton, FL, USA, pp. 5–50.
66. Benhamou CL, Lespessailles E, Jacquet G, Harba R, Jennane R, Loussot T, Tourliere D, Ohley W 1994 Fractal organization of trabecular bone images on calcaneus radiographs. J Bone Miner Res **9:**1909–1918.
67. Geraets W, Van der Stelt P, Lips P, Van Ginkel F 1998 The radio-

graphic trabecular pattern of hips in patients with hip fractures and in elderly control subjects. Bone 22:165–173.

68. Link T, Majumdar S, Konermann W, Meier N, Lin J, Newitt D, Ouyang X, Peters P, Genant H 1997 Texture analysis of direct magnification radiographs of vertebral specimens: Correlation with bone mineral density and biomechanical properties. Acad Radiol 4:167–176.

69. Lespessailles E, Roux JP, Benhamou CL, Arlot ME, Eynard E, Harba R, Padonou C, Meunier PJ 1998 Fractal analysis of bone texture on os calcis radiographs compared with trabecular microarchitecture analyzed by histomorphometry. Calcif Tissue Int 63:121–125.

70. Majumdar S, Kothari M, Augat P, Newitt DC, Link TM, Lin JC, Lang T, Lu Y, Genant HK 1998 High-resolution magnetic resonance imaging: Three-dimensional trabecular bone architecture and biomechanical properties. Bone 22:445–454.

71. Millard J, Augat P, Link TM, Kothari M, Newitt DC, Genant HK, Majumdar S 1998 Power spectral analysis of vertebral trabecular bone structure from radiographs: Orientation dependence and correlation with bone mineral density and mechanical properties. Calcif Tissue Int 63:482–489.

72. Link TM, Lin JC, Newitt D, Meier N, Waldt S, Majumdar S 1998 Computer-assisted structure analysis of trabecular bone in the diagnosis of osteoporosis. Radiologe 38:853–859.

73. Majumdar S, Link TM, Augat P, Lin JC, Newitt D, Lane NE, Genant HK 1999 Trabecular bone architecture in the distal radius using magnetic resonance imaging in subjects with fractures of the proximal femur. Magnetic Resonance Science Center and Osteoporosis and Arthritis Research Group. Osteoporos Int 10:231–239.

74. Laib A, Ruegsegger P 1999 Comparison of structure extraction methods for in vivo trabecular bone measurements. Comput Med Imaging Graph 23:69–74.

75. Cortet B, Dubois P, Boutry N, Bourel P, Cotten A, Marchandise X 1999 Image analysis of the distal radius trabecular network using computed tomography. Osteoporos Int 9:410–419.

76. Genant HK, Heck LL, Lanzl LH, Rossmann K, Vander Horst J, Paloyan E 1973 Primary hyperparathyroidism. A comprehensive study of clinical, biochemical and radiographic manifestations. Radiology 109:513–519.

77. Genant HK, Vander Horst J, Lanzl LH, Mall JC, Doi K 1974 Skeletal demineralization in primary hyperparathyroidism. Proceedings of International Conference on Bone Mineral Measurement. Washington, DC, USA, p. 177.

78. Richardson ML, Pozzi-Mucelli RS, Kanter AS, Kolb FO, Ettinger B, Genant HK 1986 Bone mineral changes in primary hyperparathyroidism. Skeletal Radiol 15:85–95.

79. Camp JD, Ochsner HC 1931 The osseous changes in hyperparathyroidism associated with parathyroid tumor: A roentgenologic study. Radiology 17:63–71.

80. Resnick D, Niwayama G 1995 Parathyroid disorders and renal osteodystrophy. In: Resnick D (ed.) Diagnosis of Bone and Joint Disorders, 3rd ed., vol. 4. W.B. Saunders Company, Philadelphia, PA, USA, pp. 2012–2075.

81. Meema HE, Meema S 1972 Microradioscopic and morphometric findings in the hand bones with densitometric findings in the proximal radius in thyrotoxicosis and in renal osteodystrophy. Invest Radiol 7:88–92.

82. Hayes CW, Conway WF 1991 Hyperparathyroidism. Radiol Clin North Am 29:85–96.

83. Steinbach HL, Gordan GS, Eisenberg E, Carne JT, Silverman S, Goldman L 1961 Primary hyperarthyroidism: A correlation of roentgen, clinical, and pathologic features. Am J Roentgenol 86:239–243.

84. Resnick D 1981 The "rugger jersey" vertebral body. Arthritis Rheum 24:1191–1194.

85. Reginato AJ, Falasca GF, Pappu R, McKnight B, Agha A 1999 Musculoskeletal manifestations of osteomalacia: Report of 26 cases and literature review. Semin Arthritis Rheum 28:287–304.

86. Kienböck R 1940 Osteomalazie, Osteoporose, Osteopsathyrose, porotische Kyphose. Fortschr Röntgenstr 61:159–166.

87. Pitt MJ 1991 Rickets and osteomalacia are still around. Radiol Clin North Am 29:97–118.

88. Kainberger F, Traindl O, Baldt M, Helbich T, Breitenseher M, Seidl G, Kovarik J 1992 renale Osteodytrophie: Spektrum der Röntgensymptomatik bei modernen Formen der Nierentransplantation und Dauerdialysetherapie. Fortschr Röntgenstr 157:501–505.

89. Adams JE 1999 Renal bone disease: Radiological investigation. Kidney Int Suppl 73:S38–S41.

90. Sundaram M 1989 Renal osteodystrophy. Skeletal Radiol 18:415–426.

91. Kriegshauser JS, Swee RG, McCarthy JT, Hauser MF 1987 Aluminum toxicity in patients undergoing dialysis: Radiographic findings and prediction of bone biobsy results. Radiology 164:399–403.

92. Murphey MD, Sartoris DJ, Quale JL, Pathria MN, Martin NL 1993 Musculoskeletal manifestations of chronic renal insufficiency. Radiographics 13:357–379.

93. Mosekilde L, Eriksen EF, Charles P 1990 Effects of thyroid hormones on bone and mineral metabolism. Endocrinol Metab Clin North Am 19:35–63.

94. Greenspan SL, Greenspan FS 1999 The effect of thyroid hormone on skeletal integrity. Ann Intern Med 130:750–758.

95. Toh SH, Claunch BC, Brown PH 1985 Effect of hyperthyroidism and its treatment on bone mineral content. Arch Intern Med 145:883–886.

96. Nuzzo V, Lupoli G, Esposito Del Puente A, Rampone E, Carpinelli A, Del Puente AE, Oriente P 1998 Bone mineral density in premenopausal women receiving levothyroxine suppressive therapy. Gynecol Endocrinol 12:333–337.

97. Chew FS 1991 Radiologic manifestations in the musculoskeletal system of miscellaneous endocrine disorders. Radiol Clin North Am 29:135–147.

98. Solomon BL, Wartofsky L, Burman KD 1993 Prevalence of fractures in postmenopausal women with thyroid disease. Thyroid 3:17–23.

99. Laan RF, Buijs WC, van Erning LJ, Lemmens JA, Corstens FH, Ruijs SH, van de Putte LB, van Riel PL 1993 Differential effects of glucocorticoids on cortical appendicular and cortical vertebral bone mineral content. Calcif Tissue Int 52:5–9.

100. Saito JK, Davis JW, Wasnich RD, Ross PD 1995 Users of low-dose glucocorticoids have increased bone loss rates: A longitudinal study. Calcif Tissue Int 57:115–119.

101. Adachi JD, Bensen WG, Hodsman AB 1993 Corticosteroid-induced osteoporosis. Semin Arthritis Rheum 22:375–384.

102. Heimann WG, Freiberger RH 1969 Avascular necrosis of the femoral and humeral heads after heigh-dosage corticosteroid therapy. N Engl J Med 263:672–674.

103. Hurel SJ, Kendall-Taylor P 1997 Avascular necrosis secondary to postoperative steroid therapy. Br J Neurosurg 11:356–358.

104. Rupp WM, McCarthy HB, Rohde TD, Blackshear PJ, Goldenberg FJ, Buchwald H 1982 Risk of osteoporosis in patients treated with long-term intravenous heparin therapy. Curr Surg 39:419–422.

105. Nelson-Piercy C 1998 Heparin-induced osteoporosis. Scand J Rheumatol Suppl 107:68–71.

106. Sackler JP, Liu L 1973 Heparin-induced osteoporosis. Br J Radiol 46:548–550.

107. Walenga JM, Bick RL 1998 Heparin-induced thrombocytopenia, paradoxical thromboembolism, and other side-effects of heparin therapy. Med Clin North Am 82:635–658.

108. Shaughnessy SG, Hirsh J, Bhandari M, Muir JM, Young E, Weitz JI 1999 A histomorphometric evaluation of heparin-induced bone loss after discontinuation of heparin treatment in rats. Blood 93:1231–1236.

109. Seeman E, Szmukler GI, Formica C, Tsalamandris C, Mestrovic R 1992 Osteoporosis in anorexia nervosa: The influence of peak bone density, bone loss, oral contraceptive use, and exercise. J Bone Miner Res 7:1467–1474.

110. Kohlmeyer L, Gasner C, Marcus R 1993 Bone mineral status of women with Marfan syndrome. Am J Med 95:568–572.

111. Smith R, Stevenson JC, Winearls CG, Woods CG, Wordsworth BP 1985 Osteoporosis of pregnancy. Lancet 1:1178–1180.

112. Hopper JL, Seeman E 1994 The bone density of twins discordant for tobacco use. N Engl J Med 330:387–392.

113. Diez A, Puig J, Serrano S, Marinoso M-L, Bosch J, Marrugat J 1994 Alcohol-induced bone disease in the absence of severe chronic liver damage. J Bone Miner Res 9:825–831.

114. Resnick D 1995 Hemoglobinopathies and other anemias. In: Resnick D (ed.) Diagnosis of Bone and Joint Disorders, 3rd ed., vol. 4. W.B. Saunders Company, Philadelphia, PA, USA, pp. 2107–2146.

115. Resnick D 1995 Plasma cell dyscrasias and dysgammaglobulinemias. In: Resnick D (ed.) Diagnosis of Bone and Joint Disorders, 3rd ed., vol. 4. W.B. Saunders Company, Philadelphia, PA, USA, pp. 2147–2189.

116. Stäbler A, Baur A, Bartl R, Munker R, Lamerz R, Reiser MF 1996 Contrast enhancement and quantitative signal analysis in MR imaging of multiple myeloma: Assessment of focal and diffuse growth patterns in marrow correlated with biopsies and survival rates. AJR Am J Roentgenol 167:1029–1036.

117. Moulopoulos LA, Dimopoulos MA 1997 Magnetic resonance imag-

ing of the bone marrow in hematologic malignancies. Blood **90:** 2127–2147.

118. Lecouvet F, Malghem J, Michaux L, Michaux J, Lehmann F, Maldague B, Jamart J, Ferrant A, Vande Berg B 1997 Vertebral compression fractures in multiple myeloma. Part II. Assessment of fracture risk with MR imaging of spinal bone marrow. Radiology **204:**201–205.

119. Lecouvet F, Van de Berg B, Maldague B, Michaux L, Laterre E, Michaux J, Ferrant A, Malghem J 1997 Vertebral compression fractures in multiple myeloma. Part I. Distribution and appearance at MR imaging. Radiology **204:**195–199.

120. Molpus WM, Pritchard RS, Walker CW, Fitzrandolph RL 1991 The radiographic spectrum of renal osteodystrophy. Am Fam Physician **43:**151–158.

121. Pitt MJ 1995 Rickets and osteomalacia. In: Resnick D (ed.) Diagnosis of Bone and Joint Disorders, 3rd ed., vol. 4. W.B. Saunders Company, Philadelphia, PA, USA, pp. 1885–1922.

122. Steinbach HL, Kolb FO, Gilfillan R 1954 A mechanism of the production of pseudofractures in osteomalacia (Milkman's syndrome). Radiology **62:**388–390.

123. Rosenberg AE 1991 The pathology of metabolic bone disease. Radiol Clin North Am **29:**19–35.

124. Smith R 1995 Idiopathic juvenile osteoporosis: Experience of twenty-one patients. Br J Rheumatol **34:**68–77.

125. Norman ME 1996 Juvenile osteoporosis. In: Favus MJ (ed.) Primer on the Metabolic Diseases and Disorders of Mineral Metabolism, 3rd ed. Lippincott-Raven, Philadelphia, PA, USA, pp. 275–278.

126. Minch CM, Kruse RW 1998 Osteogenesis imperfecta: A review of basic science and diagnosis. Orthopedics **21:**558–567.

127. Hanscom DA, Winter RB, Lutter L, Lonstein JE, Bloom BA, Bradford DS 1992 Osteogenesis imperfecta. Radiographic classification, natural history, and treatment of spinal deformities. J Bone Joint Surg Am **74:**598–616.

128. Zionts LE, Nash JP, Rude R, Ross T, Stott NS 1995 Bone mineral density in children with mild osteogenesis imperfecta. J Bone Joint Surg Br **77:**143–147.

129. Kiratli BJ 1996 Immobilization osteopenia. In: Marcus R, Feldman D, Kelsey J (eds.) Osteoporosis. Academic Press, San Diego, CA, USA, pp. 833–853.

130. Sudeck P 1901 Über die akute (reflectorische) Knochenatrophie nach entzündungen und Verletzungen an den Extremitäten und ihre klinischen Erscheinungen. Rofo Fortschr Geb Rontgenstr Neuen Bildgeb Verfahr **5:**277–307.

131. Oyen WJ, Arntz IE, Claessens RM, Van der Meer JW, Corstens FH, Goris RJ 1993 Reflex sympathetic dystrophy of the hand: An excessive inflammatory response? Pain **55:**151–157.

132. Sarangi PP, Ward AJ, Smith EJ, Staddon GE, Atkins RM 1993 Algodystrophy and osteoporosis after tibial fractures. J Bone Joint Surg Br **75:**450–452.

133. Gellman H, Keenan MA, Stone L, Hardy SE, Waters RL, Stewart C 1992 Reflex sympathetic dystrophy in brain-injured patients. Pain **51:**307–311.

134. Schwartzman RJ, McLellan TL 1987 Reflex sympathetic dystrophy: A review. Arch Neurol **44:**555–561.

135. Resnick D, Niwayama G 1995 Osteoporosis. In: Resnick D (ed.) Diagnosis of Bone and Joint Disorders, 3rd ed., vol. 4. W.B. Saunders Company, Philadelphia, PA, USA, pp. 1783–1853.

136. Todorovic Tirnanic M, Obradovic V, Han R, Goldner B, Stankovic D, Sekulic D, Lazic T, Djordjevic B 1995 Diagnostic approach to reflex sympathetic dystrophy after fracture: Radiography or bone scintigraphy? Eur J Nucl Med Mol Imaging **22:**1187–1193.

137. Leitha T, Staudenherz A, Korpan M, Fialka V 1996 Pattern recognition in five-phase bone scintigraphy: Diagnostic patterns of reflex sympathetic dystrophy in adults. Eur J Nucl Med Mol Imaging **23:**256–262.

138. Hayes CW, Conway WF, Daniel WW 1993 MR imaging of bone marrow edema pattern: Transient osteoporosis, transient bone marrow edema syndrome, or osteonecrosis. Radiographics **13:**1001–1011.

139. Boos S, Sigmund G, Huhle P, Nurbakhsch I 1993 Magnetresonanztomographie der sogenannten transitorischen Osteoporose. Primärdiagnostik und Verlaufskontrolle nach Therapie. Röfo Fortschr Geb Rontgenstr Neuen Bildgeb Verfahr **158:**201–206.

140. Trepman E, King TV 1992 Transient osteoporosis of the hip misdiagnosed as osteonecrosis on magnetic resonance imaging. Orthop Rev **21:**1089–1091,1094–1098.

141. Froberg PK, Braunstein EM, Buckwalter KA 1996 Osteonecrosis, transient osteoporosis, and transient bone marrow edema: Current concepts. Radiol Clin North Am **34:**273–291.

142. Guerra JJ, Steinberg ME 1995 Distinguishing transient osteoporosis from avascular necrosis of the hip. J Bone Joint Surg Am **77:**616–624.

143. Garton MJ, Robertson EM, Gilbert FJ, Gomersall L, Reid DM 1994 Can radiologists detect osteopenia on plain radiographs? Clin Radiol **49:**118–122.

144. Dent RV, Milne MD, Roussak NJ, Steiner G 1953 Abdominal topography in relation to senile osteoporosis of the spine. BMJ **2:**1082–1084.

145. Barnett E, Nordin BEC 1960 The radiological diagnosis of osteoporosis: A new approach. Clin Radiol **11:**166–174.

146. Urist MR 1960 Observations bearing on the problem of osteoporosis. In: Rodahl K, Nicholson JT, Brown EM Jr (eds.) Bone as a Tissue. McGraw-Hill, New York, NY, USA, pp. 18–45.

147. Kalla AA, Meyers OL, Parkyn ND, Kotze TJVW 1989 Osteoporosis screening - radiogrammetry revisited. Br J Rheumatol **28:**511–517.

148. Geusens P, Dequeker J, Verstraeten A, Nijs J 1986 Age-, sex-, and menopause-related changes of vertebral and peripheral bone: Population study using dual and single photon absorptiometry and radiogrammetry. J Nucl Med **27:**1540–1549.

149. Rosenthal DI, Gregg GA, Slovik DM, Neer RM 1987 A comparison of quantitative computed tomography to four techniques of upper extremity bone mass measurement. In: Genant HK (ed.) Osteoporosis Update 1987. Radiology Research and Education Foundation, San Francisco, CA, USA, pp. 87–93.

150. Meema HE 1991 Improved vertebral fracture threshold in postmenopausal osteoporosis by radiographic measurements: Its usefulness in selection for preventative therapy. J Bone Miner Res **6:**9–14.

151. Meema HE, Meema S 1987 Postmenopausal osteoporosis: Simple screening method for diagnosis before structural failure. Radiology **164:**405–410.

152. Jergas M, San Valentin R, Black D, Nevitt M, Palermo L, Genant HK, Cummings SR 1995 Radiogrametry of the metacarpals predicts future hip fractures. J Bone Miner Res **10:**S1;S371.

153. Jorgensen JT, Andersen PB, Rosholm A, Bjarnason NH 2000 Digital X-ray radiogrammetry: A new appendicular bone densitometric method with high precision. Clin Physiol Funct Imaging **20:**330–335.

154. Bouxsein ML, Palermo L, Yeung C, Black DM 2002 Digital X-ray radiogrammetry predicts hip, wrist and vertebral fracture risk in elderly women: A prospective analysis from the study of osteoporotic fractures. Osteoporos Int **13:**358–365.

155. Virtama P 1960 Uneven distribution of bone mineral and covering effect of non-mineralized tissue as reasons for impaired detectability of bone density from roentgenograms. Ann Med Int Fenn **49:**57–65.

156. Hodge HC, Bale WF, Warren SL, van Huysen G 1935 Factors influencing the quantitative measurement of the roentgen-ray absorption of tooth slabs. Am J Roentgenol **34:**817–838.

157. Stein I 1937 The evaluation of bone density in the roentgenogram by the use of an ivory wedge. Am J Roentgenol **37:**678–682.

158. Mack PB, O'Brian AT, Smith JM, Bauman AW 1939 A method for estimating degree of mineralization of bones from tracings of roentgenograms. Science **89:**467–469.

159. Ross P, Huang C, Davis J, Imose K, Yates J, Vogel J, Wasnich R 1995 Predicting vertebral deformity using bone densitometry at various skeletal sites and calcaneus ultrasound. Bone **16:**325–332.

160. Versluis RGJA, Petri H, Vismans FJFE, van de Ven CM, Springer MP, Papapoulos SE 2000 The relationship between phalangeal bone density and vertebral deformities. Calcif Tissue Int **66:**1–4.

161. Mussolino ME, Looker AC, Madans JH, Edelstein D, Walker RE, Lydick E, Epstein RS, Yates AJ 1997 Phalangeal bone density and hip fracture risk. Arch Intern Med **157:**433–438.

162. Mussolino ME, Looker AC, Madans JH, Langlois JA, Orwoll ES 1998 Risk factors for hip fracture in white men: The NHANES I epidemiologic follow-up study. J Bone Miner Res **13:**918–924.

163. Ekman A, Michaelsson K, Petren-Mallmin M, Ljunghall S, Mallmin H 2001 DXA of the hip and heel ultrasound but not densitometry of the fingers can discriminate female hip fracture patients from controls: A comparison between four different methods. Osteoporos Int **12:**185–191.

164. Krokowski E, Schlungbaum W 1959 Die Objektivierung der röntgenologischen Diagnose "Osteoporose". Fortschr Röntgenstr **91:** 740–746.

Chapter 30. Bone Biopsy and Histomorphometry in Clinical Practice

Robert R. Recker and M. Janet Barger-Lux

*Department of Medicine, Section of Endocrinology, Osteoporosis Research Center,
Creighton University Medical Center, Omaha, Nebraska*

INTRODUCTION

Histological examination of undecalcified transilial bone biopsy specimens has long been a valuable clinical and research tool for studying the etiology, pathogenesis, and treatment of metabolic bone diseases. In this chapter, we will:

- review briefly the underlying organization and function of bone cells;
- identify basic observations, measurements, and calculations;
- outline expected findings in a range of metabolic bone diseases;
- suggest clinical situations in which this examination can be useful; and
- describe techniques for obtaining, processing, and analyzing transilial biopsy specimens.

ORGANIZATION AND FUNCTION OF BONE CELLS

Intermediary Organization of the Skeleton

In what he termed the intermediary organization (IO) of the skeleton, Frost[1] described four discrete functions of bone cells: growth, modeling, remodeling, and fracture repair. Although each involves the same osteoclasts and osteoblasts, the coordinated outcomes differ greatly. *Growth* elongates the skeleton; *modeling* shapes it during growth; *remodeling* removes and replaces bone tissue; and *fracture repair* heals sites of structural failure.

The remodeling IO, which predominates during adult life, is the focus of this chapter. Coordinated groups of bone cells (i.e., osteoclasts, osteoblasts, osteocytes, and lining cells) comprise the basic multicellular units (BMUs) that carry out bone remodeling. Basic structural units (BSUs) are the packets of new bone that BMUs form.[2] All adult metabolic bone disease involves derangement of the remodeling IO.

Bone Cells

Osteoclasts, large-to-giant cells that are typically multinucleated, resorb bone (both its matrix, or osteoid, and mineral). They excavate shallow pits on the surface of cancellous bone, and they appear at the leading edge of tunnels ("cutting cones") in Haversian bone. Light microscopy discloses an irregular cell shape, foamy, acidophilic cytoplasm, a striated perimeter zone of attachment to the bone ("ruffled border"), and positive staining for TRACP.

Osteoblasts form new bone at sites of resorption. They produce the collagenous and noncollagenous constituents of bone matrix and participate in mineralization.[3] Under light microscopy, they appear as plump cells lined up at the surface of unmineralized osteoid. As the site matures, the cells lose their plump appearance.

Osteocytes, derived from osteoblasts, remain at the remodeling site. They reside individually in small lacunae within the mineralized bone matrix. Their cytoplasmic processes extend through a fine network of narrow canaliculi to form an interconnected network that extends throughout living bone. This network may monitor the local strain environment and/or initiate organized bone cell work in response to changes in strain.

Lining cells, also of osteoblast origin, cover cancellous and endocortical bone surfaces. By light microscopy, they appear as elongated, flattened, darkly-stained nuclei. The localization and initiation of remodeling probably involves these cells.

Bone Remodeling Process

Remodeling occurs on cancellous and haversian bone surfaces. The first step is activation of osteoclast precursors to form osteoclasts that then begin to excavate a cavity. After removal of about 0.05 mm^3 of bone tissue, the site remains quiescent for a short time. Then, activation of osteoblast precursors occurs at the site, and the excavation is refilled. The average length of time required to complete the remodeling cycle is approximately 6 months,[4] about 4 weeks for resorption and the rest for formation.

The healthy bone remodeling system accesses the required building materials within a favorable physiologic milieu to replace fully a packet of aged, microdamaged bone tissue with new, mechanically competent bone. However, overuse can overwhelm the capacity of the system to repair microdamage (the stress fractures that occur in military recruits are an example). The healthy bone remodeling system modifies bone architecture to meet changing mechanical needs. However, the system also promptly reduces the mass of underused bone (the bone loss of extended bedrest, paralysis, or space travel are examples). All bone loss occurs through bone remodeling. The bone remodeling system responds to nutritional and humoral as well as mechanical influences. Among the effects of vitamin D deficiency in adults, for example, is impaired mineralization of bone matrix. Finally, as other chapters describe, bone remodeling involves complex signaling processes between and within bone cells, and metabolic bone diseases of genetic origin involve defects at this level. Figures 1–3 present representative photomicrographs from human transilial biopsy specimens. An extensive atlas has also been published.[5]

Dr. Recker has received research funding from Merck, Novartis, Procter & Gamble, Roche, and Wyeth.

© 2003 American Society for Bone and Mineral Research

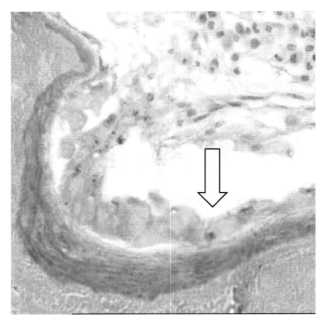

FIG. 1. A normal bone forming surface. Unmineralized osteoid is covered with plump osteoblasts, as identified by the arrow.

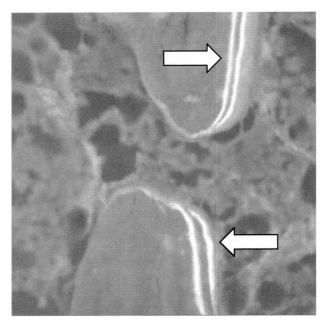

FIG. 3. The arrows identify two mineralizing surfaces with fluorescent double-labels.

BASIC OBSERVATIONS, MEASUREMENTS, AND CALCULATIONS

Bone biopsy specimens for histomorphometric examination are ordinarily obtained at the transilial site and shipped to specialized laboratories for processing and microscopic analysis. Later sections of this chapter outline these procedures. Of the dozens of measurements and calculations that have been devised, we provide here descriptions of several frequently used variables. Nomenclature is as approved by a committee of the American Society of Bone and Mineral Research.[6]

Static (Structural) Features

Core width (C.Wi) represents the thickness of the ilium (i.e., distance between periosteal surfaces, in mm) at the point of biopsy. *Cortical width* (Ct.Wi) is the combined thickness, in mm, of both cortices. *Cortical porosity* (Ct.Po) is the area of intracortical holes as percent of total cortical area.

Cancellous bone volume (BV/TV) is the percent of total marrow area (including trabeculae) occupied by cancellous bone. *Wall thickness* (W.Th) is the mean distance in μm between resting cancellous surfaces (i.e., surfaces without osteoid or Howship's lacunae) and corresponding cement lines.

Trabecular thickness (Tb.Th) is the mean distance across individual trabeculae, in μm, and *trabecular separation* (Tb.Sp) is the mean distance, also in μm, between trabeculae. *Trabecular number* (Tb.N) per mm is calculated as (BV/TV)/Tb.Th. These variables can be used to evaluate trabecular connectivity.[7] Other measures of trabecular connectivity include the ratio of nodes to free ends,[8] star volume,[9,10] and trabecular bone pattern factor (TBPf).[11]

Eroded surface (ES/BS) is the percent of cancellous surface occupied by Howship's lacunae, with and without osteoclasts. *Osteoblast surface* (Ob.S/BS) and *osteoclast surface* (Oc.S/BS) identify the percent of cancellous surface occupied by osteoblasts and osteoclasts, respectively. *Osteoid surface* (OS/BS) is the percent of cancellous surface with unmineralized osteoid, with and without osteoblasts. *Osteoid thickness* (O.Th) is the mean thickness, in μm, of the osteoid on cancellous surfaces.

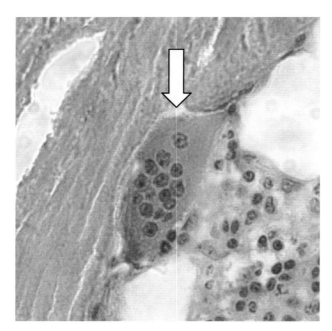

FIG. 2. A normal bone resorbing surface. The arrow locates a multinucleated osteoclast in a Howship's lacuna.

Dynamic (Kinetic) Features

A fluorochrome labeling agent, taken orally on a strict schedule before biopsy, deposits a fluorescent double-label at sites of active mineralization and allows rates of change to be determined.[12] *Mineralizing surface* (MS/BS) is the percent of cancellous surface that is mineralizing and thus labeled. The most accurate version of MS/BS includes surfaces with a double label plus one-half of those with a single label. Clear definition of MS/BS is crucial, because it is used to calculate bone formation rates, bone formation periods, and mineralization lag time.

Mineral appositional rate (MAR), is the rate (in μm/day) at which new bone mineral is being added to cancellous surfaces. MAR represents distance between labels at doubly labeled surfaces divided by the *marker interval* (span in days between the midpoints of each labeling period). This and all measurements of thickness must be corrected for obliquity (i.e., the randomness of the angle between the plane of the section and the plane of the cancellous surface) by use of a scaling factor.[13]

Activation frequency (Ac.f) is the probability that a new remodeling cycle will begin at any point on the cancellous bone surface. *Bone formation rates* (BFR/BV and BFR/BS) are estimates of cancellous bone volume (in $mm^3/mm^3/$year) and cancellous bone surface (in $mm^2/mm/$year), respectively, that are being replaced annually; BFR/BS = Ac.f $\times$ W.Th.[14] *Formation period* (FP) is the time in years required to complete a new cancellous BSU. *Mineralization lag time* (Mlt) is the interval in days between osteoid formation and mineralization. The most accurate version of Mlt is calculated as O.Th/MAR $\times$ MS/OS.

INTERPRETATION OF FINDINGS

Reference Data

In 1988, Recker et al.[4] published the results of a study to establish reference values for histomorphometric variables in postmenopausal white women. The 34 healthy subjects were evenly distributed into three age groups: 45–54, 55–64, and 65–74 years. They ranged broadly in age at menopause and in years past menopause at the time of biopsy. A comparative study of 12 blacks and 13 whites, aged 19–46 years, has also been published.[15]

In 2000, Glorieux et al.[16] reported histomorphometric data from 58 white subjects in each of five age groups: 1.5–6.9, 7.0–10.9, 11.0–13.9, 14.0–16.9, and 17.0–22.9 years. Biopsy specimens were obtained during corrective orthopedic surgeries, but the subjects had been ambulatory and otherwise healthy. The report includes within-subject coefficients of variation derived from analysis of adjacent duplicate biopsy specimens in eight subjects.

Replacement of Normal Marrow Elements

A variety of hematopoietic cells and a varying proportion of fat cells normally occupy the marrow space at the transilial biopsy site. If these normal marrow elements have been displaced by fibrous tissue (osteitis fibrosa), clumps of tumor cells, or sheets of abnormal hematopoietic cells, this change will be obvious to the histomorphometrist. The biopsy preparations described here preserve cellular detail, spatial relationships, and architectural features. However, this approach is unsuitable for hematologic diagnosis because of the time that histomorphometry laboratories require to generate a report (typically, at least 4 weeks).

Cortical Bone Deficit

Both the angle of the biopsy and site-to-site variation in cortical thickness at the biopsy site influence Ct.Wi. Nevertheless, low bone density at the lumbar spine and/or proximal femur is often reflected in low values for Ct.Wi.[17] Evidence of trabeculation of the cortex (i.e., formation of a *transitional zone* with characteristic coarse trabeculae), indicates that cortical bone, once present, has been lost.[18]

Cancellous Bone Deficit

Low BV/TV indicates a cancellous bone deficit. Generalized trabecular thinning (decreased Tb.Th) and/or complete loss of trabecular elements (poor trabecular connectivity) may contribute to this deficit. The latter finding (e.g., low Tb.N with high Tb.Sp) characterizes bone that is more fragile than its overall mass would suggest.

Altered Bone Turnover

Increased or decreased Ac.f indicates an alteration in the overall level of remodeling activity in cancellous bone.

Abnormal Osteoid Morphology

The characteristic arrangement of osteoid (collagen) fibers in lamellar and woven bone is readily apparent. Woven bone in transilial specimens is generally associated with either Paget's disease or renal osteodystrophy. It can also occur in osteitis fibrosa. In osteogenesis imperfecta, collagen abnormalities may be subtle enough to escape detection.

Accumulation of Unmineralized Osteoid

Parfitt has described the complex relationships between dynamic indices of bone formation and static indices of osteoid accumulation.[14] Increases in OS/BS, O.Th, and Mlt indicate failure of osteoid to mineralize normally. If mineralization is arrested completely, no double-label will be seen, and Mlt is unmeasurable.[19]

FINDINGS IN METABOLIC BONE DISEASE

In Table 1, we identify key histomorphometric findings that characterize representative types of metabolic bone disease. For details, we encourage the reader to consult disease-specific chapters in this volume and the current texts that we have cited.

TABLE 1. PATTERNS OF KEY HISTOMORPHOMETRIC FINDINGS THAT CHARACTERIZE SEVERAL TYPES OF METABOLIC BONE DISEASE

	Marrow spaces	Cortical bone	Cancellous bone	Bone turnover	Osteoid morphology	Osteoid mineralization
Postmenopausal osteoporosis		Cortical bone deficit with endocortical trabeculation	Cancellous bone deficit with poor trabecular connectivity	Unpredictable		
Glucocorticoid-induced osteoporosis		Cortical bone deficit	Cancellous bone deficit	Early, increased Ac.f; later, decreased Ac.f		
Primary hyperparathyroidism	Peritrabecular fibrosis may be seen	Cortical bone deficit, increased Ct.Po, endocortical trabeculation	Typically unremarkable		Woven bone may be seen	
Hypogonadism (males and females)		Cortical bone deficit	Cancellous bone deficit, sometimes with poor trabecular connectivity	Increased Ac.f		
Hypovitaminosis D osteopathy	Fibrous tissue may be seen			Early, increased Ac.f		Early, increased OS/BS; later, increased MLT and O.Th, double label may be absent
Hypophosphatemic osteopathy	Fibrous tissue may be seen					Increased MLT and O.Th; double label may be absent
Renal osteodystrophy (high turnover type)	Fibrous tissue may be seen	Endocortical trabeculation	Osteoblast, osteocyte, and trabecular abnormalities	Markedly increased remodeling activity	Woven bone may be seen	Increased OS/BS
Renal osteodystrophy (low turnover types)				Markedly decreased remodeling activity		Increased OS/BS (osteomalacic type); decreased OS/BS (adynamic type)
Renal osteodystrophy (mixed type)	Fibrous tissue may be seen		Variable BV/TV	Patchy remodeling activity	Irregular, woven bone and osteoid may be seen	Increased OS/BS and O.Th

Postmenopausal Osteoporosis

Osteoporosis in postmenopausal women is characterized by a cortical bone deficit with trabeculation of endocortical bone and a cancellous bone deficit with poor trabecular connectivity. Decreases in Tb.Th are modest; dynamic measures are unpredictable and often unremarkable.[20–21]

Glucocorticoid-Induced Osteoporosis

Early in treatment, Ac.f is increased; later, Ac.f, MAR, and MS/BS are all decreased. In femoral specimens from patients with glucocorticoid-induced osteonecrosis, abundant apoptotic osteocytes and lining cells have been reported.[22]

Primary Hyperparathyroidism

Primary hyperparathyroidism leads to a cortical bone deficit, with increased Ct.Po and trabeculation of endocortical bone.[23] Ct.Po correlates positively with fasting serum

PTH.[24] BV/TV is generally preserved, and normal cancellous bone architecture is maintained.[25,26] Osteoid with a woven appearance and peritrabecular fibrosis may also be seen.[27]

Hypogonadism

In both genders, hypogonadism increases Ac.f and leads to deficits of both cortical bone and trabecular bone. Loss of trabecular connectivity occurs at low levels of BV/TV and Tb.Th.[28]

Hypovitaminosis D Osteopathy

Vitamin D depletion of *any* etiology leads to hypovitaminosis D osteopathy (HVO). Parfitt describes three stages. In HVOi ("preosteomalacia"), Ac.f and OS/BS are increased, but O.Th is not. Accumulation of unmineralized osteoid characterizes both HVOii and HVOiii (osteomalacia), with Mlt and O.Th clearly increased (i.e., Mlt > 100 days and O.Th > 12.5 μm after correction for obliquity).[19] Some double-label can be seen in HVOii, but not in HVOiii. A cortical bone deficit also characterizes advanced HVO; secondary hyperparathyroidism is usual, and fibrous tissue in the marrow spaces is frequently seen.

Phenytoin seems to increase the vitamin D requirement, and it may have multiple effects on vitamin D metabolism.[19] Some patients on long-term phenytoin therapy develop a syndrome ("anticonvulsant osteomalacia") that includes low circulating 25-hydroxyvitamin D, a cortical bone deficit, and the histomorphometric findings of HVO.

Hypophosphatemic Osteopathy

Phosphate depletion of *any* etiology also leads to osteomalacia, with histomorphometric findings similar to those of advanced HVO.[19] These cases involve defects in renal tubular reabsorption of phosphate. Secondary hyperparathyroidism occurs variably. Transilial biopsy can be quite useful to assess the efficacy of treatment.

Gastrointestinal Bone Disease

Evidence of HVO has been reported in a variety of absorptive and digestive disorders.[29] However, these conditions also may promote deficiency of calcium and other nutrients. Malabsorption is not the only issue. For example, a calcium balance study of asymptomatic patients with celiac disease showed increased endogenous fecal calcium; the gut appeared to "weep" calcium into its lumen.[30] Bone histomorphometry may also reflect the results of treatment (i.e., corticosteroids or surgery). Parfitt describes a histomorphometric profile of low bone turnover, often with evidence of HVO and secondary hyperparathyroidism, that represents the result of multiple insults to bone health in these patients.[19]

Renal Osteodystrophy

At least three patterns of histomorphometric findings have been described among patients with end-stage renal disease (ESRD): high bone turnover with osteitis fibrosa ("hyperparathyroid bone disease"); low bone turnover (including "osteomalacic" and "adynamic" subtypes); and mixed osteodystrophy with high bone turnover, altered bone formation, and accumulation of unmineralized osteoid.[31–34]

At this time, transilial bone biopsy remains a useful "gold standard" on which to base decisions about treatment of bone disease in ESRD.[31] A dramatic example is the evaluation of bone pain and fractures in a chronic dialysis patient with hypercalcemia. If the biopsy shows high bone turnover and osteitis fibrosa, partial parathyroidectomy may be indicated. However, if the biopsy shows little turnover (little or no fluorochrome label), with or without extensive aluminum deposits, then parathyroidectomy is contraindicated, and treatment with a chelating agent may be indicated. The same biopsy can also help determine the extent of vitamin D deprivation and indicate the adequacy of vitamin D treatment.

OBTAINING THE SPECIMEN

In this section, we outline the procedures for obtaining bone biopsy specimens, processing them, and carrying out histomorphometric analysis. For greater detail, we recommend another recent publication.[35]

Fluorochrome Labeling

In clinical settings, tetracycline antibiotics are the only suitable fluorochrome labeling agents.[12] Demeclocycline (150 mg, four times daily) or tetracycline hydrochloride (250 mg, four times daily) are commonly used. The double-labeling process involves two dosing periods, and close adherence to the dosing schedule is crucial. A schedule of 3 days on, 14 days off, 3 days on, and 5 days off before biopsy (abbreviated as 3–14-3:5) produces good results, with a marker interval of 17 days.[36] Tetracyclines must be taken on an empty stomach; dairy products and calcium supplements, which interfere with tetracycline absorption, must be avoided for at least 1 h before and after each dose.

Biopsy Instrument

Specimens for histomorphometric examination require use of a trephine with inner diameter of no less than 7.5 mm. The Rochester Bone Biopsy Trephine (Medical Innovations International, Inc., Rochester, MN, USA) is a suitable instrument. The needle should be sharpened (and reconditioned, if necessary) after every three to five procedures.

Biopsy Procedure

In our institution, transilial bone biopsy is an outpatient minor surgery, with the usual procedures (e.g., the surgeon scrubs and uses a cap, mask, gown, and gloves, and the site is prepared and draped) and precautions (e.g., pulse oximetry and blood pressure monitoring). For the procedure, the patient should be off aspirin for at least 3 days and have nothing orally for 4 h. If a second biopsy is done, it should always be on the side opposite the first; there is thus a practical limit of two transilial biopsies per patient. The gowned patient lies in the supine position on the surgical table, and midazolam (2.5–5 mg) is given through a forearm intravenous catheter.

The biopsy site is about 2 cm posterior to the anterior-superior spine, which is about 2 cm inferior to the iliac crest. The skin and subcutaneous tissues on both sides of the ilium are infiltrated with local anesthetic. The periosteum is accessed by a 2-cm skin incision and blunt dissection. The trephine is inserted and advanced with steady, gentle pressure and a deliberate pace. The specimen—an intact, unfractured core with both cortices and the intervening cancellous bone—is transferred into a 20-ml screw-cap vial containing 70% ethanol.

The bony defect is then packed with Surgicel. After local pressure to facilitate hemostasis, the wound is closed with three to five stitches and covered by a pressure dressing. Follow-up care is specified clearly (i.e., dressing in place and absolutely dry for 48 h; then a daily shower is allowed; no bathing or strenuous physical activity until suture removal, 1 week after the procedure). The procedure produces localized aching for about 2 days and a small scar at the site.

Adverse Events

Patients typically describe feeling something "like a cramp" as the trephine advances, and the bone biopsy procedure described here rarely evokes pain. In the rare case in which the patient feels acute, sharp pain as the trephine passes through the marrow space, a small additional amount of intravenous midazolam can be given.

Although bleeding during the procedure is typically minimal, there is risk of bleeding in some situations (e.g., liver disease, hemodialysis, or medications that compromise hemostasis). Local bruising sometimes occurs, but hematoma is uncommon. In an early survey, physicians who were doing transilial biopsy specimens reported adverse events in 0.7% of 9131 biopsy specimens, that is, 22 with hematomas, 17 with pain for more than 7 days, 11 with transient neuropathy, 6 with wound infection, 2 with fracture, and 1 with osteomyelitis. No cases of death or permanent disability were reported.[37]

SPECIMEN PROCESSING AND ANALYSIS

Availability

Clinical pathology laboratories ordinarily do not handle undecalcified bone specimens or perform histomorphometry. However, processing and histomorphometric analysis of transilial bone biopsy specimens are available through several research laboratories that also handle clinical specimens. The specialized laboratory should be contacted before the procedure for explicit instructions on the fluorochrome labeling schedule, biopsy procedure, fixative, required patient information, shipping, etc. As noted earlier, most histomorphometry laboratories require, at minimum, 4 weeks to generate a report.

Specimen Handling and Processing

Proper fixation requires that the bone biopsy specimen remain in 70% ethanol for at least 48 h. This solution is suitable for shipping and long-term storage at room temperature. The specimen vials should be filled to capacity with 70% ethanol for shipping, handling, and storage.

Steps in laboratory processing include dehydrating, defatting, embedding, sectioning, mounting, de-plasticizing, staining, and microscopic examination.

The tissue block is sectioned parallel to the long axis of the biopsy core. Several sets of sections are obtained at 250- to 300-μm intervals, beginning 35–40% into the embedded specimen. Unstained sections 8–10 μm thick are used to examine osteoid morphology and to measure fluorochrome-labeled surfaces. Sections 5–7 μm thick stained with toluidine blue are used to measure wall thickness. Sections 5 μm thick with Goldner's stain[38] are used for other histomorphometric measurements.

Microscopy

The histomorphometric variables described earlier are derived from data gathered at the microscope. These data

include the width of both cortices and—in defined sectors of cancellous bone—volumes of bone, osteoid, and marrow; total trabecular perimeter; perimeters with features of formation (see Fig. 1) or resorption (see Fig. 2); thickness of osteoid and osteon walls; and interlabel width. Methods have been described for unbiased sampling of microscopic features.[39]

Our histomorphometry laboratory uses an interactive image analysis system (BIOQUANT True Color for Windows; Bioquant R&M Biometrics, Inc., Nashville, TN, USA). A digital camera mounted on the microscope presents the microscopic images on-screen, and measurements are made using a mouse. Fluorescent light at a wavelength of 350 nm is used to examine fluorochrome labels (see Fig. 3).

INDICATIONS FOR BONE BIOPSY AND HISTOMORPHOMETRY

The purpose of bone histomorphometry in the clinical setting is to gather information (i.e., to establish a diagnosis, clarify a prognosis, or evaluate adherence or response to treatment) on which to base informed clinical decisions. As is the case for every invasive procedure, the risk, discomfort, and expense should be proportionate to the importance of the information to be gained. Given these caveats, the number of clinical indications for this procedure is limited.

Clinicians can manage most metabolic bone diseases, including osteoporosis, without the aid of a bone biopsy. However, there are some situations in which bone biopsy after fluorochrome labeling is appropriate, as outlined in Table 2.

Bone biopsy specimens with histomorphometry have been crucial for assessing the mechanism of action, safety, and efficacy of new bone-active agents. Preclinical animal work includes serial biopsy specimens at multiple skeletal sites, using different colored fluorochrome labels (e.g., calcein or xylenol orange). Clinical trials of bisphosphonates have included subsets of patients who underwent biopsy for evaluation of bone remodeling rates and for assessment of mineralization.[40] Analysis of the biopsy specimens indicated that the bisphosphonate caused increased bone density largely by reducing the remodeling space. The data also settled two important safety concerns: whether the agent stopped remodeling completely (it did not) and whether it created a mineralization defect (it did not).

TABLE 2. SOME CLINICAL INDICATIONS FOR TRANSILIAL BONE BIOPSY*

1. When there is excessive skeletal fragility in unusual circumstances (e.g., the patient younger than age 50)
2. When a mineralizing defect is suspected (e.g., because of occult osteomalacia or treatment with anticonvulsant drugs)
3. To evaluate adherence to treatment in a malabsorption syndrome (e.g., sprue)
4. To characterize the bone lesion in renal osteodystrophy
5. To diagnose and assess response to treatment in vitamin D–resistant osteomalacia and similar disorders
6. When a rare metabolic bone disease is suspected

* Reprinted from Principles of Bone Biology, 2nd ed., Recker RR, Barger Lux MJ, Transilial bone biopsy, pp. 1625–1634, 2002, with permission from Elsevier.

Until safety and efficacy are assured, early testing of every new bone-active treatment should include bone biopsy in at least a subset of subjects. Some treatments can be predicted to fail based on the biopsy findings during treatment. An example would be continuous treatment with an agent that stops activation of remodeling and/or impairs bone formation significantly in those remodeling sites undergoing formation at the time the agent was introduced. Such an agent might harm the mechanical strength of the skeleton in the long term rather than improve it. This problem can be detected earlier by biopsy than with any other technology.

REFERENCES

1. Frost HM 1986 Intermediary Organization of the Skeleton. CRC Press, Boca Raton, FL, USA.
2. Frost HM 1973 Bone Remodeling and Its Relationship to Metabolic Bone Diseases. Charles C. Thomas, Springfield, IL, USA.
3. Marotti G, Favia A, Zallone AZ 1972 Quantitative analysis on the rate of secondary bone mineralization. Calcif Tissue Res 10:67–81.
4. Recker RR, Kimmel DB, Parfitt AM, Davies KM, Keshawarz N, Hinders S 1988 Static and tetracycline-based bone histomorphometric data from 34 normal postmenopausal females. J Bone Miner Res 3:133–144.
5. Malluche HH, Faugere MC (eds.) 1986 Atlas of Mineralized Bone Histology. Karger, New York, NY, USA.
6. Parfitt AM, Drezner MK, Glorieux FH, Kanis JA, Malluche H, Meunier PJ, Ott SM, Recker RR 1987 Bone histomorphometry: Standardization of nomenclature, symbols, and units. J Bone Miner Res 2:595–610.
7. Parfitt AM 1983 The physiologic and clinical significance of bone histomorphometric data. In: Recker RR (ed.) Bone Histomorphometry: Techniques and Interpretation. CRC Press, Boca Raton, FL, USA, pp. 143–224.
8. Garrahan NJ, Mellish RW, Compstom JE 1986 A new method for the two-dimensional analysis of bone structure in human iliac crest biopsies. J Microsc 142:341–349.
9. Vesterby A, Gundersen HJG, Melsen F 1989 Star volume of marrow space and trabeculae of the first lumbar vertebra: Sampling efficiency and biological variation. Bone 10:7–13.
10. Vesterby A, Gundersen HJG, Melsen F, Mosekilde L 1991 Marrow space star volume in the iliac crest decreases in osteoporotic patients after continuous treatment with fluoride, calcium, and vitamin D2 for five years. Bone 12:33–37.
11. Hahn M, Vogel M, Pompesius-Kempa M, Delling G 1992 Trabecular bone pattern factor: A new parameter for simple quantification of bone microarchitecture. Bone 13:327–330.
12. Frost HM 1969 Measurement of human bone formation by means of tetracycline labeling. Can J Biochem Physiol 41:331–342.
13. Schwartz MP, Recker RR 1981 Comparison of surface density and volume of human iliac trabecular bone measured directly and by applied stereology. Calcif Tissue Int 33:561–565.
14. Parfitt AM 2002 Physiologic and pathogenetic significance of bone histomorphometric data. In: Coe FL, Favus MJ (eds.) Disorders of Bone and Mineral Metabolism, 2nd ed. Lippincott Williams & Wilkins, Philadelphia, PA, USA, pp. 469–485.
15. Weinstein RS, Bell NH 1988 Diminished rates of bone formation in normal black adults. N Engl J Med 319:1698–1701.
16. Glorieux FH, Travers R, Taylor A, Bowen JR, Rauch F, Norman M, Parfitt AM 2000 Normative data for iliac bone histomorphometry in growing children. Bone 26:103–109.
17. Cosman F, Schnitzer MB, McCann PD, Parisien MV, Dempster DW, Lindsay R 1992 Relationships between quantitative histological measurements and noninvasive assessments of bone mass. Bone 13:237–242.
18. Keshawarz NM, Recker RR 1984 Expansion of the medullary cavity at the expense of cortex in postmenopausal osteoporosis. Metab Bone Dis Rel Res 5:223–228.
19. Parfitt AM 1998 Osteomalacia and related disorders. In: Avioli LV, Krane SM (eds.) Metabolic Bone Disease, 3rd ed. Academic Press, San Diego, CA, USA, pp. 327–386.
20. Kimmel DB, Recker RR, Gallagher JC, Ashok SV, Aloia JF 1990 A comparison of iliac bone histomorphometric data in post-menopausal osteoporotic and normal subjects. Bone Miner 11:217–235.
21. Recker RR, Barger-Lux MJ 2001 Bone remodeling findings in osteoporosis. In: Marcus R, Feldman D, Kelsey J (eds.) Osteoporosis, 2nd ed., vol. 2. Academic Press, San Diego, CA, USA, pp. 59–70.
22. Weinstein RS, Nicholas RW, Manolagas SC 2000 Apoptosis of osteocytes in glucocorticoid-induced osteonecrosis of the hip. J Clin Endocrinol Metab 85:2907–2912.
23. Eriksen EF 2002 Primary hyperparathyroidism: Lessons from bone histomorphometry. J Bone Miner Res 17:S2;N95–N97.
24. van Doorn L, Lips P, Netelenbos JC, Hackeng WH 1993 Bone histomorphometry and serum concentrations of intact parathyroid hormone (PTH 1–84) in patients with primary hyperparathyroidism. Bone Miner 23:233–242.
25. Parisien M, Mellish RW, Silverberg SJ, Shane E, Lindsay R, Bilezikian JP, Dempster DW 1992 Maintenance of cancellous bone connectivity in primary hyperparathyroidism: Trabecular strut analysis. J Bone Miner Res 7:913–919.
26. Uchiyama T, Tanizawa T, Ito A, Endo N, Takahashi HE 1999 Microstructure of the trabecula and cortex of iliac bone in primary hyperparathyroidism patients determined using histomorphometry and node-strut analysis. J Bone Miner Metab 17:283–288.
27. Monier-Faugere M-C, Langub MC, Malluche HH 1998 Bone biopsies: A modern approach. In: Avoli LV, Krane SM (eds.) Metabolic Bone Disease and Clinically Related Disorders, 3rd ed. Academic Press, San Diego, CA, USA, pp. 237–273.
28. Audran M, Chappard D, Legrand E, Libouban H, Baslé MF 2001 Bone microarchitecture and bone fragility in men: DXA and histomorphometry in humans and in the orchidectomized rat model. Calcif Tissue Int 69:214–217.
29. Arnala I, Kemppainen T, Kroger H, Janatuinen E, Alhava EM 2001 Bone histomorphometry in celiac disease. Ann Chir Gynaecol 90:100–104.
30. Ott SM, Tucci JR, Heaney RP, Marx SJ 1997 Hypocalciuria and abnormalities in mineral and skeletal homeostasis in patients with celiac sprue without intestinal symptoms. Endocrinol Metab 4:201–206.
31. Pecovnik Balon B, Bren A 2000 Bone histomorphometry is still the golden standard for diagnosing renal osteodystrophy. Clin Nephrol 54:463–469.
32. Parker CR, Blackwell PJ, Freemont AJ, Hosking DJ 2002 Biochemical measurements in the prediction of histologic subtype of renal transplant bone disease in women. Am J Kidney Dis 40:385–396.
33. Elder G 2002 Pathophysiology and recent advances in the management of renal osteodystrophy. J Bone Miner Res 17:2094–2105.
34. Malluche HH, Langub MC, Monier-Faugere MC 1997 Pathogenesis and histology of renal osteodystrophy. Osteoporos Int 7(Suppl 3):S184–S187.
35. Recker RR, Barger-Lux MJ 2002 Transilial bone biopsy. In: Bilezikian JP, Raisz LG, Rodan GA (eds.) Principles of Bone Biology, 2nd ed. Academic Press, San Diego, CA, USA, pp. 1625–1634.
36. Schwartz MP, Recker RR 1982 The label escape error: Determination of the active bone-forming surface in histologic sections of bone measured by tetracycline double labels. Metab Bone Dis Rel Res 4:237–241.
37. Rao DS, Matkovic V, Duncan H 1980 Transiliac bone biopsy: Complications and diagnostic value. Henry Ford Hosp Med J 28:112–118.
38. Goldner J 1938 A modification of the Masson trichrome technique for routine laboratory purposes. Am J Pathol 14:237–243.
39. Kimmel DB, Jee SS 1983 Measurements of area, perimeter, and distance: Details of data collection in bone histomorphometry. In: Recker RR (ed.) Bone Histomorphometry: Techniques and Interpretation. CRC Press, Boca Raton, FL, USA, pp. 80–108.
40. Chavassieux PM, Arlot ME, Reda C, Wei L, Yates AJ, Meunier PJ 1997 Histomorphometric assessment of the long-term effects of alendronate on bone quality and remodeling in patients with osteoporosis. J Clin Invest 100:1475–1480.

Chapter 31.   Molecular Diagnosis of Bone and Mineral Disorders

Robert F. Gagel and Gilbert J. Cote

Department of Endocrine Neoplasia and Hormonal Disorders, University of Texas M.D. Anderson Cancer Center, Houston, Texas

INTRODUCTION

Discoveries during the past 10–15 years have greatly expanded our understanding of how genetic abnormalities cause bone and mineral disorders. There are now specific genetic forms of both osteoporosis and osteosclerosis, at least four separate genetic causes of hypercalcemia, two genes that cause hypophosphatemia, and numerous examples of genetic forms of bone dysplasia. These observations have enriched our understanding of the hormonal and signal transduction pathways involved in bone formation, bone remodeling, and mineral homeostasis, and have provided new therapeutic targets for treatment of a variety of bone disorders.

Diagnostic use of this type of information has quickly made its way into the clinical practice of medicine. For example, within 3 years after the description of missense mutations in the *RET* proto-oncogene in multiple endocrine neoplasia, type 2 (MEN2), genetic testing for these mutations has replaced prior nongenetic approaches. In addition, mutational analysis of the *MEN1* gene (multiple endocrine neoplasia type 1), *RET* gene (MEN2), *HPRT2* gene (hyperparathyroidism-jaw tumor syndrome gene, which is involved in some examples of familial isolated hyperparathyroidism), and the *CASR* gene (calcium sensing receptor) can be important for evaluation of genetic hypercalcemia. This rapid acquisition of new information and its application to disease management underscore the importance of acquiring a fundamental knowledge of testing strategies and to understand the power and limitations of current approaches to genetic testing.

The single most important resource for up-to-date information related to specific genetic syndromes is provided by Online Mendelian Inheritance in Man (OMIM), available to all physicians without charge on the World Wide Web (www.ncbi.nlm.nih.gov/omim).[1] This concise but complete reference is an excellent starting point for genetic information relating to bone and mineral disorders and provides an intuitive, searchable textual database that is updated on a regular basis. For each genetic disorder, which is identified by a specific OMIM number, a detailed and well-referenced review discusses the mapping and identification of the causative gene, the spectrum of clinical presentation and management, molecular genetics, and whether animals models are available. Additional links often provide a clinical synopsis, whether genetically related disorders exist, and a detailed description of the gene involved including associated mutations. Other databases provide specific information on the availability of genetic testing and individual gene mutations. The most widely used resource for information about genetic testing is available at www.

genetests.org, a site that provides a searchable database of research and clinical sources for genetic testing, and a variety of educational materials.[2] Detailed information regarding the association of specific gene mutations with various disorders can be found at the Human Gene Mutation Database (www.hgmd.org).[3] This site provides mutation data on over 1300 genes and has direct links to several external websites including OMIM. In this chapter, our goal is to provide an overview of specific techniques used to identify mutations and to briefly discuss the advantages and disadvantages of each approach. A comprehensive list of genetic disorders of calcium and bone can be found elsewhere.

POLYMERASE CHAIN REACTION

A basic understanding of the principles underlying polymerase chain reaction (PCR) is vital to molecular genetic diagnosis. The DNA used in diagnostic studies is most commonly extracted from peripheral white blood cells and occasionally from other tissues. It is important, if possible, to obtain blood from an affected family member as well as the patient at risk. Occasionally, a DNA copy of mRNA from a specific tissue can be made by a technique called reverse transcription. Either genomic DNA or the copy of the mRNA is used as a template for PCR, a method for amplification of a selected portion of a specific DNA sequence.[4]

The specific portion of the gene of interest to be copied is targeted using small single-stranded DNA fragments that are complementary to and flank the DNA sequence of interest (oligonucleotide primers). The addition of nucleotides and a thermostabile DNA polymerase, an enzyme that synthesizes new DNA, followed by heating and cooling through 20–40 cycles, results in the formation of millions of copies of the targeted DNA (Fig. 1). Copies will be made of both parental alleles of the target DNA sequence (one derived from each parent). The sensitivity of the PCR reaction is so great that appropriate controls must be included in each amplification experiment to exclude the possibility of external DNA contamination. The amplified DNA serves as the starting material for almost all mutational analysis techniques.

GENERAL SCREENING TECHNIQUES TO DETECT MUTATIONS

There are many different strategies for identification of specific mutations. This summary will focus on four commonly used techniques and discuss the advantages and disadvantages of each (Fig. 2). Major factors for deciding which technique to use include the size of the DNA sequence to be examined, the spectrum of mutations that

---

The authors have no conflict of interest.

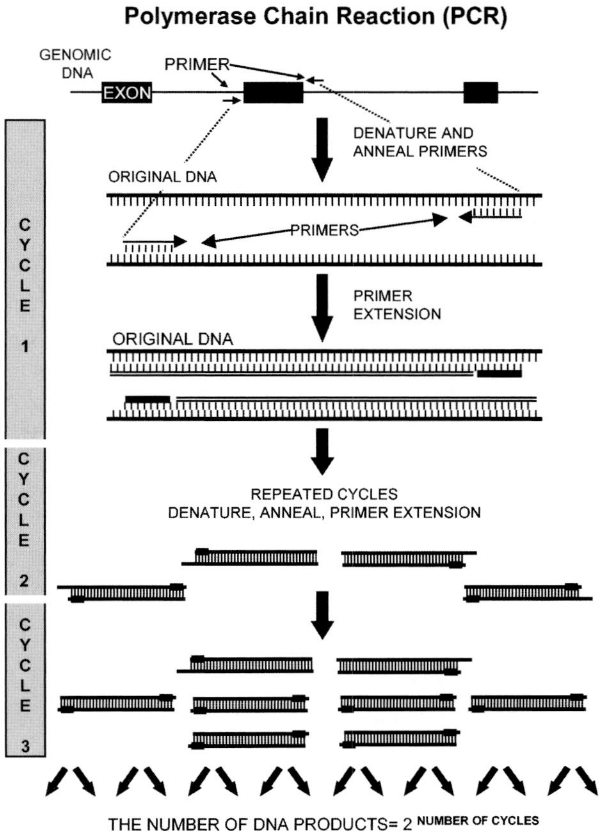

Polymerase Chain Reaction (PCR)

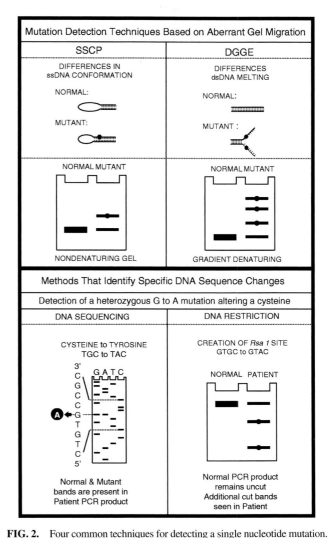

FIG. 1. PCR. DNA from the patient to be tested is denatured by heating. Oligonucleotides, which complement a small sequence flanking the targeted piece of DNA, are added to the mixture. The oligonucleotides hybridize to the target DNA and serve as a template for extension of the DNA strand by a thermostabile polymerase. The DNA is again denatured by heating, followed by a new cycle of DNA synthesis (cycle 2). In subsequent cycles, there is a logarithmic increase in the number of copies of the targeted DNA. After 20–40 cycles, most of the DNA copies are of a single size.

of DNA polymorphisms are also finding their way into mutation screening applications. Because the field is in a period of transition and the fact that for many genes com-

FIG. 2. Four common techniques for detecting a single nucleotide mutation. This figure schematically shows the results of four common methodologies used to detect a mutations. The top panels illustrate the methods of SSCP and DGGE, which detect mutations by differential migration of the normal and mutant DNA fragments in a gel. Within each panel, the fundamental mechanism or principle for each technique is diagrammed. A specific point mutation is denoted by a solid circle. In the bottom part of each panel, gel electrophoretic profiles of products derived from a normal and mutant DNA fragment analyzed by the respective technique is shown with mutant bands designated by a solid circle. SSCP separates single-stranded DNA molecules in a nondenaturing gel. The point mutation alters the mobility of the mutant band. DGGE identifies four bands—normal homoduplex, mutant homoduplex, and two additional bands that represent two variants of normal-mutant heteroduplexes. In the bottom panels, two additional methods are shown that identify specific DNA mutations. The example shown is a heterozygous G to A mutation that converts TGC (cysteine) to TAC (tyrosine). Direct manual DNA sequencing of the PCR product (bottom left panel) shows the presence of two bands at the mutated codon (G and A, respectively), indicating that one allele (PCR product) contains the normal sequence and the other the mutated sequence. The G to A substitution creates an *Rsa*I restriction site. Addition of this endonuclease to the reaction mixture that contains the normal PCR product identifies only a single electrophoretic band (bottom right panel). Addition of the same enzyme to a PCR product that contains one mutated allele results in the appearance of two new bands (bands designated by a solid circle) as well as the band derived from the normal allele.

cause the disease, access to newer equipment and technologies, whether clinical decisions will be based on the analysis, and cost. For example, mutations affecting the *collagen, type 1 α-1* gene in osteogenesis imperfecta may affect any of the greater than 50 exons in the gene, and a broad screening approach (such as single-strand conformational polymorphism, or denaturing gradient gel electrophoresis, discussed later) may provide the best approach to identify a mutation in a research setting. Identification of a potential sequence abnormality would lead to the use of a more focused approach (such as DNA sequencing, restriction endonuclease analysis).

Automation of PCR and DNA sequencing has rapidly lowered the cost of mutation analysis. This has led most commercial laboratories to adopt automated DNA sequencing as the technique of choice for detecting mutational abnormalities. Currently analysis of a single gene may cost in excess of $500; the field of genomic sequencing is rapidly evolving and there is serious discussion of utilization of techniques that could lower the cost of whole genome sequencing below $1000 during the next decade.[5] New methodologies developed to allow high throughput analysis mercial testing is unavailable, this chapter we will present a spectrum of techniques widely used in many research laboratories.

Many of the techniques for DNA analysis use gel electrophoresis. A sample containing the DNA molecules to be examined is applied to a gel (a thin layer of acrylamide or agarose), and an electrical current is applied to move the molecules along the long axis of the gel. Small differences in charge, size, or conformational state of an individual molecule can affect the mobility of the molecule (Fig. 2), making it possible to separate two pieces of DNA with a single nucleotide difference. Newer methodologies now use capillary electrophoresis or high-performance liquid chromatography (HPLC) to separate DNA fragments, or rely on fluorescence-based imaging, such as DNA melting curve analysis, to define mutations. The descriptions below focus only on gel-based methods that are still used in many research laboratories; more detailed discussion these and other protocols can be found elsewhere.[6,7]

Single-Strand Conformational Polymorphism

This technique relies on the theory that a denatured DNA molecule (one in which the two complementary strands of DNA that form the double helix are separated) forms a unique single-stranded three-dimensional structure.[6-8] The major determinants of this structure are the specific DNA sequence and internal base pairing. A single nucleotide change may result in a conformation that differs from that of the normal sequence. In many genetic disorders, an affected individual will inherit one normal and one mutated copy of a gene, which can be detected by differences in DNA mobility on nondenaturing polyacrylamide gels (Fig. 2). This technique is particularly useful for analysis of large stretches of DNA sequence when the specific mutation is not known, such as the mutations described for osteogenesis imperfecta. Manual DNA sequence analysis of such a large gene would be prohibitively expensive and time consuming; automated DNA sequencing is certainly more time effective, and access to equipment has become less of a problem with the commercialization of DNA sequencing, leaving cost the only issue. Like DNA sequencing, single-strand conformational polymorphism (SSCP) can also be automated through the incorporation of fluorescent labels, although there are no major advantages gained relative to manual approaches. A disadvantage of SSCP is that it does not identify the specific mutation and generally cannot distinguish between mutations and nucleotide polymorphisms (a change in the DNA sequence that does not alter the coding sequence of a protein). This technique cannot detect a mutation in which two copies of the mutated DNA (one from each parent) are inherited unless an external control from another patient is included in the analysis. More focused techniques, discussed later, are used to determine the nature of the DNA abnormality.

Denaturing Gradient Gel Electrophoresis

Like SSCP, this technique identifies mutations based on differences in DNA migration patterns.[6,7,9] In this method, double-stranded DNA produced by PCR is applied to a gradient gel containing urea and formamide, which results in gradient-dependent denaturation (separation of the double helix into single strands) as gel electrophoresis proceeds. Separation of the DNA strands is responsible for altering the DNA mobility. DNA denaturation is sequence dependent. Therefore, a single nucleotide change will frequently generate a specific denaturation pattern. This effect is enhanced by the addition of "GC-clamps" or stretches of GCs to a single end of the PCR product to stimulate unidirectional DNA denaturation. This is a more complex technique, requiring a period of development for optimal results. Because of these difficulties, the technique has largely been replaced by fluorescence-based examination of DNA melting profiles or denaturing HPLC in laboratories that have access to specialized equipment. Overall, denaturation methods are more sensitive than SSCP, more easily detect a single base differences, and in some cases create a mutation-specific pattern.

SPECIFIC TECHNIQUES FOR DETECTION OF DNA SEQUENCE ABNORMALITIES

Direct DNA Sequencing

Direct DNA sequencing of PCR products is the most sensitive and specific method for detection of specific mutations.[6,7,10] Direct DNA sequencing of a PCR product derived from genomic DNA permits analysis of both alleles or copies of the gene and the identification of new or unreported mutations. The disadvantages include its complexity and the difficulty of analyzing more than 200 nucleotides in a single manual sequencing reaction. Automation of DNA sequencing makes it possible to rapidly analyze larger components of the genome by incorporating newer techniques for separation of sequencing fragments, the use of overlapping PCR primers, fluorescent labels to detect product, and the use of computers to assemble a final sequence and to detect sequence variants. In a disease such as MEN2, in which more than 90% of known mutations are clustered in a small region of the *RET* proto-oncogene, this approach offers the ability to detect most mutations in a single sequencing run.[10,11]

Restriction Endonuclease Analysis

This technique provides a simple and effective method for detecting the presence or absence of mutations at a single site and is useful when a mutation creates or destroys a restriction site (defined as a sequence variation that is identified by a bacterial enzyme that cleaves the specific sequence). For example, a single nucleotide change in the sequence GTGC to GTAC would create a new restriction site for the endonuclease *Rsa*I. A PCR amplification product from a patient who inherited this mutation from a single parent would contain one normal DNA sequence and one containing the single nucleotide mutation. Addition of the restriction enzyme *Rsa*I to a PCR product from this patient would result in cleavage of the allele containing the mutant sequence into two fragments, whereas the allele containing the normal sequence would remain intact. Separation of these fragments by gel electrophoresis (Fig. 2) would show one uncut fragment representing the normal sequence and two smaller fragments representing the cleaved mutant allele. Mutations that destroy an existing restriction site provide an additional analytic challenge because it is necessary to document that the enzyme is active before concluding that the failure to cleave the DNA fragment into two pieces is caused by a mutation. To establish the activity of the enzyme, a positive control (a piece of DNA that contains the normal restriction site) is included with each analysis. This technique is used most effectively when a single DNA sequence abnormality causes all examples of the disease or in a family whose specific mutation is known.

SOURCES OF ERROR IN GENETIC TESTING

It is important that clinicians be aware of the frequency and nature of genetic testing errors.[7,11] Sample mix-up, especially in the setting of family screening where many family members share a common last name, may occur in up to 5% of analyses. These errors may occur at the time of blood drawing or during subsequent analysis or recording. A second potential source of error is contamination by DNA from individuals who harbor a disease-causing mutation. The funneling of large numbers of samples to a few laboratories for analysis of a single disease further increases the chance of contamination. The extreme sensitivity of PCR analysis makes it possible that a positive result could occur as a result of airborne contamination of a reaction tube. A third source of error is the failure to amplify both alleles, thereby resulting in the possibility of a false-negative result because only the normal allele is included in the analysis. The most common explanation for amplification failure is a random polymorphism (DNA sequence change) acting to reduce oligonucleotide primer hybridization during the PCR reaction. Other causes for amplification failure include genetic defects involving insertion, deletion, or rearrangement of DNA sequence at the site of amplification.

If genetic testing is to be used as the sole determinant for decision making in disease management, it is important for the clinician to be aware of the possibility of error and to take steps to minimize the impact on patient care. One simple approach that will eliminate the majority of these errors is to repeat each analysis, whether positive or negative, in a different laboratory on an independently obtained sample. This approach will eliminate most sample mix-up, DNA contamination, and technical errors. Sending the sample to a separate laboratory that uses a different primer set for PCR amplification will also reduce the likelihood of a single allele amplification error.

INTEGRATION OF GENETIC INFORMATION INTO CLINICAL MANAGEMENT

Genetic testing has several important clinical uses. Identification of a specific disease-causing mutation may clarify and simplify patient management. For example, the identification of a mutation of the calcium sensing receptor causative for familial hypercalcemic hypocalciuria in an individual with an atypical clinical presentation may prevent unnecessary parathyroid surgery. For other disorders, such as multiple endocrine neoplasia type 2, the identification of a specific mutation may lead to a specific action (thyroidectomy) in a child.[9,11]

In other situations, the benefits of genetic screening may be more ambiguous. The identification of a mutation in an individual with a severe and fatal form of osteogenesis imperfecta may not alter therapy for the patient; however, detection of the mutation may make prenatal genetic screening possible. Identification and categorization of these mutations are also important because gene therapy strategies, especially for single gene defects, are evolving rapidly. The discovery that mutation of a single gene can be associated with multiple disease phenotypes has also led to a rethinking of how skeletal disorders should be classified. Three major classifications have emerged based primarily either on biochemical evidence, radiographic evidence, or genetic evidence.[12,13] Each classification group serves as a unique entry point in facilitating patient diagnosis and treatment. Included in the Appendix of this Primer is a table providing an extensive listing of serum mineral and skeletal disorders and their specific genetic defects. Information in this table was primarily obtained by a keyword search of the OMIM website (discussed above). We have grouped the disorders according to serum mineral findings and followed this list with disorders grouped according to a recent International Nosology and Classification of Constitutive Disorders of Bone consensus, which is a combination of morphological findings and molecular defect.[12] A classification of many of these disorders based on gene structure and function involved is also available.[13]

An evolving area of genetic research implicates subtle DNA differences in the pathogenesis of disease.[14] For example, genetic studies examining polymorphism have identified several candidate genes that may be involved in osteoporosis, including the vitamin D receptor, the estrogen receptor, and the *collagen type I A1* gene, among others. Although the role of these polymorphisms is currently controversial, there are examples in other systems that clearly point to population-based genetic differences that may influence disease expression. The techniques for identification of these polymorphisms can use any of the methods described in Fig. 2, but automated approaches including new chip-based technologies are increasingly being used. Further characterization and clarification of the roles that these genetic polymorphisms play in disease genesis may permit us to identify high-risk populations for application of preventive strategies.

REFERENCES

1. Online Mendelian Inheritance in Man, OMIM (TM), McKusick-Nathans Institute for Genetic Medicine, Johns Hopkins University (Baltimore, MD) and National Center for Biotechnology Information, National Library of Medicine (Bethesda, MD). Available online at http://www.ncbi.nlm.nih.gov/omim/. Accessed on May 1, 2003.
2. GeneTests: Medical Genetics Information Resource. Available online at http://www.genetests.org. Accessed on May 1, 2003.
3. Krawczak M, Cooper DN 1997 The human gene mutation database. Trends Genet **13:**121–122.
4. Saiki RK, Gelfand DH, Stoffel S, Scharf SJ, Higuchi R, Horn GT, Mullis KB, Erlich HA 1988 Primer-directed enzymatic amplification of DNA with a thermostable DNA polymerase. Science **239:**487–491.
5. Pennisi E 2002 Gene researchers hunt bargains, fixer-uppers. Science **290:**735–736.

6. Myers RM, Ellenson LH, Hayashi K 1998 Detection of DNA varia-tion. In: Birren B, Green ED, Klapholz S, Myers RM, Roskams J (eds.) Genome Analysis: A Laboratory Manual, vol. 2, Detecting Genes. Cold Spring Harbor Press, New York, NY, USA, pp. 287–384.

7. Hoff AO, Cote GJ, Gagel RF 2002 Laboratory evaluation and screen-ing of genetic endocrine diseases. In: Martini L. (ed.) Modern Endo-crinology. Lippincott Williams & Wilkins, Philadelphia, PA, USA, pp. 189–220.

8. Ainsworth PJ, Surh LC, Coulter-Mackie MB 1991 Diagnostic single-strand conformational polymorphism (SSCP): A simplified non-radioisotopic method as applied to a Tay-Sachs B1 variant. Nucleic Acids Res **19:**405–406.

9. Fodde R, Losekoot M 1994 Mutation detection by denaturing gradient gel electrophoresis (DGGE). Hum Mutat **3:**83–94.

10. Khorana S, Gagel RF, Cote GJ 1994 Direct sequencing of PCR products in agarose gel slices. Nucleic Acids Res **22:**3425–3426.

11. Gagel RF, Cote GJ 2002 The role of the *RET* Proto-oncogene in multiple endocrine neoplasia Type 2. In: Bilezikian JP, Raisz LG, Rodan GA (eds.) Principles of Bone Biology, 2nd ed. Academic Press, San Diego, CA, USA, pp. 1067–1078.

12. Hall CM 2002 International nosology and classification of constitu-tional disorders of bone. Am J Med Genet **113:**65–77.

13. Superti-Furga A, Bonafe L, Rimoin DL 2001 Molecular-pathogenetic classification of genetic disorders of the skeleton. Am J Med Genet **106:**282–293.

14. Ralston SH 2002 Genetic control of susceptibility to osteoporosis. J Clin Endocrinol Metab **87:**2460–2466.

Chapter 32.   Hypercalcemia: Clinical Manifestations, Pathogenesis, Diagnosis, and Management

Meryl S. LeBoff and Katharine H. Mikulec

Department of Medicine, Division of Endocrinology, Diabetes, and Hypertension, Brigham and Women's Hospital, Harvard Medical School, Boston, Massachusetts

INTRODUCTION

Calcium plays a vital role in skeletal health, neuromuscular function, cardiac contractility, hormone secretion, blood coagulation, and other physiologic processes. Serum calcium is normally maintained at a constant level through the complex interactions of two hormones, parathyroid hormone (PTH) and vitamin D, and their target organs, the skeleton, intestines, and kidneys. Normally there is an inverse sigmoidal relationship between the serum calcium concentration and PTH release. A rise in extracellular calcium suppresses PTH release, which in turn decreases the conversion of 25-hydroxyvitamin D to 1,25-dihyroxyvitamin D in the kidneys; the net effect is a reduction in calcium resorption from bone and decreased calcium absorption from the gastrointestinal tract and kidneys. Hypercalcemia results from an alteration in these homeostatic mechanisms that leads to increased influx of calcium from the skeleton, enhanced intestinal calcium absorption, and/or reduced renal calcium clearance.

The human body contains about 1–2 kg of calcium. Ninety-nine percent of the total body calcium is in the mineral phase of bone, and the remaining 1% is distributed in the extracellular and intracellular fluids. Approximately 45% of the total calcium in the blood is bound to serum proteins, predominantly albumin, and about 10% of the calcium in blood is complexed with bicarbonate and other anions, including phosphate and citrate. The remaining 45% is the biologically active calcium ion.[1–3]

Hypoalbuminemia does not affect the ionized calcium concentration, but it does decrease the total calcium concentration. Therefore, it is necessary to correct the total calcium concentration when there are variations in serum albumin concentrations. The corrected serum calcium (CSCa) is calculated by adding 0.8 mg/dl to the total serum calcium concentration for every 1.0 g/dl by which the serum albumin concentration is <4.0 g/dl. When the serum albumin concentration is elevated, as can be seen with dehydration, it is necessary to subtract 0.8 mg/dl from the total calcium measurement for every 1.0 g/dl by which the serum albumin concentration in >4.0 g/dl.

The binding of calcium to proteins is pH dependent. Alkalosis increases protein binding, producing a decreased ionized calcium concentration. Conversely, acidosis reduces protein binding, thereby leading to a higher ionized calcium concentration. Acid-base balance does not affect the total calcium concentration. It is useful to directly measure the ionized calcium concentration for patients with marked alterations in the serum albumin concentration or acid-base balance.

CLINICAL MANIFESTATIONS

Hypercalcemia is associated with a variety of symptoms relating to the central nervous system (CNS), gastrointestinal and genitourinary tracts, and musculoskeletal and cardiovascular systems (see Table 1).[4] Patients with chronic, mild hypercalcemia, which is often caused by primary hyperparathyroidism, may not volunteer symptoms. Some may indicate that they "did not realize how poorly they felt" until after their hypercalcemia was treated. Others may experience vague neuropsychiatric changes, including difficulty with concentration, personality changes, and depression. Acute, severe hypercalcemia can present with lethargy that may progress to stupor and coma. While some patients may be lucid with a CSCa concentration of 15 mg/dl, others may be symptomatic with a CSCa concentration of 12 mg/dl. The rate of the rise in serum calcium, as well as the presence of underlying conditions (e.g., azotemia or CNS disease), may influence the severity of the CNS symptoms.

Gastrointestinal symptoms often associated with hypercalcemia include nausea, anorexia, and vomiting. Weight loss and constipation are less common. Patients with hyperparathyroid-

TABLE 1. COMMON CLINICAL PRESENTATIONS

Lethargy, stupor, coma
Personality change or psychosis
Nausea, anorexia, constipation
Peptic ulcer disease, pancreatitis
Polyuria, nephrolithiasis, nephrocalcinosis
Hypertension
Bradycardia, short QT interval, AV block
Bone pain, pathologic fractures
Muscle weakness, arthralgias

The authors have no conflict of interest.

ism have an increased risk of peptic ulcer disease. Rarely, pancreatitis may develop in severe hypercalcemia.

Hypercalcemia decreases the ability of the kidneys to concentrate urine. Polyuria, polydypsia, nocturia, and nephrogenic diabetes insipidus may develop. Anorexia in conjunction with reduced renal concentrating capacity leads to prerenal azotemia and worsening hypercalcemia; this cycle is reversed, in part, with hydration. PTH enhances renal tubular reabsorption of calcium, but despite elevated circulating levels of PTH, hypercalciuria can occur in hyperparathyroidism. In hypercalcemia caused by malignancy, granulomatous disease, and vitamin D intoxication, suppressed PTH levels contribute to the development of hypercalciuria. Nephrolithiasis may develop with sustained hypercalciuria and occurs in up to 20% of patients with hyperparathyroidism. Another complication of hypercalcemia is nephrocalcinosis, which results from the deposition of calcium salts in the corticomedullary or medullary segments of the kidney and is associated with loss of renal function.

Patients with hypercalcemia can also present with a number of musculoskeletal symptoms. Muscle weakness is a frequent symptom. Bone pain and pathological fractures may develop in patients with malignancies. Patients with hyperparathyroidism may present with arthralgias and occasionally elevated uric acid levels and gout. A rare skeletal complication of hyperparathyroidism is osteitis fibrosa cystica, which is characterized by subperiosteal resorption of the phalanges, resorption of the distal clavicle, bone cysts, and in severe disease, marrow fibrosis and anemia.

Last, cardiovascular effects of hypercalcemia include hypertension, electrocardiogram changes with shortening of the QT interval, AV blocks, bradycardia, arrhythmias, and enhanced sensitivity to digitalis.

PATHOGENESIS

In approximately 90% of patients with hypercalcemia, an elevated calcium level is most often the result of hyperparathyroidism or malignancy; longstanding hypercalcemia (>6 months) can often be documented in the former, and a clinically evident malignancy is often demonstrable in the latter.[5] In primary hyperparathyroidism, inappropriate hypersecretion of PTH and hypercalcemia are the consequence of a reduced sensitivity of the parathyroid glands to calcium (with an elevated "set-point" for calcium) and an increased parathyroid cell mass. The biochemical features of hyperparathyroidism include hypercalcemia, a low or low-normal phosphate concentration, and in some instances, hypercalciuria. Because calcium is now included on routine chemistry panels, mild disease is detected in many patients.

Familial hypocalciuric hypercalcemia (FHH) is a disorder also characterized by hypercalcemia and hypophosphatemia, but the distinguishing feature is relative hypocalciuria. FHH is caused by mutations in the calcium sensing receptor.[6] FHH is transmitted by autosomal dominant inheritance with 100% penetrance, and therefore, affected individuals may be detected at a young age. Hyperparathyroidism and FHH are discussed in detail in subsequent chapters.

Hypercalcemia of malignancy (HCM) may be associated with osteolytic metastases, humoral factors (e.g., PTH-related peptide [PTHrP], cytokines, or growth factors), or increased synthesis of vitamin D.[7-10] Tumors that produce humoral factors include squamous cell tumors of the lung, head, and neck, esophagus, and breast, renal cell, bladder, and ovarian carcinomas. PTHrP mimics many of the effects of PTH causing hypercalcemia, phosphaturia, cyclic adenosine monophosphate (cAMP) generation, and increased 1,25-dihydroxyvitamin D synthesis.[11] Ectopic production of PTH by tumor cells is extremely rare.[12,13] While PTHrP is a larger peptide than PTH, it is homologous to PTH in eight or nine of the first 13 amino acids of the amino terminus. PTHrP is expressed in many normal tissues and in fetal development. Because PTHrP levels are typically low in normal subjects, an elevation of PTHrP levels and a suppressed PTH concentration help establish the diagnosis of humoral HCM. HCM may also occur in 20–40% of patients with multiple myeloma. Tumors that produce skeletal metastases (e.g., multiple myeloma, other hematologic malignancies, and breast carcinoma) release cytokines and factors that stimulate osteoclast-mediated bone resorption (e.g., osteoclast stimulating factor, lymphotoxin, RANK ligand, TNF, transforming growth factor-α [TGF-α], interleukin (IL)-1, and IL-6).[14-16] Occasionally patients with T- and B-cell lymphomas develop hypercalcemia; here, hypercalcemia is caused by increased generation of 1,25-dihydroxyvitamin D by the neoplastic lymphoid tissue, which leads to an absorptive hypercalcemia.[17,18]

Infectious (e.g., tuberculosis, leprosy, candidiasis, histoplasmosis, coccidioidomycosis, cryptococcosis, and AIDS) and noninfectious granulomatous diseases (e.g., sarcoidosis, eosinophilic granulomas, Wegener's granulomatosis, newborn subcutaneous fat necrosis, and silicone-induced granulomatous disease) cause hypercalcemia caused by increased 1,25-dihydroxyvitamin D levels and intestinal hyperabsorption of calcium. Hypercalcemia and hypercalciuria are well-known complications of sarcoidosis, occurring in 10% and 50% of patients, respectively.[19] In sarcoidosis, there is a well-characterized extrarenal conversion of 25-hydroxyvitamin to 1,25-dihydroxyvitamin D; vitamin D intake or sun exposure can lead to hypercalcemia in these patients.[20,21]

A variety of medications can cause hypercalcemia. Vitamin D intoxication results in enhanced gastrointestinal calcium absorption and increased renal calcium excretion. The inherent suppression of PTH levels in disorders with increased 1,25-dihydroxyvitamin D and 25-hydroxyvitamin D levels may contribute to the hypercalciuria. When taken with an absorbable alkali, excessive calcium consumption can lead to milk-alkali syndrome, which is characterized by hypercalcemia, metabolic alkalosis, hypercalciuria, and renal impairment. Vitamin A can interact with the vitamin D receptor, and excess vitamin A leads to increased bone resorption, hypercalcemia, periosteal calcifications, and increased risk of hip fracture.[22,23] Thyroid hormone can increase bone turnover; triiodothyronine stimulates osteoclastic bone resorption, and thyroid hormone receptors are present on osteoblasts.[24,25] Lithium therapy acutely leads to an elevation in calcium levels and chronically to an increased set-point for PTH and parathyroid gland mass.[26,27] In renal failure, hypercalcemia may be caused by tertiary hyperparathyroidism (i.e., autonomous parathyroid

TABLE 2. CAUSES OF HYPERCALCEMIA

Hyperparathyroidism
    Adenoma
    Hyperplasia
    Carcinoma
    Tertiary hyperparathyroidism
Familial hypocalciuric hypercalcemia
Other endocrine causes
    Hyperthyroidism
    Adrenal insufficiency
    Pheochromocytoma
    VIPoma
Malignant diseases
    Osteolytic metastases
    PTHrP and other humoral factors
    Increased production of 1,25-dihydroxyvitamin D
Medications
    Thiazides
    Lithium
    Vitamin D intoxication
    Aminophylline
    Vitamin A
    Milk-alkali syndrome
    Tamoxifen (antiestrogens)
    Growth hormone
    Total parenteral nutrition
    Thyroid hormone
Granulomatous diseases: infectious
    Tuberculosis or leprosy
    Coccidiomycosis or histoplasmosis
    Cryptococcus
    Cytomegalovirus
    HIV
Granulomatous disease—noninfections
    Sarcoidosis
    Silicone
    Eosinophilic granuloma
    Wegener's granulomatosis
Miscellaneous
    Rhabdomyolysis recovery phase
    Aluminum
    William's syndrome
    Immobilization
    Renal failure (acute and chronic)

function) or aluminum bone disease, where bone is aplastic and PTH secretion is suppressed. Other causes of hypercalcemia are listed in Table 2 and detailed in subsequent chapters.

DIAGNOSIS

A careful history and physical examination are the first steps in determining the cause of hypercalcemia and will often point to a diagnosis of HCM or primary hyperparathyroidism. Simultaneous measurements of serum calcium concentration and PTH are usually the next step in the diagnostic work-up for hypercalcemia. Other useful tests include measurement of PTHrP concentration, vitamin D metabolites, and urinary calcium excretion. An elevated PTH in the setting of hypercalcemia is usually caused by primary hyperparathyroidism. FHH may also present with this biochemical picture but can be identified by a low urinary calcium excretion. If the PTH level is appropriately suppressed, further testing is necessary to establish the cause of non–PTH-mediated hypercalcemia. If malignancy or granulomatous disease is suspected, PTHrP and/or 1,25-dihydroxyvitamin D levels are diagnostically useful. In the setting of vitamin D intoxication, PTH levels are suppressed and 25-hydroxyvitamin D levels are elevated. Establishing the correct diagnosis is an essential step in the treatment of hypercalcemia.

MANAGEMENT

The management of hypercalcemia consists of diagnosing and treating the underlying pathophysiologic mechanism and decreasing the serum calcium concentration by expanding the intravascular volume, increasing urinary calcium excretion, and inhibiting bone resorption. While severe hypercalcemia can be life threatening and require immediate treatment, mild hypercalcemia is usually asymptomatic, and attention is focused on treating the underlying etiology. Patients with mild hypercalcemia (CSCa < 12 mg/dl) should be encouraged to increase their fluid intake, follow a moderate calcium diet, and if applicable, discontinue thiazide diuretics or other medications that can lead to hypercalcemia. Moderate hypercalcemia (CSCa = 12–14 mg/dl) often requires direct measures to lower the calcium concentration, especially if symptoms of hypercalcemia are present. Severe hypercalcemia (CSCa > 14 mg/dl) requires immediate treatment. However, the most common cause of severe hypercalcemia is malignancy, and the prognosis may be poor; treatment decisions must be in accordance with the patient's wishes.

Because hypercalcemia leads to dehydration, the first step in treatment is volume expansion with intravenous saline. Patients with hypercalcemia often need up to 4–6 liters of intravenous fluids during the first 24 h.[28,29] However, the rate of fluid replacement depends on the degree of dehydration and underlying comorbidities (e.g., congestive heart failure, renal insufficiency, and cirrhosis). In severe cases, careful use of loop diuretics (i.e., furosemide, bumetanide, torsemide, or ethacrynic acid) may be considered to further increase urinary calcium excretion and prevent volume overload. Loop diuretics inhibit reabsorption of sodium in the thick ascending limb and thereby inhibit passive reabsorption of calcium. (Note that thiazide diuretics increase calcium reabsorption and can exacerbate hypercalcemia, particularly in primary hyperparathyroidism; thus they must be avoided.) Loop diuretics are not necessary in most cases and should not be initiated until volume status has been restored. Volume status and electrolytes (i.e., Na, K, Mg, and Phos) need to be monitored closely. While diuresis helps increase calcium excretion, the effect tends to be modest, decreasing the calcium concentration by 1–3 mg/dl.[30] Treatments directed at inhibiting bone resorption are usually necessary to normalize serum calcium concentrations.

Inhibiting bone reabsorption with a bisphosphonate is the cornerstone of treatment. Zoledronic acid, pamidronate, and etidronate are Food and Drug Administration (FDA) approved for the treatment of HCM in adults. Bisphosphonates are poorly absorbed from the gastrointestinal tract and

Table 3. Treatments for Hypercalcemia

	Mechanism of action	Onset of action	Calcium response
Saline	Rehydration ↑ Renal calcium excretion	Hours	↓ by 1–3 mg/dl
Calcitonin	↑ Renal calcium excretion ↓ Bone resorption	Hours	↓ by 1–2 mg/dl
Etidronate	↓ Bone resorption	1–3 days	Normalizes in ≥ 60% of patients
Pamidronate	↓ Bone resorption	1–3 days	Normalizes in ≥ 70% of patients
Zoledronic acid	↓ Bone resorption	1–3 days	Normalizes in ≅ 90% of patients

thus must be given intravenously for the treatment of hypercalcemia. Etidronate, 7.5 mg/kg/day for 3–7 consecutive days, has been shown to be safe and effective treatment for HCM.[31,32] However, it has been supplanted by pamidronate and zoledronic acid, newer bisphosphonates that are more effective and cause less renal toxicity.[33–35] Pamidronate (60–90 mg) normalizes serum calcium in 70–100% of patients with HCM.[36–40] Because the calcium concentration nadir is usually seen by day 6, the dose should not be repeated until day 6 or 7. Pamidronate is generally given as a 2- to 4-h infusion and is well tolerated. Fever can occur, but it is generally mild and transient. Serum creatinine elevation has been noted in 2–3% of patients with HCM treated with pamidronate.[33,38] However, pamidronate has been used for patients with renal insufficiency (serum creatinine concentrations, 1.5–6.4 mg/dl) and for patients with end-stage renal disease on dialysis without ill effects.[41,42]

Zoledronic acid is the most potent bisphosphonate currently available and has been shown to be superior to pamidronate in the treatment of HCM.[38] In a pooled analysis of two randomized, controlled clinical trials, zoledronic acid (4 mg) normalized serum calcium concentrations in 88.4% of subjects within 10 days and pamidronate (90 mg) normalized calcium concentrations in 69.7% of subjects. The median duration of complete response was 32 days for zoledronic acid (4 mg) and 18 days for pamidronate (90 mg). Overall, adverse events were similar between zoledronic acid and pamidronate. Fever was the most common adverse event, occurring in 44.2% of subjects in the zoledronic acid (4 mg) group and 33.0% of subjects in the pamidronate (90 mg) group. Hypophosphatemia is also common but tends to be mild. Subjects with a creatinine concentration ≥4.5 mg/dl were excluded from this trial. In the zoledronic acid (4 mg) group, two (2.3%) of the subjects with HCM experienced grade 3 creatinine changes, and no subjects experienced grade 4 changes.[38] To help minimize renal injury, the infusion time has been increased from 5 minutes to 15–20 minutes, and patients should be well hydrated before infusion. If a complete response is not achieved with zoledronic acid, it is advisable to wait at least 7 days before repeating treatment.

Calcitonin has a modest, yet rapid effect on lowering serum calcium concentration in approximately 60–70% of patients with hypercalcemia. It increases urinary calcium excretion and inhibits bone resorption and can lower CSCa by 1–2 mg/dl within 2–6 h. Unfortunately, continuous exposure leads to downregulation of calcitonin receptors on osteoclasts, and most patients who initially respond to calcitonin develop tachyphylaxis with 2–3 days. It is contro-

versial whether corticosteroids prolong the response of calcitonin.[43] Salmon calcitonin is FDA approved for the treatment of hypercalcemia at an initial dose of 4 IU/kg subcutaneously or intramuscularly. If effective, it may be repeated (4–8 IU/kg every 6–12 h).

Gallium nitrate and plicamycin (Mithramycin; Fujisawa, Deerfield, IL, USA) inhibit bone resorption and have been used in the treatment of hypercalcemia. Gallium nitrate is FDA approved for the treatment of HCM and is given as a 5-day continuous infusion.[44] However, it can be nephrotoxic and has not been widely used. Plicamycin can cause hepatic toxicity, nephrotoxicity, and thrombocytopenia and is not widely available.

Corticosteroids may be useful in lowering calcium concentrations in patients with vitamin D intoxication, granulomatous disease (e.g., sarcoidosis and tuberculosis), and hematologic malignancies. Corticosteroids decrease calcitriol production and may inhibit growth of neoplastic lymphoid tissue. Intravenous hydrocortisone 100–300 mg daily (or oral prednisone 40–60 mg daily) for 3–7 days is the usual dose.[29,43] Ketoconazole, chloroquine, and hydroxychloroquine may also decrease calcitriol concentrations in patients with granulomatous disease.

Dialysis can be considered for patients with renal failure or others who cannot tolerate or do not respond to other measures. A low-calcium or calcium-free dialysate is used.[45]

Intravenous phosphate chelates calcium and decreases serum calcium within minutes. However, this therapy can be toxic because calcium-phosphate complexes may deposit in tissues and cause organ damage. This treatment is rarely necessary and should be reserved for patients with severe hypercalcemia and hypophosphatemia in whom other therapies have failed.[43] Oral phosphate may be useful in treating mild hypercalcemia caused by primary hyperparathyroidism. Oral phosphate can cause diarrhea and is generally not very effective. Serum phosphate should be maintained below 4 mg/dl.

Reduction of the dietary calcium intake is an important therapeutic intervention in disorders involving increased gastrointestinal absorption as in vitamin D intoxication, milk-alkali syndrome, and granulomatous disease. However, it is not necessary to restrict calcium intake in most patients with HCM. Patients with HCM tend to have low calcitriol concentrations and impaired calcium absorption.

An additional consideration is that bed rest can exacerbate hypercalcemia. Therefore, patients with hypercalcemia ought to be encouraged to ambulate if appropriate.

In the future, calcimimetic drugs may prove to be an effective option in the treatment of hypercalcemia, particularly for patients with primary hyperparathyroidism. Calci-mimetics act on calcium-sensing receptors and mimic the effects of extracellular calcium. These agents inhibit secretion of PTH, thereby decreasing serum calcium concentrations.[46,47]

Table 3 summarizes the treatments for hypercalcemia. Severe hypercalcemia can be life threatening and usually warrants immediate treatment. The mainstay of therapy includes intravenous fluids and intravenous bisphosphonate therapy (i.e., zoledronic acid or pamidronate). Calcitonin may be useful in combination with a bisphosphonate in the early stages of treatment to promote a faster response. Other treatments, including furosemide, dialysis, and corticosteroids, may be useful in certain cases. Efforts must be directed at identifying and treating the underlying etiology if possible.

REFERENCES

1. Aurbach GD, Marx SJ, Spiegel AM 1980 Parathyroid hormone, calcitonin, and the calciferols. In: Wilson JD, Foster DW (eds.) Williams Textbook of Endocrinology. W. B. Saunders Company, Philadelphia, PA, USA, pp. 1137–1217.
2. Heaney RP 1976 Calcium kinetics in plasma: As they apply to the measurements of bone formation and resorption rates. In: Bourne GH (ed.) Biochemistry and Physiology of Bone Calcification and Physiology. Academic Press, New York, NY, USA, pp. 105–133.
3. Tofaletti J 1982 Physiological importance of calcium complexes. In: Anghiler LJ, Tuffet-Anghileri AM (eds.) Role of Calcium in Biological Systems. CRC Press Inc., Boca Raton, FL, USA, pp. 69–78.
4. LeBoff M, Brown E 1986 Clinical disorders of calcium metabolism. In: Hare J (ed.) Signs and Symptoms in Endocrine and Metabolic Disorders. J. B. Lippincott Company, Philadelphia, PA, USA, pp. 224–238.
5. Harinck HI, Bijvoet OL, Plantingh AS, Body JJ, Elte JW, Sleeboom HP, Wildiers J, Neijt JP 1987 Role of bone and kidney in tumor-induced hypercalcemia and its treatment with bisphosphonate and sodium chloride. Am J Med 82:1133–1142.
6. Brown EM, Pollak M, Seidman CE, Seidman JG, Chou YH, Riccardi D, Hebert SC 1995 Calcium-ion-sensing cell-surface receptors. N Engl J Med 333:234–240.
7. Stewart AF, Horst R, Deftos LJ, Cadman EC, Lang R, Broadus AE 1980 Biochemical evaluation of patients with cancer-associated hypercalcemia: Evidence for humoral and nonhumoral groups. N Engl J Med 303:1377–1383.
8. Rosol TJ, Capen CC 1992 Mechanisms of cancer-induced hypercalcemia. Lab Invest 67:680–702.
9. Deftos LJ 2002 Hypercalcemia in malignant and inflammatory diseases. Endocrinol Metab 31:141–158.
10. Mundy GR 1996 Role of cytokines, parathyroid hormone, and growth factors in malignancy. In: Bilezikian J, Raisz L, Rodan G (eds.) Principles of Bone Biology. Academic Press, San Diego, CA, USA.
11. Kremer R, Sebag M, Champigny C, Meerovitch K, Hendy GN, White J, Goltzman D 1996 Identification and characterization of 1,25-dihydroxyvitamin D3-responsive repressor sequences in the rat parathyroid hormone-related peptide gene. J Biol Chem 271:16310–16316.
12. Iguchi H, Miyagi C, Tomita K, Kawauchi S, Nozuka Y, Tsuneyoshi M, Wakasugi H 1998 Hypercalcemia caused by ectopic production of parathyroid hormone in a patient with papillary adenocarcinoma of the thyroid gland. J Clin Endocrinol Metab 83:2653–2657.
13. Nussbaum SR, Gaz RD, Arnold A 1990 Hypercalcemia and ectopic secretion of parathyroid hormone by an ovarian carcinoma with rearrangement of the gene for parathyroid hormone. N Engl J Med 323:1324–1328.
14. Nagai Y, Yamato H, Akaogi K, Hirose K, Ueyama Y, Ikeda K, Matsumoto T, Fujita T, Ogata E 1998 Role of interleukin-6 in uncoupling of bone in vivo in a human squamous carcinoma coproducing parathyroid hormone-related peptide and interleukin-6. J Bone Miner Res 13:664–672.
15. Mundy GR, Martin TJ 1982 The hypercalcemia of malignancy: Pathogenesis and management. Metabolism 31:1247–1277.
16. Mundy GR, Raisz LG, Cooper RA, Schechter GP, Salmon SE 1974 Evidence for the secretion of an osteoclast stimulating factor in myeloma. N Engl J Med 291:1041–1046.
17. Seymour JF, Gagel RF 1993 Calcitriol: The major humoral mediator of hypercalcemia in Hodgkin's disease and non-Hodgkin's lymphomas. Blood 82:1383–1394.
18. Breslau NA, McGuire JL, Zerwekh JE, Frenkel EP, Pak CY 1984 Hypercalcemia associated with increased serum calcitriol levels in three patients with lymphoma. Ann Intern Med 100:1–6.
19. Studdy PR, Bird R, Neville E, James DG 1980 Biochemical findings in sarcoidosis. J Clin Pathol 33:528–533.
20. Adams JS, Fernandez M, Gacad MA, Gill PS, Endres DB, Rasheed S, Singer FR 1989 Vitamin D metabolite-mediated hypercalcemia and hypercalciuria patients with AIDS and non-AIDS associated lymphoma. Blood 73:235–239.
21. Adams JS, Singer FR, Gacad MA, Sharma OP, Hayes MJ, Vouros P, Holick MF 1985 Isolation and structural identification of 1,25-dihydroxyvitamin D3 produced by cultured alveolar macrophages in sarcoidosis. J Clin Endocrinol Metab 60:960–966.
22. Katz CM, Tzagournis M 1972 Chronic adult hypervitaminosis A with hypercalcemia. Metabolism 21:1171–1176.
23. Feskanich D, Singh V, Willett WC, Colditz GA 2002 Vitamin A intake and hip fractures among postmenopausal women. JAMA 287:47–54.
24. Burman KD, Monchik JM, Earll JM, Wartofsky L 1976 Ionized and total serum calcium and parathyroid hormone in hyperthyroidism. Ann Intern Med 84:668–671.
25. Milne M, Kang MI, Cardona G, Quail JM, Braverman LE, Chin WW, Baran DT 1999 Expression of multiple thyroid hormone receptor isoforms in rat femoral and vertebral bone and in bone marrow osteogenic cultures. J Cell Biochem 74:684–693.
26. Seely EW, Moore TJ, LeBoff MS, Brown EM 1989 A single dose of lithium carbonate acutely elevates intact parathyroid hormone levels in humans. Acta Endocrinol (Copenh) 121:174–176.
27. Mallette LE, Khouri K, Zengotita H, Hollis BW, Malini S 1989 Lithium treatment increases intact and midregion parathyroid hormone and parathyroid volume. J Clin Endocrinol Metab 68:654–660.
28. Hosking DJ, Cowley A, Bucknall CA 1981 Rehydration in the treatment of severe hypercalcemia. Q J Med 50:473–481.
29. Nussbaum SR 1993 Pathophysiology and management of severe hypercalcemia. Endocrinol Metab Clin North Am 22:343–362.
30. Suki WN, Yium JJ, Von Minden M, Saller-Hebert C, Eknoyan G, Martinez-Maldonado M 1970 Acute treatment of hypercalcemia with furosemide. N Engl J Med 283:836–840.
31. Singer FR, Ritch PS, Lad TE, Ringenberg QS, Schiller JH, Recker RR, Ryzen E 1991 Treatment of hypercalcemia of malignancy with intravenous etidronate. A controlled, multicenter study. The Hypercalcemia Study Group. Arch Intern Med 151:471–476.
32. Jacobs TP, Gordon AC, Silverberg SJ, Shane E, Reich L, Clemens TL, Gundberg CM 1987 Neoplastic hypercalcemia: Physiologic response to intravenous etidronate disodium. Am J Med 82:42–50.
33. Zojer N, Keck AV, Pecherstorfer M 1999 Comparative tolerability of drug therapies for hypercalcaemia of malignancy. Drug Saf 21:389–406.
34. Wellington K, Goa KL 2003 Zoledronic acid: A review of its use in the management of bone metastases and hypercalcaemia of malignancy. Drugs 63:417–437.
35. Berenson JR 2002 Treatment of hypercalcemia of malignancy with bisphosphonates. Semin Oncol 29(6 Suppl 2):12–18.
36. Gucalp R, Theriault R, Gill I, Madajewicz S, Chapman R, Navari R, Ahmann F, Zelenakas K, Heffernan M, Knight RD 1994 Treatment of cancer-associated hypercalcemia. Double-blind comparison of rapid and slow intravenous infusion regimens of pamidronate disodium and saline alone. Arch Intern Med 154:1935–1944.
37. Gucalp R, Ritch P, Wiernik PH, Gucalp R, Ritch P, Wiernik PH, Sarma PR, Keller A, Richman SP, Tauer K, Neidhart J, Mallette LE, Siegel R 1992 Comparative study of pamidronate disodium and etidronate disodium in the treatment of cancer-related hypercalcemia. J Clin Oncol 10:134–142.
38. Major P, Lortholary A, Hon J, Abdi E, Mills G, Menssen HD, Yunus F, Bell R, Body J, Quebe-Fehling E, Seaman J 2001 Zoledronic acid is superior to pamidronate in the treatment of hypercalcemia of malignancy: A pooled analysis of two randomized, controlled clinical trials. J Clin Oncol 19:558–567.
39. Nussbaum SR, Younger J, Vandepol CJ, Gagel RF, Zubler MA, Chapman R, Henderson IC, Mallette LE 1993 Single-dose intravenous therapy with pamidronate for the treatment of hypercalcemia of malignancy: Comparison of 30-, 60-, and 90-mg dosages. Am J Med 95:297–304.

40. Morton AR, Cantrill JA, Craig AE, Howell A, Davies M, Anderson DC 1988 Single dose versus daily intravenous aminohydroxypropylidene biphosphonate (APD) for the hypercalcaemia of malignancy. BMJ 296:811–814.

41. Machado CE, Flombaum CD 1996 Safety of pamidronate in patients with renal failure and hypercalcemia. Clin Nephrol 45:175–179.

42. Davenport A, Goel S, Mackenzie JC 1993 Treatment of hypercalcaemia with pamidronate in patients with end stage renal failure. Scand J Urol Nephrol 27:447–451.

43. Bilezikian JP 1992 Management of acute hypercalcemia. N Engl J Med 326:1196–1203.

44. Warrell RP Jr, Israel R, Frisone M, Snyder T, Gaynor JJ, Bockman RS 1988 Gallium nitrate for acute treatment of cancer-related hypercalcemia. A randomized, double-blind comparison to calcitonin. Ann Intern Med 5:669–674.

45. Koo WS, Jeon DS, Ahn SJ, Kim YS, Yoon YS, Bang BK 1996 Calcium-free hemodialysis for the management of hypercalcemia. Nephron 72:424–428.

46. Silverberg SJ, Bone HG III, Marriott TB, Locker FG, Thys-Jacobs S, Dziem G, Kaatz S, Sanguinetti EL, Bilezikian JP 1997 Short-term inhibition of parathyroid hormone secretion by a calcium-receptor agonist in patients with primary hyperparathyroidism. N Engl J Med 337:1506–1510.

47. Marx SJ 2000 Hyperparathyroid and hypoparathyroid disorders. N Engl J Med 343:1863–1875.

Chapter 33.   Primary Hyperparathyroidism

John P. Bilezikian[1,2] and Shonni J. Silverberg[1]

[1]Department of Medicine and [2]Department of Pharmacology, College of Physicians and Surgeons, Columbia University, New York, New York

INTRODUCTION

Primary hyperparathyroidism is one of the two most common causes of hypercalcemia and thus ranks high as a key diagnostic possibility in anyone with an elevated serum calcium concentration. The other common cause of hypercalcemia is malignant disease. These two causes, primary hyperparathyroidism and hypercalcemia of malignancy, account for over 90% of all patients with hypercalcemia. A much longer, complete list of potential causes of hypercalcemia is considered after the first two are ruled out, or if there is reason to believe that a different cause is likely. The differential diagnosis of hypercalcemia as well as features of hypercalcemia of malignancy are considered elsewhere in this primer. In this chapter, the clinical presentation, evaluation, and therapy of primary hyperparathyroidism are covered.

Primary hyperparathyroidism is a relatively common endocrine disease with an incidence as high as 1 in 500 to 1 in 1000.[1] Among the endocrine diseases, perhaps only diabetes mellitus and hyperthyroidism are seen more frequently. The high visibility of primary hyperparathyroidism in the population today marks a dramatic change from several generations ago, when it was considered to be a rare disorder. A 4- to 5-fold increase in incidence was noted in the early 1970s, because of the widespread use of the autoanalyzer, which provided serum calcium determinations in patients being evaluated for a set of completely unrelated complaints.[2] Recent data have suggested a decline in the incidence of primary hyperparathyroidism.[3] This may be a local phenomenon, or it may reflect a diminution of the "catch-up effect," because most cases of previously unrecognized asymptomatic disease have now been diagnosed. Primary hyperparathyroidism occurs at all ages but is most frequent in the sixth decade of life. Women are affected more often than men by a ratio of 3:1. The majority of individuals are postmenopausal women. When found in children, an unusual event, it might be a component of one of several endocrinopathies with a genetic basis, such as multiple endocrine neoplasia type I or II.

Primary hyperparathyroidism is a hypercalcemic state resulting from excessive secretion of parathyroid hormone (PTH) from one or more parathyroid glands. The disease is caused by a benign, solitary adenoma 80% of the time. A parathyroid adenoma is a collection of chief cells surrounded by a rim of normal tissue at the outer perimeter of the gland. In the patient with a parathyroid adenoma, the remaining three parathyroid glands are normal. Less commonly, primary hyperparathyroidism is caused by a pathological process characterized by hyperplasia of all four parathyroid glands. Four-gland parathyroid hyperplasia is seen in approximately 15% of patients with primary hyperparathyroidism. It may occur sporadically or in association with multiple endocrine neoplasia type I or II. A very rare presentation of primary hyperparathyroidism is parathyroid carcinoma, occurring in fewer than 0.5% of patients with hyperparathyroidism.[4] Pathological examination of the malignant tissue might show mitoses, vascular or capsular invasion, and fibrous trabeculae, but it is often not definitive. Unless gross local or distant metastases are present, the diagnosis of parathyroid cancer can be exceedingly difficult to make.

The pathophysiology of primary hyperparathyroidism relates to the loss of normal feedback control of PTH by extracellular calcium. Under virtually all other hypercalcemic conditions, the parathyroid gland is suppressed and PTH levels are low. Why the parathyroid cell loses its normal sensitivity to calcium is unknown, but in adenomas, this seems to be the major mechanism. In primary hyperparathyroidism caused by hyperplasia of the parathyroid glands, the "set point" for calcium is not changed for a given parathyroid cell: it is the increase in the number of cells that gives rise to the hypercalcemia.

The underlying cause of primary hyperparathyroidism is not known. External neck irradiation in childhood, recog-

The authors have no conflict of interest.

nized in some patients, is unlikely to be causative in the majority of patients. The molecular basis for primary hyperparathyroidism continues to be elusive.[5–10] The clonal origin of most parathyroid adenomas suggests a defect at the level of the gene controlling growth of the parathyroid cell or the expression of PTH. Patients with primary hyperparathyroidism have been discovered in whom the *PTH* gene is rearranged to a site adjacent to the *PRAD*-1 oncogene. This kind of gene rearrangement could be responsible for the altered growth properties of the abnormal parathyroid cell. Overexpression of cyclin D1, an important cell cycle regulator, is felt to have a role in the pathogenesis of some sporadic parathyroid adenomas. Loss of one copy of the *MEN1 tumor suppressor* gene located on chromosome 11 has also been seen in sporadic parathyroid adenomas. Abnormalities in the *p53 tumor suppressor* gene have not been described in primary hyperparathyroidism. Among other genes studied for a possible role in the development of sporadic parathyroid adenomas are the *calcium-sensing receptor* gene, the *vitamin D receptor* gene and *RET*. To date, such studies have not been revealing.

SIGNS AND SYMPTOMS

Classical primary hyperparathyroidism is associated with skeletal and renal complications. The skeletal disease, known historically as *osteitis fibrosa cystica*, is characterized by subperiosteal resorption of the distal phalanges, tapering of the distal clavicles, a "salt and pepper" appearance of the skull, bone cysts, and brown tumors of the long bones. Overt hyperparathyroid bone disease is now seen in less than 5% of patients in the United States with primary hyperparathyroidism.[11]

Like the skeleton, the kidney is also much less commonly involved in primary hyperparathyroidism than before. The incidence of kidney stones has declined from approximately 33% in the 1960s to 20% now. Nephrolithiasis, nevertheless, is still the most common complication of the hyperparathyroid process.[12] Other renal features of primary hyperparathyroidism include diffuse deposition of calcium-phosphate complexes in the parenchyma (nephrocalcinosis). Hypercalciuria (daily calcium excretion of >250 mg for women or >300 mg for men) is seen in up to 30% of patients. In the absence of any other cause, primary hyperparathyroidism may be associated with a reduction in creatinine clearance.

The classic neuromuscular syndrome of primary hyperparathyroidism included a definable myopathy that has virtually disappeared.[13] In its place, however, is a less well-defined syndrome characterized by easy fatigue, a sense of weakness, and a feeling that the aging process is advancing faster than it should. This is sometimes accompanied by an intellectual weariness and a sense that cognitive faculties are less sharp. In some studies, psychodynamic evaluation has appeared to reveal a distinct psychiatric profile.[14] Whether these nonspecific features of primary hyperparathyroidism are truly part and parcel of the disease process, reversible on successful parathyroid surgery, are issues that are under active investigation.[15]

Gastrointestinal manifestations of primary hyperparathyroidism have classically included peptic ulcer disease and pancreatitis. Peptic ulcer disease is not likely to be linked in a pathophysiologic way to primary hyperparathyroidism unless type I multiple endocrine neoplasia is present. Pancreatitis is virtually never seen anymore as a complication of primary hyperparathyroidism because the hypercalcemia tends to be so mild. Like peptic ulcer disease, the association between primary hyperparathyroidism and hypertension is tenuous. Although there may be an increased incidence of hypertension in primary hyperparathyroidism, it is rarely corrected or improved after successful surgery. Still other potential organ systems that in the past were affected by the hyperparathyroid state are now relegated to being archival curiosities. These include gout and pseudogout, anemia, band keratopathy, and loose teeth.

CLINICAL FORMS OF PRIMARY HYPERPARATHYROIDISM

The most common clinical presentation of primary hyperparathyroidism is characterized by asymptomatic hypercalcemia with serum calcium levels within 1 mg/dl above the upper limits of normal. Most patients do not have specific complaints and do not show evidence for any target organ complications. They have usually been discovered accidentally in the course of a routine multichannel screening test. Rarely, a patient will show serum calcium levels in the life-threatening range, so-called acute primary hyperparathyroidism or parathyroid crisis. These patients are invariably symptomatic of hypercalcemia.[16] Although this is an unusual presentation of primary hyperparathyroidism, it does occur and should always be considered in any patient who presents with acute hypercalcemia of unclear etiology.

Unusual clinical presentations of primary hyperparathyroidism include the multiple endocrine neoplasias, types I and II; familial primary hyperparathyroidism not associated with any other endocrine disorder; familial cystic parathyroid adenomatosis; and neonatal primary hyperparathyroidism.

EVALUATION AND DIAGNOSIS OF PRIMARY HYPERPARATHYROIDISM

The history and the physical examination rarely give any clear indications of primary hyperparathyroidism but are helpful because of the paucity of specific manifestations of the disease. The diagnosis of primary hyperparathyroidism is established by laboratory tests. There are two biochemical hallmarks of primary hyperparathyroidism: hypercalcemia and elevated levels of PTH. The serum phosphorus tends to be in the lower range of normal. In approximately one-third of patients, it is frankly low. The serum alkaline phosphatase activity may be elevated when bone disease is present. More specific markers of bone formation (bone-specific alkaline phosphatase, osteocalcin) and bone resorption (urinary pyridinoline, deoxypyridinoline, N-telopeptide of collagen) will be above normal when there is active bone involvement, but otherwise tend to be in the upper range of normal. The actions of PTH to alter acid-base handling in the kidney will lead, in some patients, to a small increase in the serum chloride concentration and a concomitant decrease in the serum bicarbonate concentration. Urinary calcium excretion is elevated in approximately 30% of patients. The circulating 1,25-dihydroxyvitamin D concentration is elevated in about 25% of patients with primary hyperparathyroidism,[17] although it is of little diagnostic value because 1,25-dihydroxyvitamin D levels are increased in other hypercalcemic states, such as sarcoidosis, other granulomatous diseases, and some lymphomas.[18] 25-Hydroxyvitamin D levels tend to be in the lower end of the normal range. Vitamin D deficiency or insufficiency, as reflected in lower levels of 25-hydroxyvitamin D, is being recognized in patients with primary hyperparathyroidism with increasing frequency.[19]

The lack of specific radiologic manifestations of primary hyperparathyroidism in the vast majority of patients means that X-rays are not cost-effective in the evaluation of the patient with primary hyperparathyroidism. On the other hand, bone mineral densitometry has proved to be an integral component of the evaluation because of its great sensitivity to detect early changes in bone mass. Patients with primary hyperparathyroidism tend to show a pattern of bone involvement that preferentially affects the cortical as opposed to the cancellous skeleton.[20,21] The typical pattern is a reduction in bone density of the distal third of the forearm, a site enriched in cortical bone, and relative preservation of the lumbar spine, a site enriched in cancellous bone. The hip region, best typified by the femoral neck, tends to show values intermediate between the distal radius and the lumbar spine because its composition is a more equal mixture of cortical and cancellous elements. A small subset of patients (approximately 15%) present with an atypical bone mineral density (BMD) profile, characterized by vertebral osteopenia or osteoporosis.[22] Bone densitometry has become an invaluable aspect of the evaluation of primary hyperparathyroidism because it gives a more accurate assessment of the degree of involvement of the skeleton than any other approach. This information is used to make recommendations for parathyroid surgery or for conservative medical observation (see following sections).

Measurement of the circulating PTH concentration is the most definitive way to make the diagnosis of primary hyperparathyroidism. In the presence of hypercalcemia, an elevated level of PTH virtually establishes the diagnosis. A PTH level in the mid- or upper end of the normal range in the face of hypercalcemia is also consistent with the diagnosis of primary hyperparathyroidism. Radioimmunoassays that recognize the carboxy-terminal or mid-molecule portions of the PTH molecule have been supplanted by immunoradiometric (IRMA) assays for PTH that measure the "intact" molecule.[23] The recent recognition that most commercially available IRMAs measure large carboxyterminal fragments of PTH in addition to full-length molecule PTH(1-84) has led to the development of a newer generation IRMA.[24] This newer assay measures only PTH(1-84) and may offer increased diagnostic sensitivity in primary hyperparathyroidism. The clinical usefulness of the PTH measurement in the differential diagnosis of hypercalcemia is a result both of refinements in assay techniques and of the fact that the most common other cause of hypercalcemia,

namely hypercalcemia of malignancy, is associated with suppressed levels of hormone. This is true even for the syndrome of humoral hypercalcemia of malignancy in which PTH-related peptide (PTHrP) is the major causative factor. There is no cross-reactivity between PTH and PTHrP in the IRMA assays for PTH. The only hypercalcemic disorders in which the PTH concentration might be elevated are those related to lithium or thiazide diuretic use. It is relatively easy to exclude either of these two possibilities by the history. If it is conceivable that the patient has drug-related hypercalcemia, the only secure way to make the diagnosis of primary hyperparathyroidism is to withdraw the medication and to confirm persistent hypercalcemia and elevated PTH levels 2–3 months later.

TREATMENT OF PRIMARY HYPERPARATHYROIDISM

Surgery

Primary hyperparathyroidism is cured when the abnormal parathyroid tissue is removed. While it is clear that surgery is appropriate in patients with classical symptoms of primary hyperparathyroidism, there is considerable controversy concerning the need for intervention in patients who have no clear signs or symptoms of their disease. In spring of 2002, a Workshop was conducted at the National Institutes of Health to review the available data on this group of patients. The results of that meeting[25] have led to a revision of the guidelines for management of asymptomatic primary hyperparathyroidism that were first recommended by the 1990 Consensus Development Conference on this subject. Patients are always advised to have surgery if they have symptomatic disease, such as overt bone disease, kidney stones, or if they have survived an episode of acute primary hyperparathyroidism with life-threatening hypercalcemia. Asymptomatic patients are now advised to have surgery if the serum calcium is more than 1 mg/dl above the upper limit of normal. Marked hypercalciuria (>400 mg daily excretion) or significantly reduced creatinine clearance (>30% more than age- and sex-matched controls) is another general indication for surgery. If bone mass, as determined by bone densitometry, is more than 2.5 SDs below young normal control subjects (T-score < −2.5), at any site, surgery should be recommended. Finally, the relatively young patient with primary hyperparathyroidism (under 50 years old) is at greater risk for progression of the hyperparathyroid disease process than older patients, and should be advised to undergo parathyroidectomy.[26]

Adherence to these guidelines for surgery, however, is dependent on both the physician and the patient. Some physicians will recommend surgery for all patients with primary hyperparathyroidism; other physicians will not recommend surgery unless clear-cut complications of primary hyperparathyroidism are present. Similarly, some patients cannot tolerate the idea of living with a curable disease and will seek surgery in the absence of the aforementioned guidelines. Other patients, with coexisting medical problems, may not wish to face the risks of surgery, although surgical indications are present.

Parathyroid surgery requires exceptional expertise and

experience.[27] The glands are notoriously variable in location, requiring the surgeon's knowledge of typical ectopic sites such as intrathyroidal, retroesophageal, the lateral neck, and the mediastinum. The surgeon must also be aware of the proper operation to perform. In the case of the adenoma, the other glands are ascertained to be normal and are not removed. More and more, expert parathyroid surgeons are performing this operation under local, as opposed to general, anesthesia. Recent advances in surgery have led to another approach to the patient with single gland disease. Minimally invasive parathyroidectomy (MIP) is an approach that takes advantage of successful preoperative localization by the most widely used localization modalities, technetium-99m-sestamibi and ultrasound (see below). The surgeon limits the operative field only to the small region overlying the visualized adenoma. After resection, an intraoperative PTH level is obtained. If the PTH level falls by more than 50%, the adenoma that has been removed is considered to be the only source of abnormal glandular activity and the operation is terminated. If the PTH level does not fall by more than 50%, other sources of PTH are considered, and the operation is converted to a more standardized approach. In the case of multiglandular disease, the approach is to remove all tissue save for a remnant that is left in situ or autotransplanted in the nondominant forearm. Postoperatively, the patient may experience a period of transient hypocalcemia, during which time the normal but suppressed parathyroid glands regain their sensitivity to calcium. This happens within the first few days after surgery, and it is usually not necessary to treat the postoperative patient aggressively with calcium when postoperative hypocalcemia is mild. Prolonged postoperative symptomatic hypocalcemia as a result of rapid deposition of calcium and phosphate into bone ("hungry bone" syndrome) is rarely seen today. Such patients may require parenteral calcium for symptomatic hypocalcemia. Permanent hypoparathyroidism is a potential complication of surgery in those who have had previous neck surgery or who undergo subtotal parathyroidectomy (for multiglandular disease). Another rare complication of parathyroid surgery is damage to the recurrent laryngeal nerve, which can lead to hoarseness and reduced voice volume.

A number of localization tests are available to define the site of abnormal parathyroid tissue preoperatively. Among the noninvasive tests, ultrasonography, computed tomography (CT), magnetic resonance imaging (MRI), and scintigraphy are available.[28] Radioisotopic imaging with thallium and technetium has been replaced by imaging with technetium-99m-sestamibi.[29] Sestamibi is taken up both by thyroid and parathyroid tissue but persists in the parathyroid glands. Various approaches to the use of ^{99m}Tc-sestamibi include using the imaging agent alone, and thereby depending on a difference in uptake kinetics between thyroid and parathyroid tissue; or using it in combination with ^{99}Tc-pertechnetate of 123-iodine. The use of dual isotope methods is believed by some to provide better definition of the thyroid, from which the image obtained with sestamibi can be subtracted.[30] Invasive localization tests with arteriography and selective venous sampling for PTH in the draining thyroid veins are available when noninvasive studies have not been successful.

The value of preoperative localization tests in patients about to undergo parathyroid surgery is controversial. In patients who have not had previous neck surgery, there is little evidence that such tests prevent failed operations or shorten operating time. An experienced parathyroid surgeon will find the abnormal parathyroid gland(s) over 95% of the time in the patient who has not had previous neck surgery.[27] Thus, it is hard to justify these tests in this group. On the other hand, the mere availability of these preoperative localization tests has led many endocrinologists and surgeons to begin using them.

On the other hand, in patients who have had prior neck surgery, preoperative localization can be extremely helpful, even to the expert parathyroid surgeon. The general approach is to use the noninvasive studies first. Ultrasound and radioisotope imaging are best for parathyroid tissue that is located in proximity to the thyroid, whereas CT and MRI testing are better for ectopically located parathyroid tissue. In view of the substantial incidence of false-positive studies with all the noninvasive localization procedures, confirmation with two is necessary to be confident of accurate localization. Arteriography and selective venous studies are reserved for those individuals in whom the noninvasive studies have not been successful.

In patients who undergo successful parathyroid surgery, the hyperparathyroid state is completely cured. Serum biochemistries normalize and the PTH level returns to normal. In addition, bone mass improves substantially in the first 1–3 years after surgery.[31] The increase is documented by bone densitometry. The cumulative increase in bone mass at the lumbar spine and femoral neck is approximately 12%, a rather impressive improvement, and is sustained for at least a decade after parathyroidectomy. It is particularly noteworthy that the lumbar spine, a site where PTH seems to protect from age-related and estrogen-deficiency bone loss, is a site of rapid and substantial improvement. Those patients who present with evidence of vertebral osteopenia or osteoporosis sustain an even more impressive improvement in spine bone density after cure and should therefore be routinely referred for surgery regardless of the severity of their hypercalcemia.[22]

Medical Management

Patients who are not surgical candidates for parathyroidectomy appear to do very well when they are managed conservatively.[31–32] Data on patients with primary hyperparathyroidism followed for up to a decade show that biochemical indices of disease and BMD measures of bone mass remain remarkably stable. These include serum calcium, phosphorus, PTH, 25-hydroxyvitamin D, 1,25-dihydroxyvitamin D, and urinary calcium excretion. More specific markers of bone formation and bone resorption also do not appear to change. There are several caveats to this statement, however. First, approximately 25% of patients with asymptomatic primary hyperparathyroidism will have biochemical or bone densitometric evidence of disease progression over a 10-year period. None, however, developed clinically overt complications of their disease (i.e., nephrolithiasis, fractures). Second, those under the age of 50 years have a far higher incidence of progressive disease than do older patients (approximately 65% versus 23%[26]). This supports the notion that younger patients should be referred for parathyroidectomy. Finally, today, as in the day of classical primary hyperparathyroidism, patients with symptomatic disease do poorly when observed without surgery. Thus, the data support the safety of observation without surgery in selected patients with asymptomatic primary hyperparathyroidism.

The longitudinal data on patients who do not have parathyroid surgery also support the need for medical monitoring. In those patients who do not have surgery, a set of general medical guidelines is recommended.[25] Routine medical follow-up usually includes visits twice yearly with serum calcium determinations. Yearly assessment of serum creatinine and bone densitometry at the spine, hip, and distal one-third site of the forearm is also recommended. Adequate hydration and ambulation are always encouraged. Thiazide diuretics and lithium are to be avoided if possible, because they may lead to worsening hypercalcemia. Dietary intake of calcium should be moderate. There is no good evidence that patients with primary hyperparathyroidism show significant fluctuations of their serum calcium as a function of dietary calcium intake. High calcium intakes should be avoided, however, especially in patients whose 1,25-dihydroxyvitamin D level is elevated.[33] Low-calcium diets should also be avoided because they could theoretically lead to further stimulation of PTH secretion.

We still lack an effective and safe therapeutic agent for the medical management of primary hyperparathyroidism. Oral phosphate will lower the serum calcium in patients with primary hyperparathyroidism by approximately 0.5–1 mg/dl. Phosphate seems to act by three mechanisms: interference with absorption of dietary calcium, inhibition of bone resorption, and inhibition of renal production of 1,25-dihydroxyvitamin D. Phosphate, however, is not recommended as an approach to management because of concerns related to ectopic calcification in soft tissues as a result of increasing the calcium-phosphate product. Moreover, oral phosphate may lead to an undesirable further elevation of PTH levels.[34] Gastrointestinal tolerance is another limiting feature of this approach.

In postmenopausal women, estrogen therapy has been an option.[35–37] The rationale for estrogen use in primary hyperparathyroidism is based on the known antagonism by estrogen of PTH-mediated bone resorption. Although the serum calcium concentration does tend to decline after estrogen administration (by approximately 0.5 mg/dl), PTH levels and serum phosphorous concentration do not change. Preliminary data suggest that the selective estrogen receptor modulator, raloxifene, may have a similar effect in postmenopausal women with primary hyperparathyroidism.[37]

Bisphosphonates have also been considered as a possible medical approach to primary hyperparathyroidism. Two or the original bisphosphonates, etidronate and dichloromethylene bisphosphonate, have been studied.[38–40] Although etidronate is not effective, dichloromethylene bisphosphonate temporarily reduces the serum calcium in primary hyperparathyroidism. The use of pamidronate, available exclusively as an intravenous preparation,[41] is restricted to acute hypercalcemic states associated with primary hyperparathyroidism. Alendronate may be useful to treat low

bone density in patients with primary hyperparathyroidism who choose not to have surgery.[42–46]

Finally, a more targeted approach to the medical therapy of primary hyperparathyroidism is to interfere specifically with the production of PTH. A new class of agents that alters the function of the extracellular calcium-sensing receptor offers an exciting new approach to primary hyperparathyroidism. Such agents could conceivably reduce PTH levels and thereby control the hypercalcemic state. An early clinical experience with 20 postmenopausal women who had mild primary hyperparathyroidism showed that a calcimimetic can significantly reduce PTH and serum calcium levels in this disease.[47] More recent experience with another calcimimetic that has a longer half-life has confirmed these early impressions that these agents have great potential to become the first specific medical therapy of primary hyperparathyroidism.[48]

REFERENCES

1. Silverberg SJ, Bilezikian JP 2001 Hyperparathyroidism In: Becker KL (ed.) Principles and Practice of Endocrinology and Metabolism, 3rd ed. JB Lippincott, Philadelphia, PA, USA, pp. 564–573.
2. Heath H III, Hodgson SF, Kennedy MA 1980 Primary hyperparathyroidism: Incidence, morbidity, and potential economic impact in a community. N Engl J Med 302:189–193.
3. Wermers RA, Khosla S, Atkinson EJ, Grant CS, Hodgson SF, O'Fallon WM, Melton LJ III 1998 Survival after diagnosis of PHPT: A population based study. Am J Med 104:115–122.
4. Shane E 2001 Parathyroid carcinoma. In: Bilezikian JP, Marcus R, Levine MA (eds.) The Parathyroids, 2nd ed. Raven Press, New York, NY, USA, pp. 515–526.
5. Arnold A, Shattuck TM, Mallya SM, Krebs LJ, Costa J, Gallagher J, Wild Y, Saucier K 2002 Molecular pathogenesis of primary hyperparathyroidism. J Bone Miner Res 17:N30–N36.
6. Arnold A, Kim HG, Gaz RD, Eddy RL, Fukushima Y, Byers MG, Shows TB, Kronenberg HM 1989 Molecular cloning and chromosomal mapping of DNA rearranged with the parathyroid hormone gene in parathyroid adenoma. J Clin Invest 83:2034–2040.
7. Farnebo F, Teh BT, Kytola S, Svensson A, Phelan C, Sandelin K, Thompson NW, Hoog A, Weber G, Farnebo LO, Larsson C 1998 Alterations of the MEN1 gene in sporadic parathyroid tumors. J Clin Endocrinol Metab 83:2627–2630.
8. Cetani F, Pinchera A, Pardi E, Cianferotti L, Vignali E, Picone A, Miccoli P, Viacava P, Marcocci C 1999 No evidence for mutations in the calcium-sensing receptor gene in sporadic parathyroid adenomas. J Bone Miner Res 14:878–882.
9. Pausova Z, Soliman E, Amizuka N, Janicic N, Konrad EM, Arnold A, Goltzman D, Hendy GN 1996 Role of the RET proto-oncogene in sporadic hyperparathyroidism and in hyperparathyroidism of multiple endocrine neoplasia type 2. J Clin Endocrinol Metab 81:2711–2718.
10. Hakim JP, Levine MA 1994 Absence of p53 point mutations in parathyroid adenomas and carcinoma. J Clin Endocrinol Metab 78:103–106.
11. Silverberg SJ, Bilezikian JP 2001 Clinical presentation of primary hyperparathyroidism in the United States. In: Bilezikian JP, Marcus R, Levine MA (eds.) The Parathyroids, 2nd ed. Raven Press, New York, NY, USA, pp. 349–360.
12. Silverberg SJ, Shane E, Jacobs TP, Siris ES, Gartenberg F, Seldin D, Clemens TL, Bilezikian JP 1990 Nephrolithiasis and bone involvement in primary hyperparathyroidism. Am J Med 89:327–334.
13. Turken SA, Cafferty M, Silverberg SJ, de la Cruz L, Cimino C, Lange DJ, Lovelace RE, Bilezikian JP 1989 Neuromuscular involvement in mild, asymptomatic primary hyperparathyroidism. Am J Med 87:553–557.
14. Solomon BL, Schaaf M, Smallridge RC 1994 Psychologic symptoms before and after parathyroid surgery. Am J Med 96:101–106.
15. Silverberg SJ 2002 Non-classical target organs in primary hyperparathyroidism. J Bone Miner Res 17:S1;N117–N125.
16. Fitzpatrick LA 2001 Acute primary hyperparathyroidism. In: Bilezikian JP, Marcus R, Levine MA (eds.) The Parathyroids, 2nd ed. Raven Press, New York, NY, USA, pp. 527–360.

17. Broadus AE, Horst RL, Lang R, Littledike ET, Rasmussen H 1980 The importance of circulating 1, 25-dihydroxyvitamin D in the pathogenesis of hypercalciuria and renal-stone formation in primary hyperparathyroidism. N Engl J Med 302:421–426.

18. Cox M, Haddad JG 1994 Lymphoma, hypercalcemia and the sunshine vitamin. Ann Intern Med 121:709–712.

19. Silverberg SJ, Shane E, Dempster DW, Bilezikian JP 1999 Vitamin D deficiency in primary hyperparathyroidism. Am J Med 107:561–567.

20. Silverberg SJ, Shane E, de la Cruz L, Dempster DW, Feldman F, Seldin D, Jacobs TP, Siris ES, Cafferty M, Parisien MV, Lindsay R, Clemens TL, Bilezikian JP 1989 Skeletal disease in primary hyperparathyroidism. J Bone Miner Res 4:283–291.

21. Parisien MV, Silverberg SJ, Shane E, de la Cruz L, Lindsay R, Bilezikian JP, Dempster DW 1990 The histomorphometry of bone in primary hyperparathyroidism: Preservation of cancellous bone structure. J Clin Endocrinol Metab 70:930–938.

22. Silverberg SJ, Locker FG, Bilezikian JP 1996 Vertebral osteopenia: A new indication for surgery in primary hyperparathyroidism. J Clin Endocrinol Metab 81:4007–4012.

23. Deftos LJ 2001 Immunoassays for PTH and PTHrP. In: Bilezikian JP, Marcus R, Levine MA (eds.) The Parathyroids, 2nd ed. Raven Press, New York, NY, USA, pp. 143–166.

24. Gao P, Scheibel S, D'Amour P, John MR, Rao SD, Schmidt-Gayk H, Cantor TL 2001 Development of a novel immunoradiometric assay exclusively for biologically active whole parathyroid hormone 1-84: Implications for improvement of accurate assessment of parathyroid function. J Bone Miner Res 16:605–614.

25. Bilezikian JP, Potts JT, El-Hajj Fuleihan G, Kleerekoper M, Neer R, Peacock M, Rastad J, Silverberg SJ, Udelsman R, Wells SA 2002 Summary statement from a workshop on asymptomatic primary hyperparathyroidism: A perspective for the 21st century. J Bone Miner Res 17:S2;N2–N11.

26. Silverberg SJ, Brown I, Bilezikian JP 2002 Youthfulness as a criterion for surgery in primary hyperparathyroidism. Am J Med 113:681–684.

27. Wells SA, Doherty GM 2001 The surgical management of primary hyperparathyroidism. In: Bilezikian JP, Marcus R, Levine MA (eds.) The Parathyroids, 2nd ed. Raven Press, New York, NY, USA, pp. 487–498.

28. Doppman JL 2001 Preoperative localization of parathyroid tissue in primary hyperparathyroidism. In: Bilezikian JP, Marcus R, Levine MA (eds.) The Parathyroids, 2nd ed. Raven Press, New York, NY, USA, pp. 475–486.

29. Mitchell BK, Kinder BK, Cornelius E, Stewart AF 1995 Primary hyperparathyroidism: Preoperative localization using technetium-sestamibi scanning. J Clin Endocrinol Metab 80:7–10.

30. Chen CC, Holder LE, Scovill WA, Tehan AM, Gann DS 1997 Comparison of parathyroid imaging with technetium-sestamibi subtraction, double phase sestamibi and technetium sestamibi SPECT. J Nucl Med 38:834–839.

31. Silverberg SJ, Shane E, Jacobs TP, Siris E, Bilezikian JP 1999 The natural history of treated and untreated asymptomatic primary hyperparathyroidism: A ten year prospective study. N Engl J Med 41:1249–1255.

32. Rao DS, Wilson RJ, Kleerekoper M, Parfitt AM 1988 Lack of biochemical progression or continuation of accelerated bone loss in mild asymptomatic primary hyperparathyroidism: Evidence for a biphasic disease course. J Clin Endocrinol Metab 67:1294–1298.

33. Locker FG, Silverberg SJ, Bilezikian JP 1997 Optimal dietary calcium intake in primary hyperparathyroidism. Am J Med 102:543–550.

34. Broadus AE, Magee JSI, Mallette LE, Horst RL, Lang R, Jensen RG, Gertner JM, Baron R 1983 A detailed evaluation of oral phosphate therapy in selected patients with primary hyperparathyroidism. J Clin Endocrinol Metab 56:953–1961.

35. Marcus R, Madvig P, Crim M, Pont A, Kosek J 1984 Conjugated estrogens in the treatment of postmenopausal women with hyperparathyroidism. Ann Intern Med 100:633–640.

36. Selby PL, Peacock M 1986 Ethinyl estradiol and norethindrone in the treatment of primary hyperparathyroidism in postmenopausal women. N Engl J Med 314:1481–1485.

37. McDermott MT, Perloff JJ, Kidd GS 1994 Effects of mild asymptomatic primary hyperparathyroidism on bone mass in women with and without estrogen replacement therapy. J Bone Miner Res 9:509–514.

38. Rubin MR, Lee K, Silverberg SJ 2003 Raloxifene lowers serum calcium and markers of bone turnover in primary hyperparathyroidism. J Clin Endocrinol Metab 88:1174–1178.

39. Kaplan RA, Geho WB, Poindexter C, Haussler M, Dietz GW, Pak CYC 1977 Metabolic effects of diphosphonate in primary hyperparathyroidism. J Clin Pharmacol 17:410–419.

40. Shane E, Baquiran DC, Bilezikian JP 1981 Effects of dichloromethylene disphosphonate on serum and urine calcium in primary hyperparathyroidism. Ann Intern Med 95:23–27.

41. Adami S, Mian M, Bertoldo F, Rossini M, Jayawerra P, O'Riordan JL, Lo Cascio V 1990 Regulation of calcium-parathyroid hormone feedback in primary hyperparathyroidism: Effects of bisphosphonate treatment. Clin Endocrinol (Oxf) 33:391–397.

42. Janson S, Tissell L-E, Lindstedt G, Lundberg P-A 1991 Disodium pamidronate in the preoperative treatment of hypercalcemia in patients with primary hyperparathyroidism. Surgery 110:480–486

43. Hassani S, Braunstein GD, Seibel MJ, Birckman AS, Geola F, Pekary AE, Hershman JM 2001 Alendronate therapy of primary hyperparathyroidism. Endocrinologist 11:459–464.

44. Rossini M, Gatti D, Isaia G, Sartori L, Braga V, Adami S 2001 Effects of oral alendronate in elderly patients with osteoporosis and mild primary hyperparathyroidism. J Bone Miner Res 16:113–119.

45. Parker CR, Blackwell PJ, Fairbairn KJ, Hosking DJ 2002 Alendronate in the treatment of primary hyperparathyroid-related osteoporosis: A 2-year study. J Clin Endocrinol Metab 87:4482–4489.

46. Chow CC, Chan WB, Li JK, Chan NN, Chan MH, Ko GT, Lo KW, Cockram CS 2003 Oral alendronate increased BMD in postmenopausal women with primary hyperparathyroidism. J Clin Endocrinol Metab 88:581–587.

47. Silverberg SJ, Marriott TB, Bone HG III, Locker FG, Thys-Jacobs S, Dziem G, Sanguinetti ES, Bilezikian JP 1997 Short term inhibition of parathyroid hormone secretion by a calcium receptor agonist in primary hyperparathyroidism. N Engl J Med 307:1506–1510.

48. Peacock M, Shoback DM, Greth WE, Binder TA, Graves T, Brenner RM, Turner SA, Marcus R 2001 The calcimimetic AMG073 reduces serum calcium in patients with primary hyperparathyroidism. J Bone Miner Res 16:S163.

Chapter 34.   Familial Hyperparathyroid Syndromes

Andrew Arnold

Center for Molecular Medicine and Division of Endocrinology and Metabolism, University of Connecticut School of Medicine, Farmington, Connecticut

INTRODUCTION

Compared with patients with typical, sporadically occurring primary hyperparathyroidism (HPT), individuals with recognizable familial predispositions to HPT constitute a small minority of the totality of patients with this disorder. These hereditary syndromes have been recognized as exhibiting Mendelian inheritance patterns, have been genetically elucidated to a large extent, and will be the focus of this chapter. They include multiple endocrine neoplasia types 1 and 2A, hyperparathyroid-jaw tumor syndrome, and familial isolated hyperparathyroidism. Familial (benign) hy-

The author has no conflict of interest.

pocalciuric hypercalcemia (FHH, FBH, FBHH) and neonatal severe hyperparathyroidism (NSHPT) also fall into this category, but are the subjects of a separate chapter. The extra-parathyroid manifestations present in some of the familial HPT syndromes will be mentioned but lie outside the focus of this chapter. It is worth noting that as more knowledge accumulates on genetic contributions to complex phenotypes, additional genetic loci may be identified as contributing to a less penetrant and more subtle predisposition to primary HPT in the general population.

MULTIPLE ENDOCRINE NEOPLASIA TYPE 1

Multiple endocrine neoplasia type 1 (MEN1) is a rare heritable disorder with a prevalence of around 2 per 100,000. It is classically defined as a predisposition to tumors of the parathyroids, anterior pituitary, and pancreatic islet cells, although affected patients are now known to be predisposed to many additional endocrine and nonendocrine tumors.[1,2] Primary HPT is the most penetrant component of MEN1, occurring in almost 100% of affected individuals by age 50, and is the initial manifestation of the disorder in most patients. Approximately 2% of all cases of primary HPT are caused by MEN1. Some of the other types of tumors associated with MEN1 include duodenal gastrinomas, bronchial or thymic carcinoids, gastric enterochromaffin-like tumors, adrenocortical adenomas, lipomas, angiofibromas, collagenomas, and spinal cord ependymomas.[1]

The inheritance of MEN1 follows an autosomal dominant pattern, and the molecular genetic basis is an inactivating germline mutation of the *MEN1* gene, located on chromosome band 11q13.[3] *MEN1* encodes a protein called menin, which clearly acts as a tumor suppressor but whose normal biochemical functions have not been fully established. Patients with MEN1 have typically inherited one inactivated copy of this gene from an affected parent. The actual outgrowth of a tumor requires the subsequent somatic (acquired) inactivation of the normal, remaining copy of the gene in one cell. Such a parathyroid cell, for example, would then be devoid of the *MEN1* gene's tumor suppressor function, contributing to a selective advantage over its neighbors and clonal proliferation.

Primary HPT in the setting of MEN1 has a number of different features from the common sporadic (nonfamilial) form of the disease. The male to female ratio is even in MEN1 in contrast to the female predominance of sporadic HPT. HPT in MEN1 typically presents in the second to fourth decade of life and has been found as early as age 8. Multiple gland involvement is typical in MEN1, and in most patients, three to four tumors are evident on initial neck exploration. However, these multiple tumors may vary widely in size, with an average 10:1 ratio between the largest and smallest glands.[4] An apparently inexorable drive to parathyroid tumorigenesis exists in MEN1, reflected by the impressively high rate of recurrent HPT after apparently successful subtotal parathyroidectomy (>50% after 12 years).[4] The high recurrence rate in MEN1 stands in contrast to the behavior of HPT in MEN2A, as well as sporadic primary parathyroid hyperplasia. As mentioned below, familial isolated hyperparathyroidism can manifest as an occult or variant presentation of *MEN1* mutation.

The biochemical diagnosis of primary HPT in known or suspected MEN1 is based on the finding of hypercalcemia (ionized or albumin-adjusted total calcium) with elevated (or inappropriately high) serum PTH concentrations. Once the biochemical diagnosis is established, the indications for surgical intervention are similar to those in patients with sporadic primary HPT and include symptomatic hypercalcemia, nephrolithiasis, and/or decreased bone mass, which has been observed in women with MEN1 at the age of 35.[2] Because hypercalcemia can worsen hypergastrinemia, another indication for parathyroidectomy in MEN1 is the presence of medically refractory symptoms of gastrinoma, an unusual situation given the success of pharmacotherapy for Zollinger-Ellison syndrome.

Opinions differ as to the optimal timing of surgical treatment of HPT in MEN1, and there is a dearth of useful data bearing on this question. Early presymptomatic intervention might, on one hand, lead to better long-term bone health. On the other hand, because of the high rate of recurrent HPT, a policy of deferring surgery might decrease a patient's total number of operations and thereby decrease the cumulative risk of complications.

Because of the multiplicity of parathyroid tumors in MEN1, the need to identify all parathyroid glands at surgery, and the inability of imaging tools to reliably detect all hypercellular glands, preoperative localization studies in unoperated patients are not generally indicated. For the same reason, a suspected or firm preoperative diagnosis of MEN1 should argue against performing minimally invasive parathyroidectomy. In the context of bilateral operations, however, intraoperative parathyroid hormone (PTH) measurement may be helpful.[4] In contrast, preoperative imaging/localization is useful before reoperation in patients with recurrent or persistent disease. The initial operation most frequently performed in MEN1 patients is 3.5 gland subtotal parathyroidectomy with transcervical near-total thymectomy. A parathyroid remnant of about 50 mg is usually left in situ and may be marked with a metal clip, but alternatively the remnant can be autotransplanted[2] to the forearm after intentionally complete parathyroidectomy. The efficacy of thymectomy is unproven but seems reasonable because it may cure incipient thymic carcinoids or prevent their development[5]; in addition, the thymus is a common site for parathyroid tumors in MEN1 patients with recurrent HPT. Involvement of a highly experienced parathyroid surgical team is crucial to optimal outcome.

Management of the pituitary, enteropancreatic, and other neoplastic manifestations of MEN1 are discussed in detail elsewhere.[2] It should be emphasized that MEN1-associated malignancies cause fully one-third of the deaths in MEN1 patients, and for most of these cancers, no effective prevention or cure currently exists.

Direct genetic testing for germline *MEN1* mutations is commercially available, but the indications for such testing remain under discussion.[2] It should be noted that genetic analyses, typically limited to polymerase chain reaction (PCR)-amplified coding exons, fail to detect *MEN1* mutation in 10–20% of MEN1 index patients. In contrast to the clear clinical efficacy of testing for *RET* gene mutations in MEN2, pre-symptomatic genetic diagnosis has not been established to improve morbidity or mortality in MEN1, and biochemical screening with serum calcium and PTH provides a nongenetic alternative. Thus, DNA testing is not currently determinative of important clinical interventions in MEN1, and the rationale for its use is not as well established as in MEN2.[1,2] Similarly, periodic biochemical or anatomic screening for endocrine tumor manifestations in MEN1 patients, or in family members at risk, has not been proven to enhance clinical outcomes, and whether such testing is of incremental benefit compared with careful histories and physical examinations remains to be determined. Suggested protocols for use of pre-symptomatic testing are available.[2]

MULTIPLE ENDOCRINE NEOPLASIA TYPE 2A

MEN2 is subclassified into three major clinical syndromes: MEN2A, MEN2B, and familial medullary thyroid cancer (FMTC). Of these, MEN2A is the most common (75% of MEN2 kindreds) and the only one that manifests HPT.[1,2] MEN2A is a heritable predisposition to medullary thyroid cancer (MTC), pheochromocytoma, and primary HPT. The respective frequency of these tumors in MEN2A is about 90% for MTC, 40–50% for pheochromocytoma, and 20–30% for HPT.[2] This low penetrance of HPT in MEN2A contrasts with the high penetrance found in all other familial hyperparathyroid syndromes.

MEN2A is inherited in an autosomal dominant pattern, with men and women affected in equal proportions, and the responsible genetic defect is germline mutation of the *RET* proto-oncogene on chromosome 10.[1] The RET protein is a receptor tyrosine kinase that normally transduces growth and differentiation signals in developing tissues including those derived from the neural crest. There are both differences and much overlap in the specific *RET* gene mutations underlying MEN2A and FMTC; in contrast, MEN2B is caused by entirely distinct *RET* mutations.[2] The reasons, which may include "modifier genes," for which parathyroid disease fails to develop in FMTC patients who can bear identical *RET* mutations as found in MEN2A, remain unclear but will be revealing as to the pathogenesis of HPT. Unlike the numerous different inactivating mutations of *MEN1*, which are typical of a tumor suppressor mechanism, *RET* mutations in MEN2A are limited in number, reflecting the need for specific gain-of-function changes to activate this oncogene.[1] Germline *RET* mutation is detectable in over 95% of MEN2A families. *RET* mutation at codon 634 seems to be highly associated with the expression of HPT in MEN2A.

HPT in MEN2A is often asymptomatic, and its biochemical diagnosis as well as indications for surgical treatment reflect those in sporadic primary HPT.[2] Evidence of pheochromocytoma should be sought before parathyroidectomy, and if present, the pheochromocytoma(s) should be removed before parathyroid surgery. Primary HPT in MEN2A is almost always multiglandular, but less than four clearly hypercellular glands may be present. Thus, bilateral neck exploration to identify all glands is advisable in known or suspected MEN2A, with resection of hypercellular parathyroid tissue (up to 3.5 glands) being the most common surgical approach. Issues of preoperative localization in unoperated patients are similar to MEN1. In contrast to MEN1, however, recurrent HPT is infrequent after apparently successful resection of enlarged glands, similar to the excellent long-term outcome of surgically treated patients with nonfamilial primary hyperplasia.

Intriguingly, a decreased incidence of HPT has been reported in MEN2A patients who have undergone early total thyroidectomy for cure or prevention of MTC.[6,7] Whether or not this finding is confirmed, the already low penetrance of HPT in MEN2A, and the success of its treatment, argue strongly against prophylactic total parathyroidectomy with forearm autotransplantation at the time of thyroidectomy for MTC, an approach carrying substantial risk of hypoparathyroidism.

The other major manifestations of MEN2A are MTC and pheochromocytoma. MTC, the major life-threatening manifestation of MEN2A, evolves from pre-existing parafollicular C-cell hyperplasia, and its calcitonin production provides a useful marker for monitoring tumor burden. Despite the pharmacologic properties of calcitonin, mineral metabolism is generally normal in the setting of metastatic MTC and its often dramatic hypercalcitoninemia. DNA testing for germline *RET* mutations is central to clinical management and worthy of emphasis for its role in prevention of MTC. *RET* testing is superior to immunoassay for basal or stimulated calcitonin for diagnosis of MEN2A. Molecular diagnosis allows for prophylactic or curative thyroidectomy to be performed, that is, sufficiently early in childhood as to minimize the likelihood that metastases will have occurred.[1,2]

Pheochromocytomas in MEN2A can be unilateral or bilateral, and extra-adrenal or malignant pheochromocytomas are under-represented in comparison to sporadic disease. Because undiagnosed pheochromocytoma could cause substantial morbidity or even death during thyroid or parathyroid surgery, it is important to first screen for pheochromocytoma. Different approaches to screening exist; a consensus report suggested measurement of plasma metanephrines and 24-h urinary excretion of catecholamines and metanephrines on an annual basis and supplemented by periodic imaging studies.[1,2] Laparoscopic adrenalectomy has greatly improved the management of pheochromocytoma in MEN2A, and adrenal cortical-sparing surgery may ultimately prove to be helpful in obviating the problem of adrenal insufficiency after treatment of bilateral pheochromocytoma.

HYPERPARATHYROIDISM-JAW TUMOR SYNDROME

The hyperparathyroidism-jaw tumor syndrome (HPT-JT) is a rare, autosomal dominant predisposition to primary HPT, ossifying fibromas of the mandible and maxilla, and renal manifestations including cysts, hamartomas, or Wilms tumors.[8–10] Only 28 families have been reported by a recent count.[4] HPT is the most penetrant manifestation at 80% of adults, followed by 30% for ossifying fibromas, and lower for renal lesions. As mentioned below, familial isolated hyperparathyroidism can manifest as a variant presentation of HPT-JT.

Hyperparathyroidism in HPT-JT may develop as early as the first decade or two of life. Although all parathyroids are at risk, surgical exploration may reveal a solitary parathyroid tumor rather than multigland disease, in contrast to MEN1 and MEN2A. Parathyroid neoplasms can be cystic, and while most tumors are classified as adenomas, the incidence of parathyroid carcinoma is markedly overrepresented in HPT-JT kindreds.[10] After a period of normocalcemia, treated patients may manifest recurrent HPT, and a solitary tumor asynchronously originating in a different parathyroid gland may prove responsible. The approach to monitoring and surgery in HPT-JT must take into account the predilection to parathyroid malignancy, and the finding of biochemical HPT should lead promptly to surgery. All parathyroids should be identified at operation, signs of malignancy sought, and appropriate resection of abnormal glands performed.[4]

Ossifying fibromas in HPT-JT may be large and destructive, but are often small, asymptomatic, and identified as incidental findings on dental radiographs. They are clearly distinct from the classic, osteoclast-rich "brown tumors" of severe hyperparathyroidism. Monitoring of affected or "at-risk" individuals in HPT-JT kindreds should also include attention to the associated renal abnormalities.

Germline mutation of the *HRPT2* gene is responsible for HPT-JT. *HRPT2* was first localized to chromosome 1q by linkage analysis[10] and recently identified.[11] In the initial report, the yield of *HRPT2* mutation detection in HPT-JT kindreds was about 50%.[11] Mutations of *HRPT2* are predicted to inactivate or eliminate its protein product, termed parafibromin, consistent with a tumor suppressor mechanism.[11] The identification of *HRPT2* opens the door to DNA-based carrier ascertainment and to direct examination of its role in familial HPT and parathyroid cancer.

FAMILIAL HYPOCALCIURIC HYPERCALCEMIA AND NEONATAL SEVERE HYPERPARATHYROIDISM

Familial hypocalciuric hypercalcemia (FHH) and neonatal severe hyperparathyroidism (NSHPT) are mentioned here as a reminder of their inclusion in the category of familial hyperparathyroid syndromes, but they are discussed elsewhere. Germline mutations in the *CASR* gene that cause partial or severe loss of function of the extracellular G-protein–coupled calcium receptor are a major cause of these syndromes. Genetic linkage analyses indicate that the FHH phenotype can also be caused by mutation of different genes, which have not yet been identified. As mentioned below, familial isolated hyperparathyroidism can manifest as a variant presentation of *CASR* mutation.

FAMILIAL ISOLATED HYPERPARATHYROIDISM

Familial isolated primary hyperparathyroidism (FIHPT) is a clinically defined entity, based on the absence of expression of the extra-parathyroid manifestations that characterize other familial HPT syndromes. As such, a designation of FIHPT can change with new findings in the family. Furthermore, FIHPT is genetically heterogeneous, and can be caused by variant expressions of germline mutations in *MEN1*, *HRPT2*, *CASR*, and probably other genes.[4,12,13]

Clinical monitoring and management must take into consideration the possibility that additional features of a genetically defined HPT syndrome could emerge or become detectable. For example, the heightened risk of parathyroid carcinoma must be borne in mind in FIHPT when the genetic basis is not established and *HRPT2* mutation is possible. DNA testing may prove to have a role, for example, when results might impact on the advisability of, or approach to, parathyroid surgery.

REFERENCES

1. Gagel RF, Marx SJ 2003 Multiple endocrine neoplasia. In: Larsen PR, Kronenberg HM, Melmed S, Polonsky K (eds.) Williams Textbook of Endocrinology, 10th ed. WB Saunders, Philadelphia, PA, USA, pp. 1717–1762.
2. Brandi ML, Gagel RF, Angeli A, Bilezikian JP, Beck-Peccoz P, Bordi C, Conte-Devolx B, Falchetti A, Gheri RG, Libroia A, Lips CJ, Lombardi G, Mannelli M, Pacini F, Ponder BA, Raue F, Skogseid B, Tamburrano G, Thakker RV, Thompson NW, Tomassetti P, Tonelli F, Wells SA Jr, Marx SJ 2001 Guidelines for diagnosis and therapy of MEN type 1 and type 2. J Clin Endocrinol Metab **86:**5658–5671.
3. Chandrasekharappa SC, Guru SC, Manickam P, Olufemi SE, Collins FS, Emmert-Buck MR, Debelenko LV, Zhuang Z, Lubensky IA, Liotta LA, Crabtree JS, Wang Y, Roe BA, Weisemann J, Boguski MS, Agarwal SK, Kester MB, Kim YS, Heppner C, Dong Q, Spiegel AM, Burns AL, Marx SJ 1997 Positional cloning of the gene for multiple endocrine neoplasia-type 1. Science **276:**404–407.
4. Marx SJ, Simonds WF, Agarwal SK, Burns AL, Weinstein LS, Cochran C, Skarulis MC, Spiegel AM, Libutti SK, Alexander HR Jr, Chen CC, Chang R, Chandrasekharappa SC, Collins FS 2002 Hyperparathyroidism in hereditary syndromes: Special expressions and special managements. J Bone Miner Res **17:**S2;N37–N43.
5. Gibril F, Chen YJ, Schrump DS, Vortmeyer A, Zhuang Z, Lubensky IA, Reynolds JC, Louie A, Entsuah LK, Huang K, Asgharian B, Jensen RT 2003 Prospective study of thymic carcinoids in patients with multiple endocrine neoplasia type 1. J Clin Endocrinol Metab **88:**1066–1081.
6. Gagel RF, Tashjian AH Jr, Cummings T, Papathanasopoulos N, Kaplan MM, DeLellis RA, Wolfe HJ, Reichlin S 1988 The clinical outcome of prospective screening for multiple endocrine neoplasia type 2a. An 18-year experience. N Engl J Med **318:**478–484.
7. Snow KJ, Boyd AE III 1994 Management of individual tumor syndromes. Medullary thyroid carcinoma and hyperparathyroidism. Endocrinol Metab Clin North Am **23:**157–166.
8. Mallette LE, Malini S, Rappaport MP, Kirkland JL 1987 Familial cystic parathyroid adenomatosis. Ann Intern Med **107:**54–60.
9. Jackson CE, Norum RA, Boyd SB, Talpos GB, Wilson SD, Taggart RT, Mallette LE 1990 Hereditary hyperparathyroidism and multiple ossifying jaw fibromas: A clinically and genetically distinct syndrome. Surgery **108:**1006–1013.
10. Szabo J, Heath B, Hill VM, Jackson CE, Zarbo RJ, Mallette LE, Chew SL, Besser GM, Thakker RV, Huff V, Leppert MF, Heath H 1995 Hereditary hyperparathyroidism-jaw tumor syndrome: The endocrine tumor gene HRPT2 maps to chromosome 1q21–q31. Am J Hum Genet **56:**944–950.
11. Carpten JD, Robbins CM, Villablanca A, Forsberg L, Presciuttini S, Bailey-Wilson J, Simonds WF, Gillanders EM, Kennedy AM, Chen JD, Agarwal SK, Sood R, Jones MP, Moses TY, Haven C, Petillo D, Leotlela PD, Harding B, Cameron D, Pannett AA, Hoog A, Heath H III, James-Newton LA, Robinson B, Zarbo RJ, Cavaco BM, Wassif W, Perrier ND, Rosen IB, Kristoffersson U, Turnpenny PD, Farnebo LO, Besser GM, Jackson CE, Morreau H, Trent JM, Thakker RV, Marx SJ, Teh BT, Larsson C, Hobbs MR 2002 HRPT2, encoding parafibromin, is mutated in hyperparathyroidism-jaw tumor syndrome. Nat Genet **32:**676–680.
12. Teh BT, Esapa CT, Houlston R, Grandell U, Farnebo F, Nordenskjold M, Pearce CJ, Carmichael D, Larsson C, Harris PE 1998 A family with isolated hyperparathyroidism segregating a missense MEN1 mutation and showing loss of the wild-type alleles in the parathyroid tumors. Am J Hum Genet **63:**1544–1549.
13. Simonds WF, James-Newton LA, Agarwal SK, Yang B, Skarulis MC, Hendy GN, Marx SJ 2002 Familial isolated hyperparathyroidism: Clinical and genetic characteristics of 36 kindreds. Medicine (Baltimore) **81:**1–26.

Chapter 35.   Familial Hypocalciuric Hypercalcemia

Stephen J. Marx

Metabolic Diseases Branch, National Institute of Diabetes and Digestive and Kidney Diseases, National Institutes of Health, Bethesda, Maryland

INTRODUCTION

Familial hypocalciuric hypercalcemia (FHH; also termed familial benign hypercalcemia [FBH] or familial benign hypocalciuric hypercalcemia [FBHH]) is an autosomal dominant trait with lifelong high penetrance for hypercalcemia and relative hypocalciuria.[1–3] Most cases are caused by loss-of-function mutation of the calcium-sensing receptor gene (*CASR*). The prevalence of FHH has not been established, but it is probably similar to that for multiple endocrine neoplasia type 1; each accounts for about 2% of cases with asymptomatic hypercalcemia.

CLINICAL FEATURES

Symptoms and Signs

Patients with FHH are usually asymptomatic. Occasionally, they note easy fatigue, weakness, thought disturbances, or polydipsia. Although these symptoms are common in typical primary hyperparathyroidism, they are less common and less severe in FHH. There is a low but increased incidence of relapsing pancreatitis,[1,4] and this can occasionally be severe and life threatening. The rate of peptic ulcer disease, nephrolithiasis, or even idiopathic hypercalciuria is the same as in a normal population.

Radiographs and Indices of Bone Function

Radiographs are usually normal. Nephrocalcinosis has the same incidence as in a normal population. There is an increased incidence of chondrocalcinosis (usually clinically silent) and premature vascular calcification.[1] Bone turnover is mildly increased as measured by indices of bone formation (serum bone gla-protein, serum alkaline phosphatase, or both) or by indices of bone resorption (ratio of urine hydroxyproline to creatinine).[5] Bone mass and susceptibility to fracture are normal.[2,5]

Serum Electrolytes

There is virtually 100% penetrance for hypercalcemia at all ages among FHH carriers.[1] Hypercalcemia has been documented in the first week of life.[6] Typically, the degree of hypercalcemia is similar to that in typical primary hyperparathyroidism and decreases modestly from infancy to old age.[1] Both free and bound calcium are increased, with a normal ratio of free to bound calcium.[7] The degree of hypercalcemia clusters within kindreds, with several kindreds showing very modest hypercalcemia and several showing rather severe hypercalcemia (12.5–14 mg/dl) in most affected members.[1,8] Serum magnesium is typically

in the high range of normal or modestly elevated, and serum phosphate is modestly depressed.

Renal Function Indices

Creatinine clearance is generally normal. Urinary excretion of calcium is normal, with affected and unaffected family members showing a similar distribution of values. Not surprisingly, coexistent FHH and idiopathic hypercalciuria were clearly documented in at least one individual.[1] The normal urinary calcium in the face of hypercalcemia reflects increased renal tubular reabsorption of calcium (i.e., relative hypocalciuria). The average renal tubular reabsorption of magnesium also is modestly increased. Because total urinary calcium excretion depends heavily on glomerular filtration rate, total calcium excretion is not a practical index to distinguish a case of FHH from typical primary hyperparathyroidism. The ratio of calcium clearance to creatinine clearance is calculated easily:

$$Ca_{Cl}/Cr_{Cl} = [Ca_u \times V/Ca_s]/[Cr_u \times V/Cr_s]$$
$$= [Ca_u \times Cr_s]/[Cr_u \times Ca_s]$$

where Cl is renal clearance, Ca is total calcium, Cr is creatinine, u is urine, V is volume, and s is serum. It is an empirically chosen index that corrects for most of the variation from glomerular filtration rate. This clearance ratio in FHH is one-third of that in typical primary hyperparathyroidism, and a cut-off value at 0.01 (note that all units cancel out) is helpful for diagnosis, although only in a hypercalcemic patient.

Parathyroid Function Indices

Biochemical testing of parathyroid function, including serum parathyroid hormone (PTH) and 1,25-dihydroxyvitamin D [1,25(OH)$_2$D] is usually normal, with modest elevations in 5–10% of cases.[9,10] Thus, in the presence of hypercalcemia, a normal PTH, like a low urine calcium, should raise the suspicion of FHH. Even the "normal" parathyroid function indices in the presence of lifelong hypercalcemia are inappropriate and reflect a specific role for the parathyroids in causing hypercalcemia. There is often mild parathyroid gland hyperplasia (evident only by careful measurement of gland size)[11,12] and occasional lipohyperplasia.[13]

Responses to Subtotal Versus Total Parathyroidectomy

Standard subtotal parathyroidectomy in FHH results in only a very transient lowering of serum calcium, with restoration of hypercalcemia within 1 week.[2] FHH has been a common cause of unsuccessful parathyroidectomy, accounting for 10% of unsuccessful operations in several large

---

The author has no conflict of interest.

series during the 1970s, before wider recognition of the implications of this diagnosis.[14] Total parathyroidectomy in FHH leads to low PTH, low 1,25(OH)$_2$D, and low calcium in blood, that is, chronic hypoparathyroidism. However, attempted total parathyroidectomy can fail because small amounts of residual parathyroid tissue are sufficient to sustain hypercalcemia in FHH.

A Broad Spectrum of Disorders Related to FHH

Making the Diagnosis of FHH. Family screening for FHH is valuable to establish the diagnosis (in the index case and in the family) and to start toward avoiding unnecessary parathyroidectomy in all carriers later on. Obtaining the needed family data can take many months. Because of high penetrance for hypercalcemia in FHH carriers, accurate genetic assignments can usually be made from one determination of total serum calcium (or preferably ionized or albumin-adjusted calcium). Genetic linkage testing and *CASR* mutation analysis (see below) also have occasional roles in diagnosis, particularly with an inconclusive clinical evaluation of the family or with an atypical presentation.[15] *CASR* mutation testing has been done so far only in research laboratories.

Disorders Resembling FHH

Typical Primary Hyperparathyroidism. The resemblance of typical primary hyperparathyroidism to FHH is evident and important; their distinction is the main topic of this chapter.

Autoimmune FHH. In four members of two kindreds, FHH was caused by autoantibodies against the CaS-R and was associated with other autoimmune features (thyroiditis or sprue); there was no *CASR* mutation.[16]

CASR Loss-of-Function Mutation Without FHH. One large kindred with a germline missense mutation in the *CASR* gene had a hyperparathyroid syndrome unlike FHH. There was hypercalciuria, monoclonal parathyroid adenomas, and benefit from subtotal parathyroidectomy.[17] Several other small families with *CASR* loss-of-function mutations have contained some members with features partly resembling typical primary hyperparathyroidism.[15] These families should not yet be grouped under the FHH label; however, most are likely FHH with referral bias of one outlier case.

Neonatal Severe Primary Hyperparathyroidism. Neonatal severe primary hyperparathyroidism is an unusual state of life-threatening, severe hypercalcemia with massive hyperplasia of all parathyroid glands. Most cases reflect a double dose of FHH genes.[8,18,19] This warrants early total parathyroidectomy. A similar phenotype may result from an FHH heterozygote having gestated in a normocalcemic (i.e., FHH-negative) mother, which caused superimposed intrauterine secondary hyperparathyroidism[18,20] (see below). Such a maternal contribution may resolve several weeks after birth.

PATHOPHYSIOLOGY

FHH as a Form of Primary Hyperparathyroidism

Biochemical testing has established that the parathyroid gland functions abnormally in FHH (see above). The surgically decreased gland mass can maintain the same high calcium level by increasing hormone secretion rate per unit mass of tissue. There is a selective and mild increase in glandular "setpoint" for calcium suppression of PTH secretion.[3] Depending on the definition of primary hyperparathyroidism, FHH can therefore be labeled as a form of primary hyperparathyroidism. This is even more striking for the causally related neonatal severe primary hyperparathyroidism. It is preferable to label FHH as an atypical form of primary hyperparathyroidism because of important contrasts to the more typical form associated with hypercalciuria, nephrolithiasis, markedly increased parathyroid gland mass, clear elevations of plasma PTH, and generally, excellent response to subtotal parathyroidectomy. However, some authorities prefer not to classify FHH as a form of primary hyperparathyroidism to emphasize its contrasting management needs.[21]

Independent Defect in the Kidneys

In addition to the disturbance presumed to be intrinsic to the parathyroids in FHH, there also is a disturbance intrinsic to the kidneys. The tubular reabsorption of calcium, normally increased by parathyroid hormone, is high and remains strikingly increased even after total parathyroidectomy in FHH.[22] Still the parathyroid glands sustain this hypercalcemia, virtually without contribution from increased renal resorption of calcium.

Mutations in the *CASR* Gene and Its Calcium-Sensing Receptor Protein

Most FHH cases are caused by heterozygous loss-of-function mutations in *CASR*, the gene that encodes the calcium-sensing receptor (CaS-R).[23] Its encoded CaS-R is a seven transmembrane cell-surface receptor (like adrenergic and many other G-protein–coupled receptors) that interacts with extracellular calcium ions, transducing it into an intracellular signal, its protein category products coupling to a cytoplasmic guanyl nucleotide-binding protein, but this has not yet been specifically identified. Two unusual FHH kindreds not linked to the *CASR* locus at chromosome 3q, specifically those linked to 19p or 19q, represent mutation in other unidentified genes of unknown function and likely in the same signaling pathway.[24,25] No correlation with the *CASR* mutation spectrum has been apparent among families with loss- or gain-of-function mutation (i.e., FHH, autosomal dominant hypoparathyroidism with hypercalciuria, or FHH with presumed mutation in another gene).[23,26]

MANAGEMENT

Indications for Parathyroidectomy Are Rare

Familial hypocalciuric hypercalcemia is compatible with survival into the ninth decade, and there may be normal life expectancy. Because of the generally benign course and lack of response to subtotal parathyroidectomy, virtually all patients with FHH should be advised against parathyroidectomy. In rare situations, such as (1) neonatal severe primary hyperparathyroidism resulting from a double dose of an FHH gene, (2) an adult with relapsing pancreatitis, or (3) a child or an adult with serum calcium persistently above 14 mg/dl, parathyroidectomy may be necessary. Total parathyroidectomy should be attempted in these situations.

Pharmacologic Intervention in the Typical Case

Chronic hypercalcemia in FHH has been resistant to medications (diuretics, bisphosphonates, phosphates, and estrogens). The expected availability of calcimimetic drugs acting on the CaS-R might change these considerations[27]; they have not yet been evaluated in FHH.

Sporadic Hypocalciuric Hypercalcemia

Without a positive family history, the decision about management of sporadic hypocalciuric hypercalcemia is difficult. Because there is a wide range of urine calcium values in patients with FHH and with typical primary hyperparathyroidism, an occasional patient with parathyroid adenoma will show a very low calcium-to-creatinine clearance ratio. Moreover, occasionally a patient with FHH will show a high ratio. Sporadic hypocalciuric hypercalcemia should generally be managed as typical FHH. In time, the underlying diagnosis may become evident; low morbidity in such patients, even those with undiagnosed parathyroid adenoma, should be anticipated for the same reasons that the morbidity is low in FHH. Here, detection of a *CASR* mutation can be particularly helpful. However, failure to find one does not exclude FHH, because there may be a large deletion or mutation outside the tested opened reading frame (explaining 30% falsely "normal" testing) or rarely in other FHH genes.

Pregnancy

Several pairings may cause antagonism of blood calcium regulation between fetus and mother. The affected offspring of a mother with FHH should show asymptomatic hypercalcemia. The unaffected offspring of a mother with FHH may show symptomatic hypocalcemia from reversible parathyroid suppression as a result of maternal hypercalcemia. The affected offspring of an unaffected mother may show worsened, albeit temporarily, neonatal hyperparathyroidism because of superimposed intrauterine secondary hyperparathyroidism.

CONCLUSIONS

Familial hypocalciuric hypercalcemia is an important cause of asymptomatic hypercalcemia, with greatly increasing representation at patient ages decreasing below 30 years. The index case and relatives need appropriate assessments of serum calcium and PTH and of a urinary calcium index. Subtotal parathyroidectomy virtually always would result in persistent hypercalcemia. Although mild symptoms similar to those in typical primary hyperparathyroidism are common, virtually all patients should be followed without any intervention.

REFERENCES

1. Marx SJ, Attie MF, Levine MA, Spiegel AM, Downs RW Jr, Lasker RD 1981 The hypocalciuric or benign variant of familial hypercalcemia: Clinical and biochemical features in fifteen kindreds. Medicine **60:**397–412.
2. Law WM Jr, Heath H III 1985 Familial benign hypercalcemia (hypocalciuric hypercalcemia): Clinical and pathogenetic studies in 21 families. Ann Intern Med **102:**511–519.
3. El-Hajj Fuleihan G, Brown EM, Heath H III 2002 Familial benign hypocalciuric hypercalcemia and neonatal primary hyperparathyroidism. In: Bilezikian JP, Raisz LG, Rodan GA (eds.) Principles of Bone Biology, 2nd ed. Academic Press, San Diego, CA, USA, pp. 1031–1045.
4. Davies M, Klimiuk PS, Adams PH, Lumb GA, Anderson DC 1981 Familial hypocaclciuric hypercalcemia and acute pancreatitis. BMJ **282:**1029–1031.
5. Kristiansen JH, Rodbro P, Christiansen C, Johansen J, Jensen JT 1987 Familial hypocalciuric hypercalcemia III: Bone mineral metabolism. Clin Endocrinol (Oxf) **26:**713–716.
6. Orwoll E, Silbert J, McClung M 1982 Asymptomatic neonatal familial hypercalcemia. Pediatrics **69:**109–111.
7. Marx SJ, Spiegel AM, Brown EM, Koehler JO, Gardner DG, Brennan MF, Aurbach GD 1978 Divalent cation metabolism: Familial hypocalciuric hypercalcemia versus typical primary hyperparathyroidism. Am J Med **65:**235–242.
8. Marx SJ, Fraser D, Rapoport A 1985 Familial hypocalciuric hypercalcemia: Mild expression of the gene in heterozygotes and severe expression in homozygotes. Am J Med **78:**15–22.
9. Firek AF, Kao PC, Heath H III 1991 Plasma intact parathyroid hormone (PTH) and PTH-related peptide in familial benign hypercalcemia: Greater responsiveness to endogenous PTH than in primary hyperparathyroidism. J Clin Endocrinol Metab **72:** 541–546.
10. Kristiansen JH, Rodbro P, Christiansen C, Brochner MJ, Carl J 1985 Familial hypocalciuric hypercalcemia II: Intestinal calcium absorption and vitamin D metabolism. Clin Endocrinol (Oxf) **23:**511–515.
11. Thorgeirsson U, Costa J, Marx SJ 1981 The parathyroid glands in familial hypocalciuric hypercalcemia. Hum Pathol **12:**229–237.
12. Law WM Jr, Carney JA, Heath H III 1984 Parathyroid glands in familial benign hypercalcemia (familial hypocalciuric hypercalcemia). Am J Med **76:**1021–1026.
13. Fukumoto S, Chikatsu N, Okazaki R, Takeuchi Y, Tamura Y, Murakami T, Obara T, Fujita T 2001 Inactivating mutations of calcium-sensing receptor result in parathyroid lipohyperplasia. Diagn Molec Pathol **10:**242–247.
14. Marx SJ, Stock JL, Attie MF, Downs RW Jr, Gardner DG, Brown EM, Spiegel AM, Doppman JL, Brennan MF 1980 Familial hypocalciuric hypercalcemia: Recognition among patients referred after unsuccessful parathyroid exploration. Ann Intern Med **92:**351–356.
15. Simonds WF, James-Newton LA, Agarwal SK, Yang B, Skarulis MC, Hendy GN, Marx SJ 2002 Familial isolated hyperparathyroidism: Clinical and genetic characteristics of thirty-six kindreds. Medicine **81:**1–26.
16. Kifor O, Moore FD Jr, Delaney M, Garber J, Hendy GN, Butters R, Gao P, Cantor TL, Kifor I, Brown EM, Wysolmerski J 2003 A syndrome of hypocalciuric hypercalcemia caused by autoantibodies directed at the calcium-sensing receptor. J Clin Endocrinol Metab **88:**60–72.
17. Szabo E, Carling T, Hessman O, Rastad J 2002 Loss of heterozygosity in parathyroid glands of familial hypercalcemia with hypercalciuria and point mutation in calcium receptor. J Clin Endocrinol Metab **87:**3961–3965.
18. Marx SJ, Attie MF, Spiegel AM, Levine MA, Lasker RD, Fox M 1982 An association between neonatal severe primary hyperparathyroidism and familial hypocalciuric hypercalcemia in three kindreds. N Engl J Med **306:**257–264.
19. Pollak MR, Shou YH-W, Marx SJ, Steinmann B, Cole DEC, Brandi ML, Papapoulos SE, Menko F, Hendy GN, Brown EM, Seidman CE, Seidman JG 1994 Familial hypocalciuric hypercalcemia and neonatal severe hyperparathyroidism: Effects of mutant gene dosage on phenotype. J Clin Invest **93:**1108–1112.

20. Page LA, Haddow JE 1987 Self-limited neonatal hyperparathyroidism in familial hypocalciuric hypercalcemia. J Pediatr **111**:261–264.
21. Bilezikian JP, Potts JT Jr, El-Haj Fuleihan G, Kleerekoper M, Neer R, Peacock M, Rastad J, Silverberg SJ, Udelsman R, Wells SA Jr 2002 Summary statement from a workshop on asymptomatic primary hyperparathyroidism: A perspective for the 21st century. J Bone Miner Res **17**:S2;N2–N12.
22. Attie MF, Gill RJ Jr, Stock JL, Spiegel AM, Downs RW Jr, Levine MA, Marx SJ 1983 Urinary calcium excretion in familial hypocalciuric hypercalcemia: Persistence of relative hypocalciuria after induction of hypoparathyroidism. J Clin Invest **72**:667–676.
23. Brown EM, Pollak M, Hebert SC 1998 The extracellular calcium-sensing receptor: Its role in health and disease. Ann Rev Med **49**:15–29.
24. Heath H III, Jackson CE, Otterud B, Leppert MF 1993 Genetic linkage analysis in familial benign (hypocalciuric) hypercalcemia: Evidence for locus heterogeneity. Am J Hum Genet **53**:193–200.
25. Lloyd SE, Pannett AA, Dixon PH, Whyte MP, Thakker RV 1999 Localization of familial benign hypercalcemia. Oklahoma variant (FBHOk), to chromosome 19q13. Am J Hum Genet **64**:189–195.
26. Hendy GN, D'Souza-Li L, Yang B, Canaff L, Cole DEC 2000 Mutations of the calcium-sensing receptor (CASR) in familial hypocalciuric hypercalcemia, neonatal severe hyperparathyroidism, and autosomal dominant hypocalcemia. Hum Mut **16**:281–296.
27. Antoniucci DM and Shoback D 2002 Calcimimetics in the treatment of primary hyperparathyroidism. J Bone Miner Res **17**:S2;N141–N145.

Chapter 36.   Secondary and Tertiary Hyperparathyroidism

Richard Prince

Department of Medicine, University of Western Australia, Perth, Australia

PHYSIOLOGY

Central to the understanding of the causes of secondary hyperparathyroidism (HPTH) is a detailed understanding of the physiological basis of the regulation of calcium homeostasis. It is failure in these systems that is detected biochemically as secondary HPTH. It is important to understand that parathyroid hormone (PTH) is the most important short-term initiator of defense of a reduction in the extracellular calcium concentration. Although magnesium, phosphate, and calcitriol exert regulatory influences on PTH independent of the calcium level, the principle regulator of PTH secretion is the ionized calcium concentration. The sensing system uses the calcium sensing receptor located in the plasma membrane of the parathyroid gland.[1] When this system senses a calcium level below that considered physiological a state of increased PTH secretion, secondary HPTH occurs. Thus, secondary HPTH is a condition in which the parathyroid glands are responding appropriately to a low extracellular calcium concentration. PTH acts on the organs of calcium transport to correct the defect (Fig. 1). If the increased PTH secretion cannot correct the plasma calcium, either because of a disorder within those organs or because of reduced availability of calcium, hypocalcemia can result. Thus, secondary HPTH can be associated with calcium concentrations that are within or below the population reference range.

The three major regulated sources of calcium entry and exit into the extracellular compartment are the intestine, kidney, and bone. Perspiration is another small source of calcium loss to the extracellular compartment. Calcium exchange also occurs across all cell membranes; however, in general, these fluxes of calcium have no overall effect on extracellular calcium because entry and exit from the cellular compartment are in balance. As discussed below, there are a few pathological situations where this is not so. It is clear from Fig. 1 that impairment in the balance between entry and exit of calcium from the intestine, bone, and kidney will induce secondary HPTH only when there is an overall inability of all the organs acting together to maintain a normal calcium concentration in the extracellular compartment. Secondary HPTH may be caused by a variety of disorders of the organs involved in maintenance of extracellular calcium concentrations (Table 1). It is the task of the clinician to determine the reason or reasons for the persistent error signal and correct them efficiently and elegantly.

CONSEQUENCES OF SECONDARY HPTH

Symptoms of hypocalcemia may occur if secondary HPTH fails to maintain the extracellular calcium concentration, especially in children. If the long-term absorption of calcium from the intestine and reabsorption of filtered calcium from the renal tubule is ineffective in restoring the extracellular calcium concentration, the major alternate sup-

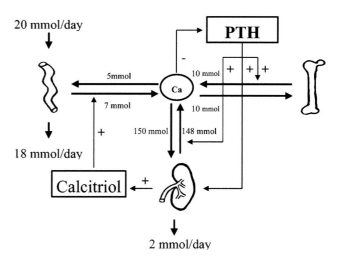

FIG. 1.   Physiology of calcium transport.

The author has no conflict of interest.

TABLE 1. DIFFERENTIAL DIAGNOSIS OF SECONDARY HPTH

Impaired intestinal calcium entry into the extracellular compartment	1) Impaired dietary calcium intake
	  Lactose intolerance
	2) Impaired dietary calcium absorption
	  i) Pancreatic disease—fat malabsorption
	  ii) Damaged enterocytes—celiac disease
	  iii) Calcium sequestration—phytates
	3) Deficiency of vitamin D
	  i) Sunlight deprivation
	  ii) Intestinal vitamin D malabsorption e.g., liver disease

Loss of calcium from the extracellular compartment	1) Bone
	  i) Growth
	  ii) Recovery postlactation
	  iii) Bisphosphonate treatment
	    Pagets disease
	    Osteoporosis
	    Bone cancer
	  iv) "Hungry bone syndrome"
	2) Lactation
	3) Kidney
	  i) Idiopathic hypercalciuria
	  ii) Increased sodium excretion
	  iii) Loop diuretics
	4) Soft tissue
	  i) Rhabdomyolysis
	  ii) Sepsis

Impaired PTH action	1) Renal failure with impaired calcitriol formation and phosphate excretion
	  i) Impaired gut calcium absorption
	  ii) Impaired parathyroid calcium sensing
	2) Pseudo-hypoparathyroidism
	  i) G-protein deficiency

ply of calcium is resorption from the skeleton. If persistent, this results in osteoporosis in adults,[2] whereas in childhood, it is associated with undermineralized osteoid defined histologically as osteomalacia.[3] Both conditions result in biomechanical insufficiency; thus, persistent secondary HPTH may result in bone pain and minimal trauma fractures.[4] It is of interest to note that, under the influence of secondary HPTH, bone is preferentially resorbed from the appendicular cortical skeleton,[5] as opposed to estrogen deficiency, where axial trabecular bone is the first target.

DIAGNOSIS OF SECONDARY HPTH

The diagnosis of secondary HPTH is best made by the measurement of a PTH concentration above the reference range at the time that a measured plasma calcium is normal or low (Tables 1 and 2). There are many excellent PTH assays now available that measure the full-length 1-84 molecule. These tests are best made on a fasting resting venous blood sample taken without a tourniquet because of its effects of increasing albumin concentrations and decreasing pH, both of which may inappropriately increase the ionized calcium concentration. The determination of the circulating calcium concentration is best undertaken by the use of an ionized calcium measurement corrected to a pH of 7.4, detected using a calcium sensitive electrode. However, the albumin corrected total calcium concentration is often used. It is especially important to definitively exclude hypercalcemia because, if present, the diagnosis is that of primary HPTH, a diagnosis that requires a radically different therapeutic approach.

A good assay of circulating 25 hydroxyvitamin D, which measures both the chole and ergocalciferol forms, is essential for the diagnosis of vitamin D deficiency.

Bone turnover markers are useful to identify increased bone turnover associated with the skeletal response to secondary HPTH.

The diagnosis of abnormalities of renal calcium handling are facilitated by the use of the relation between plasma calcium and renal calcium excretion first described by Peacock et al.[6] (Fig. 2). In secondary HPTH, the kidney usually conserves calcium by increasing renal calcium reabsorption, resulting in a low urine calcium concentration. This is a sensitive measurement of calcium deficiency. It is detected by a low urine calcium excretion relative to the plasma calcium, so that when plotted, the patient's renal calcium excretion will be to the right of the reference data. The only exception is when the kidney is the primary source of loss of calcium from the body. Under these circumstances, the renal calcium excretion is to the left of the reference data.

TABLE 2. CLINICAL HISTORY IN THE DIAGNOSIS OF SECONDARY HPTH

	Clinical features
Impaired intestinal calcium absorption	
1) Impaired dietary calcium intake	Low dairy product consumption Lactose intolerance

2) Impaired dietary calcium absorption	Pancreatic Steatorrhoea
	Enterocyte failure
	  Weight loss
	  Diarrhea
	  Iron or B_{12} deficiency
	High dietary fiber intake

3) Vitamin D deficiency	Northern or southern latitudes Lack of outdoor exposure Lack of skin exposure (personal or religious preference) Use of sun screens (skin cancer protection sun sensitivities)
Loss of calcium from the extracellular compartment	
1) Bone	Bisphosphonate treatment
2) Lactation	Recent history of weaning
3) Kidney	Kidney stones Family history Loop diuretic use
4) Soft tissue	Traumatic muscle damage Intensive care treatment Extensive burns
Impaired PTH action	
1) Renal failure	Pruritus Anemia
2) Pseudohypoparathyroidism	Albright phenotype Family history Tetany

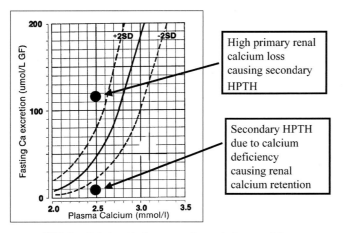

FIG. 2. Relationship between urine and plasma calcium.

INTESTINAL CAUSES OF SECONDARY HPTH

The intestine is the only external source of calcium supply to the various body compartments. There are two main sites of calcium loss that intestinal calcium absorption must replace: the kidney, through a net obligatory renal calcium loss, and the skeleton, especially during phases of growth, and also after cessation of lactation. Childhood and adolescence represent particularly important phases in intestinal calcium absorption because there is a constant flux of calcium into the growing skeleton that is exacerbated by dietary calcium deficiency, resulting in secondary HPTH, and if persistent, severe rickets.[7]

Inadequate Dietary Calcium Intake

Reliable determination of dietary calcium deficiency based on a dietary history is difficult. This is, in part, because dietary calcium requirement depends on calcium handling in the kidney and bone. In addition there is great interindividual variation in the amount of dietary calcium required to achieve calcium balance. Thus, in practice, although it may be occasionally be possible to make a positive clinical diagnosis of a low calcium intake, it is usually a diagnosis of exclusion of other causes.

It is appropriate to determine whether milk products cause abdominal symptoms, because this may be an indicator of lactose intolerance that reduces calcium intake associated with avoidance of milk products.[8] In addition, in subjects with lactose intolerance, lactose will itself induce calcium malabsorption; interestingly, in normal subjects, lactose may increase calcium absorption. Lactose intolerance predicts development of osteoporosis[9] and fracture.[8] The genetic polymorphism resulting in lactose intolerance has recently been described and presents a new diagnostic approach.[10]

Management of calcium deficiency in adults is discussed in greater detail elsewhere, but should include the use of calcium supplements in doses of at least 1200 mg of elemental calcium per day. Management in childhood is discussed elsewhere, but should include doses of calcium of at least 800 mg per day.

Dietary Calcium Malabsorption

There may be blockage of calcium absorption because of pathological processes occurring within the intestinal lumen and at the intestinal wall. In white populations, celiac disease is the most common cause of calcium malabsorption, with or without vitamin D deficiency, because of damage to the absorptive surface of the small intestine. Thus, secondary HPTH, osteoporosis, and occasionally, osteomalacia are common presenting features of celiac disease.[11]

Exocrine pancreatic failure may occur as a result of alcohol, biliary calculi, or cystic fibrosis and results in fat malabsorption. This may promote the development of nonabsorbable calcium soaps within the bowel. Associated malabsorption of fat-soluble vitamins, particularly vitamin D, can induce calcium malabsorption because of vitamin D deficiency.

Another minor cause of impaired calcium absorption is phytic acid, which may bind calcium within the bowel, thus contributing to calcium malabsorption. High-fiber diets have been recommended for various benefits on the bowel and cardiovascular system. Studies that have examined the effects of these diet on calcium consumption have not found any significant deleterious effects with moderate consumption of these foods.[12] However, high-fiber intakes can reduce calcium retention from 25% to 19%.[13]

Vitamin D Deficiency

The principle cause of vitamin D deficiency is lack of sunlight exposure, which prevents formation of vitamin D in the skin. Patients at high risk of vitamin D deficiency are those with restricted sunlight exposure by reason of Northern or Southern latitude, lack of outdoor activity, clothing restrictions, or sunscreen use. The elderly are particularly at risk. Diagnosis is best established by measuring the serum concentration of 25 hydroxyvitamin D level Secondary HPTH and increased bone turnover markers such as alkaline phosphatase are also common. Renal calcium conservation manifested by hypocalciuria is usually present.

Therapy should include increased calcium intake and sunlight exposure where possible[14] and the use of oral cholecalciferol or ergocalciferol in the dose of at least 10,000 U per week until healing has occurred. If there is impaired renal synthesis of calcitriol, one hydroxylated derivative of vitamin D should be prescribed in addition to dietary calcium supplementation.

LOSS OF CALCIUM FROM THE EXTRACELLULAR COMPARTMENT

A net loss of calcium from the extracellular compartment can occur into the skeleton, urine, breast milk during lactation, and into the soft tissue of the body. Incidentally, under circumstances of extremely low calcium intake, there can be a net loss of calcium from the bowel caused by calcium contained within pancreatic and intestinal secretions. This is called endogenous fecal calcium.

Entry of Calcium Into the Bone Compartment

A net flux of calcium into the skeletal compartment may be large enough to cause a decrease in the extracellular calcium concentration and the development of secondary HPTH, if intestinal calcium absorption and renal calcium reabsorption cannot maintain the calcium concentration. In childhood and adolescence, skeletal growth is the major cause of entry of calcium into the skeletal compartment. In adult life, the reformation of the skeleton after lactation-induced bone loss is the major physiological cause of entry of calcium into the skeletal compartment. Other causes of rapid entry of calcium into the skeleton are bisphosphonate therapy for Paget's disease,[15] osteoporosis, or cancer. In the past, this phenomena was observed with the use of estrogen in prostate cancer.[16] It may also occur after parathyroidectomy for severe primary HPTH or tertiary HPTH. The critical diagnostic factor in this setting is the low serum calcium concentration. Therapy is replacement of calcium and vitamin D as discussed above.

Entry of Calcium Into Breast Milk

During lactation, skeletal calcium is released to provide calcium for the developing and growing infant. This process does not involve extra secretion of PTH and is thus not classified as a cause of secondary HPTH, although there are many similarities. It has been suggested that PTH-related peptide secreted by the breast may be the etiological factor. At the end of lactation, the skeleton begins to regenerate, and secondary HPTH may occur if dietary calcium intake is inadequate.[17]

Entry of Calcium Into the Urine

Most commonly, hypercalciuria is associated with increased gut calcium absorption, so called absorptive hypercalciuria, usually associated with renal phosphate loss and increased synthesis of calcitriol. In this condition, although the 24-h urine calcium excretion is elevated, the fasting urine calcium excretion and PTH levels are normal. Primary renal calcium loss (renal hypercalciuria) is a hereditary disorder associated with renal stones, perhaps because of defects in renal ion transport channels. It may also be caused by excessive salt intake[18] or loop diuretic therapy,[19] both of which increase calcium loss in the urine. If these losses are not matched by increased intestinal calcium absorption, secondary HPTH and osteoporosis may occur. The diagnosis is supported by increased renal calcium excretion as assessed by an elevated 24-h and fasting urine calcium (Fig. 2).

Entry of Calcium Into Soft Tissue

Hypoxic damage to muscle or to other soft tissue will damage normal calcium transport across the plasma membrane, which allows unregulated calcium entry into cells. If rapid enough, this results in hypocalcemia and secondary HPTH.[20] Rhabdomyolysis is associated with drugs or compartment syndromes and is best diagnosed by measurement of a raised CPK, myoglobinuria, and technetium diphospho-nate isotope scan to detect the soft tissue uptake. Therapy is supportive while muscle healing occurs.

IMPAIRED PTH ACTION

Renal Failure

The role of PTH in the pathophysiology of renal failure is complex, but in essence, could be considered a state of impaired PTH action on the kidney and bone. Secondary HPTH is an early and common manifestation of chronic renal failure that may occur before clear evidence of phosphate retention. This is a treatable cause of progression of osteoporosis, especially frequent in elderly patients. Early in the course of development of renal failure, restoration of intestinal calcium absorption by increased dietary calcium and vitamin D intake either as calciferol or as calcitriol should be undertaken. In addition, dietary calcium supplementation assists in the control of phosphate concentrations in the extracellular compartment by binding phosphate in the intestine. At high concentrations, phosphate itself plays a role in the development of secondary HPTH by direct stimulation of PTH secretion.[21] Management includes a combination of dietary phosphorus restriction, phosphate binders, and dialysis to remove phosphate from the body.

Impaired PTH Signal Transduction

Failure of PTH signal transduction in the bone and kidney because of mutations in the G-protein–coupling system is an uncommon cause of secondary HPTH that is addressed elsewhere. The failure of PTH action on the bone and kidney results in hypocalcemia and appropriate secondary increases in HPTH. One manifestation of this syndrome, first described by Fuller Albright in 1934 without the benefit of a PTH assay,[22] is associated with short stature, calcific deposits in soft tissue, and one or more short metacarpals or metatarsals. The defect in G-protein signal transduction may be restricted to bone or kidney or may occur in both. If there is loss of the effect of PTH on renal phosphate handling, a high plasma phosphate and renal phosphate threshold is present. Management is aimed at correcting extracellular calcium usually with the use of calcitriol and calcium.

TERTIARY HPTH

The critical difference between secondary and tertiary HPTH is that the plasma calcium is normal or low in secondary HPTH but is elevated in tertiary HPTH. Thus, tertiary HPTH is best thought of as a variety of primary HPTH. This is because, like primary HPTH, the pathological problem in tertiary HPTH resides within the calcium sensing and PTH secretory mechanism within the parathyroid glands, resulting in constitutive overactivity of the parathyroid glands.

The difference from primary HPTH is that tertiary HPTH occurs after a prolonged period of secondary HPTH. Indeed, it has been argued that primary HPTH may occur more commonly in populations with increased prevalence of calcium and vitamin D deficiency. A specific situation in which this term is used is the hypercalcemic HPTH that occurs after the prolonged secondary HPTH of renal failure. This is caused by hyperplasia of one or more parathyroid glands. Another situation in which this term may be used is in the development of hypercalcemic HPTH after the prolonged use of phosphate supplements in patients with hypophosphatemic rickets. In this situation, the episodic increase in plasma phosphate after ingestion of the supplement is considered to induce transient hypocalcemia, which together with relative calcitriol deficiency, results in parathyroid gland hyperplasia.[23] The diagnostic and therapeutic approach is similar to that used for primary HPTH and may be associated with four-gland hyperplasia or an enlarged single gland.

REFERENCES

1. Brown E, MacLeod R 2001 Extracellular calcium sensing and extracellular calcium signaling. Physiol Rev **81:**239–297.
2. Prince RL, Dick IM, Lemmon J, Randell D 1997 The pathogenesis of age-related osteoporotic fracture: Effects of dietary calcium deprivation. J Clin Endocrinol Metab **82:**260–264.
3. Marie PJ, Pettifor JM, Ross FP, Glorieux FH 1982 Histological osteomalacia due to dietary calcium deficiency in children. N Engl J Med **307:**584–588.
4. Hoikka V, Alhava EM, Savolainen K, Parviainen M 1982 Osteomalacia in fractures of the proximal femur. Acta Orthop Scand **53:**255–260.
5. Price RI, Gutteridge DH, Stuckey BGA, Kent N, Retallack RW, Prince RL, Bhagat CI, Johnston CA, Nicholson GC, Stewart GO 1993 Rapid, divergent changes in spinal and forearm bone density following short-term intravenous treatment of Paget's disease with Pamidronate Disodium. J Bone Miner Res **8:**209–217.
6. Peacock M, Robertson WG, Nordin BE 1969 Relation between serum and urinary calcium with particular reference to parathyroid activity. Lancet **1:**384–386.
7. Thacher TD, Fischer PR, Pettifor JM, Lawson JO, Isichei CO, Reading JC, Chan GM 1999 A comparison of calcium, vitamin D, or both for nutritional rickets in Nigerian children. N Engl J Med **341:**563–568.
8. Honkanen R, Koger H, Alhava E, Tuppurainen M, Saarikoski S 1997 Lactose intolerance associated with fractures of weight-bearing bones in Finnish women aged 38–57 years. Bone **21:**473–477.
9. Finkenstedt G, Skrabal F, Gasser RW, Braunsteiner H 1986 Lactose absorption, milk consumption, and fasting blood glucose concentrations in women with idiopathic osteoporosis. BMJ **292:**161–162.
10. Kuokkanen M, Enattah NS, Oksanen A, Savilahti E, Orpana A, Jarvella II 2003 Transcriptional regulation of the lactase-phlorizin hydrolase gene by polymorphisms associated with adult-type hypolactasia. Gut **52:**647–652.
11. Selby PL, Davies M, Adams JE, Mawer EB 1999 Bone loss in celiac disease is related to secondary hyperparathyroidism. J Bone Miner Res **14:**652–657.
12. Wisker E, Nagel R, Tanudjaja TK, Feldheim W 1991 Calcium, magnesium, zinc, and iron balances in young women: Effects of a low-phytate barley-fiber concentrate. Am J Clin Nutr **54:**553–559.
13. Knox TA, Kassarjian Z, Dawson-Hughes B, Golner BB, Dallal GE, Arora S, Russell RM 1991 Calcium absorption in elderly subjects on high- and low-fiber diets: Effect of gastric acidity. Am J Clin Nutr **53:**1480–1486.
14. Chel VGM, Ooms ME, Popp-Snijders C, Pavel S, Schothorst AA, Meulemans CCE, Lips P 1998 Ultraviolet irradiation corrects vitamin D deficiency and suppresses secondary hyperparathyroidism in the elderly. J Bone Miner Res **13:**1238–1242.
15. Devlin RD, Retallack RW, Fenton AJ, Grill V, Gutteridge DH, Kent GN, Prince RL, Worth GK 1994 Long-term elevation of 1,25-dihydroxyvitamin D after short-term intravenous administration of pamidronate (aminohydroxypropylidene bisphosphonate APD) in Paget's disease of bone. J Bone Miner Res **9:**81–85.
16. Kukreja SC, Shanmugam A, Lad TE 1988 Hypocalcemia in patients with prostate cancer. Calcif Tissue Int **43:**340–345.
17. DeSantiago S, Alonso L, Halhali A, Larrea F, Isoard F, Bourges H 2002 Negative calcium balance during lactation in rural Mexican women. Am J Clin Nutr **76:**845–851.
18. Devine A, Criddle RA, Dick IM, Kerr DA, Prince RL 1995 A longitudinal study of the effect of sodium and calcium intakes on regional bone density in postmenopausal women. Am J Clin Nutr **62:**740–745.
19. Stein MS, Scherer SC, Walton SL, Gilbert RE, Ebeling PR, Flicker L, Wark JD 1996 Risk factors for secondary hyperparathyroidism in a nursing home population. Clin Endocrinol (Oxf) **44:**375–383.
20. Llach F, Felsenfeld AJ, Haussler MR 1981 The pathophysiology of altered calcium metabolism in rhabdomyolysis-induced acute renal failure. Interactions of parathyroid hormone, 25-hydroxycholcalciferol and 1, 25-dihdroxycholcalciferol. N Engl J Med **305:**117–123.
21. Estapa JC, Aguilera-Tejero E, Lopez I, Almaden Y, Rodriguez M, Felsenfeld AJ 1999 Effects of phosphate on parathyroid hormone secretion in vivo. J Bone Miner Res **14:**1848–1854.
22. Albright F, Burnett CH, Smith PH 1942 Pseudohypoparathyroidism: An example of "Seabright Bantam" syndrome. Endocrinology **30:**922–932.
23. Makitie O, Kooh SW, Sochett E 2003 Prolonged high-dose phosphate treatment: A risk factor for tertiary hyperparathyroidism in X-linked hypophosphatemic rickets. Clin Endocrinol (Oxf) **58:**163–168.

Chapter 37. Humoral Hypercalcemia of Malignancy

Mara J. Horwitz and Andrew F. Stewart

Division of Endocrinology, University of Pittsburgh School of Medicine, Pittsburgh, Pennsylvania

INTRODUCTION

The term "humoral hypercalcemia of malignancy" (HHM) describes, in broad terms, a clinical syndrome characterized by hypercalcemia caused by the secretion by a cancer of a circulating calcemic factor. The tumor typically has limited or no skeletal involvement. The term describes a classic endocrine system, with the secretory gland being the tumor and the target organs being the skeleton and the kidney. The term can be used in a general sense to describe the production by tumors of any humoral calcemic factor. For example, hypercalcemia resulting from the production of 1,25-dihydroxyvitamin D [$1,25(OH)_2D$] in patients with lymphoma and hypercalcemia resulting from ectopic secretion of parathyroid hormone (PTH) by an ovarian carcinoma would both fulfill the literal criteria for being humoral forms of hypercalcemia. These examples are discussed further at the conclusion of this chapter. As currently used, however, the term HHM describes a very specific clinical syndrome that results from the production of PTH-related protein (PTHrP). The large majority of patients with humorally

The authors have no conflict of interest.

TABLE 1. SIMILARITIES AND DIFFERENCES BETWEEN PATIENTS WITH HPT AND HHM

	HPT	HHM
Humorally mediated hypercalcemia	+	+
Increased osteoclastic bone resorption	+	+
Increased renal calcium reabsorption	+	+
Hypophosphatemia	+	+
Phosphaturia	+	+
Nephrogenous cAMP elevation	+	+
Increased plasma 1,25(OH)$_2$D	+	−
Increased osteoblastic bone formation	+	−
Increased circulating immunoreactive PTH	+	−
Increased circulating immunoreactive PTHrP	−	+
Hypercalcemia due primarily to effects on kidney and gastrointestinal tract	+	−
Hypercalcemia due primarily to effects on kidney and bone	−	+

mediated hypercalcemia have HHM. Several recent detailed reviews of the syndrome are listed at the end of this section.

The syndrome was first described in 1941, in a patient with renal carcinoma and a solitary skeletal metastasis. Subsequent studies in the 1950s and 1960s documented the humoral nature of the syndrome by showing that (1) typical patients had little or no skeletal tumor involvement and (2) the hypercalcemia and other biochemical abnormalities were reversed when the tumor was resected or treated. Evidence provided in the 1960s and 1970s suggested that the responsible factor might be either prostaglandin E$_2$, a vitamin D–like sterol, or PTH. It is now clear that none of these is responsible.

Patients with HHM account for up to 80% of patients with malignancy-associated hypercalcemia. From a clinical standpoint, patients with HHM have advanced disease with tumors that are usually obvious clinically and therefore carry a poor prognosis. As a rule, by the time hypercalcemia occurs in a patient with cancer, survival can be measured in weeks to a few months. Exceptions to this rule include small, well-differentiated endocrine tumors such as pheochromocytomas or islet cell tumors. In contrast to patients with hypercalcemia caused by skeletal involvement with cancer, who typically have breast cancer, multiple myeloma, or lymphomas, patients with HHM most often have squamous carcinomas (involving lung, esophagus, cervix, vulva, skin, or head and neck). Other tumor types commonly associated with HHM are renal, bladder, and ovarian carcinomas. Breast carcinomas may cause typical HHM, or they may lead to hypercalcemia through skeletal metastatic involvement. Finally, the subset of hypercalcemic patients with lymphomas caused by human T-cell leukemia virus I seem to have classic biochemical HHM. Certain common tumors (e.g., colon, prostate, thyroid, oat cell, and gastric carcinomas) rarely cause hypercalcemia of any type.

Biochemically and histologically, patients with HHM share certain features with patients with primary hyperparathyroidism (HPT) and differ in other respects (Table 1; Figs. 1–4). Both groups of patients have a humoral syndrome, both are hypercalcemic, and both are hy-

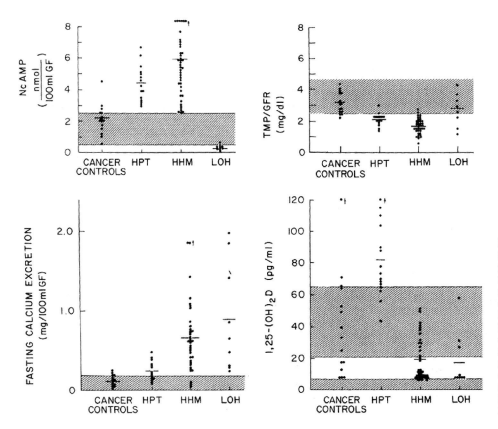

FIG. 1. Nephrogenous cAMP excretion (NcAMP), renal tubular maximum for phosphorus (TmP/GFR), fasting calcium excretion, and plasma 1,25(OH)$_2$D values in normocalcemic patients with cancer (cancer controls) and in patients with HPT, with HHM, and with hypercalcemia caused by bone metastases or local osteolytic hypercalcemia (LOH). (Adapted with permission from Stewart AF, Horst R, Deftos LJ, Cadman EC, Lang R, Broadus AE 1980 Biochemical evaluation of patients with cancer-associated hypercalcemia: Evidence for humoral and non-humoral groups. N Engl J Med 303:1377–1383.)

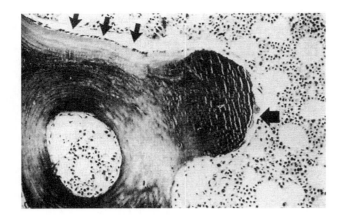

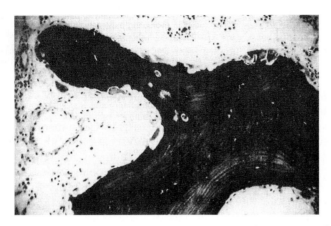

FIG. 2. Comparison of bone histology in a patient with HPT (top) and HHM (bottom). In both groups, osteoclastic activity is accelerated, although it is higher in HHM than in HPT. In HPT, osteoblastic activity and osteoid are increased, but both are markedly decreased in HHM. This uncoupling of formation from resorption in HHM plays the major rule in causing hypercalcemia. (Reproduced with permission from Stewart AF, Vignery A, Silverglate A, Ravin ND, LiVolsi V, Broadus AE, Baron R, 1982 Quantitative bone histomorphometry in humoral hypercalcemia of malignancy: Uncoupling of bone cell activity. J Clin Endocrinol Metab **55**:219–227.)

pophosphatemic and display reductions in the renal tubular phosphorus threshold. Both groups display increased nephrogenous or urinary cyclic adenosine monophosphate (cAMP) excretion, indicating an interaction of the respective humoral mediator with proximal tubular PTH receptors. Both groups display increases in osteoclastic bone resorption when bone is examined histologically (Fig. 2). Hypercalcemia in both groups result, in part, from increased distal tubular calcium reabsorption mediated by PTH and PTHrP.

In contrast, patients with HHM differ from those with HPT in two important respects (Fig. 1; Table 1). First, PTH is a potent stimulus for the renal production of $1,25(OH)_2D$. Patients with HPT therefore often show increases in circulating $1,25(OH)_2D$ and a resultant increase in calcium absorption by the intestine. In contrast, patients with HHM display reductions in serum $1,25(OH)_2D$ values and in intestinal calcium absorption. The physiology underlying this observation is uncertain, because N-terminal PTHrPs in vitro and in vivo stimulate

renal 1α-hydroxylase, the enzyme that synthesizes $1,25(OH)_2D$. Second, osteoblastic bone formation is increased and coupled to the increased bone resorption rate in patients with HPT (Fig. 2). In patients with HHM, however, osteoblastic bone formation is reduced and is therefore dissociated or uncoupled from the increased osteoclastic bone resorption (Fig. 2). The reasons for this uncoupling are also unclear, because synthetic N-terminal PTHrPs in vitro and in vivo in animals stimulate osteoblastic activity. Of course, immunoreactive PTH concentrations in plasma are elevated in patients with HPT, but they are suppressed in patients with HHM (Fig. 3). Conversely, immunoreactive PTHrP values are elevated in HHM, but they are normal in patients with HPT (Fig. 4). Preliminary studies suggested that the immunoreactive PTHrP concentration may be useful in monitoring responses to surgery, chemotherapy, or radiotherapy in patients in whom levels are elevated before therapy.

Hypercalcemia in patients with HHM has both skeletal and renal components. The skeletal component, as noted earlier, reflects increased osteoclast activity and uncoupling of osteoblasts from osteoclasts. The renal component reflects PTHrP-mediated increases in distal tubular calcium reabsorption. In addition, patients with HHM are usually volume depleted, partly as a result of their hypercalcemia, with resultant inability to concentrate the

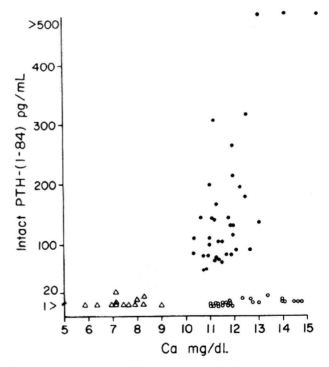

FIG. 3. Immunoreactive PTH concentration of PTH by using a two-site immunoradiometric assay for PTH(1-84) in patients with primary hyperparathyroidism (solid circles), in patients with hypoparathyroidism (open triangles), and in patients with hypercalcemia of malignancy (open circles). (Adapted with permission from Nussbaum S, Zahradnik RJ, Lavigne JR, et al. 1987 Highly sensitive two-site immunoradiometric assay of parathyrin and its clinical utility in evaluating patients with hypercalcemia. Clin Chem **33**:1364–1367.)

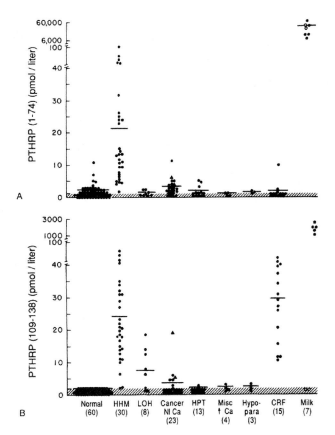

FIG. 4. Immunoreactive PTHrP values in patients with HHM and in various control groups. PTHrP values shown were obtained by using a two-site immunoradiometric assay (IRMA) directed against PTHrP(1-74) (A) and a carboxyterminal PTHrp radioimmunoassay (B). (Adapted with permission from Burtis WJ, Brady TG, Orloff JJ, et al. 1980 Immunochemical characterization of circulating PTH-related protein in patients with humoral hypercalcemia of malignancy. N Engl J Med **322:**1106–1112.)

urine, and partly as a result of poor oral fluid intake. The volume depletion leads to a reduction in the filtered load of calcium and a further reduction in the excretion of calcium.

Therapy of HHM is discussed in more detail elsewhere. Therapy should include measures aimed at (1) reducing the tumor burden, (2) reducing osteoclastic bone resorption, and (3) augmenting renal calcium clearance. Measures aimed at reducing tumor burden (surgery, radiotherapy, and chemotherapy) lead to a reduction in the circulating concentration of PTHrP. Measures aimed at inhibiting osteoclastic bone resorption (use of bisphosphonates, mithramycin, or calcitonin) may reverse hypercalcemia but have no effect on circulating PTHrP concentrations.

UNUSUAL FORMS OF HUMORAL HYPERCALCEMIA

The two broad categories of malignancy-associated hypercalcemia described in this chapter (HHM) and elsewhere (hypercalcemia caused by hematologic malignancies and solid tumors associated with extensive skeletal involvement) comprise the vast majority of patients with cancer and

hypercalcemia. It should, however, be clear that other mechanisms, although uncommon, may be encountered. For example, patients who clearly display humorally mediated hypercalcemic syndromes (i.e., hypercalcemia that is reversed by tumor resection) have been reported who do not fit into the HHM biochemical categorization described. The humoral mediator in these patients is unknown. Rare patients with renal carcinomas have been described who seem to have *bona fide* tumor secretion of prostaglandin E_2 as a cause.

Finally, it is important to emphasize that patients with cancer may develop hypercalcemia as a result of other coexisting conditions, such as primary HPT, tuberculosis, sarcoidosis, immobilization, and use of calcium-containing hyperalimentation solutions. These causes should be actively sought and corrected.

In addition to these poorly characterized syndromes, two types of malignancy-associated hypercalcemia, although rare, have been well characterized and are interesting mechanistically. These are described below.

1,25(OH)$_2$D-Secreting Lymphomas

Breslau et al. and Rosenthal et al. in 1984 described six patients with malignant lymphomas in whom circulating concentrations of 1,25(OH)$_2$D were found to be elevated, in some cases strikingly so. Seymour et al. presented a review and update of this syndrome in 1994. The elevation of plasma 1,25(OH)$_2$D is in contrast to findings in other types of malignancy-associated hypercalcemia (Fig. 1). No evidence for a role for either PTH or PTHrP has been found. Resection or medical therapy of the lymphomas reverses the hypercalcemia and reverses the elevations of 1,25(OH)$_2$D in plasma. No unifying histological theme is present among the lymphomas. Rather, lymphomas of several different subcategories are included in this group. The elevations and hypercalcemia are corrected with glucocorticoid therapy. This syndrome seems to be the malignant counterpart of sarcoidosis, with malignant lymphocytes, macrophages, or both converting diet- and sun-derived 25(OH)D to 1,25(OH)$_2$D.

Ectopic Hyperparathyroidism

From the 1940s through the 1970s, what is now called HHM was widely attributed to ectopic secretion of parathyroid hormone by malignant tumors. Terms such as "ectopic hyperparathyroidism" and "pseudohyperparathyroidism" were in common use. In the 1980s, as described earlier, it was recognized that the vast majority of cases of HHM were caused by PTHrP, and it was questioned whether "ectopic secretion of PTH" even existed. In the 1990s, this question was clearly answered. At the time of this writing, seven cases of what can be described as authentic "ectopic hyperparathyroidism" have been reported. These tumors included two small-cell carcinomas (one of the lung and one of the ovary), a squamous carcinoma of the lung, an adenocarcinoma of the ovary, a thymoma, an undifferentiated neuroendocrine tumor, and a papillary carcinoma of the thyroid. Immunoreactive PTH was found to be elevated in state-of-the-art PTH two-site assays and declined with the hypercalcemia after tumor resection. In most cases, PTH was present immunohistochemically; the tumors secreted PTH, but not PTHrP, into their culture medium in vitro; the tumors contained PTH, but not PTHrP, mRNA. In one case, PTH overexpression by an ovarian tumor resulted from a rearrangement of the *PTH* gene, which placed it under the control of an ovarian promoter. These findings make it clear that authentic ectopic secretion of PTH, although exceedingly rare, can occur. This entity should be considered in the diagnosis of patients with hypercalcemia and increased concentrations of PTH.

SUGGESTED READINGS

Humoral Hypercalcemia of Malignancy

1. Body JJ, Lortholary A, Romeiu ZG, Vigneron AM, Ford J 1999 A dose-finding study of zolendronate in hypercalcemic cancer patients. J Bone Miner Res **14:**1557–1561.
2. Bonjour J-P, Phillipe J, Guelpa G, Bisetti A, Rizzoli R, Jung A, Rosini S, Kanis JA 1988 Bone and renal components of hypercalcemia in malignancy and responses to a single infusion of clodronate. Bone **9:**123–130.
3. Budayr AA, Zysset E, Jenzer A, Thiebaud D, Ammann P, Rizzoli R, Jaquet-Muller F, Bonjour JP, Gertz B, Burckhardt P 1994 Effects of treatment of malignancy-associated hypercalcemia on serum parathyroid hormone-related protein. J Bone Miner Res **9:**521–526.
4. Everhart-Caye M, Inzucchi SE, Guinness-Henry J, Mitnick MA, Stewart AF 1995 Parathyroid hormone-related protein(1–36) is equipotent with parathyroid hormone (1–34) in humans. J Clin Endocrinol Metab **81:**199–208.
5. Godsall JW, Burtis WJ, Insogna KL, Broadus AE, Stewart AF 1986 Nephrogenous cyclic AMP, adenylate cyclase-stimulating activity, and the humoral hypercalcemia of malignancy. In: Greep RO (ed.) Recent Progress in Hormone Research, vol. 42. Academic Press, Boca Raton, FL, USA, pp. 705–750.
6. Grill V, Ho P, Body JJ, Johanson N, Lee SC, Kukreja SC, Moseley JM, Martin TJ 1991 Parathyroid hormone-related protein: Elevated levels in both humoral hypercalcemia of malignancy and hypercalcemia complicating metastatic breast cancer. J Clin Endocrinol Metab **73:**1309–1315.
7. Grill V, Murray RML, Ho PWM, Santamaria JD, Pitt P, Potts C, Jerums G, Martin TJ 1992 Circulating PTH and PTHrP levels before and after treatment of tumor induced hypercalcemia with pamidronate disodium (APD). J Clin Endocrinol Metab **74:**468–470.
8. Horwitz MJ, Tedesco MB, Gundberg C, Garcia-Ocaña A, Stewart AF 2003 Short-term, high-dose PTHrP as a skeletal anabolic agent for the treatment of postmenopausal osteoporosis. J Clin Endocrinol Metab **88:**569–575.
9. Horwitz MJ, Tedesco MB, Sereika S, Hollis B, Garcia-Ocaña A, Stewart AF 2003 Direct comparison of sustained infusion of hPTHrP(1–36) versus hPTH(1–34) on serum calcium, plasma 1,25(OH)₂ vitamin D concentrations and fractional calcium excretion in healthy human volunteers. J Clin Endocrinol Metab **88:**1603–1609.
10. Ikeda K, Ohno H, Hane M, Yokoi H, Okada M, Honma T, Yamada A, Tatsumi Y, Tanaka T, Saitoh T 1994 Development of a sensitive two-site immunoradiometric assay for parathyroid hormone-related peptide: Evidence for elevated levels in plasma from patients with adult T-cell leukemia/lymphoma and B-cell lymphoma. J Clin Endocrinol Metab **79:**1322–1327.
11. Isales C, Carcangiu ML, Stewart AF 1987 Hypercalcemia in breast cancer: A reassessment of the mechanism. Am J Med **82:**1143–1147.
12. Motokura T, Fukumoto S, Matsumoto T, Takahashi S, Fujita A, Yamashita T, Igarashi T, Ogata E 1989 Parathyroid hormone-related protein in adult T-cell leukemia-lymphoma. Ann Intern Med **111:**484–488.
13. Nagai Y, Yamato H, Akaogi K, Hirose K, Ueyama Y, Ikeda K, Matsumoto T, Fujita T, Ogata E 1998 Role of interleukin 6 in uncoupling of bone in vivo in human squamous carcinoma co-producing PTHrP and interleukin 6. J Bone Miner Res **13:**664–672.
14. Nakayama K, Fukumoto S, Takeda S, Takeuchi Y, Ishikawa T, Miura M, Hata K, Hane M, Tamura Y, Tanaka Y, Kitaoka M, Obara T, Ogata E, Matsumoto T 1996 Differences in bone and vitamin D metabolism between primary hyperparathyroidism and malignancy-associated hypercalcemia. J Clin Endocrinol Metab **81:**607–611.
15. Ralson SH, Gallagher SJ, Patel U, Campbell J, Boyle IT 1990 Cancer-associated hypercalcemia: Morbidity and mortality. Ann Intern Med **112:**499–504.
16. Skrabanek P, McPartlin J, Powell DM 1980 Tumor hypercalcemia and ectopic hyperparathyroidism. Medicine (Baltimore) **59:**262–282.
17. Stewart AF, Broadus AE 2001 Malignancy-associated hypercalcemia. In: DeGroot L, Jameson LJ (eds.) Endocrinology, 4th ed. W. B. Saunders, Philadelphia, PA, USA, pp. 1093–1100.
18. Stewart AF, Vignery A, Silvergate A, Ravin ND, LiVolsi V, Broadus AE, Baron R 1982 Quantitative bone histomorphometry in humoral hypercalcemia of malignancy: Uncoupling of bone cell activity. J Clin Endocrinol Metab **55:**219–227.

1,25(OH)₂D-Secretory Lymphomas

19. Breslau NA, McGuire JL, Zerwekh JR, Frenkel EP, Pak CYC 1984 Hypercalcemia associated with increased serum calcitrion levels in three patients with lymphoma. Ann Intern Med **100:**1–7.
20. Rosenthal NR, Insogna KL, Godsall JW, Smaldone L, Waldron JW, Stewart AF 1985 1,25 dihydroxyvitamin D-mediated humoral hypercalcemia in malignant lymphoma. J Clin Endocrinol Metab **60:**29–33.
21. Seymour JF, Gagel RF, Hagemeister FB, Dimopoulos MA, Cabanillas F 1994 Calcitriol production in hypercalcemia and normocalcemic patients with non-Hodgkin lymphoma. Ann Intern Med **121:**633–640.

Ectopic Hyperparathyroidism

22. Nussbaum SR, Gaz RD, Arnold A 1990 Hypercalcemia and ectopic secretion of PTH by an ovarian carcinoma with rearrangement of the gene for PTH. N Engl J Med **323:**1324–1328.
23. Iguchi H, Miyagi C, Tomita K, Kawauchi S, Nozuka Y, Tsuneyoshi M, Wakasugi H 1998 Hypercalcemia caused by ectopic production of parathyroid hormone in a patient with papillary adenocarcinoma of the thyroid gland. J Clin Endocrinol Metab **83:**2653–2657.

Chapter 38. Hypercalcemia in Hematologic Malignancies and in Solid Tumors Associated With Extensive Localized Bone Destruction

Gregory A. Clines and Theresa A. Guise

Division of Endocrinology and Metabolism, Department of Medicine, University of Virginia, Charlottesville, Virginia

HYPERCALCEMIA AND BONE DESTRUCTION IN MULTIPLE MYELOMA

Almost all patients with multiple myeloma have extensive bone destruction that may occur either as discrete local lesions or as diffuse involvement throughout the axial skeleton. This increased bone resorption is responsible for a number of disabling features, including susceptibility to pathological fracture, intractable bone pain, and in some patients, hypercalcemia. Approximately 80% of patients with myeloma present with the chief complaint of bone pain. Hypercalcemia occurs in between 20% and 40% of patients at some time during the course of the disease.

The bone destruction that occurs in myeloma is caused by an increase in the number and activity of osteoclasts. Myeloma cells in the marrow cavity produce cytokines that activate adjacent endosteal osteoclasts to resorb bone (Fig. 1). This was first recognized by observations on cultured human myeloma cells, which were found to release factors that stimulate osteoclast activity.[1,2] There is also evidence that the bone microenvironment promotes growth of the myeloma cells, which then enhance osteoclastogenesis and sets up the vicious cycle of bone osteolysis. Identification of myeloma-stimulating factors within the bone microenvironment has been elusive. Interleukin-6 (IL-6), produced by both osteoclasts and osteoblasts, is mitogenic and reduces apoptosis in myeloma cells.[3] Insulin-like growth factor-1 (IGF-1), produced by bone marrow stromal cells, also contributes to myeloma survival and activates a signal transduction pathway that is independent of IL-6 signaling.[4] It has been demonstrated that osteoclast activity promotes myeloma survival; severe combined immunodeficient (SCID) mice inoculated with human myeloma cells show inhibition of myeloma growth in the presence of the osteoclast inhibitors pamidronate and zoledronic acid.[5]

In contrast to the mechanisms of myeloma survival within bone, myeloma-induced osteoclastogenesis is clearer. Established cultures of human myeloma cells produce lymphotoxin, as well as other potential osteolytic factors; however, a major portion of bone-resorbing activity produced by these cells in vitro cannot be accounted for by lymphotoxin.[6] Other studies show that IL-1, IL-6, parathyroid hormone-related peptide (PTHrP), hepatocyte growth factor (HGF), and macrophage inflammatory protein-1α (MIP-1α) may also be involved in bone destruction.[7–10] Myeloma cells produce IL-6, but IL-6 is not by itself a powerful bone resorbing factor. PTHrP has been shown to be expressed in myeloma cells in some patients and increased in the plasma of some hypercalcemic patients.[9]

HGF, secreted and membrane-bound, is a product of myeloma cells and can induce osteoblast production of IL-11, which may play a role in osteolysis.[11] MIP-1α belongs to the RANTES family of chemokines. Recently, MIP-1α was found to enhance osteoclast formation induced by IL-6, PTHrP, or RANKL.[12] There was also evidence that MIP-1α directly activates early osteoclast precursors and is therefore independent of RANKL expression. In contrast to this study, one group demonstrated that MIP-1α and MIP-1β are dependent on RANKL, leading to the activation of bone marrow stromal cells.[13] It is likely that both suppositions are correct, because both groups show the presence of target MIP-1α receptors on early osteoclast precursors and stromal cells, respectively. Additionally, this molecule may have a major role in the pathogenesis of multiple myeloma as MIP-1α expression is increased in some myeloma bone marrow samples.[10] In a small study, MIP-1α neutralizing antibodies blocked osteoclast formation in bone marrow cultures treated with human myeloma bone marrow plasma[10] and were also shown to have a beneficial effect in an in vivo mouse myeloma model.[14]

Myeloma cells express the cell-surface molecule VLA-4 ($\alpha_4\beta_1$-integrin), a receptor that has affinity for fibronectin and vascular cell adhesion molecule-1 (VCAM-1). Bone

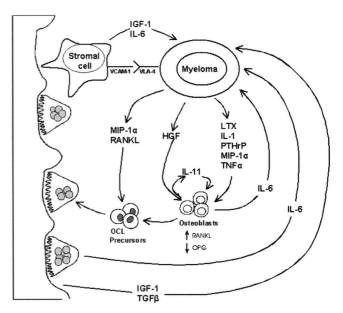

FIG. 1. Bone resorption in multiple myeloma. Numerous local factors have been identified in the bone microenvironment that contribute to increased bone resorption and osteolytic disease. IGF-1 and IL-6 secreted by bone marrow stromal cells and the VLA-4/VCAM-1 interaction increase myeloma proliferation and survival. Myeloma cells secrete factors that ultimately lead to an increase in osteoclast activity and numbers.

The authors have no conflict of interest.

marrow stromal cells express VCAM-1, thereby presumably promoting recruitment of myeloma to bone. Disruption of the VLA-4/VCAM-1 interaction in vitro results in decreased osteoclastic activity and seems to be independent of other bone microenvironment cytokines, including IL-1, IL-6, tumor necrosis factor α (TNFα), and PTHrP.[15] The VLA-4/VCAM-1 system also has a role in the regulation of RANKL and osteoprotegerin (OPG), the decoy receptor of RANKL. Cocultures of human myeloma and bone marrow stromal cells result in an increase in RANKL and a decrease in OPG expression by the stromal cells and therefore promote an environment for enhanced osteoclastogenesis. This imbalance of RANKL/OPG is inhibited in the presence of VLA-4–neutralizing antibodies.[16] A mouse model of multiple myeloma shows that an antibody inhibitor of RANKL prevents the myeloma bone destruction.[17] Increased expression RANKL in stromal cells was also found in bone marrow biopsy specimens of patients with multiple myeloma.[18] Finally, myeloma cells were recently discovered to express RANKL.[19] They could activate osteoclast precursors directly and bypass osteoblast and bone marrow stromal cell intermediaries. The difficulties in interpreting some of these results are knowing whether the in vitro behavior of the myeloma cells is the same as their behavior in vivo. Although we cannot at this time be absolutely certain of the cytokine(s) responsible for bone destruction in myeloma, it is clear that many different osteolytic factors are implicated. These factors can act directly or indirectly through RANK ligand/OPG to stimulate osteoclast activity.

Although essentially all patients with myeloma develop extensive bone destruction, less than 40% become hypercalcemic. Moreover, there is not a close correlation between the extent of bone destruction and the development of hypercalcemia.[20] The explanation is that increased bone resorption most likely leads to hypercalcemia in those patients with impaired glomerular filtration. Impairment of glomerular filtration decreases the kidney's capacity to excrete calcium and clear this from the circulation. Impairment of glomerular filtration is common in patients with myeloma[21] for a number of reasons. Probably the most important is the development of Bence Jones nephropathy, otherwise called "myeloma kidney." In this circumstance, free light-chain fragments of immunoglobin molecules (Bence Jones proteins) are filtered by the glomerulus but impair both glomerular and tubular function. Patients with myeloma may also develop azotemia, because of recurrent infections, uric acid nephropathy, and amyloidosis.

Because the mechanisms responsible for hypercalcemia are different in patients with myeloma from patients with other types of malignancy, there are subtle disparities in laboratory tests at the time of diagnosis. Because renal function is impaired, many patients with myeloma have increased serum phosphorus rather than decreased serum phosphorus, which is common with other types of hypercalcemia of malignancy. In addition, serum alkaline phosphatase, a marker of osteoblast activity, is usually not increased in patients with myeloma because there is little active new bone formation. For similar reasons, bone scans may also be negative.

HYPERCALCEMIA IN SOLID TUMORS ASSOCIATED WITH EXTENSIVE LOCALIZED BONE DESTRUCTION

The potential for tumor metastasis, especially to bone, is greater with certain types of cancers. Lung, breast, and prostate cancer all frequently metastasize to bone, and bone metastases are present in nearly all patients with advanced breast or prostate cancer. Bone is the third most common site of metastasis of solid tumors after the liver and the lung. Metastatic bone disease is generally divided into osteoblastic and osteolytic disease, but most cancers lie within a spectrum of these two extremes. Osteolytic metastases are much more common, however, and are one of the most feared complications of malignancy. They are usually destructive and are much more likely to be associated with pathological fracture and hypercalcemia. The consequences for the patient include intractable bone pain at the site of the metastasis, pathological fracture after trivial injury, nerve compression syndromes caused by obstruction of foramina (the most serious example is spinal cord compression), and hypercalcemia, when bone destruction is advanced. Once tumor cells are housed in the skeleton, curative therapy is no longer possible in most patients, only palliative therapy is available. Tumor cells metastasize most frequently to the axial skeleton, and particularly the vertebrae, pelvis, proximal ends of the long bones, and skull. It is clear that there are important properties of both the tumor cell (the seed) and the skeleton (the soil) that determine the likelihood that any particular tumor will metastasize to bone.

The mechanism by which a solitary tumor is able to escape and invade other distant structures is beginning to be understood. Once tumor cells enter the circulation, they traverse vascular organs, including the red bone marrow, where they migrate through wide-channeled sinusoids to the endosteal bone surface. Because hypercalcemia of breast cancer is associated with extensive bone metastasis in the majority of patients, understanding the mechanism for tumor cell migration to bone and subsequent bone destruction should also clarify the mechanisms by which breast cancer cells cause hypercalcemia.

The process of metastasis can be divided into four stages: escape from the primary site, homing to a particular organ or tissue, adhesion to and invasion of that structure, and propagation in a hospitable environment. The escape process is not well-defined but may involve downregulation of the adhesion protein E-cadherin. In one report, the expression of this molecule is absent in a metastatic breast cancer cell line but transfection of an E-cadherin construct results in impaired osteolysis. Interestingly, E-cadherin does not affect proliferation capacity in culture.[22] This implies that this adhesion molecule and potentially others inhibit the liberation tumor cells from the primary site.

The propensity of tumors to spread to preferred sites suggests specific molecular interactions of the tumor cells with the environment at the site of metastases. A comprehensive study to identify potential chemokine receptors in the migration of breast cancer cells to metastatic sites reported that CXCR4 is highly expressed in these cells and the ligand, stromal cell derived factor-1α (SDF-1α or CXCL12), is present in tissues that represent common sites of metastasis, including bone marrow. Moreover, neutralizing antibodies to this receptor impaired metastasis to regional lymph nodes and lung in a mouse model, but bone metastasis was not examined.[23] Another adhesion molecule, $\alpha v \beta 3$ integrin, binds the RGD peptide sequence that is found on a variety of extracellular matrix proteins and seems to be important in homing and possibly invasion of tumor cells into the bone endosteum.[24,25] The matrix metalloproteinases and urokinase also seem to have a role in cancer cell adhesion/invasion through proteolysis of the extracellular matrix.[26,27]

Significant progress has been made in the last several years elucidating the paracrine molecular interactions of breast cancer metastases with the local bone environment (Fig. 2). PTHrP is produced in excessive amounts, particularly in patients with metastatic breast cancer, but produced relatively specifically in the bone microenvironment.[28,29] The increased local PTHrP concentration drives RANKL expression and inhibits OPG secretion from osteoblasts and stromal cells and thereby activating osteoclastogenesis through RANK located on osteoclast precursors.[30] This production of PTHrP in the bone microenvironment is caused by bone-derived transforming growth factor β (TGFβ), which is released in active form as a consequence of bone resorption. Thus, the vicious cycle begins: tumor cell production of PTHrP stimulates osteoclastic bone resorption and release of more TGFβ, which in turn stimulates more tumor-produced PTHrP. This vicious cycle can be interrupted by neutralizing PTHrP effects,[29] reducing its production,[31] or by making tumor cells less susceptible to TGFβ.[32] The TGFβ signal is transduced by the p38 mitogen-activated protein kinase (MAPK) and the Smad pathways in the MDA-MB-231 breast cancer cell line. The combination of Smad dominant-negative blockade and p38 MAPK inhibition results in complete inhibition of TGFβ-stimulated PTHrP production.[33]

Tumor cells also produce a number of other important factors that lead to osteolysis. IL-6, IL-11, and vascular endothelial growth factor (VEGF) are secreted by osteolytic breast cancer cell lines from TGFβ stimulation and potentiate the effects of PTHrP on osteoclastic bone resorption.[34,35] IL-8 production correlates with an increased metastatic potential in MDA-MB-231 cells but seems to be independent of PTHrP secretion.[36] Bone-derived factors besides TGFβ also contribute to the vicious cycle. The insulin-like growth factors are released into the local bone environment during osteolysis and likely also have a role in the proliferation of bone metastases.[37,38] Extracellular calcium is also released as a consequence of osteoblastic bone resorption and stimulates tumor PTHrP production.[39,40]

HYPERCALCEMIA ASSOCIATED WITH LYMPHOMAS

Occasionally, patients with various lymphomas develop hypercalcemia.[41] This can occur in Hodgkin's disease, B-cell lymphomas, T-cell lymphomas, and Burkitt's lymphoma. In T-cell lymphomas, it is frequently associated with the human T-cell lymphotrophic virus-type I (HTLVI). This is an oncogenic type C retrovirus that is related to the

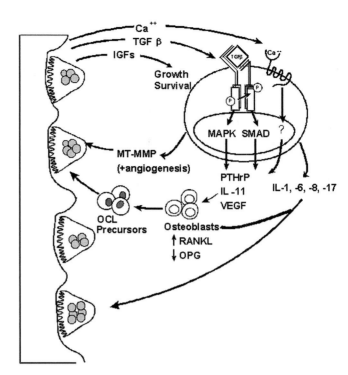

FIG. 2. Bone resorption in breast cancer osteolytic metastases. PTHrP secreted by tumor cells increases RANKL and decreases OPG activity, resulting in increased osteoclastogenesis. This escalation in bone resorption leads to higher levels of TGFβ, which activates tumor cells to produce even more PTHrP; thus, the "vicious cycle" of osteolytic bone metastases begins.

acquired immunodeficiency syndrome virus, infects certain T cells, and results in a lymphoproliferative T-cell disorder.[42] The cause of hypercalcemia and bone destruction in these lymphomas has been well characterized. In most cases, it is probably because of a bone-resorbing factor produced by the neoplastic lymphoid cells. In Japan, where hypercalcemia associated with human T-cell lymphoma virus (HTLV)-lymphoproliferative disorders is common, serum 1,25-dihydroxyvitamin D [1,25(OH)$_2$D] is not increased, but production of the PTHrP by neoplastic cells is clearly demonstrated.[43] In a few patients, hypercalcemia may be caused, at least in part, by increased 1,25(OH)$_2$D production by the lymphoid cells. Several patients with different types of lymphoma and hypercalcemia have been found to have increased serum 1,25(OH)$_2$D concentrations.[44] When measured, this has been associated with increased absorption of calcium from the intestine. Lymphoid cells transformed by inoculation with HTLV-I virus develop the capacity to synthesize 1,25(OH)$_2$D.[45] However, there has been controversy about the relative frequency of increased serum 1,25(OH)$_2$D in patients with hypercalcemia associated with lymphoproliferative disorders. One group reported that one-half of their patients had increased serum 1,25(OH)$_2$D concentrations.[46]

Hypercalcemia also occurs occasionally in other hematologic malignancies such as chronic lymphocytic leukemia, acute leukemia, and chronic myelogenous leukemia, particularly during acute blast transformation. However, the association of hypercalcemia with these disorders is unusual enough that these patients should be carefully evaluated for another cause of hypercalcemia. In most patients, if another cause is present, this will be primary hyperparathyroidism.

Treatment of hypercalcemia caused by excessive $1,25(OH)_2D$ is usually successful by reducing intestinal calcium absorption through the reduction of calcium intake, avoidance of sun exposure, and elimination of dietary vitamin D. Glucocorticoids are also effective in reducing $1,25(OH)_2D$ production.

TREATMENT OF HYPERCALCEMIA AND OSTEOLYTIC BONE DISEASE

Hypercalcemia of malignancy is a common complication of multiple myeloma and osteolytic metastases and is primarily the result of increased bone resorption. Tumor cells produce local factors within the bone microenvironment that ultimately activate osteoclasts and release calcium from bone. The initial presentation of multiple myeloma is often symptoms of hypercalcemia such as abdominal pain, muscle weakness, and polyuria; however, many patients experience the direct manifestations of osteolytic lesions such as bone pain and vertebral collapse.

The acute treatment of moderate to severe hypercalcemia of malignancy is aimed at reducing serum calcium levels within the first day of discovery. The use of volume expansion, followed by a loop diuretic once the patient is volume replete, to promote calcium excretion, can effectively lower serum calcium levels within the first 6–12 h of treatment. Salmon calcitonin also has a rapid effect by reducing bone resorption, but long-term use is limited by tachyphylaxis. Other agents such as mithramycin and gallium nitrate have been used in the past but now only rarely. These medications are nephrotoxic, and their use in the treatment of hypercalcemia is no longer recommended, because glomerular filtration is often impaired in multiple myeloma patients.

The bisphosphonates are currently the mainstay for long-term treatment of hypercalcemia and osteolytic bone disease. They have an affinity for bone surfaces undergoing active resorption and are released in the bone microenvironment during remodeling. These compounds decrease osteoclastic bone resorption by two described mechanisms. The nitrogen-substituted bisphosphonates, such as alendronate, risedronate, and zoledronic acid, are potent inhibitors of the enzyme farnesyl diphosphate synthase, thereby blocking protein isoprenylation. It is believed that the prenylation of small GTP-binding proteins are important for structural integrity of the osteoclast: without it, the osteoclasts undergo apoptosis. The non-nitrogen containing bisphosphonates, clodronate and etidronate, are less potent and also induce osteoclastic apoptosis but by a different mechanism. These bisphosphonates are metabolically incorporated into nonhydrolyzable ATP analogs that inhibit ATP-dependent intracellular enzymes. The bisphosphonates have been known to inhibit osteoclastic bone resorption for over 30 years. The Food and Drug Administration (FDA) approved their use for the treatment of myeloma osteolytic bone disease in 1995 and osteolytic bone disease caused by breast cancer in 1996.

Pamidronate and zoledronic acid are the only bisphosphonates currently FDA approved for the treatment of multiple myeloma osteolytic bone disease in the United States. A large study by Berenson et al.[47] showed that patients with stage III multiple myeloma treated with pamidronate every 4 weeks for 21 cycles had a reduction in skeletal related events (SRE), such as pathological fracture, need for radiation therapy and/or surgery for bone pain or inevitable pathological fracture, or spinal cord compression. After nine cycles of therapy, the relative risk reduction for SRE was 41%, and the number of patients needed to treat to prevent one SRE was six. Secondary endpoints of bone pain and quality of life were also significantly improved in the treatment group. A phase II trial evaluating the effective dose of zoledronic acid compared with pamidronate in patients with osteolytic lesions caused by multiple myeloma or metastatic breast cancer was published in 2001.[48] Zoledronic acid, 0.4, 2.0, or 4.0 mg, was compared with 90 mg of pamidronate administered every 4 weeks for 10 months. The primary endpoint was the need for radiation therapy to bone during the treatment period, and secondary endpoints included SRE, bone mineral density (BMD), and bone pain. The 2.0- and 4.0-mg zoledronic acid groups had an equivalent rate of radiation therapy requirement as the pamidronate arm, but the 0.4-mg zoledronic acid group underwent radiotherapy at a higher rate. A follow-up phase III trial with a similar patient population compared zoledronic acid 4 and 8 mg with pamidronate 90-mg infusion given every 3–4 weeks for 12 months.[49] SRE were the primary endpoint over 13 months. Because of decline in renal function in patients randomized to 8 mg of zoledronic acid, this dose was reduced to 4 mg. The prevalence of SRE and time to first pathological fracture was similar in all three groups, but zoledronic acid appeared to reduce the need for bone irradiation. Another high potency bisphosphonate, ibandronate, did not have benefit in regards to SRE in patients with stage II or III multiple myeloma.[50] However, further study is needed as one report using a higher dose suggested benefit.[51]

The use of bisphosphonates in the treatment of osteolytic bone disease caused by breast cancer also seems to have benefit. Two large trials have been published evaluating pamidronate in patients with stage IV breast cancer; the data were later combined to evaluate long-term benefit.[52] Patients were randomized to pamidronate 90 mg or placebo every 3–4 weeks, and the primary outcome was skeletal events per year and time to first SRE. Despite a significant number of participants not completing the study, the number of events per year in the treatment group was 2.4 compared with 3.7 in the control group. Also, the median time to the first SRE was longer in the treatment group. Zoledronic acid is also approved for the treatment of breast cancer with bone metastases with results of these studies detailed above. The oral bisphosphonate clodronate may have benefit in preventing SRE[53,54] but has not been approved for use in the United States.

Questions still remain to be answered in the use of bisphosphonates for metastatic bone disease: which is the best bisphosphonate, what is the ideal dose, for how long, how should it be administered, should it be given to patients early in the course of the disease, and most important, do these drugs have a beneficial effect on survival? Also, what are the effects of bisphosphonates on the tumor cells themselves? In experimental models, they seem to decrease breast cancer tumor burden in bone[55] and promote apoptosis in human myeloma cell lines.[56] The combination of bisphosphonates and dexamethasone in the treatment of multiple myeloma, and tamoxifen or paclitaxel for metastatic breast cancer, seems to have a synergetic effect in reducing tumor proliferation and enhancing tumor apoptosis.[57–59] Bisphosphonates may also reduce tumor burden by inhibiting angiogenesis, reducing growth factor levels in the bone microenvironment, and reducing the potential for tumor invasion.

Novel therapies for osteolytic bone disease based on inhibition of the RANK/RANKL system have been proposed, and several are in clinical trial. A phase I trial studying recombinant osteoprotegerin (AMGN-0007) in patients with multiple myeloma or bone metastases from breast cancer was recently published.[60] Participants were randomized to receive a single dose of either subcutaneous AMGN-0007 or 90 mg of intravenous pamidronate. The outcome was the urinary marker of bone resorption, N-telopeptide (NTX), at 56 days, each group showing a significant and statistically equal decrease in this surrogate marker of bone resorption. Recombinant RANK fused to the Fc region of human immunoglobulin was tested in a mouse model of multiple myeloma. Administration of this agent resulted in reduction of tumor burden and serum paraprotein presumably by saturating the cognate ligand and preventing the activation of native RANK on osteoclastic precursors.[61] A similar result was demonstrated using an antibody to MIP-1α.[14] Proteosome inhibitors have an antineoplastic effect through disruption of the mitotic cycle.[62] The proteosome inhibitor PS-341 has shown promise in early clinical studies of multiple myeloma.[63]

Because bone metastasis is such an important complication of some of the most common tumors that affect humans, understanding the cellular events involved and devising therapeutic strategies to prevent new metastasis and inhibit continued growth of established metastases are very important therapeutic goals for cancer management.

REFERENCES

1. Mundy GR, Raisz LG, Cooper RA, Schechter GP, Salmon SE 1974 Evidence for the secretion of an osteoclast stimulating factor in myeloma. N Engl J Med 291:1041–1046.
2. Mundy GR, Bertolini DB 1986 Bone destruction and hypercalcemia in plasma cell myeloma. Semin Oncol 13:291–299.
3. Bergui L, Schena M, Gaidano G, Riva M, Caligaris-Cappio F 1989 Interleukin 3 and interleukin 6 synergistically promote the proliferation and differentiation of malignant plasma cell precursors in multiple myeloma. J Exp Med 170:613–618.
4. Ferlin M, Noraz N, Hertogh C, Brochier J, Taylor N, Klein B 2000 Insulin-like growth factor induces the survival and proliferation of myeloma cells through an interleukin-6-independent transduction pathway. Br J Haematol 111:626–634.
5. Yaccoby S, Pearse RN, Johnson CL, Barlogie B, Choi Y, Epstein J 2002 Myeloma interacts with the bone marrow microenvironment to induce osteoclastogenesis and is dependent on osteoclast activity. Br J Haematol 116:278–290.
6. Garrett IR, Durie BG, Nedwin GE, Gillespie A, Bringman T, Sabatini M, Bertolini DR, Mundy GR 1987 Production of lymphotoxin, a bone-resorbing cytokine, by cultured human myeloma cells. N Engl J Med 317:526–532.
7. Bataille R, Jourdan M, Zhang X-G, Klein B 1989 Serum levels of interleukin-6, a potent myeloma cell growth factor, as a reflection of disease severity in plasma cell dyscrasias. J Clin Invest 84:2008–2011.
8. Cozzolino F, Torcia M, Aldinucci D, Rubartelli A, Miliani A, Shaw AR, Lansdorp PM, Di Guglielmo R 1989 Production of interleukin-1 by bone marrow myeloma cells. Blood 74:380–387.
9. Firkin F, Seymour JF, Watson AM, Grill V, Martin TJ 1996 Parathyroid hormone-related protein I hypercalcemia associated with haematological malignancy. Br J Haematol 94:486–492.
10. Choi SJ, Cruz JC, Craig F, Chung H, Devlin RD, Roodman GD, Alsina M 2000 Macrophage inflammatory protein 1-alpha is a potential osteoclast stimulatory factor in multiple myeloma. Blood 96:671–675.
11. Hjertner O, Torgersen ML, Seidel C, Hjorth-Hansen H, Waage A, Borset M, Sundan A 1999 Hepatocyte growth factor (HGF) induces interleukin-11 secretion from osteoblasts: A possible role for HGF in myeloma-associated osteolytic bone disease. Blood 94:3883–3888.
12. Han JH, Choi SJ, Kurihara N, Koide M, Oba Y, Roodman GD 2001 Macrophage inflammatory protein-1alpha is an osteoclastogenic factor in myeloma that is independent of receptor activator of nuclear factor kappaB ligand. Blood 97:3349–3353.
13. Abe M, Hiura K, Wilde J, Moriyama K, Hashimoto T, Ozaki S, Wakatsuki S, Kosaka M, Kido S, Inoue D, Matsumoto T 2002 Role for macrophage inflammatory protein (MIP)-1alpha and MIP-1beta in the development of osteolytic lesions in multiple myeloma. Blood 100:2195–2202.
14. Oyajobi BO, Mundy GR 2003 Receptor activator of NF-kappaB ligand, macrophage inflammatory protein-1alpha, and the proteasome. Cancer 97(Suppl 3):813–817.
15. Michigami T, Shimizu N, Williams PJ, Niewolna M, Dallas SL, Mundy GR, Yoneda T 2000 Cell-cell contact between marrow stromal cells and myeloma cells via VCAM-1 and alpha(4)beta(1)-integrin enhances production of osteoclast-stimulating activity. Blood 96:1953–1960.
16. Giuliani N, Bataille R, Mancini C, Lazzaretti M, Barille S 2001 Myeloma cells induce imbalance in the osteoprotegerin/osteoprotegerin ligand system in the human bone marrow environment. Blood 98:3527–3533.
17. Pearse RN, Sordillo EM, Yaccoby S, Wong BR, Liau DF, Colman N, Michaeli J, Epstein J, Choi Y 2001 Multiple myeloma disrupts the TRANCE/ osteoprotegerin cytokine axis to trigger bone destruction and promote tumor progression. Proc Natl Acad Sci 98:11581–11586.
18. Roux S, Meignin V, Quillard J, Meduri G, Guiochon-Mantel A, Fermand JP, Milgrom E, Mariette X 2002 RANK (receptor activator of nuclear factor-kappaB) and RANKL expression in multiple myeloma. Br J Haematol 117:86–92.
19. Sezer O, Heider U, Jakob C, Zavrski I, Eucker J, Possinger K, Sers C, Krenn V 2002 Immunocytochemistry reveals RANKL expression of myeloma cells. Blood 99:4646–4647.
20. Durie BGM, Salmon SE, Mundy GR 1981 Relation of osteoclast activating factor production to the extent of bone disease in multiple myeloma. Br J Haematol 47:21–30.
21. Harinck HIJ, Bijvoet OLM, Plantingh AST 1987 Role of bone and kidney in tumor-induced hypercalcemia and its treatment with bisphosphonate and sodium chloride. Am J Med 82:1113–1142.
22. Mbalaviele G, Dunstan CR, Sasaki A, Williams PJ, Mundy GR, Yoneda T 1996 E-cadherin expression in human breast cancer cells suppresses the development of osteolytic bone metastases in an experimental metastasis model. Cancer Res 56:4063–4070.
23. Muller A, Homey B, Soto H, Ge N, Catron D, Buchanan ME, McClanahan T, Murphy E, Yuan W, Wagner SN, Barrera JL, Mohar A, Verastegui E, Zlotnik A 2001 Involvement of chemokine receptors in breast cancer metastasis. Nature 410:50–56.
24. Sung V, Stubbs JT III, Fisher L, Aaron AD, Thompson EW 1998 Bone sialoprotein supports breast cancer cell adhesion proliferation and migration through differential usage of the alpha(v)beta3 and alpha(v)-beta5 integrins. J Cell Physiol 176:482–494.
25. Felding-Habermann B, O'Toole TE, Smith JW, Fransvea E, Ruggeri ZM, Ginsberg MH, Hughes PE, Pampori N, Shattil SJ, Saven A, Mueller BM 2001 Integrin activation controls metastasis in human breast cancer. Proc Natl Acad Sci 98:1853–1858.
26. Nelson AR, Fingleton B, Rothenberg ML, Matrisian LM 2000 Matrix metalloproteinases: Biologic activity and clinical implications. J Clin Oncol 18:1135–1149.
27. Andreasen PA, Egelund R, Petersen HH 2000 The plasminogen activation system in tumor growth, invasion, and metastasis. Cell Mol Life Sci 57:25–40.
28. Powell GJ, Southby J, Danks JA, Stillwell RG, Hayman JA, Henderson MA, Bennett RC, Martin TJ 1991 Localization of parathyroid

hormone-related protein in breast cancer metastases: Increased incidence in bone compared with other sites. Cancer Res 51:3059–3061.

29. Guise TA, Yin JJ, Taylor SD, Kumagai Y, Dallas M, Boyce BF, Yoneda T, Mundy GR 1996 Evidence for a causal role of parathyroid hormone-related protein in the pathogenesis of human breast cancer-mediated osteolysis. J Clin Invest 98:1544–1549.

30. Thomas RJ, Guise TA, Yin JJ, Elliott J, Horwood NJ, Martin TJ, Gillespie MT 1999 Breast cancer cells interact with osteoblasts to support osteoclast formation. Endocrinology 140:4451–4458.

31. Gallwitz WE, Guise TA, Mundy G 2002 Guanosine nucleotides inhibit different syndromes of PTHrP excess caused by human cancer in vitro. J Clin Invest 110:1559–1572.

32. Yin JJ, Selander K, Chirgwin JM, Dallas M, Grubbs BG, Wieser R, Massague J, Mundy GR, Guise TA 1999 TGF-beta signaling blockade inhibits PTHrP secretion by breast cancer cells and bone metastases development. J Clin Invest 103:197–206.

33. Kakonen SM, Selander KS, Chirgwin JM, Yin JJ, Burns S, Rankin WA, Grubbs BG, Dallas M, Cui Y, Guise TA 2002 Transforming growth factor-beta stimulates parathyroid hormone-related protein and osteolytic metastases via Smad and mitogen-activated protein kinase signaling pathways. J Biol Chem 277:24571–24578.

34. Kakonen SM, Kang Y, Carreon MR, Niewolna M, Kakonen RS, Chirgwin JM, Massague J, Guise TA 2002 Breast cancer cell lines selected from bone metastases have greater metastatic capacity and express increased vascular endothelial growth factor (VEGF), interleukin-11 (IL-11), and parathyroid hormone-related protein (PTHrP). J Bone Miner Res 17:S1;M060.

35. de la Mata J, Uy HL, Guise TA, Story B, Boyce BF, Mundy GR, Roodman GD 1995 Interleukin-6 enhances hypercalcemia and bone resorption mediated by parathyroid hormone-related protein in vivo. J Clin Invest 95:2846–2852.

36. Bendre MS, Gaddy-Kurten D, Mon-Foote T, Akel NS, Skinner RA, Nicholas RW, Suva LJ 2002 Expression of interleukin 8 and not parathyroid hormone-related protein by human breast cancer cells correlates with bone metastasis in vivo. Cancer Res 62:5571–5579.

37. Sachdev D, Yee D 2001 The IGF system and breast cancer. Endocrine-Related Cancer 8:197–209.

38. Yoneda T, Williams PJ, Hiraga T, Niewolna M, Nishimura R 2001 A bone-seeking clone exhibits different biological properties from the MDA-MB-231 parental human breast cancer cells and a brain-seeking clone in vivo and in vitro. J Bone Miner Res 16:1486–1495.

39. Sanders JL, Chattopadhyay N, Kifor O, Yamaguchi T, Brown EM 2001 Ca(2+)-sensing receptor expression and PTHrP secretion in PC-3 human prostate cancer cells. Am J Physiol Endocrinol Metab 281:E1267–E1274.

40. Sanders JL, Chattopadhyay N, Kifor O, Yamaguchi T, Butters RR, Brown EM 2000 Extracellular calcium-sensing receptor expression and its potential role in regulating parathyroid hormone-related peptide secretion in human breast cancer cell lines. Endocrinology 141:4357–4364.

41. Canellos GP 1974 Hypercalcemia in malignant lymphoma and leukemia. Ann NY Acad Sci 230:240–246.

42. Bunn PA Jr, Schechter GP, Jaffe E, Blayney D, Young RC, Matthews MJ, Blattner W, Broder S, Robert-Guroff M, Gallo RC 1983 Clinical course of retrovirus-associated adult T-cell lymphoma in the United States. N Engl J Med 309:257–264.

43. Motokura T, Fukumoto S, Matsumoto T, Takahashi S, Fujita A, Yamashita T, Igarashi T, Ogata E 1989 Parathyroid hormone-related protein in adult T-cell leukemia-lymphoma. Ann Intern Med 111:484–488.

44. Breslau NA, McGuire JL, Zerwekh JE, Frenkel EP, Pak CYC 1984 Hypercalcemia associated with increased serum calcitriol levels in three patients with lymphoma. Ann Intern Med 100:1–6.

45. Fetchick DA, Bertolini DR, Sarin PS, Weintraub ST, Mundy GR, Dunn JD 1986 Production of 1,25 dihydroxyvitamin D by human T-cell lymphotrophic virus-I transformed lymphocytes. J Clin Invest 78:592–596.

46. Adams JS, Fernandez M, Gacad MA, Gill PS, Endres DB, Rasheed S, Singer FR 1989 Vitamin D metabolite-mediated hypercalcemia and hypercalciuria patients with AIDS- and non-AIDS-associated lymphoma. Blood 73:235–239.

47. Berenson JR, Lichtenstein A, Porter L, Dimopoulos MA, Bordoni R, George S, Lipton A, Keller A, Ballester O, Kovacs MJ, Blacklock HA, Bell R, Simeone J, Reitsma DJ, Heffernan M, Seaman J, Knight RD 1996 Efficacy of pamidronate in reducing skeletal events in patients with advanced multiple myeloma. Myeloma Aredia Study Group. N Engl J Med 334:488–493.

48. Berenson JR, Rosen LS, Howell A, Porter L, Coleman RE, Morley W, Dreicer R, Kuross SA, Lipton A, Seaman JJ 2001 Zoledronic acid reduces skeletal-related events in patients with osteolytic metastases. Cancer 91:1191–1200.

49. Rosen LS, Gordon D, Kaminski M, Howell A, Belch A, Mackey JA, Apffelstaedt J, Hussein M, Coleman RE, Reitsma DJ, Seaman JJ, Chen BL, Ambros Y 2001 Zoledronic acid versus pamidronate in the treatment of skeletal metastases in patients with breast cancer or osteolytic lesions of multiple myeloma: A phase III, double-blind, comparative trial. Cancer J 7:377–387.

50. Menssen HD, Sakalova A, Fontana A, Herrmann Z, Boewer C, Facon T, Lichinitser MR, Singer CR, Euller-Ziegler L, Wetterwald M, Fiere D, Hrubisko M, Thiel E, Delmas PD 2002 Effects of long-term intravenous ibandronate therapy on skeletal-related events, survival, and bone resorption markers in patients with advanced multiple myeloma. J Clin Oncol 20:2353–2359.

51. Body JJ, Lichinister MR, Diehl L, Schlosser K, Pfarr E, Cavalli F, Dornoff V, Gorbunova VA, McCloskey E, Weiss J, Kanis JA 1999 Double-blind placebo-controlled trial of intravenous ibandronate in breast cancer metastatic to bone. Proc Am Soc Clin Oncol 35:575a.

52. Lipton A, Theriault RL, Hortobagyi GN, Simeone J, Knight RD, Mellars K, Reitsma DJ, Heffernan M, Seaman JJ 2000 Pamidronate prevents skeletal complications and is effective palliative treatment in women with breast carcinoma and osteolytic bone metastases: Long term follow-up of two randomized, placebo-controlled trials. Cancer 88:1082–1090.

53. Kanis JA, Powles T, Paterson AH, McCloskey EV, Ashley S 1996 Clodronate decreases the frequency of skeletal metastases in women with breast cancer. Bone 19:663–667.

54. Powles T, Paterson S, Kanis JA, McCloskey E, Ashley S, Tidy A, Rosenqvist K, Smith I, Ottestad L, Legault S, Pajunen M, Nevantaus A, Mannisto E, Suovuori A, Atula S, Nevalainen J, Pylkkanen L 2002 Randomized, placebo-controlled trial of clodronate in patients with primary operable breast cancer. J Clin Oncol 20:3219–3224.

55. Sasaki A, Boyce BF, Story B, Wright KR, Chapman M, Boyce R, Mundy GR, Yoneda T 1995 Bisphosphonate risedronate reduces metastatic human breast cancer burden in bone in nude mice. Cancer Res 55:3551–3557.

56. Shipman CM, Rogers MJ, Apperley JF, Russell RGG, Croucher PI 1997 Bisphosphonates induce apoptosis in human myeloma cell lines: A novel anti-tumor activity. Br J Haematol 98:665–672.

57. Tassone P, Forciniti S, Galea E, Morrone G, Turco MC, Martinelli V, Tagliaferri P, Venuta S 2000 Growth inhibition and synergistic induction of apoptosis by zoledronate and dexamethasone in human myeloma cell lines. Leukemia 14:841–844.

58. Jagdev SP, Croucher PI, Coleman RE 2000 Zoledronic acid induces apoptosis of breast cancer cells in vitro–evidence for additive and synergistic effects with taxol and tamoxifen. Proc Am Soc Clin Oncol 19:664a.

59. Jagdev SP, Coleman RE, Shipman CM, Rostami HA, Croucher PI 2001 The bisphosphonate, zoledronic acid, induces apoptosis of breast cancer cells: Evidence for synergy with paclitaxel. Br J Cancer 84:1126–1134.

60. Body JJ, Greipp P, Coleman RE, Facon T, Geurs F, Fermand JP, Harousseau JL, Lipton A, Mariette X, Williams CD, Nakanishi A, Holloway D, Martin SW, Dunstan CR, Bekker PJ 2003 A Phase I study of AMGN-0007, a recombinant osteoprotegerin construct, in patients with multiple myeloma or breast carcinoma related bone metastases. Cancer 97(Suppl 3):887–892.

61. Sordillo EM, Pearse RN 2003 RANK-Fc: A therapeutic antagonist for RANK-L in myeloma. Cancer 97(Suppl 3):802–812.

62. LeBlanc R, Catley LP, Hideshima T, Lentzsch S, Mitsiades CS, Mitsiades N, Neuberg D, Goloubeva O, Pien CS, Adams J, Gupta D, Richardson PG, Munshi NC, Anderson KC 2002 Proteasome inhibitor PS-341 inhibits human myeloma cell growth in vivo and prolongs survival in a murine model. Cancer Res 62:4996–5000.

63. Richardson P, Barlogie B, Berenson JR, Traynor A, Singhal S, Jagannath S, Irwin D, Rajkumar V, Srkalovic G, Alsina M, Alexanian R, Siegel D, Orlowski RZ, Kuter D, Limentani SA, Lee S, Esseltine D-E, Kauffman M, Adams J, Schenkein DP, Anderson KC 2002 A phase II multicenter study of the proteosome inhibitor bortezomib (formerly PS-341) in multiple myeloma patients with relapsed/refractory disease. Blood 100(Suppl):385.

Chapter 39. Hypercalcemia Caused by Granuloma-Forming Disorders

John S. Adams[1] and Martin Hewison[2]

[1]Division of Endocrinology, Diabetes, and Metabolism, Burns and Allen Research Institute, Cedars-Sinai Medical Center, Los Angeles, California; and [2]Division of Medical Sciences, The University of Birmingham, Queen Elizabeth Medical Center, Birmingham, United Kingdom

PATHOGENESIS

The association of dysregulated calcium homeostasis and granuloma-forming disease was established in 1939 by the work of Harrell and Fisher.[1] With the advent of automated serum chemistry testing, more recent studies indicate that mild to severe hypercalcemia is detected in 10% of patients with sarcoidosis, and up to 50% of patients will become hypercalciuric at some time during the course of their disease.[2] Vitamin D was implicated in the pathogenesis of abnormal calcium metabolism after it was appreciated that patients with sarcoidosis who had hypercalcemia or hypercalciuria (or both) absorbed high amounts of dietary calcium, and that normocalcemic patients were prone to hypercalcemia after receiving small amounts of vitamin D or ultraviolet light.[3] It has been proposed that bone resorption is also an important contributor to the pathogenesis of hypercalciuria and hypercalcemia,[4] based on the observations that a diet low in calcium seldom induces a normocalcemic state in sarcoidosis patients with moderate to severe hypercalcemia and that urinary calcium excretion often exceeds dietary calcium intake. More recent studies have demonstrated that generalized, accelerated trabecular bone loss occurs in patients with sarcoidosis before institution of steroid therapy. Rizzato et al.[5] showed that (1) bone mass was significantly decreased in patients with active sarcoidosis, (2) bone loss was most marked in patients with hypercalcemia and/or hypercalciuria, and (3) bone loss was most prominent in postmenopausal women with long-standing disease.

For many years, these and similar clinical observations suggested that hypercalcemia and/or hypercalciuria in patients with sarcoidosis resulted from a heightened sensitivity to the biological effects of vitamin D. However, the discovery that a high proportion of these patients had elevated circulating concentrations of 1,25-dihydroxyvitamin D [$1,25(OH)_2D$] indicated that the endogenous overproduction of an active vitamin D metabolite was the etiology of disordered calcium regulation in this disease. High serum $1,25(OH)_2D$ concentrations were reported in hypercalcemic patients with other granuloma-forming diseases and in patients harboring lymphoproliferative neoplasms (Table 1). In all of these disorders, there is a presumed extrarenal source for the hormone.

Four major lines of clinical evidence suggest that the endogenous extrarenal synthesis of $1,25(OH)_2D$ in some hypercalcemic/hypercalciuric patients with granulomatous disease or lymphoma is not subject to normal, physiologic regulatory influences.[24–26] First, hypercalcemic patients possess high or inappropriately elevated serum $1,25(OH)_2D$ concentrations, although serum immunoreactive parathyroid hormone levels are suppressed and serum phosphorus concentrations are relatively elevated. If $1,25(OH)_2D$ synthesis were under the trophic control of parathyroid hormone and phosphorus, then $1,25(OH)_2D$ concentrations would be low. Second, unlike in normal individuals whose serum $1,25(OH)_2D$ concentrations are not influenced by small to moderate increments of circulating 25-hydroxyvitamin D [25OHD] concentrations, serum $1,25(OH)_2D$ levels in patients with active sarcoidosis who have widespread disease and high serum angiotensin-converting enzyme activity are more likely to be hypercalciuric or hypercalcemic. Third, serum calcium and $1,25(OH)_2D$ concentrations are positively correlated to indices of disease activity; patients with sarcoidosis who have widespread disease and high serum angiotensin-converting enzyme activity are more likely to hypercalcuric or hypercalcemic. And fourth, the rate of endogenous $1,25(OH)_2D$ production, which is significantly increased in patients with sarcoidosis, is unusually sensitive to inhibition by factors (e.g., glucocorticoids) that do not influence the renal 1α-hydroxylase enzyme that catalyzes synthesis of $1,25(OH)_2D$.

CELLULAR SOURCE OF ACTIVE VITAMIN D METABOLITES

The experiments of Barbour et al.[27] proved that in sarcoidosis the source of $1,25(OH)_2D$ is extrarenal. These

TABLE 1. HUMAN DISEASE ASSOCIATED WITH 1,25-DIHYDROXIVITAMIN D–MEDIATED HYPERCALCEMIA/HYPERCALCIURIA

Granuloma-forming diseases	
Noninfectious	
Sarcoidosis	Adams et al.[6]
Silicone-induced granulomatosis	Kozeny et al.[7]
Paraffin-induced granulomatosis	Albitar et al.[8]
Berylliosis	Stoeckle et al.[9]
Wegener's	Edelson et al.[10]
Eosinophilic granuloma	Jurney[11]
Infantile fat necrosis	Cook et al.[12]
Crohn's disease	Bosch[13]
Infectious	
Tuberculosis	Gkonos et al.[14]
Candidiasis	Kantarijian et al.[15]
Leprosy	Hoffman et al.[16]
Histoplasmosis	Walker et al.[17]
Coccidiodmycosis	Parker et al.[18]
Cat-scratch disease	Bosch[19]
Malignant Lymphoproliferative disease	
B-cell lymphoma	Adams et al.[20]
Hodgkin's disease	Seymor and Gagel[21]
Lymphomatoid granulomatosis	Schienman et al.[22]
Dysgerminoma/seminoma	Grote and Hainsworth[23]

The authors have no conflict of interest.

investigators described an anephric patient with sarcoidosis, hypercalcemia, and a high serum 1,25(OH)$_2$D concentration. The elevated level of 1,25(OH)$_2$D in patients with sarcoidosis is now known to result from increased production of the steroid hormone by macrophages,[6] which make up a significant proportion of the cell population in sarcoid granulomata. The situation with lymphomas and other malignant disorders is less clear. However, recent immunohistochemical analysis of the enzyme 1α-hydroxylase in a B-cell lymphoma associated with hypercalcemia and raised circulating levels of 1,25(OH)$_2$D suggests that the tumor itself is not a source of the steroid hormone. Rather macrophages adjacent to the tumor are likely to be the major site of 1,25(OH)$_2$D synthesis.[28]

Although substrate-specificity and enzyme kinetics for the 1α-hydroxylase reaction appear to be the same for both kidney cells and macrophages,[29] the regulation of 1,25(OH)$_2$D synthesis at these sites appears to be very different. For example, the macrophage 1α-hydroxylation reaction is not induced by parathyroid hormone, but it is very sensitive to stimulation by immunoactivators such as lipopolysaccharide[29] and cytokines such as interferon-γ (IFN-γ).[30] Macrophage synthesis of 1,25(OH)$_2$D is very sensitive to inhibition by glucocorticoids,[30] chloroquine, and related analogs,[31] and the cytochrome P-450 inhibitor ketoconazole,[32] but it is refractory to inhibition by 1,25(OH)$_2$D.[30] The renal enzyme, on the other hand, is relatively insensitive to inhibition by glucocorticoids and is downregulated by 1,25(OH)$_2$D. These differences in the regulation of 1α-hydroxylase activity in the kidney and macrophages do not seem to be caused by the expression of two different gene products. Analysis of mRNA for 1α-hydroxylase in extrarenal tissues, including macrophages and keratinocytes, has revealed identity with the renal gene sequence.[33,34] Rather, it is likely that there is differential regulation of the 1α-hydroxylase gene in different cell types.[35] The renal 1α-hydroxylase is upregulated at the level of transcription by calciotropic hormones such as parathyroid hormone and calcitonin and is also subject to exquisite autoregulation by 1,25(OH)$_2$D itself.[36] In contrast, macrophage 1α-hydroxylase mRNA expression is potently stimulated by inflammatory agents such as IFN-γ and shows no feedback control in response to 1,25(OH)$_2$D.[37] The precise molecular mechanism for this remains unclear and may involve differential induction of the catabolic enzyme 24-hydroxylase.

IMMUNOACTIVITY OF 1,25(OH)$_2$D

1,25(OH)$_2$D is known to exert a potent immunoinhibitory effect on activated human lymphocytes in vitro. These actions include inhibition of lymphocyte proliferation, lymphokine production, and immunoglobulin synthesis.[38] In particular, it was suggested that 1,25(OH)$_2$D produced by the macrophage in granulomatous diseases exerts a paracrine immunoinhibitory effect on neighboring, activated lymphocytes that express receptors for the hormone and that this acts to slow an otherwise "overzealous" immune response that may be detrimental to the host.[39] The physiological significance of this has been highlighted by the recent development of 1α-hydroxylase

knockout mouse models,[40,41] which presented with multiple enlarged lymph nodes.

TREATMENT OF HYPERCALCEMIA/ HYPERCALCIURIA ASSOCIATED WITH SARCOIDOSIS

The most important factor in the successful management of disordered vitamin D metabolism of sarcoidosis is recognition of patients at risk. Those at risk include patients with (1) indices of active, widespread disease (i.e., elevated serum angiotensin-converting enzyme levels, diffuse infiltrative pulmonary disease); (2) pre-existent hypercalciuria; (3) a previous history of hypercalcemia or hypercalciuria; (4) a diet enriched in vitamin D and calcium; and (5) a recent history of sunlight exposure or treatment with vitamin D. All patients with active sarcoidosis should be screened for hypercalciuria. In a timed, fasting urine collection, a fractional urinary calcium excretion rate exceeding 0.16 mg calcium per 100 ml glomerular filtrate is considered hypercalciuria. Alternatively, 24-h urinary calcium excretion values greater than the usual normal limits for men (300 mg) and women (250 mg) are also indicative of hypercalcuria, based on a complete sample collection containing between 1.0 and 2.0 g creatinine. If the urinary calcium excretion is elevated, serum 25OHD and 1,25(OH)$_2$D concentrations should be determined as a disease marker and to judge the efficacy of therapy. Because hypercalciuria frequently precedes the development of overt hypercalcemia, the occurrence of either is an indication for therapy.

Glucocorticoids (40–60 mg prednisone or equivalent, daily) are the mainstay of therapy of disordered calcium homeostasis resulting from the endogenous overproduction of active vitamin D metabolites. Institution of glucocorticoid therapy results in a prompt decrease in the circulating 1,25(OH)$_2$D concentration (within 3 days), presumably by inhibition of macrophage 1α-hydroxylase activity. Normalization of the serum or urine calcium usually occurs within a matter of days.[25] Failure to normalize the serum calcium after 10 days of therapy suggests the coexistence of another hypercalcemic process (e.g., hyperparathyroidism or humoral hypercalcemia of malignancy). The dietary intake of calcium and vitamin D should be limited in such patients, as should sunlight (ultraviolet light) exposure. After a hypercalcemic episode, urinary calcium excretion rates should be monitored intermittently to detect recurrence.

TREATMENT OF HYPERCALCEMIA/ HYPERCALCIURIA IN OTHER DISORDERS ASSOCIATED WITH OVERPRODUCTION OF 1,25(OH)$_2$D

Glucocorticoids may also be effective in the management of vitamin D–mediated hypercalcemia or hypercalciuria associated with lymphoma or granuloma-forming diseases other than sarcoidosis. However, steroid therapy may not always be appropriate for these diseases, and consequently, alternative treatments may be necessary. Chloroquine[31,42] or hydroxychloroquine[43] and ketoconazole[32] are also capable of reducing the serum 1,25(OH)$_2$D and calcium concentration, although chloroquine and its analogs do not seem to be effective in lymphoma patients.[43] Because of the limited experience with these drugs as antihypercalcemic agents, they should be restricted to patients in whom steroid therapy is unsuccessful or contraindicated. The theoretic advantage of these agents over glucocorticoids is that correction of the serum 1,25(OH)$_2$D concentration should result in rapid recovery of at least some of the bone mineral density (BMD) lost to the disease.[44] The use of the newer bisphosphonates in blocking bone resorption in hypercalcemic/hypercalciuric patients with sarcoidosis is still unknown.

REFERENCES

1. Harrell GT, Fisher S 1939 Blood chemical changes in Boeck's sarcoid with particular reference to protein, calcium and phosphates values. J Clin Invest 18:687–693.
2. Studdy PR, Bird R, Neville E, James DG 1980 Biochemical findings in sarcoidosis. J Clin Pathol 33:528–533.
3. Bell NH, Gill JR Jr, Bartter FC 1964 On the abnormal calcium absorption in sarcoidosis: Evidence for increased sensitivity to vitamin D. Am J Med 36:500–513.
4. Fallon MD, Perry HM III, Teitelbaum SL 1981 Skeletal sarcoidosis with osteopenia. Metab Bone Dis Relat Res 3:171–174.
5. Rizzato GL, Montemurro L, Fraioli P 1992 Bone mineral content in sarcoidosis. Semin Resp Med 13:411–423.
6. Adams JS, Singer FR, Gacad MA, Sharma OP, Hayes MJ, Vouros P, Holick MF 1985 Isolation and structural identification of 1,25-dihydroxyvitamin D3 produced by cultured alveolar macrophages in sarcoidosis. J Clin Endocrinol Metab 60:960–966.
7. Kozeny GA, Barbato AL, Bansal VK, Vertuno LL, Hano JE 1984 Hypercalcemia associated with silicone-induced granulomas. N Engl J Med 311:1103–1105.
8. Albitar S, Genin R, Fen-Chong M, Schohn D, Riviere JP, Serveaux MO, Chuet C, Bourgeon B 1997 Multisystem granulomatous injuries 28 years after paraffin injections. Nephrol Dial Transplant 12:1974–1976.
9. Stoeckle JD, Hardy HL, Weber AL 1969 Chronic beryllium disease. Long-term follow-up of sixty cases and selective review of the literature. Am J Med 46:545–561.
10. Edelson GW, Talpos GB, Bone HG III 1993 Hypercalcemia associated with Wegener's granulomatosis and hyperparathyroidism: Etiology and management. Am J Nephrol 13:275–277.
11. Jurney TH 1984 Hypercalcemia in a patient with eosinophilic granuloma. Am J Med 76:527–528.
12. Cook JS, Stone MS, Hansen JR 1992 Hypercalcemia in association with subcutaneous fat necrosis of the newborn: Studies of calcium-regulating hormones. Pediatrics 90:93–96.
13. Bosch X 1998 Hypercalcemia due to endogenous overproduction of 1,25-dihydroxyvitamin D in Crohn's disease. Gastroenterology 114:1061–1065.
14. Gkonos PJ, London R, Hendler ED 1984 Hypercalcemia and elevated 1,25-dihydroxyvitamin D levels in a patient with end-stage renal disease and active tuberculosis. N Engl J Med 311:1683–1685.
15. Kantarjian HM, Saad MF, Estey EH, Sellin RV, Samaan NA 1983 Hypercalcemia in disseminated candidiasis. Am J Med 74:721–724.
16. Hoffman VN, Korzeniowski OM 1986 Leprosy, hypercalcemia, and elevated serum calcitriol levels. Ann Intern Med 105:890–891.
17. Walker JV, Baran D, Yakub N, Freeman RB 1977 Histoplasmosis with hypercalcemia, renal failure, and papillary necrosis. Confusion with sarcoidosis. JAMA 237:1350–1352.
18. Parker MS, Dokoh S, Woolfenden JM, Buchsbaum HW 1984 Hypercalcemia in coccidioidomycosis. Am J Med 76:341–344.
19. Bosch X 1988 Hypercalcemia due to endogenous overproduction of active vitamin D in identical twins with cat-scratch disease. JAMA 279:532–534.
20. Adams JS, Fernandez M, Gacad MA, Gill PS, Endres DB, Rasheed S, Singer FR 1989 Vitamin D metabolite-mediated hypercalcemia and hypercalciuria patients with AIDS- and non-AIDS-associated lymphoma. Blood 73:235–239.
21. Seymour JF, Gagel RF 1993 Calcitriol: The major humoral mediator of hypercalcemia in Hodgkin's disease and non-Hodgkin's lymphomas. Blood 82:1383–1394.
22. Scheinman SJ, Kelberman MW, Tatum AH, Zamkoff KW 1991 Hypercalcemia with excess serum 1,25 dihydroxyvitamin D in lympho-

matoid granulomatosis/angiocentric lymphoma. Am J Med Sci 301:178–181.
23. Grote TH, Hainsworth JD 1987 Hypercalcemia and elevated serum calcitriol in a patient with seminoma. Arch Intern Med 147:2212–2213.
24. Sandler LM, Winearls CJ, Fraher LJ, Clemens TL, Smith R, O'Riordan JLH 1984 Studies of the hypercalcaemia of sarcoidosis: Effect of steroids and exogenous vitamin D3 on the circulating concentrations of 1,25-dihydroxy vitamin D3. Q J Med 53:165–180.
25. Meyrier A, Valeyre D, Bouillon R, Paillard F, Battesti JP, Georges R 1985 Resorptive versus absorptive hypercalciuria in sarcoidosis: Correlations with 25-hydroxy vitamin D3 and 1,25-dihydroxy vitamin D3 and parameters of disease activity. Q J Med 54:269–281.
26. Insogna KL, Dreyer BE, Mitnick M, Ellison AF, Broadus AE 1988 Enhanced production rate of 1,25-dihydroxyvitamin D in sarcoidosis. J Clin Endocrinol Metab 66:72–75.
27. Barbour GL, Coburn JW, Slatopolsky E, Norman AW, Horst RL 1981 Hypercalcemia in an anephric patient with sarcoidosis: Evidence for extrarenal generation of 1,25-dihydroxyvitamin D. N Engl J Med 305:440–443.
28. Hewison M, Kantorovich V, Van Herle AJ, Cohan P, Zehnder D, Adams JS 2003 Vitamin D-mediated hypercalcemia in lymphoma: Evidence for hormone production by tumor-adjacent macrophages. J Bone Miner Res 18:579–582.
29. Reichel H, Koeffler HP, Bishop JE, Norman AW 1987 25-Hydroxyvitamin D3 metabolism by lipopolysaccharide-stimulated normal human macrophages. J Clin Endocrinol Metab 64:1–9.
30. Adams JS, Gacad MA 1985 Characterization of 1 alpha-hydroxylation of vitamin D3 sterols by cultured alveolar macrophages from patients with sarcoidosis. J Exp Med 161:755–765.
31. Adams JS, Diz MM, Sharma OP 1989 Effective reduction in the serum 1,25-dihydroxyvitamin D and calcium concentration in sarcoidosis-associated hypercalcemia with short-course chloroquine therapy. Ann Intern Med 111:437–438.
32. Adams JS, Sharma OP, Diz MM, Endres DB 1990 Ketoconazole decreases the serum 1,25-dihydroxyvitamin D and calcium concentration in sarcoidosis-associated hypercalcemia. J Clin Endocrinol Metab 70:1090–1095.
33. Fu GK, Lin D, Zhang MY, Bikle DD, Shackleton CH, Miller WL, Portale AA 1997 Cloning of human 25-hydroxyvitamin D-1 alpha-hydroxylase and mutations causing vitamin D-dependent rickets type 1. Mol Endocrinol 11:1961–1970.
34. Smith SJ, Rucka AK, Berry JL, Davies M, Mylchreest S, Paterson CR, Heath DA, Tassabehji M, Read AP, Mee AP, Mawer EB 1999 Novel mutations in the 1α-hydroxylase (P450c1) gene in three families with pseudovitamin D-deficiency rickets resulting in loss of functional enzyme activity in blood-derived macrophages. J Bone Miner Res 14:730–739.
35. Hewison M, Bland R, Zehnder D, Stewart PM 2000 1α-hydroxylase and the action of vitamin D. J Mol Endocrinol 25:141–148.
36. Kong XF, Zhu XH, Pei YL, Jackson DM, Holick MF 1999 Molecular cloning, characterization, and promoter analysis of the human 25-hydroxyvitamin D3-1alpha-hydroxylase gene. Proc Natl Acad Sci USA 96:6988–6993.
37. Monkawa T, Yoshida T, Hayashi M, Saruta T 2000 Identification of 25-hydroxyvitamin D3 1alpha-hydroxylase gene expression in macrophages. Kidney Int 58:559–568.
38. Hewison M, Gacad MA, Lemire J, Adams JS 2001 Vitamin D as a cytokine and hematopoietic factor. Rev Endocr Metab Disord 2:217–227.
39. Lemire JM 1995 Immunomodulatory actions of 1,25-dihydroxyvitamin D3. J Steroid Biochem Mol Biol 53:599–602.
40. Panda DK, Miao D, Tremblay ML, Sirois J, Farookhi R, Hendy GN, Goltzman D 2001 Targeted ablation of the 25-hydroxyvitamin D 1alpha -hydroxylase enzyme: Evidence for skeletal, reproductive, and immune dysfunction. Proc Natl Acad Sci USA 98:7498–7503.
41. Dardenne O, Prud'homme J, Arabian A, Glorieux FH, St-Arnaud R 2001 Targeted inactivation of the 25-hydroxyvitamin D3-1alpha-hydroxylase gene (CYP27B1) creates an animal model of pseudovitamin D-deficiency rickets. Endocrinology 142:3135–3141.
42. O'Leary TJ, Jones G, Yip A, Lohnes D, Cohanim M, Yendt ER 1986 The effects of chloroquine on serum 1,25-dihydroxyvitamin D and calcium metabolism in sarcoidosis. N Engl J Med 315:727–730.
43. Adams JS, Kantorovich V 1999 Inability of short-term, low dose hydroxychloroquine to resolve vitamin D-mediated hypercalcemia in patients with B-cell lymphoma. J Clin Endocrinol Metab 84:799–801.
44. Adams JS, Lee G 1997 Recovery of bone mineral density with resolution of exogenous vitamin D intoxication. Ann Intern Med 127:203–206.

Chapter 40. Miscellaneous Causes of Hypercalcemia

John J. Wysolmerski

Section of Endocrinology and Metabolism, Department of Internal Medicine, Yale University School of Medicine, New Haven, Connecticut

INTRODUCTION

The majority of cases of hypercalcemia are caused by disorders of parathyroid hormone (PTH) secretion, malignancy, or granulomatous disorders. Each of these situations has been discussed separately in the preceding chapters. In this chapter, we will discuss less common causes of hypercalcemia.

PSEUDOHYPERCALCEMIA

Pseudohypercalcemia refers to instances in which the measured total serum calcium is elevated, but the patient is not truly hypercalcemic. This has been described in three settings: hyperalbuminemia, increased circulating levels of an abnormal, calcium-binding immunoglobulin, and pronounced thrombocytosis.

Albumin is the primary binding protein for circulating calcium ions. Therefore, abnormalities in the concentration of albumin can lead to abnormalities in the total concentration of calcium measured in the bloodstream. Although it is widely recognized that hypoalbuminemia can lead to hypocalcemia on this basis, it is less appreciated that hyperalbuminemia can result in hypercalcemia.[1] Hyperalbuminemia principally occurs in the setting of volume contraction, and although the total calcium is elevated, the ionized calcium level is normal. Therefore, symptoms and signs of hypercalcemia are absent. Formulas have been developed to correct the calcium concentration for elevations or reductions in serum albumin, but these are not fully reliable. If knowing the true calcium concentration is important clinically, an ionized calcium level should be determined.

Abnormalities in calcium binding in the circulation have also been reported in multiple myeloma and Waldenstrom's macroglobulinemia.[2,3] These patients have an abnormal circulating immunoglobulin that binds calcium ions. In this setting, the globulin fraction, the total protein, and the total calcium levels are all elevated, but the ionized calcium level is normal. A similar situation has been reported when elevated immunoglobulins interfere with the total calcium determination by autoanalyzer. In this instance, the total calcium performed by autoanalyzer is elevated. However, both the total calcium level performed by atomic absorption and the ionized calcium level are normal. Because true hypercalcemia can complicate multiple myeloma and hyperparathyroidism has been reported to be associated with monoclonal gammopathy,[4] care must be taken not to confuse pseudohypercalcemia and true hypercalcemia in these settings. As before, the absence of all signs and symptoms of hypercalcemia coupled with a normal ionized calcium level should allow for the discrimination between these possibilities and prevent inappropriate therapy directed at pseudohypercalcemia.

The third and final situation in which pseudohypercalcemia has been described is in patients with essential thrombocythemia and platelet counts over 700,000.[5] One study reported that 15% of these patients had frank hypercalcemia when total calcium levels were measured. Ionized calcium levels were also elevated, and PTH levels were normal (not suppressed). Signs and symptoms of hypercalcemia were absent. The hypercalcemia was accompanied by hyperkalemia and resolved when platelet counts were normalized. It is thought that the hypercalcemia and hyperkalemia result from the secretion of these ions from the large number of abnormally activated platelets within the specimen tube as a clot is formed. Consistent with this thought, calcium and potassium levels have been found to improve if plasma samples are analyzed instead of serum samples. Thus, as in the previous two disorders, the elevation in serum calcium is an artifact that does not warrant specific therapy.

ENDOCRINE CAUSES OF HYPERCALCEMIA OTHER THAN HYPERPARATHYROIDISM

Thyrotoxicosis

Patients with thyrotoxicosis frequently manifest mild degrees of hypercalcemia.[6–13] It has been reported that the average calcium level rises in patients with hyperthyroidism, and up to 50% of patients with thyrotoxicosis present with serum calciums in the range of 10.5–11.5 mg/dl. A number of cases of coexistent Graves disease and hyperparathyroidism have also been reported. In this instance, the hyperthyroidism can exacerbate the degree of hypercalcemia and actually suppress the PTH values toward the normal range. However, thyrotoxicosis alone can clearly result in elevations of serum calcium. Thyroid hormone has been shown to exert direct effects on bone turnover, increasing bone resorption rates. This releases calcium into the circulation and suppresses PTH levels. Thus, patients with hyperthyroidism as a sole cause of their hypercalcemia should have low PTH and 1,25-dihydroxyvitamin D [1,25(OH)$_2$D] levels with reduced renal reabsorption of calcium. Hypercalcemia may respond to β-adrenergic blockade and is fully reversible on correction of the thyrotoxicosis.

Pheochromocytoma

Hypercalcemia can occur in patients with pheochromocytoma for two reasons.[14–16] Most commonly, the hypercalcemia is a reflection of coexistent primary hyperparathyroidism in patients with multiple endocrine neoplasia type IIa (MEN IIa). The diagnosis of pheochromocytoma should be considered before parathyroidectomy in all hypertensive patients with hyperparathyroidism. However, hypercalcemia that resolves after adrenalectomy has also been reported

The author has no conflict of interest.

in sporadic cases of pheochromocytoma, suggesting that elevations in calcium can result from factors secreted by the tumor itself. There is some evidence that catecholamines can directly affect bone turnover and thus might be the cause of hypercalcemia. However, recent experience has demonstrated that, like many other tumors of neuroendocrine origin, pheochromocytomas can secrete PTH-related protein (PTHrP) and produce hypercalcemia in a fashion identical to many carcinomas.

Adrenal Insufficiency

Hypercalcemia has been associated with adrenal insufficiency, especially in patients presenting with Addisonian crisis.[17–20] It has been seen both in patients with primary as well as secondary adrenal insufficiency. The pathophysiology is unclear. Hypercalcemia may result in part from hemoconcentration and hypovolemia, but some reports have noted increases in ionized as well as total calcium. More recent reports have described suppressed values for PTH and $1,25(OH)_2D$. It is interesting that the human homologue of stanniocalcin, a calcium-lowering agent in fish, has recently been shown to be expressed in the adrenal gland.[21] It is not yet clear if this hormone has any effects on systemic calcium metabolism in humans. Hypercalcemia responds to intravenous fluids and glucocorticoid replacement.

Islet Cell Tumors of the Pancreas

Islet cell tumors can be associated with hypercalcemia caused by the MEN I syndrome and coexistent primary hyperparathyroidism. They have also been found to secrete PTHrP and mimic the humoral hypercalcemia of malignancy (HHM) syndrome.[22–24] In addition, up to 90% of patients with islet cell tumors producing vasoactive intestinal polypeptide (VIP) develop hypercalcemia.[25–29] These patients typically present with the syndrome of watery diarrhea, hypokalemia, and achlorhydria. The pathophysiology of the hypercalcemia in this syndrome has not been fully defined. However, recent studies have demonstrated that PTH levels are suppressed during hypercalcemia, suggesting a PTH-independent mechanism. Furthermore, VIP and VIP receptors have been shown to be present in bone cells and exert effects on bone turnover in cell culture systems. Therefore, it is likely that the hypercalcemia is caused by direct effects of VIP acting on the skeleton.

Milk-Alkali Syndrome

The milk-alkali syndrome results from the ingestion of large amounts of calcium and absorbable alkali.[30–34] It was first described in the 1930s as a complication of ulcer therapy that consisted of large quantities of milk together with sodium bicarbonate. It continued to be seen commonly in the era before the introduction of H_2-blockers, when peptic ulcer disease was often treated with up to 20–26 g of calcium carbonate per day. With the introduction of nonabsorbable antacids and then H_2-blockers and proton pump inhibitors, this syndrome became rare. However, in recent years, it has become more common again because of the increasing use of calcium carbonate to treat or prevent osteoporosis. The syndrome has also been documented in betel-nut users, who sometimes mix the nuts with oyster shell calcium and alkali. A recent series from the University of Oklahoma reported that milk-alkali syndrome caused by calcium carbonate ingestion had become the third most common cause of hypercalcemia in hospitalized patients, representing 16% of hospital admissions for hypercalcemia over a 3-year survey.

The classic triad defining milk-alkali syndrome consists of hypercalcemia, systemic alkalosis, and renal insufficiency. Hypercalcemia is often severe and symptomatic, with presenting values commonly between 15 and 20 mg/dl. Renal dysfunction can vary from mild to severe, and nephrocalcinosis often exists if the syndrome has been present for some time. Other sites of soft tissue calcification, as evidenced by band keratopathy, are common as well. In the older literature, patients were generally reported to be hyperphosphatemic, but in more recent series, phosphate levels have been reported to be normal or low. This most likely reflects the shift from milk, which has a high phosphate content, as a source of calcium to calcium carbonate, which does not. Although some confusion existed in the original literature, recent measurements using modern assays have documented that PTH levels are suppressed. The diagnosis of the syndrome requires a careful history especially of over-the-counter medication use.

The pathophysiology of milk-alkali syndrome is not fully understood, but most likely represents a viscous cycle set up by the ingestion of large amounts of calcium in the setting of volume contraction, systemic alkalosis, and progressive renal insufficiency. It is unclear what the threshold for the induction of hypercalcemia from oral calcium is, but it may be as low as 2 g of calcium daily. This varies with renal function and also between different subjects. By suppressing PTH and leading to volume contraction, hypercalcemia can limit the kidney's ability to excrete bicarbonate. There may also be direct tubular effects of calcium in this regard. In turn, systemic alkalosis can impair the renal excretion of calcium, and it also favors the precipitation of calcium phosphate in the kidney and other soft tissues. The development of nephrocalcinosis then leads to progressive renal dysfunction that contributes to the inability to excrete calcium and bicarbonate. Because of volume contraction and the induction of systemic alkalosis, vomiting can precipitate the syndrome. Likewise, the use of thiazide diuretics is a risk factor because of these drugs' ability to interfere with calcium excretion and to cause volume contraction. The biochemical abnormalities are usually reversible with the discontinuation of oral calcium and alkali and with rehydration followed by forced saline diuresis. If renal failure is severe, making vigorous hydration difficult, hemodialysis against a low calcium bath has also been effective in lowering calcium levels. If the syndrome is acute, hypercalcemia and renal dysfunction resolve promptly and completely. In this setting, there can be rebound hypocalcemia and secondary hyperparathyroidism. In more chronic cases, especially if severe nephrocalcinosis is present, recovery takes longer and renal function may not completely normalize.

IMMOBILIZATION

The skeleton has the ability to sense mechanical stress and adjust bone mass to meet the physical load placed on it.[35] Although the mechanisms underlying this skeletal "mechanosensing" are not fully understood, it seems that the coupling of loading and bone turnover is accomplished primarily through the actions of osteocytes and osteoblasts. One pathological consequence of the active adjustment of bone mass to mechanical demands is that unloading of the skeleton, as happens during the weightlessness of space flight or during prolonged and complete bed rest after orthopedic or neurologic injury, leads to reductions in bone mass.[36–42] In this setting, bone loss occurs because of an uncoupling of bone turnover; one sees a simultaneous reduction in the rate of bone formation and an increase in the rate of bone resorption. This, in turn, leads to the rapid efflux of calcium from skeletal stores, the suppression of PTH and $1,25(OH)_2D$ levels, and the development of hypercalciuria. If the amount of calcium released from the skeleton exceeds the amount of calcium that can be excreted by the kidney, hypercalcemia ensues. The two main risk factors for the development of hypercalcemia during immobilization seem to be (1) an impairment in renal function and (2) an antecedent elevation in bone turnover. Possible reasons for an increased baseline rate of bone turnover include a growing skeleton as seen in children, adolescents, and young adults, hyperparathyroidism, Paget's disease of bone, and "subclinical" or mild malignancy-associated hypercalcemia. For example, 25% of children or young adults with spinal cord injury develop hypercalcemia, while it is unusual in middle-aged patients with normal renal function, despite similar degrees of immobility. Although the classic presentation is in a child or young adult with spinal cord injury, recent reports have suggested that hypercalcemia is a more common complication of stroke and hip fracture than was previously appreciated. This may be a consequence of the age-related decline of renal function in these generally older populations. Special care needs to be taken in the management of patients with hyperparathyroidism or Paget's disease who are put at bed rest, for severe elevations in serum calcium levels can occur. Hypercalcemia, if it is to occur, develops within days to weeks of complete bed rest, and if immobilization is prolonged, it can be associated with the development of upper and lower tract nephrolithiasis and osteopenia. The best treatment is the restoration of weight bearing, which normalizes calcium levels and bone turnover parameters. Passive range-of-motion exercises are not effective. If weight bearing is not possible, hydration, forced saline diuresis, and bisphosphonates have been shown to be effective at lowering calcium levels.

TOTAL PARENTERAL NUTRITION

Hypercalcemia has been reported in patients receiving total parenteral nutrition (TPN) for two reasons.[43–46] The first involves the addition of excessive amounts of calcium and/or vitamin D to the hyperalimentation fluid. This usually occurs early in the course of therapy (days to weeks) and resolves with the reduction of the amount of calcium in the TPN formula. However, there has also been at least one case report of nephrocalcinosis and hypercalcemia developing after several years of continuous TPN that responded to a reduction of the calcium content of the TPN. The second involves inadvertent aluminum toxicity derived from amino acid hydrolysates added to the hyperalimentation fluid. These patients presented after having been on TPN for months to years and were found to have hypercalcemia and low turnover osteomalacia, characteristic of aluminum bone disease. Now that aluminum has been removed from the TPN formulations, this syndrome has disappeared.

HYPERCALCEMIA SECONDARY TO MEDICATIONS

Vitamin D and Its Analogs

Hypercalcemia is a common complication of therapy with vitamin D preparations.[47–53] Vitamin D exerts effects on the intestine, skeleton, and kidney, and the hypercalcemia of vitamin D intoxication seems to be multifactorial, resulting primarily from a combination of increased gastrointestinal absorption of calcium and increased bone resorption. In the kidney, vitamin D primarily regulates the production and metabolism of calcitriol, although it has also been suggested to affect renal tubular calcium handling. Classically, patients with vitamin D intoxication present with hypercalcemia, hyperphosphatemia, and markedly elevated levels of 25-hydroxyvitamin D. Because PTH levels are appropriately suppressed and vitamin D and hypercalcemia both exert negative feedback on 1 α-hydroxylase in the proximal tubules, $1,25(OH)_2D$ levels are usually either normal or only slightly elevated. The recommended daily allowance for vitamin D is 400–800 IU per day. The amount of vitamin D required to produce hypercalcemia has been estimated to be in excess of 25,000–50,000 IU per week. Therefore, it is unusual to see vitamin D intoxication from over-the-counter nutritional supplements. However, there have been reports of hypercalcemia caused by poor quality control in the manufacture of these supplements. In these cases, the actual vitamin D content of the supplements was much higher than what was listed on the labels. There have also been outbreaks of vitamin D intoxication resulting from the accidental oversupplementation of vitamin D into cow's milk by commercial dairies. Nevertheless, the majority of cases of hypercalcemia occur in patients treated with pharmacologic doses of vitamin D or its analogs for the therapy of hypoparathyroidism, malabsorption, or renal osteodystropy. Potent vitamin D analogs have also been used in topical preparations for the treatment of psoriasis and recently for the treatment of advanced prostate cancer. The most frequent setting in which vitamin D use leads to hypercalcemia remains the treatment of secondary hyperparathyroidism complicating renal osteodystrophy. However, newer analogs of vitamin D, such as 1 α-hydroxy vitamin D_2 (Hectorol) and paricalcitol (Zemplar) seem to have less of a tendency to produce hypercalcemia. Hopefully, their deployment into the therapeutic arsenal will decrease the incidence of this complication. Treatment of vitamin D intoxication involves discontinuation of the vitamin D compound, volume expansion, and calciuresis. If hypercalcemia is severe or refractory to the above, treatment with glucocorticoids and/or bisphosphonates may be necessary. The duration of hypercalcemia after the withdrawal of the vitamin D source depends on the biological half-life of the compound used.

Vitamin A and Related Compounds

Vitamin A activates osteoclast-mediated bone resorption through mechanisms that are not well understood. The use of supplements containing vitamin A has been associated with low bone mass and fractures, and the ingestion of large doses (>50,000 IU/day) has been associated with hypercalcemia.[54–58] Like other types of "resorptive" hypercalcemia, PTH and 1,25(OH)$_2$D levels are suppressed in vitamin A intoxication. In the past, this disorder was only seen as the result of drug overdoses and in the exotic setting of arctic explorers consuming polar bear or sled-dog liver. However, more recently, hypercalcemia has been associated with the use of vitamin A analogs, such as *cis*-retinoic acid and all *trans*-retinoic acid, for the treatment of dermatologic conditions and for the therapy of neuroblastoma and hematologic malignancies.

Lithium

There have been many reports of hypercalcemia in patients receiving lithium carbonate.[59–62] The true prevalence of this disorder is uncertain, but retrospective series have suggested that hypercalcemia can occur in 5–40% of patients on the drug. Prospective studies have documented that the average serum calcium level rises in patients started on lithium. The classic presentation resembles familial hypocalciuric hypercalcemia, with elevations in calcium and PTH levels and reductions in renal calcium excretion. In fact, studies in vitro and in vivo have demonstrated that, just like FHH, the set point for calcium-regulated PTH release is shifted to the right in patients taking lithium. That is, there is an impairment of the ability of elevated calcium levels to suppress PTH release from the parathyroids. The mechanisms for this shift in Ca-PTH set point are not completely understood, but these observations suggest that lithium may somehow impair the function of the extracellular calcium-sensing receptor (CaR). There are also reports of an association between lithium use and the development of parathyroid adenomas. However, many of these cases are likely to be patients with previously mild or subclinical primary hyperparathyroidism whose hypercalcemia was worsened by the initiation of therapy with lithium. Hypercalcemia should resolve completely after the discontinuation of lithium.

Estrogens and Antiestrogens

The initiation of antiestrogens (or estrogens) has been shown to produce hypercalcemia in approximately 30% of patients with breast cancer metastatic to the skeleton.[63–66] This estrogen, or antiestrogen flare, is often associated with an increase in bone pain and seems to be related to transient increases in rates of bone resorption surrounding tumor deposits in the skeleton. The mechanisms leading to this flare are not fully understood, although recent work has suggested that estrogens and antiestrogens may modulate the production of PTHrP by breast tumors. The hypercalcemia can be treated with hydration, glucocorticoids, and bisphosphonates, and is self-limiting. The occurrence of this flare has been shown to be a good prognostic sign and may be associated with subsequent tumor regression.

Thiazide Diuretics

Thiazide diuretics enhance calcium reabsorption in the distal tubule.[67] This effect on the kidney is used therapeutically to limit urinary calcium excretion in patients with hypoparathyroidism and nephrolithiasis caused by renal calcium wasting. However, in some patients, it can produce hypercalcemia. Other mechanisms may also contribute to the development of hypercalcemia, for it has been reported in anephric patients on thiazides as well. The degree of hypercalcemia is usually mild, and it resolves rapidly on discontinuation of the drug.

Aminophylline

Mild hypercalcemia has been reported in association with the use of aminophylline and theophylline.[68] This has been observed in the setting of acute loading doses that result in drug levels that exceed the therapeutic range. It has uniformly resolved when patients are placed on maintenance therapy and levels are kept within the therapeutic range. The mechanisms causing the hypercalcemia are unknown.

Growth Hormone

Growth hormone has been used in patients with AIDS, in burn patients, and in patients in surgical intensive care units to try to reverse the catabolic state of severe illness. The use of growth hormone in this way has been reported to cause moderate degrees of hypercalcemia with serum calcium values between 11.5 and 13.5 mg/dl. The mechanisms leading to the hypercalcemia are not well defined, but serum PTH and 1,25(OH)$_2$D levels have been reported to be low.[69–71]

8-Chloro-cyclic AMP

8-Chloro-cyclic adenosine monophosphate is a protein kinase A modulator being developed as an anti-neoplastic agent. In phase I trials, hypercalcemia has been a dose-limiting toxicity. It appears that the hypercalcemia occurs, in part, because of a PTH-like induction of renal 1,25(OH)$_2$D production.[72]

Foscarnet

Foscarnet is an antiviral agent used in the treatment of patients with AIDS. It has been reported to cause both hypocalcemia and hypercalcemia through unknown mechanisms.[73]

INFLAMMATORY DISEASES

As reviewed elsewhere, granulomatous disorders such as sarcoidosis and tuberculosis can lead to hypercalcemia because of the unregulated production of $1,25(OH)_2D$ by activated macrophages. In addition, several other inflammatory conditions such as systemic lupus erythematosus, juvenile rheumatoid arthritis, and recent hepatitis B vaccination have also been reported to cause hypercalcemia.[74–77] In patients with lupus, hypercalcemia has been reported together with lymphadenopathy and pleuritis. This so-called "hypercalcemia-lymphoedema" syndrome has sometimes been associated with elevated circulating levels of PTHrP. It has also been suggested that these patients might have circulating antibodies that activate the PTH receptor. In general, the mechanisms for hypercalcemia in patients with these inflammatory disorders are ill defined.

AIDS

AIDS patients can develop hypercalcemia for a variety of reasons. As already discussed, hypoadrenalism caused by infections, granulomatous disorders such as typical and atypical mycobacterial infections, and malignancy-associated hypercalcemia caused by lymphomas can all occur. In addition, skeletal infection with HIV, HTLV-III, and/or cytomegalovirus has been reported to lead to bone resorption and hypercalcemia.[78]

RENAL FAILURE

Hypercalcemia is a common occurrence in patients with chronic renal failure on hemodialysis and can result from hyperparathyroidism, vitamin D intoxication, calcium antacid overingestion, immobilization, aluminum toxicity, or combinations of these factors. In addition, hypercalcemia is particularly common in the first year after renal transplantation. Renal bone disease and related disorders of mineral homeostasis are discussed in greater detail elsewhere.

Hypercalcemia can also occur in acute renal failure.[79–81] This has classically been described during the recovery phase from acute tubular necrosis caused by rhabdomyolysis. It has been postulated that the severe hyperphosphatemia that accompanies this syndrome leads to the deposition of calcium phosphate in soft tissues and causes hypocalcemia and secondary hyperparathyroidism. When renal function recovers, soft tissue calcium is mobilized, and there is a lag in the return of parathyroid function to normal. The combination of these two phenomena leads to transient hypercalcemia. Hypercalcemia has also been associated with granulomatous forms of interstitial nephritis caused by drug allergy.

MAMMARY HYPERPLASIA

PTHrP is produced by mammary epithelial cells during lactation, and it may play a physiologic role in either maternal or neonatal calcium metabolism during this time. There have been several reports of hypercalcemia caused by elevated circulating levels of PTHrP associated with the development of significant mammary hyperplasia in pregnant or lactating women.[82–84] This has also occurred in the setting of breast hyperplasia and inflammation caused by cyclosporin use after organ transplantation. The hypercalcemia has resolved with the resolution of the breast hyperplasia or on reduction mammoplasty.

GAUCHER'S DISEASE

One case of hypercalcemia in a patient with Gaucher's disease and acute pneumonia has been reported.[85] This patient had a normal calcium level before developing pneumonia, and the mechanisms of the elevation in calcium are unknown.

MANGANESE INTOXICATION

Workers exposed to toxic concentrations of manganese in contaminated workplaces or wells can develop severe hypercalcemia.[86,87] The mechanisms by which manganese exposure causes hypercalcemia are unknown.

END-STAGE LIVER DISEASE

Patients with end-stage chronic liver disease awaiting liver transplantation have been reported to develop hypercalcemia.[88] The mechanisms underlying the elevations in calcium are not known but are likely to be multifactorial.

PRIMARY OXALOSIS

Adults with primary oxalosis have been reported to develop severe hypercalcemia.[89,90] There seems to be increased bone resorption, perhaps because of the formation of oxalate-induced granulomas in the bone marrow. This would be consistent with the observation that PTH and $1,25(OH)_2D$ vitamin D levels are low. However, the mechanisms underlying the development of hypercalcemia are not completely understood.

REFERENCES

1. Ladenson JH, Lewis JH, McDonald JM, Slatopolsky E, Boyd JC 1978 Relationship of free and total calcium in hypercalcemic conditions. J Clin Endocrinol Metab **48:**393–397.
2. Merlini G, Fitzpatrick LA, Siris ES, Bilezikian JP, Birken S, Beychok S, Osserman EF 1984 A human myeloma immunoglobulin G binding four moles of calcium associated with asymptomatic hypercalcemia. J Clin Immunol **4:**185–196.
3. John R, Oleesky D, Issa B, Scanlon MF, Williams CP, Harrison CB, Child DF 1997 Pseudohypercalcemia in two patients with IgM paraproteinemia. Ann Clin Biochem **34:**694–696.
4. Arnulf B, Bengoufa D, Sarfati E, Toubert ME, Meignin V, Brouet JC, Fermand JP 2002 Prevalence of monoclonal gammapathy in patients with primary hyperparathyroidism: A prospective study. Arch Intern Med **162:**464–467.
5. Howard MR, Ashwell S, Bond LR, Holbrook I 2000 Artefactual serum hyperkalaemia and hypercalcaemia in essential thrombocythaemia. J Clin Pathol **53:**105–109.
6. Peerenboom H, Keck E, Kruskemper GL, Strohmeyer G 1984 The defect in intestinal calcium transport in hyperthyroidism and its response to therapy. J Clin Endocrinol Metab **59:**936–940.
7. Burman KD, Monchick JM, Earll JM, Wartofski L 1976 Ionized and total serum calcium and parathyroid hormone in hyperthyroidism. Ann Intern Med **84:**668–671.

8. Ross DS, Nussbaum SR 1989 Reciprocal changes in parathyroid hormone and thyroid function after radioiodine treatment of hyperthyroidism. J Clin Endocrinol Metab 68:1216–1219.

9. Britto JM, Fenton AJ, Holloway WR, Nicholson GC 1994 Osteoblasts mediate thyroid hormone stimulation of osteoclastic bone resorption. Endocrinology 123:169–176.

10. Rosen HN, Moses AC, Gundberg C, Kung VT, Seyedin SM, Chen T, Holick M, Greenspan SL 1993 Therapy with parenteral pamidronate prevents thyroid hormone-induced bone turnover in humans. J Clin Endocrinol Metab 77:664–669.

11. Rude RK, Oldham SB, Singer FR, Nicoloff JT 1976 Treatment of thyrotoxic hypercalcemia with propranolol. N Engl J Med 294:431–433.

12. Begis-Karup S, Wagner B, Raber W, Schneider B, Hamwi A, Waldhausl W, Vierhapper H 2001 Serum calcium in thyroid disease. Wien Klin Wochenschr 113:65–68.

13. Xiao H, Yu B, Wang S, Chen G 2002 Concomitant Graves disease and primary hyperparathyroidism: The first case report in mainland of China and literature review. Chin Med J (Engl) 115:939–941.

14. Stewart AF, Hoecker J, Segre GV, Mallette LE, Amatruda T, Vignery A 1985 Hypercalcemia in pheochromocytoma: Evidence for a novel mechanism. Ann Intern Med 102:776–779.

15. Mune T, Katakami H, Kato Y, Yasuda K, Matsukura S, Miura K 1993 Production and secretion of parathyroid hormone-related protein in pheochromocytoma: A participation of an α-adrenergic mechanism. J Clin Endocrinol Metab 76:757–762.

16. Taleda S, Elefteriou F, Levasseur R, Liu X, Zhao L, Parker KL, Armstrong D, Ducy P, Karsenty G 2002 Leptin regulates bone formation via the sympathetic nervous system. Cell 111:305–317.

17. Muls E, Bouillon R, Boelaert J, Lamberigts G, Van Imschoot S, Daneels R, De Moor P 1982 Etiology of hypercalcemia in a patient with Addison's disease. Calcif Tissue Int 34:523–526.

18. Vasikaran SD, Tallis GA, Braund WJ 1994 Secondary hypoadrenalism presenting with hypercalcaemia. Clin Endocrinol (Oxf) 41:261–265.

19. Diamond T, Thornley S 1994 Addisonian crisis and hypercalcaemia. Aust N Z J Med 24:316.

20. Wong RK, Gregory R, Lo TC 2000 A case of isolated ACTH deficiency presenting with hypercalcaemia. Int J Clin Pract 54:623–624.

21. Miura W, Mizunashi K, Kimura N, Koide Y, Noshiro T, Miura Y, Furukawa Y, Nagura H 2000 Expression of stanniocalcin in zona glomerulosa and medulla of normal human adrenal glands, and some adrenal tumors and cell lines. APMIS 108:367–372.

22. Mao C, Carter P, Schaefer P, Zhu L, Dominguez JM, Hanson DJ, Appert HE, Kim K, Howard JM 1994 Malignant islet cell tumor associated with hypercalcemia. Surgery 117:37–40.

23. Ratcliffe WA, Bowden SJ, Dunne FP, Hughes S, Emly JF, Baker JT, Pye JK, Williams CP 1994 Expression and processing of parathyroid hormone-related protein in a pancreatic endocrine cell tumour associated with hypercalcaemia. Clin Endocrinol (Oxf) 40:679–686.

24. Asa SL, Henderson J, Goltzman D, Drucker DJ 1990 Parathyroid hormone-like peptide in normal and neoplastic human endocrine tissues. J Clin Endocrinol Metab 71:1112–1118.

25. Verner JV, Morrison AB 1974 Endocrine pancreatic islet disease with diarrhea. Arch Intern Med 133:492–500.

26. Holdaway IM, Evans MC, Clarke ED 1977 Watery diarrhoea syndrome with episodic hypercalcaemia. Aust N Z J Med 7:63–65.

27. Lundgren P, Lundgren I, Mukohyama H, Lehenkari PP, Horton MA, Lerner UH 2001 Vasoactive intestinal peptide (VIP)/pituitary adenylate cyclase-activating peptide receptor subtypes in mouse calvarial osteoblasts: Presence of VIP-2 receptors and differentiation-induced expression of VIP-1 receptors. Endocrinology 142:339–347.

28. Lundberg P, Lerner UH 2002 Expression and regulatory role of receptors for vasoactive intestinal peptide in bone cells. Microsc Res Tech 58:98–103.

29. Lundberg P, Lie A, Bjurholm A, Lehenkari PP, Horton MA, Lerner UH, Ransjo M 2000 Vasoactive intestinal peptide regulates osteoclast activity via specific binding sites on both osteoclasts and osteoblasts. Bone 27:803–810.

30. Beall DP, Scofield RH 1995 Milk-alkali syndrome associated with calcium carbonate consumption. Medicine 74:89–96.

31. Orwoll ES 1982 The milk-alkali syndrome: Current concepts. Ann Intern Med 97:242–248.

32. Fiorino AS 1996 Hypercalcemia and alkalosis due to the milk-alkali syndrome: A case report and review. Yale J Biol Med 69:517–523.

33. Camidge R, Peaston R 2001 Recommended dose antacids and severe hypercalcaemia. Br J Clin Pharmacol 52:341–342.

34. Wu KD, Chuang RB, Wu FL, Hsu WA, Jan IS, Tsai KS 1996 The milk-alkali syndrome caused by betelnuts in oyster shell paste. J Toxicol 34:741–745.

35. Neuman WF 1970 Calcium metabolism in space flight. Life Sci Space Res 8:309–315.

36. Stewart AF, Adler M, Byers CM, Segre GV, Broadus AE 1982 Calcium homestasis in immobilization: An example of resorptive hypercalciuria. N Engl J Med 306:1136–1140.

37. Bergstrom WH 1978 Hypercalciuria and hypercalcemia complicating immobilization. Am J Dis Child 132:553–554.

38. Chappard D, Minaire P, Privat C, Berard E, Mendoza-Sarmiento J, Tournebise H, Basle MF, Audran M, Rebel A, Picot C, Gaud C 1995 Effects of tiludronate on bone loss in paraplegic patients. J Bone Miner Res 10:112–118.

39. Roberts D, Lee W, Cuneo RC, Wittmann J, Ward G, Flatman R, McWhinney B, Hickman PE 1998 Longitudinal study of bone turnover after acute spinal cord injury. J Clin Endocrinol Metab 83:415–442.

40. Sato Y, Kaji M, Higuchi F, Yanagida I, Oishi K, Oizumi K 2001 Changes in bone and calcium metabolism following hip fracture in elderly patients. Osteoporos Int 12:445–449.

41. Sato Y 2000 Abnormal bone and calcium metabolism in patients after stroke. Arch Phys Med Rehabil 81:117–121.

42. Massagli TL, Cardenas DD 1999 Immobilization hypercalcemia treatment with pamidronate disodium after spinal cord injury. Arch Phys Med Rehabil 80:998–1000.

43. Ott SM, Maloney NA, Klein GL, Alfrey AC, Ament ME, Coburn JW, Sherrard DJ 1983 Aluminum is associated with low bone formation in patients receiving chronic parenteral nutrition. Ann Intern Med 96:910–914.

44. Klein GL, Horst RL, Norman AW, Ament ME, Slatopolsky E, Coburn JW 1981 Reduced serum levels of 1α, 25-hydroxyvitamin D during long-term total parenteral nutrition. Ann Intern Med 94:638–643.

45. Shike M, Sturtridge WC, Tam CS, Harrison JE, Jones G, Murray TM, Husdan H, Whitewell J, Wilson DR, Jeejeebhoy KN 1981 A possible role of vitamin D in the genesis of parenteral-nutrition-induced metabolic bone disease. Ann Intern Med 95:560–568.

46. Ikema S, Horikawa R, Nakano M, Yokouchi K, Yamazaki H, Tanaka T, Tanae A 2000 Growth and metabolic disturbances in a patient with total parenteral nutrition: A case of hypercalciuric hypercalcemia. Endocr J 47(Suppl):S137–S140.

47. Haussler MR, McCain TA 1977 Basic and clinical concepts related to vitamin D metabolism and action. N Engl J Med 297:974–1041.

48. Holick MF, Shao Q, Liu WW, Chen TC 1992 The vitamin D content of fortified milk and infant formula. N Engl J Med 326:1178–1181.

49. Jacobus CH, Holick MF, Shao Q, Chen TC, Holm IA, Kolodny JM, Fuleihan GE, Seely EW 1992 Hypervitaminosis D associated with drinking milk. N Engl J Med 326:1173–1177.

50. Pettifor JM, Bikle DD, Cavalerso M, Zachen D, Kamdar MC, Ross FP 1995 Serum levels of free 1,25-dihydroxyvitamin D in vitamin D toxicity. Ann Intern Med 122:511–513.

51. Martin KJ, Gonzalez E, Lindberg JS, Taccetta C, Amdahl M, Malhotra K, Llach F 2001 Paricalcitol dosing according to body weight or severity of hyperparathyroidism: A double-blind, multicenter, randomized study. Am J Kidney Dis 38(Suppl 5):S57–S63.

52. Liu G, Oettel K, Ripple G, Staab MJ, Horvath D, Alberti D, Arzoomanian R, Mamocha R, Bruskewitz R, Mazess R, Bishop C, Bhattacharya A, Bailey H, Wilding G 2002 Phase I trial of 1 alpha-hydroxyvitamin d(2) in patients with hormone refractory prostate cancer. Clin Cancer Res 8:2820–2827.

53. Koutkia P, Chen TC, Holick MF 2001 Vitamin D intoxication associated with an over-the-counter supplement. N Engl J Med 345:66–67.

54. Valente JD, Elias AN, Weinstein GD 1983 Hypercalcemia associated with oral isotretinoin in the treatment of severe acne. JAMA 250:1899.

55. Suzumiya J, Asahara F, Katakami H, Kimuran N, Hisano S, Okumura M, Ohno R 1994 Hypercalcaemia caused by all-trans retanoic acid treatment of acute promyelocytic leukaemia: Case report. Eur J Haematol 53:126–127.

56. Bourke JF, Berth-Jones J, Hutchinson PE 1993 Hypercalcemia with topical calcipotriol. BMJ 306:1334–1335.

57. Villablanca JG, Khan AA, Avramis VI, Seeger RC, Matthay KK, Ramsay NK, Reynolds CP 1995 Phase I trial of 13-cis-retinoic acid in children with neuroblastoma following bone marrow transplantation. J Clin Oncol 13:894–901.

58. Michaëlsson K, Lithell H, Vessby B, Melhus H 2003 Serum retinal levels and the risk of fracture. N Engl J Med 348:287–294.

59. Haden ST, Stoll AL, McCormick S, Scott J, Fuleihan GE 1979 Alterations in parathyroid dynamics in lithium-treated subjects. J Clin Endocrinol Metab 82:2844–2848.

60. Rifal MA, Moles K, Harrington DP 2001 Lithium-induced hypercalcemia and parathyroid dysfunction. Psychosomatics **42**:359–361.

61. Mak TW, Shek CC, Chow CC, Wing YK, Lee S 1998 Effects of lithium therapy on bone mineral metabolism: A two-year prospective longitudinal study. J Clin Endocrinol Metab **83**:3857–3859.

62. Dwight T, Kytola S, The BT, Theodosopoulos G, Richardson AL, Philips J, Twigg S, Delbridge L, Marsh DJ, Nelson AE, Larrson C, Robinson BG 2002 Genetic analysis of lithium-associated parathyroid tumors. Eur J Endocrinol **146**:619–627.

63. Legha SS, Powell K, Buzdar AU, Blumen-Schein GR 1981 Tamoxifen-induced hypercalcemia in breast cancer. Cancer **47**:2803–2806.

64. Valentin-Opran A, Eilon G, Saez S, Mundy GR 1985 Estrogens and antiestrogens stimulate release of bone-resorbing activity in cultured human breast cancer cells. J Clin Invest **75**:726–731.

65. Funk JL, Wei H 1998 Regulation of parathyroid hormone-related protein expression of MCF-7 breast carcinoma cells by estrogen and antiestrogens. Biochem Biophy Res Commun **251**:849–854.

66. Kurebayashi J, Sonoo H 1997 Parathyroid hormone-related protein secretion is inhibited by oestradiol and stimulated by antioestrogens in KPL-3C human breast cancer cells. Br J Cancer **75**:1819–1825.

67. Porter RH, Cox BG, Heaney D, Hostetter TH, Stinebaugh BJ, Suki WN 1978 Treatment of hypoparathyroid patients with chlorthalidone. N Engl J Med **298**:577–581.

68. McPherson ML, Prince SR, Atamer E, Maxwell DB, Ross-Clunis H, Estep H 1986 Theophylline-induced hypercalcemia. Ann Intern Med **105**:52–54.

69. Knox JB, Demling RH, Wilmore DW, Sarraf P, Santos AA 1995 Hypercalcemia associated with the use of human growth hormone in an adult surgical intensive care unit. Arch Surg **130**:442–445.

70. Sakoulas G, Tritos NA, Lally M, Wanke C, Hartzband P 1977 Hypercalcemia in an AIDS patient treated with growth hormone. AIDS **11**:1353–1356.

71. Singh KP, Prasad R, Chari PS, Dash RJ 1998 Effect of growth hormone therapy in burn patients on conservative treatment. Burns **24**:733–738.

72. Saunders MP, Salisbury AJ, O'Byrne KJ, Long L, Whitehouse RM, Talbot DC, Mawer EB, Harris AL 1997 A novel cyclic adenosine monophosphate analog induces hypercalcemia via production of 1, 25-dihydroxyvitamin D in patients with solid tumors. J Clin Endocrinol Metab **83**:4044–4048.

73. Gayet S, Ville E, Durand JM, Mars ME, Morange S, Kaplanski G, Gallais H, Soubeyrand J 1997 Foscarnet-induced hypercalcemia in AIDS. AIDS **11**:1068–1070.

74. Schurman SJ, Bergstrom WH, Root AW, Souid AK, Hannah WP 1998 Interlukin 1 beta-mediated calcitropic activity in serum of children with juvenile rheumatoid arthritis. J Rheumatol **25**:161–165.

75. Cathebras P, Cartry O, Lafage-Proust MH, Lauwers A, Acquart S, Thomas T, Rousset H 1996 Arthritis, hypercalcemia and lytic bone lesions after hepatitis B vaccination. J Rheumatol **23**:558–560.

76. Deftos LJ, Burton DW, Baird SM, Terkeltaub RA 1996 Hypercalcemia and systemic lupus erythematosus. Arthritis Rheum **39**:2066–2069.

77. Berar-Yanay N, Weiner P, Magadle R 2001 Hypercalcaemia in systemic lupus erythematosus. Clin Rheumatol **20**:147–149.

78. Zaloga GP, Chernow B, Eil C 1985 Hypercalcemia and disseminated cytomegalovirus infection in the acquired immunodeficiency syndrome. Ann Intern Med **102**:331–333.

79. Llach F, Felsenfeld AJ, Haussler MR 1981 The pathophysiology of altered calcium metabolism in rhabdomyolysis-induced acute renal failure. N Engl J Med **305**:117–123.

80. Lane JT, Boudrea RJ, Kinlaw WB 1990 Disappearance of muscular calcium deposits during resolution of prolonged rhabdomyolysis-induced hypercalcemia. Am J Med **89**:523–525.

81. Wall CA, Gaffney EF, Mellotte GJ 2000 Hypercalcaemia and acute interstitial nephritis associated with omeprazole therapy. Nephrol Dial Transplant **15**:1450–1452.

82. Khosla S, van Heerden JA, Gharib H, Jackson IT, Danks J, Hayman JA, Martin TJ 1990 Parathyroid hormone-related protein and hypercalcemia secondary to massive mammary hyperplasia. N Engl J Med **322**:1157.

83. Anai T, Tomiyasu T, Arima K, Miyakawa I 1999 Pregnancy-associated osteoporosis with elevated levels of circulating parathyroid hormone-related protein: A report of two cases. J Obstet Gynaecol Res **25**:63–67.

84. Eardley KS, Wan DI, Thomas ME, Banerjee AK, Radojkovic M, Taylor JL 2002 Transplant-associated inflammatory breast disease. Nephrol Dial Transplant **17**:512–515.

85. Bryne CD, Bermann L, Cox TM 1997 Pathologic bone fractures preceded by sustained hypercalcemia in Gaucher disease. J Inherit Metab Dis **20**:709–710.

86. Chandra SV, Seth PK, Mankeshwar JK 1974 Manganese poisoning: Clinical and biochemical observations. Environ Res **7**:374–380.

87. Chandra SV, Shukla GS, Srivastava RS 1981 An exploratory study of manganese exposure to welders. Clin Toxicol **18**:407–416.

88. Gerhardt A, Greenberg A, Reilly JJ, Van Thiel DH 1987 Hypercalcemia, a complication of advanced chronic liver disease. Arch Intern Med **147**:274–277.

89. Yamaguchi K, Grant J, Noble-Jamieson G, Jamieson N, Barnes ND, Compston JE 1995 Hypercalcemia in primary oxalosis: Role of increased bone resorption and effects of treatment with pamidronate. Bone **16**:61–67.

90. Toussaint C, DePauw C, Tielmans C, Abramowicz D 1995 Hypercalcemia complicating systemic oxalosis in primary hyperoxaluria type 1. Nephrol Dial Transplant **10**(Suppl 8):17–21.

Chapter 41. Hypercalcemic Syndromes in Infants and Children

Craig B. Langman

Department of Pediatrics, Feinberg School of Medicine, Northwestern University, and Kidney Diseases Department, Children's Memorial Hospital, Chicago, Illinois

INTRODUCTION

Blood ionized calcium levels in normal infants and young children are similar to those of adults, with a mean ± 2 SD = 1.21 ± 0.13 mM. In neonates, the normal blood ionized calcium level is dependent on postnatal age.[1] In the first 72 h after birth, there is a significant decrease in the blood ionized calcium level in term newborns, from 1.4 to 1.2 mM; the decrease is exaggerated in preterm neonates.

Chronic hypercalcemia in young infants and children may not be associated with the usual signs and symptoms described elsewhere. Rather, the predominant manifestation of hypercalcemia is "failure to thrive," in which linear growth is arrested and there is lack of appropriate weight gain. Additional features of chronic hypercalcemia in children include nonspecific symptoms of irritability, gastrointestinal reflux, abdominal pain, and anorexia. Acute hypercalcemia is very uncommon in infants and children; when it occurs, its manifestations are similar to those of older children and adults, with potential alterations in the nervous system, the conduction system of the heart, and kidney functions.

WILLIAMS SYNDROME

Williams et al.[2] described a syndrome in infants with supravalvular aortic stenosis and peculiar ("elfin-like") facies; hypercalcemia during the first year of life also was noted.[3] However, the severe elevations in serum calcium initially described failed to appear with equal frequency in subsequent series of such infants. Other series of children with the cardiac lesion failed to show the associated facial dysmorphism. It is thought that there exists a spectrum of infants with some or all of these abnormalities, and a scoring system has been described to assign suspected infants as lying within or outside of the syndrome classification.[4]

Two-thirds of infants with Williams syndrome are small for their gestational age, and many are born past their expected date of birth. The facial abnormalities consist of structural asymmetry, temporal depression, flat malae with full cheeks, microcephaly, epicanthal folds, lacy or stellate irises, a short nose, long philtrum, arched upper lip with full lower lip, and small, maloccluded teeth. The vocal tone is often hoarse. Neurologic manifestations include hypotonia, hyperreflexia, and mild-to-moderate motor retardation. The personality of affected children has been described as "cocktail party," in that they are unusually friendly to strangers. Other vascular abnormalities have been described in addition to supravalvular aortic stenosis, including other congenital heart defects and many peripheral organ arterial stenoses (renal, mesenteric, and celiac).

Hypercalcemia, if initially present, rarely persists to the end of the first year of life and generally disappears spontaneously. Despite the rarity of chronic hypercalcemia, persistent hypercalciuria is not uncommon. Additionally, many of the signs and symptoms of hypercalcemia mentioned previously and in the introduction to this section have been noted in these infants. The long-term prognosis for patients with Williams syndrome seems to depend on features other than the level of blood calcium, such as the level of mental retardation and the clinical significance of the cardiovascular abnormalities. Approximately 25% of patients may have radioulnar synostosis, which may impede normal developmental milestones of fine-motor activities of the upper extremities if not recognized.[5]

A search for the gene(s) responsible for Williams syndrome localized the cardiac component, supravalvular aortic stenosis, the long arm of chromosome 7.[6] It seems that translocations of the *elastin* gene may be responsible for isolated or familial supravalvular aortic stenosis,[7,8] whereas a heterozygous microdeletion of chromosome 7q11.23, which encompasses the *elastin* gene,[9] produces Williams syndrome. Rarely, it may involve a defect of chromosome 11 [del(11)(q13.5q14.2)] or chromosome 22 [r(22)p11→q13)].[10]

Despite the potential localization of the disorder of the deletion of the elastin locus on chromosome 7, the pathogenesis of the disorder remains unknown, although many studies focused on disordered control of vitamin D metabolism. Previous studies of affected children demonstrated increased circulating levels of 25-hydoxyvitamin D after vitamin D administration,[11] increased levels of calcitriol (1,25-dihydroxyvitamin D [1,25(OH)$_2$D]) during periods of hypercalcemia[12] but not during normocalcemia,[13,14] or diminished levels of calcitonin during calcium infusion.[15] Although excess administration of vitamin D to pregnant rabbits may produce an experimental picture not dissimilar to that in humans with Williams syndrome, the overwhelming majority of children with Williams syndrome are not the result of maternal vitamin D intoxication.

IDIOPATHIC INFANTILE HYPERCALCEMIA

In the early 1950s in England, Lightwood[16] reported a series of infants with severe hypercalcemia. Epidemiologic investigations revealed that the majority of affected infants were born to mothers ingesting foods heavily fortified with vitamin D. The incidence of the disease declined dramatically with reduction of vitamin D supplementation. Other cases have been described without previous exposure to excessive maternal vitamin D intake, and the incidence of idiopathic infantile hypercalcemia (IIH) has remained fixed

The author has no conflict of interest.

over the past 20 years. Affected infants have polyuria, increased thirst, and the general manifestations of hypercalcemia previously noted. Severely affected neonates may have cardiac lesions similar to those seen in Williams syndrome and may even manifest the dysmorphic features of those infants and children. The distinction between the two syndromes remains problematic.[17] Other clinical manifestations include chronic arterial hypertension, strabismus, inguinal hernias, musculoskeletal abnormalities (disordered posture and mild kyphosis), and bony abnormalities (radio-ulnar synostosis and dislocated patella). Hyperacusis is present in the majority of affected children with IIH, but not Williams syndrome, and it is persistent.

As in Williams syndrome, disordered vitamin D metabolism with increased vitamin D sensitivity with respect to gastrointestinal transport of calcium has been posited as the cause of this disorder,[18] although the data are conflicting. We identified seven consecutive children with IIH in whom the presence of an elevated level of N-terminal parathyroid hormone-related protein (PTHrP) was demonstrated at the time of hypercalcemia.[19] Its familial occurrence has been described.[20] Furthermore, in five of these children who achieved normocalcemia, the levels of PTHrP normalized or were immeasurably low, and in one child with persistent hypercalcemia, the level of PTHrP remained elevated. No other nonmalignant disorder of childhood that we have examined, including two children with hypercalcemia from Williams syndrome, has had elevated levels of PTHrP, although a report of an infantile fibrosarcoma and hypercalcemia demonstrated PTHrP production from the soft-tissue tumor.[21] In contrast to the hypercalcemia of Williams syndrome, the level of blood calcium in IIH remains elevated for a prolonged period in the most severely affected children. After relief of the hypercalcemia, persistent hypercalciuria has been noted.[22] Therapy includes the use of glucocorticoids to reduce gastrointestinal absorption of calcium, as well as the avoidance of vitamin D and excess dietary calcium.

FAMILIAL HYPOCALCIURIC HYPERCALCEMIA

This disorder also is called familial benign hypercalcemia and has been recognized since 1972[23] as a cause of elevated total and serum ionized calcium. The onset of the change in calcium is commonly before age 10 years and was described in newborns.[24]

NEONATAL PRIMARY HYPERPARATHYROIDISM

Primary hyperparathyroidism is uncommon in neonates and children,[25] with less than 100 cases reported. Additionally, only 20% of cases occur in children younger than 10 years. Hypercalcemia in the first decade of life may more likely be caused by the other disorders discussed in this chapter. The presenting clinical manifestations are weakness, anorexia, and irritability, which are seen in a multitude of pediatric disorders. The association with other endocrine disorders occurs with decreased frequency in young children with primary hyperparathyroidism. Histological examination of the parathyroid glands show that 20–40% of affected children may have hyperplasia rather than the more typical adenoma in older individuals.

However, the neonate may show one unusual form of hyperparathyroidism. Neonatal severe primary hyperparathyroidism is now known to result from inheritance of two mutant alleles associated with the *calcium-sensing receptor* gene on chromosome 3.[26] Extreme elevations of serum calcium (total calcium ≥ 20 mg/dl; blood ionized calcium levels ≥ 3 mM) is a hallmark of the disorder, and emergency total surgical parathyroidectomy is required for life-saving reasons. An attempt to salvage one of the parathyroid glands and perform autotransplantation is suggested for such infants. Certain heterozygous inactivating mutations in the *extracellular calcium-receptor* gene may still produce neonatal hypercalcemia,[27] leading to the conclusion that even the heterozygous state has important clinical implications for the neonate.

JANSEN SYNDROME

Jansen syndrome[28–31] presents in neonates with hypercalcemia and skeletal radiographs that resemble a rachitic condition. It is a form of metaphyseal dysplasia, and after infancy, the radiographic condition evolves into a more typical picture, with resultant mottled calcifications in the distal end of the long bones. These areas represent patches of partially calcified cartilage protruding into the diaphyseal portion of bone. The skull and spine may be affected also. The hypercalcemia appears to be lifelong.

Biochemical findings in patients with Jansen syndrome are consistent with primary hyperparathyroidism, but there are no measurable levels of PTH or PTHrP. The disorder results from a defect in the gene for the PTH/PTH-like protein receptor. One of three different amino acid substitutions produces a mutant receptor that is capable of auto-activation in the absence of ligand. This produces unopposed PTH/PTH-like protein actions in such patients and thereby explains the absence of circulating levels of either hormone. Such patients seem to be at risk for the development of the complications of hyperparathyroidism in the adult years. However, other patients have been given the diagnosis of Jansen syndrome without either hypercalcemia or the finding of a mutation in the gene for the PTH/PTHrP receptor.

MISCELLANEOUS DISORDERS

Subcutaneous Fat Necrosis

Michael et al.[32] reported the association of significant birth trauma with fat necrosis in two small-for-gestational-age infants who subsequently developed severe hypercalcemia (serum calcium > 15 mg/dl) and violaceous discoloration in pressure sites. Histological examination of the affected pressure sites in such patients demonstrated both an inflammatory, mononuclear cell infiltrate and crystals that contain calcium. We also noted hypercalcemia in several children with subcutaneous fat necrosis associated with major trauma or disseminated varicella. The mechanism of the hypercalcemia is unknown, but it may be related to mildly elevated levels of $1,25(OH)_2D$[33] or excess prostaglandin E production.[34] The prognosis for infants and children with subcutaneous fat necrosis depends on the duration of the hypercalcemia. Reductions in serum calcium have been noted with the use of exogenous corticosteroids, saline, and furosemide diuresis, and the avoidance of excess dietary calcium and vitamin D. Recurrence of hypercalcemia has not been seen.

Hypophosphatasia

This disorder is discussed in detail elsewhere and is mentioned here only for completeness. Severe infantile hypophosphatasia is associated with markedly elevated serum calcium levels and a reduction in circulating alkaline phosphatase, increase in urinary phosphoethanolamine, and elevated serum pyridoxal-5-phosphate concentrations. The use of calcitonin in a neonate with hypercalcemia was reported as beneficial to long-term outcome.[35]

Sarcoidosis and Other Granulomatous Disorders of Childhood

Thirty percent to 50% of children with the autoimmune disorder sarcoidosis[36] manifest hypercalcemia, and an additional 20–30% show hypercalciuria with normocalcemia. Many of the presenting manifestations of children with sarcoidosis may be related to the presence of hypercalcemia. A recent report of hypercalcemia in twin children with cat-scratch disease,[37] a granulomatous disorder resulting from infection with *Bartonella henselae*, shows that the granuloma may represent a source of $1,25(OH)_2D$ production that leads to the hypercalcemia. Successful therapy of these disorders reduces the circulating levels of that hormone to normal.

Limb Fracture

Isolated weight-bearing limb fracture[38] that requires immobilization for even several days may be associated with elevated blood ionized calcium levels and hypercalciuria in young children and adolescents. Although prolonged immobilization itself commonly produces hypercalcemia and hypercalciuria, the occurrence after short-term bed rest in children probably reflects their more rapid skeletal turnover.

Vitamin D (or Vitamin D Metabolite)

Hypervitaminosis D (vitamin D intoxication) produces symptomatic hypercalcemia. In childhood, vitamin D intoxication has been seen after excessively prolonged feeding of premature infants with a vitamin D–fortified formula,[39] after ingestion of improperly fortified dairy milk,[40,41] and in children receiving therapeutic vitamin D or vitamin D metabolites.[42]

An outbreak of hypercalcemia in eight patients was reported from the incorrect dosing of dairy milk with vitamin D,[40] and in addition, a defect was found in the concentrate used to fortify the milk (containing cholecalciferol rather than the expected ergocalciferol). These same investigators extended their measurements of the vitamin D content to both commercial dairy milks and fortified infant formulas, and they found that only 29% of the milks and formulas contained a vitamin D content within 20% of the stated amount.[41] These studies suggest that improved monitoring of the fortification process is mandatory and may explain the rare finding of clinical vitamin D deficiency in children drinking fortified milk.

Children with renal osteodystrophy are commonly treated with 1,25-dihydroxyvitamin D_3 [$1,25(OH)_2D_3$] and develop hypercalcemia once every 12–15 treatment months, whereas the use of 25-hydroxyvitamin D_3 is associated with a lower incidence of hypercalcemia. Children with frank hypocalcemic disorders treated with $1,25(OH)_2D_3$ develop hypercalcemia at one-third the frequency of children with renal osteodystrophy treated with any vitamin D metabolite.[42] Treatment with the parent vitamin D compound is associated with the production of hypercalcemia similar to the rate produced with calcitriol. However, the hypercalcemia associated with vitamin D is prolonged 4- to 6-fold compared with hypercalcemia with metabolite therapy because of retention in body fat stores.

Prostaglandin E

Bartter syndrome may result from one of several mutations in the genes for various sodium-linked chloride transporters.[43] A neonatal form may produce a marked increase in prostaglandin E production and lead to hypercalcemia, in part, from excessive bone resorption.[44] Such a disturbance in bone also may contribute to the hypercalcemia seen in neonates who receive prostaglandin E infusions for congenital cardiovascular diseases that mandate patency of the fetal ductus arteriosus.

Congenital Lactase Deficiency

In one study, it was noted that 7 of 10 infants with congenital lactase deficiency manifested hypercalcemia within the first 3 months of life and was associated with renal medullary nephrocalcinosis.[45] A lactose-free diet was associated with return of elevated serum calcium levels to normal. The mechanism of the hypercalcemia remains unclear but may reflect the known effects of lactose to promote direct calcium absorption through the intestine.

REFERENCES

1. Specker BL, Lichtenstein P, Mimouni F, Gormley C, Tsang RC 1986 Calcium-regulating hormones and minerals from birth to 18 months of age: A cross-sectional study. II. Effects of sex, rage, age, season and diet on serum minerals, parathyroid hormone and calcitonin. Pediatrics **77:**891–896.
2. Williams JCP, Barratt-Boyes BG, Lower JB 1961 Supravalvular aortic stenosis. Circulation **24:**1311–1316.
3. Black JA, Bonham Carter RE 1984 Association between aortic stenosis and facies of severe infantile hypercalcemia. Lancet **2:**745–748.
4. Preus M 1984 The Williams syndrome: Objective definition and diagnosis. Clin Genet **25:**422–428.
5. Charvat KA, Hornstein L, Oestreich AE 1991 Radio-ulnarsynostosis in Williams syndrome: A frequently associated anomaly. Pediatr Radiol **21:**508–510.
6. Ewart AK, Morris CA, Ensing GJ, Loker J, Moore C, Leppert M, Keating M 1993 A human vascular disorder, supravalvular aortic stenosis, maps to chromosome 7. Proc Natl Acad Sci USA **90:**3226–3230.

7. Curran ME, Atkinson DL, Ewart AK, Morris CA, Keppert MF, Keating MT 1993 The elastin gene is disrupted by a translocation associated with supravalvular aortic stenosis. Cell 73:159–168.
8. Ewart AK, Jin W, Atkinson D, Morris CA, Keating MT 1994 Supravalvular aortic stenosis associated with a deletion disrupting the elastin gene. J Clin Invest 93:1071–1077.
9. Perez Jurado LA, Peoples R, Kaplan P, Hamel BC, Francke U 1996 Molecular definition of the chromosome 7 deletion in Williams syndrome and parent-of-origin effects on growth. Am J Hum Genet 59:781–792.
10. Joyce CA, Zorich B, Pike SJ, Barber JC, Dennis NR 1996 Williams-Beuren syndrome: Phenotypic variability and deletions of chromosomes 7, 11 and 22 in a series of 52 patients. J Med Genet 33:986–992.
11. Taylor AB, Stern PH, Bell NH 1982 Abnormal regulation of circulating 25OHD in the Williams syndrome. N Engl J Med 306:972–975.
12. Garabedian M, Jacqz E, Guillozo H, Grimberg R, Guillot M, Gagnadoux MF, Broyer M, Lenoir G, Balsan S 1985 Elevated plasma 1,25(OH)₂D₃ concentrations in infants with hypercalcemia and an elfin facies. N Engl J Med 312:948–952.
13. Martin NDT, Snodgrass GJAI, Makin HLJ, Cohen RD 1986 Letter. N Engl J Med 313:888–889.
14. Chesney RW, DeLuca HF, Gertner JM, Genel M 1986 Letter. N Engl J Med 313:889–890.
15. Culler FL, Jones KL, Deftos LJ 1985 Impaired calcitonin secretion in patients with Williams syndrome. J Pediatr 107:720–723.
16. Lightwood RL 1952 Idiopathic hypercalcemia with failure to thrive. Arch Dis Child 27:302–303.
17. Martin NDT, Snodgras GJAI, Cohen RD 1984 Idiopathic infantile hypercalcemia: A continuing enigma. Arch Dis Child 59:605–613.
18. Aarskog D, Asknes L, Markstead T 1981 Vitamin D metabolism in idiopathic infantile hypercalcemia. Am J Dis Child 135:1021–1025.
19. Langman CB, Budayr AA, Sailer DE, Strewler GJ 1992 Nonmalignant expression of parathyroid hormone-related protein is responsible for idiopathic infantile hypercalcemia. J Bone Miner Res 7:593S.
20. McTaggart SJ, Craig J, MacMillan J, Burke JR 1999 Familial occurrence of idiopathic infantile hypercalcemia. Pediatr Nephrol 13:668–671.
21. Michigami T, Yamato H, Mushiake S, Nakayama M, Yoneda A, Satomura K, Imura K, Ozono K 1996 Hypercalcemia associated with infantile fibrosarcoma producing parathyroid hormone-related protein. J Clin Endocrinol Metab 81:1090–1095.
22. Pronicka E, Rowinska E, Kulzycka H, Lukaszkiewicz J, Lorenc R, Janas R 1997 Persistent hypercalciuria and elevated 25-hydroxyvitamin D₃ in children with infantile hypercalcemia. Pediatr Nephrol 11:2–6.
23. Foley TP Jr, Jarrison HC, Arnaud CD, Harrison HE 1972 Familial benign hypercalcemia. J Pediatr 81:1060–1067.
24. Marx SJ, Attie MF, Spiegel AM, Levine MA, Lasker RD, Fox M 1982 An association between neonatal severe primary hyperparathyroidism and familial hypocalciuric hypercalcemia. N Engl J Med 306:257–264.
25. Bernulf J, Hall K, Sjogren I, Werner I 1970 Primary hyperparathyroidism in children. Acta Pediatr 59:249–258.
26. Pollak MR, Chou YH, Marx SJ, Steinmann B, Cole DE, Brandi ML, Papapoulos SE, Menko FH, Hendy GN, Brown EM 1994 Familial hypocalciuric hypercalcemia and neonatal severe hyperparathyroidism: Effects of mutant gene dosage on phenotype. J Clin Invest 93:1108–1112.
27. Cole DE, Janicic N, Salisbury SR, Hendy GN 1997 Neonatal severe hyperparathyroidism, secondary hyperparathyroidism and familial hypocalciuric hypercalcemia: Multiple different phenotypes associated with an inactivating Alu insertion mutation of the calcium-sensing receptor gene. Am J Hum Genet 71:202–210.
28. Frame B, Poznanski AK 1980 Conditions that may be confused with rickets. In: Deluca HR, Anast CN (eds.) Pediatric Diseases Related to Calcium. Elsevier, New York, NY, USA, pp. 269–289.
29. Schipani E, Kruse K, Jüppner H 1995 A constitutively active mutant PTH-PTHrp receptor in Jansen-type metaphyseal chondrodysplasia. Science 268:98–100.
30. Schipani E, Langman CB, Parfitt AM, Jensen GS, Kikuchi S, Kooh SW, Cole WG, Juppner H 1996 Two different constitutively active PTH/PTHrP receptor mutations cause Jansen-type metaphyseal chondrodysplasia. N Engl J Med 335:708–714.
31. Schipani E, Langman C, Hunzelman J, Le Merrer M, Loke KY, Dillon MJ, Silve C, Jüppner H 1999 A novel parathyroid hormone (PTH)/PTH-related peptide receptor mutation in Jansen's metaphyseal chondrodysplasia. J Clin Endocrinol Metab 84:3052–3057.
32. Michael AF, Hong R, West CD 1962 Hypercalcemia in infancy. Am J Dis Child 104:235–244.
33. Sharata H, Postellon DC, Hashimoto K 1995 Subcutaneous fat necrosis, hypercalcemia and prostaglandin E. Pediatr Dermatol 12:43–47.
34. Kruse K, Irle U, Uhlig R 1993 Elevated 1, 25-dihydroxyvitamin D serum concentrations in infants with subcutaneous fat necrosis. J Pediatr 122:460–463.
35. Barcia JP, Strife CF, Langman CB 1997 Infantile hypophosphatasia: Treatment options to control acute hypercalcemia and chronic bone demineralization. J Pediatr 130:825–828.
36. Jasper PL, Denny FW 1968 Sarcoidosis in children. J Pediatr 73:499–512.
37. Bosch X 1998 Hypercalcemia due to endogenous overproduction of vitamin D in identical twins with cat-scratch disease. JAMA 279:532–534.
38. Rosen JF, Wolin DA, Finberg L 1978 Immobilization hypercalcemia after single limb fractures in children and adolescents. Am J Dis Child 132:560–564.
39. Nako Y, Fukushima N, Tomomasa T, Nagashima K, Kuroume T 1993 Hypervitaminosis D after prolonged feeding with a premature formula. Pediatrics 92:862–864.
40. Jacobus CH, Holick MF, Shao Q, Chen TC, Holm IA, Kolodny JM, Fuleihan GE, Seely EW 1992 Hypervitaminosis D associated with drinking milk. N Engl J Med 326:1173–1177.
41. Holick MF, Shao Q, Liu WW, Chen TC 1992 The vitamin D content of fortified milk and infant formula. N Engl J Med 326:1178–1181.
42. Chan JCM, Young RB, Alon U, Manunes P 1983 Hypercalcemia in children with disorders of calcium and phosphate metabolism during long-term treatment with 1, 25(OH)₂D. Pediatrics 72:225–233.
43. Karolyi L, Koch MC, Grzeschik KH, Seyberth HW 1998 The molecular genetic approach to Bartter's syndrome. J Mol Med 76:317–325.
44. Welch TR 1997 The hyperprostaglandin E syndrome: A hypercalciuric variation of Bartter syndrome. J Bone Miner Res 12:1753–1754.
45. Saarela T, Simila S, Koivisto M 1995 Hypercalcemia and nephrocalcinosis in patients with congenital lactase deficiency. J Pediatr 127:920–923.

Chapter 42. Hypocalcemia: Pathogenesis, Differential Diagnosis, and Management

Rajesh V. Thakker

Nuffield Department of Clinical Medicine, Botnar Research Centre, Nuffield Orthopaedic Centre, University of Oxford, Headington, Oxford, United Kingdom

INTRODUCTION

Hypocalcemia, which is frequently encountered in adult and pediatric medicine, has many causes (Table 1) that can be broadly subdivided into two groups according to whether the hypocalcemia is associated with low serum parathyroid hormone (PTH) concentrations (i.e., hypoparathyroidism) or with high PTH concentrations (i.e., secondary hyperparathyroidism). These hypocalcemic diseases are considered separately in subsequent chapters, and this chapter will review the general principles that determine calcium homeostasis and apply to the differential diagnosis and management of hypocalcemia.

CALCIUM HOMEOSTASIS, PATHOGENESIS, AND DIFFERENTIAL DIAGNOSIS OF HYPOCALCEMIA

The total body content of calcium in a normal adult is 1000 g, and over 99% of this is within the crystal structure of bone mineral and less than 1% is in the soluble form in the extracellular and intracellular fluid compartments. In the extracellular fluid (ECF) compartment, about 50% of the total calcium is ionized, and the rest is principally bound to albumin or complexed with counter-ions. The ionized calcium concentrations range from 1.00 to 1.25 mM, and the total serum calcium concentration ranges from 2.20 to 2.60 mM (8.8–10.4 mg/dl), depending on the laboratory. Measurements of ionized calcium, which has the main regulatory role, are not often undertaken because the methods are difficult and variable and thus a total serum calcium concentration is the usual estimation. However, the usual 2:1 ratio of total to ionized calcium may be disturbed by disorders such as metabolic acidosis, which reduces calcium binding by proteins; metabolic alkalosis, which increases calcium binding by proteins; or by changes in protein concentration, for example, starvation, cirrhosis, dehydration, venous stasis, or multiple myeloma. In view of this, total serum calcium concentrations are adjusted, or "corrected," to a reference albumin concentration; thus, the corrected serum calcium may be expressed to a reference albumin concentration of 41 g/liter (4.1 g/dl), and for every 1 g/liter (1.0 g/dl) of albumin above or below the reference value, the calcium is adjusted by ±0.016 mM (0.064 mg/dl), respectively. For example, a total serum calcium of 2.10 mM (8.4 mg/dl) with an albumin concentration of 35 g/liter (3.5 g/dl) would be equivalent to a corrected serum calcium of 2.20 mM (8.8 mg/dl), thereby correcting the initial apparent hypocalcemic value to a normal value.

The extracellular concentration of calcium is closely regulated within the narrow physiological range that is optimal for the normal cellular functions affected by calcium in many tissues. This regulation of extracellular calcium takes place through complex interactions (Fig. 1) at the target organs of the major calcium-regulating hormone—parathyroid hormone (PTH)—and vitamin D and its active metabolites, for example, 1,25-dihydroxyvitamin D $[1,25(OH)_2D]$. The parathyroid glands secrete PTH at a rate that is appropriate to, and dependent on, the prevailing extracellular calcium ion concentration. Thus, hypocalcemic diseases may arise because of a destruction of the parathyroids or because of a failure of parathyroid gland development, PTH secretion, or PTH-mediated actions in target tissues. These diseases may therefore be classified as being caused by a deficiency of PTH, a defect in the PTH receptor (i.e., the PTH/PTHrP receptor), or an insensitivity to PTH caused by defects downstream of the PTH-PTHrP receptor (Fig. 1). The diseases may be inherited, and molecular genetic studies have identified many of the underlying genetic abnormalities (Table 2).

CLINICAL FEATURES AND INVESTIGATIONS

The clinical presentation of hypocalcemia (serum calcium < 2.20 mM or 8.8 mg/dl) ranges from an asymptomatic biochemical abnormality to a severe, life-threatening condition. In mild hypocalcemia (serum calcium 2.00–2.20 mM or 8.0–8.8 mg/dl), patients may be asymptomatic. Those with more severe (serum calcium < 1.9 mM or 7.6 mg/dl) and long-term hypocalcemia may develop acute symptoms of neuromuscular irritability (Table 3); ectopic calcification (e.g., in the basal ganglia, which may be associated with extrapyramidal neurological symptoms); subcapsular cataract; papilledema; and abnormal dentition. Investigations should be directed at confirming the presence of hypocalcemia and establishing the cause.

The causes of hypocalcemia (Table 1) can be classified according to whether serum PTH concentrations are low (i.e., hypoparathyroid disorders) or high (i.e., disorders associated with secondary hyperparathyroidism). The most common causes of hypocalcemia are hypoparathyroidism, a deficiency or abnormal metabolism of vitamin D, acute or chronic renal failure, and hypomagnesemia. In *hypoparathyroidism*, serum calcium is low, phosphate is high, and PTH is undetectable; renal function and concentrations of the 25-hydroxy and 1,25-dihydroxy metabolites of vitamin D are usually normal. The features of *pseudohypoparathyroidism* are similar to those of hypoparathyroidism except for PTH, which is markedly increased. In *chronic renal failure*, which is the most common cause of hypocalcemia, phosphate is high and alkaline phosphatase, creatinine, and PTH are elevated; 25-hydroxyvitamin D_3 is normal and 1,25-dihydroxyvitamin D_3 is low. In *vitamin D deficiency osteomalacia*, serum calcium and phosphate are low, alka-

The author has no conflict of interest.

Table 1. Causes of Hypocalemia

LOW PARATHYROID HORMONE LEVELS
(HYPOPARATHYROIDISM)
- Parathyroid agenesis
  - Isolated or part of complex developmental anomaly (e.g., DiGeorge syndrome)
- Parathyroid destruction
  - Surgery*
  - Radiation
  - Infiltration by metastases or systemic disease (e.g., hemochromatosis, amyloidosis, sarcoidosis, Wilson's disease, thalassaemia)
- Autoimmune
  - Isolated
  - Polyglandular (type 1)*
- Reduced parathyroid function (i.e., parathyroid hormone secretion)
  - Parathyroid hormone gene defects
  - Hypomagnesemia*
  - Neonatal hypocalcemia (may be associated with maternal hypercalcaemia)
  - Hungry bone disease (post-parathyroidectomy)
  - Calcium-sensing receptor mutations

HIGH PARATHYROID HORMONE LEVELS (SECONDARY
HYPERPARATHYROIDISM)
- Vitamin D deficiency*
  - As a result of nutritional lack,* lack of sunlight,* malabsorption,* liver disease or acute or chronic renal failure*
- Vitamin D resistance (rickets)
  - As a result of renal tubular dysfunction (Fanconi's syndrome), or vitamin D receptor defects
- Parathyroid hormone resistance (e.g., pseudohypoparathyroidism, hypomagnesemia)
- Drugs
  - Calcium chelators (e.g., citrated blood transfusions, phosphate, cow's milk is rich in phosphate)
  - Inhibitors of bone resorption (e.g., bisphosphonate, calcitonin, plicamycin, gallium nitrate, cisplatinum, doxorubicin)
  - Altered vitamin D metabolism (e.g., phenytoin, ketaconazole)
  - Foscarnet
- Miscellaeneous
  - Acute pancreatitis
  - Acute rhabdomyolysis
  - Massive tumor lysis
  - Osteoblastic metastases (e.g., from prostate or breast carcinoma)
  - Toxic shock syndrome
  - Hyperventilation
  - Acute severe illness

* Most common causes.

line phosphatase and PTH are elevated, renal function is normal, and 25-hydroxyvitamin D_3 is low. The most common artifactual cause of hypocalcemia is hypoalbuminemia, such as occurs in liver disease.

MANAGEMENT OF ACUTE HYPOCALCEMIA

The management of acute hypocalcemia depends on the severity of the hypocalcemia, the rapidity with which it

developed, and the degree of neuromuscular irritability (Table 3). Treatment should be given to symptomatic patients (e.g., with seizures or tetany) and asymptomatic patients with a serum calcium of less than 1.90 mM (7.6 mg/dl) who may be at high risk of developing complications. The preferred treatment for acute symptomatic hypocalcemia is calcium gluconate, 10 ml 10% wt/vol (2.20 mmol or 90 mg of calcium) intravenously, diluted in 50 ml of 5% dextrose or 0.9% sodium chloride and given by slow injection (>5

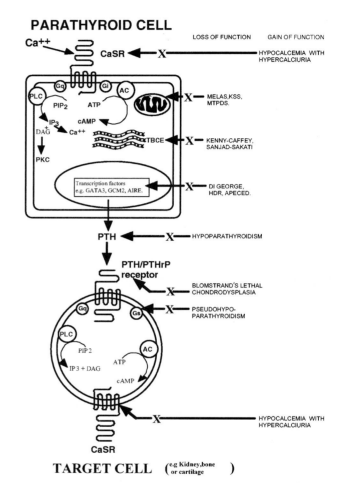

FIG. 1. Schematic representation of some of the components involved in calcium homeostasis. Alterations in extracellular calcium are detected by the calcium-sensing receptor (CaSR), which is a 1078 amino acid G-protein–coupled receptor. The PTH/PTHrP receptor, which mediates the actions of PTH and PTHrP, is also a G-protein–coupled receptor. Thus, Ca^{2+}, PTH, and PTHrP involve G-protein–coupled signaling pathways, and interaction with their specific receptors can lead to activation of Gs, Gi, and Gq, respectively. Gs stimulates adenylylcyclase (AC), which catalyzes the formation of cyclic adenosine monophosphate (cAMP) from adenosine triphosphate (ATP). Gi inhibits AC activity. cAMP stimulates protein kinase A (PKA), which phosphorylates cell-specific substrates. Activation of Gq stimulates phospholipase C (PLC), which catalyzes the hydrolysis of the phosphoinositide (PIP_2) to inositol triphosphate (IP_3), which increases intracellular calcium, and diacylglycerol (DAG), which activates protein kinase C (PKC). These proximal signals modulate downstream pathways, which result in specific physiological effects. Abnormalities in several genes, which lead to mutations in proteins in these pathways, have been identified in specific disorders of calcium homeostasis (Table 2). (Adapted with permission from Thakker RV 2000 Parathyroid disorders, molecular genetics and physiology. In: Morris PJ, Wood WC, eds. Oxford Textbook of Surgery. Oxford University Press, Oxford, UK, pp. 1121–1129.)

TABLE 2. HYPOPARATHYROID DISEASES AND THEIR CHROMOSOMAL LOCATIONS

Disease	Inheritance	Gene product	Chromosomal location
Isolated hypoparathyroidism	Autosomal dominant	PTH	11p15*
	Autosomal recessive	PTH, GCMB	11p15*, 6p23-24*
	X-linked recessive	Unknown	Xq26-27
Hypocalcaemic hypercalciuria	Autosomal dominant	CaSR	3q21.1
Hypoparathyroidism associated with polyglandular autoimmune syndrome (APECED)	Autosomal recessive	AIRE-1	21q22.3
Hypoparathyroidism associated with KSS, MELAS and MTPDS	Maternal	Mitochondrial genome	
Hypoparathyroidism associated with complex congenital syndromes			
DiGeorge	Autosomal dominant	rnex40‡ nex2.2-nex3‡ UDF1L TBX1‡	22q11/10p
HDR syndrome	Autosomal dominant	GATA3	10p13-14
Blomstrand lethal chondrodysplasia	Autosomal recessive	PTH/PTHrPR	3p21.1-p22
Kenney-Caffey	Autosomal recessive	TBCE	1q43-44
Barakat	Autosomal recessive†	Unknown	?
Lymphoedema	Autosomal recessive	Unknown	?
Nephropathy, nerve deafness	Autosomal dominant†	Unknown	?
Nerve deafness without renal dysplasia	Autosomal dominant	Unknown	?
Sanjad-Sakati (Dysmorphology, growth failure)	Autosomal recessive	TBCE	1q43-44
Pseudohypoparathyroidism (type Ia)	Autosomal dominant parentally imprinted	Gsα	20q13.2-13.3
Pseudohypoparathyroidism (type Ib)	Autosomal dominant parentally imprinted	Gsα	20q13.2-13.3

MELAS, mitochondrial encephalopathy, lactic acidosis and stroke like episodes; MTPDS, mitochondrial trifunctional protein deficiency syndrome; AIRE-1, autoimmune regulator 1; HDR, hypoprathyroidism, deafness, renal dysplasia; GCMB, glial cells missing B; GATA3, third member of family of transcription factors that bind to DNA sequence motif GATA; TBCE, tubulin specific chaperone E; KSS, Kearns Sayre syndrome.

* Mutations identified only in some families.
† Most likely inheritance shown.
‡ Most likely candidate genes.
?, Location not known.

minutes); this can be repeated as required to control symptoms. Serum calcium should be assessed regularly. Continuing hypocalcemia may be managed acutely by administration of a calcium gluconate infusion; for example, dilute 10 ampoules of calcium gluconate, 10 ml 10% wt/vol (22.0 mmol or 900 mg of calcium), in 1 liter of 5% dextrose or 0.9% sodium chloride, start infusion at 50 ml/h, and titrate to maintain serum calcium in the low normal range. Generally, 0.30–0.40 mmol/kg or 15 mg/kg of elemental calcium infused over 4–6 h increases serum calcium by 0.5–0.75 mM (2–3 mg/dl). If hypocalcemia is likely to persist, oral vitamin D therapy (see below) should also be commenced. It is important to note that, in hypocalcemic patients who are also hypomagnesemic, the hypomagnesemia must be corrected before the hypocalcemia will resolve. This may occur in the post-parathyroidectomy period or in those with alcoholism or severe malabsorption. While acute hypocalcemia is being treated, investigations to establish the underlying cause (Table 1) should be undertaken, and the appropriate treatment should be initiated.

TABLE 3. HYPOCALCEMIC CLINICAL FEATURES OF NEUROMUSCULAR IRRITABILITY

Paraesthesia, usually of fingers, toes and circumoral regions
Tetany, carpopedal spasm, muscle cramps
Chvostek's sign*
Trousseau's sign†
Seizures of all types (i.e., focal or petit mal, grand mal, or syncope)
Prolonged QT interval on ECG
Laryngospasm
Bronchospasm

* Chvostek's sign is twitching of the circumoral muscles in response to gentle tapping of the facial nerve just anterior to the ear; it may be present in 10% of normal individuals.
† Trousseau's sign is carpal spasm elicited by inflation of a blood pressure cuff to 20 mmHg above the patient's systolic blood pressure for 3 minutes.

MANAGEMENT OF PERSISTENT HYPOCALCEMIA

The two major groups of drugs available for the treatment of hypocalcemia are supplemental calcium, about 10–20 mmol (400–800 mg) calcium every 6–12 h, and vitamin D preparations. Patients with hypoparathyroidism seldom require calcium supplements after the early stages of stabilization on vitamin D. A variety of vitamin D preparations have been used. These include vitamin D_3 (cholecalciferol) or vitamin D_2 (ergocalciferol), 25,000–100,000 U (1.25–5 mg/day); dihydrotachysterol (now seldom used), 0.25–1.25

mg/day; alfacalcidol (1α-hydroxycholecalciferol), 0.25–1.0 μg/day; and calcitriol (1,25-dihydroxycholecalciferol), 0.25–2.0 μg/day. In children, these preparations are prescribed in doses based on body weight. Cholecalciferol and ergocalciferol are the least expensive preparations, but they have the longest durations of action and may result in prolonged toxicity. The other preparations, which do not require renal 1α-hydroxylation, have the advantage of shorter half-lives and thereby minimize the risk of prolonged toxicity. Calcitriol is probably the drug of choice because it is the active metabolite, and unlike alfacalcidol, does not require hepatic 25-hydroxylation. However, in patients with low serum 25-hydroxyvitamin D concentrations caused by vitamin D deficiency, the treatment of choice is a parent vitamin D compound such as cholecalciferol or ergocalciferol. Close monitoring (at about 1- to 2-week intervals) of the patient's serum and urine calcium are required initially and at 3- to 6-month intervals once stabilization is achieved. The aim is to avoid hypercalcemia, hypercalciuria, nephrolithiasis, and renal failure. It should be noted that hypercalciuria may occur in the absence of hypercalcemia.

SUGGESTED READINGS

1. Bilezikian JP, Thakker RV 1998 Hypoparathyroidism. Curr Opin Endocrinol Diabetes **4:**427–432.
2. Deftos LJ 1998 Clinical Essentials of Calcium and Skeletal Disorders, 1st ed. Professional Communications Inc., Caddo, OK, USA.
3. Thakker RV, Jüppner H 2001 Genetic disorders of calcium homeostasis caused by abnormal regulation of parathyroid hormone secretion or responsiveness. In: DeGroot LJ, Jameson JL (eds.) Endocrinology, 4th ed. WB Saunders Company, Philadelphia, PA, USA, pp. 1062–1074.
4. Marx SJ 2000 Hyperparathyroid and hypoparathyroid disorders. N Engl J Med **343:**1803–1875.
5. Thakker RV 2000 Parathyroid disorders, molecular genetics and physiology. In: Morris PJ, Wood WC (ed.) Oxford Textbook of Surgery. Oxford University Press, Oxford, UK, pp. 1121–1129.

Chapter 43. Hypoparathyroidism

David Goltzman and David E.C. Cole

[1]*Department of Medicine, McGill University and McGill University Health Centre, Montreal, Quebec, Canada; and [2]Departments of Laboratory Medicine and Pathobiology, Medicine, and Pediatrics (Genetics), University of Toronto, Toronto, Ontario, Canada*

INTRODUCTION

Hypoparathyroidism is a clinical disorder that manifests when the parathyroid hormone (PTH) produced by the parathyroid gland is insufficient to maintain extracellular fluid (ECF) calcium in the normal range or when adequate circulating concentrations of PTH are unable to function optimally in target tissues to maintain normal ECF calcium levels. The causes of hypoparathyroidism (Table 1) can be classified broadly as (1) failure of parathyroid gland development, (2) destruction of the parathyroid glands, (3) reduced parathyroid gland function because of altered PTH production or secretion, and (4) impaired PTH action. The common aspect of these conditions is the presence of reduced, biologically active PTH. This results in characteristic clinical and laboratory features, which may be influenced, however, by the specific pathogenetic mechanism.

CLINICAL MANIFESTATIONS

The acute clinical signs and symptoms of hypoparathyroidism of any etiology include evidence of latent or overt increased neuromuscular irritability caused by hypocalcemia. The acute symptoms are more likely to occur during times of increased demand on the calcium homeostatic system (pregnancy and lactation, the menstrual cycle, and states of alkalosis). Chronically, patients may manifest muscle cramps, pseudopapilledema, extrapyramidal signs, mental retardation, and personality disturbances, as well as cataracts, dry rough skin, coarse brittle hair, alopecia, and abnormal dentition. The dental abnormalities may include defects caused by enamel hypoplasia, defects in dentin, shortened premolar roots, thickened lamina dura, delayed tooth eruption, and increased frequency of dental caries. Occasionally, patients may be edentulous. Finally, some patients may be diagnosed only after a low serum calcium is detected on routine blood screening.

LABORATORY ABNORMALITIES

The biochemical hallmarks of hypoparathyroidism are hypocalcemia and hyperphosphatemia in the presence of normal renal function. Serum calcium concentrations are often 6–7 mg/dl (1.50–1.75 mM) and serum phosphorus levels are 6–9 mg/dl (1.93–2.90 mM). In most instances, an ionized calcium concentration of less than 4 mg/liter (1.0 mM) is also observed. Serum concentrations of immunoreactive PTH are low or undetectable, except in cases of PTH resistance where they are elevated or high normal. Serum concentrations of 1,25(OH)$_2$D are usually low or low-normal, but alkaline phosphatase activity is unchanged. The 24-h urinary excretion of calcium is reduced, despite the fact that the fractional excretion of calcium is increased because the filtered load is low, because of the hypocalcemia induced by decreased intestinal calcium absorption and diminished bone resorption. Nephrogenous cyclic AMP excretion is low and renal tubular reabsorption of phosphorus is elevated. Urinary cyclic AMP and phosphorus excretion both increase markedly after administration of exogenous

The authors have no conflict of interest.

TABLE 1. PATHOGENETIC CLASSIFICATION OF HYPOPARATHYROIDISM

I. Abnormal parathyroid gland development
  Isolated hypoparathyroidism
    X-linked (#307700)*
    Autosomal recessive (#241400)
      GCMB mutation (#603716)
  DiGeorge syndrome (#188400)
    Velocardiofacial (VCF) syndrome (#192430)
      DiGeorge Critical Region 1 - 22q11.2 (#602054)
    Barakat (HDR) syndrome - 10p (#146255 & #256340)
      DiGeorge Critical Region 2 - 10p13–14 (#601362)
        GATA3 haploinsufficiency (#131320)
  Hypoparathyroidism with short stature, mental retardation, and
    seizures
    Sanjat-Sakati syndrome (#241410)
    Kenny-Caffey syndrome Type I (#244460)
      TBCE mutations (#604934)
  Mitochondrial neuromyopathies
    Kearns-Sayre syndrome (#530000)
    Pearson syndrome (#557000)
    tRNA-Leu mutations (#590050)
  Long-chain hydroxyacyl-CoA dehydrogenase deficiency (#600890)
II. Destruction of the parathyroid glands
  Surgical
  Polyglandular autoimmune disease (APECED) (#240300)
    AIRE mutations (#607358)
  Radiation
  Metal overload (iron, copper)
  Granulomatous infiltration
  Neoplastic invasion
III. Decreased parathyroid gland function due to altered PTH production
    or secretion
  Primary
    Autosomal dominant (#146200)
      Calcium-sensing receptor mutations (#145980)†
      PTH mutation (#168450.0001)
    Autosomal recessive
      PTH mutation (#168450.0002)
  Secondary
    Maternal hyperparathyroidism
    Hypomagnesemia
IV. Impaired parathyroid hormone action
  Hypomagnesemia
  Pseudohypoparathyroidism

* Numbers are from Online Mendelian Inheritance in Man, http://www.ncbi.nlm.nih.gov/entrez/query.fcgi?db=OMIM, accessible by browsing the web using the search team >OMIM=.

† De novo mutations are common in sporadic hypoparathyroidism.

bioactive PTH except in PTH-resistant states. If hypoparathyroidism presenting at birth or in early childhood is not otherwise explained, serum magnesium should be measured. If serum magnesium is low, a more complete assessment of magnesium metabolism is warranted.

Calcification of the basal ganglia or other intracranial structures may be detected on routine radiographs or by enhanced imaging (computed tomography [CT] scan or magnetic resonance imaging [MRI]), and electroencephalographic changes may be present. These are occasionally the only clinical evidence of disease. Detection of limited parathyroid gland reserve may rarely require an ethylenediaminetetraacetate (EDTA) or citrate infusion study, which should only be conducted under close supervision.

CAUSES OF HYPOPARATHYROIDISM

Abnormal Parathyroid Gland Development

Congenital agenesis or hypoplasia of the parathyroid glands can produce hypoparathyroidism that manifests in the newborn period. Most often, this occurs as isolated or sporadic hypoparathyroidism, and would have previously been considered idiopathic. There is now evidence that de novo activating mutations of the calcium-sensing receptor gene account for a number of these cases (see below).

Familial isolated hypoparathyroidism may show autosomal recessive or X-linked inheritance patterns. Examples of the latter are rare. However, linkage analysis of the few affected families has narrowed the X-chromosome locus to the Xq26–27 region. Recently, an autosomal recessive form of familial isolated hypoparathyroidism has been attributed to mutations of the GCMB (Glial Cells Missing B) gene, which encodes a nuclear transcription factor predominantly expressed in the parathyroid gland and apparently critical for its development.

Maldevelopment of the parathyroid gland more often occurs as a feature of various malformation syndromes. When other structures derived from the third and fourth branchial pouches are involved, thymic aplasia with immunodeficiency and congenital conotruncal cardiac anomalies are typically present. Originally called the DiGeorge syndrome, this phenotype is now known to include a wide range of congenital anomalies, including distinctive facial features, cleft lip/palate, oropharyngeal anomalies, and other forms of congenital heart disease. In most cases, a microdeletion of chromosome 22 in the region of 22q11.21-q11.23 is the cause. Detection of the microdeletion by fluorescence in situ hybridization (FISH) is diagnostic, but a negative result does not exclude the possibility of a 22q abnormality. Individuals with the velocardiofacial (VCF or Schprintzen) syndrome also have microdeletions of 22q, and it is now believed the two conditions overlap. Haploinsufficiency of a transcription factor gene, Tbx1, has been implicated as the common molecular defect; there are no human examples to date of specific Tbx1 mutations causing the DiGeorge phenotype. The possibility that other candidate genes or modifiers may be important is being vigorously pursued.

The clinical overlap has led to increasing use of the term, 22q11 syndrome, to include the varying phenotypes associated with the chromosomal microdeletion. In the VCF subgroup, anatomical anomalies of the pharynx are prominent, and hypernasal speech caused by abnormal pharyngeal musculature with or without cleft palate is typical. In most patients, some degree of intellectual deficit is present, and there is strong predisposition to psychotic illness (schizophrenia or bipolar disorder) in adolescents and adults. A number of web sites (http://www.vcfsef.org/ or http://www.geneclinics.org/profiles/22q11deletion/details.html) provide regularly updated information on this common and complex group of disorders.

Hypoparathyroidism is a part of the Barakat or HDR (Hypoparathyroidism, nerve Deafness, and Renal dysplasia) syndrome. Deletions of two non-overlapping regions of chromosome 10p contribute to a DiGeorge-like phenotype (the DiGeorge critical region II on 10p13–14) and the HDR syndrome (10p14–10pter). Deletion mapping studies in HDR patients defined a region containing the *GATA3* gene that encodes a zinc finger transcription factor involved in vertebrate embryonic development. Microdeletions leading to GATA3 haploinsufficiency and point mutations in the gene itself have been identified in various HDR kindreds. Thus, GATA3 appears essential for normal embryonic development of the parathyroids, auditory system, and kidney.

All patients with otherwise unexplained persistent hypoparathyroidism in childhood should be karyotyped (±FISH for 22q11 or 10p microdeletions) and evaluated for other occult anomalies, including subclinical cardiac disease, renal dysplasia, hearing abnormalities, and gastrointestinal maldevelopment. Conversely, because the hypoparathyroidism may be very mild, transient, or greatly delayed in onset, demonstration of decreased parathyroid reserve in an otherwise healthy individual with a suspected syndrome may require provocative testing. Evidence of dominant inheritance may depend on detailed examination to identify other features (conotruncal cardiac anomalies, renal dysplasia, decreased cell-mediated immunity, etc.) in first-degree relatives of the index case. Although many cases with the DiGeorge phenotype are the result of de novo deletions, autosomal dominant inheritance is not uncommon, and such families require detailed genetic counseling and follow-up. Other karyotypic abnormalities have been reported occasionally in patients with the DiGeorge phenotype, raising the possibility that other genetic loci are yet to be identified. The DiGeorge phenotype has been described as part of the CHARGE association (*c*oloboma of the iris, *h*eart disease, choanal *a*tresia, *r*etarded growth and development, *g*enital anomalies, and *e*ar anomalies) and may be seen as phenocopies in cases of diabetic embryopathy, fetal alcohol syndrome, and fetal retinoid embryopathy.

The *Sanjat-Sakati syndrome* is an autosomal recessive disorder of congenital hypoparathyroidism associated with short stature, mental retardation, and seizures. Described in Middle Eastern kindreds, it has been localized to chromosome 1q43–44 along with a recessive form of *Kenny-Caffey syndrome*, a condition dominated by radiologic findings that include calvarial hyperostosis and marked tubular stenosis of the long bones. The relationship between mutations of the *TBCE* (*t*ubulin-specific *c*haperone *E*) gene, which encodes a protein required for folding of α-tubulin and its heterodimerization with β-tubulin, and hypoparathyroidism is unexpected, and further studies will undoubtedly offer new insights into parathyroid gland biology.

Hypoparathyroidism is also a variable component of the neuromyopathies caused by mitochondrial gene defects. Among the clinical conditions are the *Kearns-Sayre syndrome* (ophthalmoplegia, retinal degeneration, and cardiac conduction defects), the *Pearson marrow pancreas syndrome* (lactic acidosis, neutropenia, sideroblastic anemia, and pancreatic exocrine dysfunction), and mitochondrial encephalomyopathy. The molecular defects range from large deletions of the mitochondrial genomes in an extensive range of tissues (Pearson syndrome) to single base-pair mutations in one of the transfer RNA genes found only in a restricted range of cell types (mitochondrial encephalomyopathy). Because renal magnesium wasting is frequently

seen in these conditions, a readily reversible form of hypocalcemic hypoparathyroidism caused by hypomagnesemia should also be considered.

Another unusual myopathy associated with an inborn error of fatty acid oxidation (*L*ong-*C*hain *H*ydroxy*A*cyl*C*o*A* *D*ehydrogenase deficiency [LCHAD]) may also be accompanied by hypoparathyroidism. This condition manifests as nonketotic hypoglycemia, cardiomyopathy, hepatic dysfunction, and developmental delay, and is associated with maternal fatty liver of pregnancy.

Destruction of the Parathyroid Glands

The most common cause of hypoparathyroidism in adults is surgical excision of or damage to the parathyroid glands as a result of total thyroidectomy for thyroid cancer, radical neck dissection for other cancers, or repeated operations for primary hyperparathyroidism. Transient and reversible hypocalcemia after parathyroid surgery may be caused by (1) edema or hemorrhage into the parathyroids, (2) "hungry bone syndrome" caused by severe hyperparathyroidism, or (3) postoperative hypomagnesemia. Prolonged hypocalcemia, which may develop immediately, or weeks to years after neck surgery, suggests permanent hypoparathyroidism. The incidence of this condition after neck exploration for primary hyperparathyroidism is usually less than 5%. In patients with a higher risk of developing permanent hypoparathyroidism, such as those with primary parathyroid hyperplasia or with repeated neck explorations required to identify an adenoma, parathyroid tissue may be autotransplanted into the brachioradialis or sternocleidomastoid muscle at the time of parathyroidectomy or cryopreserved for subsequent transplantation, as necessary.

Rarely, hypoparathyroidism has also been described in a small number of patients who receive extensive radiation to the neck and mediastinum. It is also reported in metal overload diseases such as hemochromatosis (iron), thalassemia (iron) and Wilson's disease (copper), and in neoplastic or granulomatous infiltration of the parathyroid glands. In view of the fact that permanent hypoparathyroidism will only occur if all four parathyroid glands are affected, these are unusual causes of hypoparathyroidism.

Hypoparathyroidism may also occur as a presumed autoimmune disorder either alone or in association with other endocrine deficiency states. Antibodies directed against parathyroid tissue can be detected in 33% of patients with isolated disease and 41% of patients with hypoparathyroidism and other endocrine deficiencies. The genetic etiology of the autosomal recessive polyglandular disorder, APECED (*A*utoimmune *P*olyglandular *C*andidiasis *E*ctodermal *D*ystrophy syndrome)—also known as AP1 (*A*utoimmune *P*olyglandular syndrome, type1)—has been traced to mutations of the autoimmune regulator (*AIRE*) gene on chromosome 21q22.3, which encodes a unique protein with characteristics of a transcription factor. This protein is expressed predominantly in immunologically related tissues, especially the thymus, and functional loss leads to breakdown of immune tolerance to organ-specific self-antigens. In this condition, the most common associated manifestations are mucocutaneous candidiasis (65–75%) and Addison's disease (55–60%). Adrenal insufficiency occurs in only 10% of all patients with hypoparathyroidism and moniliasis in only 15%, so that their presence together should suggest polyglandular deficiency. Hypoparathyroidism, either as an isolated autoimmune disorder or as part of APECED, may present between 6 months and 20 years of age (average age, 7–8 years). Candidiasis may affect the skin, nails, and mucous membranes of the mouth and vagina and is often intractable. Addison's disease can mask the presence of hypoparathyroidism or may manifest only in improvement of the hypoparathyroidism with a reduced requirement for calcium and vitamin D. By diminishing gastrointestinal absorption of calcium and increasing renal calcium excretion, glucocorticoid therapy for the adrenal insufficiency may exacerbate the hypocalcemia and could prove lethal if introduced before the hypoparathyroidism is recognized.

In addition to Addison's disease and moniliasis, hypoparathyroidism in APECED may be associated with multiple autoimmune endocrinopathies, including insulin-dependent diabetes mellitus, primary hypogonadism, and autoimmune thyroiditis, as well as ectodermal dysplasia, keratoconjunctivitis, pernicious anemia, chronic active hepatitis, steatorrhea (malabsorption resembling celiac disease), alopecia (totalis or areata), and vitiligo. Pernicious anemia and diabetes mellitus usually develop after hypoparathyroidism.

Reduced Parathyroid Gland Function Caused by Altered Regulation

Altered regulation of parathyroid gland function may be primary or secondary. Secondary causes include maternal hyperparathyroidism and hypomagnesemia. The infant of a mother with primary hyperparathyroidism generally develops hypocalcemia within the first 3 weeks of life, but it may occur up to 1 year after birth. Although therapy may be required acutely, the disorder is usually self-limited. Hypomagnesemia caused by defective intestinal absorption or renal tubular reabsorption of magnesium may impair secretion of PTH and in this way contribute to hypoparathyroidism. Magnesium replacement will correct the hypoparathyroidism.

Primary alterations of parathyroid gland secretion are most commonly caused by activating mutations of the calcium-sensing receptor (CASR) gene on chromosome 3q13.3-q21. These mutations, which decrease set-point for calcium or otherwise increase the sensitivity to ECF calcium concentrations, cause a functional hypoparathyroid state with hypocalcemia and hypercalciuria. When the mutations are transmitted through several generations, the clinical picture is one of familial isolated autosomal dominant hypocalcemia. Not infrequently, however, sporadic disease has been shown to arise from de novo activating mutations. The consequence of the activated parathyroid gland, CASR is chronic suppression of PTH secretion, while the activated CASR receptor in kidney induces hypercalciuria, which exacerbates the hypocalcemia. In many instances, however, the degree of hypocalcemia and hypercalciuria may be mild and well-tolerated. For subjects without symptoms, the greatest threat can be excessive intervention with vitamin D. However, individuals who are aware of the condition are more likely to identify early, nonspecific signs and symptoms of hypocalcemia and can avert the sudden, unexpected onset of more serious manifestations, such as tetany and seizures. Because of the therapeutic implications, molecular studies to identify CASR mutations are now recommended for all cases of sporadic isolated hypoparathyroidism.

Isolated hypoparathyroidism has also been found with a single base substitution in exon 2 of the PTH gene. This mutation in the signal sequence of PTH apparently impedes conversion of pre-pro-PTH to pro-PTH, thereby reducing normal production of the mature hormone. In another family with autosomal recessive isolated hypoparathyroidism, the entire exon 2 of the PTH gene was deleted. This exon contains the initiation codon and a portion of the signal sequence required for peptide translocation at the endoplasmic reticulum in the process of generating a mature secretory peptide.

Impaired PTH Action

Although in theory a bioinactive form of PTH could be synthesized and secreted by the parathyroid gland, this has not been documented. Rather, ineffective PTH action seems to be caused by peripheral resistance to the hormone's effects. Such resistance may occur secondary to hypomagnesemia or as a primary disorder (pseudohypoparathyroidism).

THERAPY

The major goal of therapy in all hypoparathyroid states is to restore serum calcium and phosphorus as close to normal as possible. The main pharmacologic agents available are supplemental calcium and vitamin D preparations. Phosphate binders and thiazide diuretics may be useful ancillary agents. The major impediment to restoration of normocalcemia is the development of hypercalciuria with a resulting predilection for renal stone formation. With the loss of the renal calcium-retaining effect of PTH, the enhanced calcium absorption of the gut induced by vitamin D therapy results in an increased filtered load of calcium that is readily cleared through the kidney. Consequently, urinary calcium excretion frequently increases in response to vitamin D supplementation well before serum calcium is normalized. It is often necessary, or even desirable, to aim for a low normal serum calcium concentration to prevent chronic hypercalciuria. Avoidance of hypercalciuria is probably most important for patients with hypercalciuric hypocalcemia caused by activating mutations of the CASR gene and thiazides may be the preferred treatment. Hydrochlorothiazide therapy (25–100 mg/day in adults to 0.5–2.0 mg/kg/day in children) has been effective in reducing the vitamin D requirement, but potassium supplementation is necessary to offset the thiazide-induced hypokalemia.

If serum calcium is normalized, and the serum phosphorus remains greater than 6 mg/dl (1.93 mM), a nonabsorbable antacid may be added to reduce the hyperphosphatemia and prevent metastatic calcification. Dairy products, which are high in phosphate, should be avoided, and calcium should be administered in the form of supplements. Generally, at least 1 g/day of elemental calcium is required.

A variety of vitamin D preparations may be used including (1) vitamin D_3 or D_2, 25,000–100,000 IU (1.25–5 mg) per day; (2) dihydrotachysterol, 0.2–1.2 mg per day; (3) 1-α-hydroxyvitamin D_3, 0.5–2.0 μg per day; or (4) calcitriol [1,25$(OH)_2D_3$], 0.25–1.0 μg day. Although vitamin D_3 and D_2 are the least expensive forms of therapy, they have the longest duration of action and can result in prolonged toxicity. The other preparations listed above all have the advantage of shorter half-lives and no requirement for renal 1-α-hydroxylation, which is impaired in hypoparathyroidism. Dihydrotachysterol is rarely used today, however, and calcitriol is probably the treatment of choice. In children, these preparations should be prescribed on a body weight basis. Close monitoring of urine calcium, serum calcium, and serum phosphate are required in the first month or so, but follow-up at 3- to 6-month intervals may be adequate once stable laboratory values are reached.

SUGGESTED READINGS

1. Bergada I, Schiffrin A, Abu Srair H, Kaplan P, Dornan J, Goltzman D, Hendy GN 1988 Kenny syndrome: Description of additional abnormalities and molecular studies. Hum Genet 80:39–42.
2. Daw SC, Taylor C, Kraman M, Call K, Mao J, Schuffenhauer S, Meitinger T, Lipson T, Goodship J, Scambler P 1996 A common region of 10p deleted in diGeorge and velocardiofacial syndromes. Nat Genet 13:458–460.
3. Ding C, Buckingham B, Levine MA 2001 Familial isolated hypoparathyroidism caused by a mutation in the gene for the transcription factor GCMB. J Clin Invest 108:1215–1220.
4. Gidding SS, Minciotti AL, Langman CB 1988 Unmasking of hypoparathyroidism in familial partial DiGeorge syndrome by challenge with disodium edetate. N Engl J Med 319:1589–1591.
5. Gottlieb S, Driscoll DA, Punnett HH, Sellinger B, Emanuel BS, Budarf ML 1998 Characterization of 10p deletions suggests two non-overlapping regions contribute to the DiGeorge syndrome phenotype. Am J Hum Genet 62:495–498.
6. Harvey JN, Barnett D 1992 Endocrine dysfunction in Kearns-Sayre syndrome. Clin Endocrinol (Oxf) 37:97–103.
7. HRD/Autosomal Recessive Kenny-Caffey Syndrome Consortium 2002 Mutation of TBCE causes hypoparathyroidism-retardation-dysmorphism and autosomal recessive Kenny-Caffey syndrome. Nat Genet 32:448–452.
8. Illum F, Dupont E 1985 Prevalence of CT-detected calcification in the basal ganglia in idiopathic hypoparathyroidism and pseudohypoparathyroidism. Neuroradiology 27:32–37.
9. Lienhardt A, Bai M, Lagarde JP, Rigaud M, Zhang Z, Jiang Y, Kottler ML, Brown EM, Garabedian M 2001 Activating mutations of the calcium-sensing receptor: Management of hypocalcemia. J Clin Endocrinol Metab 86:5313–5323.
10. Mallette L 1988 Synthetic human parathyroid hormone 1–34 fragment for diagnostic testing. Ann Intern Med 109:800–802.
11. Mumm S, Whyte MP, Thakker RV, Buetow KH, Schlessinger D 1997 mtDNA analysis shows common ancestry in two kindreds with X-linked recessive hypoparathyroidism and reveals a heteroplasmic silent mutation. Am J Hum Genet 60:153–159.
12. Muroya K, Hasegawa T, Ito Y, Nagai T, Isotani H, Iwata Y, Yamamoto K, Fujimoto S, Seishu S, Fukushima Y, Hasegawa Y, Ogata T 2001 GATA3 abnormalities and the phenotypic spectrum of HDR syndrome. J Med Genet 38:374–380.
13. Okano O, Furukawa Y, Morii H, Fujita T 1982 Comparative efficacy of various vitamin D metabolites in the treatment of various types of hypoparathyroidism. J Clin Endocrinol Metab 55:238–243.
14. Parkinson DB, Thakker RV 1992 A donor splice site mutation in the parathyroid hormone gene is associated with autosomal recessive hypoparathyroidism. Nat Genet 1:149–152.
15. Pollak MR, Brown EM, Estep HL, McLaine PN, Kifor O, Park J, Hebert SC, Seidman CE, Seidman JG 1994 Autosomal dominant hypocalcemia caused by a Ca^{2+}-sensing receptor gene mutation. Nat Genet 8:303–307.
16. Rude RK 1997 Hypocalcemia and hypoparathyroidism. Curr Ther Endocrinol Metab 6:546–551.
17. Sato K, Hasegawa Y, Nakae J, Nanao K, Takahashi I, Tajima T, Shinohara N, Fujieda K 2002 Hydrochlorothiazide effectively reduces urinary calcium excretion in two Japanese patients with gain-of-function mutations of the calcium-sensing receptor gene. J Clin Endocrinol Metab 87:3068–3073.
18. Seneca S, DeMeirleir L, DeSchepper J, Balduck N, Jochmans K, Liebaers I, Lissens W 1997 Pearson marrow pancreas syndrome: A molecular study and clinical management. Clin Genet 51:338–342.
19. Sherwood LM, Santora AC 1994 Hypoparathyroid states in the differential diagnosis of hypocalcemia. In: Bilezikian JP, Marcus R, Levine MA (eds.) The Parathyroids. Raven Press, New York, NY, USA, pp. 747–752.
20. Stalmans I, Lambrechts D, De Smet F, Jansen S, Wang J, Maity S, Kneer P, Von Der Ohe M, Swillen A, Maes C, Gewillig M, Molin DG, Hellings P, Boetel T, Haardt M, Compernolle V, Dewerchin M, Plaisance S, Vlietinck R, Emanuel B, Gittenberger-De Groot AC, Scambler P, Morrow B, Driscol DA, Moons L, Esguerra CV, Carmeliet G, Behn-Krappa A, Devriendt K, Collen D, Conway SJ, Carmeliet P 2003 VEGF: A modifier of the del22q11 (DiGeorge) syndrome? Nat Med 9:173–182.

Chapter 44.   Parathyroid Hormone Resistance Syndromes

Michael A. Levine

Division of Pediatrics, Cleveland Clinic Foundation, Cleveland, Ohio; and Department of Pediatrics, The Johns Hopkins University School of Medicine, Baltimore, Maryland

INTRODUCTION

The term *pseudohypoparathyroidism* (PHP) describes a group of disorders characterized by biochemical hypoparathyroidism (i.e., hypocalcemia and hyperphosphatemia), increased secretion of parathyroid hormone (PTH), and target tissue unresponsiveness to the biological actions of PTH.

In the initial description of PHP, Albright et al. focused on the failure of patients with this syndrome to show either a calcemic or a phosphaturic response to administered parathyroid extract.[1] These observations provided the basis for the hypothesis that biochemical hypoparathyroidism in PHP was due not to a deficiency of PTH but rather to resistance of the target organs, bone, and kidney to the biological actions of PTH. Thus, the pathophysiology of PHP differs fundamentally from true hypoparathyroidism, in which PTH secretion rather than PTH responsiveness is defective.

The author has no conflict of interest.

The initial event in the expression of PTH action is binding of the hormone to specific heptahelical receptors that are located on the plasma membrane of target cells. Because the native and cloned receptors for PTH[2] also bind parathyroid hormone-related protein (PTHrP) with equivalent affinity, they are termed PTH/PTHrP receptors. The PTH/PTHrP receptor (also termed the type 1 PTH receptor) is a member of a superfamily of receptors that are coupled by heterotrimeric (α, β, γ) guanine nucleotide binding regulatory proteins (G proteins) to signal effector molecules that are localized to the inner surface of the plasma membrane. These receptors share a common predicted topology that includes seven transmembrane α-helices, hence their description as heptahelical receptors. PTH binding is followed rapidly by the generation of a variety of second messengers, including cyclic adenosine monophosphate (cAMP), inositol 1,4,5-trisphosphate and diacylglycerol, and cytosolic calcium, indicating that a single class of PTH/PTHrP receptors can couple not only to G_s to stimulate adenylyl cyclase, but also to G_q and G_{11}, albeit with lesser affinity, to stimulate phospholipase C. The best-characterized mediator of PTH action is cAMP, which rapidly activates protein kinase A. The relevant target proteins that are phosphorylated by protein kinase A and the precise actions of these proteins have not yet been fully characterized, but include enzymes, ion channels, and proteins that regulate gene expression. In contrast to the well-recognized effects of the second messenger cAMP in bone and kidney cells, the physiological importance of the phospholipase C signaling pathway in these PTH target tissues has not yet been established.

PATHOGENESIS OF PHP

Characterization of the molecular basis for PHP commenced with the observation that cAMP mediates many of the actions of PTH on kidney and bone and that administration of biologically active PTH to normal subjects leads to a significant increase in the urinary excretion of nephrogenous cAMP.[3] The PTH infusion test remains the most reliable test available for the diagnosis of PHP and enables distinction between the several variants of the syndrome (Fig. 1). Thus, patients with PHP type 1 fail to show an appropriate increase in urinary excretion of both cAMP and phosphate,[3] whereas subjects with the less common type 2 form show a normal increase in urinary cAMP excretion but have an impaired phosphaturic response.[4]

PHP Type 1

The blunted nephrogenous cAMP response to exogenous PTH in subjects with PHP type 1 first suggested that PTH resistance is caused by a defect in the hormone-sensitive signal transduction pathway that activates adenylyl cyclase in renal tubule cells. Adenylyl cyclase is under dual regulatory control: relevant hormones, cytokines, and neurotransmitters interact with heptahelical receptors that are coupled either through G_s or G_i to stimulate or inhibit catalytic activity, respectively.

Early studies of the transmembrane signal transduction

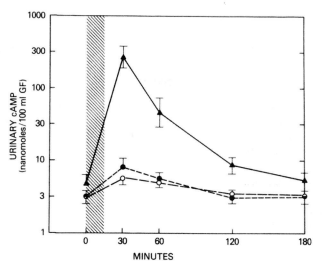

FIG. 1. cAMP excretion in urine in response to the intravenous administration of bovine parathyroid extract (300 USP units) from 9:00 to 9:15 a.m. The peak response in normals (▲) is 50- to 100-fold times basal; patients with PHP type Ia (●) or PHP type Ib (○) show only a 2- to 5-fold response.

system for PTH in subjects with PHP type 1 revealed that most patients had an approximately 50% reduction in expression or function of the α subunit of G_s ($G\alpha_s$), the signaling protein that couples PTH/PTHrP receptors to stimulation of adenylyl cyclase, in membranes from a variety of cell types.[5,6] These studies provide a biochemical basis for distinguishing two groups of patients with PHP type 1: patients with $G\alpha_s$ deficiency are classified as PHP type 1a, whereas patients with normal levels of $G\alpha_s$ are classified as PHP type 1b. Comprehensive studies of endocrine function in patients with PHP type 1a have demonstrated that these patients have resistance not only to PTH but also to additional hormones, including thyroid-stimulating hormone (TSH), gonadotropins, glucagon, calcitonin, and growth hormone–releasing hormone, whose receptors interact with G_s to stimulate adenylyl cyclase.[7–12] By contrast, subjects with PHP type 1b show hormone resistance that is limited to PTH.

PHP Type 1a. In addition to hormone resistance, patients with PHP type 1a (OMIM 30080, 103580) also manifest a peculiar constellation of developmental and somatic defects that are collectively termed Albright's hereditary osteodystrophy (AHO).[1,13] The AHO phenotype consists of short stature, round faces, obesity, brachydactyly, and subcutaneous ossifications, but dental defects[14] and sensory-neural abnormalities may also be present.[15] The subsequent identification of individuals with AHO who lacked apparent hormone resistance led Albright et al. to propose the rather awkward term pseudopseudohypoparathyroidism (pseudo-PHP) to describe this normocalcemic variant of PHP.[16] Subjects with pseudo-PHP have a normal urinary cAMP response to PTH,[3,17] which distinguishes them from occasional patients with PHP type 1a who maintain normal serum calcium levels without treatment.[18] Pseudo-PHP is genetically related to PHP type 1a.[13] Within a given kindred, some affected members will have only AHO (i.e., pseudo-PHP), while others will have hormone resistance as well (i.e., PHP type 1a), despite equivalent functional deficiency of $G\alpha_s$ in tissues that have been analyzed.[17] It therefore seems reasonable to use the term AHO to simplify description of these two variants of the same syndrome[13] and to acknowledge the common clinical and biochemical characteristics that patients with PHP type 1a and pseudo-PHP share.

$G\alpha_s$ deficiency in patients with AHO results from heterozygous inactivating mutations in the *GNAS1* gene, a complex gene that maps to 20q13.3.[19] $G\alpha_s$ is encoded by 13 exons, with four forms generated by the inclusion (52 kDa) or exclusion (45 kDa) of exon 3 and by using alternative splice sites in intron 3.[20] Additional complexity in the processing of the *GNAS1* gene arises from the use of alternative first exons that generate novel transcripts. One promoter, located approximately 47 kb upstream of $G\alpha_s$, encodes the neuroendocrine secretory protein NESP55, a chromogranin-like protein, and is translated from a transcript that contains sequences derived from exon 2–13 of *GNAS1* in the 3′ untranslated region.[21,22] Accordingly, NESP55 shares no protein homology with $G\alpha_s$. A second alternative first exon, termed XL, is located 11 kb further downstream and generates a transcript with two overlapping open reading frames that encode $XL\alpha_s$ and ALEX (the alternative gene product encoded by the XL exon).[23] Both proteins are translated from the same mRNA, are interacting cofactors, and are specifically expressed in neuroendocrine cells. $XL\alpha_s$ is a large $G\alpha_s$ isoform ($\approx$78 kDa), which consists of an N-terminal half encoded by the >1 kb exon XL plus a C-terminal half encoded by exons 2–13 of $G\alpha_s$.[24,25] $XL\alpha_s$ is able to interact with $\beta\gamma$ chains through sequences in the carboxy-terminal region of the XL domain, which shows high homology to the exon 1–encoded portion of $G\alpha_s$ that promotes binding to $\beta\gamma$ dimers.[26,27] $XL\alpha_s$ is targeted to the plasma membrane[26] and can activate adenylyl cyclase[27]; however, the native receptors that interact with $XL\alpha_s$ in vivo are presently unknown.[27] By contrast, recent expression studies have demonstrated that $XL\alpha_s$ can interact with cloned receptors for PTH and a variety of other hormones in vitro.[28] ALEX is encoded by the second open reading frame in the XL exon 1, which starts 32 nucleotides downstream of the start codon for the XL domain and is terminated by a stop codon exactly at the end of the XL exon.[23]

A third alternative first exon of *GNAS1*, exon 1A, generates a transcript that lacks an initiator ATG; it is unlikely that any protein is translated from this mRNA.

Molecular studies of DNA from subjects with AHO have disclosed a variety of *GNAS1* gene mutations[9,29–36] that account for autosomal dominant inheritance of the disorder. Although most gene mutations impair expression of $G\alpha_s$ mRNA, in some subjects, abnormal forms of $G\alpha_s$ mRNA are produced that encode dysfunctional $G\alpha_s$ proteins.[37–40] Although private mutations have been found in nearly all of the kindreds studied, a 4-base deletion in exon 7 has been detected in multiple families,[41–46] and an unusual missense mutation in exon 13 (A366S) has been identified in two unrelated young boys,[47] suggesting that these two regions may be genetic "hot spots."

These studies confirm the molecular defect in AHO, but they do not explain the striking variability in biochemical and clinical phenotype. Why do some $G\alpha_s$-coupled pathways show reduced hormone responsiveness (e.g., PTH, TSH, gonadotropins), whereas other pathways are clinically unaffected (adrenocorticotropic hormone [ACTH] in the adrenal and vasopressin in the renal medulla). Perhaps even more intriguing is the paradox of why some subjects with $G\alpha_s$ deficiency have hormone resistance (PHP type 1a), whereas others may lack hormone resistance (pseudo-PHP) or physical features of AHO altogether.[48] These observations, when considered in the context of studies showing that the number of G_s molecules in cell membranes greatly exceeds the number of either receptor or adenylyl cyclase molecules,[49] raise issue with the hypothesis that a 50% deficiency of $G\alpha_s$ can impair hormone responsiveness. Indeed, in vitro studies of tissues and cells from subjects with PHP type 1a have often demonstrated normal hormonal responsiveness despite a 50% reduction in $G\alpha_s$ expression.[50]

Several observations now suggest that genomic imprinting of *GNAS1* can provide a molecular basis for the variable phenotypes that arise from identical *GNAS1* gene defects. First, clinical genetic studies have documented that PHP type 1a and pseudo-PHP frequently occur in the same family but are not present in the same generation. Second, analysis of published pedigrees has indicated that in nearly all cases maternal transmission of $G\alpha_s$ deficiency leads to PHP type 1a, whereas paternal transmission of the defect leads to pseudo-PHP.[17,46,51,52] These findings are inconsistent with stochastic models in which chance determines phenotype or interactive models in which a second gene is interactive with the defective *GNAS1* gene. Rather, a more tenable explanation for variable AHO phenotypes is that *GNAS1* expression is modified by tissue-specific genomic imprinting.[52] Genomic imprinting is a phenomenon by which the two copies of some genes are differentially expressed depending on the sex of the parent of origin. Genomic imprinting has been implicated in the molecular pathophysiology of a number of human disorders that affect growth, development, or endocrine function, including Prader-Willi/Angelman syndromes, transient neonatal diabetes, and PHP.[53] The *GNAS1* gene, as well as the syntenic murine *Gnas* gene located on a region of distal chromosome 2, produces a variety of sense and antisense transcripts that exhibit reciprocal imprinting.[54] Three unique, alternative first exons, and their respective promoters, are located upstream of the *GNAS1* exon 1, and each has a differentially methylated region (DMR) that correlates with parent-of-origin specific allelic transcription. NESP55 is expressed exclusively from the maternal allele and shows methylation of the DMR on the paternal allele. By contrast, the XL exon, which is only 11 kb downstream, is paternally expressed and shows methylation of the DMR on the maternal allele.[25,55] The exon 1A DMR is only 2 kb downstream from XL and is similarly methylated on the maternal allele and expressed from only the paternal allele.[56] Despite the reciprocal imprinting in both the paternal and maternal directions of the *GNAS1* gene, expression of $G\alpha_s$ appears to be biallelic in most tissues that have been examined.[25,55,57] However, predominant monoallelic expression from the maternally derived allele has been documented in tissues (e.g., murine renal proximal tubule[58,59]; human pituitary[9,60]; human thyroid[8,9]; and human ovary[9] that are associated with hormone resistance.

Recent analyses of heterozygous *Gnas* knockout mice confirm that $G\alpha_s$ expression is preferentially derived from the maternal allele in some tissues (e.g., renal cortex) and from both alleles in other tissues (e.g., renal medulla).[58] Accordingly, mice that inherit the defective *Gnas* gene maternally express that allele preferentially in imprinted tissues, such as the PTH-sensitive renal proximal tubule, resulting in a near absence of functional $G\alpha_s$ protein. By contrast, the 50% reduction in $G\alpha_s$ expression that occurs in nonimprinted tissues, which express both *Gnas* alleles, may account for more variable and moderate hormone resistance in these sites.

In AHO, inherited *GNAS1* gene mutations reduce expression or function of $G\alpha_s$ protein. By contrast, postzygotic somatic mutations in the *GNAS1* gene that enhance activity of the protein are found in many autonomous endocrine tumors[61-64] and affected tissues of patients with the McCune-Albright syndrome.[65,66] These mutations lead to constitutive activation of adenylyl cyclase and result in proliferation and autonomous hyperfunction of hormonally responsive cells. Not surprisingly, in most cases, *GNAS1* activating mutations occur on the maternally derived allele, which is preferentially expressed in imprinted tissues and would, therefore, be expected to result in a more severe clinical phenotype.[60] The clinical significance of $G\alpha_s$ activity as a determinant of hormone action is further emphasized by the description by Iiri et al.[47] of two unrelated males with both precocious puberty and PHP type 1a. These two subjects had identical *GNAS1* mutations in exon 13 (A366S) that resulted in a temperature-sensitive form of $G\alpha_s$. This $G\alpha_s$ is constitutively active in the cooler environment of the testis while being rapidly degraded in other tissues at normal body temperature. Thus, different tissues in these two individuals could show hormone resistance (to PTH and TSH), hormone responsiveness (to ACTH), or hormone-independent activation (to LH).

PHP type 1b. The characteristics of PHP type 1a contrast sharply with those of PHP type 1b (OMIM 603233), a less common and clinically distinct variant of PHP type 1. Although most cases of PHP type 1b seem to be sporadic, familial cases have been described in which transmission of the defect is consistent with an autosomal dominant pattern.[67] Subjects with PHP type 1b lack features of AHO, show decreased responsiveness to PTH as the only manifestation of hormone resistance, and have normal $G\alpha_s$ activity in accessible tissues.[29] Despite renal resistance to PTH, subjects with PHP type 1b who have elevated levels of PTH often manifest skeletal lesions similar to those that occur in patients with hyperparathyroidism.[68]

Specific resistance of target tissues to PTH and normal activity of $G\alpha_s$ first suggested decreased expression or function of the PTH/PTHrP receptor as the cause for hormone resistance in PHP type 1b. Early studies showed that cultured fibroblasts from some PHP type 1b patients accumulated less cAMP in response to PTH[69] and contained decreased levels of mRNA encoding the PTH/PTHrP receptor.[70] Subsequent studies failed to disclose mutations in the coding exons[71] and promoter regions[72] of the PTH/PTHrP receptor gene or its mRNA,[73] and mice[74] and humans[75] that are heterozygous for inactivation of the gene encoding the PTH/PTHrP receptor do not manifest PTH resistance or hypocalcemia. These studies provided compelling evidence that the PTH/PTHrP receptor was not the primary defect in PHP type 1b and encouraged consideration of other components of the PTH signal transduction pathway. Recently, genetic linkage analyses of PHP type 1b kindreds have mapped PHP type 1b to the *GNAS1* locus.[76-78] The nucleotide sequence of the coding exons and flanking intron-exon boundaries of the *GNAS1* gene is normal in patients with PHP type 1b, but an epigenetic defect that results in switching of the maternal *GNAS1* allele to a paternal pattern of methylation for exon 1A is a consistent finding in sporadic and familial PHP type 1b.[56,76,79] Similarly, in one patient with a syndrome that closely resembles PHP type 1b, deficiency of $G\alpha_s$ was ascribed to paternal uniparental disomy of *GNAS1*, such that little or no expression of $G\alpha_s$ would occur in imprinted tissues in which only the maternal allele is transcribed.[79] It is conceivable that loss of maternal-specific methylation of the exon 1A DMR converts this allele to a "paternal" one, with consequent effects on transcription of $G\alpha_s$ in imprinted tissues that are similar to those in paternal uniparental disomy. Thus, the defect in PHP type 1b would result in severe deficiency of functional $G\alpha_s$ in some imprinted tissues, such as the renal proximal tubules, thereby leading to hormone resistance. The genetic defect(s) that account for the loss of the maternal imprint (epigenotype) is presently unknown.

PHP type 1c. In rare instances, patients with PHP type 1 and features of AHO show resistance to multiple hormones in the absence of a demonstrable defect in G_s or G_i.[7] The nature of the lesion in such patients is unclear, but it has been proposed that the defect is related to some other general component of the receptor-adenylyl cyclase system, such as the catalytic unit.[80] However, recent molecular studies now suggest that these patients have *GNAS1* mutations that result in functional defects of $G\alpha_s$ that are not apparent in the in vitro assays presently available.[36]

PHP Type 2

PHP type 2 is a heterogeneous disorder without a clear genetic or familial basis. In these patients, renal resistance to PTH is manifested by a reduced phosphaturic response to administration of PTH, despite a normal increase in urinary cAMP excretion.[4] These observations suggest that the PTH receptor-adenylyl cyclase complex functions normally to increase nephrogenous cAMP in response to PTH and are consistent with a model in which PTH resistance arises from an inability of intracellular cAMP to activate downstream targets. Although no supportive data are yet available, a defect in cAMP-dependent protein kinase A has been proposed as a potential candidate.[4] However, such a lesion might be expected to produce the contrasting phenotype noted in Carney complex, a developmental disorder in which mutations in the *PRKAR1A* gene, which codes for the type 1A regulatory subunit of protein kinase A, leads to generalized activation of protein kinase A and diverse endocrine tumors.[81,82] Given the restricted biochemical defect in PHP type 2 and the relatively few cases identified recently, it seems more likely that PTH resistance in these patients results from severe and unsuspected deficiency of vitamin D.[83]

PTH Inhibitor as a Cause of PTH Resistance

Several studies have reported an apparent dissociation between circulating levels of immunoreactive and bioactive PTH in patients with PHP type 1. Despite high levels of immunoreactive PTH, the levels of bioactive PTH in many patients with PHP type 1 have been found to be within the normal range when measured in vitro with highly sensitive cytochemical bioassay systems. Furthermore, plasma from many of these patients has been shown to diminish the biological activity of exogenous PTH in these in vitro bioassays.[84] Although the identity of this putative inhibitor or antagonist is unknown, one potential candidate is the N-terminally truncated PTH fragment, hPTH(7-84), which can inhibit the calcemic actions of hPTH(1-34) or hPTH(1-84) through a nonclassical PTH receptor.[85] Circulating levels of PTH(7-84) immunoreactivity are elevated in patients with PHP type 1a and 1b, and the proportion of PTH(7--84)-like fragments to biologically active PTH(1-84) is increased.[86] Although it is conceivable that circulating hPTH(7-84)-like fragments may contribute to PTH resistance in some patients with PHP, it is likely that these circulating antagonists arise as a consequence of sustained secondary hyperparathyroidism and do not have a significant role in the primary pathophysiology of the disorder.

DIAGNOSIS OF PHP

A diagnosis of PHP should be considered in an individual who has functional hypoparathyroidism (i.e., hypocalcemia and hyperphosphatemia) and an elevated plasma concentration of immunoreactive PTH. Because hypomagnesemia is associated with reduced responsiveness to PTH, it is important to measure serum concentrations of magnesium in these subjects. Moreover, similar biochemical features may occur in some patients who have severe vitamin D deficiency.[83] Although hypocalcemia is usually the presenting feature of PHP, unusual initial manifestations of PHP include neonatal hypothyroidism, unexplained cardiac failure, Parkinson's disease, and spinal cord compression.[15]

The diagnosis of PHP (or pseudo-PHP) may also be suspected based on clinical features of AHO. However, several features of AHO, for example, obesity, round face, brachydactyly, and mental retardation, are common to other disorders (Prader-Willi syndrome, acrodysostosis, Ullrich-Turner syndrome) that are often associated with chromosomal defects. A growing number of reports have described small terminal deletions of chromosome 2q in patients with variable AHO-like phenotypes. Terminal deletion of 2q37 [del(2)(q37.3)] is the first consistent karyotypic abnormality that has been documented in patients with an AHO-like syndrome.[87,88] These patients have normal endocrine function and normal $G_{s\alpha}$ activity, however.[88] Thus, high-resolution chromosome analysis, biochemical/molecular analysis, and careful physical and radiological examination are essential in discriminating between these phenocopies and AHO.

The classical tests for PHP, the Ellsworth-Howard test and later modifications by Chase et al.,[3] involved the administration of 200–300 USP units of purified bovine PTH or parathyroid extract. Although these preparations are no longer available, the synthetic hPTH(1-34) peptide has been approved for human use, and several protocols for its use in the differential diagnosis of hypoparathyroidism have been developed.[89,90] These protocols are based on intravenous infusion of the peptide, but similar results may be obtained following subcutaneous injection of hPTH(1-34).[91] The patient should be fasting, supine except for voiding, and hydrated (250 ml of water hourly from 6 a.m. to 12:00 p.m.). Two control urine specimens are collected before 9:00 a.m. Synthetic human PTH(1-34) peptide (5 U [0.625 μg]/kg body weight to a maximum of 200 U or 25 μg) is administered intravenously from 9:00 to 9:15 a.m., and experimental urine specimens are collected from 9:00 to 9:30 a.m., 9:30 to 10:00 a.m., 10:00 to 11:00 a.m., and 11:00 a.m. to 12:00 p.m. Blood samples should be obtained at 9:00 and 11:00 a.m. for measurement of serum creatinine and phosphorous concentrations. Urine samples are analyzed for cAMP, phosphorous, and creatinine concentrations, and results are expressed as nanomoles of cAMP per 100 ml GF and TmP/GFR. Normal subjects and patients with hormonopenic hypoparathyroidism usually display a 10- to 20-fold increase in urinary cAMP excretion, whereas patients with PHP type 1 (types 1a and 1b), regardless of their serum calcium concentration, will show a markedly blunted response (Fig. 1). Thus, this test can distinguish patients with so-called "normocalcemic" PHP (i.e., patients with PTH resistance who are able to maintain normal serum calcium levels without treatment) from subjects with pseudo-PHP (who will have a normal urinary cAMP response to PTH.[3,17] The urinary cAMP and phosphate responses to PTH are dependent on the endogenous serum PTH and calcium levels,[92] and treatment with vitamin D to normalize serum calcium levels may normalize the phosphaturic response to PTH in patients with PHP type 1. Recent studies indicate that measurement of plasma cAMP[93] or plasma 1,25-dihydroxyvitamin D[94] after infusion of hPTH(1-34) may also differentiate PHP type 1 from other causes of hypoparathyroidism.

The presence of classical features of AHO and multihormonal resistance are diagnostic of PHP type 1a, but patients who lack obvious AHO have been found to have mutations in the *GNAS1* gene. Further testing (e.g., *GNAS1* gene analysis) may be required, and several reference laboratories now offer appropriate services. By contrast, genetic testing for PHP type 1b is still considered a research test and will require documentation of either an imprinting defect within the *GNAS1* gene or biallelic expression of transcripts encoded by exon 1a.[76,78,79,95]

The diagnosis of PHP type 2, a much rarer entity, is less straightforward. Documentation of elevated serum PTH and basal urinary (or nephrogenous) cAMP is a prerequisite for a definitive diagnosis of PHP type 2.[4] These subjects have a normal urinary cAMP response to infusion of PTH but characteristically fail to show a phosphaturic response. Unfortunately, interpretation of the phosphaturic response to PTH is often complicated by random variations in phosphate clearance, and it is sometimes not possible to classify a phosphaturic response as normal or subnormal regardless of the criteria used. More perplexing yet is the observation that biochemical findings that resemble PHP type 2 have been found in patients with various forms of vitamin D deficiency. In these patients, marked hypocalcemia is accompanied by hyperphosphatemia due presumably to an acquired dissociation between the amount of cAMP generated in the renal tubule and its effect on phosphate clearance.

TREATMENT

The basic principles of treatment of hypocalcemia in PHP are essentially those outlined for the treatment of hormonopenic hypoparathyroidism. Therapy is directed at maintaining a low- to mid-normal serum calcium concentration, thereby controlling symptoms of tetany while avoiding hypercalciuria. Patients with PHP require lower doses of vitamin D and have less risk of treatment-related hypercalciuria than patients with hypoparathyroidism. Treatment with calcium and vitamin D usually decreases the elevated serum phosphate to a high normal level because of a favorable balance between increased urinary phosphate excretion and decreased intestinal phosphate absorption. In general, phosphate binding gels such as aluminum hydroxide are not necessary.

Estrogen therapy and pregnancy have particularly interesting effects on the maintenance of normocalcemia in patients with PHP. Estrogen therapy may reduce serum levels of calcium in women with PHP[96] or hypoparathyroidism.[97] In addition, symptomatic hypocalcemia may also occur in some women at the time of the menses, when estrogen levels are low, with the cause remaining unknown.[98] Paradoxically, during the high estrogen state of pregnancy, some patients with PHP have required less, or no,[99] vitamin D to maintain normal serum concentrations of calcium owing to physiological increases in serum concentration of $1,25(OH)_2D_3$.[99] After delivery, serum calcium and $1,25(OH)_2D_3$ levels typically decrease, and PTH rises.[96] As placental synthesis of 1,25-dihydroxyvitamin D is not compromised in patients with PHP,[99] it appears that the placenta may contribute to the maintenance of normocalcemia during pregnancy. By contrast, patients with hypoparathyroidism may require treatment with larger amounts of vitamin D and calcium in the latter half of pregnancy.[100]

Patients with PHP type 1a will frequently manifest resistance to other hormones in addition to PTH and may display clinical evidence of hypothyroidism, gonadal dysfunction, or growth hormone deficiency. The basic principles used in the treatment of primary hypothyroidism apply to therapy of hypothyroidism in patients with PHP type 1a, as do approaches for the evaluation and treatment of growth hormone deficiency.

REFERENCES

1. Albright F, Burnett CH, Smith PH 1942 Pseudohypoparathyroidism: An example of "Seabright-Bantam syndrome." Endocrinology **30:** 922–932.
2. Schipani E, Karga H, Karaplis AC, Potts JT Jr, Kronenberg HM, Segre GV, Abou-Samra AB, Juppner H 1993 Identical complementary deoxyribonucleic acids encode a human renal and bone parathyroid hormone (PTH)/PTH-related peptide receptor. Endocrinology **132:**2157–2165.
3. Chase LR, Melson GL, Aurbach GD 1969 Pseudohypoparathyroidism: Defective excretion of 3′, 5′-AMP in response to parathyroid hormone. J Clin Invest **48:**1832–1844.
4. Drezner MK, Neelon FA, Lebovitz HE 1973 Pseudohypoparathyroidism type II: A possible defect in the reception of the cyclic AMP signal. N Engl J Med **280:**1056–1060.
5. Levine MA, Downs RW Jr, Singer MJ Jr, Marx SJ, Aurbach GD, Spiegel AM 1980 Deficient activity of guanine nucleotide regulatory protein in erythrocytes from patients with pseudohypoparathyroidism. Biochem Biophys Res Commun **94:**1319–1324.
6. Farfel Z, Brickman AS, Kaslow HR, Brothers VM, Bourne HR 1980 Defect of receptor-cyclase coupling protein in pseudohypoparathyroidism. N Engl J Med **303:**237–242.
7. Levine MA, Downs RW Jr, Moses AM, Breslau NA, Marx SJ, Lasker RD, Rizzoli RE, Aurbach GD, Spiegel AM 1983 Resistance to multiple hormones in patients with pseudohypoparathyroidism. Association with deficient activity of guanine nucleotide regulatory protein. Am J Med **74:**545–556.
8. Germain-Lee EL, Ding CL, Deng Z, Crane JK, Saji M, Ringel MD, Levine MA 2002 Paternal imprinting of Galpha(s) in the human thyroid as the basis of TSH resistance in pseudohypoparathyroidism type 1a. Biochem Biophys Res Commun **296:**62–72.
9. Mantovani G, Ballare E, Giammona E, Beck-Peccoz P, Spada A 2002 The gsalpha gene: Predominant maternal origin of transcription in human thyroid gland and gonads. J Clin Endocrinol Metab **87:**4736–4740.
10. Germain-Lee EL, Groman J, Crane JL, Jan de Beur SM, Levine MA 2003 Growth hormone deficiency in pseudohypoparathyroidism type 1a: Another manifestation of multi-hormone resistance. J Clin Endocrinol Metab (in press).
11. Kaji M, Umeda K, Ashida M, Tajima T 2001 A case of pseudohypoparathyroidism type 1a complicated with growth hormone deficiency: Recovery of growth hormone secretion after vitamin D therapy. Eur J Pediatr **160:**679–681.
12. Vlaeminck-Guillem V, D'herbomez M, Pigny P, Fayard A, Bauters C, Decoulx M, Wemeau JL 2001 Pseudohypoparathyroidism Ia and hypercalcitoninemia. J Clin Endocrinol Metab **86:**3091–3096.
13. Mann JB, Alterman S, Hills AG 1962 Albright's hereditary osteodystrophy comprising pseudohypoparathyroidism and pseudopseudohypoparathyroidism with a report of two cases representing the complete syndrome occurring in successive generations. Ann Intern Med **56:**315–342.
14. Gomes MF, Camargo AM, Sampaio TA, Graziozi MA, Armond MC 2002 Oral manifestations of Albright hereditary osteodystrophy: A case report. Rev Hosp Clin Fac Med Sao Paulo **57:**161–166.
15. Levine MA 1998 Hypoparathyroidism and pseudohypoparathyroidism. In: Avioli LV, Krane SM (eds.) Metabolic Bone Disease. Academic Press, San Diego, CA, USA.
16. Albright F, Forbes AP, Henneman PH 1952 Pseudopseudohypoparathyroidism. Trans Assoc Am Physicians **65:**337–350.
17. Levine MA, Jap TS, Mauseth RS, Downs RW, Spiegel AM 1986 Activity of the stimulatory guanine nucleotide-binding protein is reduced in erythrocytes from patients with pseudohypoparathyroidism and pseudopseudohypoparathyroidism: Biochemical, endocrine, and genetic analysis of Albright's hereditary osteodystrophy in six kindreds. J Clin Endocrinol Metab **62:**497–502.
18. Drezner MK, Haussler MR 1979 Normocalcemic pseudohypoparathyroidism. Am J Med **66:**503–508.
19. Levine MA, Modi WS, OBrien SJ 1991 Mapping of the gene encoding the alpha subunit of the stimulatory G protein of adenylyl cyclase (GNAS1) to 20q13.2–q13.3 in human by in situ hybridization. Genomics **11:**478–479.
20. Kozasa T, Itoh H, Tsukamoto T, Kaziro Y 1988 Isolation and characterization of the human Gs alpha gene. Proc Natl Acad Sci USA **85:**2081–2085.
21. Leitner B, Lovisetti-Scamihorn P, Heilmann J, Striessnig J, Blakely RD, Eiden LE, Winkler H 1999 Subcellular localization of chromogranins, calcium channels, amine carriers, and proteins of the exo-

cytotic machinery in bovine splenic nerve. J Neurochem **72**:1110–1116.

22. Ischia R, Lovisetti-Scamihorn P, Hogue-Angeletti R, Wolkersdorfer M, Winkler H, Fischer-Colbie R 1997 Molecular cloning and characterization of NESP55, a novel chromogranin-like precursor of a peptide with 5-HT1B receptor antagonist activity. J Biol Chem **272**:11657–11662.

23. Klemke M, Kehlenbach RH, Huttner WB 2001 Two overlapping reading frames in a single exon encode interacting proteins–a novel way of gene usage. EMBO J **20**:3849–3860.

24. Kehlenbach RH, Matthey J, Huttner WB 1994 XLαs is a new type of G protein. Nature **372**:804–808.

25. Hayward BE, Kamiya M, Strain L, Moran V, Campbell R, Hayashizaki Y, Bonthron DT 1998 The human GNAS1 gene is imprinted and encodes distinct paternally and biallelically expressed G proteins. Proc Natl Acad Sci USA **95**:10038–10043.

26. Pasolli HA, Klemke M, Kehlenbach RH, Wang Y, Huttner WB 2000 Characterization of the extra-large G protein alpha -subunit XLalpha s. I. Tissue distribution and subcellular localization. J Biol Chem **275**:33622–33632.

27. Klemke M, Pasolli HA, Kehlenbach RH, Offermanns S, Schultz G, Huttner WB 2000 Characterization of the extra-large G protein alpha -subunit XLalpha s. II. Signal transduction properties. J Biol Chem **275**:33633–33640.

28. Bastepe M, Gunes Y, Perez-Villamil B, Hunzelman J, Weinstein LS, Juppner H 2002 Receptor-mediated adenylyl cyclase activation through XLalpha(s), the extra-large variant of the stimulatory G protein alpha-subunit. Mol Endocrinol **16**:1912–1919.

29. Jan de Beur SM, Levine MA 2001 Pseudohypoparathyroidism: Clinical, biochemical, and molecular features. In: Bilezikian JP, Marcus R, Levine MA (eds.) The Parathyroids: Basic and Clinical Concepts. Academic Press, San Diego, CA, USA, pp. 807–826

30. Ishikawa Y, Tajima T, Nakae J, Nagashima T, Satoh K, Okuhara K, Fujieda K 2001 Two mutations of the Gsalpha gene in two Japanese patients with sporadic pseudohypoparathyroidism type Ia. J Hum Genet **46**:426–430.

31. de Sanctis L, Romagnolo D, Olivero M, Buzi F, Maghnie M, Scire G, Crino A, Baroncelli GI, Salerno M, Di Maio S, Cappa M, Grosso S, Rigon F, Lala R, de Sanctis C, Dianzani I 2003 Molecular analysis of the GNAS1 gene for the correct diagnosis of Albright hereditary osteodystrophy and pseudohypoparathyroidism. Pediatr Res **53**:749–755.

32. Pohlenz J, Ahrens W, Hiort O 2003 A new heterozygous mutation (L338N) in the human Gsalpha (GNAS1) gene as a cause for congenital hypothyroidism in Albright's hereditary osteodystrophy. Eur J Endocrinol **148**:463–468.

33. Rickard SJ, Wilson LC 2003 Analysis of GNAS1 and overlapping transcripts identifies the parental origin of mutations in patients with sporadic Albright hereditary osteodystrophy and reveals a model system in which to observe the effects of splicing mutations on translated and untranslated messenger RNA. Am J Hum Genet **72**:961–974.

34. Farfel Z 2002 Pseudohypoparathyroidism: A multitude of mutations in the stimulatory G protein alpha subunit (Gsalpha). J Pediatr Endocrinol Metab **15**:255–257.

35. Lim SH, Poh LK, Cowell CT, Tey BH, Loke KY 2002 Mutational analysis of the GNAS1 exons encoding the stimulatory G protein in five patients with pseudohypoparathyroidism type 1a. J Pediatr Endocrinol Metab **15**:259–268.

36. Linglart A, Carel JC, Garabedian M, Le T, Mallet E, Kottler ML 2002 GNAS1 lesions in pseudohypoparathyroidism Ia and Ic: Genotype phenotype relationship and evidence of the maternal transmission of the hormonal resistance. J Clin Endocrinol Metab **87**:189–197.

37. Schwindinger WF, Miric A, Zimmerman D, Levine MA 1994 A novel Gsα mutant in a patient with Albright hereditary osteodystrophy uncouples cell surface receptors from adenylyl cyclase. J Biol Chem **269**:25387–25391.

38. Warner DR, Gejman PV, Collins RM, Weinstein LS 1997 A novel mutation adjacent to the switch III domain of G(S alpha) in a patient with pseudohypoparathyroidism. Mol Endocrinol **11**:1718–1727.

39. Warner DR, Weng G, Yu S, Matalon R, Weinstein LS 1998 A novel mutation in the switch 3 region of Gsalpha in a patient with Albright hereditary osteodystrophy impairs GDP binding and receptor activation. J Biol Chem **273**:23976–23983.

40. Wu WI, Schwindinger WF, Aparicio LF, Levine MA 2001 Selective resistance to parathyroid hormone caused by a novel uncoupling mutation in the carboxyl terminus of Gαs: A cause of pseudohypoparathyroidism Type Ib. J Biol Chem **276**:165–171.

41. Weinstein LS, Gejman PV, de Mazancourt P, American N, Spiegel AM 1992 A heterozygous 4-bp deletion mutation in the G_sα gene (GNAS1) in a patient with Albright hereditary osteodystrophy. Genomics **13**:1319–1321.

42. Yu S, Yu D, Hainline BE, Brener JL, Wilson KA, Wilson LC, Oude-Luttikhuis ME, Trembath RC, Weinstein LS 1995 A deletion hot-spot in exon 7 of the Gs alpha gene (GNAS1) in patients with Albright hereditary osteodystrophy. Hum Mol Genet **4**:2001–2002.

43. Ahmed SF, Dixon PH, Bonthron DT, Stirling HF, Barr DG, Kelnar CJ, Thakker RV 1998 GNAS1 mutational analysis in pseudohypoparathyroidism. Clin Endocrinol (Oxf) **49**:525–531.

44. Yokoyama M, Takeda K, Iyota K, Okabayashi T, Hashimoto K 1996 A 4-base pair deletion mutation of Gs alpha gene in a Japanese patient with pseudohypoparathyroidism. J Endocrinol Invest **19**:236–241.

45. Walden U, Weissortel R, Corria Z, Yu D, Weinstein L, Kruse K, Dorr HG 1999 Stimulatory guanine nucleotide binding protein subunit 1 mutation in two siblings with pseudohypoparathyroidism type 1a and mother with pseudopseudohypoparathyroidism. Eur J Pediatr **158**:200–203.

46. Nakamoto JM, Sandstrom AT, Brickman AS, Christenson RA, Van Dop C 1998 Pseudohypoparathyroidism type Ia from maternal but not paternal transmission of a Gsalpha gene mutation. Am J Med Genet **77**:261–267.

47. Iiri T, Herzmark P, Nakamoto JM, Van Dop C, Bourne HR 1994 Rapid GDP release from Gs alpha in patients with gain and loss of endocrine function. Nature **371**:164–168.

48. Miric A, Vechio JD, Levine MA 1993 Heterogeneous mutations in the gene encoding the alpha subunit of the stimulatory G protein of adenylyl cyclase in Albright hereditary osteodystrophy. J Clin Endocrinol Metab **76**:1560–1568.

49. Levis MJ, Bourne HR 1992 Activation of the alpha subunit of Gs in intact cells alters its abundance, rate of degradation, and membrane avidity. J Cell Biol **119**:1297–1307.

50. Levine MA 1996 Pseudohypoparathyroidism. In: Bilezikian JP, Raisz LG, Rodan GA (eds.) Principles of Bone Biology. Academic Press, San Diego, CA, USA, pp. 853–876.

51. Wilson LC, Oude Luttikhuis ME, Clayton PT, Fraser WD, Trembath RC 1994 Parental origin of Gs alpha gene mutations in Albright's hereditary osteodystrophy. J Med Genet **31**:835–839.

52. Davies SJ, Hughes HE 1993 Imprinting in Albright's hereditary osteodystrophy. J Med Genet **30**:101–103.

53. Polychronakos C, Kukuvitis A 2002 Parental genomic imprinting in endocrinopathies. Eur J Endocrinol **147**:561–569.

54. Weinstein LS 2001 The stimulatory G protein alpha-subunit gene: Mutations and imprinting lead to complex phenotypes. J Clin Endocrinol Metab **86**:4622–4626.

55. Hayward BE, Moran V, Strain L, Bonthron DT 1998 Bidirectional imprinting of a single gene: GNAS1 encodes maternally, paternally, and biallelically derived proteins. Proc Natl Acad Sci USA **95**:15475–15480.

56. Liu J, Yu S, Litman D, Chen W, Weinstein LS 2000 Identification of a methylation imprint mark within the mouse Gnas locus. Mol Cell Biol **20**:5808–5817.

57. Campbell R, Gosden CM, Bonthron DT 1994 Parental origin of transcription from the human GNAS1 gene. J Med Genet **31**:607–614.

58. Yu S, Yu D, Lee E, Eckhaus M, Lee R, Corria Z, Accili D, Westphal H, Weinstein LS 1998 Variable and tissue-specific hormone resistance in heterotrimeric Gs protein alpha-subunit (Gsalpha) knockout mice is due to tissue-specific imprinting of the gsalpha gene. Proc Natl Acad Sci USA **95**:8715–8720.

59. Schwindinger WF, Lawler AM, Gearhart JD, Levine MA 1998 A murine model of Albright hereditary osteodystrophy. Endocrinology Society abstract no. 480.

60. Hayward BE, Barlier A, Korbonits M, Grossman AB, Jacquet P, Enjalbert A, Bonthron DT 2001 Imprinting of the G(s)alpha gene GNAS1 in the pathogenesis of acromegaly. J Clin Invest **107**:R31–R36.

61. Landis CA, Masters SB, Spada A, Pace AM, Bourne HR, Vallar L 1989 GTPase inhibiting mutations activate the alpha chain of Gs and stimulate adenylyl cyclase in human pituitary tumours. Nature **340**:692–696.

62. Fragoso MC, Latronico AC, Carvalho FM, Zerbini MC, Marcondes JA, Araujo LM, Lando VS, Frazzatto ET, Mendonca BB, Villares SM 1998 Activating mutation of the stimulatory G protein (gsp) as a

putative cause of ovarian and testicular human stromal Leydig cell tumors. J Clin Endocrinol Metab 83:2074–2078.

63. Gorelov VN, Gyenes M, Neser F, Roher HD, Goretzki PE 1996 Distribution of Gs-alpha activating mutations in human thyroid tumors measured by subcloning. J Cancer Res Clin Oncol 122:453–457.

64. O'Sullivan C, Barton CM, Staddon SL, Brown CL, Lemoine NR 1991 Activating point mutations of the gsp oncogene in human thyroid adenomas. Mol Carcinog 4:345–349.

65. Schwindinger WF, Francomano CA, Levine MA 1992 Identification of a mutation in the gene encoding the alpha subunit of the stimulatory G protein of adenylyl cyclase in McCune-Albright syndrome. Proc Natl Acad Sci USA 89:5152–5156.

66. Weinstein LS, Shenker A, Gejman PV, Merino MJ, Friedman E, Spiegel AM 1991 Activating mutations of the stimulatory G protein in the McCune-Albright syndrome. N Engl J Med 325:1688–1695.

67. Winter JSD, Hughes IA 1980 Familial pseudohypoparathyroidism without somatic anomalies. Can Med Assoc J 123:26–31.

68. Kidd GS, Schaaf M, Adler RA, Lassman MN, Wray HL 1980 Skeletal responsiveness in pseudohypoparathyroidism: A spectrum of clinical disease. Am J Med 68:772–781.

69. Silve C, Suarez F, el Hessni A, Loiseau A, Graulet AM, Gueris J 1990 The resistance to parathyroid hormone of fibroblasts from some patients with type Ib pseudohypoparathyroidism is reversible with dexamethasone. J Clin Endocrinol Metab 71:631–638.

70. Suarez F, Lebrun JJ, Lecossier D, Escoubet B, Coureau C, Silve C 1995 Expression and modulation of the parathyroid hormone (PTH)/PTH-related peptide receptor messenger ribonucleic acid in skin fibroblasts from patients with type Ib pseudohypoparathyroidism. J Clin Endocrinol Metab 80:965–970.

71. Schipani E, Weinstein LS, Bergwitz C, Iida-Klein A, Kong XF, Stuhrmann M, Kruse K, Whyte MP, Murray T, Schmidtke J, Van Dop C, Brickman AS, Crawford JD, Potts JTJ, Kronenberg HM, Abou-Samra AB, Segre GV, Juppner H 1995 Pseudohypoparathyroidism type Ib is not caused by mutations in the coding exons of the human parathyroid hormone (PTH)/PTH-related peptide receptor gene. J Clin Endocrinol Metab 80:1611–1621.

72. Bettoun JD, Minagawa M, Kwan MY, Lee HS, Yasuda T, Hendy GN, Goltzman D, White JH 1997 Cloning and characterization of the promoter regions of the human parathyroid hormone (PTH)/PTH-related peptide receptor gene: Analysis of deoxyribonucleic acid from normal subjects and patients with pseudohypoparathyroidism type 1b. J Clin Endocrinol Metab 82:1031–1040.

73. Fukumoto S, Suzawa M, Takeuchi Y, Kodama Y, Nakayama K, Ogata E, Matsumoto T, Fujita T 1996 Absence of mutations in parathyroid hormone (PTH)/PTH-related protein receptor complementary deoxyribonucleic acid in patients with pseudohypoparathyroidism type Ib. J Clin Endocrinol Metab 81:2554–2558.

74. Lanske B, Karaplis AC, Lee K, Luz A, Vortkamp A, Pirro A, Karperien M, Defize LK, Ho C, Mulligan RC, Abou-Samra AB, Juppner H, Segre GV, Kronenberg HM 1996 PTH/PTHrP receptor in early development and Indian hedgehog-regulated bone growth. Science 273:663–666.

75. Jobert AS, Zhang P, Couvineau A, Bonaventure J, Roume J, Le Merrer M, Silve C 1998 Absence of functional receptors for parathyroid hormone and parathyroid hormone-related peptide in Blomstrand chondrodysplasia. J Clin Invest 102:34–40.

76. Bastepe M, Pincus JE, Sugimoto T, Tojo K, Kanatani M, Azuma Y, Kruse K, Rosenbloom AL, Koshiyama H, Juppner H 2001 Positional dissociation between the genetic mutation responsible for pseudohypoparathyroidism type Ib and the associated methylation defect at exon A/B: Evidence for a long-range regulatory element within the imprinted GNAS1 locus. Hum Mol Genet 10:1231–1241.

77. Juppner H, Schipani E, Bastepe M, Cole DE, Lawson ML, Mannstadt M, Hendy GN, Plotkin H, Koshiyama H, Koh T, Crawford JD, Olsen BR, Vikkula M 1998 The gene responsible for pseudohypoparathyroidism type Ib is paternally imprinted and maps in four unrelated kindreds to chromosome 20q13.3. Proc Natl Acad Sci USA 95:11798–11803.

78. Jan de Beur SM, O'Connell JR, Peila R, Cho J, Deng Z, Kam S, Levine MA 2003 The pseudohypoparathyroidism type 1b locus is linked to a region including GNAS1 at 20q13.3. J Bone Miner Res 18:424–433.

79. Bastepe M, Lane AH, Juppner H 2001 Paternal uniparental isodisomy of chromosome 20q–and the resulting changes in GNAS1 methylation–as a plausible cause of pseudohypoparathyroidism. Am J Hum Genet 68:1283–1289.

80. Barrett D, Breslau NA, Wax MB, Molinoff PB, Downs RW Jr 1989

81. Kirschner LS, Carney JA, Pack SD, Taymans SE, Giatzakis C, Cho YS, Cho-Chung YS, Stratakis CA 2000 Mutations of the gene encoding the protein kinase A type I-alpha regulatory subunit in patients with the Carney complex. Nat Genet 26:89–92.

82. Stratakis CA, Miller WR, Severin E, Chin KV, Bertherat J, Amieux PS, Eng C, Kammer GM, Dumont JE, Tortora G, Beaven MA, Puck TT, Jan de Beur SM, Weistein LS, Cho-Chung YS 2002 Protein-kinase a and human disease: The core of cAMP-dependent signaling in health and disease. Horm Metab Res 34:169–175.

83. Rao DS, Parfitt AM, Kleerekoper M, Pumo BS, Frame B 1985 Dissociation between the effects of endogenous parathyroid hormone on adenosine 3′, 5′-monophosphate generation and phosphate reabsorption in hypocalcemia due to vitamin D depletion: An acquired disorder resembling pseudohypoparathyroidism type II. J Clin Endocrinol Metab 61:285–290.

84. Loveridge N, Fischer JA, Nagant de Deuxchaisnes C, Dambacher MA, Tschopp F, Werder E, Devogelaer JP, De Meyer R, Bitensky L, Chayen J 1982 Inhibition of cytochemical bioactivity of parathyroid hormone by plasma in pseudohypoparathyroidism type I. J Clin Endocrinol Metab 54:1274–1275.

85. Divieti P, John MR, Juppner H, Bringhurst FR 2002 Human PTH-(7–84) inhibits bone resorption in vitro via actions independent of the type 1 PTH/PTHrP receptor. Endocrinology 143:171–176.

86. Hatakeyama Y, Mizunashi K, Furukawa Y, Yabuki S, Sato Y, Igarashi T 2003 Plasma levels of parathyroid hormone (1–84) whole molecule and parathyroid hormone (7–84)-like fragments in pseudohypoparathyroidism type I. J Clin Endocrinol Metab 88:2250–2255.

87. Wilson LC, Leverton K, Oude Luttikhuis ME, Oley CA, Flint J, Wolstenholme J, Duckett DP, Barrow MA, Leonard JV, Read AP, Trembath RC 1995 Brachydactyly and mental retardation: An Albright hereditary osteodystrophy-like syndrome localized to 2q37. Am J Hum Genet 56:400–407.

88. Phelan MC, Rogers RC, Clarkson KB, Bowyer FP, Levine MA, Estabrooks LL, Severson MC, Dobyns WB 1995 Albright hereditary osteodystrophy and del(2)(q37.3) in four unrelated individuals. Am J Med Genet 58:1–7.

89. Mallette LE, Kirkland JL, Gagel RF, Law WM Jr, Heath H III 1988 Synthetic human parathyroid hormone-(1–34) for the study of pseudohypoparathyroidism. J Clin Endocrinol Metab 67:964–972.

90. Bhatt B, Burns J, Flanner D, McGee J 1988 Direct visualization of single copy genes on banded metaphase chromosomes by nonisotopic in situ hybridization. Nucleic Acids Res 16:3951–3961.

91. Lindsay R, Nieves J, Henneman E, Shen V, Cosman F 1993 Subcutaneous administration of the amino-terminal fragment of human parathyroid hormone-(1–34): Kinetics and biochemical response in estrogenized osteoporotic patients. J Clin Endocrinol Metab 77:1535–1539.

92. Stone MD, Hosking DJ, Garcia-Himmelstine C, White DA, Rosenblum D, Worth HG 1993 The renal response to exogenous parathyroid hormone in treated pseudohypoparathyroidism. Bone 14:727–735.

93. Stirling HF, Darling JA, Barr DG 1991 Plasma cyclic AMP response to intravenous parathyroid hormone in pseudohypoparathyroidism. Acta Paediatr Scand 80:333–338.

94. Miura R, Yumita S, Yoshinaga K, Furukawa Y 1990 Response of plasma 1,25-dihydroxyvitamin D in the human PTH(1–34) infusion test: An improved index for the diagnosis of idiopathic hypoparathyroidism and pseudohypoparathyroidism. Calcif Tissue Int 46:309–313.

95. Liu J, Litman D, Rosenberg MJ, Yu S, Biesecker LG, Weinstein LS 2000 A GNAS1 imprinting defect in pseudohypoparathyroidism type IB. J Clin Invest 106:1167–1174.

96. Breslau NA, Zerwekh JE 1986 Relationship of estrogen and pregnancy to calcium homeostasis in pseudohypoparathyroidism. J Clin Endocrinol Metab 62:45–51.

97. Verbeelen D, Fuss M 1979 Hypercalcemia induced by estrogen withdrawal in vitamin D-treated hypoparathyroidism. BMJ 1:522–523.

98. Mallette LE 1992 Case report: Hypoparathyrodisim with menses-associated hypocalcemia. Am J Med Sci 304:32–37.

99. Zerwekh JE, Breslau NA 1986 Human placental production of 1 alpha, 25-dihydroxyvitamin D3: Biochemical characterization and production in normal subjects and patients with pseudohypoparathyroidism. J Clin Endocrinol Metab 62:192–196.

100. Caplan RH, Beguin EA 1990 Hypercalcemia in a calcitriol-treated hypoparathyroid woman during lactation. Obstet Gynecol 76:485–489.

New form of pseudohypoparathyroidism with abnormal catalytic adenylate cyclase. Am J Physiol 257:E277–E283.

Chapter 45. Neonatal Hypocalcemia

Thomas O. Carpenter

Department of Pediatrics, Yale University School of Medicine, New Haven, Connecticut

CALCIUM METABOLISM IN THE PERINATAL PERIOD

Mineralization of the fetal skeleton is provided by active calcium transport from mother to fetus across the placenta, such that the fetus is relatively hypercalcemic compared with the mother. The rate-limiting step in calcium transport is apparently a calcium pump in the basal membrane (fetus-directed side) of the trophoblast. The net effect of this system is to maintain a 1:1.4 (mother:fetus) calcium gradient throughout gestation,[1] providing ample mineral for the demands of mineralization of the skeleton, particularly late in gestation. Evidence in the pregnant ewe suggests that a mid-region fragment of parathyroid hormone–related peptide (PTHrP) may play a role in the regulation of this function. Other studies in murine models indicate that PTH also plays a role in maintaining serum calcium levels in the fetus. At term, the fetus is hypercalcemic, is likely to have elevated circulating calcitonin, and may have low levels of PTH compared with maternal circulation. An abrupt transition to autonomous regulation of mineral homeostasis occurs at partum. The abundant placental supply of calcium is removed, and the circulating calcium level begins to fall, reaching a nadir within the first 4 days of life, and subsequently rising to normal adult levels in the second week of life.

HYPOCALCEMIC SYNDROMES IN THE NEWBORN PERIOD

Manifestations of neonatal hypocalcemia are variable and may not correlate with the magnitude of depression in the circulating ionized calcium level. As in older people, increased neuromuscular excitability (tetany) is a cardinal feature of newborn hypocalcemia. Generalized or focal clonic seizures, jitteriness, irritability, and frequent twitches or jerking of limbs are seen. Hyperacusis and laryngospasm may occur. Nonspecific signs include apnea, tachycardia, tachypnea, cyanosis, and edema; vomiting has also been reported. Neonatal hypocalcemia may be classified by its time of onset; differences in etiology are suggested by "early" occurring hypocalcemia as contrasted with that occurring "late" (Table 1).[2]

Early Neonatal Hypocalcemia

Early neonatal hypocalcemia occurs during the first 3 days of life, usually between 24 and 48 h, and characteristically is seen in premature infants, infants of diabetic mothers, and asphyxiated infants. The premature infant normally has an exaggerated postnatal depression in circulating calcium, dropping lower and earlier than in the term infant. Total calcium levels may drop below 7.0 mg/dl, but the

proportional drop in ionized calcium is less and may explain the lack of symptoms in many premature infants with total calcium in this range.

It is widely believed that maturation of parathyroid secretion in response to low serum calcium levels is particularly delayed in premature infants. Early studies have variably reported normal, elevated, or impaired secretion of PTH in prematures during citrate-induced hypocalcemia. Conflict also exists regarding the action of PTH in the newborn. A several day delay in the phosphaturic effect of PTH in both term and preterm infants has been described; resultant hyperphosphatemia may decrease serum calcium. The premature infant's exaggerated rise in calcitonin may provoke hypocalcemia. A role for vitamin D and its metabolites in early neonatal hypocalcemia is less convincing.

The infant of the diabetic mother (IDM) also shows an exaggerated postnatal drop in the circulating calcium level compared with other infants of comparable maturity. As in premature infants, the decrease is not entirely explained by a fall in ionized calcium concentrations. The pregnant diabetic tends to have lower circulating PTH and magnesium levels; the IDM has lower circulating magnesium and PTH, but normal calcitonin. Abnormalities in vitamin D metabolism do not seem to play a role in the development of hypocalcemia in the IDM. IDMs who maintain optimal glycemic control during pregnancy have a decreased incidence of hypocalcemia compared with infants of mothers with less regulated blood sugar levels; however, the incidence of hypocalcemia even with optimal maternal glycemic control is greater than control infants of mothers without diabetes.[3] One preventative strategy, administration of intramuscular magnesium to IDMs, failed to show a reduction in the incidence of hypocalcemia.[4]

Early hypocalcemia occurs in asphyxiated infants; calcitonin response is augmented, and PTH levels are elevated. Infants of pre-eclamptic mothers and postmature infants with growth retardation develop early hypocalcemia and are prone to hypomagnesemia.

Late Neonatal Hypocalcemia

The presentation of hypocalcemic tetany between 5 and 10 days of life is termed "late" neonatal hypocalcemia. The incidence of this disorder is greater in full-term that in premature infants and is not correlated with birth trauma or asphyxia. Affected children may have received cow's milk or cow's milk formula, which may have considerably more phosphate than human milk. Hyperphosphatemia is associated with late neonatal hypocalcemia and may reflect (1) inability of the immature kidney to efficiently excrete phosphate; (2) dietary phosphate load; or (3) transiently low levels of circulating PTH. Others have noted an association between late neonatal hypocalcemia and modest maternal vitamin D insufficiency. An increased occurrence of late neonatal hypocalcemia in winter has also been noted.

Hypocalcemia associated with magnesium deficiency

Dr. Carpenter has served as a consultant for Merck.

TABLE 1. NEONATAL HYPOCALCEMIA

	Characteristics	Mechanism
Early:	Onset within first 3–4 days of life; seen in infants of diabetic mother, perinatal asphyxia, pre-eclampsia	Uncertain; possible exaggerated post-natal calcitonin surge or decrease in parathyroid response
Late:	Onset days 5–10 of life, seen in winter, in infants of mother with marginal vitamin D intake; associated with dietary phosphate load	Possible transient parathyroid dysfunction; hypomagnesemia in some cases; calcium malabsorption
Other:		
Congenital hypoparathyroidism	Usually present after first 5 days of life with overt tetany; associated with 22q- syndromes	
"Late-late" hypocalcemia	Presents in premature at 2–4 months; associated with skeletal hypomineralization and inadequate dietary mineral or vitamin D intake	
Infants of hyperparathyroid mothers	May present as late as 1 year of age; mother possibly undiagnosed	
Ionized hypocalcemia (with normal total calcium)	In exchange transfusion with citrated blood products, lipid infusions, or alkalosis	
Phosphate load	Can be severe after administration of phosphate enemas	
Osteopetrosis	Defective mobilization of skeletal calcium related to severely impaired osteoclastic resorption	
Magnesium-wasting	Familial disorders of renal Mg wasting may result in refractory hypocalcemia in infancy	

may present as late neonatal hypocalcemia. Severe hypomagnesemia (circulating levels less that 0.8 mg/dl) may occur in congenital defects of intestinal magnesium absorption or renal tubular reabsorption. Transient hypomagnesemia of unknown etiology is associated with a less severe decrease in circulating magnesium (between 0.8 and 1.4 mg/dl). Hypocalcemia frequently complicates hypomagnesemic states because of impaired secretion of PTH. Impaired PTH responsiveness has also been demonstrated as an inconsistent finding in magnesium deficiency. Hypomagnesemia with secondary hypocalcemia (and hypocalciuria) has been recently identified to be caused by homozygous mutations in TRPM6, a bifunctional protein found in renal and intestinal epithelia.[5] The protein acts as both a divalent cation channel and has receptor-like protein kinase activity. Hypocalcemia in this setting is refractory to therapy unless correction of magnesium levels is attained, and usually presents at several weeks of age. Mutations in a renal tubular paracellular transport protein, CLDN16, also can cause hypomagnesemia and hypocalcemia, associated with hypercalciuria.[6]

Other Causes of Neonatal Hypocalcemia

Symptomatic neonatal hypocalcemia may occur within the first 3 weeks of life in infants born to mothers with hyperparathyroidism. Presentation at 1 year of age has also been reported. Serum phosphate is often greater than 8 mg/dl; symptoms may be exacerbated by feeding cow's milk or other high phosphate formulas. The proposed mechanism for the development of neonatal hypocalcemia in the infant of the hyperparathyroid mother is as follows: maternal hypercalcemia occurs secondary to hyperparathyroidism, resulting in increased calcium delivery to the fetus and fetal hypercalcemia, which inhibits fetal parathyroid secretion. The infant's oversuppressed parathyroid is not able to maintain normal calcium levels postpartum. Hypomagnesemia may be observed in the infant of the hyperparathyroid mother. Maternal hyperparathyroidism has been diagnosed after hypocalcemic infants have been identified.

"Late-late" neonatal hypocalcemia has been used in reference to premature infants who develop hypocalcemia with poor bone mineralization within the first 3–4 months of life. These infants tend to have an inadequate dietary supply of mineral and/or vitamin D.

The previously discussed forms of neonatal hypocalcemia are generally found to be of a transient nature. More rarely, hypocalcemia that is permanent is detected in the newborn period and caused by congenital hypoparathyroidism. Isolated absence of the parathyroids may be inherited in X-linked or autosomal recessive fashion. Hypocalcemia may occur secondary to activating mutations of the parathyroid calcium-sensing receptor.[7] Congenital hypoparathyroidism also occurs as the DiGeorge anomaly, classically the triad of hypoparathyroidism, T-cell incompetence caused by a partial or absent thymus, and conotruncal heart defects (e.g., tetralogy of Fallot, truncus arteriosus) or aortic arch abnormalities. These structures are derived from the embryologic third and fourth pharyngeal pouches; the usual sporadic occurrence reflects developmental abnormalities of these structures, which can be seen in association with microdeletions of chromosome 22q11.2.[8] Other defects may variably occur in this broad spectrum field defect, including other midline anomalies such as cleft palate and facial dysmorphism, or the vello-cardio-facial syndrome. Individuals with various phenotypic features of this syndrome have come to attention in late childhood or in adolescence with the onset of symptomatic hypocalcemia.[9] Presumably "partial" hypoparathyroidism in these individuals was not apparent early in life because of the mild nature of the partial defect. On the other hand, at least one of these individuals had transient hypocalcemia in the newborn period.

Severe hypocalcemia has been induced in the newborn period when phosphate enema preparations have been administered.[10] The phosphate load resulting from this inappropriate measure can result in extreme hyperphosphatemia, life-threatening hypocalcemia, and hypomagnesemia. Diarrhea associated with rotavirus infection in the newborn frequently results in hypocalcemia.[11]

© 2003 American Society for Bone and Mineral Research

Hypocalcemia in the newborn period may be the presenting manifestation of malignant infantile osteopetrosis, in which resorption of bone is defective, thereby compromising the maintenance of normal serum calcium levels. The Kenny-Caffey syndrome is a congenital anomaly associated with hypoparathyroidism, growth retardation, and medullary stenosis of tubular bones. Several reports of mitochondrial and fatty acid oxidation disorders have described hypoparathyroidism as a rare associated feature. Such disorders include the Kearns-Sayre syndrome, mitochondrial trifunctional protein deficiency, and long chain fatty acyl Co-A dehydrogenase (LCHAD) deficiency.[12,13] No mechanism for the hypoparathyroidism in any of these metabolic conditions has been clearly identified. Resistance to PTH in infancy has also been described in association with propionic acidemia.[14]

Decreases in the ionized fraction of the circulating calcium occur in infants undergoing exchange transfusions with citrated blood products or receiving lipid infusions. Citrate and fatty acids form complexes with ionized calcium, reducing the free calcium compartment. Alkalosis secondary to adjustments in ventilatory assistance may provoke a shift of ionized calcium to the protein-bound compartment. It should be pointed out that appropriate collection of sample for performance of ionized calcium levels may require anaerobic collection from a free-flowing vessel and prompt sample handling for accurate results; given these requirements, measurement of ionized calcium may be difficult to obtain under routine circumstances in small children.

TREATMENT OF NEONATAL HYPOCALCEMIA

Early neonatal hypocalcemia may be asymptomatic, and the necessity of therapy may be questioned in such infants. Most authors recommend that early neonatal hypocalcemia be treated when the circulating concentration of total serum calcium is less the 5–6 mg/dl (1.25–1.50 mM; or of ionized calcium less than 2.5–3 mg/dl, 0.62–0.72 mM) in the premature infant and when total serum calcium is less than 6–7 mg/dl (1.50–1.75 mM) in the term infant. Emergency therapy of acute tetany consists of intravenous (never intramuscular) calcium gluconate (10% solution) given slowly (less than 1 ml per minute). A dose of 1–3 ml will usually arrest convulsions. Doses should generally not exceed 20 mg/kg body weight and may be repeated up to four times per 24 h. After successful management of acute emergencies, maintenance therapy may be achieved by intravenous administration of 20–50 mg of elemental calcium per kg body weight per 24 h. Calcium glubionate is a commonly used oral supplement. Management of late neonatal tetany should include low-phosphate formula such as Similac PM 60/40, in addition to calcium supplements. A calcium:phosphate ratio of 4:1 has been recommended. Monitoring generally reveals that therapy can be discontinued after several weeks.

When hypomagnesemia is a causal feature of the hypocalcemia, magnesium administration may be indicated. Magnesium sulfate is given intravenously using cardiac monitoring or intramuscularly as a 50% solution at a dose of 0.1–0.2 ml/kg. One or two doses may treat transient hypomagnesemia: a dose may be repeated after 12–24 h. Patients with primary defects in magnesium metabolism require long-term oral magnesium supplements.

The place of vitamin D in the management of transient hypocalcemia is less clear. Daily supplementation of 400–800 U of vitamin D has been suggested for all premature infants as a preventative measure. Patients with normal intestinal absorption who develop "late-late" hypocalcemia with vitamin D deficiency rickets should respond within 4 weeks to 1000–2000 U of daily oral vitamin D. Such patients should receive a total of at least 40 mg of elemental calcium/kg body weight/day. In the various forms of persistent congenital hypoparathyroidism, long-term treatment with vitamin D (or its therapeutic metabolites) are used; the preferred agent is calcitriol for these purposes at our center.

REFERENCES

1. Kohlmeier L, Marcus R 1995 Calcium disorders of pregnancy. Endocrinol Metab Clin North Am **24:**15–39.
2. Hillman LS, Haddad JG 1982 Hypocalcemia and other abnormalities of mineral homeostasis during the neonatal period. In: Heath DA, Marx SJ (eds.) Calcium Disorders: Clinical Endocrinology, Butterworths International Medical Reviews. Butterworths, London, UK, pp. 248–276.
3. Jimenez-Moleon JJ, Bueno-Cavanillas A, Luna-del-Castillo JD, Garcia-Martin M, Lardelli-claret P, Galvez-Vargas R 2002 Impact of different levels of carbohydrate intolerance on neonatal outcomes classically associated with gestational diabetes mellitus. Eur J Obstet Gynecol Reprod Biol **102:**36–41.
4. Mehta KC, Kalkwarf HJ, Mimouni F, Khoury J, Tsang RC 1998 Randomized trial of magnesium administration to prevent hypocalcemia in infants of diabetic mothers. J Perinatol **18:**352–356.
5. Schlingmann KP, Weber S, Peters M, Niemann Nejsum L, Vitzhum H, Klingel K, Kratz M, Haddad E, Ristoff E, Dinour D, Syrrou M, Nielsen S, Sassen M, Waldegger S, Seyberth HW, Konrad M 2002 Hypomagnesemia with secondary hypocalcemia is caused by mutations in TRPM6, a new member of the TRPM gene family. Nat Genet **31:**166–170.
6. Simon DB, Lu Y, Choate KA, Velazquez H, Al-Sabban E, Praga M, Casari G, Bettinelli A, Colussi G, Rodriguez-Soriano J, McCredie D, Milford D, Sanjad S, Lifton RP 1999 Paracellin-1, a renal tight junction protein required for paracellular Mg^{2+} resorption. Science **285:**103–106.
7. Watanabe T, Bai M, Lane CR, Matsumoto S, Minamitani K, Minagawa M, Niimi H, Brown EM, Yasuda T 1998 Familial hypoparathyroidism: Identification of a novel gain of function mutation in transmembrane domain 5 of the calcium-sensing receptor. J Clin Endocrinol Metab **83:**2497–2502.
8. Webber SA, Hatchwell E, Barber JC, Daubeney PE, Crolla JA, Salmon AP, Keeton BR, Temple IK, Dennis NR 1996 Importance of microdeletions of chromosomal region 22q11 as a cause of selected malformations of the ventricular outflow tracts and aortic arch: A three-year prospective study. J Pediatr **129:**26–32.
9. Sykes KS, Bachrach LK, Siegel-Bartelt J, Ipp M, Kooh SW, Cytrynbaum C 1997 Velocardiofacial syndrome presenting as hypocalcemia in early adolescence. Arch Pediatr Adolesc Med **151:**745–747.
10. Walton DM, Thomas DC, Aly HZ, Short BL 2000 Morbid hypocalcemia associated with phosphate enema in a six-week-old infant. Pediatrics **106:**E37.
11. Foldenauer A, VossbeckS, Pohlandt F 1998 Neonatal hypocalcaemia associated with rotavirus diarrhoea. Eur J Pediatr **157:**838–842.
12. Tyni T, Rapola J, Palotie A, Pihko H 1997 Hypoparathyroidism in a patient with long-chain 3-hydroxyacyl-coenzyme A dehydrogenase deficiency caused by the G1528C mutation. J Pediatr **131:**766–768.
13. Dionisi-Vici C, Garavaglia B, Burlina AB, Bertini E, Saponara I, Sabetta G, Taroni F 1996 Hypoparathyroidism in mitochondrial trifunctional protein deficiency. J Pediatr **129:**159–162.
14. Griffin TA, Hostoffer RW, Tserng KY, Lebovitz DJ, Hoppel CL, Mosser JL, Kaplan D, Kerr DS 1996 Parathyroid hormone resistance and B cell lymphopenia in propionic acidemia. Acta Paediatr **85:**875–878.

Chapter 46.   Miscellaneous Causes of Hypocalcemia

Robert W. Downs, Jr.

Division of Endocrinology and Metabolism, Department of Internal Medicine, Virginia Commonwealth University School of Medicine, Richmond, Virginia

INTRODUCTION

The complete differential diagnosis of hypocalcemic disorders is extensive and is reviewed in a previous chapter. Other chapters in this text have covered in detail the important aspects of hypoparathyroidism, pseudohypoparathyroidism, disorders of vitamin D deficiency, and vitamin D metabolism, and special consideration has been given to neonatal hypocalcemia and to magnesium depletion as an important cause of hypocalcemia.

This chapter will deal with other "miscellaneous," but not necessarily less common, causes of hypocalcemia.

HYPOALBUMINEMIA

The ionized or free fraction of serum calcium is physiologically important for cellular function, and low ionized calcium is responsible for the symptoms of hypocalcemia. However, we most often measure *total* serum calcium, of which about one-half is bound to proteins, mostly to albumin. Significant changes in serum protein concentrations can sometimes cause large changes in total serum calcium concentration without affecting the important ionized calcium fraction. Thus, in malnourished and ill individuals, hypoalbuminemia is the most common cause of a low total serum calcium measurement, and such patients do not have symptoms or clinical signs of ionized hypocalcemia.

There are a number of "rule of thumb" correction formulas that can be used to estimate whether low total serum calcium can be attributed simply to low albumin or serum protein. The most widely used is based on the fact that, at normal pH, each gram of albumin is capable of binding approximately 0.8 mg of calcium:

"Corrected Calcium" = Measured Total Calcium

+ [0.8 × (4.0 − Measured Albumin)]

None of these formulas are entirely satisfactory, however,[1] and particularly in ill patients or when there are symptoms or signs that could be caused by hypocalcemia, it is important to consider direct measurement of ionized calcium if the clinical situation warrants.[2] The problem is that direct measurement of ionized calcium is not a straightforward laboratory test, and careful attention must be paid to ensure the reliability of the measurement.[3]

LABORATORY ERROR

It should be obvious that laboratory test results suggesting hypocalcemia can only be dependable if sample collection and handling is correct. Nevertheless, it is worth emphasizing that if the serum calcium is significantly abnormal in a patient who is asymptomatic, consideration of the reliability of the data itself is worthwhile as part of the evaluation of the hypocalcemia. There have been reports of apparently "severe" hypocalcemia in cases in which blood is mistakenly collected in tubes containing EDTA.[4]

ALTERATIONS IN BOUND CALCIUM

In addition to the binding of calcium to albumin and plasma proteins, about 5% of circulating calcium is complexed with inorganic anions. There are a number of situations in which increases in the concentration of anions or changes in calcium binding caused by changes in pH result in a shift between bound and ionized calcium.

Hyperphosphatemia is a common cause of significant hypocalcemia. Rapid increases in serum phosphorus concentrations can occur in the setting of exogenous phosphate administration by oral, rectal, or intravenous routes. Hypocalcemia has been reported after phosphate enemas, particularly in children.[5,6] Even short courses of oral sodium phosphate can cause symptomatic hypocalcemia in adults who may have underlying asymptomatic vitamin D deficiency or magnesium depletion or significant renal insufficiency preventing normal elimination of phosphorus.[7] Patients who have impaired ability to mobilize calcium from skeletal stores could also be at increased risk for the development of hypocalcemia after phosphate administration.[8] Hyperphosphatemia can also cause hypocalcemia as a result of release of phosphate from endogenous tissue stores in patients who have rhabdomyolysis and the tumor lysis syndrome.[9] The causes of hyperphosphatemia and its management are reviewed in detail elsewhere.

Infusion of citrate will complex calcium and lead to acute decreases in ionized calcium concentrations. This is well-recognized for massive transfusion with citrated blood products, particularly in the setting of liver transplantation, in which the citrate may not be readily metabolized.[10] Citrate is also used during plasma exchange and during apheresis, and monitoring of citrate delivery and steps to prevent hypocalcemic toxicity during plasmapheresis are important.[11,12] Interestingly, even small volume blood transfusion has been associated with the precipitation of hypocalcemic symptoms in patients with pre-existing untreated asymptomatic hypocalcemia.[13]

Because albumin binds calcium, it is possible that infusion of albumin could lower ionized calcium. This is generally not a problem for the usual small 100-ml volumes of 25% albumin administered to patients on medical wards,[14] but can be a problem during infusion of larger volumes of colloid during therapeutic plasma exchange, a problem that can be ameliorated by use of an alternate non-calcium binding colloid.[11]

The author has no conflict of interest.

INCREASED OSTEOBLASTIC ACTIVITY

Bone formation and resorption are usually tightly coupled, but in certain circumstances, osteoblastic activity may be so great that hypocalcemia occurs. Two situations in which this occurs are during healing of bone disease after parathyroidectomy ("hungry-bones syndrome") and in the presence of widespread osteoblastic metastases.

In most patients with relatively mild hyperparathyroidism, surgical removal of an abnormal parathyroid gland results in mild transient hypocalcemia caused by suppression of the remaining normal parathyroid glands, but prompt recovery to normal serum calcium concentrations is expected. In other patients with more severe hyperparathyroidism who have evidence for significant bone disease, hypocalcemia and hypophosphatemia persist despite recovery of parathyroid hormone secretion from the remaining normal glands. The distinction between hungry bones and postoperative hypoparathyroidism is based on the persistently low serum phosphorus concentration in patients with hungry bones and on normal or even high concentrations of parathyroid hormone. Individuals with pre-existing vitamin D deficiency accompanying their primary hyperparathyroidism seem to be at greater risk for hungry bones, or at least the presence of lasting hypocalcemia leads to the discovery of the underlying vitamin D deficiency. Patients may require treatment with calcium and vitamin D to enhance intestinal calcium absorption for weeks and even months, until the bone heals.[15,16]

Avid uptake of calcium by osteoblastic metastatic lesions can also cause hypocalcemia. Prostate cancer metastases are commonly osteoblastic and are frequently associated with this syndrome, but other cancers can also cause hypocalcemia by this mechanism.[17,18] A recent prospective study of patients with advanced prostate cancer found that 57% of patients with proven bone metastases had elevated circulating concentrations of parathyroid hormone, suggesting that mild secondary hyperparathyroidism caused by osteoblastic metastases could be more common than generally recognized.[19]

ACUTE ILLNESS

Hypocalcemia is quite common in severely ill patients. In many, changes in serum proteins are responsible for the majority of the change in serum calcium, and ionized calcium remains normal. This seems to be the case for much of the mild hypocalcemia that often accompanies surgical procedures.[20] However, there clearly are patients who develop significant ionized hypocalcemia during severe illness. Because serum proteins are often abnormal in these patients, ionized calcium determination is often required to appropriately diagnose and treat these individuals.

Hypocalcemia is common in acute pancreatitis and is one of the prognostic signs indicative of overall poor outcome. Free fatty acids seem to be generated by the actions of pancreatic enzymes, and these complex with calcium to form insoluble soaps. In addition, the inflammatory process may be associated with other systemic mediators, although it is not clear whether elevations of these mediators are causally related to the hypocalcemia. Patients with acute pancreatitis may often have other factors contributing to the development of hypocalcemia, such as hypomagnesemia, malabsorption with vitamin D deficiency, and hypoalbuminemia.[21,22]

Hypocalcemia in the setting of other acute illnesses, particularly bacterial sepsis, is a very poor prognostic sign. The mechanism of hypocalcemia in sepsis remains unclear. PTH secretion appears to be appropriately increased, but the degree of hypocalcemia has been found to be inversely correlated with TNF-α and interleukin-6 (IL-6) activity, so it may be that circulating cytokines play a role in the development of the hypocalcemia.[23]

Patients with AIDS and hypocalcemia may have a distinct pathophysiology. After adjusting for hypoalbuminemia, hypocalcemia is present in AIDS patients more commonly than in control hospital outpatients (6.5% versus 1.1% in one study). AIDS patients may have concomitant vitamin D deficiency or hypomagnesemia and do seem to lack an entirely normal parathyroid hormone secretory response for the degree of hypocalcemia.[24] CD4 is expressed in parathyroid glands, so there is the possibility that a lack of parathyroid hormone reserve could be related to HIV infection of parathyroid cells.[25]

MEDICATIONS

In patients who appear to have drug-related hypocalcemia, the presence of symptomatic hypocalcemia should prompt a complete evaluation for other underlying abnormalities of calcium regulatory hormones. A common theme that runs through many of the case reports of patients who have symptomatic hypocalcemia induced by medications and during acute illness is that the development of hypocalcemia often leads to the discovery of previously unrecognized vitamin D deficiency or hypoparathyroidism.

During aggressive treatment of patients who have hypercalcemia, potent antiresorptive medications that interfere with mobilization of calcium from skeletal stores can cause hypocalcemia. Even when care is used, there may be a brief phase of transient hypocalcemia after successful reduction of the serum calcium until parathyroid hormone secretion recovers from suppression. If treatment is particularly zealous, osteoclastic activity may be more profoundly decreased, and hypocalcemia can be long-lasting. In addition, patients with malignancy may have other problems, such as hypomagnesemia or vitamin D deficiency, which can be unmasked during aggressive intravenous bisphosphonate treatment.[26]

Mild asymptomatic hypocalcemia occurs occasionally in patients with osteoporosis or Paget's disease who are treated with oral or intravenous bisphosphonates, and this is not usually a clinical problem. However, patients who have unrecognized hypoparathyroidism or vitamin D deficiency can develop more severe symptomatic hypocalcemia during bisphosphonate therapy.[27–30] In addition, the recent availability of highly potent and long-lasting bisphosphonates such as zoledronate suggests the possibility that clinically significant hypocalcemia might occur in patients receiving frequent treatment, even in the absence of underlying disorders of mineral metabolism.

Long-term anticonvulsant therapy with phenytoin or phenobarbital is associated with an increased risk for osteomalacia and hypocalcemia. Institutionalized patients seem most likely to be affected,[31] and ambulatory outpatients who have adequate calcium and vitamin D intake have a fairly low risk for this complication.

Medications that cause hypomagnesemia, such as amphotericin B, furosemide, cyclosporine, and cisplatin can provoke hypokalemia.[32] Medications that contain calcium-binding properties can precipitate hypocalcemia. Fosphenytoin provides a large phosphate load.[33] Foscarnet, an antiviral antibiotic used primarily in patients with AIDS, is a pyrophosphate analog that complexes calcium and magnesium.[34] Intravenous contrast agents containing EDTA were previously reported to cause hypocalcemia but are less widely used now.

Antineoplastic agents seem capable of causing hypocalcemia in some patients even when a tumor lysis syndrome does not occur.[35] It may be that effective treatment of patients who have bone lesions then allows healing of bones with a hungry-bones effect, and this has been reported in several patients who have prostate cancer treated with estramustine.[36]

Finally, symptomatic hypocalcemia has been reported in patients receiving magnesium as tocolytic therapy for premature labor.[37] Increases in magnesium are known to suppress parathyroid hormone secretion, probably through effects on the calcium-sensing receptor, but it is not clear why some patients are more susceptible to this complication.

REFERENCES

1. Ladenson JH, Lewis JW, Boyd JC 1978 Failure of total calcium corrected for protein, albumin, and pH to correctly assess free calcium status. J Clin Endocrinol Metab **46**:986–993.
2. Koch SM, Warters RD, Melhorn 2002 The simultaneous measurement of ionized and total calcium and ionized and total magnesium in intensive care unit patients. J Crit Care **17**:203–205.
3. Burnett RW, Christiansen TF, Covington AK, Fogh-Andersen N, Kulpmann WR, Lewenstam A, Maas AHJ, Muller-Plathe O, Sachs C, Andersen OS, VanKessel AL, Zijlstra WG 2000 IFCC recommended reference method for the determination of the substance concentration of ionized calcium in undiluted serum, plasma, or whole blood. Clin Chem Lab Med **38**:1301–1314.
4. Naguib MT, Evans N 2002 Combined false hyperkalemia and hypocalcemia due to specimen contamination during routine phlebotomy. South Med J **95**:18–20.
5. Walton DM, Thomas DC, Aly HZ, Short BL 2000 Morbid hypocalcemia associated with phosphate enema in a six-week old infant. Pediatrics **106**:E37.
6. Helikson MA, Parham WA, Tobias JD 1997 Hypocalcemia and hyperphosphatemia after phosphate enema use in a child. J Pediatr Surg **32**:1244–1246.
7. Boivin MA, Kahn SR 1998 Symptomatic hypocalcemia from oral sodium phosphate: A report of two cases. Am J Gastroenterol **93**:2577–2579.
8. Campisi P, Badhwar V, Morin S, Trudel JL 1999 Postoperative hypocalcemic tetany caused by fleet phosphosoda preparation in patient taking alendronate sodium: Report of a case. Dis Colon Rectum **42**:1499–1501.
9. Akmal M, Bishop JE, Telfer N, Norman AW, Massry SG 1986 Hypocalcemia and hypercalcemia in patients with rhabdomyolysis with and without acute renal failure. J Clin Endocrinol Metab **63**:137–142.
10. Wu AH, Bracey A, Bryan-Brown CW, Harper JV, Burritt MF 1987 Ionized calcium monitoring during liver transplantation. Arch Pathol Lab Med **111**:935–938.
11. Weinstein R 2001 Hypocalcemic toxicity and atypical reactions in therapeutic plasma exchange. J Clin Apheresis **16**:210–211.
12. Kishimoto M, Ohto H, Shikama Y, Kikuta A, Kimijima I, Takenoshita S 2002 Treatment for the decline of ionized calcium levels during peripheral blood progenitor cell harvesting. Transfusion **42**:1340–1347.
13. Niven MJ, Zohar M, Shimoni Z, Glick J 1998 Symptomatic hypocal-cemia precipitated by small-volume blood transfusion. Ann Emerg Med **32**:498–501.
14. Erstad BL, Richards H, Rose S, Nakazato P, Fortune J 1999 Influence of 25% human serum albumin on total and ionized calcium concentrations in vivo. Crit Care **3**:117–121.
15. Brasier AR, Nussbaum SR 1988 Hungry bone syndrome: Clinical and biochemical predictors of its occurrence after parathyroid surgery. Am J Med **84**:654–660.
16. Savazzi GM, Allegri L 1993 The hungry bone syndrome: Clinical problems and therapeutic approaches following parathyroidectomy. Eur J Med **2**:363–368.
17. Riancho JA, Arjona R, Valle R, Sanz J, Gonzalez-Macias J 1989 The clinical spectrum of hypocalcemia associated with bone metastases. J Intern Med **226**:449–452.
18. Chap LI, Mirra J, Ippolito V, Rentschler R, Rosen P 1997 Miliary osteosarcomatosis with associated hypocalcemia. Am J Clin Oncol **20**:505–508.
19. Murray RML, Grill V, Crinis N, Ho PWM, Davison J, Pitt P 2001 Hypocalcemia and normocalcemic hyperparathyroidism in patients with advanced prostate cancer. J Clin Endocrinol Metab **86**:4133–4138.
20. Lepage R, Legare G, Racicot C, Brossard J-H, Lapointe R, Dagenais M, D'Amour P 1999 Hypocalcemia induced during major and minor abdominal surgery in humans. J Clin Endocrinol Metab **84**:2654–2658.
21. Agarwal N, Pitchumoni CS 1993 Acute pancreatitis: A multisystem disease. Gastroenterologist **1**:115–128.
22. Ammori BJ, Barclay GR, Larvin M, McMahon MJ 2003 Hypocalcemia in patients with acute pancreatitis: A putative role for systemic endotoxin exposure. Pancreas **26**:213–217.
23. Lind L, Carlstedt F, Rastad J, Stiernstrom H, Stridsberg M, Ljunggren O, Wide L, Larsson A, Hellman P, Ljunghall S 2000 Hypocalcemia and parathyroid hormone secretion in critically ill patients. Crit Care Med **28**:93–99.
24. Kuehn EW, Anders HJ, Bogner JR, Obermaier J, Goebel FD, Schlondorff D 1999 Hypocalcemia in HIV infection and AIDS. J Intern Med **245**:69–73.
25. Hellman P, Karlsson PA, Klareskog L, Ridefelt P, Bjerneroth G, Rastad J 1996 Expression and function of a CD-4 like molecule in parathyroid tissue. Surgery **120**:985–992.
26. Champallou C, Basuyau JP, Veyret C, Chinet P, Debled M, Chevrier A, Grongnet MH, Brunelle F 2003 Hypocalcemia following pamidronate administration for bone metastases of solid tumor: Three clinical case reports. J Pain Symptom Manage **25**:185–190.
27. Schussheim DH, Jacobs TP, Silverberg SJ 1999 Hypocalcemia associated with alendronate. Ann Intern Med **130**:329.
28. Kashyap AS, Kashyap S 2000 Hypoparathyroidism unmasked by alendronate. Postgrad Med J **76**:417–419.
29. Rosen CJ, Brown S 2003 Severe hypocalcemia after intravenous bisphosphonate therapy in occult vitamin D deficiency. N Engl J Med **348**:1503–1504.
30. Stuckey BG, Lim EM, Kent GN, Ward LC, Gutteridge DH 2001 Bisphosphonate therapy for Paget's disease in a patient with hypoparathyroidism: Profound hypocalcemia, rapid response, and prolonged remission. J Bone Miner Res **16**:1719–1723.
31. Schmitt BP, Nordlund DJ, Rodgers LA 1984 Prevalence of hypocalcemia and elevated serum alkaline phosphatase in patients receiving chronic anticonvulsant therapy. J Fam Pract **18**:873–877.
32. Marcus N, Garty BZ 2001 Transient hypoparathyroidism due to amphotericin B-induced hypomagnesemia in a patient with beta-thalassemia. Ann Pharmacother **35**:1042–1044.
33. Keegan MT, Bondy LR, Blackshear JL, Lanier WL 2002 Hypocalcemia-like electrocardiographic changes after administration of fosphenytoin. Mayo Clin Proc **77**:584–586.
34. Huycke MM, Naguib MT, Stroemmel MM, Blick K, Monti K, Martin-Munley S, Kaufman C 2000 A double-blind placebo-controlled crossover trial of intravenous magnesium sulfate for foscarnet-induced ionized hypocalcemia and hypomagnesemia in patients with AIDS and cytomegalovirus infection. Antimicrob Agents Chemother **44**:2143–2148.
35. Kidu Y, Okamura T, Tomikawa M, Yamamoto M, Shiraishi M, Okada Y, Kimura T, Sugimachi K 1996 Hypokalemia associated with 5-flurouracil and low dose leucovorin in patients with advanced colorectal or gastric carcinomas. Cancer **78**:1794–1797.
36. Park DS, Sellin RV, Tu SM 2001 Estramustine-related hypocalcemia in patients with prostate carcinoma and osteoblastic metastases. Urology **58**:105xii–105xv.
37. Mayan H, Hourvitz A, Schiff E, Farfel Z 1999 Symptomatic hypocalcemia in hypermagnesemia-induced hypoparathyroidism during magnesium tocolytic therapy—possible involvement of the calcium sensing receptor. Nephrol Dial Transplant **14**:1764–1766.

Chapter 47. Magnesium Depletion and Hypermagnesemia

Robert K. Rude

Division of Endocrinology, University of Southern California, Los Angeles, California

HYPOMAGNESEMIA/MAGNESIUM DEPLETION

Magnesium (Mg) depletion, as determined by low serum Mg levels, is present in approximately 10% of patients admitted to city hospitals, and as many as 65% of patients in an intensive care unit have been reported to be hypomagnesemic. Hypomagnesemia and/or Mg depletion is usually caused by losses of Mg from either the gastrointestinal tract or the kidney, as outlined in Table 1.

Causes of Magnesium Depletion

The Mg content of upper intestinal tract fluids is approximately 1 mEq/liter. Vomiting and nasogastric suction therefore may contribute to Mg depletion. The Mg content of diarrheal fluids and fistulous drainage are much higher (up to 15 mEq/liter), and consequently, Mg depletion is common in acute and chronic diarrhea, regional enteritis, ulcerative colitis, and intestinal and biliary fistulas. Malabsorption syndromes caused by nontropical sprue, radiation injury resulting from therapy for disorders such as carcinoma of the cervix, and intestinal lymphangiectasia may also result in Mg deficiency. Steatorrhea and resection or bypass of the small bowel, particularly the ileum, often results in intestinal Mg loss or malabsorption. Last, acute severe pancreatitis is associated with hypomagnesemia, which may be because of the clinical problem causing the pancreatitis, such as alcoholism, or the saponification of Mg in necrotic parapancreatic fat. A primary defect in intestinal Mg absorption, which presents early in life with hypomagnesemia, hypocalcemia, and seizures, has been described as an autosomal recessive disorder linked to chromosome 9q22. This disorder seems to be caused by mutations in *TRPM6*, which expresses a protein involved with active intestinal Mg transport.

Excessive excretion of Mg into the urine may be the basis of Mg depletion. Renal Mg reabsorption is proportional to tubular fluid flow, as well as to sodium and calcium excretion. Therefore, chronic parenteral fluid therapy, particularly with saline, and volume expansion states such as primary aldosteronism and hypercalciuric states may result in Mg depletion. Hypercalcemia have been shown to decrease renal Mg reabsorption, probably mediated by calcium binding to the calcium-sensing receptor in the thick ascending limb of Henle and decreasing transepithelial voltage, and is probably the cause of renal Mg wasting and hypomagnesemia observed in many hypercalcemic states. Osmotic diuresis caused by glucosuria will result in urinary Mg wasting. Diabetes mellitus is probably the most common clinical disorder associated with Mg depletion.

An increasing list of drugs is becoming recognized as causing renal Mg wasting and Mg depletion. The major site of renal Mg reabsorption is at the loop of Henle; therefore,

diuretics such as furosemide and ethacrynic acid have been shown to result in marked Mg wasting. Aminoglycosides have been shown to cause a reversible renal lesion that results in hypermagnesemia and hypomagnesemia. Similarly, amphotericin B therapy has been reported to result in renal Mg wasting. Other renal Mg-wasting agents include cisplatin, cyclosporin, tacolimus, and pentamidine. A rising blood alcohol level has been associated with hypermagnesemia and is one factor contributing to Mg depletion in chronic alcoholism. Metabolic acidosis caused by diabetic ketoacidosis, starvation, or alcoholism may also result in renal Mg wasting.

Several renal Mg wasting disorders have been described that may be genetic or sporadic. One form, which is autosomal recessive, results from mutations in the *paracellin-1* gene on chromosome 3. This disorder is characterized by low serum Mg as well as hypercalciuria and nephrocalcinosis. Another autosomal dominant form of isolated renal Mg wasting and hypomagnesemia has been linked to chromosome 11q23 and identified as a mutation on the $Na^+,K^{(+)}$-ATPase γ-subunit of gene *FXYD2*. Gitelman's

TABLE 1. CAUSES OF MG DEFICIENCY

Gastrointestinal disorders
  Prolonged nasogastric suction/vomiting
  Acute and chronic diarrhea
  Intestinal and biliary fistulas
  Malabsorption syndromes
  Extensive bowel resection or bypass
  Acute hemorrhagic pancreatitis
  Protein-calorie malnutrition
  Primary hypomagnesemia (neonatal)
Renal loss
  Chronic parenteral fluid therapy
  Osmotic diuresis (glucose, urea, manitol)
  Hypercalcemia
  Alcohol
  Diuretics (furosemide, ethacrynic acid)
  Aminoglycosides
  Cisplatin
  Cyclosporin
  Amphotericin B
  Pentamidine
  Tacolimus
  Metabolic acidosis
  Renal disorders with Mg wasting
  Primary hypomagnesemia
Endocrine and metabolic disorders
  Diabetes mellitus (glycosuria)
  Phosphate depletion
  Primary hyperparathyroidism (hypercalcemia)
  Hypoparathyroidism (hypercalciuria, hypercalcemia due to
    overtreatment with vitamin D)
  Primary aldosteronism
  Hungry bone syndrome
  Chronic renal disease
  Excessive lactation

Dr. Rude has served as a consultant for Blaine Pharmaceuticals.

syndrome (familial hypokalemia-hypomagnesemia syndrome) is an autosomal recessive disorder caused by a genetic defect of the thiazide-sensitive NaCl cotransporter gene on chromosome 16.

Hypomagnesemia may accompany a number of other disorders. Phosphate depletion has been shown experimentally to result in urinary Mg wasting and hypomagnesemia. Hypomagnesemia may also accompany the "hungry bone" syndrome, a phase of rapid bone mineral accretion in subjects with hyperparathyroidism or hyperthyroidism after surgical treatment. Finally, chronic renal tubular, glomerular, or interstitial diseases may be associated with renal Mg wasting. Rarely, excessive lactation may result in hypomagnesemia.

Manifestations of Magnesium Depletion

Because Mg depletion is usually secondary to another disease process or to a therapeutic agent, the features of the primary disease process may complicate or mask Mg depletion. A high index of suspicion is therefore warranted.

Neuromuscular hyperexcitability may be the presenting complaint. Latent tetany, as elicited by positive Chvostek's and Trousseau's signs, or spontaneous carpal-pedal spasm may be present. Frank generalized seizures may also occur. Although hypocalcemia often contributes to the neurological signs, hypomagnesemia without hypocalcemia has been reported to result in neuromuscular hyperexcitability. Other signs may include vertigo, ataxia, nystagmus, and athetoid and choreiform movements as well as muscular tremor, fasciculation, wasting, and weakness.

Electrocardiographic abnormalities of Mg depletion in humans include prolonged P-R interval and Q-T interval. Mg depletion may also result in cardiac arrhythmias. Supraventricular arrhythmias including premature atrial complexes, atrial tachycardia, atrial fibrillation, and junctional arrhythmias have been described. Ventricular premature complexes, ventricular tachycardia, and ventricular fibrillation are more serious complications. In some studies, but not all, Mg administration to patients with acute myocardial infarction has been shown to decrease the mortality rate.

A common laboratory feature of Mg depletion is hypokalemia. During Mg depletion, there is loss of potassium from the cell with intracellular potassium depletion as well as an inability of the kidney to conserve potassium. Attempts to replete the potassium deficit with potassium therapy alone are not successful without simultaneous Mg therapy. This biochemical feature may be a contributing cause of the electrocardiologic findings and cardiac arrhythmias discussed above.

Hypocalcemia is a common manifestation of moderate to severe Mg depletion. The hypocalcemia may be a major contributing factor to the increased neuromuscular excitability often present in Mg-depleted patients. The pathogenesis of hypocalcemia is multifactorial. In normal subjects, acute changes in the serum Mg concentration will influence parathyroid hormone (PTH) secretion in a manner similar to calcium. That is, an acute fall in serum Mg stimulates PTH secretion while hypermagnesemia inhibits PTH secretion. During chronic and severe Mg depletion, however, PTH secretion is impaired. The majority of patients will have

serum PTH concentrations that are undetectable or inappropriately normal for the degree of hypocalcemia. Some patients, however, may have serum PTH levels above the normal range that may reflect early magnesium depletion. Regardless of the basal circulating PTH concentration, an acute injection of Mg stimulates PTH secretion as illustrated in Fig. 1. Impaired PTH secretion, therefore, seems to be a major factor in hypomagnesemia-induced hypocalcemia. Hypocalcemia in the presence of normal or elevated serum PTH concentrations also suggests end-organ resistance to PTH. Patients with hypocalcemia caused by Mg depletion have both renal and skeletal resistance to exogenously administered PTH as manifested by subnormal urinary cyclic adenosine monophosphate (cAMP) and phosphate excretion and diminished calcemic response. This renal and skeletal resistance to PTH is reversed after several days of Mg therapy. The basis for the defect in PTH secretion and PTH end-organ resistance is unclear but may be because of a defect in the adenylate cyclase and/or phospholipase C second messenger systems, because they are important in PTH secretion and mediating PTH effects in kidney and bone. Magnesium is necessary for the activity of the G-proteins in both enzyme systems. Magnesium is also

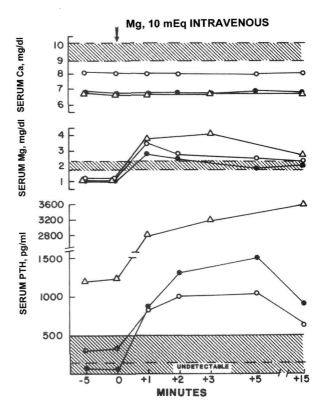

FIG. 1. Effect of an intravenous injection of 10 mEq magnesium on the serum concentration of calcium, magnesium, and iPTH in hypocalcemic magnesium-deficient patients with undetectable (●), normal (○), or elevated (△) levels of iPTH. Shaded area represents the range of normal for assay. Broken line for the iPTH assay represents the level of detectability. The magnesium injection resulted in a marked rise in PTH secretion within 1 minute in all three patients. (Reproduced with permission from Rude RK 1989 Parathyroid function in magnesium deficiency. In: Itokawa V, Durlach J, eds., Magnesium in Health and Disease. John Libby and Co., London, UK, pp. 317–321).

TABLE 2. SUGGESTED PROTOCOL FOR USE OF MAGNESIUM TOLERANCE TEST

I. Collect baseline 24-h urine for magnesium/creatinine ratio.*

II. Infuse 0.2 mEq (2.4 mg) elemental magnesium per kilogram lean body weight in 50 ml 5% dextrose over 4 h.

III. Collect urine (starting with infusion) for magnesium and creatinine for 24 h.

IV. Percentage magnesium retained is calculated by the following formula:

$$\%Mg\ retained = \left[1 - \frac{\text{Postinfusion 24-h urine Mg} - \frac{\text{Preinfusion urine Mg/creatinine} \times \text{Postinfusion urine creatinine}}{\text{Total elemental Mg infused}}}{}\right] \times 100$$

V. Criteria for Mg deficiency:
>50% retention at 24 h = definite deficiency
>25% retention at 24 h = probable deficiency

* A fasting shorter timed-urine (2-h spot) may be used.

necessary for substrate formation (MgATP) as well as being an allosteric activator of adenylate cyclase.

Clinically, patients with hypocalcemia caused by Mg depletion are resistant not only to PTH, but also to calcium and vitamin D therapy. The vitamin D resistance may be caused by impaired metabolism of vitamin D because serum concentrations of 1,25-dihydroxyvitamin D are low.

Diagnosis of Magnesium Depletion

Measurement of the serum Mg concentration is the most commonly used test to assess Mg status. The normal serum Mg concentration ranges from 1.5 to 1.9 mEq/liter (1.8–2.2 mg/dl), and a value less than 1.5 mEq/liter usually indicates Mg depletion. Mg is principally an intracellular cation, and only approximately 1% of the body Mg content is in the extracellular fluid compartments. The serum Mg concentration therefore may not reflect the intracellular Mg content. Because vitamin D and calcium therapy are relatively ineffective in correcting the hypocalcemia, there must be a high index of suspicion for the presence of Mg depletion. Patients with Mg depletion severe enough to result in hypocalcemia are usually significantly hypomagnesemic. However, occasionally, patients may have normal serum Mg concentrations. Magnesium deficiency in the presence of a normal serum Mg concentration has been demonstrated by measuring intracellular Mg (in lymphocytes or muscle biopsy), or by whole body retention of infused Mg. Therefore, hypocalcemic patients who are at risk for Mg depletion, but who have normal serum Mg levels, should receive a trial of Mg therapy. The Mg tolerance test (or retention test) seems to be an accurate means of assessing Mg status. Correlations with skeletal muscle Mg content and Mg balance studies have been shown. This test seems to be discriminatory in patients with normal renal function; however, its usefulness may be limited if the patient has a renal Mg wasting disorder or is on a medication that induces renal Mg wasting. A suggested protocol for the Mg tolerance test is shown in Table 2.

Therapy

Patients who present with signs and symptoms of Mg depletion should be treated with Mg. These patients will usually be hypomagnesemic and/or have an abnormal Mg tolerance test. The extent of the total body Mg deficit is impossible to predict, but it may be as high as 200–400 mEq. Under these circumstances, parenteral Mg administration is usually indicated. An effective treatment regimen is the administration of 2 g MgSO$_4 \cdot$ 7H$_2$O (16.2 mEq Mg) as a 50% solution every 8 h intramuscularly. Because these injections can be painful, a continuous intravenous infusion of 48 mEq over 24 h may therefore be preferred and is better tolerated. Either regimen will usually result in a normal to slightly elevated serum Mg concentration. Despite the fact that PTH secretion increases within minutes after beginning Mg administration, the serum calcium concentration may not return to normal for 3–7 days. This probably reflects slow restoration of intracellular Mg. During this period of therapy, serum Mg concentration may be normal, but the total body deficit may not yet be corrected. Magnesium should be continued until the clinical and biochemical manifestations (hypocalcemia and hypokalemia) of Mg depletion are resolved.

Patients who are hypomagnesemic and have seizures or an acute arrhythmia may be given 8–16 mEq of Mg as an intravenous injection over 5–10 minutes followed by 48 mEq iv per day. Ongoing Mg losses should be monitored during therapy. If the patient continues to lose Mg from the intestine or kidney, therapy may have to be continued for a longer duration. Once repletion has been accomplished, patients usually can maintain a normal Mg status on a regular diet. If repletion is accomplished and the patient cannot eat, a maintenance dose of 8 mEq should be given daily. Patients who have chronic Mg loss from the intestine or kidney may require continued oral Mg supplementation. A daily dose of 300–600 mg of elemental Mg may be given; however, they should be given in divided doses to avoid the cathartic effect of Mg.

Caution should be taken during Mg therapy in patients with any degree of renal failure. If a decrease in glomerular filtration rate exists, the dose of Mg should be halved, and the serum Mg concentration must be monitored daily. If hypermagnesemia ensues, therapy must be stopped.

HYPERMAGNESEMIA

Magnesium intoxication is not a frequently encountered clinical problem, although mild to moderate elevations in the serum Mg concentration may be seen in as many as 12% of hospitalized patients.

Symptomatic hypermagnesemia is virtually always caused by excessive intake or administration of Mg salts. The majority of patients with hypermagnesemia have concomitant renal failure. Hypermagnesemia is usually seen in patients with renal failure who are receiving Mg as an antacid, enema, or infusion. Hypermagnesemia is also sometimes seen in acute renal failure in the setting of rhabdomyolysis.

Large amounts of oral Mg have rarely been reported to cause symptomatic hypermagnesemia in patients with normal renal function. The rectal administration of Mg for purgation may result in hypermagnesemia. Mg is a standard form of therapy for pregnancy-induced hypertension (pre-eclampsia and eclampsia) and may cause Mg intoxication in the mother as well as in the neonate. Ureteral irrigation with hemiacidrin (Renacidin; Guardian Laboratories, Hauppauge, NY, USA) has been reported to cause symptomatic hypermagnesemia in patients with and without renal failure. Modest elevations in the serum Mg concentration may be seen in familial hypocalcemic hypercalcemia, lithium ingestion, and during volume depletion.

Signs and Symptoms

Neuromuscular symptoms are the most common presenting problem of Mg intoxication. One of the earliest demonstrable effects of hypermagnesemia is the disappearance of the deep tendon reflexes. This is reached at serum Mg concentrations of 4–7 mEq/liter. Depressed respiration and apnea caused by paralysis of the voluntary musculature may be seen at serum Mg concentrations in excess of 8–10 mEq/liter. Somnolence may be observed at levels as low as 3 mEq/liter and above.

Moderate elevations in the serum Mg concentration of 3–5 mEq/liter result in a mild reduction in blood pressure. High concentrations may result in severe symptomatic hypotension. Mg can also be cardiotoxic. At serum Mg concentrations greater than 5 mEq/liter, electrocardiographic findings of prolonged P-R intervals as well as increased QRS duration and QT interval are seen. Complete heart block, as well as cardiac arrest, may occur at concentrations greater than 15 mEq/liter.

Hypermagnesemia causes a fall in the serum calcium concentration. The hypocalcemia may be related to the suppressive effect of hypermagnesemia on PTH secretion or to hypermagnesemia-induced parathyroid hormone end-organ resistance. A direct effect of Mg on decreasing the serum calcium is suggested by the observation that hypermagnesemia causes hypocalcemia in hypoparathyroid subjects as well.

Other nonspecific manifestations of Mg intoxication include nausea, vomiting, and cutaneous flushing at serum levels of 3–9 mEq/liter.

Therapy

The possibility of Mg intoxication should be anticipated in any patient receiving Mg, especially if the patient has a reduction in renal function. Mg therapy should merely be discontinued in patients with mild to moderate elevations in the serum Mg level. Excess Mg will be excreted by the kidney, and any symptoms or signs of Mg intoxication will resolve. Patients with severe Mg intoxication may be treated with intravenous calcium. Calcium will antagonize the toxic effects of Mg. This antagonism is immediate, but transient. The usual dose is an infusion of 100–200 mg of elemental calcium over 5–10 minutes. If the patient is in renal failure, peritoneal dialysis or hemodialysis against a low dialysis Mg bath will rapidly and effectively lower the serum Mg concentration.

SUGGESTED READINGS

1. Rude RK 2001 Magnesium metabolism. In: Becker KL (ed.) Principles & Practice of Endocrinology & Metabolism. J. B. Lippincott Co, Philadelphia, PA, USA, pp. 350–354.
2. Rude RK 2001 Magnesium homeostasis. In: Bilezikian JB, Raisz L, Rodan G (eds.) Principles of Bone Biology, 2nd ed. Academic Press, San Diego, CA, USA, pp. 339–358.
3. Rude RK 2001 Magnesium deficiency in parathyroid function. In: Bilezikian JP (ed.) The Parathyroids. Raven Press, New York, NY, USA, pp. 763–777.
4. Vetter T, Lohse MJ 2002 Magnesium and the parathyroid. Curr Opin Nephrol Hypertens 11:403–410.
5. Quamme GA 1997 Renal magnesium handling: New insights in understanding old problems. Kidney Int 52:1180–1195.
6. Simon DB, Lu Y, Choate KA, Velazquez H, Al-Sabban E, Praga M, Casari G, Bettinelli A, Colussi G, Rodriquez-Soriano J, McCredle D, Milford D, Sanjad S, Lifton RP 1999 Paracellin-1, a renal tight junction protein required for paracellular Mg(2+) resorption. Science 285:103–106.
7. Praga M, Vara J, Gonzalez-Parra E, Andres A, Alamo C, Araque A, Ortiz A, Rodicio JL 1995 Familial hypomagnesemia with hypercalciuria and nephrocalcinosis. Kidney Int 47:1419–1425.
8. Meij IC, Saar K, van den Heuvel LPWJ, Nuernberg G, Vollmer M, Hjildebrant F, Reis A, Monnens LAH, Knoers NVAM 1999 Hereditary isolated renal magnesium loss maps to chromosome 11q23. Am J Hum Genet 64:180–188.
9. Simon DB, Nelson-Williams C, Bia MJ, Ellison D, Karet FE, Molina AM, Vaara I, Iwata F, Cushner HM, Koolen M, Gainza FJ, Gitleman HJ, Liofton RP 1996 Gitelman's variant of Bartter's syndropme, inherited hypokalaemic alkalosis, is caused by mutations in the thiazide-sensitive Na-Cl cotransporter. Nat Genet 12:24–30.
10. Kantorovich V, Adams JS, Gaines JE, Guo X, Pandian MR, Cohn DH, Rude RK 2002 Genetic heterogeneity in familial renal magnesium wasting. J Clin Endocrinol Metab 87:612–617.
11. Schlingmann KP, Weber S, Peters M, Nejsum LN, Vitzthum H, Klingel K, Kratz M, Haddad E, Ristoff E, Dinour D, Surrou M, Nielsen S, Sassen M, Waldegger S, Seyberth HW, Konrad M 2002 Hypomagnesemia with secondary hypocalcemia is caused by mutations in TRPM6, a new member of the TRPM gene family. Nat Genet 31:166–170.
12. Kondrad M, Weber S 2003 Recent advances in molecular genetics of hereditary magnesium-losing disorders. J Am Soc Nephrol 14:249–260.
13. Woods KL, Fletcher S 1994 Long-term outcome after intravenous magnesium sulphate in suspected acute myocardial infarction: The second Leicester intravenous magnesium intervention trial (Limit-2). Lancet 343:816–819.
14. ISIS-4 1995 A randomized factorial trial assessing early oral captopril, oral mononitratre, and intravenous magnesium sulphate in 58, 050 patients with suspected acute myocardial infarction. Lancet 245:669–682.
15. Fassler CA, Rodriguez RM, Badesch DB, Stone WJ, Marini JJ 1985 Magnesium toxicity as a cause of hypotension and hypoventilation: Occurrence in patients with normal renal function. Arch Intern Med 145:1604–1606.
16. Cholst IN, Steinberg SF, Trooper PJ, Fox HE, Segre GV, Bilezikian JP 1984 The influence of hypermagnesemia on serum calcium and parathyroid hormone levels in human subjects. N Engl J Med 310:1221–1225.

Chapter 48. Hyperphosphatemia and Hypophosphatemia

Keith A. Hruska[1] and Eleanor D. Lederer[2]

[1]Departments of Pediatrics, Medicine, and Cell Biology, Washington University School of Medicine, St. Louis, Missouri; and [2]Department of Medicine/Nephrology, University of Louisville, and Renal Department, University of Louisville Affiliated Hospitals, Louisville, Kentucky

INTRODUCTION

The mechanisms for sensing and regulating serum phosphate concentration are not understood. The bulk of total body phosphate (85%) is in the bone as part of the mineralized extracellular matrix. This phosphate pool is accessible, albeit in a somewhat limited fashion. Phosphate is a predominantly intracellular anion with an estimated concentration of approximately 100 mM, most of which is either complexed or bound to proteins or lipids. Serum phosphate concentration varies with age, time of day, fasting state, and season. It is higher in children than adults. Phosphate levels exhibit a diurnal variation, with the highest phosphate level occurring near noon. Serum phosphate concentration is regulated by diet, hormones, and physical factors such as pH. Importantly, because phosphate moves in and out of cells under several influences, the serum concentration of phosphate may not reflect true phosphate stores.

HYPERPHOSPHATEMIA

Serum inorganic phosphorus (Pi) concentrations are generally maintained at 2.5–4.5 mg/dl or 0.75–1.45 mM in adults, whereas hyperphosphatemia is not present in children unless serum Pi levels are greater than 6 or 7 mg/dl. Hyperphosphatemia may be the consequence of an increased intake of Pi, a decreased excretion of Pi, or translocation of Pi from tissue breakdown into the extracellular fluid[1] (Table 1). Because the kidneys are able to excrete phosphate very efficiently over a wide range of dietary intakes, hyperphosphatemia most frequently results from renal insufficiency and the attendant inability to excrete Pi.

Etiology and Pathogenesis

Increased Intake. Hyperphosphatemia can be the consequence of an *increased intake* or administration of Pi. Intravenous administration of 1–2 g of Pi during the treatment of Pi depletion or hypercalcemia can cause hyperphosphatemia, especially in patients with underlying renal insufficiency. Hyperphosphatemia may also result from overzealous use of oral phosphates or of phosphate-containing enemas because phosphate can be absorbed passively from the colon through paracellular pathways. Administration of vitamin D and its metabolites in pharmacologic doses may be responsible for the development of hyperphosphatemia, although suppression of PTH and hypercalcemia-induced renal failure are important pathogenetic factors in this setting.

Impaired Excretion. Clinically, hyperphosphatemia occurs most commonly as a result of impaired excretion caused by renal failure. During the early and middle stages of *chronic renal insufficiency*, phosphate balance is maintained by a progressive reduction in tubular Pi transport leading to increased Pi excretion by the remaining nephrons and a maintenance of normal renal Pi clearance.[2] In advanced renal insufficiency, the fractional excretion of Pi may be as high as 60–90% of the filtered load of phosphate. However, when the number of functional nephrons becomes too diminished (glomerular filtration rate usually <20 ml/min) and dietary intake is constant, Pi balance can no longer be maintained by reductions of tubular reabsorption, and hyperphosphatemia develops.[2] When hyperphosphatemia develops, the filtered load of Pi per nephron increases and Pi excretion rises. As a result, Pi balance and renal excretory rate is reestablished, but at a higher serum Pi level.

Defects in renal excretion of Pi in the absence of renal failure may be primary, as in *pseudohypoparathyroidism* or *tumoral calcinosis*.[3,4] The latter is usually seen in young black males with ectopic calcification around large joints and is characterized by increased tubular reabsorption of calcium, Pi, and normal responses to parathyroid hormone (PTH).[5] Secondary tubular defects include *hypoparathyroidism*[6] and high blood levels of growth hormone.[7] Serum phosphorus values are normally elevated in children compared with adults. Finally, bisphosphonates such as Didronel (disodium etidronate), pamidronate, or alendronate may cause hyperphosphatemia. The mechanisms of action are unclear, but they may involve cellular phosphate redistribution and decreased renal excretion.[8]

TABLE 1. CAUSES OF HYPERPHOSPHATEMIA

Increased intake
  Oral administration—NeutraPhos
  Rectal—Fleets phosphosoda enemas
  Intravenous—sodium or potassium phosphate
Decreased renal excretion
  Childhood
  Renal insufficiency/failure—acute or chronic
  Hypoparathyroidism
  Pseudohypoparathyroidism
  Acromegaly
  Bisphosphonates
  Tumoral calcinosis
Transcellular shift from intracellular to extracellular spaces
  Catabolic states
  Fulminant hepatitis
  Hyperthermia
  Rhabdomyolysis—crush injuries or nontraumatic
  Cytotoxic therapy—tumor lysis
  Hemolytic anemia
  Acute leukemia
  Acidosis—metabolic or respiratory
Artifactual

The authors have no conflict of interest.

Transcellular Shift. Transcellular shift of Pi from cells into the extracellular fluid compartment may lead to hyperphosphatemia, as seen in conditions associated with increased catabolism or tissue destruction (e.g., systemic infections, fulminant hepatitis, severe hyperthermia, crush injuries, nontraumatic rhabdomyolysis, and cytotoxic therapy for hematologic malignancies such as acute lymphoblastic leukemia and Burkitts lymphoma[1]. In the *"tumor lysis syndrome,"* serum Pi levels typically rise within 12 days after initiation of treatment. The rising serum Pi concentration often is accompanied by hypocalcemia, hyperuricemia, hyperkalemia, and renal failure. Patients with *diabetic ketoacidosis* commonly have hyperphosphatemia at the time of presentation despite total body Pi depletion. Insulin, fluid, and bicarbonate therapy is accompanied by a shift of Pi back into cells and the development of hypophosphatemia. In lactic acidosis, hyperphosphatemia likely results from tissue hypoxia with a breakdown of ATP to AMP and Pi.

Hyperphosphatemia may be artifactual when hemolysis occurs during the collection, storage, or processing of blood samples.

Clinical Consequences of Hyperphosphatemia

The most important short-term consequences of hyperphosphatemia are hypocalcemia and tetany, which occur most commonly in patients with an increased Pi load from any source, exogenous or endogenous. By contrast, soft tissue calcification and secondary hyperparathyroidism are long-term consequences of hyperphosphatemia that occur mainly in patients with renal insufficiency and decreased renal Pi excretion.

Hypocalcemia and Tetany. With rapid elevations of serum Pi, hypocalcemia and tetany may occur with serum Pi concentrations as low as 6 mg/dl, a level that, if reached more slowly, has no detectable effect on serum calcium. Hyperphosphatemia, in addition to its effect on the calcium × phosphate ion product with resultant calcium deposition in soft tissues, also inhibits the activity of 1α-hydroxylase in the kidney, resulting in a lower circulating level of 1,25-dihydroxyvitamin D_3. This further aggravates hypocalcemia by impairing intestinal absorption of calcium and inducing a state of skeletal resistance to the action of PTH.

Phosphate-induced hypocalcemia is common in patients with acute or chronic renal failure and usually develops slowly. Tetany is uncommon unless a superimposed acid-base disorder produces an abrupt rise in plasma pH that acutely lowers the serum ionized calcium concentration. Profound hypocalcemia and tetany are occasionally observed during the early phase of the "tumor lysis" syndrome and rhabdomyolysis.

Soft Tissue Calcification. Extraskeletal calcification associated with hyperphosphatemia is usually seen in patients with chronic kidney failure (CKD), diabetes, and severe atherosclerosis. Recent basic and clinical research studies have led to new theories concerning the pathogenesis and the consequences of this phenomenon. Several inhibitors of calcification have been discovered, including osteoprotegerin,[9] osteopontin,[10,11] matrix Gla protein,[12] and the klotho gene product.[13] These substances constitute an inherent defense against heterotopic mineralization that is breached in the disease environment. In the setting of CKD, hyperphosphatemia has been identified as a major factor contributing to the forces favoring mineralization.[14] In contrast to the breach of defense theory of vascular calcification, there is significant evidence that the vascular smooth muscle cells undergo a transformation from a smooth muscle to an osteoblast phenotype, manifested by the expression of osteoblast-specific gene products such as osteocalcin cbfal and osterix[15–18] and by the deposition of calcium. Experimental models have suggested that elevated phosphate alone may trigger this transformation.[19–22] The finding of vascular calcification and the role of hyperphosphatemia has more than academic significance. Calcification of the endothelium including the large blood vessels, coronary arteries, and heart valves in renal failure patients is associated with a high morbidity and mortality from systolic hypertension, congestive heart failure, coronary artery disease, and myocardial infarction.[23–30] Another manifestation of vascular calcification, calciphylaxis, is also associated with hyperphosphatemia and carries a poor prognosis.[31–33]

Occasionally, an acute rise in serum Pi (e.g., during Pi treatment for hypercalcemia) may lead to soft tissue calcification in clinical settings besides those mentioned in the preceding paragraph. The blood vessels, skin, cornea (band keratopathy), and periarticular tissues are common sites of calcium precipitation.

Secondary Hyperparathyroidism and Renal Osteodystrophy. Hyperphosphatemia caused by renal failure also plays a critical role in development of secondary hyperparathyroidism and renal osteodystrophy. Several mechanisms contribute to these complications, including hyperphosphatemia-induced hypocalcemia through physical-chemical interactions, hyperphosphatemia-induced hypocalcemia through inhibition of vitamin D synthesis, and hyperphosphatemia-stimulated PTH secretion. In patients with advanced renal failure, the enhanced phosphate load from PTH-mediated osteolysis may ultimately become the dominant influence on serum phosphorus levels. This phenomenon may account for the correlation between serum phosphorus levels and the severity of osteitis fibrosa cystica in patients maintained on chronic hemodialysis. Hyperphosphatemia also plays a critical role in the development of vascular calcification as discussed above.[21] There may be a direct relationship between defective orthotopic mineralization (bone formation) in CKD and increased heterotopic mineralization.[19,34–36] Our data[34,37] and that of Price et al.[38] and Morishita et al.[19] suggest that increasing bone formation will lower phosphate levels and diminish vascular calcification in CKD.

Treatment

Correction of the pathogenetic defect should be the primary aim in the treatment of hyperphosphatemia. When hyperphosphatemia is due solely to increased intake, discontinuation of supplemental phosphate and maintenance of adequate volume for diuresis is generally sufficient because the kidneys will promptly excrete the excess. In the uncommon circumstance of significant hyperphosphatemia caused by transcellular shift, treatment should be dictated by the underlying cause. For example, hyperphosphatemia that accompanies diabetic ketoacidosis will resolve with insulin therapy, as insulin stimulates cellular uptake of phosphate. On the other hand, hyperphosphatemia seen with tumor lysis, rhabdomyolysis, or other conditions characterized by massive cell death or injury should be treated as an excess phosphate load, albeit endogenous instead of exogenous. Limitation of phosphate intake and enhanced diuresis will generally resolve this cause of hyperphosphatemia, provided renal function is adequate.

When renal insufficiency is present, however, the most effective way to treat hyperphosphatemia is to reduce dietary Pi intake and to add phosphate-binding agents. Because Pi is present in almost all foodstuffs, rigid dietary phosphate restriction requires a barely palatable diet that few patients can accept. However, dietary Pi can be reduced to 800-1000 mg/day with modest protein restriction. A predialysis level of 4.5–5.0 mg/dl is reasonable and allows some room for removal of phosphorus with dialysis while avoiding severe postdialysis hypophosphatemia. To achieve this, the addition of phosphate binders to reduce intestinal absorption of dietary Pi is required. Aluminum hydroxide or aluminum carbonate, when administered to patients with renal failure over the long-term, has been shown to result in aluminum toxicity with encephalopathy, osteomalacia, proximal myopathy, and anemia. Therefore, calcium salts replaced aluminum salts as first-line Pi binders.[39–41] However, calcium salts contribute to the calcium phosphate ion product, and massive calcium intake is often required to maintain serum phosphorus in the target range. Elevated calcium phosphorus products and the calcium load induced increase in the serum calcium contribute to the development of vascular calcification.[42] Therefore, newer Pi binders have been introduced such as sevelamer hydrochloride.[43] This resin has an improved safety profile over calcium salts, and as a binding resin, it also binds cholesterol and low-density lipoproteins (LDLs), leading to improved lipid profiles in patients with end-stage kidney disease (ESKD).[44] Calcium acetate and aluminum carbonate are equally potent and bind more Pi than equivalent amounts of calcium carbonate or citrate. sevelamer binds calcium equally to calcium carbonate, but the large doses required to maintain serum phosphorus, the pill sizes, and gastrointestinal side effects make compliance a difficult issue with the sole use of sevelamer. In addition, cost of the agent has limited coverage in some instances. Therefore, the prescription of an effective Pi-binding regimen is a complex issue for ESKD patients at the present time. In general, treatment is started with 1 g of calcium carbonate with each meal to treat any tendency to hypocalcemia, and sevelamer is added in increasing doses until the target serum phosphorus is achieved. This regimen is as effective as increasing Ca salts which are gradually increased up to 8–12 g daily. Calcium acetate may be preferred over calcium carbonate to limit Ca intake as increased dose of phosphate binding is required.

Either of these regimens effectively controls serum Pi in about two-thirds of patients on chronic dialysis.[40] Calcium salts tend to increase serum calcium levels, and if hypercalcemia (>11 mg/dl) develops, calcium carbonate should not be increased further and a switch to sevelamer or reduction in dialysate calcium should be considered. If aluminum gels are used, calcium citrate must not be taken concomitantly, because citrate markedly increases the absorption of aluminum. Maximal Pi binding occurs when phosphate binder is taken with a meal rather than 2 h afterward. Magnesium-containing antacids are also effective phosphate binders; however, their use in renal failure is limited because intestinal absorption of magnesium can lead to magnesium toxicity. Newer lanthanide- and iron-based phosphorus binders are in the mid- to late stages of clinical trials.

The treatment of chronic hyperphosphatemia secondary to hypoparathyroidism occasionally requires that phosphate binders be added to the other therapeutic agents.

HYPOPHOSPHATEMIA

Hypophosphatemia is defined as an abnormally low concentration of inorganic phosphate in serum or plasma. Hypophosphatemia does not necessarily indicate total body Pi depletion because only 1% of the total body Pi is found in extracellular fluids. Conversely, serious Pi depletion may exist in the presence of a normal or even elevated serum Pi concentration. Moderate hypophosphatemia, defined as a serum Pi concentration between 2.5 and 1 mg/dl, is not uncommon, and is usually not associated with signs or symptoms. Severe hypophosphatemia, defined as serum phosphorus levels below 1.0 mg/dl, is often associated with clinical signs and symptoms that require therapy. Approximately 2% of hospital patients have levels of serum Pi below 2 mg/dl according to some estimates. Hypophosphatemia is encountered more frequently among alcoholic patients, and up to 10% of patients admitted to hospitals because of chronic alcoholism are hypophosphatemic.

Pathogenesis of Hypophosphatemia

Three types of pathophysiologic abnormalities can cause hypophosphatemia and total body Pi depletion: decreased intestinal absorption of Pi, increased urinary losses of this ion, and a shift of Pi from extracellular to intracellular compartments. Combinations of these disturbances are common.[45,46] The causes and mechanisms of moderate hypophosphatemia are shown in Table 2; the clinical conditions associated with severe hypophosphatemia are shown in Table 3.

Decreased Intake

Impaired Gastrointestinal Absorption. Severe hypophosphatemia and phosphate depletion may result from vigorous use of oral antacids, which bind phosphate, usually for peptic ulcer disease.[47] Patients so treated may develop osteomalacia and severe skeletal symptoms caused by phosphorus deficiency. Intestinal malabsorption can cause hypophosphatemia and phosphate depletion through malabsorption of Pi and vitamin D and through increased urinary

TABLE 2. CAUSES OF MODERATE HYPOPHOSPHATEMIA
AND/OR PHOSPHATE DEPLETION

Decreased intestinal absorption
  Antacid abuse
  Vitamin D deficiency
  Malabsorption
  Starvation—famine, anorexia nervosa, alcoholism
Increased urinary losses
  Hyperparathyroidism
  Renal tubular defects—Fanconi, post-transplant, hypomagnesemia,
    fructose intolerance
  Abnormalities of Vitamin D metabolism
    X-linked hypophosphatemic rickets
    Vitamin D–dependent rickets
    Vitamine D deficiency
  Oncogenic osteomalacia
  Alcoholism
  Diabetic ketoacidosis
  Metabolic or respiratory acidosis
  Respiratory alkalosis
  Drugs: calcitonin, diuretics, glucocorticoids, bicarbonate, β agonists
  Extracellular fluid volume expansion
Transcellular shift from the extracellular to the intracellular space
  Nutritional repletion—refeeding syndrome
  Respiratory alkalosis
  Recovery from metabolic acidosis, commonly diabetic ketoacidosis
  Recovery from hypothermia
  Sepsis, especially gram negative bacteremia
  Salicylate intoxication
  Sugars—glucose, fructose, glycerol
  Insulin therapy
  Blast crisis in leukemia
  "Hungry-bone" syndrome after parathyroidectomy

Pi losses resulting from secondary hyperparathyroidism induced by calcium malabsorption.

Alcohol and Alcohol Withdrawal. Alcohol abuse is a common cause of severe hypophosphatemia (Table 3)[48,49] because of both poor intake and excessive losses. Poor intake results from dietary deficiencies, the use of antacids, and vomiting. Patients with alcoholism have also been shown to have a variety of defects in renal tubular function, including a decrease in threshold for phosphate excretion, which are reversible with abstinence. Ethanol enhances urinary Pi excretion, and marked phosphaturia tends to occur during episodes of alcoholic ketoacidosis. Because such patients often eat poorly, ketonuria is common. Repeated episodes of ketoacidosis catabolize organic phosphates within cells and cause phosphaturia by mechanisms analogous to those seen in diabetic ketoacidosis. Chronic alcoholism may also cause magnesium deficiency and hypomagnesemia, which may in turn, cause phosphaturia and Pi depletion, especially in skeletal muscle.

Nutritional Repletion: Oral, Enteral, and Parenteral Nutrition. Nutritional repletion of the malnourished patient implies the provision of sufficient calories, protein, and other nutrients to allow accelerated tissue accretion. In the course of this process, cellular uptake and use of Pi increase. When insufficient amounts of Pi are provided, an acute state of severe hypophosphatemia and intracellular Pi depletion with serious clinical and metabolic consequences can occur.[50,51] This type of hypophosphatemia has been observed in malnourished patients receiving parenteral nutrition and after refeeding of prisoners of war.

Increased Losses

Primary Hyperparathyroidism. This is a common entity in clinical medicine.[52] PTH is secreted in excess of the physiologic needs for mineral homeostasis owing either to adenoma or hyperplasia of the parathyroid glands. This results in decreased phosphorus reabsorption by the kidney, and the urinary losses of phosphorus result in hypophosphatemia. The degree of hypophosphatemia varies considerably because mobilization of phosphorus from stimulation of skeletal remodeling in part mitigates the hypophosphatemia. Secondary hyperparathyroidism associated with normal renal function has been observed in patients with gastrointestinal abnormalities resulting in calcium malabsorption. Such patients may have low levels of serum calcium and phosphorus.[53] In these patients, the hypocalcemia is responsible for increased release of PTH. Decreased intestinal absorption of phosphorus as a result of the primary gastrointestinal disease may contribute to the decrement in the levels of the serum phosphorus. In general, these patients have urinary losses of phosphorus that are out of proportion to the hypophosphatemia in contrast to patients with predominant phosphorus malabsorption and no secondary hyperparathyroidism in whom urinary excretion of phosphorus is low.

Renal Tubular Defects. Several conditions characterized by either single or multiple tubular ion transport defects have been characterized in which phosphorus reabsorption is decreased. In Fanconi syndrome, patients excrete not only an increased amount of phosphorus in the urine but also increased quantities of amino acids, uric acid, and glucose, resulting in hypouricemia and hypophosphatemia.[54] There are other conditions in which an isolated defect in the renal tubular transport of phosphorus has been found (e.g., in fructose intolerance, an autosomal recessive disorder). After renal transplantation, an acquired renal tubular defect may be responsible for the persistence of hypophosphatemia in

TABLE 3. RISK FACTORS FOR SEVERE HYPOPHOSPHATEMIA
AND/OR PHOSPHATE DEPLETION

Alcohol withdrawal
Nutritional repletion in at risk patients
  Anorexia nervosa and other eating disorders
  Starvation due to famine, neglect, alcoholism, malabsorption,
    prisoners of war
  AIDS and other chronic infections
  Massive weight loss for morbid obesity
Treatment of diabetic ketoacidosis
Critical illness
  Sepsis
  Post-trauma
  Extensive burns

some patients. Studies in patients after transplantation[55,56] suggest that a phosphatonin may be responsible for post-transplant hypophosphatemia. The hypophosphatemia is important because recent studies implicate it in the osteoblast failure contributing to the development of osteoporosis.[57]

Vitamin D and its metabolites play an important role in phosphorus homeostasis.[58,59] Vitamin D promotes intestinal absorption of calcium and phosphorus, and it is necessary to maintain the normal mineralization and remodeling processes of bone. In addition, vitamin D metabolites have important actions in the control of renal tubular ion transport. Vitamin D–deficient rickets (when the deficiency occurs in children) or osteomalacia (when the deficiency occurs in adults) may result in severe deformities of the skeleton. Hypophosphatemia is the most frequent biochemical alteration associated with this metabolic abnormality.

X-Linked Hypophosphatemic Rickets and Autosomal Dominant Hypophosphatemic Rickets. These disorders are characterized by hypophosphatemia, decreased reabsorption of phosphorus by the renal tubule, decreased absorption of calcium and phosphorus from the gastrointestinal tract, and varying degrees of rickets or osteomalacia.[60] Patients with the disorders exhibit normal or reduced levels of 1,25-dihydroxycholecalciferol (should be elevated because of the hypophosphatemia) and reduced Na-phosphate transport in the proximal tubule in the face of severe hypophosphatemia. The gene for X-linked hypophosphatemia (XLH) is not the Pi transport protein itself, which maps to chromosome 5[61] in humans and which exhibits a normal function in isolated brush border membrane preparations from animal models of XLH rickets.[62] The genetic defect for this disorder is in a gene termed *PHEX*,[63] which encodes for a neutral endopeptidase presumed to be responsible for degradation of a group of new hormones identified as systemic phosphaturic factors, "phosphatonins."[64] The defective PHEX gene product in XLH rickets permits "phosphatonin" to inhibit renal phosphate absorption, despite persistent hypophosphatemia. Several phosphatonins have been identified in oncogenic osteomalacia by genetic screening techniques.[65–68] One of them, fibroblast growth factor (FGF)23,[65] is a PHEX substrate[69] and has recently been identified as the causal substance in autosomal dominant hypophosphatemic rickets (ADHR).[70] A mutation in FGF23 that blocks its proteolytic processing from the proform of the hormone to the mature protein prevents its processing by PHEX and leads to increased circulating proFGF23 levels that lead to the ADHR syndrome.[65] Recent studies have demonstrated that FGF23 levels are elevated in patients with XLH.[71] Thus, defective proteolytic cleavage of FGF23 by PHEX is the pathogenesis of XLH.

Vitamin D–Dependent Rickets. This is a recessively inherited form of vitamin D–refractory rickets associated with hypophosphatemia, hypocalcemia, elevated levels of serum alkaline phosphatase, and sometimes, generalized amino aciduria and severe bone lesions. There are two main forms of the syndrome. Type I is an inborn error in conversion of 25-hydroxyvitamin D to 1,25-dihydroxyvitamin D caused by deficiency of the renal 1-hydroxylase enzyme.[72] This condition responds to very large doses of vitamin D_2 and D_3 but to normal doses of 1,25-dihydroxyvitamin D_3. Type II is characterized by an end-organ resistance to 1,25-dihydroxyvitamin D_3 caused by an abnormal vitamin D receptor.[73,74] Plasma levels of 1,25-dihydroxyvitamin D_3 are elevated. Large pharmacologic doses of 1,25-dihydroxyvitamin D_3 are required for treatment of this syndrome.

Oncogenic Osteomalacia. This entity is characterized by hypophosphatemia in association with mesenchymal tumors.[75,76] The patients exhibit osteomalacia on histomorphologic examination of bone biopsy specimens, renal wasting of phosphorus, and markedly reduced levels of 1,25-dihydroxyvitamin D_3. The existence of a possible circulating humoral factor has long been suspected and is supported by the identification of tumor products from patients with hemangiopericytoma that inhibit renal phosphate transport[77] and recent genetic screens of tumors associated with hypophosphatemia compared with those without.[65–68] Two novel new hormones have been discovered by these studies. The first, FGF23, is the etiologic agent in XLH and ADHR discussed above. Physiologic secretion of FGF23 is unknown, but its circulating levels are maintained low by the function in PHEX. Production of FGF23 by the oncogenic osteomalacic tumors overwhelms PHEX activity leading to the syndrome. Thus, FGF23 is the first hormone discovered that is produced in the bone and functions to regulate renal and intestinal phosphate transport.

The second new hormone regulating phosphate transport in the kidney is a member of the secreted frizzled related protein family (sFrp). Recent studies have shown that sFrp4 is a phosphatonin in some cases of oncogenic osteomalacia.[67,68,78] The secreted frizzled related proteins are decoy receptors and inhibitors of Wnt signaling. The frizzled proteins are the receptors for the Wnt family of developmental morphogens along with the co-receptor, LDL receptor related protein 5 (Lrp5).[79] Lrp5 is a member of the Lrp family, which are promiscuous endocytic receptors.[80] Lrp2 is megalin, which is involved in endocytosis of the vitamin D–binding protein in the proximal tubule and delivery of 25OHD$_3$ for production of calcitriol.[81] Lrp5 is a divergent family member, and its main function seems to be as the co-receptor with the frizzled family for the Wnts.[79] Lrp5 has been identified as the nonsyndromic high bone mass gene,[82] showing the critical nature of Wnt signaling in bone anabolism, and setting the pathophysiologic stage for interference with Wnt signaling by sFrp4, to decrease bone formation, and as a phosphatonin, to increase Pi excretion. SFrp4 is widely expressed, including in the kidney, and disease states increase its production (Surendran and Hruska, unpublished data), potentially leading to a mechanism whereby CKD inhibits bone formation and contributes to renal osteodystrophy.

Miscellaneous Urinary Losses. Abnormalities in tubular handling of phosphate have also been implicated in the genesis of severe hypophosphatemia induced by hypokalemia, hypomagnesemia, systemic acidosis, hypothyroidism, and humoral hypercalcemia of malignancy. During the recovery phase from severe burns, hypophosphatemia may occur secondary to massive diuresis with phosphaturia.

Transcellular Shift

Diabetes Mellitus. Patients with well-controlled diabetes mellitus do not have excessive losses of phosphate. However, in the presence of hyperglycemia, polyuria, and acidosis, Pi is lost through the urine in excessive amounts. In ketoacidosis, intracellular organic components tend to be broken down, releasing a large amount of Pi into the plasma, which is subsequently lost in the urine.[83] This process, combined with the enhanced osmotic Pi diuresis secondary to glycosuria, ketonuria, and polyuria, may cause large urinary losses of Pi and subsequent depletion. The plasma Pi is usually normal or slightly elevated in the ketotic patient despite the excessive urinary losses because of the continuous large shift of Pi from the cells into the plasma. With insulin, fluids, and correction of the ketoacidosis, however, serum and urine Pi may fall sharply. Despite the appearance of hypophosphatemia during treatment, previously well-controlled patients with diabetic ketoacidosis of only a few days duration almost never have serious phosphorus deficiency. Serum Pi rarely falls below 1.0 mg/dl in these patients. Administration of Pi-containing salts does not improve glucose use, nor does it reduce insulin requirements or the time for recovery from ketoacidosis. Thus, Pi therapy should be reserved for patients with serum Pi concentration <1.0 mg/dl.

Respiratory Alkalosis. Intense hyperventilation for prolonged periods may depress serum Pi to values below 1.0 mg/dl.[84] This is important in patients with alcoholic withdrawal because of attendant hyperventilation. A similar degree of alkalemia induced by infusion of bicarbonate depresses Pi concentration only mildly. The combined hypophosphatemic effects of respiratory and metabolic alkalosis may be pronounced. Severe hypophosphatemia is common in patients with extensive burns. It usually appears within several days after the injury. Phosphorus is virtually undetectable in the urine. Hypophosphatemia may result from transductive losses, respiratory alkalosis, or other factors.

Leukemia. Advanced leukemia that is markedly proliferative (blast crisis), with total leukocyte counts above 100,000, has been associated with severe hypophosphatemia. This would seem to result from excessive phosphorus uptake into rapidly multiplying cells.[85]

Clinical Effects of Severe Hypophosphatemia

Severe hypophosphatemia with phosphorus deficiency may cause widespread disturbances. There are at least eight well-established effects of severe hypophosphatemia (Table 4). The signs and symptoms of severe hypophosphatemia may be related to a decrease in 2,3-diphosphoglycerate in

TABLE 4. CONSEQUENCES OF SEVERE HYPOPHOSPHATEMIA

Red blood cell dysfunction—hemolysis, tissue hypoxia
Leukocyte dysfunction—increased susceptibility to infection
Platelet dysfunction—thrombocytopenia, hemorrhage
CNS dysfunction—encephalopathy, seizures, delirium, coma, paresthesias
Skeletal muscle dysfunction—weakness, respiratory failure, rhabdomyolysis
Cardiac muscle dysfunction—cardiomyopathy, congestive heart failure
Bone disease—osteomalacia/rickets
Metabolic acidosis

the red cell. This change is associated with increased affinity of hemoglobin for oxygen and therefore tissue hypoxia. There is also a decrease in tissue content of ATP, and consequently, a decrease in the availability of energy-rich phosphate compounds for cell function.

Central Nervous System

Some patients with severe hypophosphatemia display symptoms compatible with metabolic encephalopathy.[86–88] They may display, in sequence, irritability, apprehension, weakness, numbness, paresthesia, dysarthria, confusion, obtundation, seizures, and coma. In contrast to delirium tremens, the syndrome does not include hallucinations. Patients with very severe hypophosphatemia may show diffuse slowing of their electroencephalogram.

Hematopoietic System

A decrease in the red cell content of 2,3-diphosphoglycerate and ATP leads to increased rigidity, and in rare instances, hemolysis.[89] Hemolysis is usually provoked by unusual stress on the metabolic requirements of the red cell, such as severe metabolic acidosis or infection. When hemolysis has occurred, ATP content has invariably been depressed. Leukocyte/macrophage dysfunction can be demonstrated in vitro using Pi-depleted cells.[90] Suggestion that a predisposition to infection commonly seen in patients on intravenous hyperalimentation may be partly related to hypophosphatemia remains to be proven. Hypophosphatemia impairs granulocyte function by interfering with ATP synthesis. In experimental hypophosphatemia, there is an increase in platelet diameter, suggesting shortened platelet survival, and also a marked acceleration of platelet disappearance from the blood. These lead to thrombocytopenia and a reactive megakaryocytosis. In addition, there is an impairment of clot retraction and a hemorrhagic tendency, especially involving gut and skin.

Musculoskeletal System

Myopathy and Rhabdomyolysis. Muscle tissue requires large amounts of high-energy bonds (ATP, creatine phosphate) and oxygen for contraction, for maintenance of membrane potential, and for other functions. Pi deprivation induces muscle cell injury characterized by a decrease in intracellular Pi and an increase in water, sodium, and chloride. An apparent relationship between hypophosphatemia and alcoholic myopathy has been observed in chronic alcoholism.[91] The muscular clinical manifestations of Pi deficiency syndrome include myalgia, objective weakness, and myopathy with pathological findings of intracellular edema and a subnormal resting muscle membrane potential on electromyography. In patients with pre-existing Pi deficiency who develop acute hypophosphatemia, rhabdomyolysis might occur.[92] Hypophosphatemia and phosphate deficiency may be associated with creatine phosphokinase elevations in blood.

Bone. Skeletal defects have been reported in association with Pi depletion of different causes. These are discussed in detail elsewhere. Suffice it to say here that phosphate depletion is associated with rickets in children and osteomalacia in adults. However, the discovery of the phosphatonins, especially FGF23, show that osteomalacia is more that just hypophosphatemia decreasing mineralization, but rather impaired osteoblast function caused by the actions of FGF23 or the inhibition of Wnt signaling by sFrp4 that contribute directly to impaired mineralization.

Cardiovascular System

Severe hypophosphatemia has been associated with a cardiomyopathy characterized by a low cardiac output, a decreased ventricular ejection velocity, and an elevated left ventricular end-diastolic pressure.[93] A decrease in myocardial content of inorganic phosphorus, ATP, and creatinine phosphate seems to underlie the impairment in myocardial contractibility.[94] During phosphorus depletion, blood pressure may be low and the pressor response to naturally occurring vasoconstrictor agonists such as norepinephrine or angiotensin II is reduced.

Renal Effects of Hypophosphatemia and Phosphate Depletion

Severe hypophosphatemia and phosphate depletion affect the balance and serum concentrations of various electrolytes. Hypophosphatemia and phosphate depletion may produce changes in cardiovascular function (described above) and alterations in renal hemodynamics that affect renal tubule transport processes and renal cell metabolism. These disturbances are listed in Table 5.[1]

Tubular Transport

Calcium. A marked increase in urinary calcium excretion occurs during phosphate depletion proportional to the severity of phosphate depletion and the degree of hypophosphatemia.[95]

Phosphate. Dietary Pi restriction and Pi depletion is associated with enhanced renal tubular reabsorption of Pi.[87,96] Urinary excretion of Pi declines within hours after the reduction in its dietary intake, and Pi virtually disappears from the urine within 12 days. The changes in renal tubular reabsorption of Pi occur before detectable falls in the serum

TABLE 5. RENAL EFFECTS OF HYPOPHOSPHATEMIA

Decreased glomerular filtration rate
Metabolic abnormalities
    Decreased gluconeogenesis
    Insulin resistance
    Hypoparathyroidism, reduced urinary cAMP
    Increased production of 1,25 dihydroxyvitamin D3
Transport abnormalities
    Hypercalciuria
    Decreased proximal tubular sodium transport
    Hypermagnesiuria
    Hypophosphaturia
    Bicarbonaturia
    Glycosuria

Pi. The adaptation to a reduction in Pi supply is a direct response of the proximal tubule, rendering this nephron segment resistant to most phosphaturic stimuli, including PTH.[96] Acutely, Pi depletion causes an increase in the apical membrane expression of sodium-phosphate cotransporters likely by insertion of pre-existing transporter proteins from an endosomal pool.[97–100] Chronically, the increase in transporter expression is also accomplished by the synthesis of new transporter proteins. The adaptation to reduced Pi supply is independent of cellular responses to PTH. The signaling mechanisms responsible for adaptation are unknown.

Metabolic Acidosis. Severe hypophosphatemia with Pi deficiency may result in metabolic acidosis through three mechanisms.[101,102] First, severe hypophosphatemia is generally associated with a proportionate reduction of Pi excretion in the urine, thereby limiting hydrogen excretion as a titratable acid. Second, if Pi buffer is inadequate, acid secretion depends on production of ammonia and its conversion to ammonium ion. Ammonia production is severely depressed in Pi deficiency. The third mechanism is that of decreased renal tubular reabsorption of bicarbonate.

Treatment

The appropriate management of hypophosphatemia and Pi depletion requires identification of the underlying causes, treatment with supplemental Pi when necessary, and prevention of recurrence of the problem by correcting the underlying causes. The symptoms and signs of Pi depletion can vary, are nonspecific, and are usually seen in patients with multiple problems such as those encountered in intensive care unit settings. This makes it difficult to identify Pi depletion as the cause of clinical manifestations and Pi depletion is frequently overlooked.

Mild hypophosphatemia secondary to redistribution, with plasma Pi levels higher than 2 mg/dl, is transient and requires no treatment. In cases of moderate hypophosphatemia, associated with Pi depletion (serum Pi higher than 1.0 mg/dl in adults or 2.0 mg/dl in children), Pi supplementation should be administered in addition to treating the cause of hypophosphatemia. Milk is an excellent source of phosphorus, containing 1 g (33 mM) of inorganic phosphorus per liter. Skimmed milk may be better tolerated than whole milk, especially in children and malnourished patients because of concomitant lactose or fat intolerance. Alternatively, potassium phosphate tablets (which contain 250 mg of Pi per tablet as a sodium or potassium salt) may be given. Oral Pi can be given in a dose up to 3 g/day (i.e., three tablets of Neutraphos every 6 h). The serum Pi level rises by as much as 1.5 mg/dl, 60–120 minutes after ingestion of 1000 mg of Pi. A phosphosoda enema solution, composed of buffered sodium phosphate, may also be used in a dose of 15–30 ml three or four times daily.

Severe hypophosphatemia with serum levels lower than 0.5 mg/dl occurs only when there is cumulative net loss of more than 3.3 g of Pi. If asymptomatic, oral replacement with a total of 6–10 g of Pi (1–3 g of Pi per day) over a few days is usually sufficient. Symptomatic hypophosphatemia indicates that net Pi deficit exceeds 10 g. In these cases, 20 g of Pi is given spread over 1 week (up to 3 g/day). Patients with Pi deficiency tolerate substantially larger doses of oral Pi without side effects, such as diarrhea, than do normal subjects. However, patients with severe symptomatic hypophosphatemia who are unable to eat may be safely treated intravenously with 1 g of Pi delivered in 1 liter of fluid over 8–12 h. This is usually sufficient to raise serum Pi level to 1.0 mg/dl. It is unusual for hypophosphatemia to cause metabolic disturbances at serum Pi >1.0 mg/dl; therefore, full parenteral replacement is neither necessary nor desirable.

Treatment with phosphate can result in diarrhea, hyperphosphatemia, hypocalcemia, and hyperkalemia. These side effects can be prevented by paying careful attention to phosphorus dosages.

Prevention

The most effective approach to hypophosphatemia is prevention of predisposing conditions. Patients on total parenteral nutrition should receive a daily maintenance dose of Pi amounting to 1000 mg in 24 h, with increases as required by the clinical and metabolic states. Alcoholic patients and malnourished patients receiving intravenous fluids, particularly those containing glucose, should receive Pi supplementation, particularly if hypophosphatemia is observed.

REFERENCES

1. Hruska K, Slatopolsky E 1996 Disorders of phosphorus, calcium, and magnesium metabolism. In: Schrier RW, Gottschalk CW (ed.) Diseases of the Kidney. Little, Brown and Co., Boston, MA, USA.
2. Slatopolsky E, Robson AM, Elkan I, Bricker NS 1968 Control of phosphate excretion in uremic man. J Clin Invest 47:1865–1874.
3. Albright R, Burnett CH, Smith PH 1942 Pseudohypoparathyroidism: An example of Seabright Bantam Syndrome. Endocrinology 30:922.
4. Mitnick PD, Goldbarb S, Slatopolsky E, Lemann JJ, Gray RW, Agus ZS 1980 Calcium and phosphate metabolism in tumoral calcinosis. Ann Intern Med 92:482–487.
5. Lufkin EG, Wilson DM, Smith LH, Bill NJ, DeLuca HF, Dousa TP, Knox FG 1980 Phosphorus excretion in tumoral calcinosis: Response to parathyroid hormone and acetazolamide. J Clin Endocrinol Metab 50:648–653.
6. Parfitt AJ 1972 The spectrum of hypoparathyroidism. J Clin Endocrinol Metab 34:152–158.
7. McConnell TH 1971 Fatal hypocalcemia from phosphate absorption from laxative preparation. JAMA 216:147–148.
8. Walton RJ, Russell RG, Smith R 1975 Changes in the renal and extrarenal handling of phosphate induced by disodium etidronate (EHDP) in man. Clin Sci Mol Med 49:45–56.
9. Bucay N, Sarosi I, Dunstan CR, Morony S, Tarpleyl J, Capparelli C, Scully S, Tan HL, Xu W, Lacey DL, Boyle WJ, Simonet WS 1998 Osteoprotegerin-deficient mice develop early onset osteoporosis and arterial calcification. Genes Dev 12:1260–1268.
10. Jono S, Peinado C, Giachelli CM 2000 Phosphorylation of osteopontin is required for inhibition of vascular smooth muscle cell calcification. J Biol Chem 275:20197–20203.
11. Demer LL, Tintut Y 1999 Osteopontin: Between a rock and a hard plaque. Circ Res 84:250–252.
12. Luo G, Ducy P, McKee MD, Pinero GJ, Loyer E, Behringer RR, Karsenty G 1997 Spontaneous calcification of arteries and cartilage in mice lacking matrix GLA protein. Nature 386:78–81.
13. Kawaguchi H, Manabe N, Miyaura C, Chikuda H, Nakamura K, Kuro-o M 1999 Independent impairment of osteoblast and osteoclast differentiation in klotho mouse exhibiting low-turnover osteopenia. J Clin Invest 104:229–237.
14. Block GA, Port FK 2000 Re-evaluation of risks associated with hyperphosphatemia and hyperparathyroidism in dialysis patients: Recommendations for a change in management. Am J Kidney Dis 35:1226–1237.
15. Demer L 1997 Lipid hypothesis of cardiovascular calcification. Circulation 95:297–298.
16. Tintut Y, Parhami F, Bostrom K, Jackson SM, Demer LL 1998 cAMP stimulates osteoblast-like differentiation of calcifying vascular cells. J Biol Chem 273:7547–7553.
17. Tintut Y, Parhami F, Le V, Karsenty G, Demer LL 1999 Inhibition of osteoblast-specific transcription factor Cbfal by the cAMP pathway in osteoblastic cells. Ubiquitin/proteasome-dependent regulation. J Biol Chem 274:28875–28879.
18. Bostrom K, Watson KE, Stanford WP, Demer LL 1995 Atherosclerotic calcification: Relation to developmental osteogenesis. Am J Cardiol 75:88B–91B.
19. Morishita K, Shirai A, Kubota M, Katakura Y, Nabeshima Y, Takeshige K, Kamiya T 2001 The progression of aging in klotho mutant mice can be modified by dietary phosphorus and zinc. J Nutr 131:3182–3188.
20. Steitz SA, Speer MY, Curinga G, Yang H-Y, Haynes P, Aebersold R, Schinke T, Karsenty G, Giachelli CM 2001 Smooth muscle cell phenotypic transition associated with calcification. Circ Res 89: 1147–1154.
21. Jono S, McKee MD, Murry CE, Shioi A, Nishizawa Y, Mori K, Morii H, Giachelli CM 2000 Phosphate regulation of vascular smooth muscle cell calcification. Circ Res 87:e10–e17.
22. Chen NX, O'Neill KD, Duan D, More SM 2002 Phosphorus and uremic serum up-regulate osteopontin expression in vascular smooth muscle cells. Kidney Int 62:1724–1731.
23. Blacher J, Guerin AP, Pannier B, Marchais SJ, London GM 2001 Arterial calcifications, arterial stiffness, and cardiovascular risk in end-stage renal disease. Hypertension 38:938–942.
24. Chertow GM, Burke SK, Raggi P 2002 Sevelamer attenuates the progression of coronary and aortic calcification in hemodialysis patients. Kidney Int 62:245–252.
25. Cozzolino M, Dusso AS, Slatopolsky E 2001 Role of calcium-phosphate product and bone-associated proteins on vascular calcification in renal failure. J Am Soc Nephrol 12:2511–2516.
26. Fatica RA, Dennis VW 2002 Cardiovascular mortality in chronic renal failure: Hyperphosphatemia, coronary calcification, and the role of phosphate binders. Cleve Clin J Med 69:S21–S27.
27. Iribarren C, Sidney S, Sternfeld B, Browner WS 2000 Calcification of the aortic arch: Risk factors and association with coronary heart disease, stroke, and peripheral vascular disease. JAMA 283:2810–2815.
28. Newman AB, Naydeck BL, Sutton-Tyrrell K, Edmmundowicz D, O'Leary D, Kronmal R, Burke GL, Kuller LH 2002 Relationship between coronary artery calcification and other measures of subclinical cardiovascular disease in older adults. Arterioscler Thromb Vasc Biol 22:1674–1679.
29. Raggi P, Boulay A, Chasan-Taber S, Amin N, Dillon M, Burke SK, Chertow GM 2002 Cardiac calcification in adult hemodialysis patients. A link between end-stage renal disease and cardiovascular disease? J Am Coll Cardiol 39:695–701.
30. Reslerova M, Moe SM 2003 Vascular calcification in dialysis patients: Pathogenesis and consequences. Am J Kidney Dis 41:S96–S99.
31. Ahmed S, O'Neill KD, Hood AF, Evan AP, Moe SM 2001 Calci-

phylaxis is associated with hyperphosphatemia and increased osteopontin expression by vascular smooth muscle cells. Am J Kidney
Dis 37:1267–1276.

32. Block GA 2001 Control of serum phosphorus: Implications for coronary artery calcification and calcific uremic arteriolopathy (calciphylaxis). Curr Opin Nephrol Hypertens 10:741–747.

33. Wilmer WA, Magro CM 2002 Calciphylaxis: Emerging concepts in
prevention, diagnosis, and treatment. Semin Dial 15:172–86.

34. Lund RJ, Huq N, Davies MR, Hruska KA 2002 Efficacy of BMP-7
treatment of adynamic renal osteodystrophy. J Am Soc Nephrol
13:578A.

35. Bucay N, Sarosi I, Dunstan CR, Morony S, Tarpley J, Capparelli C,
Scully S, Tan HL, Xu W, Lacey DL, Boyle WJ, Simonet WS 1998
Osteoprotegerin-deficient mice develop early onset osteoporosis and
arterial calcification. Genes Dev 12:1260–1268.

36. Hak AE, Pols HAP, van Hemert AM, Hofman A, Witteman JCM
2000 Progression of aortic calcification is associated with metacarpal
bone loss during menopause: A population-based longitudinal study.
Arterioscler Thromb Vasc Biol 20:1926–1931.

37. Davies MR, Lund RJ, Hruska KA 2003 BMP-7 is an efficacious
treatment of vascular calcification in a murine model of atherosclerosis and chronic renal failure. J Am Soc Nephrol 14:1559–1567.

38. Price PA, June HH, Buckley JR, Williamson MK 2001 Osteoprotegerin inhibits artery calcification induced by Warfarin and by Vitamin
D. Arterioscler Thromb Vasc Biol 21:1610–1616.

39. Moriniere PH, Roussel A, Tahira Y, de Fremont JP, Maurel G,
Jaudon MC, Gueris J, Fournier A 1982 Substitution of aluminum
hydroxide by high doses of calcium carbonate in patients on chronic
hemodialysis: Disappearance of hyperaluminaemia and equal control
of hyperparathyroidism. Proc Eur Dial Transplant Assoc 19:784–
787.

40. Slatopolsky E, Weerts C, Lopez S 1986 Calcium carbonate is an
effective phosphate binder in dialysis patients. N Engl J Med 315:
157.

41. Slatopolsky E, Weerts C, Norwood K, Giles K, Fryer P, Finch J,
Windus D, Delmez J 1989 Long-term effects of calcium carbonate
and 2.5 mEq/liter calcium dialysate on mineral metabolism. Kidney
Int 36:897–903.

42. Chertow GM, Burke SK, Dillon MA, Slatopolsky E 1999 Long-term
effects of sevelamer hydrochloride on the calcium x phosphate product and lipid profile of haemodialysis patients. Nephrol Dial Transplant 14:2907–2914.

43. Chertow GM, Burke SK, Lazarus JM, Stenzel KH, Wombolt D,
Goldberg D, Bonventre JV, Slatopolsky E 1997 Polyalylamine hydrochloride (RenaGel): A noncalcemic phosphate binder for the
treatment of hyperphosphatemia in chronic renal failure. Am J Kidney Dis 29:66–71.

44. Slatopolsky E, Burke SK, Dillon MA 1999 RenaGel, a nonabsorbed
calcium and aluminum-free phosphate-binder, lowers serum phosphorus and parathyroid hormone. Kidney Int 55:299–307.

45. Knochel JP 1977 The pathophysiology and clinical characteristics of
severe hyperphosphatemia. Arch Intern Med 137:203–220.

46. Kreisberg RA 1977 Phosphorus deficiency and hypophosphatemia.
Hosp Pract (Hosp Ed) 12:121–128.

47. Shields HM 1978 Rapid fall of serum phosphorus secondary to
antacid therapy. Gastroenterology 75:1137–1141.

48. Larsson L, Rebel K, Sorbo B 1983 Severe hypophosphatemia-a
hospital survey. Acta Med Scand 214:221–223.

49. Ryback RS, Eckardt MJ, Pautler CP 1980 Clinical relationships
between serum phosphorus and other blood chemistry values in
alcoholics. Arch Intern Med 140:673–677.

50. Juan D, Elrazak MA 1979 Hypophosphatemia in hospitalized patients. JAMA 242:163–164.

51. Betro MG, Pain RW 1972 Hypophosphatemia and hyperphosphatemia in a hospital population. BMJ 1:273–276.

52. Arnaud CD, Clar OH 1983 Primary hyperparathyroidism. In: Krieger
DT, Bardin CW (ed.) Current Therapy in Endocrinology 1983–1984.
Decker and Mosby, Philadelphia, PA, USA, pp. 270–277.

53. Glikman RM 1985 Malabsorption. Pathophysiology and diagnosis.
In: Wyngaarden JB, Smith LHJ (ed.) Cecil's Textbook of Medicine,
17th ed. Saunders, Philadelphia, PA, USA, pp. 710–719.

54. Roth KS, Foreman JW, Segal S 1981 The Fanconi syndrome and
mechanisms of tubular dysfunction. Kidney Int 20:705–716.

55. Rosenbaum RW, Hruska KA, Korkor A, Anderson C, Slatopolsky E
1981 Decreased phosphate reabsorption after renal transplantation:
Evidence for a mechanism independent of calcium and parathyroid
hormone. Kidney Int 19:568–578.

56. Green J, Debby H, Lederer E, Levi M, Zajicek H, Bick T 2001

57. Rojas E, Carlini RG, Clesca P, Arminio A, Zuniaga O, de Elguezabal
K, Weisinger JR, Hruska KA, Bellorin-Font E 2003 The pathogenesis
of post-transplant osteodystrophy as detected by early alterations in
bone remodeling. Kidney Int 63:1915–1923.

58. Gray RW, Caldas AE, Wilz DR, Lemann J Jr, Smith GA, DeLuca HF
1978 Metabolism and excretion of ^{3}H-1,25(OH)$_2$ vitamin D$_3$ in
healthy adults. J Clin Endocrinol Metab 46:756–750.

59. Gray RW, Wilz DR, Caldas AE, Lemann JJ 1977 The importance of
phosphate in regulating plasma 1,25(OH)$_2$ vitamin D levels in humans: Studies in healthy subjects, in calcium-stone formers and in
patients with primary hyperparathyroidism. J Clin Endocrinol Metab
45:299–306.

60. Econs MJ, Francis F 1997 Positional cloning of the PEX gene: New
insights into the pathophysiology of X-linked hypophosphatemic
rickets. Am J Physiol 273:F489–F498.

61. Kos CH, Tihy F, Econs MJ, Murer H, Lemieux N, Tenenhouse HS
1994 Localization of a renal sodium phosphate cotransporter gene to
human chromosome 5q35. Genomics 19:176–77.

62. Nesbitt T, Econs MJ, Byun JK, Martel J, Tenenhouse HS, Drezner
MK 1995 Phosphate transport in immortalized cell cultures from the
renal proximal tubule of normal and Hyp mice: Evidence that the
HYP gene locus product is an extrarenal factor. J Bone Miner Res
10:1–7.

63. The Hyp Consortium 1995 A gene (PEX) with homologies to endopeptidases is mutated in patients with X-linked hypophosphatemic
rickets. Nat Genet 11:130–136.

64. Econs MJ, Drezner MK 1994 Tumor-induced osteomalacia: Unveil-
ing a new hormone. N Engl J Med 330:1645–1649.

65. Shimada T, Mizutani S, Muto T, Yoneya T, Hino R, Takeda S,
Takeuchi Y, Fujita T, Fukumoto S, Yamashita T 2001 Cloning and
characterization of FGF23 as a causative factor of tumor-induced
osteomalacia. Proc Natl Acad Sci USA 98:6500–6505.

66. White KE, Jonsson KB, Carn G, Hampson G, Spector TD, Mannstadt
M, Lorenz-Depiereux B, Miyauchi A, Yang IM, Ljunggren O, Meitinger T, Strom TM, Juppner H, Econs MJ 2001 The autosomal
dominant hypophosphatemic rickets (ADHR) gene is a secreted
polypeptide overexpressed by tumors that cause phosphate wasting.
J Clin Endocrinol Metab 86:497–500.

67. Kumar R 2002 New insights into phosphate homeostasis: Fibroblast
growth factor 23 and frizzled-related protein-4 are phosphaturic factors derived from tumors associated with osteomalacia. Curr Opin
Nephrol Hypertens 11:547–553.

68. Jan de Beur SM, Finnegan RB, Vassiliadis J, Cook B, Barberio D,
Estes S, Manavalan P, Petroziello J, Madden SL, Cho JY, Kumar R,
Levine MA, Schiavi SC 2002 Tumors associated with oncogenic
osteomalacia express genes important in bone and mineral metabolism. J Bone Miner Res 17:1102–1110.

69. Bowe AE, Finnegan R, Jan de Beur SM, Cho J, Levine MA, Kumar
R, Schiavi SC 2001 FGF-23 inhibits renal tubular phosphate transport
and is a PHEX substrate. Biochem Biophys Res Commun 284:977–
981.

70. The ADHR Consortium, Group 1: White KE, Evans WE, O'Riordan
JLH, Speer MC, Econs JJ; Group 2: Lorenz-Depiereux B, Grabowski
M, Meitinger T, Strom TM 2000 Autosomal dominant hypophosphatemic rickets is associated with mutations in FGF23. Nat Genet
26:345–348.

71. Jonsson KB, Zahradnik R, Larsson T, White KE, Hampson G,
Miyauchi A, Ljunggren O 2002 FGF-23 is a circulating factor that is
elevated in oncogenic osteomalacia and X-linked hypophosphatemic
rickets. J Bone Miner Res 17:S1;S158.

72. Fraser D, Kooh SW, Kind HP, Holick MF, Tanaka Y, DeLuca HF
1973 Pathogenesis of hereditary vitamin-D-dependent rickets. An
inborn error of vitamin D metabolism involving defective conversion
of 25-hydroxyvitamin D to 1alpha, 25-dihydroxyvitamin D. N Engl
J Med 289:817–822.

73. Liberman UA, Eil C, Marx SJ 1983 Resistance of 1,25 dihydroxyvitamin D. Associated with heterogeneous defects in cultured skin
fibroblasts. J Clin Invest 71:192–200.

74. Malloy PJ, Hochberg Z, Pike JW, Feldman D 1989 Abnormal binding of vitamin D receptors to deoxyribonucleic acid in a kindred with
vitamin D-dependent rickets, type II. J Clin Endocrinol Metab 68:
263–269.

75. Parker MS, Klein I, Haussler MR, Mintz DH 1981 Tumor-induced
osteomalacia: Evidence of a surgically correctable alteration in vitamin D metabolism. JAMA 245:492–493.

76. Sweet RA, Males JL, Hamstra AJ, DeLuca HF 1980 Vitamin D metabolite-levels in oncogenic osteomalacia. Ann Intern Med **93:** 279–270.

77. Cai Q, Hodgson SF, Kao PC, Lennon VA, Klee GG, Zinsmiester AR, Kumar R 1994 Brief report: Inhibition of renal phosphate transport by a tumor product in a patient with oncogenic osteomalacia. N Engl J Med **330:**1645–1649.

78. Schiavi SC, Moe OW 2002 Phosphatonins: A new class of phosphate-regulating proteins. Curr Opin Nephrol Hypertens **11:** 423–430.

79. Niehrs C 2001 Solving a sticky problem. Nature **413:**787–788.

80. Schneider WJ, Young SG 1999 Genetics and molecular biology. Curr Opin Lipidol **10:**85–87.

81. Leheste JR, Melsen F, Wellner M, Jansen P, Schlichting U, Renner-Müller I, Andreassen TT, Wolf E, Bachmann S, Nykjaer A, Willnow TE 2002 Hypocalcemia and osteopathy in mice with kidney-specific megalin gene defect. FASEB Journal **17:**247–249.

82. Little RD, Carulli JP, DelMastro RG, Dupuis J, Osborne M, Folz C, Manning SP, Swain PM, Zhao S-C, Eustace B, Lappe MM, Spitzer L, Zweier S, Braunschweiger K, Benchekroun Y, Hu X, Adair R, Chee L, Fitzgerald MG, Tulig C, Caruso A, Tzellas N, Bawa A, Franklin B, McGuire S, Nogues X, Gong G, Allen KM, Anisowicz A, Morales AJ, Lomedico PT, Recker SM, Van Eerdewegh P, Recker RR, Johnson ML 2002 A mutation in the LDL receptor-related protein 5 gene results in the autosomal dominant high-bone-mass trait. Am J Hum Genet **70:**11–19.

83. Seldin DW, Tarail R 1950 The metabolism of glucose and electrolytes in diabetic acidosis. J Clin Invest **29:**552–565.

84. Mostellar ME, Tuttle EPJ 1964 Effects of alkalosis on plasma concentration and urinary excretion of urinary phosphate in man. J Clin Invest **43:**138–149.

85. Zamkoff KW, Kirshner JJ 1980 Marked hypophosphatemia associated with acute myelomonocytic leukemia: Indirect evidence of phosphorus uptake by leukemic cells. Arch Intern Med **140:**1523–1524.

86. Lotz M, Ney R, Bartter FC 1964 Osteomalacia and debility resulting from phosphorus depletion. Trans Assoc Am Physicians **77:**281–295.

87. Lotz M, Zisman E, Bartter FC 1968 Evidence for a phosphorus-depletion syndrome in man. N Engl J Med **278:**409–415.

88. Prins JG, Schrijver H, Staghouwer JM 1973 Hyperalimentation, hypophosphatemia and coma. Lancet **1:**1253–1254.

89. Jacob HS, Amsden T 1971 Acute hemolytic anemia and rigid red cells in hypophosphatemia. N Engl J Med **285:**1446–1450.

90. Craddock PR, Yawata Y, Van Santen L, Gilberstadt S, Silvis S, Jacob HS 1974 Acquired phagocyte dysfunction: A complication of the hypophosphatemia of parental hyperalimentation. N Engl J Med **290:**1403–1407.

91. Knochel JP, Bilbrey GL, Fuller TJ 1975 The muscle cell in chronic alcoholism: The possible role of phosphate depletion in alcoholic myopathy. Ann NY Acad Sci **252:**274–286.

92. Knochel JP, Barcenas C, Cotton JR, Fuller TJ, Haller R, Carter NW 1978 Hypophosphatemia and rhabdomyolysis. J Clin Invest **62:** 1240–1246.

93. Darsee JR, Nutter DO 1978 Reversible severe congestive cardiomyopathy in three cases of hypophosphatemia. Ann Intern Med **89:**867–870.

94. Fuller TJ, Nichols WW, Brenner BJ, Peterson JC 1978 Reversible depression in myocardial performance in dogs with experimental phosphorus deficiency. J Clin Invest **62:**1194–1190.

95. Coburn JW, Massry SG 1970 Changes in serum and urinary calcium during phosphate depletion: Studies on mechanisms. J Clin Invest **49:**1073–1087.

96. Steele TH, Stromberg BA, Larmore CA 1976 Renal resistance to parathyroid hormone during phosphorus deprivation. J Clin Invest **58:**1461–1464.

97. Levi M, Lotscher M, Sorribas V, Custer M, Arar M, Kaissling B, Murer H, Biber J 1994 Cellular mechanisms of acute and chronic adaptation of rat renal P(i) transporter to alterations in dietary P(i). Am J Physiol **267:**F900–F908.

98. Lotscher M, Wilson P, Nguyen S, Kaissling B, Biber J, Murer H 1996 New aspects of adaptation of rat renal Na-Pi cotransporter to alterations in dietary phosphate. Kidney Int **49:**1012–1018.

99. Lotscher M, Kaissling B, Biber J, Murer H, Levi M 1997 Role of microtubules in the rapid regulation of renal phosphate transport in response to acute alterations in dietary phosphate content. J Clin Invest **99:**1302–1312.

100. Ritthaler T, Traebert M, Lotscher M, Biber J, Murer H, Kaissling B 1999 Effects of phosphate intake on distribution of type II Na/P$_i$ cotransporter mRNA in rat kidney. Kidney Int **55:**976–983.

101. Dominguez JH, Gray RW, Lemann JJ 1976 Dietary phosphate deprivation in women and men: Effects on mineral and acid balances, parathyroid hormone and the metabolism of 25-OH-vitamin D. J Clin Endocrinol Metab **43:**1056–1068.

102. O'Donovan DJ, Lotspeich WD 1966 Activation of kidney mitochondrial glutaminase by inorganic phosphate and organic acids. Nature **212:**930–932.

Chapter 49. Epidemiology of Osteoporosis

Cyrus Cooper

MRC Environmental Epidemiology Unit, University of Southampton, Southampton General Hospital, Southampton, United Kingdom

INTRODUCTION

Osteoporosis is currently defined as a systemic skeletal disorder characterized by low bone mass and micro architectural deterioration of bone tissue, with a consequent increase in bone fragility and susceptibility to fracture.[1] Clinically, osteoporosis is recognized by the occurrence of characteristic low trauma fractures, which typically arise at the hip, spine, and distal forearm. Historical approaches to the definition of osteoporosis have varied in their focus on bone density and the occurrence of fracture. The advantage of a fracture based definition is that fracture is a discrete event, which can be diagnosed using a simple algorithm. The disadvantage of this approach is that the diagnosis is delayed in some subjects who are clearly at increased risk of future fracture. As a consequence, a World Health Organization (WHO) study group was convened in 1994 with the objective of incorporating both bone mass and fracture into a simple stratified definition of osteoporosis.[2] This definition is summarized in Table 1 and designates osteoporosis at a bone density value more than 2.5 SDs below the young adult mean value. Whether defined densitometrically, or as the fracture burden, osteoporosis is undoubtedly a major public health problem. Around 20% of all postmenopausal women in western countries would meet the WHO criteria for osteoporosis, and around 1.3 million fractures in the United States each year are attributable to the disorder. Although the WHO definition remains the most widely used current approach to defining osteoporosis, the absence of a threshold in the relationship between bone density and the future risk of fracture, coupled with the difficulty of adopting the WHO value as a universal therapeutic threshold, has led to a recent reappraisal of diagnostic approaches. The most likely future outcome will be a modification in our interpretation of bone densitometry, such that the result is expressed as an absolute risk of future fracture over a particular period of time, say 10 years. This risk could then be estimated in the light of other historical risk factors, most importantly previous fracture history, and modified to varying degrees by the host of therapeutic interventions currently available to physicians and their patients.

FRACTURE EPIDEMIOLOGY

Incidence and Prevalence

It is estimated that around 40% of U.S. white women and 13% of U.S. white men 50 years of age will experience at least one clinically apparent fragility fracture in their lifetimes (Table 2).[3] However, taking into account sites other than the hip, spine, and distal forearm, the lifetime risk among women aged 50 years might be as high as 70%.[4] Estimates for the British population are around 20% lower. The medical costs of osteoporosis and its attendant fractures have been estimated in the United States to be $17.9 billion per annum, with hip fractures accounting for one-third of the total. In England and Wales, hip fracture patients alone take up 20% of orthopedic beds, with an estimated cost for all osteoporotic fractures of £1.7 billion per annum.[5] Furthermore, the overall burden on public health is set to increase dramatically over the next 60 years because of the steep predicted increase in the proportion of elderly people in the population.

Fracture incidence in the community is bimodal, with peaks in youth and in the very elderly. In young people, fractures of the long bones predominate, usually after substantial trauma, more frequently in males than females. None of these fractures seem to be related to osteoporosis. As the forces involved are substantial, the question of bone strength rarely arises. Over the age of 35 years, overall fracture incidence in women climbs steeply, so that rates become twice those in men. Hip and distal forearm fractures are the main contributors to this later peak, which also

TABLE 1. DIAGNOSTIC CATEGORIES FOR OSTEOPOROSIS BASED ON WHO CRITERIA

Category	Definition by bone density
Normal	A value for BMD that is not more than 1 SD below the young adult mean value
Osteopenia	A value for BMD that lies between 1 and 2.5 SD below the young adult mean value
Osteoporosis	A value for BMD that is more than 2.5 SD below the young adult mean value
Severe osteoporosis (established)	A value for BMD more than 2.5 SD below the young adult mean value in the presence of one or more fragility fractures

World Health Organization 1994.

The author has no conflict of interest.

Table 2. Estimated Lifetime Risk of Fracture in 50-Year-Old White Men and Women

	Lifetime risk	
Fracture site	Men (%)	Women (%)
Hip fracture	6.0	17.5
Clinically diagnosed vertebral fracture	5.0	15.6
Distal forearm fracture	2.5	16.0
Any of the above	13.1	39.7

Adapted from J Bone Miner Res 1992;**7**:1005–1010 with permission of the American Society for Bone and Mineral Research.

Prevalence of Vertebral Deformity EVOS

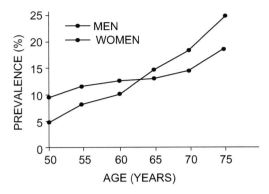

FIG. 2. Prevalence of vertebral deformity by sex. Data derived from the European Vertebral Osteoporosis Survey. (Reproduced from J Bone Miner Res 1996;**11**:1011–1019 with permission of the American Society for Bone and Mineral Research.)

includes proximal humeral, pelvic, and proximal tibial fractures.

The classical epidemiological hallmarks of these fractures were recognized over a century ago.[6] Incidence rates increase with age; rates are higher among women than men, and fracture is associated with moderate trauma at sites containing large amounts of trabecular bone. There are, however, substantial differences in the incidence patterns of these fractures by age and sex, which emphasize the varying contributions of bone strength and trauma to their pathogenesis.

Hip Fracture. In most populations, hip fracture incidence rates increase exponentially with age (Fig. 1). Above 50 years of age, there is a female to male incidence ratio of approximately two to one.[7] Overall, about 98% of all hip fractures occur among people aged 35 years and above, and 80% occur in women (because there are more elderly women than men). Worldwide, there were an estimated 1.66 million hip fractures in 1990,[8] about 1.19 million in women and 463,000 in men. Femoral neck bone strength declines with age in both sexes and is less in women than men. Over a lifetime, bone mineral density (BMD) of the femoral neck declines an estimated 58% in women and 39% in men, while BMD of the intertrochanteric region of the proximal femur falls about 53% and 35% in women and men, respectively.[9] Most hip fractures occur after a fall

Age-Related Fractures

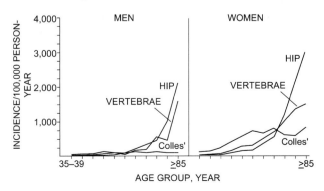

FIG. 1. Age-specific incidence rates for hip, vertebral, and distal forearm fractures in men and women. Data derived from the population of Rochester, Minnesota.

from standing height or less in men or women with reduced bone strength. The risk of falling increases with age and is higher in elderly women than elderly men. Hip fractures show marked seasonality in their incidence, tending to occur more frequently in the winter in temperate countries. However, the majority of hip fractures occur indoors and not as a result of slipping on icy pavements. Therefore, it is hypothesized that the seasonality may be caused by hypothermia impairing neuromuscular coordination or wintertime deficiency of sunlight and vitamin D. The combination of inexorable bone loss and increasing frequency of falls would seem to suggest that hip fractures are an inevitable consequence of aging. In fact, incidence rates vary substantially from one population to another. Hip fractures occur less frequently in nonwhites than whites, although there are differences within populations of a given gender or race. In Europe, hip fracture rates vary more than 7-fold from one country to another.[10] These variations imply an important role of environmental factors in the incidence of hip fractures. However, factors studied so far, such as variation in activity levels, obesity, cigarette smoking, alcohol consumption, or migration status, have not explained these trends. Further research is needed to identify the important environmental factors.

Vertebral Fracture. Elucidating the epidemiology of vertebral fractures has proved difficult for two reasons. First, a significant proportion of vertebral fractures are asymptomatic, and radiographic surveys of the general population are required to generate valid estimates of prevalence. Furthermore, there has been difficulty in achieving consensus as to the definition of vertebral deformities from lateral thoracolumbar radiographs.[11] Morphometric and semiquantitative visual techniques have now evolved for use in large epidemiological surveys and use of these techniques in Europe has improved our understanding of the epidemiology of prevalent and incident deformities.[11] In the European Vertebral Osteoporosis Study (EVOS), 15,570 men and women aged 50–79 years were enrolled from population registers in 36 countries.[12] The overall prevalence of morphometrically defined vertebral deformity in men and women was 12%. The prevalence increased in both sexes with age, but the curve was steeper in women (Fig. 2). There were substantial variations observed between countries, with the highest rates in Scandinavian countries. Some of these variations were explained by physical activity levels and body mass index (BMI) differences. Strong associations were identified between the number of vertebral deformities and the prevalence of reported back pain and height loss.[13] Data for the incidence of morphometrically defined vertebral deformities have recently been obtained from 3-year follow-up of this large European cohort.[14] This study suggests an annual incidence for new radiographic vertebral deformities of around 1% among women aged 65 and 0.5% among men of the same age. Although there was evidence of geographic variation in the incidence of radiographic vertebral deformities, with higher rates in Scandinavia, the geographic north-south gradient was much less marked than that observed for hip fracture.

Incidence rates for clinically diagnosed vertebral fractures have also been obtained in North America and Europe. In Rochester, Minnesota, the incidence of clinically ascertained vertebral deformities was around 30% of the rate for all radiographic deformities, suggesting that around 1 in 3 incidence deformities come to clinical attention.[15] This is a considerably higher proportion than that obtained in a recent epidemiological study from England and Wales.[16] This used the General Practice Research Database, which contains the computerized medical records of around 6% of all adults resident in the United Kingdom. Over the period of 1988–1998, 103,052 men and 119,317 women sustained a fracture over 21 million person-years of follow-up. The incidence of clinically diagnosed vertebral fractures in this cohort was only 8% of the figure estimated for incidence radiographic vertebral deformities. Although the clinically diagnosed incidence rate in general practice is likely to represent an underestimate of all patients with vertebral deformities who come to clinical attention, the data suggest that substantial numbers of elderly men and women with radiographic vertebral deformities (who are already at increased risk of future fractures) remain unidentified.

Distal Forearm Fracture. Distal forearm fractures almost always follow a fall on the outstretched arm. Most of these fractures are of the Colles' type, with displacement of the distal radial segment. They display a different pattern of incidence to that of hip and vertebral fractures. In white women, incidence increases linearly from age 40 to 65 years; thereafter, the rate of increase is less pronounced. In earlier studies, the incidence rate after age 70 years appeared to stabilize completely, whereas in more recent data, rates continue to increase gently. In men, incidence remains constant between age 20 and 80 years. Consequently, the majority of distal forearm fractures occur in women (age-adjusted female to male ratio of 4 to 1), and around one-half occur among women aged 65 years and over. The reason for the plateau in female incidence above the age of 65 years is

unknown, although it may be related to a change in the pattern of falls with advancing age, perhaps because of a slower gait or a loss of neuromuscular protective reflexes. Alternatively, it may relate to a postmenopausal cessation of cortical bone loss at the forearm. As with hip fractures, there is a winter peak in distal forearm fracture incidence,[17] but the winter peak in wrist fractures is more pronounced and more clearly related to falls outdoors during periods of icy weather.[8] The epidemiology characteristics of distal forearm fracture appear to be changing over the last decade. In recent studies,[16,18] the apparent plateau in female incidence rates with advancing age shows marked attenuation; distal forearm fracture rates continue to rise in women between ages 65 and 80 years, albeit with an age-related increase that is not as steep as that observed for hip fracture. This change suggests that the characteristics of falls which predispose to wrist fracture (the ability to stretch out the arm to protect against a fall) may have altered in the recent past.

Other Age-Related Fractures. The incidence rates of proximal humeral, pelvic, rib, clavicle, and scapula fractures also rise steeply with age and are greater in women than men. These are in marked contrast to the incidence patterns observed for fractures of the tibia, fibula, ankle, foot, and skull. Proximal humeral fractures typically occur after a fall from standing height or less, but severe trauma might occur in a greater proportion of proximal tibial and pelvic fractures. There is also direct evidence from noninvasive assessments of BMD that these fractures are related to this risk factor.[19]

Clustering of Fractures in Individuals

Epidemiological studies suggest that patients with different types of fragility fractures are at increased risk of developing other types of fracture. For example, the presence of a previous vertebral deformity leads to a 7- to 10-fold increase in the risk of subsequent vertebral deformities.[20] This is a comparable level of increased risk to that seen for individuals who have sustained one hip fracture to then sustain a second hip fracture. Furthermore, data from Rochester, Minnesota, suggest that the risk of a hip fracture is increased 1.4-fold in women and 2.7-fold in men after the occurrence of a distal forearm fracture.[21] This is an age-related phenomenon in women, such that those aged over 70 years at the time of their distal forearm fracture had a 1.6-fold increase in their risk of hip fracture, but those aged less than 70 years had no increased risk of future hip fracture. Vertebral fractures were significantly increased at all ages after a distal forearm fracture: 5.2-fold in women (95% CI, 4.5–5.9) and 10.7-fold in men (95% CI, 6.7–16.3). Similarly, people with radiologically diagnosed vertebral deformities have an increased risk of limb fracture over subsequent follow-up. In a population-based retrospective cohort study in Rochester, Minnesota,[22] 802 men and women were followed forward over 4349 person-years to identify 896 incident fractures. Relative to incidence rates in the community, there was a 2.8-fold increase in the risk of any fracture, which was greater in men (standardized incidence ratio 4.2; 95% CI, 3.2–5.3) than women (standardized incidence ratio 2.7; 95% CI, 2.4–3.0). The estimated cumulative incidence of any fracture after 10 years was 70%. The greatest increase in risk was for subsequent fractures of the axial skeleton, in particular a 12.6-fold increase (95% CI, 11–14) in additional vertebral fractures. There was a lesser increase in most limb fractures, including a 2.3-fold increase (95% CI, 1.8–2.9) in hip fractures and a 1.6-fold increase (95% CI, 1.0–2.4) in distal forearm fractures. The equivalent increases in subsequent fracture risk were observed whether the initial vertebral fracture was attributed to severe or moderate trauma. These data show that vertebral fractures represent an important risk factor for fractures in general, not just those of the spine and hip. They also suggest that the risk of a future hip fracture among those with clinically diagnosed vertebral fractures is not as high as the risk of subsequent vertebral deformities. The predictive capacity is, however, sufficient to continue to justify the cost-effective use of a prevalent vertebral deformity in any therapeutic algorithm that aims to prevent hip fractures. However, the correspondence between different fractures is sufficiently disparate to suggest that there is not a uniform etiological model for fractures at all sites. Fractures at any one site are influenced by both the patterns of involutional bone loss and the patterns of external trauma experienced at that site and the influences on both of these are heterogeneous at different skeletal sites.

Time Trends and Future Projections

The financial and health-related costs of osteoporosis can only rise in future generations. Life expectancy is increasing around the globe, and the number of elderly individuals is rising in every geographic region. There are an estimated 323 million individuals aged 65 years or over at present, and this number is expected to reach 1555 million by the year 2050.[23] The demographic changes alone can be expected to cause the number of hip fractures occurring among people aged 35 years and over throughout the world to increase from 1.66 million in 1990 to 6.26 million in 2050. Using current estimates for hip fracture incidence from various parts of the world, it can be calculated that around one-half of all hip fractures among elderly people in 1990 took place in Europe and North America. By 2050, the rapid aging of the Asian and Latin American populations will result in the European and North American contribution falling to only 25%, with over one-half of all hip fractures occurring in Asia.[23] It is clear, therefore, that osteoporosis will truly become a global problem over the next half century and that measures are urgently required to avert this trend.

Such projections would be worsened by the increases in hip fracture incidence seen in some countries even after adjustment for growth in the elderly population. Although age-adjusted rates appear to have leveled off in the northern region of the United States,[24,25] in parts of Sweden,[26,27] and in Great Britain,[28] rates in Hong Kong rose substantially between 1966 and 1985.[29] Based on current trends, hip fractures might increase in the United Kingdom from 46,000 in 1985 to 117,000 in 2016.[30] In Australia, they could rise from 10,150 in 1986 to 18,550 in 2011, with a doubling in the cost of care in constant dollars from $38 to $69 million annually.[31] Health authorities in Finland ex-

pect to see a 38% increase in the number of hip fractures between 1938 and 2010 and a 71% increase in the hospital bed-days needed to care for these patients; construction of those beds could cost FIM 250 million with an additional operating expense of FIM 100 million annually.[32]

There are three broad explanations for these trends. First, they might reflect the influence of some increasingly prevalent risk factor for osteoporosis or for falling. Time trends for a number of such risk factors, including oophorectomy, estrogen replacement therapy, cigarette smoking, alcohol consumption, and dietary calcium intake, do not match those observed for hip fractures.[24] Physical activity, however, appears to be a likely candidate. There is ample epidemiologic evidence linking inactivity to the risk of hip fracture,[33–35] whether this effect is mediated through bone density, the risk of falls, or both. Furthermore, some of the steepest secular trends have been observed in Asian countries such as Hong Kong, which have witnessed dramatic reductions in customary activity levels of their populations in recent decades.[29]

A second possible explanation for the secular changes is that the elderly population is becoming increasingly frail. The prevalence of disability is known to rise with age and to be greater among women at any age than among men.[36] Because many of the contributory disorders to this frailty are independently associated with osteoporosis and the risk of falling,[37] this tendency might have contributed to the secular increases in western nations during earlier decades of this century.

Finally, the trends could arise from a cohort phenomenon: some adverse influence on bone mass or falling risk that acted at an earlier time, but is now manifesting as rising incidence in successive generations of the elderly. Generational effects explain some of the secular trends in adult height during this century. Similar effects on the skeleton are likely. Indeed, it has been speculated that the increase in height led to a secular trend toward longer hip axis length, which may increase the risk of hip fracture.[38]

Incidence rates for fractures at other skeletal sites have also risen during the last half century. Studies from Malmö, Sweden, have suggested age-specific secular increases for distal forearm, ankle, proximal humeral, and vertebral fractures.[39] In many instances, these trends appeared in men as well as women. The observation for vertebral fractures is particularly important as it points to an increasing prevalence of osteoporosis, rather than falling, as a general explanation for these trends. Recent data from the northern United States confirmed increases in the incidence of clinically diagnosed vertebral fractures among postmenopausal women until the early 1960s, with a plateau in rates thereafter.[15] As with the Swedish data, these rate changes paralleled those observed for hip fractures in the same population.

Table 3 shows the projections for the number of hip fractures throughout Europe in 2000, 2020, and 2050, assuming constant incidence rates over that period. The demographic changes alone will account for an almost 3-fold increase in the number of hip fractures among both men and women. Table 4 illustrates the impact of a 1% annual increase in the age-adjusted incidence of hip fracture over this period. It shows that the projections for hip fracture

TABLE 3. EUROPEAN PROJECTIONS FOR HIP FRACTURE[11]

Year	No. of hip fractures ($\times 10^3$)	
	Male	Female
2000	88	326
2020	139	456
2050	230	742

European Community 1998.

based on demographic changes alone would almost double with each percentage point increase in age-adjusted rates. Finally, Table 4 illustrates the current estimates for the impact of osteoporosis related fractures throughout Europe. The cost of these fractures would currently be estimated at around UK £10 billion.

Geography

There are considerable geographical variations in the age- and sex-standardized discharge rates after hip fractures in the United Kingdom[40] and in the United States.[25] In the United Kingdom, the variation could not be explained by differences in water fluoride content or by dietary consumption of calcium (assessed from a national food survey). In the United States, there is a north-south gradient of fracture risk with a cluster of high incidence in the southeast. An association was detected between hip fracture incidence and southerly latitude, socioeconomic deprivation, proportion of agricultural land, reduced sunlight exposure, and soft, fluoridated water supply. Differences in body weight, smoking, and alcohol consumption do not reveal parallel geographic trends.[41]

International comparisons of fracture incidence reveal a more consistent pattern, but one in which ethnic group plays a major part (Fig. 3). Wherever these have been examined, hip fracture rates are higher among whites than among blacks. Within Negroid populations, both in South Africa and in North America, rates in men and women are similar. Urbanization in certain parts of Africa has led to an increase in hip fracture incidence, but even recently derived urban African rates for hip fracture are considerably lower than those found in western whites.[42] The highest recorded rates of hip fracture, after age-adjustment, come from Sweden and the northern United States. Rates in southern Europe and Israel are substantially lower, and there is a conver-

TABLE 4. WORLDWIDE PROJECTIONS FOR HIP FRACTURE

	No. of hip fractures ($\times 10^6$)			
	Stable incidence		1% annual increase	
Year	Male	Female	Male	Female
1990	0.3	0.3	0.3	0.9
2000	0.4	1.1	0.5	1.2
2025	0.8	1.8	1.1	2.6
2050	1.4	3.1	2.5	5.7

Derived from Gullberg et al. Osteoporosis Int 1997 7:407.

TABLE 5. IMPACT OF OSTEOPOROSIS-RELATED FRACTURES IN EUROPE

	Hip	Spine	Wrist
Lifetime risk (%)			
Women	14	11	13
Men	3	2	2
Cases/year	400,000	270,000	330,000
Hospitalization (%)	100	2–10	22
Relative survival	0.83	0.82	1.00

Costs: all sites combined ~ UK £10 billion.

gence of female and male rates.[7] This sex ratio reaches unity in Oriental populations such as in Hong Kong and Singapore, where rates overall are intermediate between those found in whites and blacks. The reasons for these ethnic patterns are uncertain, but bone density appears to be greater in blacks than whites during middle life; blacks may manifest a greater resistance to the bone resorptive effects of parathyroid hormone and 1,25 dihydroxyvitamin D_3; and body composition studies in black women report greater muscle and fat mass, suggesting a possible reduction in fractures through a reduction in the likelihood and severity of falls in later life.

MORTALITY AND MORBIDITY

Mortality

Mortality patterns have been studied for the three most frequent osteoporotic fractures. Survival rates 5 years after hip and vertebral fractures were found in Rochester, Minnesota, to be around 80% of those expected for men and women of similar age without fractures.[43] Mortality after Colles' fracture is not thought to deviate from the expected rate.

Hip Fracture. Hip fracture mortality is higher for men than for women, increases with age,[43] and is greater for those with coexisting illnesses and poor prefracture functional status. There are about 31,000 excess deaths within 6

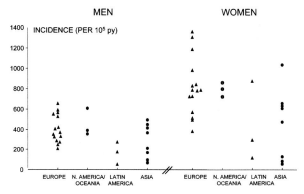

FIG. 3. Geographic variation in hip fracture incidence. (Adapted from J Bone Miner Res 2002;17:1237–1244 with permission of the American Society for Bone and Mineral Research.)

months of the approximately 300,000 hip fractures that occur annually in the United States. About 8% of men and 3% of women >50 years of age die while hospitalized for their fractures. At 1 year after hip fracture, mortality is 36% for men and 21% for women and is much higher in older men. One French study reported that 21% of hip fracture patients studied died within 3 months of their fracture, and mortality was twice as high in men as women.[44] Two years after hip fracture, mortality rates become comparable with people of the same age without hip fractures, although higher rates persist longer among the elderly and among men. The interaction of acute injury or surgery with comorbid conditions may contribute substantially to the excess mortality early after hip fracture. Both high levels of comorbidity and the presence of mental confusion during hospitalization are associated with an increased risk of dying after a hip fracture.[44]

Vertebral Fracture. Excess mortality after vertebral fracture appears to increase progressively after diagnosis of the fracture. Impaired survival is more pronounced for vertebral fractures that follow mild or moderate, rather than severe, trauma. Survival at 5 years appears to be worse for men (72%) than for women (84%). Among patients with vertebral fractures secondary to mild or moderate trauma, only a small proportion (8%) can be attributed to osteoporosis. The pattern of divergence between observed and expected survival suggests that the fractures are less the cause of death than an indicator of the presence of comorbid pathology and that it is the comorbidity that is responsible for the observed increased risk of death. There are an estimated 263,000 vertebral fractures annually in white U.S. citizens followed within 6 months by about 11,000 excess deaths.

Morbidity

In the United States, about 7% of survivors of all types of fragility fractures have some degree of permanent disability, and 8% require long-term nursing home care. Overall, a 50-year-old U.S. white woman has a 13% chance of experiencing fracture-related functional decline after any fracture.[45] However, the greatest fracture-attributable morbidity arises from hip fracture.

Hip Fracture. Inability to walk after a hip fracture makes this a particularly disabling event with a pronounced effect on quality of life. Hip fractures invariably require hospitalization. The degree of functional recovery after a hip fracture is age-dependent. In the United States, the proportion of hip fracture patients who were discharged from hospital to nursing homes was 14% for those aged 50–55 years, but 55% of those aged >90 years and the length of stay was also related to age.[46] One year after hip fracture, 40% of patients are still unable to walk independently, 60% require assistance in at least one essential activity of daily living (e.g., dressing, bathing), and 80% are unable to perform at least one instrumental activity of daily living (e.g., driving, shopping). Prefracture status is a strong predictor of outcome. In the United States, for example, about 25% of formerly independent people become at least partially dependent, 50% of those who were dependent prefracture are admitted to nursing homes, and those who were in nursing homes predictably remain there.

Vertebral Fracture. The clinical impact of a single vertebral fracture may be minimal, but the effects of multiple fractures are cumulative, leading to acute and chronic back pain, limitation of physical activity, progressive kyphosis, and loss of height.[13] These, in turn, lead to a loss of functional capacities and an inability to take part in recreational activities, which leads to social isolation, depression, and low self-esteem. Pain and fear of additional fractures cause decreased physical activity, exacerbating further the underlying osteoporosis and leading to an increased risk of further fractures.

Distal Forearm Fracture. Distal forearm fractures are not associated with increased mortality, but they do cause significant morbidity. One study showed that only 50% of patients report good functional recovery 1-year postfracture, and 1% become dependent.[47] The poor recovery results from long-term complications such as reflex sympathetic dystrophy, neuropathy, and post-traumatic arthritis.

CONCLUSION

This review has shown that osteoporosis is a major public health problem because of its association with fracture. It is now possible to predict future risk of fracture by measuring BMD with noninvasive techniques. The relationship between BMD and fracture is comparable with that between blood pressure and stroke, so that fracture risk can be assessed from a definition of osteoporosis using bone mass and past history of fracture. Because some of the risk factors for peak bone mass, involutional bone loss, and fracture are now characterized, coupled with innovative agents that are capable of retarding bone loss, it is becoming possible to generate preventive strategies, both for the entire population and those at the highest risk.

REFERENCES

1. Consensus Development Conference 1993 Diagnosis, prophylaxis and treatment of osteoporosis. Am J Med 94:646–650.
2. World Health Organisation 1994 Assessment of Fracture Risk and Its Application to Screening for Postmenopausal Osteoporosis. World Health Organization, Geneva, Switzerland, pp. 1–129.
3. Melton LJ, Chrischilles EA, Cooper C, Lane AW, Riggs BL 1992 How many women have osteoporosis? J Bone Miner Res 7:1005–1010.
4. Cooper C 1997 The crippling consequences of fractures and their impact on quality of life. Am J Med 103:12S–19S.
5. Department of Health Advisory Group on Osteoporosis 1994 Report. Department of Health, London, UK, pp. 1–86.
6. Cooper AP 1892 A Treatise on Dislocations and Fractures of the Joints. John Churchill, London, UK.
7. Melton LJ 1988 Epidemiology of fractures. In: Riggs BL, Melton LJ (eds.) Osteoporosis: Etiology, Diagnosis and Management. Raven Press, New York, NY,USA, pp. 133–154.
8. Cooper C, Melton LJ 1992 Epidemiology of osteoporosis. Trends Endocrinol Metab 3:224–229.
9. Cooper C, Melton LJ 1996 Magnitude and impact of osteoporosis and fractures. In: Marcus R, Feldman D, Kelsey J (eds.) Osteoporosis. Academic Press, San Diego, CA, USA, pp. 419–434.

10. Johnell O, Gullberg B, Allander E, Kanis J 1992 The apparent incidence of hip fracture in Europe: A study of national register sources. Osteoporos Int **2:**298–302.

11. Cooper C 1999 The epidemiology of osteoporosis. Osteoporos Int **10**(Suppl 2)**:**S2–S8.

12. O'Neill TW, Felsenberg D, Varlow J, Cooper C, Kanis JA, Silman AJ 1996 The prevalence of vertebral deformity in European men and women: The European Vertebral Osteoporosis Study. J Bone Miner Res **11:**1010–1018.

13. Ismail AA, Cooper C, Felsenberg D, Varlow J, Kanis JA, Silman AG, O'Neill TW, the European Vertebral Osteoporosis Study Group 1999 Number and type of vertebral deformities: Epidemiological characteristics and relation to back pain and height loss. Osteoporos Int **9:**206–213.

14. The European Prospective Osteoporosis Study (EPOS) Group 2002 Incidence of vertebral fracture in Europe: Results from the European Prospective Osteoporosis Study (EPOS). J Bone Miner Res **17:**716–724.

15. Cooper C, Atkinson EJ, O'Fallon WM, Melton LJ 1992 Incidence of clinically diagnosed vertebral fractures: A population-based study in Rochester, Minnesota, 1985–1989. J Bone Miner Res **7:**221–227.

16. van Staa TP, Dennison EM, Leufkens HGM, Cooper C 2001 Epidemiology of fractures in England and Wales. Bone **29:**517–522.

17. Ralis ZA 1981 Epidemic of fractures during periods of snow and ice. BMJ **282:**603–605.

18. O'Neill TW, Cooper C, Finn JD, Lunt M, Purdie D, Reid DM, Rowe R, Woolf AD, Wallace A on behalf of the UK Colles' Fracture Study Group 2001 Incidence of distal forearm fracture in British men and women. Osteoporos Int **12:**555–558.

19. Seeley DG, Browner WS, Nevitt MC, Genant HK, Scott JC, Cummings SR 1991 Which fractures are associated with low appendicular bone mass in elderly women? Ann Intern Med **115:**837–842.

20. Ross PD, Davis JW, Epstein RS 1991 Pre-existing fractures and bone mass predict vertebral fracture incidence in women. Ann Intern Med **114:**919–923.

21. Cuddihy MT, Gabriel SE, Crowson CS, O'Fallon WM, Melton LJ III 1999 Forearm fractures as predictors of subsequent osteoporotic fractures. Osteoporos Int **9:**469–475.

22. Melton LJ, Atkinson EJ, Cooper C, O'Fallon WM, Riggs BL 1999 Vertebral fractures predict subsequent fractures. Osteoporos Int **10:**214–221.

23. Cooper C, Campion G, Melton LJ 1992 Hip fractures in the elderly: A worldwide projection. Osteoporos Int **2:**285–289.

24. Melton LJ, O'Fallon WM, Riggs BL 1987 Secular trends in the incidence of hip fractures. Calcif Tissue Int **41:**57–64.

25. Jacobsen SJ, Goldberg J, Miles TP, Brody JA, Stiers W, Rimm AA 1990 Regional variation in the incidence of hip fracture among white persons aged 65 years and older in the United States, 1984–7. Am J Epidemiol **133:**996–1004.

26. Naessen T, Parker R, Persson I, Zack M, Adami HO 1989 Time trends in incidence rates of first hip fracture in the Uppsala Health Care Region, Sweden, 1965–1983. Am J Epidemiol **130:**289–299.

27. Rehnberg L, Nungu S, Olerud C 1992 The incidence of femoral neck fractures in women is decreasing. Acta Orthop Scand **63:**92–93.

28. Spector TD, Cooper C, Lewis AF 1990 Recent changes in hip fracture incidence in England and Wales 1968–85. BMJ **300:**1178–1184.

29. Lau EMC, Cooper C, Wickham C, Donnan S, Barker DJP 1990 Hip fracture in Hong Kong and Britain. Int J Epidemiol **19:**1119–1121.

30. Royal College of Physicians 1989 Fractured neck of femur: Prevention and management. Summary and recommendations of a report of the Royal College of Physicians. J Roy Coll Physicians Lond **23:**8–12.

31. Lord SR, Sinnett PF 1986 Femoral neck fractures: Admissions, bed use, outcome and projections. Med J Aust **145:**493–496.

32. Simonen O 1988 Epidemiology and socio-economic aspects of osteoporosis in Finland. Ann Chir Gynaecol Suppl **77:**173–175.

33. Cooper C, Barker DJP, Wickham C 1988 Physical activity, muscle strength and calcium intake in fracture of the proximal femur in Britain. BMJ **297:**1443–1446.

34. Lau E, Donnan S, Barker DJ, Cooper C 1988 Physical activity and calcium intake in fracture of the proximal femur in Hong Kong. BMJ **297:**1441–1443.

35. Wickham C, Walsh K, Cooper C, Barker BJP, Margetts BM, Morris J, Bruce S 1989 Dietary calcium, physical activity, and risk of hip fracture: A prospective study. BMJ **299:**889–892.

36. McAlindon TE, Cooper C, Dieppe PA 1992 Knee pain and disability in the elderly. Br J Rheumatol **31:**189–192.

37. Wickham C, Cooper C, Margetts BM, Barker DJP 1989 Muscle strength, activity, housing and the risk of falls in elderly people. Age Ageing **18:**47–51.

38. Reid IR, Chin K, Evans MC, Jones JG 1994 Relation between increase in length of hip axis in older women between 1950s and 1990s and increase in age-specific rates of hip fracture. BMJ **309:**508–509.

39. Obrant KJ, Bengner U, Johnell O, Nilsson BE, Sernbo I 1989 Increasing age-adjusted risk of fragility fractures: A sign of increasing osteoporosis in successive generations? Calcif Tissue Int **44:**157–167.

40. Cooper C, Wickham C, Lacey R, Barker DJP 1990 Water fluoride content and fracture of the proximal femur. J Epidemiol Community Health **44:**17–19.

41. Melton LJ 1993 Epidemiology of Age Related Fractures in the Osteoporotic Syndrome: Detection, Prevention and Treatment. Raven Press, New York, NY, USA, pp. 17–18.

42. Adebajo AO, Cooper C, Evans JG 1991 Fracture of the hip and distal forearm in West Africa and the United Kingdom. Age Ageing **20:**435–438.

43. Cooper C, Atkinson EJ, Jacobsen SJ, O'Fallon WM, Melton LJ 1993 Population-based study of survival following osteoporotic fractures. Am J Epidemiol **137:**1001–1005.

44. Baudoin C, Fardellone P, Bean K, Ostertag-Ezembe A, Hervy F 1996 Clinical outcomes and mortality after hip fracture. Bone **18:**S149–S157.

45. Chrischilles EA, Butler CD, Davis CS, Wallace RB 1991 A model of lifetime osteoporosis impact. Arch Intern Med **151:**2026–2032.

46. Office of Technology Assessment of the United States 1993 Hip fracture outcomes in people aged 50 and over. In: Mortality, Service Use, Expenditures, and Long-term Functional Impairment. U.S. Government Printing Office, Washington, DC, USA. OTA-BP-H-120.

47. Kaukonen JP, Karaharju EO, Porras M, Luthje P, Jakobsson A 1988 Functional recovery after fractures of the distal forearm. Ann Chir Gynaecol Suppl **77:**27–31.

Chapter 50.   Pathogenesis of Postmenopausal Osteoporosis

Richard Eastell

Bone Metabolism Group, Section of Human Metabolism, Division of Clinical Sciences (North), University of Sheffield, South Yorkshire, United Kingdom

INTRODUCTION

Osteoporosis-related fractures result from a combination of decreased bone mineral density (BMD) and a deterioration in bone microarchitecture. A BMD below average for age can be considered a consequence of inadequate accumulation of bone in young adult life (low peak bone mass) or of excessive rates of bone loss. The microarchitectural changes occur with the bone loss but will be considered separately.

DETERMINANTS OF PEAK BONE MASS

The increase in bone mass that occurs during childhood and puberty results from a combination of growth of bone at the endplates (endochondral bone formation) and of change in bone shape (modeling). The rapid increase in bone mass at puberty is associated with an increase in sex hormone levels and the closure of the growth plates. Within 3 years of menarche, there is little further increase in bone mass. The small increase in BMD over the next 5–15 years is a consequence of periosteal apposition (modeling). The resulting peak bone mass is achieved by the age of 20–30 years old.

Genetic factors are the main determinants of peak bone mass.[1] This has been shown by studies made on twins or on mother–daughter pairs. Hereditability appears to account for about 50–85% of the variance in bone mass, depending on the skeletal site. It is likely that several genes regulate bone mass, each with a modest effect, and likely candidates include the genes for type I collagen (*COL1A1*) and for the vitamin D receptor.[1] The nongenetic factors include low calcium intake during childhood, low body weight at maturity, at 1 year of life, sedentary lifestyle, and delayed puberty. Each of these results in decreased bone mass.

BONE LOSS

Mechanisms

Bone loss occurs in the postmenopausal woman as a result of an increase in the rate of bone remodeling and an imbalance between the activity of osteoclasts and osteoblasts. Bone remodeling occurs at discrete sites within the skeleton and proceeds in an orderly fashion with bone resorption always being followed by bone formation, a phenomenon referred to as "coupling." In cortical and cancellous bone the sequence of bone remodeling is similar.[2] The quiescent bone surface is converted to activity ("origination"), and the osteoclasts resorb bone ("progression"), forming a cutting cone (cortical bone) or a trench (cancellous bone). The osteoblasts synthesize bone matrix that subsequently mineralizes. The sequence takes up to 8 months. If the processes of bone resorption and bone formation are not matched, there is "remodeling imbalance." In postmenopausal women, this imbalance is magnified by the increase in the rate of initiation of new bone remodeling cycles ("activation frequency").

Remodeling imbalance results in irreversible bone loss. There are two other causes of irreversible bone loss, referred to as "remodeling errors." First is the excavation of overlarge haversian spaces in cortical bone.[3] Radial infilling is regulated by signals from the outermost osteocytes and is generally no more than 90 μm. Hence, large external diameters, which may simply occur randomly, lead to large central haversian canals, which then accumulate with age, leading to increased cortical porosity. In a similar way, osteoclast penetration of trabecular plates, or severing of trabecular beams, removes the scaffolding needed for osteoblastic replacement of resorbed bone. In both ways, random remodeling errors tend to reduce both cancellous and cortical bone density and structural integrity.

Causes

Estrogen Deficiency. Bone loss in the postmenopausal woman occurs in two phases.[4] There is a phase of rapid bone loss that lasts for 5 years (about 3%/year in the spine). Subsequently, there is lower bone loss that is more generalized (about 0.5%/year at many sites). This slower phase of bone loss affects men, starting at about 55 years of age.

The major mechanism of the rapid phase of bone loss in women is estrogen deficiency. The circulating level of estradiol decreases by 90% at the time of the menopause. Estrogen either alone or in combination with progestins can prevent the bone loss in postmenopausal women and thus prevent or minimize about 50% of the bone lost during a woman's lifetime. The decision to use estrogen plus progestin must consider the several potential adverse events that may accompany the use of this regimen.

The major effect of estrogen deficiency is on bone, where it increases activation frequency and may contribute to the remodeling imbalance. The exact mechanism of action of estrogen on bone is unclear. Estrogen may act partly through the osteoblast (e.g., increased synthesis of insulin-like growth factor I, osteoprotegerin, and transforming growth factor β) and partly through monocytes in the bone marrow environment (e.g., decreased synthesis of interleukin 1 and tumor necrosis factor α). This modulation of locally active growth factors and cytokines mediates the effects of estrogen on osteoblasts and osteoclasts. Thus, a greater increase in cytokines (e.g., interleukin 1) in response to estrogen deficiency may account for the more rapid bone loss in some women.

Estrogen deficiency may be a determinant of bone loss in men.[4] Decreased BMD has been reported in men with an inactivating mutation of the genes for the estrogen receptor or for aromatase (the enzyme that converts androgens to

The author has no conflict of interest.

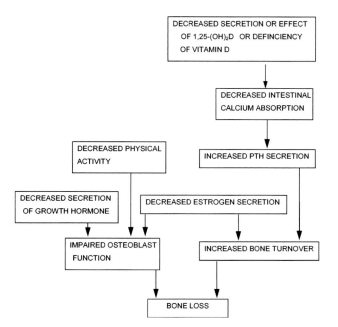

FIG. 1. Proposed mechanism for age-related bone loss in women.[5] Note how estrogen deficiency probably results in both increased bone turnover and remodeling imbalance.[4]

estrogens). In older men, estrogen levels correlate more closely with BMD than testosterone levels. In men with osteoporosis, estradiol (but not testosterone) levels have been reported to be decreased.

Aging. The slow phase of bone loss is attributed to age-related factors such as an increase in parathyroid hormone (PTH) levels and osteoblast senescence (Fig. 1). An increase in PTH levels (and action) occurs in both men and women with aging.[5] PTH levels correlate with biochemical markers of bone turnover, and both may be returned to those found in young adults by the intravenous infusion of calcium.[4] The increase in PTH results from decreased renal calcium reabsorption and decreased intestinal calcium absorption. The latter may result from vitamin D deficiency (e.g., in the housebound elderly), decreased 1-α hydroxylase activity in the kidney, resulting in decreased synthesis of 1,25(OH)2 vitamin D or resistance to vitamin D. Whatever the cause, a diet high in calcium returns both PTH and bone turnover markers to levels found in healthy young adults.

It has been proposed that the age-related increase in PTH could result from indirect effects of estrogen deficiency.[4] This proposal is based on the following evidence. In older women treated with estrogen, (1) there is a decrease in bone turnover markers and PTH levels, (2) there is an increase in calcium absorption, possibly mediated by an increase in 1,25(OH)2 vitamin D, (3) there is an increase in the PTH-independent calcium reabsorption in the kidney, and (4) there is a decrease in the parathyroid secretory reserve.

Accelerating Factors. A number of diseases and drugs are clearly related to accelerated bone loss, and these are described elsewhere. Their effects are superimposed on those

described above. Thus, a patient starting on corticosteroid therapy is more likely to have an osteoporosis-related fracture if she has low BMD resulting from low peak bone mass and the accelerated bone loss of the menopause.

Identification of Mechanism of Bone Loss in an Individual. In a woman presenting with osteoporosis at the age of 70 years, it is often possible to identify several reasons for the low BMD (Fig. 2). Some of these may be identified from a history (early menopause, drugs that accelerate bone loss), but some cannot be identified in retrospect (low peak bone mass, rapid losers).

OTHER DETERMINANTS OF BONE STRENGTH

Bone Geometry

Bone geometry has a major effect on fracture risk.[3] One example is hip axis length, the distance from the lateral surface of the trochanter to the inner surface of the pelvis, along the axis of the femoral neck. Short hip axis length results in an architecturally stronger structure for any given bone density. This is probably the reason why Japanese and other Orientals have about one-half the hip fracture rate of whites, despite similar bone density values. Likewise, large vertebral body end-plate areas result in lower spine pressure values for individuals of the same body size. Those with small vertebral bodies are thus more likely to fracture. Such geometric factors both contribute to individual fracture risk and explain a substantial portion of the population level variance in fracture rate. In each situation, however, the ultimate pathogenesis of the fracture is the fall and the force sustained by the bone on impact.

Fatigue Damage

Fatigue damage consists of ultramicroscopic rents in the basic bony material, resulting from the inevitable bending

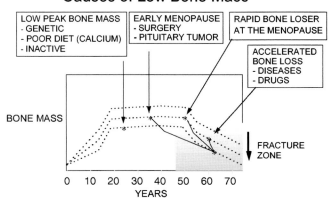

FIG. 2. Causes of low BMD in postmenopausal women. BMD reaches a peak between ages 20 and 30 years and then is followed by a rapid phase of bone loss at the menopause lasting 5 years, followed by a slower phase of bone loss. Bone loss in a 65-year-old woman may have a single cause (as shown here) or there may be several causes contributing to the low BMD.

© 2003 American Society for Bone and Mineral Research

that occurs when a structural member is loaded.[3] Fatigue damage is the principal cause of failure in mechanical engineering structures; its prevention is the responsibility of the remodeling apparatus, which detects and removes fatigue-damaged bone. Fractures related to fatigue damage occur whenever the damage occurs faster than remodeling can repair it or whenever the remodeling apparatus is defective. March fractures and the fractures of radiation necrosis are well-recognized examples of fractures caused by these two mechanisms. Fatigue damage definitely occurs in normal bone, under ordinary usage, although it is less certain as to precisely what role it may play in predisposing to osteoporotic fracture. Furthermore, there is suggestive evidence for certain fractures (notably hip) that remodeling repair may be defective specifically at the site that ultimately fractures. Why remodeling surveillance or effectiveness might fail locally is not known. Nevertheless, it is clear that such failure would lead to accumulation of fatigue damage, and therefore, to local weakening of bone.

Loss of Trabecular Connectivity

Bone structures loaded vertically, such as the vertebral bodies and femoral and tibial metaphyses, derive a substantial portion of their structural strength from a system of horizontal, cross-bracing trabeculae, which support the vertical elements and limit lateral bowing and consequent snapping under vertical loading. Severance of such trabecular connections is known to occur preferentially in postmenopausal women and is considered to be a major reason for the large female/male preponderance of vertebral osteoporosis. That long, unsupported vertical trabeculae are susceptible to fracture is reflected in the extraordinarily high prevalence of trabecular fracture callus sites in vertebral bodies examined at autopsy, typically 200–450 healing or healed fractures per vertebral body. While many of these will be well enough healed at any given time to be structurally competent, others will be fresh and structurally weak. Such fractures are asymptomatic, and their accumulation both reflects the impact of lost trabecular connections and greatly weakens the cancellous structure of the vertebral body. The incident fracture prediction ability of prior vertebral fractures is probably due in part to the presence of such otherwise undetected trabecular defects. That is why prior fracture seems to predict future fracture even when bone density is relatively high. The reason for preferential osteoclastic severance of horizontal trabeculae is not known. It is sometimes attributed to overaggressive osteoclastic resorption, but that seems more descriptive than explanatory.

REFERENCES

1. Ralston SH 2002 Genetic control of susceptibility to osteoporosis. J Clin Endocrinol Metab **87:**2460–2466.
2. Parfitt AM, Mundy GR, Roodman GD, Hughes DE, Boyce BF 1996 A new model for the regulation of bone resorption, with particular reference to the effects of bisphosphonates. J Bone Miner Res **11:**150–159.
3. Seeman E 2002 Pathogenesis of bone fragility in women and men. Lancet **359:**1841–1850.
4. Riggs BL, Khosla S, Melton LJ III 1998 A unitary model for involutional osteoporosis: Estrogen deficiency causes both type I and type II osteoporosis in postmenopausal women and contributes to bone loss in aging men. J Bone Miner Res **13:**763–773.
5. Eastell R 2002 Osteoporosis. In: Wass JAH, Shalet SM (eds.) Oxford Text Book of Endocrinology and Diabetes. Oxford University Press, Oxford, UK, pp. 65–675.

Chapter 51.   Assessment of Fracture Risk. Who Should Be Screened?

John A. Kanis

Centre for Metabolic Bone Diseases (WHO Collaborating Centre), University of Sheffield Medical School, Sheffield, United Kingdom

INTRODUCTION

The internationally agreed description of osteoporosis is a systemic disease characterized by low bone mass and microarchitectural deterioration of bone tissue, with a consequent increase in bone fragility and susceptibility to fracture.[1] The diagnosis thus centers on the assessment of bone mass and quality. There are no satisfactory clinical tools available to assess bone quality independently of bone density; therefore, for practical purposes, the diagnosis of osteoporosis depends on the measurement of skeletal mass, as assessed by measurements of bone mineral density (BMD).

From this perspective, the aim of treatment in osteoporosis is to increase BMD and thereby decrease the risk of fracture. Strategies for changing bone mass may be based on a global approach, where the intention is to shift the distribution of BMD in the whole population (e.g., by the promotion of exercise, smoking cessation, or manipulating dietary intake of calcium). However, evidence for the efficacy of such approaches is lacking, and their feasibility has never been tested.[2] The alternative approach is the "high-risk" strategy, whereby segments of the population most at risk are targeted for intervention (e.g., mass population screening of women at the time of the menopause).

There are many reasons why population screening is not feasible at present with the use of BMD tests. A particular problem is that the sensitivity (detection rate of the test to predict fracture) is low over most reasonable assumptions so

The author has no conflict of interest.

that the impact of screening on the societal burden of fracture would be low.[3] For this reason, the identification of patients has been based on a case finding strategy based on the identification of individuals at high risk.

CURRENT CASE-FINDING STRATEGIES

The identification of risk factors for fracture has been widely used in case-finding strategies. In such schemes, patients are identified based on clinical risk factors. Examples include a family history of fragility fracture, a previous fragility fracture, low body mass index (BMI), and the long-term use of corticosteroids. Patients so identified are referred for BMD measurements, and intervention offered if BMD falls below a given threshold. Current guidelines in Europe suggest that intervention should be offered in those individuals subsequently shown to have osteoporosis (i.e., a T-score of −2.5 SDs or less). [2,4] In the United States, the National Osteoporosis Foundation (NOF) recommends a less stringent threshold of −2.0 SDs in the absence of significant risk factors and −1.5 SDs in the presence of risk factors.[5] These case-finding strategies are conservative. Individuals must have one of the chosen risk factors before they are referred for a BMD test. Moreover, the vast majority of fractures will occur in those individuals who are never assessed.

The clinical significance of osteoporosis lies not in bone mass, but in the fractures that arise with their attendant morbidity and mortality. The ultimate aim of assessment is, therefore, to characterize fracture risk. Although bone mass is an important component of the risk of fracture, other abnormalities occur in the skeleton that contribute to fragility. In addition, a variety of nonskeletal factors, such as the liability to fall and force of impact, contribute to fracture risk. Because BMD forms but one component of fracture risk, accurate assessment of fracture risk should ideally take into account other readily measured indices of fracture risk that add information over and above that provided by BMD. Against this background, a growing view is that the assessment of fracture risk should encompass all aspects of risk and that intervention should not be guided solely based on BMD. [6,7] There is a distinction to be made, therefore, between diagnosis of osteoporosis and the assessment of fracture risk, which in turn implies a distinction between diagnostic and intervention thresholds. This chapter reviews the extent that this can be achieved in clinical practice.

BMD

The cornerstone for the diagnosis of osteoporosis lies in the assessment of BMD. In 1994, an expert panel of the World Health Organization recommended thresholds of BMD in women to define osteoporosis[3,8] that have been widely accepted.[9–11] Osteoporosis in postmenopausal white women is defined as a value for BMD more than 2.5 SDs below the young average value (i.e., a T-score of < −2.5 SDs). Severe osteoporosis (established osteoporosis) uses the same threshold but in the presence of one or more fragility fracture. The preferred site for diagnostic purposes is BMD measurements made at the hip[6]; however, in my

TABLE 1. PROPORTION (%) OF WHITE WOMEN WITH OSTEOPOROSIS BY AGE ADJUSTED TO 1990 U.S. WHITE WOMEN DEFINED AS A BONE MASS BELOW 2.5 SDs OF THE YOUNG ADULT REFERENCE RANGE AT THE SPINE, HIP, OR MIDRADIUS[3,8]

Age range (years)	Any site*	Hip alone
30–39	0	0
40–49	0	0
50–59	14.8	3.9
60–69	21.6	8.0
70–79	38.5	24.5
80+	70.0	47.5
≥50	30.3	16.2

* Hip, spine, or forearm.

own view, the femoral neck is preferable.[6] For men, the same threshold used for women is appropriate, because for any given BMD, the age-adjusted fracture risk is more or less the same.[12–15]

The diagnostic threshold identifies about 16% of postmenopausal women as having osteoporosis when measurements using DXA are made at the hip[3,8] and approximates the remaining lifetime risk of hip fracture at the age of 50 years (Table 1).

The diagnostic use of the T-score cannot be used interchangeably with different techniques and at different sites, because the same T-score derived from different sites and techniques yields different information on fracture risk.[16] For example, in women 60 years of age, the average T-score ranges from −0.7 to −2.5 SDs, depending on the technique used and site measured. Reasons include differences in the gradients of fracture risk prediction, in the population SDs, and in the apparent rates of bone loss with age. A further problem is that intersite correlations, although usually of statistical significance, are inadequate for predictive purposes in individuals; this gives rise to errors of misclassification.[17] This does not mean that other sites and other techniques cannot be used for risk assessment—only that the performance characteristics of the different techniques differ.

The causation of fracture is multifactorial, and the risk of fracture rises continuously with decreasing BMD. There is therefore no cut-off for BMD that will accurately distinguish those who will or will not fracture. Thus, an important use of BMD measurements is to assess fracture probability so that this information can be combined with other clinical input to aid decision-making for intervention.

ASSESSMENT OF RISK

The use of bone mass measurements for prognosis depends on accuracy. Accuracy in this context is the ability of the measurement to predict fracture. In general, all absorptiometric techniques have high specificity but low sensitivity, which vary with the cut-off chosen to designate high risk (the definitions of risk used are summarized in Table 2). Many cross-sectional prospective population studies indicate that the risk for fracture increases by a factor of 1.5–3.0 for each SD decrease in BMD (Table 3).[18] The ability of

© 2003 American Society for Bone and Mineral Research

TABLE 2. DEFINITION OF RISK

Term	Manner used
Absolute risk	Probability
Gradient of risk	Increase in fracture risk per SD decrease in bone mineral density
Population relative risk	Ratio of risk of those with a risk factor compared with the general population of the same age and sex
Probability of fracture	The likelihood of fracture in individuals without fracture over a defined interval (e.g., 10-year hip fracture probability). Computed from the risk of death and risk of first fracture.
Relative risk	Ratio of risk: usually risk in a population with a risk factor compared with those without a risk factor
Remaining lifetime (risk) probability of fracture	Likelihood of a first fracture from a specified age over the remaining lifetime
Risk	A generic term usually shorthand for incidence

BMD to predict fracture is comparable with the use of blood pressure measurements to predict stroke and significantly better than serum cholesterol to predict myocardial infarction. [10,18,19] Accuracy is improved by site-specific measurements (see Table 3), so that for forearm fractures, the risk might ideally be measured at the forearm, and for hip fracture prediction, measurements should be made at the hip. In the immediate postmenopausal population, measurements at any site (hip, spine, or wrist) predict any osteoporotic fracture equally well, with a gradient of risk of approximately 1.5 per SD decrease in BMD.

The highest gradient of risk is found at the hip to predict hip fracture where the gradient of risk is 2.6. Thus, an individual with a T-score of -3 SDs at the hip would have a 2.6,[3] or greater than 15-fold higher risk, than an individual with a T-score of 0 SD. By contrast, the same T-score at the spine would yield much lower risk estimate—approximately a 4-fold increase (1.6).[3] This emphasizes the importance of accuracy or gradient of risk in the categorization of fracture risk.

Despite these performance characteristics, it should be recognized that, just because BMD is normal, there is no guarantee that a fracture will not occur—only that the risk is decreased. Conversely, if BMD is in the osteoporotic range, fractures are more likely but not invariable. At the age of 50 years, the proportion of women with osteoporosis who will fracture their hip, spine, or forearm or proximal humerus in the next 10 years (i.e., positive predictive value) is approximately 45%. The detection rate for these fractures (sensitivity) is, however, low, and 96% of such fractures would occur in women without osteoporosis.[20] The low sensitivity is one of the reasons why widespread population-based screening is not recommended in women at the time of the menopause.

FRACTURE PROBABILITY

Fracture risk is commonly expressed as a relative risk, but this has different meanings in different contexts. In the case of bone density measurements, gradients of risk are used (e.g., a 2.6-fold increase in hip fracture risk for each SD decrease in BMD). For risk factors, risk is commonly expressed as the risk in individuals with a risk factor compared with the risk in those without the risk factor. To combine risks, these risk estimates need to be expressed in a uniform manner (e.g., the risk relative to the population risk). Algorithms are now available for this computation.[20,21] Nevertheless, the use of population relative risks is problematic. For example, at a given BMD, the relative risk of fracture decreases with age (because more of the population has osteoporosis).[21] This is confusing for clinicians because the absolute risk of fractures increases with age. For this and other reasons mentioned below, there has been interest in expressing risk in absolute terms—namely the probability or likelihood of fractures over a given period of time.

The absolute risk of fracture depends on age and life expectancy, as well as the current relative risk. In general, remaining lifetime risk of fracture increases with age up to the age of 70 years or so. Thereafter, probability plateaus and then decreases because the risk of death with age outstrips the increase in incidence of fracture with age. Estimates of lifetime risk are of value in considering the burden of osteoporosis in the community and the effects of intervention strategies. For several reasons, they are less relevant for assessing risk of individuals in whom treatment might be envisaged. First, treatments are not presently given for a lifetime, due variably to side effects of continued treatment (e.g., hormone replacement treatment) or low continuance (most treatments). Moreover, the feasibility of lifelong interventions has never been tested, either using high risk or global strategies. Second, the predictive value of low BMD and some other risk factors for fracture risk is attenuated over time.[22] Finally, the confidence in estimates decreases with time because of the uncertainties concerning future mortality trends.[23] For this reason, the International Osteoporosis Foundation (IOF), NOF, and WHO recommend that risk of fracture should be expressed as a short-term absolute risk (i.e., probability over a 10-year interval).[7] The period of 10 years covers the likely duration of treatment and the benefits that may continue once treatment is stopped.

A further advantage of using absolute fracture probability in risk assessment is that it standardizes the output from the multiple techniques and sites used for the assessment of risk. The estimated probability will of course depend on the

TABLE 3. AGE-ADJUSTED RELATIVE INCREASE IN RISK OF FRACTURE (WITH 95% CI) IN WOMEN FOR EVERY 1 SD DECREASE IN BMD (ABSORPTIOMETRY) BELOW THE MEAN VALUE FOR AGE[18]

Site of measurement	Forearm fracture	Hip fracture	Vertebral fracture	All fractures
Distal radius	1.7 (1.4–2.0)	1.8 (1.4–2.2)	1.7 (1.4–2.1)	1.4 (1.3–1.6)
Femoral neck	1.4 (1.4–1.6)	2.6 (2.0–3.5)	1.8 (1.1–2.7)	1.6 (1.4–1.8)
Lumbar spine	1.5 (1.3–1.8)	1.6 (1.2–2.2)	2.3 (1.9–2.8)	1.5 (1.4–1.7)

TABLE 4. TEN-YEAR PROBABILITY OF CLINICALLY APPARENT SPINE FRACTURE IN SWEDISH MEN AND WOMEN
BY AGE AND T-SCORE AT THE FEMORAL NECK[25]

Age (years)	T-score						
	+1	0	−1	−2.0	−2.5	−3.0	−4.0
Men							
50	0.5	0.9	1.5	2.5	3.2	4.1	6.9
55	0.6	1.0	1.7	2.9	3.8	5.0	8.5
60	0.7	1.1	1.9	3.1	3.9	5.0	8.1
65	0.9	1.4	2.2	3.4	4.2	5.3	8.3
70	1.1	1.8	2.9	4.7	6.0	7.6	12.2
75	1.1	1.9	3.3	5.6	7.2	9.4	15.6
80	1.3	2.1	3.4	5.5	6.9	8.7	13.7
85	1.2	1.9	2.9	4.4	5.4	6.7	10.1
Women							
50	0.4	0.6	1.1	2.0	2.6	3.5	6.1
55	0.4	0.7	1.4	2.5	3.4	4.6	8.3
60	0.6	1.0	1.9	3.4	4.6	6.1	11.0
65	0.8	1.4	2.6	4.7	6.2	8.3	14.6
70	0.8	1.6	2.9	5.5	7.4	10.0	18.0
75	0.7	1.3	2.5	5.0	6.9	9.5	17.9
80	0.7	1.2	2.4	4.6	6.3	8.7	16.1
85	0.6	1.1	2.1	4.0	5.5	7.5	13.6

performance characteristics (e.g., gradient of risk) provided by any technique at any one site. Moreover, it also permits the presence or absence of risk factors other than BMD to be incorporated as a single metric. This is important because there are many risk factors that give information over and above that provided by BMD. The most important of these is age.

AGE AND BMD

The same T-score with the same technique at any one site has a different significance at different ages. Fracture risk is much higher in the elderly than in the young.[24] This is because age contributes to risk independently of BMD. Indeed, from knowledge of the relationship between BMD and fracture risk, it would be predicted that fracture risk might increase 4-fold between the ages of 50 and 80 years. In reality, for hip fracture, the risk increases 30-fold, indicating that over a lifetime, changes in age are approximately 7-fold more important than changes in BMD. This highlights the importance of taking age into account when interpreting information from BMD tests.

At the threshold for osteoporosis (T-score = −2.5 SDs), the 10-year probability of hip fracture ranges from 1.4% to 10.5% in men and women.[25] Any difference in probability between men and women is not marked because the same BMD carries a similar risk in both sexes. The relationship between T-score and spine fracture probability is shown in Table 4.[25] At any given T-score, there is approximately a 2- to 3-fold increase in probability with age between the ages of 50 and 85 years. For any given age, there is approximately a 4- to 5-fold increase in probability between a T-score of 0 and −2.5 SDs. Thus, the consideration of age and BMD together increases the range of risk that can be identified.

CLINICAL RISK FACTORS

A large number of additional risk factors for fracture have been identified. In general, risk scores based on clinical risk factors show relatively poor specificity and sensitivity in predicting either BMD or fracture risk.[26–34] For the purposes of risk assessment, interest lies in those factors that contribute significantly to fracture risk over and above that provided by BMD measurements or age (Table 5), because, as for age and BMD, they enhance a case-finding strategy by increasing the dynamic range of risk stratification. A caveat is that some risk factors are not amenable to particular treatments; therefore, the relationship between absolute probability of fracture and reversible risk is important. Li-

TABLE 5. RISKS FOR OSTEOPOROTIC FRACTURES THAT CAN BE USED IN CASE FINDING

Age*
Premature menopause
Primary or secondary amenorrhea
Primary and secondary hypogonadism in man
Previous fragility fracture*
Glucocorticoid therapy*
Family history of hip fracture*
Low body weight*
Cigarette smoking*
Excessive alcohol consumption
Prolonged immobilization
Secondary causes of osteoporosis
Low BMD (or ultrasound)
High bone turnover*
Poor visual acuity*
Neuromuscular disorders*

* These characteristics capture aspects of fracture risk over and above that provided by BMD.

TABLE 6. RISK OF HIP FRACTURE ASSOCIATED WITH EVER USE OF CORTICOSTEROIDS COMPARED WITH NEVER USE ACCORDING TO AGE, WITH AND WITHOUT ADJUSTMENT FOR BMD[37]

Age (years)	Without BMD		With BMD	
	RR	95% CI	RR	95% CI
50	3.47	0.99–12.21	4.42	1.26–15.49
55	3.47	1.25–9.60	4.15	1.50–11.49
60	3.26	1.47–7.24	3.71	1.67–8.23
65	2.69	1.40–5.16	2.98	1.55–5.74
70	2.22	1.26–3.91	2.44	1.37–4.36
75	2.16	1.37–3.41	2.22	1.35–3.63
80	2.25	1.53–3.30	2.13	1.39–3.27
85	2.42	1.59–3.67	2.48	1.58–3.89

ability to falls is an appropriate example where the risk of fracture is high, but treatment with agents affecting bone metabolism may have little effect on risk. Other risk factors, including a prior fragility fracture and exposure to glucocorticoids, contribute to a risk that is responsive to intervention.[26]

Glucocorticoids are an important cause of osteoporosis and fractures.[35,36] Bone loss is believed to be most rapid in the first few months of treatment, and it affects both axial and appendicular sites. Loss is most marked at the spine, where cancellous bone predominates. The fracture risk conferred by the use of corticosteroids is, however, not solely dependent on bone loss, and BMD-independent risks have been identified.[37] In a recent meta-analysis, the relative risk of hip fracture was increased 2.1- to 4.4-fold, depending on age (Table 6).

Many studies indicate that history of fragility fracture is an important risk factor for further fracture.[38] Fracture risk is approximately doubled in the presence of a prior fracture. The increase in risk is even more marked for a vertebral fracture following a previous spine fracture. For example, the presence of two or more prevalent vertebral fractures was associated with a 12-fold increase in fracture risk for any given BMD.[39] A recent meta-analysis showing risks according to the site of a prior fracture is given in Table 7.[38] These risks are not adjusted for BMD. In general, adjustment for BMD would decrease the relative risk by 10–20%.[5]

TABLE 7. META-ANALYSIS OF THE RISK OF FRACTURE IN WOMEN WITH A PRIOR FRACTURE AT THE SITES SHOWN

Site of prior fracture	Risk of subsequent fracture at			
	Hip	Spine	Forearm	Minor fracture
Hip	2.3	2.5	1.4	1.9
Spine	2.3	4.4	1.4	1.8
Forearm	1.9	1.7	3.3	2.4
Minor fracture	2.0	1.9	1.8	1.9

(Adapted from J Bone Miner Res 2000;**15**:721–739 with permission of the American Society for Bone and Mineral Research.)

TABLE 8. TEN-YEAR PROBABILITY OF FRACTURE IN MEN AND WOMEN FROM SWEDEN ACCORDING TO AGE AND THE RISK (RR) RELATIVE TO THE AVERAGE POPULATION[20]

RR	Age (years)			
	50	60	70	80
Hip fracture				
Men				
1	0.8	1.3	3.7	9.5
2	1.7	2.5	7.2	17.9
3	2.5	3.7	10.6	25.3
4	3.3	4.9	13.8	31.8
Women				
1	0.6	2.4	7.9	18.0
2	1.1	4.8	15.1	32.0
3	1.7	7.0	21.7	42.9
4	2.3	9.3	27.7	51.6
Hip, clinical spine, humeral, or Colles' fracture				
Men				
1	3.3	4.7	7.0	12.6
2	6.5	9.1	13.5	23.1
3	9.6	13.3	19.4	13.9
4	12.6	17.3	24.9	39.3
Women				
1	5.8	9.6	16.1	21.5
2	11.3	18.2	29.4	37.4
3	16.5	26.0	40.0	49.2
4	21.4	33.1	49.5	58.1

BIOCHEMICAL ASSESSMENT OF FRACTURE RISK

Bone markers are increased after menopause, and in several studies, the rate of bone loss varies according to the marker value.[40] Thus, a potential clinical application of biochemical indices of skeletal metabolism is in assessing fracture risk. Prospective studies have shown an association of osteoporotic fracture with indices of bone turnover independent of BMD in women at the time of the menopause and elderly women.[41–43] In elderly women with values for resorption markers exceeding the reference range for premenopausal women, fracture risk is increased approximately 2-fold after adjusting for BMD. These studies suggest that a combined approach using BMD with indices of bone turnover may improve fracture prediction in postmenopausal women.[44]

INTEGRATING RISK FACTORS

How can the combined knowledge of the presence or absence of risk factors, BMD, and age be factored into estimates of fracture probability? The general relationship between relative risk and 10-year probability of hip fracture is shown in Table 8.[20] For example, a woman at the age of 60 years has, on average, a 10-year probability of hip fracture of 2.4% (see Table 8). In the presence of a prior fragility fracture, this risk is increased approximately 2-fold, and the probability increases to 4.8%. The example combines age, sex, and prior fracture history. It is also possible to combine BMD and risk factors. Consider, for example, the same woman aged 60 years, but with a T-score of −2

TABLE 9. TEN-YEAR HIP FRACTURE PROBABILITY (%) ACCORDING TO AGE AND RISK RELATIVE TO THE GENERAL FEMALE POPULATION AT WHICH INTERVENTION IS COST EFFECTIVE[48]

Age (years)	RR	Probability (%)
50	3.9	1.37
55	2.4	2.14
60	1.5	3.18
65	1.0	4.14
70	1.0	5.60*
75	1.0	8.8*
80	1.0	13.0*
85	1.0	17.4*
90	1.0	21.0*

* Ten-year probability of the general population.

SDs. The low BMD gives a 10-year hip fracture probability of 3.4% (see Table 4), but approximately doubles to 6.8% because of a history of a previous fracture. It is also possible to combine population relative risks (i.e., the risk compared with the risk of the general population of the same age and sex). For example, a woman aged 60 years with a T-score of −2.5 SDs has a relative risk of hip fracture of 1.9. In a woman of the same age exposed to corticosteroids, the relative risk is 2.1 adjusted for BMD. The combined relative risk in the presence of both risk factors (osteoporosis plus corticosteroid use) is 4.0 (2.1 × 1.9), corresponding to a 10-year hip fracture probability of 9.3%.

The integration of risk factors is not new and has been successfully applied in the management of coronary heart disease.[45]

There are, however, a number of problems to be resolved before all BMD independent risk factors can be used together. Although corticosteroid treatment confers a risk over and above that afforded by age and BMD, as does a prior fragility fracture, the relationship between corticosteroid use and prior fragility fracture has not yet been explored. Until these interrelationships are established and validated on an international basis, the use of multiple risk factors must be used cautiously.

INTERVENTION THRESHOLDS

Of all osteoporotic fractures, hip fracture confers the greatest morbidity and economic consequences and has been the subject of much research. When hip fracture alone is considered, a 10-year probability of 10% or more provides a cost-effective threshold for women in Sweden.[46] However, many fractures other than hip fracture also contribute to morbidity, particularly in the young, in whom hip fractures are rare. An approach to integrating all osteoporotic fractures is to weight the incidence of osteoporotic fractures at different ages according to their morbidity assessed as disutility (i.e., the cumulative loss in quality of life). For example, in terms of disutility, four vertebral fractures might equate to one hip fracture.[47] When the incidence by age is weighted in this way, the morbidity from osteoporotic fractures at the age of 50 years is approximately 5-fold greater than that caused by hip fracture at this

age. Conversely, at the age of 80 years, the ratio is approximately 1.2. On the assumption that the relationship between morbidity from hip fracture and from other fractures is proportional to the costs of hip fracture and other fractures, intervention thresholds can be established based on cost utility. When account is taken of other fractures, the threshold for hip fracture probability at which interventions become cost effective decreases, particularly in younger individuals (Table 9).[48] Women with a probability of hip fracture above the thresholds given in Table 9 can be offered intervention that is cost effective. These thresholds for intervention correspond to a BMD value that lies between −2 and −3 SDs over all ages (in the absence of other risk factors; Fig. 1).[26] This threshold is (fortuitously perhaps) close to the diagnostic threshold. Thus, intervention can be recommended in individuals with a diagnosis of osteoporosis and with higher BMD in the presence of other independent risk factors.

OPTIMIZATION OF CASE-FINDING STRATEGY

It is evident that the consideration of multiple risk factors improves risk stratification of individuals so that those above a given threshold can be offered treatment. The interrelationship between BMD, age, and other independent risk factors is now established, although the relationship between the clinical risk factors has yet to be formalized.

The value of pharmacologic agents in decreasing fracture risk has been best quantified in those identified based on low BMD. Indeed, for some interventions, treatment of individuals without osteoporosis may yield less in terms of fracture dividends, but in other studies, individuals with osteopenia respond to treatment with the same relative risk reduction.

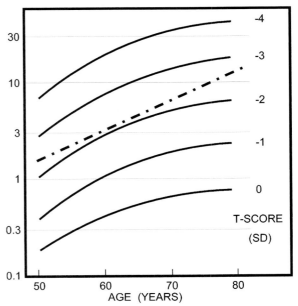

PROBABILITY (%)

FIG. 1. Ten-year probability of hip fracture in Swedish women according to T-scores assessed at the femoral neck by DXA. The diagonal dotted line denotes the probability at which interventions are cost effective.[26]

In this regard, the question arises whether patients identified based on clinical risk factors alone have a risk identified that would be amenable to therapeutic manipulation. Although risk factors such as a prior fragility fracture are "independent" of BMD, they are not totally independent in the sense that patients identified based on fragility fracture do have low BMD. Moreover, patients selected only based on fracture have been shown to respond to therapeutic intervention with bisphosphonates. Thus, individuals selected based on clinical risk factors are likely to have a low BMD. If this assumption is accepted, then the following strategy can be envisaged. The first step is an assessment of fracture probability that is based solely on clinical risk factors. This is expected to identify three groups of individuals. The first are those at very high risk above an intervention threshold in whom a BMD test would not alter their classification. These patients can be offered treatment irrespective of BMD. In practice, BMD might be measured so that response to treatment can be monitored. A second group is comprised of individuals who, based on clinical risk factor assessment, have a very low probability of osteoporotic fracture, so low that the estimate of BMD would not alter their stratification to be above a given level of risk. An intermediate group are those in whom fracture probability is close to an intervention threshold where the probability is high that a BMD test might recategorize individuals at high risk to low risk (or vice versa). The formalization of this approach is not yet complete, but preliminary evidence from a variety of prospectively studied cohorts suggests that a minority of individuals would require a BMD test on this basis.

CONCLUSIONS

The diagnosis of osteoporosis centers on the assessment of BMD at the hip using DXA. However, other sites and validated techniques can be used for fracture prediction. Several clinical risk factors contribute to fracture risk independently of BMD. These include age, prior fragility fracture, premature menopause, a family history of hip fracture, and the use of oral corticosteroids. The use of these risk factors in conjunction with BMD improves sensitivity of fracture prediction without adverse effects on specificity.

In the absence of validated population screening strategies, a case-finding strategy is recommended based on the assessment of fracture probability using clinical risk factors, and where appropriate, additional testing such as BMD. Because of the multiple techniques available for fracture risk assessment and the multiple fracture outcomes, the desirable measurement to determine intervention thresholds is 10-year probability of fracture. Many treatments can be given cost effectively to men and women where hip fracture probability over 10 years ranges from 2% to 20%, depending on age.

REFERENCES

1. Anonymous 1993 Consensus development conference: Diagnosis, prophylaxis and treatment of osteoporosis. Am J Med **94:**646–650.
2. Royal College of Physicians 1999 Clinical Guidelines for the Prevention and Treatment of Osteoporosis. Royal College of Physicians, London, UK.
3. World Health Organisation 1994 Assessment of Fracture Risk and Its Application to Screening for Postmenopausal Osteoporosis. Technical Report Series 843. World Health Organization, Geneva, Switzerland.
4. Kanis JA, Delmas P, Burckhardt P, Cooper C, Torgerson D on behalf of the European Foundation for Osteoporosis and Bone Disease 1997 Guidelines for diagnosis and management of osteoporosis. Osteoporos Int **7:**390–406.
5. National Osteoporosis Foundation 1998 Analyses of the effectiveness and cost of screening and treatment strategies for osteoporosis: A basis for development of practice guidelines. Osteoporos Int **8**(Suppl 4)**:**1–88.
6. Kanis JA, Glüer CC for the Committee of Scientific Advisors, International Osteoporosis Foundation 2000 An update on the diagnosis and assessment of osteoporosis with densitometry. Osteoporos Int **11:**192–202.
7. Kanis JA, Black D, Cooper C, Dargent P, Dawson-Hughes B, De Laet C, Delmas P, Eisman J, Johnell O, Jonsson B, Melton L, Oden A, Papapoulos S, Pols H, Rizzoli R, Silman A, Tenenhouse A, International Osteoporosis Foundation, National Osteoporosis Foundation 2002 A new approach to the development of assessment guidelines for osteoporosis. Osteoporos Int **13:**527–536.
8. Kanis JA, Melton LJ, Christiansen C, Johnston CC, Khaltaev N 1994 The diagnosis of osteoporosis. J Bone Miner Res **9:**17–1141.
9. Committee for Proprietary Medicinal Products (CPMP) 1997 Note for Guidance on Involutional Osteoporosis in Women. European Agency for the Evaluation of Medicinal Products, London, UK.
10. World Health Organisation 1998 Guidelines for Preclinical Evaluation and Clinical Trials in Osteoporosis. World Health Organization, Geneva, Switzerland.
11. Liu Z, Piao J, Pang L, Qing X, Nan S, Pan Z, Guo Y, Wang X, Li F, Liu J, Cheng X 2002 The diagnostic criteria for primary osteoporosis and the incidence of osteoporosis in China. J Bone Miner Metab **20:**181–189.
12. Kanis JA, Johnell O, Oden A, De Laet C, Mellstrom D 2001 Diagnosis of osteoporosis and fracture threshold in men. Calcif Tissue Int **69:**218–221.
13. DeLaet CEDH, Van Hout BA, Burger H, Hofman A, Weel AEAM, Pols HAP 1998 Hip fracture prediction in elderly men and women: Validation in the Rotterdam Study. J Bone Miner Res **13:**1587–1593.
14. Ross P, Huang C, Davis J, Imose K, Yates J, Vogel J, Wasnich R 1995 Predicting vertebral deformity using bone densitometry at various skeletal sites and calcaneous ultrasound. Bone **16:**325–332.
15. Lunt M, Felsenberg D, Reeve J, Benevolenskaya L, Cannata J, Dequeker J 1997 Bone density variation and its effect on risk of vertebral deformity in men and women studied in thirteen European Centres: The EVOS Study. J Bone Miner Res **12:**1883–1894.
16. Faulkner KG, von Stetten E, Miller P 1999 Discordance in patient classification using T-scores. J Clin Densitom **2:**343–350.
17. Arlot ME, Sornay-Rendu E, Garnero P, Vey-Marty B, Delmas PD 1997 Apparent pre- and postmenopausal bone loss evaluated by DXA at different skeletal sites in women: The OFELY cohort. J Bone Miner Res **12:**683–690.
18. Marshall D, Johnell O, Wedel H 1996 Meta-analysis of how well measures of bone mineral density predict occurrence of osteoporotic fractures. BMJ **312:**1254–1259.
19. Cooper C, Aihie A 1994 Osteoporosis: Recent advances in pathogenesis and treatment. Q J Med **87:**203–209.
20. Kanis JA, Johnell O, Oden A, De Laet C, Jonsson B, Dawson A 2001 Ten year risk of osteoporotic fracture and the effect of risk factors on screening strategies. Bone **30:**251–258.
21. Kanis JA, Johnell O, Oden A, Jonsson B, Dawson A, Dere W 2000 Risk of hip fracture in Sweden according to relative risk: An analysis applied to the population of Sweden. Osteoporos Int **11:**120–127.
22. Kanis JA, Johnell O, Oden A, Jonsson B, DeLaet C, Dawson A 2000 Prediction of fracture from low bone mineral density measurements overestimates risk. Bone **26:**387–391.
23. Oden A, Dawson A, Dere W, Johnell O, Jonsson B, Kanis JA 1999 Lifetime risk of hip fracture is underestimated. Osteoporos Int **8:**599–603.
24. Hui SL, Slemenda CW, Johnston CC 1998 Age and bone mass as predictors of fracture in a prospective study. J Clin Invest **81:**1804–1809.
25. Kanis JA, Johnell O, Oden A, Dawson A, De Laet C, Jonsson B 2001 Ten year probabilities of osteoporotic fractures according to BMD and diagnostic thresholds. Osteoporos Int **12:**989–995.
26. Kanis JA 2002 Diagnosis of osteoporosis and assessment of fracture risk. Lancet **359:**1929–1936.
27. Johnell O, Gullberg B, Kanis JA, Allander E, Elffors L, Dequeker J,

Dilsen G, Gennari C, Lopez Vaz A, Lyritis G, Mazzuoli G, Minavet L, Passuri L, Perez-Ceno R, Repado A, Ribut C 1995 Risk factors for hip fracture in European women: The MEDOS Study. J Bone Miner Res **10**:1802–1815.

28. Cummings SR, Nevitt MC, Browner WS, Stone K, Fox KM, Ensrud KE, Cauley J, Black D, Vogt TM 1995 Risk factors for hip fracture in white women. N Engl J Med **332**:767–773.

29. Compston JE 1992 Risk factors for osteoporosis. Clin Endocrinol (Oxf) **36**:223–224.

30. Ribot C, Pouilles JM, Bonneu M, Tremollieres F 1992 Assessment of the risk of postmenopausal osteoporosis using clinical risk factors. Clin Endocrinol (Oxf) **36**:225–228.

31. Kanis J, Johnell O, Gullberg B, Allander E, Elffors L, Ranstam J, Dequeker J, Dilsen G, Gennari C, Vaz AL, Lyritis G, Mazzuoli G, Miravet L, Passeri M, Perez Cano R, Rapado A, Ribot C 1999 Risk factors for hip fracture in men from southern Europe: The MEDOS study. Osteoporos Int **9**:45–54.

32. Nguyen T, Sambrook SP, Kelly P, Jones G, Freund J, Eisman J 1993 Prediction of osteoporotic fractures by postural instability and bone density. BMJ **307**:1111–1115.

33. Poor G, Atkinson EJ, O'Fallon WM, Melton LJ III 1995 Predictors of hip fractures in elderly men. J Bone Miner Res **10**:1900–1907.

34. Kanis JA, McCloskey EV 1996 Evaluation of the risk of hip fracture. Bone **18**(Suppl 3):127–132.

35. Van Staa TP, Leufkens HGM, Abenhaim L, Zhang B, Cooper C 2001 Use of oral corticosteroids and risk of fractures. J Bone Miner Res **15**:993–1000.

36. Van Staa TP, Leufkens HGM, Cooper C 2002 The epidemiology of corticosteroid-induced osteoporosis: A meta-analysis. Osteoporos Int **13**:777–787.

37. Johnell O, De Laet C, Oden A, Johansson H, Melton LJ, Eisman J, Reeve J, Tenenhouse A, McCloskey EV, Kanis JA 2001 Oral corticosteroids increase fracture risk independently of BMD. Osteoporos Int **13**(Suppl 1):S13.

38. Klotzbuecher CM, Ross PD, Landsman PB, Abbot TA, Berger M 2000 Patients with prior fractures have increased risk of future fractures: A summary of the literature and statistical synthesis. J Bone Miner Res **15**:721–739.

39. Ross PD, Genant HK, Davis JW, Miller PD, Wasnich RD 1993 Predicting vertebral fracture incidence from prevalent fractures and bone density among non black, osteoporotic women. Osteoporos Int **3**:120–126.

40. Delmas PD 2000 The use of biochemical markers of bone turnover in the management of post-menopausal osteoporosis. Osteoporos Int **11**(Suppl 6):S1–S76.

41. Garnero P, Sornay-Rendu E, Claustrat B, Delmas PD 2000 Biochemical markers of bone turnover, endogenous hormones and the risk of fractures in postmenopausal women. The Ofely study. J Bone Miner Res **15**:1526–1536.

42. Garnero P, Hauser E, Chapuy MC, Marcelli C, Grandjean H, Muller C, Cormier C, Breard G, Meunier PJ, Delmas PD 1996 Markers of bone turnover predict hip fractures in elderly women. The EPIDOS prospective study. J Bone Miner Res **11**:1531–1538.

43. Hansen M, Overgaard K, Riis B, Christiansen C 1991 Role of peak bone mass and bone loss in postmenopausal osteoporosis: 12 year study. BMJ **303**:961–964.

44. Johnell O, Oden A, DeLaet C, Garnero P, Delmas PD, Kanis JA 2002 Biochemical indices of bone turnover and the assessment of fracture probability. Osteoporos Int **13**:523–526.

45. Dyslipidaemia Advisory Group on behalf of the Scientific Committee of the National Heart Foundation of New Zealand 1996 National Heart Foundation clinical guidelines for the assessment and management of dyslipidaemia. N Z Med J **109**:224–232.

46. Kanis JA, Dawson A, Oden A, Johnell O, De Laet C, Jonsson B 2001 Cost-effectiveness of preventing hip fracture in the general female population. Osteoporos Int **12**:356–361.

47. Kanis JA, Oden A, Johnell O, Jonsson B, De Laet C, Dawson A 2001 The burden of osteoporotic fractures: A method for setting intervention thresholds. Osteoporos Int **12**:417–427.

48. Kanis JA, Johnell O, Oden A, De Laet C, Oglesby A, Jonsson B 2002 Intervention thresholds for osteoporosis. Bone **13**:26–31.

Chapter 52. Role of Physical Activity in the Regulation and Maintenance of Bone

Everett L. Smith

Department of Population Health Sciences, University of Wisconsin-Madison, Madison, Wisconsin

INTRODUCTION

Osteoporosis is a major public health crisis in the elderly, manifested by the presence of low bone mineral content (BMC), decreased skeletal integrity, and an increased risk of fractures. Physical activity has been shown to be a contributor in the prevention and maintenance of skeletal integrity and thus a factor in the strategy to reduce fractures in later life. While skeletal development is clearly under genetic control,[1] diet and physical activity have been shown to significantly influence bone growth and development. Although the effect of mechanical loading on bone has long been acknowledged, only in the past two decades have the cellular mechanisms by which it affects BMC, structural characteristics and strength, been extensively investigated. While the cellular control mechanisms are not yet completely defined, the response of bone cells and thus skeletal structure have now been sufficiently delineated, so that physical activity may be dosed with reasonable certainty and the loaded skeletal segment will respond.

Both cross-sectional and longitudinal investigations in which the level and type of physical activity has been well documented show a positive effect of physical activity. Numerous studies have shown an increase in bone mineral density (BMD) or reduction of bone loss in both humans[2,3] and animals[4] with exercise or mechanical loading of sufficient intensity. Animal studies have demonstrated loading thresholds and an increased bone mass proportional to the applied load.[5–7] Mechanical loading stimulated transformation of lining cells to osteoblasts[8,9] and changes in the levels of c-*fos* and mRNA, indicative of increased cell metabolism and proliferation[10] and an increased level of prostaglandin production proportional to the load.[7,11,12]

Physical activity as a loading mechanism in the skeleton is critical in the strategies to reduce the incidence of osteoporosis in the elderly. These strategies include (1) growing a larger skeleton, (2) maintaining a strong skeleton into

---

The author has no conflict of interest.

maturity and old age, and (3) minimizing bone loss after the age of 50 and menopause.

GROWING A LARGER SKELETON DURING CHILDHOOD

The risk of developing osteoporosis may be initiated during childhood when the full skeletal development (peak bone mass) is inhibited by poor diet and inactivity. If this is true, a clearly defined quality physical activity and dietary program for children should enhance skeletal development. Fuchs et al.[13] conducted a 7-month physical activity program where 89 prepubescent children age 5.9–9.8 years were randomized into jumping (25 boys and 20 girls) and control groups (26 boys and 18 girls). Those in the jumping group participated in a 3 day per week program of 100 jumps off of a 61-cm-high step, while the control group participated in a stretching program. The two-foot landing of the jump group induced a ground reaction force of about eight times body weight. There was no difference between the control and jumping groups in anthropometric characteristics before or after the 7-month program. However, the jumping group significantly increased ($p = 0.001$) their BMC by 4.5% at the femur neck and 3.1% at the lumbar spine compared with controls. A 14-month follow-up measurement with no jumping showed that the jumpers continued to have a 4% greater BMC at the femur neck but showed no difference from the controls at the lumbar spine. Singh et al.,[14] using growing rats trained to jump to an elevated platform 40 times a day for 4 weeks, showed a significant increase in periosteal diameter, which was maintained after stopping the jumping program for 4 weeks.

Increased bone formation in the humerus was observed in competitive tennis players. Kontulainen et al.[15] divided 64 nationally ranked competitive racquet-sports players into those who started playing premenarche and those that had started 1 year after menarche. Those that had started premenarche showed a greater BMC in the loaded humerus than in the nonloaded humerus (19.6%), whereas those that started postmenarche showed a smaller difference (9.4%). Bass et al.[16] measured BMC in the loaded and nonloaded arms of 47 competitive female tennis players ages 8–17 years. The humerus was 11–14% greater in the loaded arm compared with the nonloaded arm. In addition to the greater differences in bone mass in the younger-starting subjects, Bass et al.[16] and Kontulainen et al.[15] observed different patterns of humeral response in those women who started before or after puberty. The subjects who started at the younger ages had a greater diameter resulting in an increased BMC, whereas those who started after puberty tended to have bone mass increases as the result of endocortical formation. The periosteal growth potentially results in a lifelong larger skeleton providing greater resistance to fracture and periosteal remodeling.

GROWING A STRONGER SKELETON

Bone strength depends on four major components: BMC, geometric structure at the macro- and microarchitectural levels, quality of tissue, and level of microdamage. Strength is affected by the relative proportions and geometric organization of the organic and inorganic components of bone. The quantity of inorganic substance or BMC or BMD has frequently been used as a surrogate for bone strength.[17] Those persons with values greater than 1.4 g/cm^2 for the spine and hip have a fracture prevalence of only about 1% per 1000 person-years. If BMD is less than 0.6, fracture prevalence is about 55% per 1000 person-years for the spine and about 18% for the hip.[18] However, there is a large overlap between those with and without fractures. Absorptiometry does not take into account microarchitectural changes or the quality of bone tissue, both of which are significant components of bone strength.[19,20]

Mechanical loading improves bone quality and quantity. Smith and Gilligan[21] investigated the impact of exercise and diet on 1-year-old hens. The hens were randomly assigned to either an exercise group that jogged on a motor-driven treadmill at 7 mph 5 days a week for 5 weeks or to a sedentary group. The hens were further divided within each group to normal or half-normal dietary calcium. BMC was measured by single photon absorptiometry at baseline and at 5 and 8 weeks. At the end of 5 weeks, the hens in the low calcium group had significantly lower BMC than did those on the normal calcium diet. All hens were returned to a normal calcium diet for 3 weeks before death. No significant difference in BMC was observed between the groups at the end of the 8-week study. In contrast to BMC, the ultimate breaking strength of the tibia was 12–14% greater in the exercised hens than in the nonexercising hens. Smith hypothesized that geometric structure, microarchitecture, and collagen fiber organization were different between the sedentary and exercised hens, resulting in a bone more resistant to fracture. Robling et al.[22] demonstrated a greater increase in ultimate strength than BMC in response to exercise. The right ulnas of female rats were subjected to 360 loading cycles per day (either as one uninterrupted bout or four bouts of 90 cycles each). The loaded bones had greater biomechanical measures of resistance to fracture (e.g., 64–87% in ultimate force) but only a 5–12% increase in BMC. Geometric changes on the medial and lateral sections of the ulna were observed, placing new mineral content at the critical areas of the bone, resulting in greater strength with minimal BMC changes. The explanation for minimal increases in BMC induced by physical activity may relate to the fact that physical activity increases strength first by internal architectural change and then by adding BMC. If results from exercising animals are projected to the human model, it may indicate that for each percentage increase of BMC induced by physical activity, there would be a 7–12% increase in strength. This increase in skeletal strength caused by physical activity may explain why there is an overlap between fracture and nonfracture subjects with similar BMC. Increased skeletal strength induced by exercise can be contrasted with the differential response in strength induced with a parathyroid hormone intervention by Sato et al.,[23] in which they observed a 36% increase in BMC and an increase in strength of 50%. Although both Robling et al. with loading and Sato et al. with parathyroid hormone achieved an increase in BMC, the resultant strength per unit of BMC was greater in the loaded animals. The increased strength in the loaded bone was a result of bone formation along the lines of strain and was site specific, whereas the increase in strength with parathyroid hormone was the result of a general bone formation. Srinivasan et al.,[24] using the same wave form and load intensity at varied intervals, found that mechanical loads applied once per second for 100 cycles per day was less osteogenic than the same load intensity applied 10 times over the same 100 s but with a 10-s rest period between loads in a tibia mouse model. These experiments indicate that the bone becomes desensitized even within 100 cycles, and the maximal response for a given load may be obtained in shorter loading cycles with a rest period between cycles. Srinivasan et al.[24] also used an avian ulna model and found that inserting rest periods between each load cycle significantly enhanced periosteal response (22% labeled surface) compared with continuous cycles (3.8% versus 1.6% in controls). These load cycle results confirm the earlier work of Rubin and Lanyon,[25] suggesting that bone becomes desensitized, with no further response by increasing the number from 36 to 1800 consecutive cycles at 1 Hz.

New horizons in mechanical stimulation of bone have been introduced by Rubin et al., in which high frequencies in the 30-Hz range with a very low-level strain (0.3 g) have introduced an increase in trabecular bone. There were not, however, significant cortical increases. Coupled with the load experiments using a 10-s pause and the significance of Rubin et al.[26] high hertz low load, new opportunities are now open to design osteoporosis-specific physical activity protocols to stimulate bone cell formation along the lines of strain thus reducing fracture risk with minimal therapeutic risk in older subjects.

SKELETAL STRENGTH AND MAINTAINENCE AFTER PEAK MATURITY

"Use it or lose it" applies to all aspects of the human body—the mind, muscle, and cardiovascular and skeletal systems. If one is put on bed rest or reduces physical activity, every system will decline in function and increase in weakness.[27,28] Numerous cross-sectional studies have shown that those persons that maintain physical activity over their lifespan also maintain a higher BMC and reduced risk of fracture. Feskanich et al.,[29] using the Nurses Health Study Cohort of registered nurses in 11 states of the United States, studied the relationship of walking with hip fracture in postmenopausal women ages 40–77 years. The total population of 61,200 was evaluated for total hours spent walking, and those that walked at least 4 h/wk had a 41% lower risk of hip fracture. Feskanich et al. [29] concluded that moderate levels of activity such as walking are associated with substantially lower risk of hip fracture in postmenopausal women. Wiswell et al.[30] concluded that hip and spine BMD are maintained in 40- to 80-year-old master runners, even with moderate decreases in training. They suggested that the minimal threshold of mileage for bone maintenance was below the average mileage of these runners.

Smith et al.[31] showed that physical activity can increase BMC even at a very late age. Women in a nursing home (mean age, 81 years) who participated in a chair exercise

program for 36 months, 3 days per week, increased BMC of the radius by 3.29%, whereas the control group lost 2.29%. Similarly, Jessup et al.[32] found that training of older women (mean age, 69 years) for 32 weeks improved not only BMD of the femoral neck but also improved sense of balance. The exercise group participated in three sessions/week of supervised strength training and walking, stair climbing and balance exercises for 32 weeks. Both exercise and control groups were provided calcium and vitamin D. The studies support the concept that physical activity in a mature person will assist in skeletal maintenance, while physical activity in early children will permit the development of a larger skeleton.

SKELETAL INTEGRITY COMPROMISED

The skeleton's integrity can be compromised by over- or underuse, such as in basic training of military recruits or athletic training, or inactivity at any age, bed rest, or loss of gravity in space travel. A number of researchers[33,34] have reported a high level of stress fracture (4–14%) in male and female military recruits during basic training. It was determined that those with a history of regular exercise and greater muscular strength had a lower risk of fracture, suggesting the importance of regular physical activity before starting an intense training program.

Highly competitive female athletes have an associated increase in the prevalence of exercise amenorrhea and oligomenorrhea[35,36] and a lower BMC at the hip and spine compared with matched controls for age, height, and weight. The implication is that the estrogen deficiency induced by exercise caused an increased bone turnover and modulated the loading threshold,[37] resulting in a lower BMC. Robinson et al.[38] compared the impact of estrogen deficiency on BMC at the hip and spine, in college runners, gymnasts, and controls. The presence of amenorrhea and oligomenorrhea in the runners was 30%, in the gymnasts 47%, and in the controls 0%. When Robinson et al.[38] adjusted for estimated bone size, lumbar spine, and femoral neck, the apparent bone mineral densities were highest in the gymnasts and lowest in the runners. Robinson concluded that, although the gymnasts had a greater incidence of amenorrhea and oligomenorrhea, their greater BMC with high impact loading in gymnastic participation had a greater osteogenic effect than the increased resorption induced by amenorrhea. It is clear from the articles reviewed that the type of loading is important in skeletal response to loading. Bone cells lose sensitivity after 100 cycles. However, runners often train at three to five times body weight at about 1 or 2 Hz for 3600–5400 cycles per exercise bout using the same load pattern. If the bone only responds to the first 100 cycles, the osteogenic stimulus is not as strong as the resorptive stimuli from estrogen deficiency. While the gymnasts are equally estrogen deficient, their bone loading pattern is 10–14 times body weight performed at about 1–2 Hz over 60–90 cycles with a rest period between loading sequences. This regimen seems to maximize the osteogenic stimuli, having a positive formation balance over the estrogen deficiency resorptive stimuli.[39]

Bed rest can cause devastating atrophy of trabecular and

cortical bone.[27] Os calcis BMC declined 25–45% during 18–24 weeks of bed rest, with a slower rate but still significant loss in nonweight bearing bones,[40] and spine bone mineral declined 1–2% per week in patients hospitalized for scoliosis surgery.[41,42] LeBlanc et al.[28] reported that total body, lumbar spine, femoral neck, trochanter, tibia, and calcaneus BMD declined significantly with 17 weeks of bed rest and that only the calcaneus rebounded significantly within 6 months of reambulation.

The skeleton is a dynamic tissue well suited for the balance between its multiple functions of mechanical support, protection, and mineral reservoir. Hormonal homeostasis is clearly defined in the maintenance of blood chemistry from organ of origin to cell receptor. The homeostasis of bone response to mechanical loading as a cause and effect relationship is on the threshold of emergence in the maintenance of skeletal integrity. The most effective strategies for the future will be the merger of physical activity and drug therapy to eliminate osteoporosis by maximizing peak skeletal development at maturity and then maintaining skeletal integrity throughout the life span.

REFERENCES

1. Rubin LA, Hawker GA, Peltekova VD, Fielding LJ, Ridout R, Cole DE 1999 Determinants of peak bone mass: Clinical and genetic analyses in a young female Canadian cohort. J Bone Miner Res 14:633–643.
2. Dalsky GP, Stocke KS, Ehsani AA, Slatopolsky E, Lee WC, Birge SJ Jr 1988 Weight-bearing exercise training and lumbar bone mineral content in postmenopausal women. Ann Intern Med 108:824–828.
3. Smith EL, Gilligan C, McAdam M, Ensign CP, Smith PE 1989 Deterring bone loss by exercise intervention in premenopausal and postmenopausal women. Calcif Tissue Int 44:312–321.
4. Raab DM, Crenshaw TD, Kimmel DB, Smith EL 1991 A histomorphometric study of cortical bone activity during increased weight-bearing exercise. J Bone Miner Res 6:741–749.
5. Rubin CT, Lanyon LE 1985 Regulation of bone mass by mechanical strain magnitude. Calcif Tissue Int 37:411–417.
6. Turner CH, Forwood MR, Rho JY, Yoshikawa T 1994 Mechanical loading thresholds for lamellar and woven bone formation. J Bone Miner Res 9:87–97.
7. Raab-Cullen DM, Akhter MP, Kimmel DB, Recker RR 1994 Periosteal bone formation stimulated by externally induced bending strains. J Bone Miner Res 9:1143–1152.
8. Pead MJ, Suswillo R, Skerry TM, Vedi S, Lanyon LE 1988 Increased 3H-uridine levels in osteocytes following a single short period of dynamic bone loading in vivo. Calcif Tissue Int 43:92–96.
9. Boppart MD, Kimmel DB, Yee JA, Cullen DM 1998 Time course of osteoblast appearance after in vivo mechanical loading. Bone 23:409–415.
10. Raab-Cullen DM, Thiede MA, Petersen DN, Kimmel DB, Recker RR 1994 Mechanical loading stimulates rapid changes in periosteal gene expression. Calcif Tissue Int 55:473–478.
11. Jones DB, Nolte H, Scholubbers JG, Turner E, Veltel D 1991 Biochemical signal transduction of mechanical strain in osteoblast-like cells. Biomaterials 12:101–110.
12. Reich KM, Frangos JA 1993 Protein kinase C mediates flow-induced prostaglandin E2 production in osteoblasts. Calcif Tissue Int 52:62–66.
13. Fuchs RK, Bauer JJ, Snow CM 2001 Jumping improves hip and lumbar spine bone mass in prepubescent children: A randomized controlled trial. J Bone Miner Res 16:148–156.
14. Singh R, Umemura Y, Honda A, Nagasawa S 2002 Maintenance of bone mass and mechanical properties after short-term cessation of high impact exercise in rats. Int J Sports Med 23:77–81.
15. Kontulainen S, Sievanen H, Kannus P, Pasanen M, Vuori I 2002 Effect of long-term impact-loading on mass, size, and estimated strength of humerus and radius of female racquet-sports players: A peripheral quantitative computed tomography study between young and old starters and controls. J Bone Miner Res 17:2281–2289.
16. Bass SL, Saxon L, Daly RM, Turner CH, Robling AG, Seeman E, Stuckey S 2002 The effect of mechanical loading on the size and shape of bone in pre-, peri-, and postpubertal girls: A study in tennis players. J Bone Miner Res 17:2274–2280.
17. Turner CH, Robling AG 2003 Designing exercise regimens to increase bone strength. Exerc Sport Sci Rev 31:45–50.
18. Riggs BL, Melton LJ III 1986 Involutional osteoporosis. N Eng J Med 314:1676–1686.
19. Recker RR 1989 Low bone mass may not be the only cause of skeletal fragility in osteoporosis. Proc Soc Exper Biol Med 191:272–274.
20. Recker RR 1993 Architecture and vertebral fracture. Calcif Tissue Int 53(Suppl 1):S139–S142.
21. Smith EL, Gilligan C 1996 Dose-response relationship between physical loading and mechanical competence of bone. Bone 18(Suppl 1):455–505.
22. Robling AG, Hinant FM, Burr DB, Turner CH 2002 Shorter, more frequent mechanical loading sessions enhance bone mass. Med Sci Sports Exerc 34:196–202.
23. Sato M, Zeng GQ, Turner CH 1997 Biosynthetic human parathyroid hormone (1–34) effects on bone quality in aged ovariectomized rats. Endocrinology 138:4330–4337.
24. Srinivasan S, Weimer DA, Agans SC, Bain SD, Gross TS 2002 Low-magnitude mechanical loading becomes osteogenic when rest is inserted between each load cycle. J Bone Miner Res 17:1613–1620.
25. Rubin CT, Lanyon LE 1984 Regulation of bone formation by applied dynamic loads. J Bone Joint Surg Am 66:397–402.
26. Rubin C, Turner AS, Bain S, Mallinckrodt C, McLeod K 2001 Anabolism. Low mechanical signals strengthen long bones. Nature 412:603–604.
27. Bloomfield SA 1997 Changes in musculoskeletal structure and function with prolonged bed rest. Med Sci Sports Exerc 29:197–206.
28. LeBlanc A, Marsh C, Evans H, Johnson P, Schneider V, Jhingran S 1985 Bone and muscle atrophy with suspension of the rat. J Appl Physiol 58:1669–1675.
29. Feskanich D, Willett W, Colditz G 2002 Walking and leisure-time activity and risk of hip fracture in postmenopausal women. JAMA 288:2300–2306.
30. Wiswell RA, Hawkins SA, Dreyer HC, Jaque SV 2002 Maintenance of BMD in older male runners is independent of changes in training volume or VO(2)peak. J Gerontol A Biol Sci Med Sci 57:M203–M208.
31. Smith EL Jr, Reddan W, Smith PE 1981 Physical activity and calcium modalities for bone mineral increase in aged women. Med Sci Sports Exerc 13:60–64.
32. Jessup JV, Horne C, Vishen RK, Wheeler D 2003 Effects of exercise on bone density, balance, and self-efficacy in older women. Biol Res Nurs 4:171–180.
33. Beck TJ, Ruff CB, Shaffer RA, Betsinger K, Trone DW, Brodine SK 2000 Stress fracture in military recruits: Gender differences in muscle and bone susceptibility factors. Bone 27:437–444.
34. Lappe JM, Stegman MR, Recker RR 2001 The impact of lifestyle factors on stress fractures in female Army recruits. Osteoporos Int 12:35–42.
35. Drinkwater BL, Bruemner B, Chesnut CH III 1990 Menstrual history as a determinant of current bone density in young athletes. JAMA 263:545–548.
36. Marcus R, Cann C, Madvig P, Minkoff J, Goddard M, Bayer M, Martin M, Gaudiani L, Haskell W, Genant H 1985 Menstrual function and bone mass in elite women distance runners. Endocrine and metabolic features. Ann Intern Med 102:158–163.
37. Frost HM 1999 On the estrogen-bone relationship and postmenopausal bone loss: A new model. J Bone Miner Res 14:1473–1477.
38. Robinson TL, Snow-Harter C, Taaffe DR, Gillis D, Shaw J, Marcus R 1995 Gymnasts exhibit higher bone mass than runners despite similar prevalence of amenorrhea and oligomenorrhea. J Bone Miner Res 10:26–35.
39. Helge EW, Kanstrup IL 2002 Bone density in female elite gymnasts: Impact of muscle strength and sex hormones. Med Sci Sports Exerc 34:174–180.
40. Hulley SB, Vogel JM, Donaldson CL, Bayers JH, Friedman RJ, Rosen SN 1971 The effect of supplemental oral phosphate on the bone mineral changes during prolonged bed rest. J Clin Invest 50:2506–2518.
41. Krolner B, Toft B 1983 Vertebral bone loss: An unheeded side effect of therapeutic bed rest. Clin Sci 64:537–540.
42. Hansson TH, Roos BO, Nachemson A 1975 Development of osteopenia in the fourth lumbar vertebra during prolonged bed rest after operation for scoliosis. Acta Orthop Scand 46:621–630.

Chapter 53.   Effect of Estrogen on Bone

J. Christopher Gallagher

Creighton University Medical Center, Bone Metabolism Unit, Omaha, Nebraska

PATHOGENESIS OF MENOPAUSAL BONE LOSS

Recent advances in basic bone biology have shown that estrogen deficiency is associated with an increase in the monocyte secretion of cytokines interleukin (IL)-1, IL-6, and TNF macrophage colony stimulating factor (M-CSI).[1] Marrow stromal cells also secrete more of the cytokines IL-I, IL-6, M-CSF, and granulocyte M-CSF (GM-CSF), together with an important cytokine RANK ligand. The increased cytokine activity results in the recruitment and activation of more osteoclasts and a decrease in osteoprotegerin (OPG), which acts as a decoy receptor for RANKL. OPG is a very potent antiresorptive agent. The result of all the increased cytokine activity is increased bone resorption. Estrogen treatment reverses this process within 4 weeks.

ESTROGEN DEFICIENCY AND BONE MASS

The main impact of estrogen deficiency is on trabecular bone of the skeleton. Because trabecular bone has a much larger surface area than cortical bone, there is a more rapid (7-fold) decrease in trabecular bone than cortical bone as demonstrated by quantitative computerized tomography measurements. The difference between cortical and trabecular bone loss is only two to three times less using DXA because this test measures both types of bone at the same time. Apart from menopause, any disease, illness, or factor that produces estrogen deficiency will cause bone loss. Common examples are amenorrhea from eating disorders, excess athletic activity, chemotherapy, or drugs such as gonadotrophin releasing hormone (GnRH) agonists for the treatment of endometriosis and medroxyprogesternine acetate (Depo-Provera) for birth control. Some women have fewer menstrual cycles each year associated with hypoestrogenicity and have lower bone density. Some of these causes of estrogen deficiency are transient, and bone density recovers after withdrawal of therapy. The average age of menopause is around 51 years of age, so menopause before this age causes menopausal bone loss earlier. This is especially important in women who have early menopause. It has been estimated that early menopause—before age 40 years—occurs in 0.9% of women (400,000 women) annually.[2]

For example, a woman who has menopause at the age of 37 years will have bone loss advanced 14 years compared with an average woman. By the time that person reaches 51 years of age, her bone density will be equivalent to a 65-year-old woman who underwent menopause at the average time. A study of women who had early menopause (between 33 and 43 years of age) were shown to have a bone mineral density (BMD) that was 1.0 T-score (approximately 12–14%) lower compared with women of similar age who had menopause at the normal age of 51 years.[3]

DIAGNOSIS OF OSTEOPOROSIS IN THE POSTMENOPAUSAL WOMAN

As bone loss continues after menopause and with aging, the decrease in bone mass or bone density starts to become more critical in leading to fractures. Forearm fractures are the first manifestation of postmenopausal bone loss, and their incidence peaks in the fifth decade. The World Health Organization produced criteria for categorizing the severity of different levels of BMD (Table 1).[4]

In support of these recommendations, a recent prospective study of about 200,000 women[5] showed a direct correlation between the baseline BMD T-score at any peripheral bone site and the incident fracture rate. Using a T-score of −1.0 as reference, women with T-scores of −2.0 to −2.5 had fracture rates 2.5 times higher, T-scores of −2.5 to −3.0 had fracture rates 3 times higher, and T-scores of −3.0 to −3.5 had a 4-fold higher fracture rate. This study provides strong evidence that peripheral measurements predict future fracture risk, although the false positive and negative rates for these tests are about 30%.

The National Osteoporosis Foundation[6] has suggested the following guidelines for postmenopausal women.

1. Counsel all women on risk factors for osteoporosis.
2. Perform BMD tests on all postmenopausal women with one or more risk factors.
3. Perform BMD tests on all women older than 65 years of age.
4. Consider treatment if the T-score is below −2.0 or below −1.5 with risk factors.

Common risk factors for postmenopausal osteoporosis are female gender; early menopause; history of fracture as an adult; white, Asian, or Hispanic ethnicities; osteoporosis in a first-degree relative; low body weight (<127 lbs); poor health/frailty or recurrent falls; and certain lifestyle factors—high caffeine intake (~300 mg/day; three cups coffee/day), cigarette smoking, low calcium intake (<800 mg/day), and low physical activity.

PREVENTION OF BONE LOSS WITH ESTROGEN THERAPY OR HORMONE THERAPY

Effect on BMD

A recent meta analysis of all estrogen therapy (ET) and hormone (HT) trials performed up to 1999 included 57

TABLE 1. WHO CRITERIA FOR DIAGNOSIS OF BONE STATUS

T-score	Classification
Above 1.0	Normal
−1.0 to −2.5	Osteopenia or low bone mass
Below −2.5	Osteoporosis
Below −2.5 + fractures	Severe osteoporosis

Dr. Gallagher has received grants, served as a consultant, and been a speaker for Pfizer, Orgaron, and Wyeth.

trials: 31 blinded and 26 open studies.[7] There were 70 dose groups, about one-half being Premarin 0.625 mg or oral Estradiol (Wyeth Pharmaceuticals) 2 mg. Approximately 10,000 women were included in these trials.

The weighted mean increase in bone density in HT/ET-treated women compared with the placebo group was 5.5% (spine), 3.0% (forearm), and 2.5% (femoral neck) after year 1 and 6.8% (spine), 4.5% (forearm), and 4.1% (femoral neck) after year 2.

Effect of ET/HT in Osteoporosis Prevention or Treatment Trials

There was no difference in the response to ET/HT. The mean increase in BMD at 1 year in the prevention studies was 4.9% (spine), 3.0% (forearm), and 2.4% (femoral neck), whereas in treatment trials, the change was 7.7% (spine), 3.3% (forearm), and 3.5% (femoral neck); these were not significantly different. After 2 years of treatment, the mean increase in BMD in the prevention studies was 6.9% (spine), 4.5% (forearm), and 4.0% (femoral neck) compared with 5.65% (spine), forearm (not available), and 4.7% (femoral neck).

Analysis of the different doses of ET/HT shows a difference in the BMD response on low-dose estrogen (equivalent to Premarin 0.3 mg) compared with high dose (equivalent to 0.9 mg Premarin). The mean increase in BMD on low dose HT/ET compared with placebo was 3.9% (spine), 3.1% (forearm), and 2% (femoral neck), whereas the increase in BMD on high dose compared with placebo was 8.0% (spine), 4.5% (forearm), and 4.7% (femoral neck).

Since that meta-analysis, there have been another 12 double-blind placebo-controlled randomized trials that add about another 4000 patients for analysis. Most trials lasted 2 years, although some were 3 years. In the HT trials, women were between the ages of 45 and 60 years. Most were within 5 years of menopause, some were hysterectomized; otherwise, progestins were added.[8–15] There were three ET-only trials.[16–18]

In general, the increase in spine BMD relative to placebo was similar to that reported in the meta-analysis. The mean increase on all doses was 6.1% (spine), 3.5% (total hip), and 3.5% (femoral neck) after 2 years.

Effect of Estrogen in Older Women

There have been two double-blind randomized placebo-controlled studies of bone in women in their seventh decade that used Premarin 0.625 mg.[19,20] In the former study of 489 elderly women, there was an increase of 6% in spine BMD, 5% in total hip BMD, and 4% in femoral neck BMD compared with placebo. In the latter study of 143 women,[20] Premarin 0.625 mg increased spine BMD by 6.6%, femoral neck BMD by 3.2%, and total hip BMD by 3.1% compared with placebo. In the same study, another group randomized to alendronate 10 mg showed identical changes to that of Premarin in BMD, and in those 140 women, the increase in spine BMD of 8.3% was significantly higher.

In a double-blind placebo-controlled study of 125 elderly women, a lower dose of Premarin 0.3 mg plus calcium and 25-hydroxyvitamin D showed a significant increase in spine

BMD of 3.5% compared with −0.35% on calcium/vitamin D. There was no significant treatment difference in femoral neck BMD.[21]

Effect of ET/HT on Bone Markers

In three transdermal studies with variable doses,[8,9,18] urine C-telopeptides (CTx) showed a dose-related decline at 2 years. In the first two studies, the decrease in urine CTx was about 40% on 25 μg and 45% on 50 μg; the decrease in the higher doses was similar, 65% on 75 μg and 67% on 100 μg. There was no difference in spine BMD between 75- and 100-μg doses either. In the other study,[18] there was a similar decrease in urine CTx by about 50% on 50 μg and 50% on 100 μg transdermal estradiol. Serum osteocalcin also showed a good dose response on ET/HT: a decrease of about 10% on 25 μg, 30% on 50 μg, 40% on 75 μg, and 45% on 100 μg. The third study,[18] using a different method, showed a decline of 15% on 50 μg and 30% on 100 μg. In a dose-ranging study of Premarin, serum osteocalcin showed a decrease of about 20% on 0.3 mg, 32% on 0.45 mg, and 32% on 0.625 mg. Urine N telopeptides (NTx) decreased about 40% on 0.3 mg, 48% on 0.45 mg, and 49% on 0.625 mg. Bone markers did not discriminate between 0.45- and 0.625-mg doses; however, spine BMD showed a clearer dose response.

Dose Response of ET/HT on the Spine

Evaluation of the response of spine BMD to the estrogen dose is complicated in many studies by the addition of a progestin, which is known to have a additive effect to that of ET on BMD.

Transdermal Estrogens. Five of the studies used transdermal estradiol either alone[13,16,17] or transdermal estradiol with dydrogesterone if the women had a uterus.[8,9] The average increase in spine BMD compared with placebo was 7.6% on 100 mg, 7.3% on 75 mg, 6.3% on 50 mg, and 3.9% on 25 mg.

Oral ET/HT. There are three studies of 17β-estradiol, 1- and 2-mg doses, in combination with a progestin.[10,12,13,22] The increase in spine density on 1 mg compared with placebo was 6.5%, and on 2 mg was 7.5%. There has been only one new study on conjugated equine estrogens (CEE; Premarin).[14] It was a study of 822 women who had a mean age of 52 years and who were 3 years past menopause. There were seven treatment groups and one placebo group. There were three unopposed estrogen doses of Premarin 0.3, 0.45, and 0.625 mg and four opposed doses using medroxyprogesterone acetate (MPA), and the study lasted 2 years. In the groups on 0.625 CEE, there was a dose response on spine BMD. Compared with placebo, spine BMD on the 0.625-mg dose was 4.9% higher, on 0.45 mg CEE, it was 4.5% higher, and on 0.3 mg, it was 3.8% higher. On combination with MPA, spine BMD in all groups was significantly higher by about 1%.

Dose Response on the Hip. ET (Premarin) increased total hip BMD 3–3.5% and HT (Premarin + MPA) increased it

2.5–3.7% above placebo. ET (Premarin) increased femoral neck BMD 3.5–3.6% and the HT (Premarin + MPA) increased femoral neck BMD 1.5–3.5% above placebo.

Examination of all the responses in spine BMD to ET/HT suggests that the higher doses can be grouped as 2 mg 17β-estradiol (+norethisterone acetate [NETA]) and 100 mg transdermal patch. The medium doses are 1 mg 17β-estradiol (+NETA), the 50 mg transdermal patch, and 0.625 mg CEE, and the lower doses are CEE 0.3 mg, oral 17β-estradiol 0.5 mg, and 25 mg transdermal patch. The doses of Premarin 0.45 mg and the 37.5 μg patch would have to be classified as doses intermediate between low and medium. There is only one small trial on the 37.5 μg patch.

Using this classification of doses for ET/HT compared with placebo, the increases in spine BMD were 7.9% (high dose), 6.4% (medium), 3.3% (low-medium), and 3.9% (low). For total hip BMD, it was 4.6%, 3.7%, 3.0%, and 2.4%, respectively. For femoral neck BMD, it was 4.1%, 3.2%, 2.3%, and 2.7%, respectively.

The response to estrogen depends on the degree of bone resorption at the onset of treatment, the number of years since menopause, the length of the trial (larger changes at 3 years than 1 or 2 years), the addition of calcium supplements/vitamin D, age, dose and type of estrogen, the addition of certain progestins, and the adjustment of BMD for other covariates (e.g., baseline BMD, smoking, and the precision of the BMD measurement relative to the change in BMD).

Discontinuation of Estrogen

Two recent studies[23,24] followed the discontinuation of estrogen in elderly women who were treated for 3 years with Premarin 0.625 mg. In both studies, there was rapid loss of bone, most of it occurring within the first year. This implies that discontinuation of estrogen could be a clinical problem in older women or women with low BMD, and the rapid loss of bone will probably lead to new fractures unless another antiresorptive therapy is added immediately after discontinuing ET/HT. Therefore, women who discontinue estrogen after several years of treatment should undergo central measurement of BMD by DXA, and those at risk, as defined above, should be treated with an antiresorptive agent. In a follow-up of a younger cohort of women in their mid-fifties from the PEPI study treated for 3 years with Premarin 0.625 mg, there was no rapid bone loss after discontinuing HT,[25] although other studies of younger women have noticed rapid bone loss.[26–28]

Combinations Therapy with ET/HT

There have been several large studies where estrogen was combined with other agents. Although it is now common to give calcium to all women in trials, a review of older studies before this was a common practice compared 11 trials where ET/HT was given alone with 20 trials where calcium was added to the ET/HT. The analysis showed that adding calcium supplementation to estrogen therapy increased spine BMD by 2% and femoral neck BMD by 1.5% compared with ET/HT alone.[29] Other agents combined with ET/HT have been alendronate,[20] risedronate,[30] and calcit-

riol.[19] In all studies, the combination of two agents produced a 2% higher spine BMD than the single agent and a 1% higher hip BMD and a faster response in BMD. In addition, the biochemical markers of bone resorption showed further suppression in combination therapy. These studies suggest that neither alendronate 10 mg daily nor Premarin 0.625 mg completely suppress bone resorption on their own. However, because the extra gain in BMD is small in combination therapy, this clinical regimen should only be used in certain circumstances, such as initiation of therapy in a new patient with very low BMD (T-score < 3.5), a new fracture in a patient already on single therapy, or in a patient who is losing bone on single therapy. There are no fracture data to support the use of combination therapy.

Effect of Estrogen on Fractures

The results of the recent WHI trial[31] compared 8102 women on placebo with 8506 on HT (Premarin 0.625 mg + MPA 2.5 mg). After 5.2 years, there was a 23% reduction in all osteoporotic fractures (excluding hip, spine, skull, fingers, toes, sternum) with a relative risk (RR) of 0.77 (95% CI, 0.69–0.86; or adjusted 95% CI, 0.63–0.94), a 34% reduction in hip fracture RR of 0.66 (95% CI, 0.45–0.98; or adjusted 95% CI, 0.33–1.33), and a 34% decrease in vertebral fracture RR of 0.66 (95% CI, 0.44–0.98; or adjusted 95% CI, 0.32–1.34).

A meta analysis by Torgerson and Bell-Syer[32] looked at the effect of ET/HT on nonvertebral fractures. It included data from 22 trials. There was a reduction in fractures in the ET/HT groups with an RR of 0.73 (95% CI, 0.56–0.94). If the women were divided into two groups, younger and older than 60 years of age, the RR was 0.67 (95% CI, 0.49–0.55) for the younger group and RR was 0.88 (95% CI, 0.77–1.08) for the older group, suggesting that prevention of early bone loss is more effective.

In two prospective placebo-controlled studies of early postmenopausal women, HT significantly reduced the incidence of fracture RR of 0.29 (95% CI, 0.10–0.90) after 4.5 years of treatment,[33] and in a 5-year study, the incidence of forearm fractures was reduced, RR of 0.45 (95% CI, 0.22–0.90).[34]

Several cohort studies reported a significant reduction in hip fractures on ET/HT; in seven studies, the relative risk of hip fractures decreased by an average of 39% with an average RR of 0.61. All but one study was significant. Similar findings are seen for ET/HT reducing forearm fractures by an average of 54% with an average RR of 0.46. All studies were significant. Two studies clearly showed that the nearer to menopause that ET/HT was started, the better the effect.

SUMMARY

ET/HT is an effective antiresorptive agent for preventing postmenopausal bone loss. In addition, there is convincing evidence now that ET/HT reduces all types of osteoporotic fractures, including hip fractures. Recent trials show that in the past we have used doses of ET/HT that were larger than necessary, and that in the great majority of women, we can use low-dose regimens with periodic BMD measurements to provide reassurance that bone loss is stabilized.

REFERENCES

1. Pacifici R 1996 Estrogen, cytokines, and pathogenesis of postmenopausal osteoporosis. J Bone Miner Res **11**:1043–1051.
2. Coulam CB, Adamson SC, Annegers JF 1986 Incidence of premature ovarian failure. Obstet Gynecol **67**:604–606.
3. Pouilles JM, Tremollieres F, Bonneu M, Ribot C 1994 Influence of early age at menopause on vertebral bone mass. J Bone Miner Res **9**:311–315.
4. World Health Organization Study Group 1994 Assessment of fracture risk and its application to screening for postmenopausal osteoporosis. World Health Organ Tech Rep Ser **843**:1–129.
5. Siris ES, Miller PD, Barrett-Connor E, Faulkner KG, Wehren LE, Abbott TA, Berger ML, Santora AC, Sherwood LM 2001 Identification and fracture outcomes of undiagnosed low bone mineral density in postmenopausal women: Results from the National Osteoporosis Risk Assessment. JAMA **286**:2815–2822.
6. National Osteoporosis Foundation 1998 Physicians Guide to Prevention and Treatment of Osteoporosis. National Osteoporosis Foundation.
7. Wells G, Tugwell P, Shea B, Guyatt G, Peterson J, Zytaruk N, Robinson V, Henry D, O'Connell D, Cranney A 2002 Meta-analyses of therapies for postmenopausal osteoporosis. V. Meta-analysis of the efficacy of hormone replacement therapy in treating and preventing osteoporosis in postmenopausal women. Endocr Rev **23**:529–539.
8. Delmas PD, Pornel B, Felsenberg D, Garnero P, Hardy P, Pilate C, Dain MP 1999 Bone. A dose-ranging trial of a matrix transdermal 17beta-estradiol for the prevention of bone loss in early postmenopausal women. International Study Group. Bone **24**:517–523.
9. Cooper C, Stakkestad JA, Radowicki S, Hardy P, Pilate C, Dain MP, Delmas PD 1999 Matrix delivery transdermal 17beta-estradiol for the prevention of bone loss in postmenopausal women. The International Study Group. Osteoporos Int **9**:358–366.
10. Lees B, Stevenson JC 2001 The prevention of osteoporosis using sequential low-dose hormone replacement therapy with estradiol-17 beta and Dydrogesterone. Osteoporos Int **12**:251–258.
11. Bunyavejchevin S, Limpaphayom KK 2001 The metabolic and bone density effects of continuous combined 17-beta estradiol and noresthisterone acetate treatments in Thai postmenopausal women: A double-blind placebo-controlled trial. J Med Assoc Thai **84**:45–53.
12. Delmas PD, Confavreux E, Garnero P, Fardellone P, de Vernejoul MC, Cormier C, Arce A 2000 Combination of low doses of 17 beta-estradiol and norethisterone acetate prevents bone loss and normalizes bone turnover in postmenopausal women. Osteoporos Int **11**:177–187.
13. Bjarnason NH, Byrjalsen I, Hassager C, Haarbo J, Christiansen C 2000 Low doses of estradiol in combination with gestodene to prevent early postmenopausal bone loss. Am J Obstet Gynecol **183**:550–560.
14. Lindsay R, Gallagher JC, Kleerekoper M, Pickar JH 2002 Effect of lower doses of conjugated equine estrogens with and without medroxyprogesterone acetate on bone in early postmenopausal women. JAMA **287**:2668–2676.
15. McKeever C, McIlwain H, Greenwald M, Gupta N, Jayawardene S, Huels G, Roberts M 2000 An estradiol matrix transdermal system for the prevention of postmenopausal bone loss. ClinTher **22**:845–857.
16. Weiss SR, Ellman H, Dolker M 1999 A randomized controlled trial of four doses of transdermal estradiol for preventing postmenopausal bone loss. Obstet Gynecol **94**:330–336.
17. Notelovitz M, John VA, Good WR 2002 Effectiveness of Alora estradiol matrixtransdermal delivery system in improving lumbar bone mineral density in healthy, postmenopausal women. Menopause **9**:343–353.
18. Arrenbrecht S, Boermans AJ 2002 Effects of transdermal estradiol delivered by a matrix patch on bone density in hysterectomized, postmenopausal women: A 2-year placebo-controlled trial. Osteoporos Int **13**:176–183.
19. Gallagher JC, Fowler SE, Detter JR, Sherman SS 2001 Combination treatment with estrogen and calcitriol in the prevention of age-related bone loss. J Clin Endocrinol Metab **86**:3618–3628.
20. Bone HG, Greenspan SL, McKeever C, Bell N, Davidson M, Downs RW, Emkey R, Meunier PJ, Miller SS, Mulloy AL, Recker RR, Weiss SR, Heyden N, Musliner T, Suryawanshi S, Yates AJ, Lombardi A 2000 Alendronate and estrogen effects in postmenopausal women with low bone mineral density. Alendronate/Estrogen Study Group. J Clin Endocrinol Metab **85**:720–726.
21. Recker RR, Davies KM, Dowd RM, Heaney RP 1999 The effect of low-dose continuous estrogen and progesterone therapy with calcium and vitamin D on bone in elderly women. A randomized, controlled trial. Ann Intern Med **130**:897–904.
22. Giske LE, Hall G, Rud T, Landgren 2002 The effect of 17β-estradial at doses of 0.5, 1, and 2 mg compared with placebo on early postmenopausal bone loss in hysterectomized women. Osteoporos Int **13**:309–316.
23. Gallagher JC, Rapuri PB, Haynatzki G, Detter JR 2002 Effect of discontinuation of estrogen, calcitriol, and the combination of both on bone density and bone markers. J Clin Endocrinol Metab **87**:4914–4923.
24. Greenspan SL, Emkey RD, Bone HG, Weiss SR, Bell NH, Downs RW, McKeever C, Miller SS, Davidson M, Bolognese MA, Mulloy AL, Heyden N, Wu M, Kaur A, Lombardi A 2002 Significant differential effects of alendronate, estrogen, or combination therapy on the rate of bone loss after discontinuation of treatment of postmenopausal osteoporosis. A randomized, double-blind, placebo-controlled trial. Ann Intern Med **137**:875–883.
25. Greendale GA, Espeland M, Slone S, Marcus R, Barrett-Connor E 2002 Bone mass response to discontinuation of long-term hormone replacement therapy: Results from the Postmenopausal Estrogen/Progestin Interventions (PEPI) Safety Follow-up Study. Arch Intern Med **162**:665–672.
26. Tremollieres FA, Pouilles JM, Ribot C 2001 Withdrawal of hormone replacement therapy is associated with significant vertebral bone loss in postmenopausal women. Osteoporos Int **12**:385–390.
27. Horsman A, Nordin BEC, Crilly RG 1979 Effect of bone on withdrawal of estrogen therapy. Lancet **2**:33.
28. Lindsay R, Hart DM, Forrest C, Baird C 1980 Prevention of spinal osteoporosis in oophorectomised women. Lancet **2**:1151–1154.
29. Nieves JW, Komar L, Cosman F, Lindsay R 1998 Calcium potentiates the effect of estrogen and calcitonin on bone mass: Review and analysis. Am J Clin Nutr **67**:18–24.
30. Harris ST, Eriksen EF, Davidson M, Ettinger MP, Moffett AH Jr, Baylink DJ, Crusan CE, Chines AA 2001 Effect of combined risedronate and hormone replacement therapies on bone mineral density in postmenopausal women. J Clin Endocrinol Metab **86**:1890–1897.
31. Writing group for the Women's Health Initiative Investigator 2002 Risks and benefits of estrogen plus progestin in healthy postmenopausal women. JAMA **288**:321–333.
32. Torgerson DJ, Bell-Syer SE 2001 Hormone replacement therapy and prevention of nonvertebral fractures: A meta-analysis of randomized trials. JAMA **285**:2891–2897.
33. Komulainen MH, Kroger H, Tuppurainen MT, Heikkinen AM, Alhava E, Honkanen R, Saarikoski S 1998 HRT and Vit D in prevention of non-vertebral fractures in postmenopausal women: A 5 year randomized trial. Maturitas **31**:45–54.
34. Mosekilde L, Beck-Nielsen H, Sorensen OH, Nielsen SP, Charles P, Vestergaard P, Hermann AP, Gram J, HansenTB, Abrahamsen B, Ebbesen EN, Stilgren L, Jensen LB, Brot C, Hansen B, Tofteng CL, Eiken P, Kolthoff 2000 Hormonal replacement therapy reduces forearm fracture incidence in recent postmenopausal women: Results of the Danish Osteoporosis Prevention Study. Maturitas **36**:181–193.

Chapter 54. Clinical Use of Selective Estrogen Receptor Modulators and Other Estrogen Analogs

Pierre D. Delmas

Claude Bernard University of Lyon, INSERM Research Unit 403, Lyon, France

INTRODUCTION

The concept of selective estrogen receptor modulators (SERMs) is derived from the observation that tamoxifen, an effective adjuvant therapy of breast cancer that has an anti-estrogenic effect on breast tissue, has estrogen-like effects on the skeleton and on lipoproteins. Thus, an estrogen-like compound that binds with high affinity to the estrogen receptor (ER) could have either estrogen agonist or antagonist activity according to the type of estrogen-responsive tissue. Although the molecular basis for tissue-specific actions of SERMs is not yet fully understood, recent advances in the field of ER biology has led to new insights in their mechanism of action. The ER ligand-binding domain has been recently crystallized, and its structure has been studied without bound ligand and after binding to either 17β estradiol or to raloxifene,[1] a SERM that has undergone extensive clinical investigation. Although both compounds bind the same site of the ER, raloxifene induces conformational changes of surrounding sites that differ from those induced by 17β estradiol, resulting in an inability of the activating function-2 (AF-2) to activate the ER element-driven gene transcription.[1] The recent discovery of a second ER isoform, $ER\beta$, that has a tissue distribution distinct from ER, probably also contributes to the tissue specificity of action of SERMs,[2,3] as well as the potential role of tissue specific transcription factors interacting with the ER-ligand complex.[4] Numerous coactivators and corepressors that modulate receptor function have been identified, with an expression that may be different in various target tissues. Finally, there might be gene-specific pathways for ER-mediated gene transcription that do not depend on the classical ERE sequence.[5] The molecular mechanisms of action of SERMs have been recently reviewed.[6]

The clinical interest in SERMs is linked to the limitations of hormone replacement therapy (HRT). Long-term HRT is associated with an increase in bone mineral density (BMD) and a decrease in skeletal fragility[7] and with an improvement of the plasma lipoprotein profile that was thought to result into a reduced incidence of coronary heart disease. Unfortunately, evidence derived from placebo-controlled trials suggest that HRT increases cardiovascular events in postmenopausal women both in secondary[8,9] and primary[10] prevention trials. Long-term compliance to HRT is limited by side effects such as uterine bleeding and the fear of breast cancer, the risk of which increases after prolonged treatment. Although tamoxifen has an excellent benefit/risk ratio as an adjuvant treatment of breast cancer, its use in healthy postmenopausal women is questionable because of its associated increased risk of endometrial cancer. A SERM that would have an estrogen agonist activity on the skeleton

without having some of the undesirable estrogen actions on tissues such as the endometrium, the breast, and the cardiovascular system would represent a major advance for the management of postmenopausal women. There are several synthetic compounds, most of them nonsteroidal, that have both estrogen agonist and estrogen antagonist activities in vitro and in animal models. They can be classified as triphenylethylenes (tamoxifen, toremifene, droloxifene, and idoxifene), chroman (levormeloxifene) benzothiophenes (raloxifene and LY 35 3381), and others. We will only review the clinical effects of newly developed SERMs on major tissue targets, with reference to the effects of tamoxifen.

EFFECTS OF SERMs ON THE SKELETON

Tamoxifen has a protective effect on bone in postmenopausal women.[11] In women with breast cancer who were on average 10 years postmenopausal, tamoxifen 20 mg/day prevented bone loss at the lumbar spine over 2 years, while the rate of bone loss at the radius was not different from the placebo group.[12] In younger women who had menopause induced by the chemotherapy of breast cancer, we found that tamoxifen only halved the rate of bone loss at the spine and hip, contrasting with no bone loss in those receiving a new bisphosphonate-risedronate with or without tamoxifen.[13] These data suggest that tamoxifen acts as a partial estrogen agonist on bone. Its effects on osteoporotic fractures is not adequately documented. In the National Surgical Adjuvant Breast and Bowel Project (NSABP) P-1 Study involving over 13,000 women with increased risk of breast cancer randomized to tamoxifen or placebo for up to 5 years, there was a nonsignificant decrease of hip, vertebral, and wrist Colle's fractures.[14] Because the population was not selected based on a low BMD, the number of fracture events was quite low, and therefore the study was underpowered to show a reduction of osteoporotic fractures.

Raloxifene is the first SERM to be available worldwide for the treatment of osteoporosis. In a multicentric European study, 600 early postmenopausal women were randomized to raloxifene 30, 60, or 120 mg/day or to placebo.[15] Raloxifene prevented bone loss at all skeletal sites and at all doses, with a 2.4% increase in BMD at the lumbar spine and total hip over placebo at 2 years and 2% in the total body with the daily dose of 60 mg. Bone turnover decreased to premenopausal levels, with a reduction of the markers of bone formation (serum osteocalcin and bone specific alkaline phosphatase) of 23% and 15%, respectively, and a reduction of 34% of the urinary excretion of type I collagen C-telopeptide (CTX), a sensitive index of bone resorption.[15]

The effect of raloxifene (60 and 120 mg/day) on fracture risk has been evaluated in a large placebo-controlled study—the MORE study—including 7705 postmenopausal

---

The author has no conflict of interest.

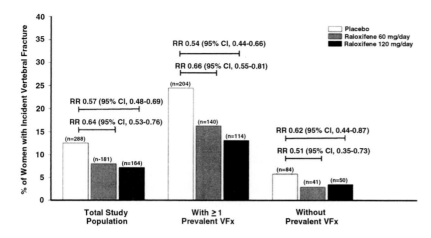

FIG. 1. The cumulative proportion of women with at least one incident vertebral fracture at 4 years. Women with or without prevalent vertebral fractures, and who had a baseline and any follow-up radiograph, were treated with placebo or raloxifene (60 or 120 mg/day; $n = 6828$). The numbers above each bar indicates the number of women in each group who had a new vertebral fracture. (Adapted from J Clin Endocrinol Metab **87**:3609–3617 with permission from The Endocrine Society.)

women with osteoporosis with or without vertebral fractures at baseline.[16] All patients were supplemented daily with calcium (500 mg) and vitamin D (400 IU). At 36 months, the risk of new vertebral fractures defined by vertebral morphometry was reduced in both groups receiving raloxifene with a relative risk (RR) of 0.7 (95% CI, 0.5–0.8) with 60 mg and 0.5 (95% CI, 0.4–0.7) with 120 mg. The reduction was significant both in women with and without prevalent vertebral fractures. With the recommended daily dose of 60 mg, the RRs were 0.7 (0.6–0.9) and 0.5 (0.3–0.7) in women with and without prevalent vertebral fractures, respectively. Overall, there was no difference in the incidence of fractures in the 120-mg raloxifene group and in the 60-mg group (5.4% versus 6.6%, respectively). There was, however, a lower incidence of vertebral fractures with the highest dose (120 mg) in women with but not in women without prevalent vertebral fractures. There was a 60% reduction in the occurrence of clinical vertebral fracture that was already significant (−62%) after 1 year of treatment, and that was significant both for mild and moderate/severe fractures.[17] In contrast, there was no significant decrease in the rate of nonvertebral fracture with raloxifene at either

dose (RR 0.9; 95% CI, 0.8–1.1). The results of a 12-month blinded extension of the MORE study was recently published.[18] The 4-year culmination risks (RRs) for one or more new vertebral fractures were 0.64 (95% CI, 0.53, 0.76) with raloxifene 60 mg and 0.57 (97% CI, 0.48, 0.69) with raloxifene 120 mg/day (Fig. 1). In year 4 alone, the reduction of vertebral fracture was significant and not different from the first 3 years, with a RR of 0.62 (0.41, 0.96) and 0.50 (0.26, 0.98) in patients with and without prevalent vertebral fractures, respectively, treated with raloxifene 60 mg/day (Fig. 2). The nonvertebral fracture risk was not significantly reduced (RR 0.93; 95% CI, 0.81, 1.06).[18]

The increase in BMD at various skeletal sites and the reduction of bone turnover observed in the MORE study were of magnitude comparable with that observed in the prevention study.[15] The discrepancy between the modest increase in BMD and the substantial decrease in fracture rate raises the intriguing hypothesis that the antifracture efficacy of raloxifene (and perhaps of other SERMs) may only be partly related to its effect on BMD. When the change in hip BMD during treatment is plotted versus vertebral fracture incidence using a logistic regression

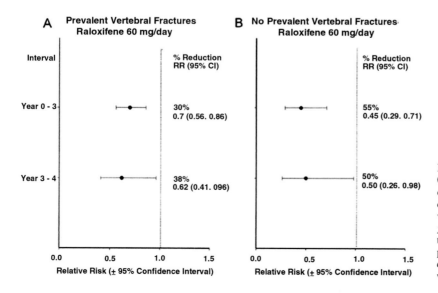

FIG. 2. Relative risks of new vertebral fractures in years 0–3 and in year 4. Analyses for years 0–3 were based on cumulative proportions using Pearson's χ^2 test. The percentage of women in each group who experienced new vertebral fractures in year 4 was analyzed using Pearson's χ^2 test. (A) Women with prevalent vertebral fractures treated with raloxifene 60 mg/day and (B) women with no prevalent vertebral fractures treated with raloxifene 60 mg/day. (Adapted from J Clin Endocrinol Metab **87**:3609–3617 with permission from The Endocrine Society.)

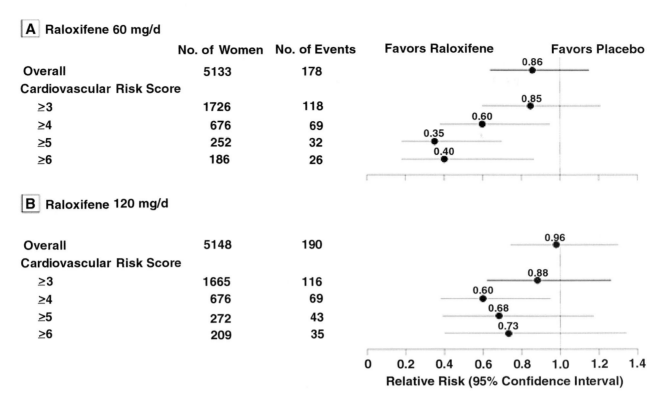

FIG. 3. Relative risk of any cardiovascular events compared by raloxifene and placebo. (JAMA 2002:**287**:847–857 with permission from the American Medical Association)

model, it seems that fracture reduction is greater than predicted by changes in BMD that explained only 4% of the observed fracture risk reduction.[19] Interestingly, the fracture reduction is partly related to decreased bone turnover assessed by changes in serum osteocalcin during treatment.[20] In a study in which osteoporotic women were randomized to raloxifene, alendronate, both, or placebo, the combination reduced bone turnover more than either drug alone, resulting in greater BMD increment, but whether this difference reflects better fracture risk reduction is unknown.[21]

The effects on bone turnover of two other SERMs, idoxifene and levormeloxifene, have been reported.[22,23] Two other SERMs (basedoxifene and lasofoxifene) are under clinical development, with phase III trials currently running.

EFFECTS OF SERMs ON LIPOPROTEINS AND CARDIOVASCULAR DISEASES

Tamoxifen reduces the serum levels of total and low-density lipoprotein (LDL)-cholesterol[24] and may reduce the risk of coronary heart disease in postmenopausal women with breast cancer.[25] In the NSABP P-1 study, however, there was no difference between tamoxifen and placebo-treated women for the incidence of myocardial infarction and of events related to ischemic heart disease regardless of age.[14] There was a trend for an increase in the risk of stroke.

In all osteoporosis prevention and treatment studies,[15,16] raloxifene induced a dose-dependent decrease of serum total and LDL-cholesterol (averaging 11% with 60 mg) without significant change in high-density lipoprotein (HDL)-cholesterol or triglycerides. In a 6-month randomized, placebo- and HRT-controlled trial with cardiovascular markers as a primary endpoint, raloxifene was also found to increase the HDL2 subfraction of cholesterol and to decrease plasma fibrinogen without significantly changing plasminogen activator inhibitor-1 (PAI-1) levels.[26]

Although the overall effect of SERMs on plasma lipoproteins is consistent with a beneficial effect, plasma lipids and coagulation factors are not reliable surrogate markers of cardiovascular disease. Experimental models of atherogenesis in monkeys and rabbits fed with a high-cholesterol diet suggest a protective effect of 17β estradiol and phytoestrogens against the development of the atherosclerotic plaque that is independent, at least in part, of their effects on plasma lipids[27]; this was not confirmed by a recent clinical trial.[10] The effect of raloxifene in these models is controversial.[28,29] The effects of various SERMs on in vitro models of vascular functions are also studied with reference to 17β estradiol. Eventually, the potentially beneficial effects of SERMs will have to be documented in clinical trials with adequate clinical endpoint(s). In the MORE study, raloxifene did not significantly affect the risk of cardiovascular events in the overall cohort but did significantly reduce the risk of cardiovascular event in a subset of 1035 women with increased cardiovascular risk at baseline (RR 0.60; 95% CI, 0.38–0.95 for both doses of raloxifene)[30] (Fig. 3). The effects of raloxifene on coronary heart disease morbidity and mortality will be assessed in 10,000 postmenopausal women at increased risk of cardiovascular disease (Raloxifene Use in the Heart [RUTH] study).[31]

EFFECTS OF SERMs ON THE BREAST

Tamoxifen is an effective adjuvant therapy in advanced breast cancer and in reducing tumor recurrence and prolonging survival when administered after surgery in stages I and II disease. It also reduces the incidence of contralateral breast cancer.[32,33] The NSABP P-1 study showed that tamoxifen given at 20 mg/day for 5 years reduces the risk of breast cancer by 49% in women considered to be at high risk because of their age (60 years or more), of a history of lobular carcinoma in situ, or because of combined clinical risk factors including first degree relatives with breast cancer, nulliparity, or age at first childbirth, age of menarche, number of breast biopsy specimens and pathological diagnostic of atypical hyperplasia. The reduction was more pronounced for women 60 years or older (-55%) than 49 years or younger (-44%) and was significant only for ER-positive tumors (-69%).[14] Although two European studies were published that did not find such a reduction[34,35]-probably for methodological reasons such as the size and type of population studied-the NSABP P-1 trial clearly opens the way for primary prevention of breast cancer in high risk patients with tamoxifen or eventually with another SERM that would have the same antiproliferative effect on the breast but a better safety profile.

In the MORE study, raloxifene induced a marked reduction of both invasive and noninvasive breast cancer cases, detected with annual mammograms, with a RR of 0.30 (95% CI 0.2–0.6).[36] At 4 years, 61 invasive breast cancer cases were reported and confirmed, resulting in a 72% risk reduction with raloxifene (RR 0.28; 95% CI 0.17, 0.46). The reduction of ER positive invasive breast cancer was reduced by 84% (RR 0.16; 95% CI 0.09, 0.30).[37] As the magnitude of the reduction may not be the same in a population of women at high risk of breast cancer, a head-to-head comparison of raloxifene with tamoxifen for prevention of breast cancer (STAR study) is running, that will enroll 22,000 women.

EFFECTS OF SERMs ON THE UTERUS

Tamoxifen increases the endometrial thickness evaluated by transvaginal ultrasonography (TVU)[38] and significantly increases the risk of endometrial adenocarcinoma.[39] In the NSABP P-1 trial, the RR in tamoxifen users was 2.5 and reached 4 in women over the age of 50 years. Thus, a careful evaluation of new SERMs on the genital tract is critical in determining their safety profile. The overall analysis of all phase III trials of raloxifene showed no increase of endometrial thickness (but a small increase in the number of patients with endometrial cavity fluid) by TVU, no increased incidence of proliferative or hyperplastic endometrium on biopsy specimens, and a nonsignificant decrease of the risk of endometrial cancer, although the total number of cases is still low. Clinically, there was no increase in vaginal bleeding and spotting with raloxifene compared with placebo.[36,38] Thus, in contrast to tamoxifen, raloxifene has

no estrogen agonist activity on the endometrium, and its clinical use does not require a specific gynecologic surveillance.

OVERALL SAFETY OF SERMs

Because of its size, the NSABP P-1 trial provides useful information on the safety profile of tamoxifen.[14] There was an age-related increase of deep venous thrombosis (RR 1.60; 95% CI, 0.91–2.86) and pulmonary embolism (RR 3.01; 95% CI, 1.15–9.27). In addition to the increased risk of endometrial cancer, tamoxifen use was associated with a significant increase of vaginal discharge, hot flushes, and unexpectedly, of cataracts (RR 1.14) and of surgery for cataracts (RR 1.57). Conversely, there was no increased risk of colon, ovarian, and liver cancer, or of mental depression. The safety profile of raloxifene is well documented in the MORE study.[16] The magnitude of the increased risk of venous thrombosis and pulmonary embolism is of comparable magnitude to that observed with tamoxifen and with HRT, suggesting similar mechanisms. The risk seems to be highest in the first 6 months of therapy. This vascular event is quite uncommon in postmenopausal women, so that the absolute attributable risk under raloxifene is low. Thromboembolic disease, including deep venous thrombosis or pulmonary embolism, occurred significantly more frequently with raloxifene (1.44, 3.32, and 3.63 events per 1000 woman-years for placebo, raloxifene 60 mg, or raloxifene 120 mg/day, respectively) during 4 years of the MORE study.[37] HRT has been suggested to be associated with a reduced risk of Alzheimer disease, but this interesting hypothesis has not been confirmed in a recent prospective controlled study.[40] The safety of SERMs on cognitive functions has to be established. There are some preclinical data suggesting that raloxifene acts as an estrogen agonist on the brain, and it is reassuring that no deterioration of cognitive functions assessed by a battery of tests has been detected so far in the MORE study that includes a large number of elderly women. Actually, there was a trend toward less decline in raloxifene-treated women of two tests of vertebral memory and attention compared with placebo-treated women.[41]

Other adverse events were uncommon and benign and did not lead to treatment discontinuation, including flu syndrome (involving 2% more of patients on raloxifene 60 mg than on placebo), hot flushes (approximately 3.3% more on raloxifene), and leg cramps (an excess of less than 2% with raloxifene over placebo). Thus, data available today indicate a favorable safety profile of raloxifene with only one serious—but uncommon—side effect (venous thromboembolism, with an RR similar or lower than that of HRT).

TIBOLONE

Tibolone is a synthetic steroid that acts on the estrogen, progesterone, and androgen receptor either directly or indirectly through its metabolites, with a different pattern according to the target tissue. Tibolone prevents bone loss in early and late postmenopausal women,[42,43] but its effects on fracture incidence have not been studied. Tibolone reduces menopausal symptoms, seems to be neutral on the

TABLE 1. SUMMARY OF EFFECTS OF HRT, RALOXIFENE, AND TIBOLONE ON TARGET TISSUES FROM PUBLISHED LITERATURE

	HRT	Raloxifene	Tibolone
Menopausal symptoms	+	0/−	+
Prevention of bone loss	+	+	+
Prevention of fractures	+	+	?
Bleeding/endometrium	−	0	0/−
Breast cancer	−	+	?
Cardiovascular risk	−	+*	?

+, beneficial effect; 0, neutral; −, negative effect.
* In high-risk patients.

endometrium,[44] and does not induce breast tenderness, but its overall effect on the uterus and the breast should be studied in large and long-term placebo-controlled studies. Its effects on cardiovascular disease is unknown. Its effects in postmenopausal women have been recently reviewed.[45] Table 1 compares the clinical effects of HRT, raloxifene, and tibolone on major target organs.

CONCLUSION AND PERSPECTIVES

Raloxifene, the first of the second generation of SERMs to be widely available, represents a significant improvement over tamoxifen. It prevents postmenopausal bone loss and reduces the incidence of vertebral fractures and of new breast cancer cases in osteoporotic patients, without stimulating the endometrium. The extension of the MORE study for an additional 4 years (CORE) will provide additional information on efficacy and safety. In early postmenopausal women, raloxifene is not an alternative to HRT in those who have severe hot flushes. It remains to be demonstrated if the beneficial effect on cardiovascular disease risk observed in osteoporotic women is confirmed in the RUTH study. Because of the multiplicity of the potential target organs (i.e., all ER responsive tissues), the development of long-term use of SERMs in postmenopausal women is challenging. One fundamental question is to know if the dose response curve of new SERMs on the ER is the same or differs in various estrogen responsive tissue (in which it may act as an estrogen agonist or antagonist), because this will determine the choice of the dose providing the best benefit/risk profile. In conclusion, SERMs represent a new and promising class of agents for the management of postmenopausal women, with a scope that goes far beyond the prevention and treatment of osteoporosis. Finally, the recent observation that estrogens may play a crucial role in bone metabolism of men and that SERMs prevent bone loss and induce prostatic atrophy in orchidectomized male rats[46] raises the possibility that they also may be of interest for the treatment of elderly men.

REFERENCES

1. Brzozowski AM, Pike AC, Dauter Z, Hubbard RE, Bonn T, Engstrom O, Ohman L, Greene GL, Gustafsson JA, Carlquist M 1997 Molecular basis of agonism and antagonism in the oestrogen receptor. Nature 389:753–758.
2. Giguere V, Tremblay A, Tremblay GB 1998 Estrogen receptor beta: Re-evaluation of estrogen and antiestrogen signaling. Steroids 63:335–339.
3. Paech K, Webb P, Kuiper GG, Nilsson S, Gustafsson J, Kushner PJ, Scanlan TS 1997 Differential ligand activation of estrogen receptors ERalpha and ERbeta at AP1 sites. Science 277:1508–1510.
4. White R, Parker MG 1998 Molecular mechanisms of steroid hormone action. Endocr Relat Cancer :1–13.
5. Elgort MG, Zou A, Marschke KB, Allegretto EA 1996 Estrogen and estrogen receptor antagonists stimulate transcription from the human retinoic acid receptor-alpha 1 promoter via a novel sequence. Mol Endocrinol 10:477–487.
6. Lonard DM, Smith CL 2002 Molecular perspectives on selective estrogen receptor modulators (SERMs): Progress in understanding their tissue-specific agonist and antagonist actions. Steroids 67:15–24.
7. Delmas PD 1997 Hormone replacement therapy in the prevention and treatment of osteoporosis. Osteoporos Int 7:S3–S7.
8. Hulley S, Grady D, Bush T, Furberg C, Herrington D, Riggs B, Vittinghoff E 1998 Randomized trial of estrogen plus progestin for secondary prevention of coronary heart disease in postmenopausal women. Heart and Estrogen/progestin Replacement Study (HERS) Research Group. JAMA 280:605–613.
9. Grady D, Herrington D, Bittner V, Blumenthal R, Davidson M, Hlatky M, Hsia J, Hulley S, Herd A, Khan S, Newby LK, Waters D, Vittinghoff E, Wenger N 2002 Cardiovascular disease outcomes during 6.8 years of hormone therapy: Heart and Estrogen/progestin Replacement Study follow-up (HERS II). JAMA 288:49–57.
10. Rossouw JE, Anderson GL, Prentice RL, LaCroix AZ, Kooperberg C, Stefanick ML, Jackson RD, Beresford SA, Howard BV, Johnson KC, Kotchen JM, Ockene J 2002 Risks and benefits of estrogen plus progestin in healthy postmenopausal women: Principal results from the Women's Health Initiative randomized controlled trial. JAMA 288:321–333.
11. Turken S, Siris E, Seldin D, Flaster E, Hyman G, Lindsay R 1989 Effects of tamoxifen on spinal bone density in women with breast cancer. J Natl Cancer Inst 81:1086–1088.
12. Love RR, Mazess RB, Barden HS, Epstein S, Newcomb PA, Jordan VC, Carbone PP, DeMets DL 1992 Effects of tamoxifen on bone mineral density in postmenopausal women with breast cancer. N Engl J Med 326:852–856.
13. Delmas PD, Balena R, Confravreux E, Hardouin C, Hardy P, Bremond A 1997 Bisphosphonate risedronate prevents bone loss in women with artificial menopause due to chemotherapy of breast cancer: A double-blind, placebo- controlled study. J Clin Oncol 15:955–962.
14. Fisher B, Costantino JP, Wickerham DL, Redmond CK, Kavanah M, Cronin WM, Vogel V, Robidoux A, Dimitrov N, Atkins J, Daly M, Wieand S, Tan-Chiu E, Ford L, Wolmark N 1998 Tamoxifen for prevention of breast cancer: Report of the National Surgical Adjuvant Breast and Bowel Project P-1 Study. J Natl Cancer Inst 90:1371–1388.
15. Delmas PD, Bjarnason NH, Mitlak BH, Ravoux AC, Shah AS, Huster WJ, Draper M, Christiansen C 1997 Effects of raloxifene on bone mineral density, serum cholesterol concentrations, and uterine endometrium in postmenopausal women. N Engl J Med 337:1641–1647.
16. Ettinger B, Black DM, Mitlak BH, Knickerbocker RK, Nickelsen T, Genant HK, Christiansen C, Delmas PD, Zanchetta JR, Stakkestad J, Gluer CC, Krueger K, Cohen FJ, Eckert S, Ensrud KE, Avioli LV, Lips P, Cummings SR 1999 Reduction of vertebral fracture risk in postmenopausal women with osteoporosis treated with raloxifene: Results from a 3-year randomized clinical trial. Multiple Outcomes of Raloxifene Evaluation (MORE) Investigators. JAMA 282:637–645.
17. Siris E, Adachi JD, Lu Y, Fuerst T, Crans GG, Wong M, Harper KD, Genant HK 2002 Effects of raloxifene on fracture severity in postmenopausal women with osteoporosis: Results from the MORE study. Multiple Outcomes of Raloxifene Evaluation. Osteoporos Int 13:907–913.
18. Delmas PD, Ensrud KE, Adachi JD, Harper KD, Sarkar S, Gennari C, Reginster JY, Pols HA, Recker RR, Harris ST, Wu W, Genant HK, Black DM, Eastell R 2002 Efficacy of raloxifene on vertebral fracture risk reduction in postmenopausal women with osteoporosis: Four-year results from a randomized clinical trial. J Clin Endocrinol Metab 87:3609–3617.
19. Sarkar S, Mitlak BH, Wong M, Stock JL, Black DM, Harper KD 2002 Relationships between bone mineral density and incident vertebral fracture risk with raloxifene therapy. J Bone Miner Res 17:1–10.
20. Bjarnason NH, Sarkar S, Duong T, Mitlak B, Delmas PD, Christiansen C 2001 Six and twelve month changes in bone turnover are related to reduction in vertebral fracture risk during 3 years of raloxifene treatment in postmenopausal osteoporosis. Osteoporos Int 12:922–930.
21. Johnell O, Scheele WH, Lu Y, Reginster JY, Need AG, Seeman E

2002 Additive effects of raloxifene and alendronate on bone density and biochemical markers of bone remodeling in postmenopausal women with osteoporosis. J Clin Endocrinol Metab **87**:985–992.

22. Delmas PD, Garnero P, McDonald B 1998 Idoxifene reduces bone turnover in osteopenic postmenopausal women. Bone **23**:S494.

23. Alexandersen P, Riis BJ, Stakkestad JA, Delmas PD, Christiansen C 2001 Efficacy of levormeloxifene in the prevention of postmenopausal bone loss and on the lipid profile compared to low dose hormone replacement therapy. J Clin Endocrinol Metab **86**:755–760.

24. Chang J, Powles TJ, Ashley SE, Gregory RK, Tidy VA, Treleaven JG, Singh R 1996 The effect of tamoxifen and hormone replacement therapy on serum cholesterol, bone mineral density and coagulation factors in healthy postmenopausal women participating in a randomised, controlled tamoxifen prevention study. Ann Oncol **7**:671–675.

25. McDonald CC, Alexander FE, Whyte BW, Forrest AP, Stewart HJ 1995 Cardiac and vascular morbidity in women receiving adjuvant tamoxifen for breast cancer in a randomised trial. The Scottish Cancer Trials Breast Group. BMJ **311**:977–980.

26. Walsh BW, Kuller LH, Wild RA, Paul S, Farmer M, Lawrence JB, Shah AS, Anderson PW 1998 Effects of raloxifene on serum lipids and coagulation factors in healthy postmenopausal women. JAMA **279**:1445–1451.

27. Clarkson TB, Cline JM, Williams JK, Anthony MS 1997 Gonadal hormone substitutes: Effects on the cardiovascular system. Osteoporos Int **7**:S43–S51.

28. Bjarnason NH, Haarbo J, Byrjalsen I, Kauffman RF, Christiansen C 1997 Raloxifene inhibits aortic accumulation of cholesterol in ovariectomized, cholesterol-fed rabbits. Circulation **96**:1964–1969.

29. Clarkson TB, Anthony MS, Jerome CP 1998 Lack of effect of raloxifene on coronary artery atherosclerosis of postmenopausal monkeys. J Clin Endocrinol Metab **83**:721–726.

30. Barrett-Connor E, Grady D, Sashegyi A, Anderson PW, Cox DA, Hoszowski K, Rautaharju P, Harper KD 2002 Raloxifene and cardiovascular events in osteoporotic postmenopausal women: Four-year results from the MORE (Multiple Outcomes of Raloxifene Evaluation) randomized trial. JAMA **287**:847–857.

31. Mosca L, Barrett-Connor E, Wenger NK, Collins P, Grady D, Kornitzer M, Moscarelli E, Paul S, Wright TJ, Helterbrand JD, Anderson PW 2001 Design and methods of the Raloxifene Use for The Heart (RUTH) study. Am J Cardiol **88**:392–395.

32. Group EBCTC 1998 Tamoxifen for early breast cancer: An overview of the randomised trials. Lancet **351**:1451–1467.

33. Osborne CK 1998 Tamoxifen in the treatment of breast cancer. N Engl J Med **339**:1609–1618.

34. Veronesi U, Maisonneuve P, Costa A, Sacchini V, Maltoni C, Robertson C, Rotmensz N, Boyle P 1998 Prevention of breast cancer with tamoxifen: Preliminary findings from the Italian randomised trial among hysterectomised women. Italian Tamoxifen Prevention Study. Lancet **352**:93–97.

35. Powles T, Eeles R, Ashley S, Easton D, Chang J, Dowsett M, Tidy A, Viggers J, Davey J 1998 Interim analysis of the incidence of breast cancer in the Royal Marsden Hospital tamoxifen randomised chemoprevention trial. Lancet **352**:98–101.

36. Cummings SR, Eckert S, Krueger KA, Grady D, Powles TJ, Cauley JA, Norton L, Nickelsen T, Bjarnason NH, Morrow M, Lippman ME, Black D, Glusman JE, Costa A, Jordan VC 1999 The effect of raloxifene on risk of breast cancer in postmenopausal women: Results from the MORE randomized trial. Multiple Outcomes of Raloxifene Evaluation. JAMA **281**:2189–2197.

37. Cauley JA, Norton L, Lippman ME, Eckert S, Krueger KA, Purdie DW, Farrerons J, Karasik A, Mellstrom D, Ng KW, Stepan JJ, Powles TJ, Morrow M, Costa A, Silfen SL, Walls EL, Schmitt H, Muchmore DB, Jordan VC 2001 Continued breast cancer risk reduction in postmenopausal women treated with raloxifene: 4-year results from the MORE trial. Multiple outcomes of raloxifene evaluation. Breast Cancer Res Treat **65**:125–134.

38. Kedar RP, Bourne TH, Powles TJ, Collins WP, Ashley SE, Cosgrove DO, Campbell S 1994 Effects of tamoxifen on uterus and ovaries of postmenopausal women in a randomised breast cancer prevention trial. Lancet **343**:1318–1321.

39. Sasco AJ 1996 Tamoxifen and menopausal status: Risks and benefits. Lancet **347**:761–762.

40. Shumaker SA, Legault C, Thal L, Wallace RB, Ockene JK, Hendrix SL, Jones BN, Assaf AR, Jackson RD, Kotchen JM, Wassertheil-Smoller S, Wactawski-Wende J for the WHIMS Investigators 2003 Estrogen plus progestin and the incidence of dementia and mild cognitive impairment in postmenopausal women. JAMA **289**:2651–2662.

41. Yaffe K, Krueger K, Sarkar S, Grady D, Barrett-Connor E, Cox DA, Nickelsen T 2001 Cognitive function in postmenopausal women treated with raloxifene. N Engl J Med **344**:1207–1213.

42. Bjarnason NH, Bjarnason K, Haarbo J, Rosenquist C, Christiansen C 1996 Tibolone: Prevention of bone loss in late postmenopausal women. J Clin Endocrinol Metab **81**:2419–2422.

43. Berning B, Kuijk CV, Kuiper JW, Bennink HJ, Kicovic PM, Fauser BC 1996 Effects of two doses of tibolone on trabecular and cortical bone loss in early postmenopausal women: A two-year randomized, placebo-controlled study. Bone **19**:395–399.

44. Johannes EJ 1997 Tibolone: Vaginal bleeding and the specific endometrial response in postmenopausal women. Gynecol Endocrinol **11**:25–30.

45. Modelska K, Cummings S 2002 Tibolone for postmenopausal women: Systematic review of randomized trials. J Clin Endocrinol Metab **87**:16–23.

46. Ke HZ, Qi H, Chidsey-Frink KL, Crawford DT, Thompson DD 2001 Lasofoxifene (CP-336, 156) protects against the age-related changes in bone mass, bone strength, and total serum cholesterol in intact aged male rats. J Bone Miner Res **16**:765–773.

Chapter 55. Bisphosphonates for Treatment of Osteoporosis

Nelson B. Watts

University of Cincinnati Bone Health and Osteoporosis Center, Cincinnati, Ohio

INTRODUCTION

Bisphosphonates are made up of two phosphonic acids joined to a carbon, plus two side chains, designated R^1 and R^2 (Fig. 1). The P-C-P structure acts as a "bone hook" that causes these compounds to bind avidly to hydroxyapatite crystals on bone surfaces, particularly at sites of active bone remodeling. Because of their affinity for bone, bisphosphonates are used for nuclear bone scintigraphy.

The R^1 side chain determines the binding affinity of the compound. The R^2 side chain determines the antiresorptive potency. Modification of these side chains allows for a variety of agents (Table 1). Bisphosphonates have been evaluated as therapeutic agents in a variety of diseases and conditions in addition to osteoporosis, especially those characterized by increased bone remodeling. Examples include

Dr. Watts has received research/consultant support from Abbott Labs, Amgen, Aventis, Eli Lilly & Company, Merck, Novartis, Procter & Gamble Pharmaceuticals, Inc., and Wyeth.

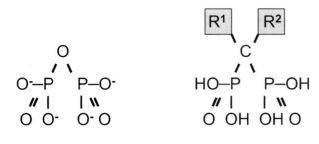

PYROPHOSPHATE   BISPHOSPHONATE

FIG. 1. Structure of pyrophosphate and geminal bisphosphonates. (Reprinted from The Osteoporotic Syndrome, Avioli L, Bisphosphonate therapy for postmenopausal osteoporosis, pp. 121–132, 2000 with permission from Elsevier.)

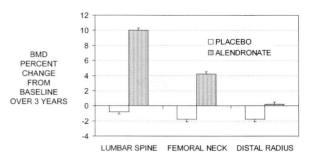

FIG. 2. After 3 years, mean percent change ($\pm$SE) in bone mineral density measured by DXA in the placebo group (open bars) and 10 mg alendronate group (dark bars) in women with established postmenopausal osteoporosis (Reprinted from American Journal of Medicine, 101, Tucci JR, Tonino RP, Emkey RD, Peverly CA, Kher U, Santora AC, Effect of three yeras of oral alendronate treatment in postmenopausal women with osteoporosis, pp. 488–501, 1996 with permission from Elsevier.)

heterotopic ossification, fibrous dysplasia, osteogenesis imperfecta, Paget's disease of bone, hypercalcemia due to a variety of causes, bone loss due to a variety of causes, destructive arthropathy, and skeletal involvement with metastatic cancer or multiple myeloma.

MECHANISMS OF ACTION

Bisphosphonates reduce osteoclastic bone resorption. The net result is an increase in bone mineral density (BMD) and a decrease in bone turnover markers. Non–nitrogen-containing bisphosphonates (e.g., etidronate, clodronate; see Table 1) do so by producing toxic analogs of ATP that cause cell death.[1] Nitrogen-containing compounds (e.g., alendronate, risedronate, and others; see Table 1) interfere with protein prenylation by inhibiting farnesyl pyrophosphatase, an enzyme in the HMG-CoA reductase pathway.[2] Inhibition of this enzyme prevents post-translational prenylation of guanosine triphosphate (GTP)-binding proteins, which leads to reduced resorptive activity of osteoclasts and accelerated apoptosis (programmed cell death).

Bisphosphonates have proven efficacy for prevention of bone loss caused by aging, estrogen deficiency, and glucocorticoid use, and for prevention of fractures in women with postmenopausal osteoporosis and in women and men with glucocorticoid-induced osteoporosis. Two bisphosphonates, alendronate and risedronate, are currently approved by the U.S. Food and Drug Administration (FDA) for use in

TABLE 1. STRUCTURES OF BISPHOSPHONATES IN GENERAL CLINICAL USE IN NORTH AMERICA

	R^1	R^2
Non–nitrogen-containing compounds		
etidronate	OH	CH_3
clodronate	Cl	Cl
tiludronate	H	SC_6H_3Cl
Nitrogen-containing compounds		
pamidronate	OH	$CH_2CH_2NH_2$
alendronate	OH	$CH_2CH_2CH_2NH_2$
risedronate	OH	CH_2-3-pyridinyl
zoledronate	OH	$CH_2C_3N_2H_3$

(Reprinted from Clinics in Geriatric Medicine, Siris E, Bisphosphonate treatment for osteoporosis, pp. 395–414, 2003 with permission from Elsevier.)

osteoporosis. There have been recent meta-analyses of their effect on fractures in postmenopausal osteoporosis.[3,4] Several others are on the market for other indications, and sometimes used "off label" for treatment of osteoporosis.

BISPHOSPHONATES APPROVED FOR USE IN OSTEOPOROSIS

Alendronate

Alendronate, a nitrogen-containing bisphosphonate (Table 1), was the first bisphosphonate approved by the FDA (in 1995) for use in osteoporosis. In the pivotal phase III study, which involved almost 1000 postmenopausal women who had osteoporosis (low BMD), treatment with alendronate increased BMD in the spine and hip. The optimal dose of alendronate for BMD effect appears to be 10 mg daily.[5] BMD continued to increase over 7[6] and 10 years[7] of treatment, and appeared to be maintained for at least 2 years after the drug was stopped after 5 years of treatment.[6,7] The increase in BMD with alendronate (and with other bisphosphonates) is greatest and occurs earliest at the spine, is less at the hip, and is minimal at the forearm (Fig. 2). Alendronate also reduces bone turnover markers by 50–70%.

The Vertebral Fracture Arm of the Fracture Intervention Trial (FIT) was the first prospective study to show a reduction in fractures with any agent. Women with prevalent vertebral fractures ($n = 2027$) received either alendronate (5 mg daily for 2 years, 10 mg daily for 1 year) or placebo. The incidence of new fractures was reduced by approximately 50% with alendronate treatment compared with placebo (47% for radiographic vertebral fractures, 48% for wrist fractures, and 51% for hip fractures; Fig. 3).[8] In a pooled analysis of two trials, the risk of clinical vertebral fractures was reduced after 1 year of treatment with alendronate.[9] In addition to reducing fracture risk, therapy with alendronate has been shown to reduce days of decreased activity, days in bed, and use of hospital services.[10]

In recently menopausal women, alendronate (5 mg daily) was shown to prevent bone loss at the spine and hip through at least 5 years of treatment.[11] In men with osteoporosis (either idiopathic or caused by hypogonadism), alendronate (10 mg daily) for 2 years produced BMD changes similar to

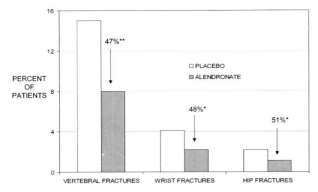

FIG. 3. Percent of placebo patients (open bars) and alendronate-treated patients (shaded bars) in the Vertebral Fracture Arm of the Fracture Intervention Trial (FIT) having new fractures after 3 years of treatment. **$p < 0.001$, *$p < 0.05$. (Adapted from Lancet, 19, Black DM et al., Randomised trial of effect of alendronate on risk of fracture in women with existing vertebral fractures, pp. 1535–1541, 1996, with permission of Elsevier.)

those seen in postmenopausal osteoporosis; the data suggest a reduction of vertebral fractures.[12] In a study of 477 men and women receiving corticosteroid therapy, alendronate significantly improved spine and hip BMD over 48 weeks.[13]

The recommended dose of alendronate for prevention of postmenopausal osteoporosis is 5 mg daily (or 35 mg once weekly). The recommended dose for treatment of post-menopausal osteoporosis is 10 mg daily or 70 mg once weekly. The once-weekly regimen of alendronate has been shown to have similar effects on BMD and bone turnover markers as daily dosing[14] and was approved by the FDA in September 2000. For treatment of corticosteroid-induced osteoporosis, the indicated dose is 5 mg daily for men and for estrogen-replete women and 10 mg daily for postmenopausal women who are not taking estrogen. "Off label" use for prevention of corticosteroid-induced osteoporosis and for prevention and treatment of various secondary forms of osteoporosis is common.

Risedronate

Risedronate has a nitrogen molecule in a pyridinyl ring in the R^2 position (Table 1). Risedronate increases BMD by 3–6% and reduces bone turnover markers by 40–60%. Risedronate has been shown to reduce vertebral fractures by 41% and 49% in two 3-year pivotal studies including over 3600 women with prevalent vertebral fractures.[15,16] Radiographic new vertebral fractures were significantly reduced after only 1 year of treatment[15] (Fig. 4), and clinical vertebral fractures were significantly reduced after just 6 months.[17] Nonvertebral fractures, a secondary end-point, were reduced significantly (by 39%) in the North American risedronate trial.[15] The antifracture effect of risedronate has been shown to continue through 5 years of treatment.[18]

The risedronate Hip Intervention Program (HIP), which enrolled almost 9500 women, is the largest prospective, randomized trial of osteoporosis therapy to date and the only prospective study in which reduction of hip fracture was the primary end-point(s). Treatment with risedronate

over 3 years produced a significant 30% overall reduction in hip fractures, and in a subset of women with low bone mass, a 40% reduction.[19] In a subset of elderly women who were enrolled in the trial because they had clinical risk factors for fractures (but not necessarily low bone mass), risedronate did not show a benefit. This suggests that patients with nonskeletal factors for hip fracture need different management than anti-osteoporosis medication.

Risedronate has been shown to prevent bone loss in recently menopausal women,[20] and in a post hoc analysis of pooled data, to reduce the risk of new vertebral fractures in women with low bone mass but without prevalent vertebral fractures.[21] Risedronate has been shown to prevent corticosteroid-induced bone loss in patients beginning corticosteroid therapy[22] and to increase BMD in patients who have been treated with glucocorticoids (in this study, prior glucocorticoid treatment was for an average of 5 years).[23] A significant 70% reduction in the incidence of new vertebral fractures was found in a post hoc analysis of pooled data from these trials.[24]

Risedronate is approved by the FDA for prevention and treatment of postmenopausal osteoporosis and for prevention and treatment of corticosteroid-induced osteoporosis. The approved dose is 5 mg daily or 35 mg once weekly; the once-weekly regimen has been shown to have similar effects on BMD and bone turnover compared with daily dosing.[25]

OTHER BISPHOSPHONATES IN CLINCAL USE

Etidronate

Etidronate was the first bisphosphonate to be studied in osteoporosis. Etidronate may impair mineralization of new bone if given continuously, so an intermittent cyclical regimen (400 mg daily for 14 days every 3 months) has been used for treatment of osteoporosis. The studies with cyclical etidronate in women with postmenopausal osteoporosis showed an increase in BMD, but were not powered to show a benefit on fracture.[26,27] However, they suggested a decrease in the risk of vertebral fractures, especially among high-risk patients, that has been reinforced by postmarketing data.[28] Treatment with intermittent cyclical etidronate

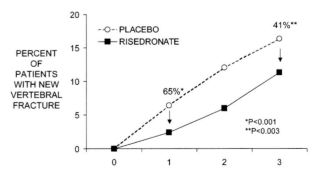

FIG. 4. Percent of placebo patients (open circles, dashed line) and risedronate 5 mg patients (closed squares, solid line) in the North American Vertebral Effectiveness of Risedronate Therapy (VERT) study having new vertebral fractures. *$p < 0.001$, **$p < 0.003$. (JAMA 1999:**282**:1344–1352 with permission from the American Medical Association)

therapy has been shown to prevent bone loss in recently menopausal women[29] and glucocorticoid-induced osteoporosis.[30] A small, open study has shown increases in bone density in osteoporotic men treated with etidronate. Etidronate is generally well tolerated and seems safe through at least 7 years of treatment.[31] Etidronate is not approved in the United States for use in osteoporosis, but it is approved in Canada and many European countries. It is available in the United States for other indications. Because of its good tolerability and relatively low cost, etidronate is sometimes used "off label" in the United States for patients who cannot tolerate other oral bisphosphonates.

Pamidronate

Pamidronate (sometimes called APD, for aminopropylidene diphosphonate) is approved by the FDA for treatment of hypercalcemia of malignancy and Paget's disease of bone. Pamidronate administered intravenously has been shown to increase BMD or prevent bone loss in patients with postmenopausal osteoporosis,[32] in recently menopausal women, and in patients with corticosteroid-induced osteoporosis.[33] A typical regimen is an initial dose of pamidronate 90 mg iv, with subsequent doses of 30 mg every third month. The 30-mg dose can be infused over about 60 minutes.[34] Pamidronate is not approved in the United States for use in osteoporosis. It is used "off label" for patients who cannot tolerate or cannot absorb oral bisphosphonates.

Zoledronate

Zoledronate (or zoledronic acid) contains two nitrogens in the R^2 position, and is the most potent bisphosphonate currently available. It is approved by the FDA for treatment of hypercalcemia of malignancy and metastatic bone disease. In a phase II trial of women with postmenopausal osteoporosis, a single intravenous 4-mg dose of zoledronate increased bone mass and resulted in a sustained reduction in bone turnover that lasted at least 12 months.[35] Large-scale phase III trials to evaluate the antifracture effect of intravenous zoledronate are currently under way.

Other Bisphosphonates

There have been some small trials of clodronate for treatment of osteoporosis, but there is not enough data to judge its effectiveness. Tiludronate (given orally) and ibandronate (given intravenously, 1 mg every third month) failed to show a fracture benefit in large trials, perhaps because the doses chosen were not optimal. Clodronate is not available in the United States. In Europe and Canada, where it is available, clodronate is used mainly for treatment of hypercalcemia of malignancy. Tiludronate is approved by the FDA for treatment of Paget's disease. Ibandronate is not approved for clinical use.

DOSING, SIDE EFFECTS, SAFETY ISSUES

Bisphosphonates taken orally are poorly absorbed under ideal conditions. Typically, less than 1% of an administered dose is absorbed. Absorption is completely abolished in the presence of divalent cations and most foods. All bisphosphonates must be taken in the fasting state; for most, a prolonged fast is required (generally an overnight fast), with nothing but water orally for at least 30 minutes. To minimize the chance of esophageal irritation, the tablet should be taken with 8 oz of water (to be certain the tablet passes through the esophagus), and the patient should remain upright (seated or standing) until after eating (to avoid reflux of drug into the esophagus). Patients who cannot remain upright, who have active upper gastrointestinal symptoms, or who have delayed esophageal emptying (e.g., strictures, achalasia, or severe dysmotility) should not take alendronate, and other bisphosphonates should be used with caution in such situations.

Etidronate does not seem to cause upper gastrointestinal symptoms that occur with some nitrogen-containing bisphosphonates. Occasionally, etidronate causes diarrhea, which, if it occurs, it typically mild. As is true for other bisphosphonates, etidronate must be taken on an empty stomach (with water only). However, etidronate can be taken between meals (2 h before and 2 h after eating) or during the night.

About one-third of patients receiving their first intravenous dose of nitrogen-containing bisphosphonate experience acute-phase reactions (fever, myalgias, lymphopenia, etc.),[36–38] but these rarely recur with repeated administration. Pretreatment with histamine blockers, anti-pyretics, or corticosteroids may reduce these symptoms.

The only route of elimination for bisphosphonates is renal excretion, but little information is available on dosing in patients who have impaired renal function. Renal toxicity may occur with rapid intravenous administration. Other side effects include eye reactions (uveitis, scleritis, episcleritis, and conjunctivitis), which have been reported with a frequency of about 1:1000, mainly with intravenous pamidronate. With rapid parenteral administration of bisphosphonates, hypocalcemia may occur; however, it is infrequent and usually mild. Pancreatitis has been reported with alendronate.[39]

Optimal effectiveness of bisphosphonates requires that patients engage in weight-bearing exercise and have adequate calcium and vitamin D nutrition. Bisphosphonates are contraindicated in patients with hypocalcemia.

RELATIVE EFFICACY, SAFETY, AND TOLERABILITY

Bisphosphonates seem to produce greater increases in BMD than other antiresorptive drugs, but not as great as teriparatide.[40] However, changes in BMD account for relatively little of the effect of bisphosphonates on vertebral fractures.[41] Reduction in bone turnover may provide a better indication of fracture reduction.[42] There are no head-to-head trials comparing bisphosphonates with regard to fracture efficacy or comparing a bisphosphonate with any other drug with a fracture end-point. Bisphosphonates are the only approved agents that have been shown to reduce the risk of hip fractures.[43] Both alendronate and risedronate were well tolerated in clinical trials. However, daily dosing of alendronate was associated with upper gastrointestinal side effects (e.g., heartburn, pain on swallowing, etc.) in about 10% of patients. Daily dosing with risedronate might be better tolerated, but, because once weekly dosing of both agents is well tolerated, this no longer seems to be an important issue.

There has also been concern that potent antiresorptive agents, such as bisphosphonates, might turn off remodeling completely, leading to "frozen bone." There is no evidence that this actually occurs with the doses used clinically. There are some studies that show increased microcracks but preserved biomechanical properties in dogs treated with very high doses of bisphosphonates, but without compromise of bone strength. Fracture healing in patients treated with bisphosphonates does not seem to be a problem.

USE OF BISPHOSPHONATES IN COMBINATION WITH OTHER AGENTS

Mechanisms of action differ for different antiresorptive drugs, which offers the possibility that combining two agents might produce greater benefit than a single agent. Combining a bisphosphonate with calcitonin, estrogen, or raloxifene is probably safe. Several studies have shown that combining a bisphosphonate with estrogen or raloxifene produces greater change in BMD than a single agent alone. None of these studies was large enough to determine if there was a greater reduction in fracture risk with combination therapy. Using two agents together obviously increases the cost and probably increases the occurrence of side effects. For these reasons, combination therapy with antiresorptive drugs should probably be reserved for patients who have severe osteoporosis and perhaps for those who fail to respond to a single drug.[44] Combining an anabolic agent (e.g., teriparatide) with a bisphosphonate is more appealing than the simultaneous use of two antiresorptive medications, but the only antiresorptive agent that has been studied with PTH thus far is estrogen.

SUMMARY AND CONCLUSIONS

Bisphosphonates are the best studied of all agents for the prevention of bone loss and the reduction in fractures. They increase BMD, primarily at the lumbar spine, but also at the proximal femur. In patients who have established osteoporosis, they reduce the risk of vertebral fractures, and are the only agents currently approved for treatment of osteoporosis shown in prospective trials to reduce the risk of hip fractures. Bisphosphonates reduce the risk of fracture quickly. The risk of radiographic vertebral deformities is reduced after 1 year of treatment with risedronate.[15] The risk of clinical vertebral fractures is reduced after 1 year of treatment with alendronate[9] and just 6 months of treatment with risedronate.[17] BMD continues to increase through 10 years of treatment.[7] The antifracture effect of risedronate has been shown to continue through 5 years of treatment.[18] For all these reasons, bisphosphonates are the agents of choice for most patients with osteoporosis.

Alendronate and risedronate are approved by the FDA for prevention of bone loss in recently menopausal women, for treatment of postmenopausal osteoporosis, and for prevention (risedronate) and treatment (alendronate and risedronate) of glucocorticoid-induced osteoporosis. Alendronate is also approved for treatment of osteoporosis in men. Other bisphosphonates (etidronate for oral use, pamidronate and zoledronate for intravenous infusion) are also available and can be used "off label" for patients who cannot tolerate approved agents. Although bisphosphonates combined with estrogen or raloxifene produce greater gains in bone mass compared with monotherapy, the use of two antiresorptive agents in combination cannot be recommended because the benefit on fracture risk has not been demonstrated and because of increased cost and side effects. Use of bisphosphonates in combination with teriparatide has not been studied.

REFERENCES

1. Frith JC, Monkkonen J, Blackburn GM, Russell RG, Rogers MJ 1997 Clodronate and liposome-encapsulated clodronate are metabolized to a toxic ATP analog, adenosine 5′ (beta, gamma-dichloromethylene) triphosphate, by mammalian cells in vitro. J Bone Miner Res 12:1358–1367.
2. Rogers MJ, Frith JC, Luckman SP, Coxon FP, Benford HL, Monkkonen J, Auriola S, Chilton KM, Russell RG 1999 Molecular mechanisms of action of bisphosphonates. Bone 24(Suppl 5):73S–79S.
3. Cranney A, Wells G, Willan A, Griffith L, Zytaruk N, Robinson V, Black D, Adachi J, Shea B, Tugwell P, Guyatt, Osteoporosis Methodology Group, The Osteoporosis Research Advisory Group 2002 Meta-analysis of alendronate for the treatment of postmenopausal women. Endocr Rev 23:508–516.
4. Cranney A, Tugwell P, Adachi J, Weaver B, Zytaruk N, Papaioannou A, Robinson V, Shea B, Wells G, Guyatt G, Osteoporosis Methodology Group, The Osteoporosis Research Advisory Group 2002 Meta-analysis of risedronate for the treatment of postmenopausal osteoporosis. Endocr Rev 23:517–523.
5. Liberman UA, Weiss SR, Broll J, Minne HW, Quan H, Bell NH, Rodriguez-Portales J, Downs RW Jr, Dequeker J, Favus M 1995 Effect of oral alendronate on bone mineral density and the incidence of fractures in postmenopausal osteoporosis. N Engl J Med 333:1437–1443.
6. Tonino RP, Meunier PJ, Emkey R, Rodriguez-Portales JA, Menkes CJ, Wasnich RD, Bone HG, Santora AC, Wu M, Desai R, Ross PD 2000 Skeletal benefits of alendronate: 7-year treatment of postmenopausal osteoporotic women. J Clin Endocrinol Metab 85:3109–3115.
7. Emkey R, Reid I, Mulloy A, Correa-Rotter R, Favus M, Bone H, Gupta J, LaMotta A, Santora A 2002 Ten-year efficacy and safety of alendronate in the treatment of osteoporosis in postmenopausal women. J Bone Miner Res 17:S139.
8. Black DM, Cummings SR, Karpf DB, Cauley JA, Thompson DE, Nevitt MC, Bauer DC, Genant HK, Haskell WL, Marcus R, Ott SM, Torner JC, Quandt SA, Reiss TF, Ensrud KE 1996 Randomised trial of effect of alendronate on risk of fracture in women with existing vertebral fractures. Lancet 348:1535–1541.
9. Black DM, Thompson DE, Bauer DC, Ensrud K, Musliner T, Hochberg MC, Nevitt MC, Suryawanshi S, Cummings SR 2000 Fracture risk reduction with alendronate in women with osteoporosis: The Fracture Intervention Trial. J Clin Endocrinol Metab 85:4118–4124.
10. Nevitt MC, Thompson DE, Black DM, Rubin SR, Ensrud K, Yates AJ, Cummings SR 2000 Effect of alendronate on limited-activity days and bed-disability days caused by back pain in postmenopausal women with existing vertebral fractures. Arch Intern Med 160:77–85.
11. Ravn P, Weiss SR, Rodriguez-Portales JA, McClung MR, Wasnich RD, Gilchrist NL, Sambrook P, Fogelman I, Krupa D, Yates AJ, Daifotis A, Fuleihan GE 2000 Alendronate in early postmenopausal women: Effects on bone mass during long-term treatment and after withdrawal. J Clin Endocrinol Metab 85:1942–1947.
12. Orwoll E, Ettinger M, Weiss S, Miller P, Kendler D, Graham J, Adami S, Weber K, Lorenc R, Pietschmann P, Vandormael K, Lombardi A 2000 Alendronate for the treatment of osteoporosis in men. N Engl J Med 343:604–610.
13. Saag KG, Emkey R, Schnitzer TJ, Brown JP, Hawkins F, Goemaere S,

Thamsborg G, Liberman UA, Delmas PD, Malice MP, Czachur M, Daifotis A 1998 Alendronate for the prevention and treatment of glucocorticoid-induced osteoporosis. N Engl J Med 339:292–299.

14. Schnitzer T, Bone HG, Crepaldi G, Adami S, McClung M, Kiel D, Felsenberg D, Recker RR, Tonino RP, Roux C, Pinchera A, Foldes AJ, Greenspan SL, Levine MA, Emkey R, Santora AC Jr, Kaur A, Thompson DE, Yates J, Orloff JJ 2000 Alendronate 70 mg once weekly is therapeutically equivalent to alendronate 10 mg daily for treatment of postmenopausal osteoporosis. Aging Clin Exp Res 12:1–12.

15. Harris ST, Watts NB, Genant HK, McKeever CD, Hangartner T, Keller M, Chesnut CH III, Brown J, Eriksen EF, Hoseyni MS, Axelrod DW, Miller PD 1999 Effects of risedronate treatment on vertebral and nonvertebral fractures in women with postmenopausal osteoporosis - A randomized controlled trial. JAMA 282:1344–1352.

16. Reginster J, Minne HW, Sorensen OH, Hooper M, Roux C, Brandi ML, Lund B, Ethgen D, Pack S, Roumagnac I, Eastell R 2000 Randomized trial of the effects of risedronate on vertebral fractures in women with established postmenopausal osteoporosis. Osteoporos Int 11:83–91.

17. Watts NB, Adami S, Chesnut C 2002 Risedronate reduces the risk of clinical vertebral fractures in just 6 months. J Bone Miner Res 17:S407.

18. Sorensen OH, Crawford GM, Mulder H, Hosking DJ, Gennari C, Mellstrom D, Pack S, Wenderoth D, Cooper C, Reginster JY 2003 Long-term efficacy of risedronate: A 5-year placebo-controlled clinical experience. Bone 32:120–126.

19. McClung MR, Geusens P, Miller PD, Zippel H, Bensen WG, Roux C, Adami S, Fogelman I, Diamond T, Eastell R, Meunier PJ, Reginster JY 2001 Effect of risedronate on the risk of hip fracture in elderly women. N Engl J Med 344:333–340.

20. Fogelman I, Ribot C, Smith R, Ethgen D, Sod E, Reginster JY 2000 Risedronate reverses bone loss in postmenopausal women with low bone mass: Results from a multinational, double-blind, placebo-controlled trial. J Clin Endocrinol Metab 85:1895–1900.

21. Heaney RP, Zizic TM, Fogelman I, Olszynski WP, Geusens P, Kasibhatla C, Alsayed N, Isaia G, Davie MW, Chesnut CH III 2002 Risedronate reduces the risk of first vertebral fracture in osteoporotic women. Osteoporosis Int 13:501–505.

22. Cohen S, Levy RM, Keller M, Boling E, Emkey RD, Greenwald M, Zizic TM, Wallach S, Sewell KL, Lukert BP, Axelrod DW, Chines AA 1999 Risedronate therapy prevents corticosteroid-induced bone loss - A twelve-month, multicenter, randomized, double-blind, placebo-controlled, parallel-group study. Arthritis Rheum 42:2309–2318.

23. Reid DM, Hughes RA, Laan RF, Sacco-Gibson NA, Wenderoth DH, Adami S, Eusebio RA, Devogelaer JP 2000 Efficacy and safety of daily risedronate in the treatment of corticosteroid-induced osteoporosis in men and women: A randomized trial. J Bone Miner Res 15:1006–1013.

24. Wallach S, Cohen S, Reid DM, Hughes RA, Hosking DJ, Laan RF, Doherty SM, Maricic M, Rosen C, Brown J, Barton I, Chines AA 2000 Effects of risedronate treatment on bone density and vertebral fracture in patients on corticosteroid therapy. Calcif Tissue Int 67:277–285.

25. Brown JP, Kendler DL, McClung MR, Emkey RD, Adachi JD, Bolognese MA, Li Z, Balske A, Lindsay R 2002 The efficacy and tolerability of risedronate once a week for the treatment of postmenopausal osteoporosis. Calcif Tiss Int 71:103–111.

26. Storm T, Thamsborg G, Steiniche T, Genant HK, Sorensen OH 1990 Effect of intermittent cyclical etidronate therapy on bone mass and fracture rate in women with postmenopausal osteoporosis. N Engl J Med 322:1265–1271.

27. Watts NB, Harris ST, Genant HK, Wasnich RD, Miller PD, Jackson RD, Licata AA, Ross P, Woodson GC, Yanover MJ, Misiw WJ, Kohse I, Rao MB, Steiger P, Richmond B, Chesnut CH 1990 Intermittent cyclical etidronate treatment of postmenopausal osteoporosis. N Engl J Med 323:73–79.

28. van Staa TP, Abenhaim L, Cooper C 1998 Use of cyclical etidronate and prevention of non-vertebral fractures. Br J Rhematol 37:87–94.

29. Herd RJ, Balena R, Blake GM, Ryan PJ, Fogelman I 1997 Prevention of early menopausal bone loss by cyclical etidronate therapy: A 2-year, double-blind, placebo-controlled study. Am J Med 103:92–99.

30. Adachi JD, Bensen WG, Brown J, Hanley D, Hodsman A, Josse R, Kendler DL, Lentle B, Olszynski W, Ste-Marie LG, Tenenhouse A, Chines AA 1997 Intermittent etidronate therapy to prevent corticosteroid-induced osteoporosis. N Engl J Med 337:382–387.

31. Miller PD, Watts NB, Licata AA, Harris ST, Genant HK, Wasnich RD, Ross PD, Jackson RD, Hoseyni MS, Schoenfeld SL, Valent DJ, Chesnut CH III 1997 Cyclical etidronate in the treatment of postmenopausal osteoporosis: Efficacy and safety after 7 years of treatment. Am J Med 103:468–476.

32. Peretz A, Body JJ, Dumon JC, Rozenberg S, Hotimski A, Praet JP, Moris M, Ham H, Bergmann P 1996 Cyclical pamidronate infusions in postmenopausal osteoporosis. Maturitas 25:69–75.

33. Boutsen Y, Jamart J, Esselinckx W, Devogelaer JP 2001 Primary prevention of glucocorticoid-induced osteoporosis with intravenous pamidronate and calcium: A prospective controlled 1-year study comparing a single infusion, an infusion given once every 3 months, and calcium alone. J Bone Miner Res 16:104–112.

34. Tyrrell CJ, Collinson M, Madsen EL, Ford JM, Coleman T 1994 Intravenous pamidronate: Infusion rate and safety. Ann Oncol 5:S27–S29.

35. Reid IR, Brown JP, Burckhardt P, Horowitz Z, Richardson P, Trechsel U, Widmer A, Devogelaer JP, Kaufman JM, Jaeger P, Body JJ, Brandi ML, Broell J, Di Micco R, Genazzani AR, Felsenberg D, Happ J, Hooper MJ, Ittner J, Leb G, Mallmin H, Murray T, Ortolani S, Rubinacci A, Saaf M, Samsioe G, Verbruggen L, Meunier PJ 2002 Intravenous zoledronic acid in postmenopausal women with low bone mineral density. N Engl J Med 346:653–661.

36. Adami S, Bhalla AK, Dorizzi R, Montesanti F, Rosini S, Salvagno G, Lo Cascio V 1987 The acute phase response after bisphosphonate administration. Calcif Tissue Int 41:326–331.

37. Gallacher SJ, Ralston SH, Patel U, Boyle IT 1989 Side-effects of pamidronate. Lancet 2:42–43.

38. Zojer N, Keck AV, Pecherstorfer M 1999 Comparative tolerability of drug therapies for hypercalcaemia of malignancy. Drug Saf 21:389–406.

39. Cadario B 2002 Alendronate: Suspected pancreatitis. Can Med Assoc J 166:86–87.

40. Body JJ, Gaich GA, Scheele WH, Kulkarni PM, Miller PD, Peretz A, Dore RK, Correa-Rotter R, Papaioannou A, Cumming DC, Hodsman A 2002 A randomized double-blind trial to compare the efficacy of teriparatide [recombinant human parathyroid hormone (1–34)] with alendronate in postmenopausal women with osteoporosis. J Clin Endocrinol Metab 87:4528–4535.

41. Delmas PD 2002 Different effects of antiresorptive therapies on vertebral and nonvertebral fractures in postmenopausal osteoporosis. Bone 30:14–17.

42. Eastell R, Barton I, Hannon RA, Garnero P, Chines A, Pack S, Delmas P 2002 Antifracture efficacy of risedronate: Prediction by change in bone resorption markers. J Bone Miner Res 16:S1;S163.

43. Cranney A, Guyatt G, Griffith L, Wells G, Tugwell P, Rosen C, Osteoporosis Methodology Group, The Osteoporosis Research Advisory Group 2002 Summary of meta-analyses of therapies for postmenopausal osteoporosis. Endocr Rev 23:570–578.

44. Compston JE, Watts NB 2002 Combination therapy for postmenopausal osteoporosis. Clin Endocrinol (Oxf) 56:565–569.

45. Watts NB 2003 Bisphosphonate treatment of osteoporosis. In: Siris E (ed.) Clinics in Geriatric Medicine. Saunders, Philadelphia, PA, USA, pp. 395–414.

46. Tucci JR, Tonino RP, Emkey RD, Peverly CA, Kher U, Santora AC Jr 1996 Effect of three years of oral alendronate treatment in postmenopausal women with osteoporosis. Am J Med 101:488–501.

Chapter 56.   Calcitonin Therapy for Osteoporosis

Stuart L. Silverman[1] and Charles H. Chesnut III[2]

[1]Department of Medicine and Rheumatology, UCLA School of Medicine and Cedars-Sinai Medical Center, Beverly Hills, California;
and [2]Department of Radiology and Medicine, Osteoporosis Research Group, University of Washington
Medical Center, Seattle, Washington

INTRODUCTION

Calcitonin, a 32 amino acid peptide secreted by the C-cells in the thyroid and by the ultimobranchial gland in submammals, was originally identified as a hypocalcemic factor present in bovine serum.[1] It exerts its hypocalcemic effects by directly inhibiting osteoclast resorption. It is currently available as a parenteral or nasal spray (NS-CT) formulation.

BASIC PHARMACOLOGY

Calcitonin inhibits bone resorption by osteoclasts.[2] Inhibition of osteoclastic bone resorption by calcitonin is mediated in part by binding to osteoclast receptors. After exposure to calcitonin in vitro, osteoclasts undergo flattening of their ruffled borders and withdraw from sites of active bone resorption. In the continued presence of calcitonin, escape from the inhibitory action of calcitonin may occur, possibly as a result of antibodies[3] or downregulation of receptors.[4]

The exact physiologic role of calcitonin in calcium homeostasis and skeletal metabolism in humans is not known.

Calcitonin knockout mice have been found to develop osteopenia. The exact mechanism is not known.[5]

EFFECTS OF CALCITONIN ON BONE MINERAL DENSITY

Postmenopausal Women

There are three small randomized clinical trials of injectable calcitonin on bone mineral density (BMD) in the treatment of osteoporosis[6] and two randomized clinical trials in the prevention of osteoporosis.[6] There are 12 published randomized clinical trials on the efficacy of nasal calcitonin on BMD for the prevention and treatment of postmenopausal osteoporosis.[6] In late postmenopausal women (greater than 5 years postmenopause), nasal calcitonin increased lumbar spine BMD by an average of 1–2%, significant over 2 years. There was no significant effect at cortical bone sites such as hip or forearm.

Men

There is an increase in lumbar BMD with nasal calcitonin in men.[7] There are no data with fracture as an endpoint.

Glucocorticoid-Induced Osteoporosis

A few small studies indicate that injectable calcitonin may reduce the rate of bone loss in lumbar spine and radius in patients both initiating and receiving corticosteroid therapy.[8] Data on bone loss prevention are conflicting with NS-CT. There are no data with fracture as an endpoint.

EFFECTS OF CALCITONIN ON FRACTURE

Data on the efficacy of injectable calcitonin on fracture are limited.[9,10] There have been no randomized controlled trials with injectable calcitonin using vertebral fracture as the primary endpoint.

There have been two randomized controlled trials on the efficacy of nasal calcitonin on fracture.[11,12] Both have shown vertebral fracture efficacy. None have shown hip fracture efficacy.

PROOF

The PROOF trial (Prevent Recurrence of Osteoporotic Fracture)[11] was designed to assess the efficacy of NS-CT in the prevention of vertebral fractures. A total of 1255 postmenopausal women with lumbar spine BMD T-scores of < -2 (78% with prevalent vertebral fracture) were randomized to placebo nasal spray: 100, 200, or 400 IU NS-CT. All patients received 1000 mg calcium and 400 IU vitamin D.

In the women with prevalent vertebral fractures receiving 200 IU NS-CT, there was a 36% reduction in the risk of new vertebral fracture (relative risk [RR] = 0.64, 0.43–0.96) compared with placebo nasal spray (Fig. 1). In the entire cohort receiving 200 IU NS-CT, there was a 33% reduction in the risk of new vertebral fracture compared with placebo. There was no significant fracture reduction with the other two doses of NS-CT.

The PROOF study was not powered to examine the occurrence of hip fracture; however, when the data from the

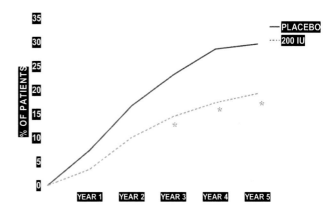

FIG. 1.   Cumulative percent of patients with new vertebral fractures by year in PROOF (patients with 1–5 prevalent vertebral fractures). *$p < 0.05$ vs. placebo.

Dr. Chesnut and Dr. Silverman have received research grants and served as speakers for Novartis.

100 and 200 IU doses were pooled, there was a 68% reduction in the risk of hip fracture compared with placebo.

BMD increased at the lumbar spine from baseline in all treatment groups over the 5 years of the trial (1.0–1.5%, $p = 0.01$), with no loss of bone at the hip. There was significant decrease in bone resorption as measured by serum C-telopeptide in the 200- and 400-IU groups at 1 year (about 25%, $p < 0.05$), with persistence of effect through 5 years.

Although no dose response for reduction of vertebral fracture risk was seen across doses in the intent-to-treat analysis, there was a significant fracture reduction with 400 IU in the valid completer analysis at 3 years.

Post Hoc Stratification Analysis of PROOF

A post hoc stratification analysis in older women showed a 53% reduction in the risk of vertebral fracture in women over age 70 and a 59% reduction in women over age 75.[13]

BONE QUALITY VERSUS QUANTITY: THE QUEST STUDY

The PROOF study demonstrated only a modest effect of NS-CT on BMD and bone turnover, yet NS-CT was associated with significant vertebral fracture reduction. This finding suggested that the therapeutic effect on fracture reduction is mediated through effects on bone quality rather than on bone quantity. The QUEST study (quantitative effects of salmon calcitonin therapy; C. Chesnut, personal communication, 2002) is a 2-year prospective placebo-controlled trial that is examining the effects of NS-CT on bone microarchitecture. Preliminary results suggest an increase in trabecular number and maintenance of trabecular spacing and thickness with NS-CT compared with placebo.

EFFECTS OF CALCITONIN IN PAGET'S DISEASE

Calcitonin injection is indicated for the treatment of symptomatic Paget's disease of bone.[14] The effectiveness of calcitonin salmon injection has been demonstrated in individuals with moderate to severe disease characterized by involvement with elevated serum alkaline phosphatase and urinary hydroxyproline excretion. In these patients, more than 30% reduction in biochemical markers were observed with similar decreases in pain.

ANALGESIC EFFECTS

Salmon calcitonin, both injectable and nasal, is unique among osteoporosis therapies in that it has an analgesic effect on the bone pain of acute vertebral fracture.[15] This analgesic effect is most pronounced in the first weeks after vertebral fracture, with a decrease in analgesic consumption by 3 days. Calcitonin also relieves bone pain in Paget's disease and bony metastasis.[14] Salmon calcitonin may have a role in the management of acute vertebral fracture by decreasing analgesic dependence and decreasing immobilization.[16]

CLINICAL USE

Indications

Salmon calcitonin is indicated for treatment of osteoporosis in postmenopausal women at least 5 years after the menopause and may be of particular benefit in the elderly (>70 years). Salmon calcitonin may be considered for its analgesic efficacy.

Administration

Administration of salmon calcitonin should be 200 IU of nasal calcitonin daily in alternating nostrils or 100 IU salmon calcitonin parenterally. Calcitonin should always be accompanied by optimal calcium and vitamin D.

Adverse Effects

Side effects with nasal calcitonin are minimal.[11] In the PROOF study, the only significant side effect was rhinitis. For parenteral calcitonin, facial flushing and/or nausea and vomiting can occur.

Monitoring

The increase in lumbar spine BMD with calcitonin is modest as is the reduction in bone markers. BMD should be monitored at 2 years to assure no significant loss.

CONCLUSIONS

Treatment with calcitonin should be considered for older women with osteoporosis on multiple medications or those who fail to respond or cannot tolerate other treatments. Treatment with calcitonin should be considered as a treatment option in the management of acute vertebral fractures because of its analgesic effect and reduction of vertebral fracture risk.

REFERENCES

1. Azria M, Copp SH, Zanelli JM 1995 25 years of salmon calcitonin: From synthesis to therapeutic use. Calcif Tissue Int **57:**405–408.
2. Chambers TJ, Moore A 1983 The sensitivity of isolated osteoclasts to morphological transformation by calcitonin. J Clin Endocrinol Metab **57:**819–824.
3. Singer FR, Aldred JP, Neer RM, Krane SM, Potts JT, Bloch KJ 1972 An evaluation of antibodies and clinical resistance to salmon calcitonin. J Clin Invest **51:**2331–2338.
4. Takahashi S, Goldring S, Katz M, Hilsenbeck S, Williams R, Roodman GD 1995 Downregulation of calcitonin receptor mRNA expression by calcitonin during human osteoclast-like cell differentiation. J Clin Invest **95:**167–171.
5. Hoff AO, Thomas M, Cote GJ 1998 Generation of a calcitonin knockout mouse model. Bone **23:**1062.
6. Silverman SL 2002 Calcitonin. In: Cummings SR, Cosman F, Jamal SA (eds.) Osteoporosis: An evidence based guide to prevention and management. American College of Physicians, Philadelphia, PA, USA, pp. 197–208.
7. Trovas GP, Lyritis GP, Galanos A, Raptou P, Constantelou E 2002 A randomized trial of nasal spray salcitonin in men with idiopathic osteoporosis: Effects on bone mineral density and bone markers. J Bone Miner Res **17:**521–527.
8. Reid IR 2002 Glucocorticoid induced osteoporosis. In: Cummings SR, Cosman F, Jamal SA (eds.) Osteoporosis: An Evidence Based Guide

to Prevention and Management. American College of Physicians, Philadelphia, PA, USA, pp. 223–240.

9. Rico H, Revilla M, Hernandez ER, Villa LF, Alvarez de Buergo M 1995 Total and regional bone mineral content and fracture rate in postmenopausal osteoporosis treated with salmon calcitonin. A prospective study. Calcif Tissue Int 47:209–214.

10. Kanis JA, Johnell O, Gullberg B, Allander E, Dilsen G, Gennari C, Lopes Vaz AA, Lyritis GP, Mazzuoli G, Miravet L 1992 Evidence for efficacy of drugs affecting bone metabolism in preventing hip fracture. BMJ 305:1124–1128.

11. Chesnut CH, Silverman S, Andriano K, Genant H, Gimona A, Harris S, Kiel D, LeBoff M, Maricic M, Miller P, Moniz C, Peacock M, Richardson P, Watts N, Baylink D for the PROOF study group 2000 A randomized trial of nasal spray calcitonin in postmenopausal women with established osteoporosis. The Prevent Recurrence of Osteoporotic Fractures Study. Am J Med 109:267–276.

12. Overgaard K, Hansen MA, Jensen SB, Christiansen C 1992 Effect of calcitonin given intranasally on bone mass and fracture rates in established osteoporosis. A dose response study. BMJ 305:556–561.

13. Silverman SL, Chesnut C, Baylink D, Gimona A, Adriano K, Mindeholm L 2001 Salmon calcitonin nasal spray (SCNS) is effective and safe in older osteoporotic women—results from the PROOF study. J Bone Miner Res 16:S1;S530.

14. Singer FR, Krane SM 1990 Paget's disease of bone. In: Avioli L, Krane SM (eds.) Metabolic Bone Disease and Clinically Related Disorders. WB Saunders, Philadelphia, PA, USA, pp. 588–595.

15. Silverman SL, Azria M 2002 The analgesic role of calcitonin following osteoporotic fracture. Osteoporos Int 13:858–867.

16. Lyritis GP, Tsakalakos N, Magiasis B, Karachalios T, Yiatzides A, Tsekoura M 1991 Analgesic effect of salmon calcitonin in osteoporotic vertebral fractures: A double-blind placebo-controlled study. Calcif Tissue Int 49:369–372.

Chapter 57.   Teriparatide [rhPTH(1-34)] and Future Anabolic Treatments for Osteoporosis

Jonathan Reeve

University Department of Medicine, Addenbrooke's Hospital, Cambridge, United Kingdom

INTRODUCTION

Patients who present with osteoporotic fractures do so typically only after they have lost around one-half of the cancellous bone in the spine[1] and one-third or more elsewhere. Patients who enroll in clinical trials often have fracture rates an order of magnitude greater than non-osteoporotic population-based controls. Our experience with licensed agents that reduce bone resorption (bisphosphonates, estrogens and selective estrogen receptor modulators [SERMS], calcitonins, and calcitriol) is that bone density does indeed increase slowly for 1 or 2 years and then plateaus. Therefore, these antiresorbers rarely normalize the bone density of such patients, but nevertheless, reduce spine fractures by 30–50%. So treatment, while demonstrably effective, does not reduce to control levels the risk of fracture. Moreover, one class of treatment that is no longer used, the so called anabolic steroids (e.g., nandrolone), behaved more like antiresorbers than anabolic treatments in their effects on bone. One genuinely anabolic therapy for osteoporosis, teriparatide [rhPTH(1-34)], has recently received a license from the Food and Drug Administration (FDA) in the United States, and a similar European license has been granted. A second so-called anabolic agent, strontium ranelate, has just completed phase III clinical trials, and peer-reviewed publications on its antifracture efficacy are anticipated. It is therefore timely to review the current data on the effectiveness of parathyroid hormone (PTH) therapy.

PTH AND RELATED COMPOUNDS

The first indications that PTH injections could have anabolic, not just catabolic, action on the skeleton emerged 70 years ago.[2–4] One of the first investigators, Edith Bülbring, encouraged John Parsons to recommence work on PTH's anabolic effects. Eventually, three European teams collaborated with John Potts and his colleagues, who had recently sequenced and synthesized the N-terminal region of PTH in the first clinical trial of hPTH(1-34), the amino terminal fragment of the human PTH molecule in osteoporosis. The results of this work were encouraging: bone formation was greatly increased and iliac trabecular bone volume seemed to increase in proportion to the formative response.[5] Later studies showed that the anabolic effects of hPTH(1-34) on bone depended on discontinuous exposures to transiently high blood levels of hPTH(1-34) and were lost if the hPTH(1-34) was given continuously.[6] Sustained increases in hPTH(1-34) levels led to a hyperparathyroid-like state of raised plasma calcium and increased bone resorption.

BIOLOGICAL BASIS OF PTH'S THERAPEUTIC ACTION

PTH exerts many of its most important biological actions on bone through the PTH1 receptor it shares with the PTH-related protein (PTHrP). The intracellular consequences of interactions of PTH with its receptor can modulate concentrations of cyclic adenosine monophosphate (cAMP) and the activity of cAMP-dependent protein kinase (PKA); however, one consequence of this can be that proliferation of osteoblasts is inhibited. Protein kinase C (PKC) is involved in the proliferation response, but the role of intermittent PTH stimulation in PKC pathways still requires clarification.[7] Stimulation of phospholipase C also occurs, which modulates the intracellular concentrations of calcium ions, diacyl glycerol, and hydrogen ions; also, insulin-like growth factor (IGF)-1 may be involved in coupling PTH-stimulated bone resorption to subsequent bone formation.

Dr. Reeve serves as consultant for Eli Lilly and Company and Procter & Gamble.

TABLE 1. SUMMARY OF KEY TRIALS ON THE EFFECTS OF hPTH THERAPY IN PATIENTS

Trial	Active agent	Duration of treatment	Treatment regimen	Disease treated	Key outcome measure(s)	Trial category	Key references
Multicenter trial of hPTH(1-34)	Synthetic hPTH(1-34)	6 months (most subjects)	DI	"Idiopathic" osteoporosis M + F	Iliac TBV	Patients were own controls	(5)
Sequential hPTH and nasal calcitonin (Hanover)	Synthetic hPTH(1-38) calcitonin NS	14 months	DI/altCT	"Idiopathic" osteoporosis	QCT spine + iliac TBV	Patients were own controls	(33)
Multi-outcome trial of hPTH(1-34) and estrogen	hPTH(1-34)	12 months	DI	Postmenopausal osteoporosis	QCT spine, DPA spine, iliac TBV	Patients were own controls	(13, 34)
Effect of hPTH(1-34) in acute estrogen suppression	hPTH(1-34)	12 months	DI	Endometriosis, treated with GnRH agonist (nafarelin)	DXA spine and hip	RCT	(19)
Sequential hPTH$^{+/-}$ parenteral calcitonin (Ontario)	hPTH(1-34)	24 months	DI, 1 28-day cycle per 3 months	Postmenopausal osteoporosis	DXA spine/ proximal femur	RCT to compare efficacy of additional CT	(35)
RCT in estrogenized women with osteoporosis (New York)	hPTH(1-34)	36 months	DI	Postmenopausal osteoporosis	DXA spine/ proximal femur	RCT to compare efficacy of adding hPTH treatment	(36)
Trial of different weekly doses of hPTH (Japan)	hPTH(1-34)	12 months	Weekly injections, 3 doses	Radiographically defined osteoporosis	DXA spine	Multicenter RCT	(37)
Fracture Prevention Trial	rhPTH(1-34), teriparatide	19 months (11 months in men)	DI, 20 or 40 microg	Untreated vertebral fracture osteoporosis	Vertebral and nonvertebral fractures	Multicenter RCT	(12, 17)

DI, daily injections; DI/alt, CT daily injections alternating with calcitonin; TBV, trabecular bone volume; QCT, quantitative computed tomography; RCT, randomized controlled trial; DPA, dual photon absorptometry.

Increased osteoclastic resorption driven by PTH infused continuously is believed to be a consequence of communication of the cells lining quiescent bone surfaces or other stromal cells with osteoclast precursors through RANK signaling. Further events that are more typical of the effects of daily injections include the recruitment of quiescent bone lining cells to the osteoblastic phenotype, with prevention of programmed cell death (apoptosis) of osteoblasts prolonging their effective lifespan. This augments the capacity of osteoblasts to form new bone.[6]

EFFECTS OF PTH IN ANIMALS

In the last 20 years, there has been a tremendous revival in rat studies on the effects of PTH treatment, and these have recently been reviewed.[6] Nearly all have shown intermittently dosed PTH, usually as hPTH(1-34), to have a positive effect on bone mass, size, structure, and strength. This has now been confirmed in a large animal study.[8]

From these rat studies, PTH seemed to have considerable potential when given intermittently, having proved itself capable of increasing trabecular bone mass at all skeletal sites and of maintaining or improving trabecular connectivity. At the same time, PTH has increased cortical thickness by adding bone both at the endocortical surface and also at the biomechanically more important periosteal surface. Furthermore, PTH has been able to increase bone structural strength, including material strength, at all skeletal sites tested (vertebrae, tibial metaphyseal and cortical bone, femoral cortical bone, and femoral neck). Also, all animal models (young, growing intact rats; mature ovariectomized rats; orchidectomized rats; aged, osteopenic rats; and cynomolgus monkeys) have responded in an equally positive manner. PTH treatment improved the structure as well as the amount of cancellous bone in ovariectomized monkeys.

CLINICAL STUDIES

PTH as hPTH(1-34) or hPTH(1-38) has been trialed in postmenopausal osteoporosis, in idiopathic osteoporosis in men, in glucocorticoid osteoporosis, and in the prevention of the bone loss that is a consequence of suppression of estrogen synthesis in endometriosis when treated with GnRH agonists (Table 1). It can be confidently predicted that PTH will now be studied as a treatment for other forms of osteoporosis, because there was no obvious difference in responsiveness between these different groups. However, the FDA license for teriparatide strongly discourages its use in children, in patients with Paget's disease of bone, or in patients with low bone mass caused by hyperparathyroidism because of a theoretically increased risk of skeletal neoplasia uncovered during a safety study undertaken in rats.

EFFECTS OF hPTH ON BONE AND OTHER ORGANS

A single subcutaneous injection of hPTH(1-34) causes a very brief peak of plasma PTH bioactivity followed by a rather longer effect on maximal renal transport for phosphate, which is nevertheless no longer evident 6–8 h after injection.[6] As a result, endogenous PTH is mildly suppressed over 24 h. In the long term, no tachyphylaxis occurs, with the generation of similar amounts of nephrogenous cAMP at the beginning and end of long-term treatment. Treatment with hPTH(1-38) had substantial effects on iliac cancellous bone remodeling within 1 month of the start of therapy[9]; however, at later stages in treatment, there were either smaller increments (at 6 months) or minimal changes (at 1 year) in remodeling, while the wall thicknesses of new packets of cancellous bone were increased.[10]

By 6 months of treatment with hPTH(1-34) alone, rates of ^{47}Ca estimated bone mineralization increased substantially in many patients,[5] and this could be tracked by the biochemical marker plasma osteocalcin.[11] Daily injections also increase spinal bone mass. Until the recent study of Neer et al.,[12] all the data on the spinal response to treatment had been obtained in patients given some form of cotherapy. Reeve et al.[13] found that, when combined with estrogens, daily hPTH(1-34) injections increased vertebral body cancellous bone without changing cortical or posterior element mineral content. Consequently, quantitative computed tomography (QCT) revealed increases in spinal bone density that were about twice as large in relative terms as observed with DXA, because the latter technique does not differentiate cancellous from the surrounding cortical bone.

Now that DXA and QCT densitometry can be used to measure more precisely bone density in the proximal femur, new data have appeared showing that daily hPTH therapy increases bone density in the total hip region in parallel with spinal increases.[11,12,14] However, the size of the response is smaller in relative terms than in the spine. In a QCT study, Cann et al. were able to show that the cortical bone also expanded, perhaps because of subperiosteal bone formation,[15] as has been seen in animal studies.

ANTIFRACTURE EFFICACY USING DAILY rhPTH(1-34) (TERIPARATIDE)

The best clinical test of the effectiveness of treatment on the biomechanical competence of bone is a randomized control trial of its antifracture efficacy. In the Fracture Prevention Trial of Neer et al., over 1600 postmenopausal women with prior vertebral fracture were randomly assigned to receive 20 or 40 mg of PTH [rhPTH(1-34)] placebo.[12] These were administered daily by the women themselves as subcutaneous injections using a pen-like device resembling an insulin pen used by diabetics.

New vertebral fractures were identified radiologically, and nonvertebral fractures were recorded with the help of medical and radiological records. The trial was interrupted

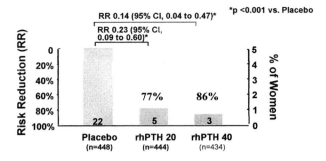

FIG. 1. Effect of rhPTH(1-34) treatment on multiple spinal fractures. (Reproduced with the permission from the Massachusetts Medical Society N Engl J Med 2001:**344**:1434–1441.)

after a mean duration of 21 months because of concerns over some long-term treatments studies being undertaken in parallel in rats. Notwithstanding the truncation of treatment, the effectiveness against fractures of teriparatide exceeded prior expectations, with the two treatment groups combined having a relative risk of vertebral fracture of 33% (i.e., a 3-fold reduction) and of nonvertebral fracture of 47% (a 2-fold reduction) compared with the control group.[12] Figure 1 shows the strength of the effect against multiple vertebral fractures, which have more impact on quality of life than single fractures. The cumulative plots of nonvertebral fractures versus months since randomization suggested that the antifracture efficacy began to take effect for nonspine fractures after the eighth month of treatment. In further analysis, patient's age had little influence on the effectiveness of treatment, and the more severe cases had a similar proportionate reduction in risk to the less severe.[16]

In a study of male osteoporosis, 437 men were randomly assigned similarly to 20 or 40 mg of PTH or placebo, and the median drug exposure was 11 months, after which the men were observed off PTH treatment for a further 18 months.[17] Essentially, there were few if any differences in the response to treatment of these male patients, many but not all of whom were hypogonadal, compared with the postmenopausal women of Neer et al.[12] In these men, the reduction in risk of any vertebral fracture over a total 3-year observation period was reported as similar to that in women studied both during treatment and for up to 18 months after discontinuation of treatment.[18] In the women,[18] the effectiveness of prior treatment was such that the relative risk of a vertebral fracture was reduced by over 40% during 18 months of post-treatment follow-up.

Another interesting study has been published in which hPTH(1-34) was shown to prevent or reverse bone loss provoked by gonadotrophin releasing hormone (GnRH) agonist treatment of endometriosis.[19] This was not, however, powered to study antifracture efficacy.

hPTH GIVEN WITH OTHER AGENTS

Over the past 15 years, efforts have been made, by adding a second agent, to develop subcutaneous injection regimens that improve protection to the peripheral skeleton while preserving the anabolic effect on the spine. The impetus for these studies was that hPTH(1-34), when used alone, did not seem to increase gastrointestinal absorption of calcium,[5] although more recent work has shown that total body calcium does increase in the long term. These trials of modified or cotherapy now are of somewhat historical interest in light of the better than expected results of the Neer trial in preventing nonspine fractures. Nevertheless, they might also be of interest in the context of protecting the patient after PTH therapy is stopped, so they are reported briefly. Three approaches were used. The first was to add calcitriol to promote calcium absorption.[20] The second aimed also to control bone resorption with the combination of PTH and estrogen in postmenopausal women.[11,21] No randomized trial of cotherapy was adequately powered to test reliably the antifracture efficacy of hPTH(1-34) in such contexts; however, the study of Cosman et al., which used hPTH(1-34) in already estrogenized postmenopausal women, actually found a statistically significant effect.[21] Also, hPTH(1-34) with estrogen cotherapy was used to reverse the bone loss associated with therapeutic glucocorticoid therapy.[14] In two histological analyses,[10,22], the later of which used sophisticated three-dimensional (3-D) technology, hPTH plus estrogen therapy was associated with increased connectivity of iliac cancellous bone in addition to trabecular thickening.

The third approach was to give PTH cyclically. Cycle lengths have varied; in short, the longer the cycle and the more sustained the individual courses of PTH, the more effect was observed. In summary, none of these regimens seem to have obvious potential as competitors to the regimen of 20 μg/day teriparatide given alone for 18 months.[6]

LOCALLY ADMINISTERED PTH PEPTIDES

Interest is also awakening in the generation of PTH locally in orthopedic procedures[23] or in using systemic PTH to enhance implant fixation.[24] Currently, such studies are still at the experimental stage. Competing approaches still also experimental are to use mitogenic agents such as osteoblast stimulating factor 1 incorporated into implantable scaffolds.[25] Also experimental is the use of adenoviruses for carrying the gene for bone morphogenetic protein 2 (BMP-2) to achieve spinal fusions.

EFFECTS OF COMING OFF hPTH TREATMENT

A large body of animal data suggests that bone acquired during PTH treatment tends to be lost when it is discontinued.[6] The Fracture Prevention Trial investigators have been collecting bone density and fracture data to determine whether this "off" effect is sufficiently serious to warrant continued treatment with an antiresorber after PTH is stopped. Both Reeve et al.[11] and Cosman et al.[21] found that continuing hormone replacement therapy (HRT) used in cotherapy with PTH after the PTH was stopped was associated with negligible bone loss in the 1–3 years subsequently. Rittmaster et al.[26] started alendronate therapy after PTH was stopped. Eriksen et al.[18] has suggested that the antifracture efficacy of teriparatide used alone continues

after the cessation of treatment, even if an antiresorber is not prescribed (after the Fracture Prevention Trial was stopped, physicians had prescribing freedom). Further follow-up and analysis is awaited with interest.

WHEN DOES AN ANABOLIC AGENT MAKE SENSE?

The data of Marcus et al.[16] suggest that, when working within given resource limits, more fractures could be prevented in absolute terms if more severely affected and older patients with osteoporosis (and fair life expectancy) were preferentially treated with teriparatide. This is because age, low bone density, and prior fractures are the major positive determinants of fracture risk in untreated patients. Looked at another way, patients at only moderately increased risk of an osteoporotic fracture might consider that a once weekly oral bisphosphonate or a daily SERM should provides the natural first choice of antifracture protective agent, given the current state of our knowledge of the relative effectiveness of the various licensed agents available.

However, such an ideal scenario, in which the patient is identified early before risk has increased by an order of magnitude, as is seen commonly in randomized trial participants, is not as common as would be desirable. Cooper et al. found that, in Minnesota, only about one-third of patients with a spine fracture were identified clinically; therefore, the two-thirds of patients with a 4-fold or greater increase in future fracture risk were unaware of their vulnerability.[27] In Britain, it can be inferred that only about 1 in 13 patients with at least one spine fracture are identified in primary medical care.[28,29] Consequently, many such patients, when they do come to attention, are at very high risk of future fractures.

Currently, bisphosphonate treatments for spinal osteoporosis have been available for some years, and substantial numbers of treated patients are experiencing fractures despite bisphosphonate therapy (about 50% of those who would suffer similarly without treatment). Physicians and patients will naturally consider after a fracture event while on treatment whether to change to a second line treatment such as teriparatide.

The numbers are substantial. With white postmenopausal women at the age of 65 having a 10% or greater risk of a new vertebral fracture every 10 years,[28] and this risk being increased 7-fold in those who already have a fracture,[28] candidate patients for a second line treatment on the perceived failure of bisphosphonate therapy could after 3 years be 3% of those with pre-existing osteoporosis and 20% of those with severe osteoporosis and a pretreatment spine fracture.

SAFETY OF TERIPARATIDE

In the study of Neer et al., there were few side effects attributable to the treatment at the approved dose of 20 μg/day apart from transient mild hypercalcemia in a minority and a tendency for a rise in uric acid levels: neither had apparent clinical sequelae. However, the planned 3-year treatment duration was truncated abruptly in this and the

Orwoll study because of the appearance of osteosarcomas in a strain of Fisher rats given long-term teriparatide from an early age, in some, but not all, animals at very high doses compared with those used in humans. Previously, no association had been reported of osteosarcoma and hyperparathyroidism, primary or secondary; no case of sarcoma has been reported in the over 2000 patients treated with parathyroid peptides in clinical trials so far. Nevertheless, these data require that clinicians act cautiously, and the FDA has approved teriparatide for human use with restrictions to protect patients thought potentially vulnerable, including all children and adolescents. The possible explanations for the observations seen so far in Fisher rats have been thoroughly discussed by Tashjian and Chabner.[30] A further rat study is being prepared for publication; in the meantime, the view is surely correct that although several factors limit our ability to extrapolate the published rat findings to humans these preclinical data should not be dismissed as clinically irrelevant and should be factored into the drug's profile of benefits versus risks.

FUTURE ALTERNATIVE ANABOLIC THERAPIES

Other activators of the PTH receptor(s) under development for possible human use include rhPTH(1-84), this being the intact molecule secreted by the parathyroid gland in man and the fragment of rhPTHrP(1-36). So far, only short-term phase I or phase II studies not powered to detect an effect against fractures are available for these molecules.

Strontium ranelate provides an interesting alternative approach. The preclinical and clinical data are not consistent concerning its effects on the absolute rate of bone formation; however, it does seem that the strontium ion is incorporated into the hydroxyapatite crystalline structure and also binds to its surface. The effect is to prevent the osteoclasts from resorbing bone efficiently, and this occurs without impeding the ability of the osteoblasts to make new bone. Thus, a favorable balance is induced between bone formation and bone resorption and DXA-measured bone density increases. Part of this increase is artifactual, being caused by the higher atomic weight of strontium than calcium. This can only be adjusted for if the strontium content of bone is known, a harder task than is sometimes admitted because of the complex dynamics of long-term equilibration of strontium with calcium, as studied previously in the context of fall-out radiation exposure. Ultimately, the effectiveness of strontium ranelate in safely preventing fractures will determine whether it goes forward for consideration for a license. Although no peer-reviewed report has appeared at the time of writing, a preliminary communication suggests that in a dose of 2 g/day, strontium ranelate prevents both hip and spine fractures in women with postmenopausal osteoporosis.[31]

Other approaches to increasing bone formation are at a less advanced stage. They include the development of statins that reportedly increase BMP-2 and bone formation in growing rodents,[32] but through their actions on the mevalonate pathway could also modulate osteoclast function analogously to the nitrogen-containing bisphosphonates. Current statins are thought to be limited in their applicability by being optimized for liver rather than bone uptake. Growth hormone has been studied extensively in clinical trials, but currently it seems that because it does not greatly improve the balance between bone formation and resorption its role is limited in osteoporosis.

It is likely that many other approaches to increasing bone formation and thereby inducing a favorable bone balance will develop out of the current ferment of interest in the basic biology of osteoblast induction and regulation in bone. However, bringing these anticipated developments into clinical use will be a process taking us toward the end of the present decade.

REFERENCES

1. Kröger HPJ, Lunt M, Reeve J, Dequeker J, Adams JE, Birkenhäger JC, Diaz Curiel M, Felsenberg D, Hyldstrup L, Kotzki P, Laval-Jeantet A-M, Lips P, Louis O, Perez Cano R, Reiners C, Ribot C, Ruegsegger P, Schneider P, Braillon P, Pearson J 1999 Bone density reduction in various measurement sites in men and women with osteoporotic fractures of spine and hip: The European Quantitation of Osteoporosis (QAO) Study. Calcif Tissue Int **64:**191–199.
2. Bauer E, Aub J, Albright F 1929 Studies of calcium and phosphorus metabolism. V. A study of the bone trabeculae as a readily available reserve supply of calcium. J Exp Med **49:**145–162.
3. Pugsley LI, Selye H 1933 The histological changes in the bone responsible for the action of parathyroid hormone on the calcium metabolism of the rat. J Physiol **79:**113–117.
4. Bülbring E 1931 Über die Beziehungen zwischen Epithelkörperchen, Calciumstoffwechsel und Knochenwachstum. Arch Exp Path Pharm **162:**209–248.
5. Reeve J, Meunier PJ, Parsons JA, Bernat M, Bijvoet OLM, Courpron P, Edouard C, Klenerman L, Neer RM, Renier JC, Slovik DM, Vismans FJFE, Potts JT Jr 1980 The anabolic effect of human parathyroid hormone fragment (hPTH 1–34) therapy on trabecular bone in involutional osteoporosis: Report of a multi-centre trial. Br Med J **280:**1340–1344.
6. Mosekilde L, Reeve J 2001 Treatment with PTH Peptides. In: Marcus R, Feldman D, Kelsey J (eds.) Osteoporosis, 2nd ed., vol. 2. Academic Press, New York, NY, USA, pp. 725–746.
7. Swarthout J, D'Alonzo R, Selvamurugan N, Partridge N 2002 Parathyroid hormone-dependent signaling pathways regulating genes in bone cells. Gene **282:**1–17.
8. Jerome CP, Johnson CS, Vafai HT, Kaplan KC, Bailey J, Capwell B, Fraser F, Hansen L, Ramsay H, Shadoan M, Lees CJ, Thomsen JS, Mosekilde AL 1999 Effect of treatment for 6 months with human parathyroid hormone (1–34) peptide in ovariectomized cynomolgus monkeys (Macaca fascicularis). Bone **25:**301–309.
9. Hodsman AB, Steer BM 1993 Early histomorphomorphic changes in response to parathyroid hormone therapy in osteoporosis: Evidence for de novo bone formation on quiescent cancellous surfaces. Bone **14:** 523–527.
10. Bradbeer JN, Arlot ME, Meunier PJ, Reeve J 1992 Treatment of osteoporosis with parathyroid peptide (hPTH 1–34) and oestrogen: Increase in volumetric density of iliac cancellous bone may depend on reduced trabecular spacing as well as increased thickness of packets of newly formed bone. Clin Endocrinol **37:**282–289.
11. Reeve J, Mitchell A, Tellez M, Hulme P, Green JR, Wardley-Smith B, Mitchell R 2001 Treatment with parathyroid peptides and estrogen replacement for severe post-menopausal vertebral osteoporosis: Long-term effects on spine and femur and determinants of magnitude of response. J Bone Miner Metab **19:**102–114.
12. Neer RM, Arnaud CD, Zanchetta JR, Prince R, Gaich GA, Reginster JY, Hodsman AB, Eriksen EF, Ish-Shalom S, Genant HK, Wang O, Mitlak BH, Mellstrom D, Oefjord ES, Marcinowska-Sucherowierska E, Salmi J, Gaspar L, Mulder H, Halse J, Sawicki AZ 2001 Recombinant human PTH (1–34) fragment [rhPTH] reduces the risk of spine and non-spine fractures in post-menopausal osteoporosis. N Engl J Med **344:**1434–1441.
13. Reeve J, Davies UM, Hesp R, McNally E, Katz D 1990 Human parathyroid peptide treatment of osteoporosis substantially increases spinal trabecular bone (with observations on the effects of sodium fluoride therapy). Br Med J **301:**314–318,477.
14. Lane NE, Sanchez S, Modlin GW, Genant HK, Pierini E, Arnaud CD

1998 Parathyroid hormone treatment can reverse corticosteroid-induced osteoporosis—results of a randomised controlled clinical trial. J Clin Invest 102:1627–1633.

15. Cann CE, Roe EB, Sanchez SD, Arnaud CD 1999 PTH effects in the femur: Envelope-specific responses by 3DQCT in postmenopausal women. J Bone Miner Res 14:S1;S137.

16. Marcus R, Wang OH, Satterwhite J, Mitlak B 2003 The skeletal response to teriparatide is largely independent of age, initial bone mineral density, and prevalent vertebral fractures in postmenopausal women with osteoporosis. J Bone Miner Res 18:18–23.

17. Orwoll E, Scheele W, Paul S, Adami S, Syversen U, Diez-Perez A, Kaufman JM, Clancy A, Gaich G 2003 The effect of teriparatide [human parathyroid hormone (1–34)] therapy on bone density in men with osteoporosis. J Bone Miner Res 18:9–17.

18. Eriksen EF, Lindsay R, Scheele WH, Clancy AD, Mitlak BH 2001 Incident vertebral fractures during an 18-month observation period following discontinuation of recombinant human parathyroid hormone (1–34) use in postmenopausal women with osteoporosis. Osteoporos Int 12(Suppl 2):S46.

19. Finkelstein JS, Klibanski A, Arnold AL, Toth TL, Hornstein MD, Neer RM 1998 Prevention of estrogen deficiency-related bone loss with human parathyroid hormone-(1–34): A randomised trial. J Am Med Assoc 280:1067–1073.

20. Slovik DM, Rosenthal DI, Doppelt SH, Potts JT Jr, Daly M, Campbell JA, Neer RM 1986 Restoration of spinal bone in osteoporotic men by treatment with human parathyroid hormone (1–34) and 1,25-dihydroxyvitamin. J Bone Miner Res 1:377–381.

21. Cosman F, Nieves J, Woelfert L, Formica C, Gordon S, Shen V, Lindsay R 2001 Parathyroid hormone added to established hormone therapy: Effects on vertebral fracture and maintenance of bone mass after parathyroid hormone withdrawal. J Bone Miner Res 16:925–931.

22. Dempster DW, Cosman F, Kurland ES, Zhou H, Nieves J, Woelfert L, Shane E, Plavetic K, Muller R, Bilezikian J, Lindsay R 2001 Effects of daily treatment with parathyroid hormone on bone microarchitecture and turnover in patients with osteoporosis: A paired biopsy study. J Bone Miner Res 16:1846–1853.

23. Bonadio J, Smiley E, Patil P, Goldstein S 1999 Localised, direct plasmid gene delivery in vivo: Prolonged therapy results in reproducible tissue regeneration. Nat Med 5:753–759.

24. Skripitz R, Aspenberg P 2001 Implant fixation enhanced by intermittent treatment with parathyroid hormone. J Bone Joint Surg Br 83:437–440.

25. Yang X, Tare RS, Partridge KA, Roach HI, Clarke NM, Howdle SM, Shakesheff KM, Oreffo RO 2003 Induction of human osteoprogenitor chemotaxis, proliferation, differentiation, and bone formation by osteoblast stimulating factor-1/pleiotrophin: Osteoconductive biomimetic scaffolds for tissue engineering. J Bone Miner Res 18:47–57.

26. Rittmaster RS, Bolognese M, Ettinger MP, Hanley DA, Hodsman AB, Kendler DL, Rosen CJ 2000 Enhancement of bone mass in osteoporotic women with parathyroid hormone followed by alendronate. J Clin Endocrinol Metab 85:2129–2134.

27. Cooper C, Atkinson EJ, O'Fallon WM, Melton LJ III 1992 Incidence

of clinically diagnosed vertebral fractures: A population-based study in Rochester, Minnesota, 1985–1989. J Bone Miner Res 7:221–227.

28. Felsenberg D, Silman AJ, Lunt M, Armbrecht G, Ismail AA, Finn JD, Cockerill WC, Banzer D, Benevolenskaya LI, Bhalla A, Bruges Armas J, Cannata JB, Cooper C, Dequeker J, Eastell R, Felsch B, Gowin W, Havelka S, Hoszowski K, Jajic I, Janott J, Johnell O, Kanis JA, Kragl G, Lopes Vaz A, Lorenc R, Lyritis G, Masaryk P, Matthis C, Miazgowski T, Parisi G, Pols HAP, Poor G, Raspe HH, Reid DM, Reisinger W, Scheidt-Nave C, Stepan JJ, Todd CJ, Weber K, Woolf AD, Yershova OB, Reeve J, O'Neill TW 2002 Incidence of vertebral fractures in Europe: Results from the European Prospective Osteoporosis Study (EPOS). J Bone Miner Res 17:716–724.

29. van Staa TP, Dennison EM, Leufkens HGM, Cooper C 2001 Epidemiology of fractures in England and Wales. Bone 29:517–522.

30. Tashjian AH Jr, Chabner BA 2002 Commentary on clinical safety of recombinant human parathyroid hormone 1–34 in the treatment of osteoporosis in men and postmenopausal women. J Bone Miner Res 17:1151–1161.

31. Reginster JY, Sawicki A, Devogelaer JP, Padrino JM, Kaufman JM, Doyle DV, Fardellone P, Graham J, Felsenberg D, Tulassay Z, Soren-Sen OH, Luisetto G, Rizzoli R, Blotman F, Phenekos C, Meunier PJ 2002 Strontium Ranelate reduces the risk of hip fractures in women with postmenopausal osteoporosis. Osteoporos Int 13(Suppl 3):S14.

32. Mundy G, Garrett R, Harris S, Chan J, Chen D, Rossini G, Boyce B, Zhao M, Gutierrez G 1999 Stimulation of bone formation in vitro and in rodents by statins. Science 286:1946–1949.

33. Hesch R-D, Busch U, Prokop M, Delling G, Rittinghaus E-F 1989 Increase of vertebral density by combination therapy with pulsatile 1–38hPTH and sequential addition of calcitonin nasal spray in osteoporotic patients. Calcif Tissue Int 44:176–180.

34. Reeve J, Bradbeer JN, Arlot ME, Davies UM, Green JR, Hampton L, Edouard C, Hesp R, Hulme P, Ashby JP, Zanelli JM, Meunier PJ 1991 hPTH 1–34 treatment of osteoporosis with added hormone replacement therapy: Biochemical, kinetic and histological responses. Osteoporos Int 1:162–170.

35. Hodsman A, Fraher L, Watson P, Ostbye T, Stitt L, Adachi J, Taves D, Drost D 1997 A randomized controlled trial to compare the efficacy of cyclical parathyroid hormone versus cyclical parathyroid hormone and sequential calcitonin to improve bone mass in postmenopausal women with osteoporosis. J Clin Endocrinol Metab 82:620–628.

36. Lindsay R, Nieves J, Formica C, Henneman E, Woelfert L, Shen V, Dempster DW, Cosman F 1997 Randomised controlled study of effect of parathyroid hormone on vertebral-bone mass and fracture incidence among postmenopausal women on oestrogen with osteoporosis. Lancet 350:550–555.

37. Fujita T, Inoue T, Morii H, Morita R, Norimatsu H, Orimo H, Takahashi HE, Yamamoto K, Fukunaga M 1999 Effect of an intermittent weekly dose of human parathyroid hormone (1–34) on osteoporosis: A randomised double-masked prospective study using three dose levels. Osteoporos Int 9:296–306.

Chapter 58.   Calcium and Vitamin D

Bess Dawson-Hughes

Jean Mayer USDA Human Nutrition Research Center on Aging, Tufts University, Boston, Massachusetts

INTRODUCTION

Calcium is required for the bone formation phase of bone remodeling. Typically, about 5 mmol (200 mg) of calcium is removed from the adult skeleton and replaced each day. To supply this, one would need to consume about 600 mg of

calcium, because calcium is not very efficiently absorbed. Calcium also affects bone mass through its impact on the remodeling rate. An inadequate intake of calcium results in reduced calcium absorption, a lower circulating ionized calcium concentration, and an increased secretion of parathyroid hormone (PTH), a potent bone-resorbing agent. A high remodeling rate leads to bone loss; it is also an independent risk factor for fracture.[1] Dietary calcium at sufficiently high levels, usually 1000 mg per day or more, lowers the bone remodeling rate by about 10–20% in older men

Dr. Dawson-Hughes served on the scientific advisory boards for Eli Lilly, GlaxoSmithKline, and Procter & Gamble. In addition, she also served on the speakers bureau for Aventis, Eli Lilly, and Procter & Gamble.

and women,[2-5] and the degree of suppression seems to be dose related.[5] The reduction in remodeling rate accounts for the increase in bone mineral density (BMD) that occurs in the first 12–18 months of treatment with calcium.

With aging, there is a decline in calcium absorption efficiency in men and women.[6] This may be related to loss of intestinal vitamin D receptors or resistance of these receptors to the action of $1,25(OH)_2D$.[7] Diet composition, season, and race also influence calcium absorption efficiency.

Vitamin D is acquired from the diet and from skin synthesis on exposure to ultraviolet B rays. The best clinical indicator of vitamin D status is the serum 25-hydroxyvitamin D (25OHD) level. Serum 25OHD levels are lower in individuals using sunscreens and in those with more pigmented skin. Season is an important determinant of vitamin D levels. In much of the temperate zone, skin synthesis of vitamin D does not occur during the winter. Consequently, 25OHD levels fall in the winter and early spring.[8] Serum PTH levels vary inversely with 25OHD levels. These cyclic changes are not benign. Bone loss from the spine[9] and femoral neck[10] is greater in the winter/spring, when 25OHD levels are lowest (and PTH levels are highest), than in the summer/fall, when 25OHD levels are highest (and PTH levels are lowest).

Serum 25OHD levels decline with aging for several reasons. There is less efficient skin synthesis of vitamin D with aging as a result of an age-related decline in the amount of 7-dehydrocholesterol, the precursor to vitamin D, in the epidermal layer of skin.[11] Also, older individuals as a group spend less time outdoors. There does not seem to be an impairment in the intestinal absorption of vitamin D with aging.[12]

IMPACT ON BMD

Calcium and vitamin D support bone growth in children and adolescents and lower rates of bone loss in adults and the elderly. A recent meta-analysis of 15 trials found that calcium alone in adults caused positive mean percentage BMD changes from baseline of 1.7% at lumbar spine, 1.6% at the hip, and 1.9% at the distal radius.[13] In one trial, the effects of calcium from food (milk powder) and supplement sources on changes in BMD in older postmenopausal women were compared and found to be similar.[14] Supplementation with vitamin D also reduces rates of bone loss in older adults,[15] as does supplementation with both calcium and vitamin D.[4] To sustain the reduced turnover rate and higher bone mass induced by increased calcium and vitamin D intakes, the higher intakes need to be maintained.[16]

IMPACT ON FRACTURE RATES

Several small studies have examined the impact of calcium on fracture rates. The recent Shea meta-analysis of these studies[13] found that calcium alone (versus placebo) tended to lower risk of vertebral fractures (relative risk [RR] 0.77; CI, 0.54–1.09) but not nonvertebral fractures (RR 0.86; CI, 0.43–1.72). The studies in this analysis range from 18 months to 4 years in duration.

The effect of supplemental vitamin D on fracture incidence has been examined in several large trials. One study was positive, finding that annual subcutaneous injections of vitamin D lowered all clinical fractures,[17] but others found no effect of vitamin D in doses of 300[18] or 400 IU per day[19,20] on fracture rates at any skeletal site.

Supplementation with calcium and vitamin D together (in doses of 500-1200 mg of calcium and 700–800 IU of vitamin D) significantly reduced all clinical fractures,[4,21,22] and more importantly, reduced hip fracture rates.[21] The consistently positive effects of combined calcium and vitamin D supplementation were probably related to the fact that higher doses of vitamin D (compared with the vitamin D intervention studies described above) were used and/or to the concurrent use of calcium.

ROLE IN PHARMACOTHERAPY

In recent randomized, controlled trials testing the antifracture efficacy of the antiresorptive therapies alendronate,[23] risedronate,[24] raloxifene,[25] and calcitonin,[26] and the anabolic drug, PTH(1-34),[27] calcium and vitamin D were given to both the control and intervention groups. This allows one to define the impact of these drugs in calcium- and vitamin D-replete patients and to conclude that any efficacy of the drugs is beyond that associated with calcium and vitamin D alone. Based on the evidence that follows, however, one can't conclude that these drugs would have the same efficacy in calcium- and vitamin D–deficient patients. In a comparative analysis of the impact of estrogen on BMD in early postmenopausal women who did and did not take calcium supplements, Nieves et al.[28] found that the BMD gains at the spine, hip, and forearm were several-fold greater in the women who increased their calcium intakes than in those who took estrogen without added calcium. From this, it seems that calcium enables estrogen to be more effective in building BMD. In the Mediterranean Osteoporosis Study (MEDOS) in southern Europe,[29] use of nasal calcitonin was associated with a nonsignificant decrease in vertebral fracture risk (RR = 0.78) as was use of calcium alone (RR = 0.82). Use of calcitonin and calcium together, however, was associated with a significant reduction in vertebral fracture risk (RR = 0.63), suggesting that the effects of calcium and this antiresorptive therapy are additive. Little information is available on a potential interaction of other osteoporosis treatments with calcium intake. One can certainly infer that an adequate calcium intake is essential for an optimal response to treatment with the bone-building drug, PTH(1-34). Little direct evidence is available of an interaction of vitamin D with pharmacotherapy, but because vitamin D works in concert with calcium, adequate vitamin D status is very likely to be an important component of the therapy.

INTAKE REQUIREMENTS

Calcium intake recommendations vary enormously worldwide. Recommendations by the U.S. National Academy of Sciences (NAS) are among the highest. The NAS recommended intakes of calcium are as follows: ages 1–3 years, 500 mg; 4–8 years, 800 mg; 9–18 years, 1300 mg;

19–50 years, 1000 mg; and 51+ years, 1200 mg per day.[30] Lower calcium intakes would likely be adequate for populations with lower intakes of salt and protein.

Among females in the United States, fewer than 1 in 10 up to the age of 70 years and fewer than 1 in 100 over that age meet the calcium requirement through their diets.[31] Among males, no more than 25% in any age group has an adequate calcium intake from the diet.[31] Without major dietary changes, most of the American population will need to rely on fortified foods and supplements to meet calcium requirements. Calcium from calcium carbonate, the most commonly used supplement, is better absorbed when taken with a meal.[32,33] Absorption from all supplements is more efficient in single doses of 500 mg or less.[34] Thus, individuals requiring more than 500 mg per day from supplements should take it in divided doses. The safe upper limit for calcium set by the NAS is 2500 mg per day.[30]

The vitamin D intake recommendations of the NAS are as follows: up to age 50 years, about 200 IU; 51–70 years, 400 IU; and 71+ years, 600 IU per day.[30] These recommendations are based on the amount of vitamin D needed to maximally suppress PTH secretion. However, for reasons that are not entirely clear, variability in this end-point is very large across study populations. Several studies have placed the 25OHD level needed for maximal PTH suppression in the range of 75–110 nM,[8,35–37] whereas another places it as low as 25 nM.[38] In the future, it will be important to have more data on other measures of vitamin D adequacy such as BMD and change in BMD. The currently recommended vitamin D intake of 600 IU per day for men and women age 71 and older is not adequate to bring most of the elderly population to 25OHD levels of 75–80 nM. To meet this target, vitamin D intakes of 1000 IU per day or higher would be needed. The safe upper limit for vitamin D was set at 2000 IU per day.[30]

In conclusion, adequate intakes of calcium and vitamin D are essential preventative measures and essential components of any therapeutic regimen for osteoporosis. Many men and women will need supplements, and supplementation with both calcium and vitamin D gives more consistent benefit than supplementation with either nutrient alone.

REFERENCES

1. Garnero P, Hausherr E, Chapuy MC, Marcelli C, Grandjean H, Muller C, Cormier C, Breart G, Meunier PJ, Delmas PD 1996 Markers of bone resorption predict hip fracture in elderly women: The EPIDOS Prospective Study. J Bone Miner Res 11:1531–1538.
2. Riis B, Thomsen K, Christiansen C 1987 Does calcium supplementation prevent postmenopausal bone loss? A double-blind, controlled clinical study. N Engl J Med 316:173–177.
3. Chevalley T, Rizzoli R, Nydegger V, Rapin CH, Michel JP, Vasey H, Bonjour JP 1994 Effects of calcium supplements on femoral bone mineral density and vertebral fracture rate in vitamin-D-replete elderly patients. Osteoporos Int 4:245–252.
4. Dawson-Hughes B, Harris SS, Krall EA, Dallal GE 1997 Effect of calcium and vitamin D supplementation on bone density in men and women 65 years of age or older. N Engl J Med 337:670–676.
5. Elders PJ, Netelenbos JC, Lips P, van Ginkel FC, Khoe E, Leeuwenkamp OR, Hackeng WH, van der Stelt PF 1991 Calcium supplementation reduces vertebral bone loss in perimenopausal women: A controlled trial in 248 women between 46 and 55 years of age. J Clin Endocrinol Metab 73:533–540.
6. Bullamore JR, Wilkinson R, Gallagher JC, Nordin BE, Marshall DH 1970 Effect of age on calcium absorption. Lancet 2:535–537.
7. Ebeling PR, Sandgren ME, DiMagno EP, Lane AW, DeLuca HF, Riggs BL 1992 Evidence of an age-related decrease in intestinal responsiveness to vitamin D: Relationship between serum 1,25-dihydroxyvitamin D3 and intestinal vitamin D receptor concentrations in normal women. J Clin Endocrinol Metab 75:176–182.
8. Krall EA, Sahyoun N, Tannenbaum S, Dallal GE, Dawson-Hughes B 1989 Effect of vitamin D intake on seasonal variations in parathyroid hormone secretion in postmenopausal women. N Engl J Med 321:1777–1783.
9. Dawson-Hughes B, Dallal GE, Krall EA, Harris S, Sokoll LJ, Falconer G 1991 Effect of vitamin D supplementation on wintertime and overall bone loss in healthy postmenopausal women. Ann Intern Med 115:505–512.
10. Dawson-Hughes B, Harris SS, Krall EA, Dallal GE, Falconer G, Green CL 1995 Rates of bone loss in postmenopausal women randomly assigned to one of two dosages of vitamin D. Am J Clin Nutr 61:1140–1145.
11. MacLaughlin J, Holick MF 1985 Aging decreases the capacity of human skin to produce vitamin D3. J Clin Invest 76:1536–1538.
12. Harris SS, Dawson-Hughes B 2002 Plasma vitamin D and 25OHD responses of young and old men to supplementation with vitamin D3. J Am Coll Nutr 21:357–362.
13. Shea B, Wells G, Cranney A, Zytaruk N, Robinson V, Griffith L, Ortiz Z, Peterson J, Adachi J, Tugwell P, Guyatt G VII 2002 Meta-Analysis of calcium supplementation for the prevention of postmenopausal osteoporosis. Endocr Rev 23:552–559.
14. Prince R, Devine A, Dick I, Criddle A, Kerr D, Kent N, Price R, Randell A 1995 The effects of calcium supplementation (milk powder or tablets) and exercise on bone density in postmenopausal women. J Bone Miner Res 10:1068–1075.
15. Ooms ME, Roos JC, Bezemer PD, van der Vijgh WJ, Bouter LM, Lips P 1995 Prevention of bone loss by vitamin D supplementation in elderly women: A randomized double-blind trial. J Clin Endocrinol Metab 80:1052–1058.
16. Dawson-Hughes B, Harris SS, Krall EA, Dallal GE 2000 Effect of withdrawal of calcium and vitamin D supplements on bone mass in elderly men and women. Am J Clin Nutr 72:745–750.
17. Heikinheimo RJ, Inkovaara JA, Harju EJ, Haavisto MV, Kaarela RH, Kataja JM, Kokko AM, Kolho LA, Rajala SA 1992 Annual injection of vitamin D and fractures of aged bones. Calcif Tissue Int 51:105–110.
18. Komulainen MH, Kroger H, Tuppurainen MT, Heikkinen AM, Alhava E, Honkanen R, Saarikoski S 1998 HRT and Vit D in prevention of non-vertebral fractures in postmenopausal women; a 5 year randomized trial. Maturitas 31:45–54.
19. Lips P, Graafmans WC, Ooms ME, Bezemer PD, Bouter LM 1996 Vitamin D supplementation and fracture incidence in elderly persons. A randomized, placebo-controlled clinical trial. Ann Intern Med 124:400–406.
20. Meyer HE, Smedshaug GB, Kvaavik E, Falch JA, Tverdal A, Pedersen JI 2002 Can vitamin D supplementation reduce the risk of fracture in the elderly? A randomized controlled trial. J Bone Miner Res 17:709–715.
21. Chapuy MC, Arlot ME, Duboeuf F, Brun J, Crouzet B, Arnaud S, Delmas PD, Meunier PJ 1992 Vitamin D3 and calcium to prevent hip fractures in the elderly women. N Engl J Med 327:1637–1642.
22. Chapuy MC, Pamphile R, Paris E, Kempf C, Schlichting M, Arnaud S, Garnero P, Meunier PJ 2002 Combined calcium and vitamin D3 supplementation in elderly women: Confirmation of reversal of secondary hyperparathyroidism and hip fracture risk. The Decalyos II study. Osteoporos Int 13:257–264.
23. Black DM, Cummings SR, Karpf DB, Cauley JA, Thompson DE, Nevitt MC, Bauer DC, Genant HK, Haskell WL, Marcus R, Ott SM, Torner JC, Quandt SA, Reiss TF, Ensrud KE 1996 Randomised trial of effect of alendronate on risk of fracture in women with existing vertebral fractures. Fracture Intervention Trial Research Group. Lancet 348:1535–1541.
24. Harris STM, Watts NBM, Genant HKM, McKeever CDM, Hangartner TP, Keller MM, Chesnut CHI, Brown JM, Eriksen EFM, Hoseyni MSP, Axelrod DWM, Miller PDM 1999 Effects of risedronate treatment on vertebral and nonvertebral fractures in women with postmenopausal osteoporosis: A randomized controlled trial. JAMA 282:1344–1352.
25. Ettinger BM, Black DMP, Mitlak BHM, Knickerbocker RKP, Nickelsen TM, Genant HKM, Christiansen CM, Delmas PDM, Zanchetta JRM, Stakkestad JM, Gluer CCP, Krueger KM, Cohen FJM, Eckert SP, Ensrud KEMM, Avioli LVM, Lips PM, Cummings SRM 1999 Reduction of vertebral fracture risk in postmenopausal women with

osteoporosis treated with raloxifene: Results from a 3-year randomized clinical trial. JAMA **282**:637–645.

26. Chesnut CH, Silverman SM, Andriano KP, Genant HM, Gimona AM, Harris SM, Kiel DM, LeBoff MM, Maricic MM, Miller PM, Moniz CM, Peacock MM, Richardson PM, Watts NM, Baylink DM 2000 A randomized trial of nasal spray salmon calcitonin in postmenopausal women with established osteoporosis: The prevent recurrence of osteoporotic fractures study. Am J Med **109**:267–276.

27. Neer RM, Arnaud CD, Zanchetta JR, Prince R, Gaich GA, Reginster JY, Hodsman AB, Eriksen EF, Ish-Shalom S, Genant HK, Wang O, Bruce HM 2001 Effect of parathyroid hormone (1–34) on fractures and bone mineral density in postmenopausal women with osteoporosis. N Engl J Med **344**:1434–1441.

28. Nieves JW, Komar L, Cosman F, Lindsay R 1998 Calcium potentiates the effect of estrogen and calcitonin on bone mass: Review and analysis. Am J Clin Nutr **67**:18–24.

29. Johnell O, Gullberg B, Kanis JA, Allander E, Elffors L, Dequeker J, Dilsen G, Gennari C, Lopes VA, Lyritis G 1995 Risk factors for hip fracture in European women: The MEDOS Study. Mediterranean Osteoporosis Study. J Bone Miner Res **10**:1802–1815.

30. Standing Committee on the Scientific Evaluation of Dietary Reference Intakes 1997 Dietary reference intakes. In: Dietary Reference Intakes: Calcium, Phosphorus, Magnesium, Vitamin D, and Fluoride. National Academy Press, Washington, DC, USA, pp. 21–37.

31. Nusser SM, Carriquiry AL, Dodd KW, Fuller WA 1996 A semiparametric transformation approach to estimating usual daily intake distributions. J Am Stat Assoc **91**:1440–1449.

32. Heaney RP, Smith KT, Recker RR, Hinders SM 1989 Meal effects on calcium absorption. Am J Clin Nutr **49**:372–376.

33. Recker RR 1985 Calcium absorption and achlorhydria. N Engl J Med **313**:70–73.

34. Harvey JA, Zobitz MM, Pak CY 1988 Dose dependency of calcium absorption: A comparison of calcium carbonate and calcium citrate. J Bone Miner Res **3**:253–258.

35. Peacock M 1998 Effects of calcium and vitamin D insufficiency on the skeleton. Osteoporos Int **8**(Suppl 2):S45–S51.

36. Chapuy MC, Preziosi P, Maamer M, Arnaud S, Galan P, Hercberg S, Meunier PJ 1997 Prevalence of vitamin D insufficiency in an adult normal population. Osteoporos Int **7**:439–443.

37. Dawson-Hughes B, Harris SS, Dallal GE 1997 Plasma calcidiol, season, and serum parathyroid hormone concentrations in healthy elderly men and women. Am J Clin Nutr **65**:67–71.

38. Lips P, Wiersinga A, van Ginkel FC, Jongen MJ, Netelenbos JC, Hackeng WH, Delmas PD, van der Vijgh WJ 1988 The effect of vitamin D supplementation on vitamin D status and parathyroid function in elderly subjects. J Clin Endocrinol Metab **67**:644–650.

Chapter 59. Nutrition and Osteoporosis

Robert P. Heaney

Creighton University, Omaha, Nebraska

INTRODUCTION

Nutrition plays a role in pathogenesis, prevention, and treatment of osteoporosis.[1] The nutrients known with certainty to be important are calcium, vitamin D, and protein. Phosphorus, certain trace minerals (manganese, copper, and zinc), and vitamins C and K, while involved in bone health generally, are less certainly involved in osteoporosis. Bone cells, of course, are as dependent on total nutrition—including all the vitamins and trace minerals—as are all other cells and tissues. However, current bone mass and bone strength are dependent on cell activity extending back in time over a several-year period. Hence, acute nutrient deficiencies, while undoubtedly impairing current cellular competence, tend to have less effect on overall bone strength, which is the concern in this primer. The major exceptions to this generalization are the nutrients, calcium, vitamin D, and protein.

CALCIUM

Calcium is the principal cation of bone mineral. Bone constitutes a very large nutrient reserve for calcium, which over the course of evolution, acquired a secondary, structural function that explains its importance for osteoporosis. Bone strength varies as the approximate second power of bone structural density. Accordingly, any decrease in bone mass produces a corresponding decrease in bone strength. While reserves are designed to be used in times of need,

such use would normally be temporary. Sustained drawing on the reserves depletes them and reduces bone strength.

Bone mass is ultimately determined by the genetic program as modified by mechanical loading. However, the genetic potential cannot be reached or maintained if dietary calcium intake is insufficient. The aggregate total of bone resorptive activity, as noted elsewhere in this volume, is controlled systemically by parathyroid hormone, which in turn responds to the demands of extracellular fluid calcium ion maintenance, not to the need for bone mass. Whenever absorbed calcium intake is insufficient to meet either the demands of growth or the drain of cutaneous and excretory losses, resorption will be stimulated and bone mass will be reduced.

The intake of calcium that is optimal for growth and adult maintenance has been estimated at a National Institutes of Health (NIH) Consensus Conference in 1994[2] to be 800-1000 mg/day during childhood, 1200–1500 mg/day from age 12–24, 1000 mg/day from age 25 to time of estrogen deprivation or age 65 (whichever comes first), and 1500 mg/day thereafter. These intakes are specific for North America. A recommended dietary allowance (RDA) is a value for a population and is intended to be an intake at or above the actual requirement of 90–95% of the individuals making up the population. (Thus, many individuals could have intakes below the RDA, which would still be fully adequate for their personal needs. Conventionally, nutritionists have considered as cause for concern only individual values less than two-thirds of the RDA.) An optimal intake value, by contrast, applies to individuals.

Harmonizing the NIH optimal intakes[2] and the Institute

The author has no conflict of interest.

of Medicine (IOM) recommendations[3] results in the following composite RDA estimates for various ages and states: ages 1–3, 600 mg; 4–8, 1000 mg; 9–18, 1600 mg; 19–50, 1200 mg; 50+, 1400 mg; and pregnancy and lactation over age 19, 1200 mg.

The specific applicability of these values to North America reflects the effect of other nutrients on the calcium requirement and hence is a function of the total diet of the North American population. Diets high in protein and sodium and low in potassium, such as are typical of the developed nations, increase urinary calcium loss and tend thereby to increase the calcium intake requirement. For low intakes of sodium and with small body size, such as might be found in certain Third World environments, the adult calcium requirement for bone maintenance can be less than 500 mg/day. This is part of the reason why requirements seem to vary across countries and cultures.

Low-calcium intakes in childhood are associated with increased risk of fracture both later in life and even in adolescence.[1,4,5] Calcium intakes are positively correlated with bone mass at all ages, but most especially in old age when the requirement rises and the calcium intake tends to drop (thereby widening the gap between supply and demand). Calcium supplementation reduces both bone loss and fracture rate in the elderly.[6–12] Only in the few years immediately after estrogen withdrawal at menopause is calcium without much effect.[12] This is largely because bone loss then is due mainly to estrogen deficiency, not to nutrient deficiency. But even then, calcium greatly augments the bone-sparing effect of estrogen replacement.[13] The abnormal parathyroid secretory physiology, high circulating parathyroid hormone (PTH) levels, and elevated biomarkers for bone resorption typical of the elderly are all reversible with a high-calcium intake.[14] These hallmarks of the aging calcium economy, once considered caused by aging itself, are now recognized as manifestations of calcium privation. Thus, low calcium intakes are often pathogenetic for osteoporosis.

Optimal prophylaxis is provided by meeting the NIH/IOM recommendations, either with natural foods (principally dairy products, tofu, a few greens, and a few crustaceans) or with such calcium-fortified foods as may be available locally (e.g., fortified fruit juices, bread, breakfast cereals, and so forth). Calcium-rich foods, especially milk, tend to be less expensive per calorie than the calcium-poor foods they would displace in the diet. Calcium ingested in this way has a negative cost, and hence such dietary change has a very favorable cost–benefit relationship.

Supplements may also be indicated. Most calcium salts exhibit similar bioavailability.[15–17] Calcium carbonate is the salt most widely used in the United States. Like all calcium sources (including food), supplements should be taken with meals to ensure optimal absorption. Even for relatively less soluble salts such as the carbonate or phosphate, gastric acid is not necessary if the supplement is taken with food. Brand name or chewable products have proved over the years to be the most reliable.

Calcium is also of critical importance as cotherapy in the prevention and treatment of established osteoporosis. Estrogen prophylaxis exhibits a two to three times larger protective effect when taken with supplemental calcium than when taken alone.[13,18] Agents capable of substantially increasing bone mass (such as teriparatide and fluoride) cannot achieve their full effect if calcium intake is limiting. Agents with a preferential trophic effect for axial cancellous bone will actually take bone from other regions of the skeleton to meet the needs of new bone formation in the central skeleton when ingested calcium is not adequate. Because of poor absorption efficiency common in the elderly and in many patients with osteoporosis, therapeutic calcium intakes should be above the maintenance figure for older adults of 1400 mg/day, possibly 2000–2500 mg/day. Unless the number and variety of available calcium-fortified foods increases substantially, supplements will be the obvious choice here.

VITAMIN D

Vitamin D is important for bone, certainly for its role in facilitating calcium absorption and osteoclastic resorption, but probably for other reasons as well. Serum 25(OH)D levels, which are the best clinical indicators of vitamin D nutritional status, decline with age. This is due mainly to decreased solar exposure and to decreased efficiency of vitamin D synthesis in skin. Best current estimate of the lower limit of the healthy range for serum 25(OH)D is ~32 ng/ml (80 nM),[19,20] substantially higher than laboratory reference ranges.

Vitamin D supplementation in the elderly reduces fractures of all types.[21] It takes about 500–600 IU/day to maintain 25(OH)D levels in healthy young males deprived of solar exposure, and the requirement may be even higher in the elderly. Given what is known of cutaneous production from solar exposure at various ages, oral intake of vitamin D should be about 200 IU up to age 50, 400 IU from 50 to 70, and 600–800 IU above age 70. Oral intakes are typically much less than these recommendations. Accordingly, suboptimal 25(OH)D levels are found in a majority of adults living in North America and Northern Europe.[22] If individuals succeed in raising their calcium intakes through increased milk consumption, they will at the same time improve their vitamin D status, because fluid milks in the United States and Canada are fortified with vitamin D at a level of 100 IU per serving.

PROTEIN

One-half the volume of the extracellular material of bone consists of protein. Because of cross-links and other post-translational modifications, many of the constituent amino acids cannot be recycled. Hence bone turnover requires a continuing input of fresh dietary protein. Protein, once considered harmful for bone because of its tendency to increase urinary calcium loss, is now recognized as an important co-factor for bone health along with calcium. In the Framingham cohort, age-related bone loss was inversely related to protein intake,[23] and in a calcium intervention trial, bone gain occurred only in subjects with the highest protein intake.[24] Finally, adequacy of protein intake is a major factor determining outcome after hip fracture.[25] Patients with hip fracture are commonly malnourished, enter the hospital with low serum albumin levels, and typically become more severely hypoproteinemic during hospitalization. Serum albumin levels are the single best predictor of survival or death after hip fracture.[26] Protein supplementation of hip fracture patients has been shown to improve outcome dramatically (fewer deaths, less permanent institutionalization, more return to independent living).[25,27] Unfortunately, most hospital standards of care for hip fracture patients lack a nutritional component.

PHOSPHORUS

Phosphorus intake is generally above the RDA in North Americans; hence, phosphorus depletion is not common. (There has even been some concern expressed that there is too much phosphorus in the American diet. That is probably not correct.) Moreover, low phosphorus intakes are relatively common among the elderly (i.e., 10–15% of women over 60 ingest under two-thirds of the RDA). Whether such low intakes directly contribute to the problem of osteoporosis is not known, but it is unlikely. Nevertheless, phosphate is just as important a component of bone mineral as is calcium. When serum inorganic phosphorus (P_i) levels are low, bone mineralization will be limited by phosphate depletion in the microenvironment of the mineralizing front. Depending on serum P_i, this may occur before calcium is locally depleted. It is probable that osteoblast function is compromised by such low ambient phosphate concentrations. This relationship may become important when patients with low phosphorus intakes are given large calcium supplements and placed on anabolic agents (such as teriparatide). The calcium supplements, if given as the carbonate or citrate salts, will bind most or all of the ingested food phosphorus,[28] thereby limiting the bone gain potentially achievable with anabolic agents. A calcium phosphate supplement obviates this problem.

VITAMINS AND TRACE MINERALS

Vitamins C and K and the minerals manganese, copper, and zinc are necessary cofactors for enzymes involved in the synthesis or post-translational modification of various constituents of bone matrix. When these micronutrients are deficient in the diets of growing animals, various bone lesions develop.[29] Bone fragility has been reported with manganese deficiency in one human patient, and a bony lesion resembling osteoporosis occurs in sheep with copper deficiency. However, it is not known whether acquired adult deficiencies of any of these minerals in humans play a role in pathogenesis or treatment of osteoporosis. One randomized trial involving supplementation with manganese, copper, and zinc produced suggestive, but not conclusive, evidence of some benefit when these minerals were added to a calcium supplementation regimen.[30]

Vitamin C and copper are necessary for collagen cross-linking, and bony defects are well recognized as a part of the scurvy syndrome. However, apart from general nutritional considerations, there is no known role for vitamin C in osteoporotic bony fragility, and a role for copper remains unclear.

Vitamin K is necessary for the γ-carboxylation of three bone matrix proteins, a step necessary for their binding to hydroxyapatite. Osteocalcin is the best studied of these. Circulating serum osteocalcin is commonly undercarboxylated in patients with osteoporosis, especially those with hip fracture, and the defect responds to modest doses of vitamin K.[31] There is also suggestive evidence that vitamin K may reduce urinary calcium loss in patients with osteoporosis. Low vitamin K intakes have been linked to hip fracture in both the Framingham[32] and Nurses' Health Study cohorts.[33] In the former, the linkage was to fracture, not bone mineral density (BMD), suggesting a role of vitamin K in repair of fatigue damage. However, in the Framingham offspring cohort, a weak association of vitamin K intake and BMD was found.[34] The extent to which these differences and associations are causal, or are instead simply markers for the general debility and global malnutrition common in elderly patients with osteoporosis, is not known. Vitamin K deficiency is, however, easily treatable and, if some component of the fragility of the elderly is caused by inadequate intakes of vitamin K, that component of the fracture burden could be inexpensively eliminated.

REFERENCES

1. Heaney RP 2001 Nutrition and risk for osteoporosis. In: Marcus R, Feldman D, Kelsey J (eds.) Osteoporosis, 2nd ed., vol. 2. Academic Press, San Diego, CA, USA, pp. 513–532.
2. NIH Consensus Conference 1994 Optimal calcium intake. JAMA **272:**1942–1948.
3. Food and Nutrition Board, Institute of Medicine 1997 Calcium. In: Dietary Reference Intakes for Calcium, Magnesium, Phosphorus, Vitamin D, and Fluoride. National Academy Press, Washington, DC, USA, pp. 71–145.
4. Chan GM, Hess M, Hollis J, Book LS 1984 Bone mineral status in childhood accidental fractures. Am J Dis Child **138:**569–570.
5. Goulding A, Cannan R, Williams SM, Gold EJ, Taylor RW, Lewis-Barned NJ 1998 Bone mineral density in girls with forearm fractures. J Bone Miner Res **13:**143–148.
6. Chapuy MC, Arlot ME, Duboeuf F, Brun J, Crouzet B, Arnaud S, Delmas PD, Meunier PJ 1992 Vitamin D₃ and calcium to prevent hip fractures in elderly women. N Engl J Med **327:**1637–1642.
7. Chevalley T, Rizzoli R, Nydegger V, Slosman D, Rapin C-H, Michel J-P, Vasey H, Bonjour J-P 1994 Effects of calcium supplements on femoral bone mineral density and vertebral fracture rate in vitamin D-replete elderly patients. Osteoporos Int **4:**245–252.
8. Recker RR, Hinders S, Davies KM, Heaney RP, Stegman MR, Kimmel DB, Lappe JM 1996 Correcting calcium nutritional deficiency prevents spine fractures in elderly women. J Bone Miner Res **11:**1961–1966.
9. Reid IR, Ames RW, Evans MC, Gamble GD, Sharpe SJ 1993 Effect of calcium supplementation on bone loss in postmenopausal women. N Engl J Med **328:**460–464.
10. Aloia JF, Vaswani A, Yeh JK, Ross PL, Flaster E, Dilmanian FA 1994 Calcium supplementation with and without hormone replacement therapy to prevent postmenopausal bone loss. Ann Intern Med **120:**97–103.
11. Dawson-Hughes B, Harris SS, Krall EA, Dallal GE 1997 Effect of calcium and vitamin D supplementation on bone density in men and women 65 years of age or older. N Engl J Med **337:**670–676.
12. Dawson-Hughes B, Dallal GE, Krall EA, Sadowski L, Sahyoun N, Tannenbaum S 1990 A controlled trial of the effect of calcium supplementation on bone density in postmenopausal women. N Engl J Med **323:**878–883.
13. Nieves JW, Komar L, Cosman F, Lindsay R 1998 Calcium potentiates the effect of estrogen and calcitonin on bone mass: Review and analysis. Am J Clin Nutr **67:**18–24.
14. McKane WR, Khosla S, O'Fallon WM, Robins SP, Burritt MF, Riggs BL 1996 Role of calcium intake in modulating age-related increases in parathyroid function and bone resorption. J Clin Endocrinol Metab **81:**1699–1703.

15. Heaney RP, Recker RR, Weaver CM 1990 Absorbability of calcium sources: The limited role of solubility. Calcif Tissue Int **46:**300–304.
16. Heaney RP, Dowell MS, Barger-Lux MJ 1999 Absorption of calcium as the carbonate and citrate salts, with some observations on method. Osteoporos Int **9:**19–23.
17. Heaney RP, Dowell MS, Bierman J, Hale CA, Bendich A 2001 Absorbability and cost effectiveness in calcium supplementation. J Am Coll Nutr **20:**239–246.
18. Davis JW, Ross PD, Johnson NE, Wasnich RD 1995 Estrogen and calcium supplement use among Japanese-American women: Effects upon bone loss when used singly and in combination. Bone **17:**369–373.
19. Chapuy M-C, Preziosi P, Maamer M, Arnaud S, Galan P, Hercberg S, Meunier PJ 1997 Prevalence of vitamin D insufficiency in an adult normal population. Osteoporos Int **7:**439–443.
20. Heaney RP, Dowell MS, Hale CA, Bendich A 2003 Calcium absorption varies within the reference range for serum 25-hydroxyvitamin D. J Am Coll Nutr **22:**142–146.
21. Heikinheimo RJ, Inkovaara JA, Harju EJ, Haavisto MV, Kaarela RH, Kataja JM, Kokko AM-L, Kolho LA, Rajala SA 1992 Annual injection of vitamin D and fractures of aged bones. Calcif Tissue Int **51:**105–110.
22. Thomas MK, Lloyd-Jones DM, Thadhani RI, Shaw AC, Debraska DJ, Kitch BT, Vamvakas EC, Dick IM, Prince RL, Finkelstein JS 1998 Hypovitaminosis D in medical inpatients. N Engl J Med **338:**777–783.
23. Hannan MT, Tucker KL, Dawson-Hughes B, Cupples LA, Felson DT, Kiel DP 2000 Effect of dietary protein on bone loss in elderly men and women: The Framingham Osteoporosis Study. J Bone Miner Res **15:**2504–2512.
24. Dawson-Hughes B, Harris SS 2002 Calcium intake influences the association of protein intake with rates of bone loss in elderly men and women. Am J Clin Nutr **75:**773–779.
25. Delmi M, Rapin CH, Bengoa JM, Delmas PD, Vasey H, Bonjour JP 1990 Dietary supplementation in elderly patients with fractured neck of the femur. Lancet **335:**1013–1016.
26. Rico H, Revilla M, Villa LF, Hernandez ER, Fernandez JP 1992 Crush fracture syndrome in senile osteoporosis: A nutritional consequence. J Bone Miner Res **7:**317–319.
27. Bastow MD, Rawlings J, Allison SP 1983 Benefits of supplementary tube feeding after fractured neck of femur. BMJ **287:**1589–1592.
28. Heaney RP, Nordin BEC 2002 Calcium effects on phosphorus absorption: Implications for the prevention and co-therapy of osteoporosis. J Am Coll Nutr **21:**239–244.
29. Heaney RP 1993 Nutritional factors in osteoporosis. Annu Rev Nutr **13:**287–316.
30. Strause L, Saltman P, Smith K, Andon M 1991 The role of trace elements in bone metabolism. In: Burckhardt P, Heaney RP (eds.) Nutritional Aspects of Osteoporosis. Raven Press, New York, NY, USA, pp. 223–233.
31. Vermeer C, Jie K-S G, Knapen MHJ 1995 Role of vitamin K in bone metabolism. Annu Rev Nutr **15:**1–22.
32. Feskanich D, Weber P, Willett WC, Rockett H, Booth SL, Colditz GA 1999 Vitamin K intake and hip fractures in women: A prospective study. Am J Clin Nutr **69:**74–79.
33. Booth SL, Tucker KL, Chen H, Hannan MT, Gagnon DR, Cupples LA, Wilson PW, Ordovas J, Schaefer EJ, Dawson-Hughes B, Kiel DP 2000 Dietary vitamin K intakes are associated with hip fracture but not with bone mineral density in elderly men and women. Am J Clin Nutr **71:**1201–1208.
34. Booth SL, Broe KE, Gagnon DR, Tucker KL, Hannan MT, McLean RR, Dawson-Hughes B, Wilson PW, Cupples LA, Kiel DP 2003 Vitamin K intake and bone mineral density in women and men. Am J Clin Nutr **77:**512–516.

Chapter 60.   Evaluation of Postmenopausal Osteoporosis

Susan L. Greenspan[1] and Marjorie M. Luckey[2]

[1]Division of Endocrinology, University of Pittsburgh, Pittsburgh, Pennsylvania; and
[2]Saint Barnabus Arthritis and Rheumatic Disease Center, Livingston, New Jersey

INTRODUCTION

Osteoporosis is the most common disorder of bone mineral metabolism and affects up to 40% of postmenopausal women. It is considered a silent disease because approximately two-thirds of vertebral fractures are asymptomatic.[1,2] By the time a woman has her first osteoporotic fracture, she may have already lost 30% of her bone mass. Therefore, the goal in evaluating postmenopausal women is to identify those who are at risk for an osteoporotic fracture, to classify the degree of bone loss, and to exclude secondary causes of bone loss. For those who are diagnosed with this disease, preventive measures are recommended, and therapeutic alternatives are prescribed if clinically indicated.

PEAK BONE MASS AND BONE LOSS

The bone mass of a postmenopausal woman is determined by the development of her peak bone mass and the presence of factors causing bone loss in adulthood.[3] Peak bone mass is usually achieved between age 25 and 30 years for women and is primarily determined by genetic factors.

For instance, black and Hispanic women have a higher peak bone mass than white or Asian women. Men have a higher peak bone mass than women. Multiple genes, such as the vitamin D receptor allele, estrogen receptor genes, collagen receptor genes, and the high bone mass gene, *LRP-5*, may be associated with development of peak bone mass. Additional factors such as gonadal steroids, timing of puberty, growth hormone, calcium intake, and exercise are important in the development of peak bone mass.

The causes of bone loss in adult women are multifactorial, because bone mass is influenced by calcium intake, vitamin D, physical activity, and body weight. During the first 10 years of menopause, estrogen deficiency may cause losses of 20–30% in cancellous bone and 5–10% in cortical bone.[4] However, women continue to lose bone throughout the remainder of their lives, and bone loss is often accelerated after the mid-seventies. In addition, a variety of conditions and medications may precipitate bone loss (see SECONDARY CAUSES OF BONE LOSS).

RISK FACTORS FOR OSTEOPOROSIS AND FRACTURES

Epidemiologic studies have examined the risk factors that are associated with low bone mass and hip fractures. As

---

The authors have no conflict of interest.

© 2003 American Society for Bone and Mineral Research

TABLE 1. MAJOR RISK FACTORS FOR OSTEOPOROSIS [NATIONAL OSTEOPOROSIS FOUNDATION][5]

Major risk factors for osteoporosis and related fractures in postmenopausal women
  Personal history of fracture as an adult
  History of fragility fracture in a first degree relative
  Low body weight (< approximately 127 lbs.)
  Current smoking
Additional risk factors
  Caucasian race
  Advanced age
  Female sex
  Dementia
  Estrogen deficiency (early menopause [age < 45 years] or bilateral ovariectomy; prolonged premenopausal amenorrhea [>1 year])
  Low calcium intake (lifelong)
  Alcoholism
  Impaired eyesight despite adequate correction
  Inadequate physical activity
  Poor health/frailty

outlined by the National Osteoporosis Foundation, major risk factors for osteoporosis and related fractures include a personal history of fracture as an adult, a history of fragility fracture in a first degree relative, low body weight, current smoking, and use of oral corticosteroid therapy (Table 1[5]). Risk factors for hip fracture were examined by the Study of Osteoporotic Fractures, which followed 9704 postmenopausal women over 65 years of age (Table 2[6]). The investigators determined that many factors contribute independently to the risk of fracture, including age, history of maternal hip fracture, low body weight, height, poor health, previous hyperthyroidism, poor depth perception, tachycardia, previous fracture, low bone mass, and benzodiazepines (Table 2). Other studies have found that a sideways fall, low bone mass, and increased biochemical markers of bone turnover are independent contributors to the risk of hip fracture.[7,8] Pre-existing fractures double to quadruple the risk of a subsequent osteoporotic fracture.

TABLE 2. MAJOR RISK FACTORS FOR HIP FRACTURES[6–8]

Risk factors for hip fracture
  Age
  Maternal history of hip fracture
  Weight loss
  Tall height at age 25
  Poor health
  Previous hyperthyroidism
  Use of long-acting benzodiazepines
  Use of anticonvulsants
  Current caffeine intake (per 190 mg/day)
  Inability to rise from a chair
  Poor depth perception
  Poor contrast sensitivity (vision)
  Pulse >80 beats per minute
  Previous fracture since age 50
  Sideways fall
  Low bone mass
  Low body mass index
  Increased markers of bone resorption

TABLE 3. RELATIVE RISK OF FRACTURE FOR 1 SD DECREASE IN BMD[9]*

Site	Hip fracture	Vertebral fracture
Distal radius	1.8	1.7
Proximal radius	2.1	2.2
Calcaneus	2.0	2.4
Spine	1.6	2.3
Femoral neck	2.6	1.8

* Meta-analysis of 11 prospective cohort studies, with 90,000 person-years observation and greater than 2000 fractures.

BONE MINERAL DENSITY

Bone mineral density (BMD) is the single best predictor of osteoporotic fracture risk. Prospective studies suggest that a decrease of 1 SD in bone mass at the spine, hip, or wrist is associated with an approximate doubling of fracture risk (Table 3[9]). BMD can be assessed with a variety of techniques, including DXA, single X-ray absorptiometry (SXA), quantitative computed tomography (QCT), and calcaneal ultrasonometry.[10] The International Society for Clinical Densitometry (ISCD) recommends that bone mass of the spine (L1–L4) be assessed as well as bone mass of the hip (femoral neck, total hip, and trochanter[11]). The lowest value of these areas should be used in classifying bone mass according to World Health Organization (WHO) criteria. Women with a BMD less than −2.5 SDs are classified as osteoporotic.[12,13] Women who are normal have a BMD at −1.0 SD and above. Those with BMD between −1.0 and −2.5 SDs are classified as osteopenic. Although the WHO guidelines were based on BMD data from postmenopausal white women, these cut-off values are also commonly used for Hispanic and black women. These WHO T-score criteria are not applicable to "peripheral devices" (equipment that assesses bone mass of the finger or heel).

Clinicians should base their management not only on bone mass, but other risk factors. The risk of fracture increases significantly with the cumulative effect of multiple risk factors (Fig. 1). For example, women with very low bone mass and multiple risk factors are at significantly higher risk of fracture than those with low bone mass and no risk factors. In addition to bone mass, there are several clinical risk factor algorithms available to predict which patients have osteoporosis or are at risk of fracture. However, none have been shown to have the associated predictive fracture risk of BMD.

WHO SHOULD BE MEASURED

Guidelines established by the National Osteoporosis Foundation (NOF) suggest that all women over the age of 65 have bone mass assessments, because the rate of fracture and number of osteoporotic women in this age group are significant.[5] The NOF also suggests that bone mass be measured in postmenopausal women up to 65 years who have one or more risk factors (Table 4). In addition, women should be assessed if they are considering therapy for osteoporosis or if they present with fractures (to confirm the diagnosis).

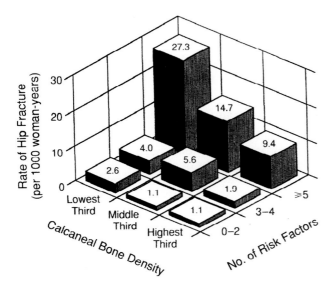

FIG. 1. Annual risk of hip fracture according to the number of risk factors and the age-specific calcaneal bone density. The risk factors are as follows: age ≥80 years; maternal history of hip fracture; any fracture (except hip fracture) since the age of 50; fair, poor, or very poor health; previous hyperthyroidism; anticonvulsant therapy; current long-acting benzodiazepine therapy; current weight less than at the age of 25; height at the age of 25 ≥168 cm; caffeine intake more than the equivalent of 2 cups of coffee per day; on feet ≤4 h per day; no walking for exercise; inability to rise from chair without using arms; lowest quartile (SD > 2.44) of depth perception; lowest quartile (≤0.70 U) of contrast sensitivity; and pulse rate >80 per minute. (Reproduced with permission from the Massachusetts Medical Society N Engl J Med 1995:**332:**767–773.)

In 2002, the U.S. Preventive Health Task Force issued recommendations for bone mass testing (Table 4[14]). The panel suggested that all women over 65 years and women between 60 and 65 years who have risk factors should have BMD assessments. They did not make recommendations for postmenopausal women under 60 years.

Currently, Medicare (applicable only in the United States) covers BMD testing for individuals 65 years and older with estrogen deficiency, individuals with vertebral abnormalities, those who are on or are planning to initiate long-term glucocorticoid therapy, patients with primary hyperparathyroidism, and patients who are being monitored to assess the efficacy of an approved osteoporosis therapy (Table 4[15]).

The current recommendation of the ISCD is to consider monitoring therapy with bone mass measurements every 1–2 years at the same facility with the same device that was previously used. The Bone Mass Measurement Act covers follow-up after a 2-year interval for Medicare patients.

SECONDARY CAUSES OF BONE LOSS

The diagnosis of osteoporosis can be made with a BMD test or after an acute clinical fracture. However, secondary causes of bone loss need to be evaluated. The true prevalence of secondary osteoporosis in women is unknown. In published studies from referral centers, approximately 50% of women with low bone density have a history of other disorders or medications known to cause bone loss.[16–18] In

addition, these studies report that 20–30% of women who present with osteoporosis have an occult secondary cause of bone loss that was identified only by laboratory testing.[17–20] The list of secondary causes of osteoporosis can be separated into the following: (1) endocrine disorders, (2) gastrointestinal disorders, (3) bone marrow and connective tissue disorders, (4) renal disorders, (5) miscellaneous disorders, and (6) medications associated with bone loss (Table 5).

Endocrine Disorders

The most common endocrine disorders that cause bone loss include hyperparathyroidism and hyperthyroidism. Both conditions are more common in elderly women than young women. Hyperparathyroidism has been shown to be associated with significant bone loss at cortical sites, such as the forearm and hip, but also causes trabecular bone loss in a small subset of women with this disease. Excessive production of parathyroid hormone (PTH) causes increased bone resorption and turnover in addition to hypercalcemia. After treatment of hyperparathyroidism, vertebral bone mass improves significantly. Patients can be screened with serum calcium and PTH to exclude hyperparathyroidism. Grave's disease and other causes of hyperthyroidism have been associated with fractures and bone loss, especially at sites of cortical bone. The etiology of this bone loss is caused by an increase in bone resorption. Serum thyroid stimulating hormone is the single best test to exclude hyperthyroidism, which can present silently in older women.

Other endocrine disorders that can cause secondary bone loss are conditions that lead to hypogonadism, hyperprolactinemia, acromegaly, Cushing's syndrome, eating disorders (anorexia and bulimia if the latter is associated with low body mass index [BMI]), and type 1 diabetes. Vitamin D insufficiency and deficiency are common causes of low

TABLE 4. WHO SHOULD BE TESTED

National Osteoporosis Foundation[5]
1. All women age 65 and older regardless of risk factors
2. All postmenopausal women under age 65 years who have one or more risk factors for osteoporotic fracture (other than being white, postmenopausal, and female)
3. Postmenopausal women who are considering therapy for osteoporosis, if BMD testing would facilitate the decision
4. Postmenopausal women who present with fractures (to confirm the diagnosis and determine disease severity
U.S. Preventive Services Task Force[14]
1. Postmenopausal women age 65 years and older
2. Postmenopausal women age 60–64 years with a risk factor (weight <70 kg; estrogen deficiency)
Medicare Coverage for BMD—Bone Mass Act*
1. Estrogen deficient women at clinical risk for osteoporosis
2. Individuals with vertebral abnormalities
3. Individuals receiving, or planning to receive, long-term corticosteroid therapy
4. Individuals with primary hyperparathyroidism
5. Individuals being monitored to assess the response or efficacy of an approved osteoporosis drug therapy.

* Applies only to the United States.

Table 5. Secondary Causes of Low Bone Mass

Endocrine disorders	Renal disorders
Female hypogonadism	Hypercalciuria
Hyperprolactinemia	Renal osteodystrophy
Hypothalamic amenorrhea	Renal tubular acidosis
Anorexia nervosa	Miscellaneous disorders
Premature and primary ovarian	Amyloidosis
failure	Idiopathic scoliosis
Hyperthyroidism	Immobilization
Hyperparathyroidism	Multiple sclerosis
Hypercortisolism	Porphyria
Vitamin D insufficiency,	Weight loss
deficiency, resistance	Medications associated with low
Gastrointestinal disorders	bone mass
Bariatric surgery	Alcohol
Chronic obstructive jaundice	Aluminum
Hemochromatosis	Anticonvulsants
Malabsorption syndromes	Chemotherapy/
Celiac sprue	immunosuppressive
Inflammatory bowel disease	agents
Other cirrhoses	Corticosteroids
Primary biliary cirrhosis	Cyclosporine
Subtotal gastrectomy	Excess thyroid hormone
Bone marrow disorders	Gonadotropin-releasing
AIDS/HIV	hormone agonists
Gaucher's disease	Heparin
Hemophilia	Lithium
Hemochromatosis	Smoking
Leukemia and lymphoma	Tamoxifen (premenopausal
Metastatic carcinoma	women)
Multiple myeloma	Total parenteral nutrition
Systemic mastocytosis	
Thalassemia	
Connective tissue disorders	
Ankylosing spondylitis	
Ehler-Danlos syndrome	
Homocystinuria	
Marfan's syndrome	
Osteogenesis imperfecta	
Rheumatoid arthritis	

bone mass, with a reported prevalence of 16–18% in women presenting with low bone density or fractures.[20,21] Without vitamin D, osteoid cannot be mineralized and calcium absorption is decreased. Patients with vitamin D deficiency (25-hydroxyvitamin D < 20 ng/dl) may present with normal levels of calcium and increased serum PTH and hypocalciuria. 25-hydroxyvitamin D level is the most reliable screen for this. A bone biopsy is rarely indicated to exclude osteomalacia.

Gastrointestinal Disorders

Gastrointestinal disorders can cause bone loss through malabsorption or liver disease. Such conditions include subtotal gastrectomy, bariatric surgery, malabsorption syndromes (e.g., celiac sprue, ulcerative colitis, Crohn's disease), primary biliary cirrhosis, other types of cirrhosis, chronic obstructive jaundice, and hepatitis. Liver function tests are needed to evaluate hepatic status. A low albumin level may be seen with malabsorption, coupled with hypocalciuria. Celiac sprue may be subtle, leading to calcium

malabsorption, often without other symptoms or findings associated with generalized malabsorption. The only indication of its presence may be hypocalciuria in association with elevated levels of serum tissue transglutaminase. A small bowel biopsy may be needed for verification.

Bone Marrow and Connective Tissue Disorders

Bone marrow disorders can mimic osteoporotic bone loss and result in fractures. Elderly patients with anemia who present with height loss or a fracture should have a clinical and laboratory evaluation for multiple myeloma, lymphoma, and leukemia. Elderly patients can be screened for myeloma with a urine or serum protein electrophoresis. In addition, patients with metastatic cancer can present with an osteoporotic fracture. Infiltrative disorders include systemic mastocytosis (generally presenting with pruritus, flushing, urticaria, and hypotension), which can be identified with focal radiologic abnormalities; a small number of patients present with generalized osteopenia. Histocytosis generally presents in childhood with focal radiologic abnormalities. Connective tissue diseases, including osteogenesis imperfecta, Ehler-Danlos syndrome, Marfan's syndrome, and homocystinuria, can present with low bone mass. Autoimmune-related disorders that are associated with low bone mass include rheumatoid arthritis and ankylosing spondylitis.

Renal Disorders

Significant renal disease can lead to renal osteodystrophy. In addition, idiopathic hypercalciuria and renal tubular acidosis are associated with low bone mass. Patients with renal tubular acidosis have metabolic acidosis and hypercalciuria.

Miscellaneous Disorders

Immobilization and weight loss are associated with loss of bone mass. Furthermore, patients undergoing bone marrow, heart, liver, kidney, or lung transplantation have significant bone loss, caused by the corticosteroid therapy, immobilization, immunosuppressive agents, and poor nutritional status.

Drugs Associated With Bone Loss

The list of medications associated with bone loss is extensive (Table 5). Corticosteroids are well known to cause bone loss because of suppression of osteoblastic function, increased osteoclast-mediated bone loss, inhibition of intestinal calcium absorption, and secondary hyperparathyroidism. In addition, excess use of corticosteroids may cause hypogonadism, which may accelerate bone loss. Studies have shown that as little as 2.5 mg of oral prednisone per day can produce bone loss, but a minimum dose has not been established. It is clear that the higher the dose and the greater the duration of treatment, the greater the bone loss. Some studies suggest that even inhaled glucocorticoids may be associated with bone loss.

Anticonvulsants have also been associated with high

turnover osteoporosis. Phenobarbital, phenytoin, and carbamazepine are the most commonly used anticonvulsants that can increase bone loss, due primarily to increased metabolism and clearance of vitamin D.

Excess thyroid hormone has been shown to cause bone loss. Thyroid hormone replacement is common in postmenopausal women. Up to 10% of elderly women may be on thyroid hormone replacement. However, only *excess* use of thyroid hormone has been associated with significant bone loss in postmenopausal, but not in premenopausal, women.

Other medications that contribute to bone loss include aluminum, anticoagulants, cyclosporine, excess vitamin A, gonadotropin releasing hormone agonists, heparin, and lithium. Tamoxifen, a selective estrogen receptor modulator, leads to bone loss only in premenopausal women.

Alcoholism and smoking also contribute to bone loss.

WORK-UP FOR SECONDARY CAUSES OF BONE LOSS

Although many secondary causes of osteoporosis can be identified in the medical history, others will remain undetected without laboratory testing. The reported prevalence of occult disorders ranges from 11% to 63%, depending, in part, on the extent of the laboratory evaluation.[16,17,19,20,22] There are currently no established guidelines for the most cost-effective evaluation to exclude secondary causes of bone loss in patients without an obvious etiology. A recent study examined 173 postmenopausal osteoporotic women without a history of diseases or medications known to affect bone mineral metabolism.[17] Evaluation in this study included a complete blood count, chemistry profile, 24-h urinary calcium, serum 25-hydroxyvitamin D, and serum PTH. Thirty-two percent of women were discovered to have previously unsuspected disorders of bone and mineral metabolism. Hypercalciuria was found in 9.8% of subjects, malabsorption in 8.1%, primary or secondary hyperparathyroidism in 6.9%, and severe vitamin D deficiency (25-hydroxyvitamin D < 12 ng/ml) in 4.1%. Among osteoporotic women on thyroid replacement, 29% had a suppressed thyroid-stimulating hormone (TSH). This study suggested a laboratory evaluation strategy, which included measurements of 24-h urinary calcium, serum calcium, and PTH for all women and TSH for women on thyroid hormone replacement. Such a strategy would have been sufficient to correctly identify 85% of the cases of secondary osteoporosis. If serum 25-hydroxyvitamin D is added to the evaluation, 98% of patients with an occult disorder would have been identified as well as an additional 16% of women who had less severe, but clinically significant vitamin D deficiency (25-hydroxyvitamin D, 13–20 ng/ml).[23] Although a 24-h urine collection may be onerous to some patients and the results influenced by incomplete collection and variations in dietary sodium and protein intake, 34% of the occult disorders identified in the above study would have been missed without this measurement.

In bone mineral densitometry, the "Z-score" represents the SDs from the mean for individuals of the same age and gender. Although a Z-score within the normal range (±2 SDs) does not rule out an occult disorder,[16,17] a very low Z-score heightens the possibility that another disorder is contributing to bone loss. The ISCD has recommended that patients with a Z-score lower than −2.0 SDs have a thorough evaluation for secondary causes of bone loss. In addition to a thorough history and physical examination, the routine laboratory evaluation discussed above should be augmented with a serum or urine protein electrophoresis (SPEP or UPEP) to rule out multiple myeloma, and a tissue transglutaminase may be needed to exclude celiac sprue. In some patients, a 24-h urinary free cortisol should be collected to assess the possibility of Cushing's syndrome.

Bone biopsy is rarely indicated, except for a formal evaluation for osteomalacia. Patients who present with back pain should be considered for vertebral X-rays to assess for an osteoporotic versus a pathological fracture. Bone mineral densitometry software is available to assess vertebral fractures through a technique known as Instant Vertebral Assessment.[24] While this is not as sensitive as an X-ray, it can examine vertebral compression fractures without the radiation exposure of a standard X-ray.

BIOCHEMICAL INDICES OF BONE MINERAL METABOLISM

In addition to bone mass, the rate of bone turnover may be assessed with biochemical markers of bone turnover.[25] They provide a dynamic assessment of skeletal activity, but do not provide information on the density of the skeleton. Osteoclast function can be assessed with markers of bone resorption, including N-telopeptide crosslinked collagen type 1 (NTx), deoxypyridinoline (Dpd), and C-telopeptide crosslinked collagen type 1 (CTx). Osteoblastic activity can be assessed through a variety of markers, including osteocalcin, bone specific alkaline phosphatase (BSAP), and amino-terminal propeptide of type 1 collagen (P1NP). While many of these assessments are measured in clinical research investigations, they are still under evaluation for use in clinical practice. High bone turnover has been shown to be an independent risk factor for fracture. Patients with a normal bone density and a high rate of resorption are at risk for fracture. However, resorption markers are more often used to assess medication compliance. A decrease in resorption markers should occur approximately 3 months after initiation of therapy.

SUMMARY

The evaluation of postmenopausal osteoporosis includes an assessment of risk factors for bone loss and determination of bone mass measurements of the hip and spine. Patients without an obvious secondary cause of bone loss should have a general evaluation, including serum calcium, serum parathyroid hormone, serum 25-hydroxyvitamin D, and 24-h urinary calcium and serum TSH if they are on thyroid hormone replacement. However, patients who have a Z-score that is 2 or more SDs below the age-matched mean should have a more comprehensive evaluation for a secondary and potentially reversible cause of bone loss.

REFERENCES

1. Ray N, Chan J, Melton L 1997 Medical expenditures of the treatment of osteoporotic fractures in the United States in 1995: Report from the National Osteoporosis Foundation. J Bone Miner Res **12:**24–35.

2. Cooper C, Atkinson EJ, O'Fallon WM, Melton LJ III 1992 Incidence of clinically diagnosed vertebral fractures: A population-based study in Rochester, Minnesota, 1985–1989. J Bone Miner Res 7:221–227.
3. Seeman E 2002 Pathogenesis of bone fragility in women and men. Lancet 259:1841–1850.
4. Riggs BL, Khosla S, Melton LJ III 1998 A unitary model for involutional osteoporosis: Estrogen deficiency causes both type I and type II osteoporosis in postmenopausal women and contributes to bone loss in aging men. J Bone Miner Res 13:763–773.
5. Anonymous 1998 Physician's Guide To Prevention and Treatment of Osteoporosis. National Osteoporosis Foundation, Washington, DC, USA, pp. 1–38.
6. Cummings SR, Nevitt MC, Browner WS, Stone K, Fox KM, Ensrud KE, Cauley J, Black D, Vogt TM 1995 Risk factors for hip fractures in white women. N Engl J Med 23:767–773.
7. Greenspan SL, Myers ER, Maitland LA, Resnick NM, Hayes WC 1994 Fall severity and bone mineral density as risk factors for hip fracture in ambulatory elderly. JAMA 271:128–133.
8. Garnero P, Hausherr E, Chapuy MC, Marcelli C, Grandjean H, Muller C, Cormier C, Breart G, Meunier PJ, Delmas PD 1996 Markers of bone resorption predict hip fracture in elderly women: The EPIDOS Prospective Study. J Bone Miner Res 11:1531–1538.
9. Marshall D, Johnell O, Wedel H 1996 Meta-analysis of how well measures of bone mineral density predict occurrence of osteoporotic fractures. BMJ 312:1254–1259.
10. Cummings SR, Bates D, Black DM 2002 Clinical use of bone densitometry: Scientific review. 288:JAMA 1889–1897.
11. Hamdy RC, Petak SM, Lenchik L 2002 Which central dual X-ray absorptiometry skeletal sites and regions of interest should be used to determine the diagnosis of osteoporosis? J Clin Densitom 5(Suppl):S11–S17.
12. Kanis JA for the WHO Study Group 1994 Assessment of fracture risk and its application to screening for postmenopausal osteoporosis: Synopsis of a WHO report. Osteoporos Int 4:368–381.
13. Kanis JA 2003 Diagnosis of osteoporosis and assessment of fracture risk. Lancet 359:1929–1936.
14. US Preventive Services Task Force 2002 Screening for osteoporosis in postmenopausal women: Recommendations and rationale. Ann Intern Med 137:526–528.
15. Anonymous 1998 Medicare coverage of and payments for bone mass measurements. Federal Register 63:34321–34325.
16. Deutschmann HA, Weger M, Weger W, Kotanko P, Deutschmann MJ, Skrabal F 2002 Search for occult secondary osteoporosis: Impact of identified possible risk factors on bone mineral density. J Intern Med 252:389–397.
17. Tannenbaum C, Clark J, Schwartzman K, Wallenstein S, Lapinski R, Meier D, Luckey M 2002 Yield of laboratory testing to identify secondary contributors to osteoporosis in otherwise healthy women. J Clin Endocrinol Metab 87:4431–4437.
18. Fitzpatrick LA 2002 Secondary causes of osteoporosis. Mayo Clin Proc 77:453–468.
19. Caplan GA, Scane AC, Francis RM 1994 Pathogenesis of vertebral crush fractures in women. J R Soc Med 87:200–202.
20. Freitag A, Barzel U 2002 Differential diagnosis of osteoporosis. Gerontology 48:98–102.
21. Haden ST, Fuleihan GE, Angell JE, Cotran NM, LeBoff MS 1999 Calcidiol and PTH levels in women attending an osteoporosis program. Calcif Tissue Int 64:275–279.
22. Heaney RP 2000 Vitamin D: How much do we need, and how much is too much? Osteoporos Int 11:553–555.
23. Luckey MM, Tannenbaum C 2003 Authors' response: Recommended testing in patients with low bone density. J Clin Endocrinol Metab 88:1405.
24. Greenspan SL, von Stetten E, Emond SK, Jones L, Parker RA 2001 Instant vertebral assessment: A noninvasive DXA technique to avoid misclassification and clinical mismanagement of osteoporosis. J Clin Densitom 4:373–380.
25. Miller PD, Baran DT, Bilezikian JP, Greenspan SL, Lindsay R, Riggs BL, Rosen CJ, Watts NB 1999 Practical clinical application of biochemical markers of bone turnover: Consensus of an expert panel. J Clin Densitom 2:323–342.

Chapter 61. Osteoporosis in Men

Eric S. Orwoll

Bone and Research Unit, Oregon Health Sciences University, Portland, Oregon

INTRODUCTION

Osteoporosis in men was generally unrecognized 20 years ago, but it is now the source of much discussion and very active research. Efforts devoted to the issue have been productive. There is now a much greater understanding of the disorder, and effective diagnostic, preventive, and treatment strategies have been developed. Moreover, the study of osteoporosis in men has revealed male–female differences that in turn have fostered a greater understanding of bone biology in general. Here these issues are considered and recommendations are made for the clinical management of men confronted with the disorder.

SKELETAL DEVELOPMENT

Bone mass accumulation in males occurs gradually during childhood and accelerates dramatically during adolescence. Peak bone mass is closely tied to pubertal development, and male–female differences in the skeleton appear during adolescence.[1] Peak bone mass is achieved somewhat later in boys than girls, and whereas trabecular bone accumulation is similar in boys and girls, boys generally develop thicker cortices and larger bones than do girls, even when adjusted for body size. These differences may provide important biomechanical advantages that could in part underlie the lower fracture risk observed in men later in life. The reasons for these sexual differences in skeletal development are unclear but could be related to differences in sex steroid action (androgens seem to stimulate periosteal bone formation and bone expansion), growth factor concentrations, mechanical forces exerted on bone (for instance by greater muscle action or activity), etc.

EFFECTS OF AGING ON THE SKELETON IN MEN

As in women, aging is associated with large changes in bone mass and architecture in men.[2] Trabecular bone loss (for instance in the vertebrae and proximal femur) occurs during mid-life and accelerates in later life. The magnitude of these changes is similar, but probably slightly less, than

---

Dr. Orwoll serves as a consultant for Eli Lilly and Enzon, Merck, NPS, Procter & Gamble, and Roche.

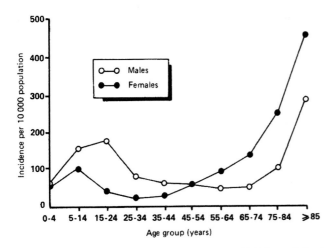

FIG. 1. Average annual fracture incidence rate per 10,000 population in Leicester, UK, by age group and sex.

those in women. Endocortical loss with resulting cortical thinning also takes place in long bones, but that process seems to be somewhat mitigated by a concomitant increase in periosteal bone expansion that tends to preserve the breaking strength of bone.[3] The increase in periosteal bone formation that occurs in men may be greater than that in women and has been postulated to contribute to the lower fracture risk observed in older men.

FRACTURE EPIDEMIOLOGY

Fractures are common in men. The data concerning fractures are derived primarily from the study of white populations. In them, the incidence of fracture is bimodal, with a peak of fracture incidence in adolescence and young adulthood, a lower incidence in middle age, and a dramatic increase after the age of 70 years (Fig. 1).[4] The types of fractures sustained in younger and older men are different, with long bone fractures being common in the young, whereas vertebral and hip fracture predominate in the elderly. These differences suggest that the etiologies of fractures at these two periods of life are distinct. In younger men, trauma may play a larger role, whereas in older men, skeletal fragility is a major factor. The increase in fracture incidence in older men is as dramatic as the similar increase that occurs in women, but it begins 5–10 years later in life. This delay, combined with the longer life expectancy in women, probably is the major explanation for the greater burden of osteoporotic fractures in women. The age-adjusted incidence of hip fracture in men is one-third to one-half that in women, and 20–25% of hip fractures occur in men.[2] The consequences of fracture in men are at least as great as in women, and in fact, elderly men seem to be more likely to die and to suffer disability than women after a hip fracture. Men suffer much lower rates of other long bone fractures than do women.[5] There is less information concerning vertebral fracture epidemiology in men, but the age-adjusted incidence seems to be approximately 50% that in women.[6] In younger men, the prevalence of vertebral fracture is actually higher in men than in women, probably

in part the result of higher rates of spinal trauma experienced by men. Although there are inadequate data, the epidemiology of fracture seems to be dramatically influenced by both race and geography.[7,8] For instance, black men have a much lower likelihood of fractures than whites, and Asian men have a lower likelihood of suffering hip fracture than whites. Much more information is needed concerning these differences and their causation.

Fractures in men are related to a variety of risk factors. Inherent skeletal fragility makes fracture more likely. This trait is most commonly measured as reduced bone mineral density (BMD), but almost certainly has other components (bone geometry, material properties, etc.). Aging and a previous history of fracture are independently associated with a higher probability of future fracture, and men of lower weight and those at risk for falling have a higher fracture risk.[2,9]

CAUSES OF OSTEOPOROSIS IN MEN

The causation of osteoporosis in men is commonly heterogeneous, and most osteoporotic men have several factors that contribute to the disease. One-half to two-thirds of men with osteoporosis have secondary osteoporosis—or that associated with other medical conditions, medications, or lifestyle factors that result in bone loss and fragility (Table 1).[2,7] The most important include alcohol abuse, glucocorticoid excess, and hypogonadism. An important fraction of osteoporotic men, however, have idiopathic disease.

- Idiopathic osteoporosis. Osteoporosis of unknown etiology can present in men of any age,[10] but is most dramatic in younger men who are otherwise unlikely to be affected. Several possible contributors have been identified. Most prominent among them are genetic factors, because bone density and the risk of fracture are highly heritable. The specific genes that may be responsible are uncertain.
- Hypogonadism. Sex steroids are clearly important for

TABLE 1. CAUSES OF OSTEOPOROSIS IN MEN

Primary
Aging
Idiopathic
Secondary
Hypogonadism
Glucocorticoid excess
Alcoholism, tobacco abuse
Renal insufficiency
Gastrointestinal, hepatic disorders; malabsorption
Hyperparathyroidism
Hypercalciuria
Anticonvulsants
Thyrotoxicosis
Chronic respiratory disorders
Anemias, hemoglobinopathies
Immobilization
Osteogenesis imperfecta
Homocystinuria
Systemic mastocytosis
Neoplastic diseases
Rheumatoid arthritis

skeletal health in men, both during growth and the attainment of peak bone mass as well as the maintenance of bone strength in adults.[10] Hypogonadism is associated with low BMD, the development of hypogonadism results in increased bone remodeling and rapid bone loss, and hormone replacement increases bone density in hypogonadal men. One of the most important causes of severe hypogonadism is androgen deprivation therapy for prostate cancer. In that situation, bone loss is rapid. Gonadal function also declines with age in men, and it has been postulated that the decline may be related to age-related bone loss and fracture risk. This hypothesis has not been adequately tested.

- The relative roles of estrogens and androgens in skeletal physiology in men are uncertain.[11–13] Estrogen is essential for normal bone development in young men, as evidenced by the immature development and low bone mass in men with aromatase deficiency and their reversal with estrogen therapy. Moreover, estrogen is correlated with bone remodeling, BMD, and rate of BMD loss in older men, apparently more strongly than is testosterone. However, testosterone is independently related to indices of bone resorption and formation and may stimulate periosteal bone formation.[14–16] The relative roles of estrogen and androgen must be better defined.

EVALUATION OF OSTEOPOROSIS IN MEN

Guidelines for the evaluation of osteoporosis in men are not well validated but there are several recommendations that can be made confidently.

Bone Density Measurements

There are important sexual differences in skeletal biology that could influence the measurement of bone density. In particular, bone size is larger in men. Areal measures of BMD assessment (e.g., DXA) do not completely consider differences in bone volume, and there is a resultant size-induced artifact. In this light, it is useful to independently consider BMD measures in men and women.

The interpretation of BMD measures in men has been controversial. The World Health Organization definition of osteoporosis was developed to categorize fracture risk in women but is frequently used for similar purposes in men. Most commonly, these definitions are based on young normal male reference populations (i.e., T-scores are calculated in SDs from the mean of young normal men). In fact, the relationship between BMD and fracture risk in men has not been adequately investigated. Some data suggest that the risk of future fracture is similar in men and women at the same *absolute* level of BMD, leading to the recommendation that the definition of osteoporosis should be the same in men and women (i.e., T-scores for both men and women calculated in SDs from the mean of young *females*). However, the usefulness of using that approach isn't yet clear. Moreover, using a young female reference population (a lower absolute level of BMD than in young men) results in more stringent criteria for osteoporosis, and many fewer men over age 50 years are identified as being at risk

TABLE 2. EVALUATION OF OSTEOPOROSIS IN MEN—LABORATORY TESTS

Serum calcium, phosphorus, creatinine, alkaline phosphatase, liver function tests
Complete blood count (protein electrophoresis in those over 50 years)
Serum 25(OH) vitamin D and parathyroid hormone
Serum testosterone and luteinizing hormone
24-h urine calcium and creatinine
Targeted diagnostic testing in men with signs, symptoms, or other indications of secondary disorders

When an etiology is not apparent after the above, additional testing may be appropriate: thyroid function tests, 24-h urine cortisol, biochemical indices of remodeling.

($\approx 5\%$)—a result that doesn't seem to be appropriate given the frequency of fragility fractures in older men. Therefore, it is more apt to use criteria based on young male reference populations to identify men who deserve diagnostic evaluation and consideration for therapy, at least until the longitudinal studies are available to better define the BMD–fracture risk relationship in men.

In light of the prevalence of osteoporosis and the high incidence of fractures in men, bone density measures are performed too infrequently. Two groups of men clearly would benefit from BMD testing. First, those over the age of 50 who have suffered a fracture (except with high trauma) including those with vertebral deformity. Younger men who suffer low trauma fractures should also be assessed. Second, men who have known secondary causes of bone loss should have BMD determined. These include men treated with glucocorticoids or other medications associated with osteoporosis, with hypogonadism of any cause, and with alcoholism. Many other risk factors may also prompt BMD measures (Table 1). Screening BMD measures in older men have been recommended (e.g., over age 70),[17] but the effectiveness of this approach hasn't been formally evaluated.

Men who have been selected for androgen ablation therapy deserve special note. Men starting high-dose glucocorticoid therapy present the same challenges and should be similarly managed. When antiandrogen (or glucocorticoid) therapy is begun, a BMD measure is appropriate. If it is normal, routine preventative measures are appropriate. Because rapid bone loss occurs in these men, a repeat BMD measurement should be done in 1–2 years. If BMD is reduced at the onset of therapy, more aggressive preventive measures should be considered (e.g., bisphosphonate therapy). In men with osteoporosis even before antiandrogen (or glucocorticoid) therapy is begun, pharmacologic preventive approaches are recommended.

Whether bone density measurements in men should be interpreted using a male specific reference range or using the same reference range used in women has been controversial. Until adequate data are available to confidently link fracture risk to BMD measures in men, the use a male-specific reference ranges is suggested. This provides a better estimate of the prevalence of fracture in men.

The clinical evaluation of men found to have low bone density should include a careful history and physical examination designed to identify any factors that may contribute to deficits in bone mass. Careful attention should be paid to

TABLE 3. RANDOMIZED, PLACEBO-CONTROLLED TREATMENT TRIALS IN MEN WITH OSTEOPOROSIS

Reference	Therapy	Patients	Treatment duration	BMD change from baseline	Comment
Orwoll et al.[18]	Alendronate 10 mg/day	241 men with idiopathic osteoporosis	24 months	Lumbar spine ⇧ 7.1% Femoral neck ⇧ 2.5%	Reduction in vertebral fracture risk in treated men
Kurland et al.[22]	PTH(1-34) 400 IU/day	23 men with idiopathic osteoporosis	18 months	Lumbar spine ⇧ 13.5% Femoral neck ⇧ 2.9%	
Trovas et al.[23]	Calcitonin nasal 200 IU/day	28 men with idiopathic osteoporosis	12 months	Lumbar spine ⇧ 7.1% Femoral neck no change	
Orwoll et al.[19]	Teriparatide 20 μg/day	437 men with idiopathic osteoporosis	11 months	Lumbar spine ⇧ 5.9% Femoral neck ⇧ 1.5%	

lifestyle factors, nutrition (especially calcium and vitamin D nutrition), activity level, and family history. Any previous fracture history should be identified, and fall risk should be assessed. This information should be used to formulate recommendations for prevention and treatment.

Laboratory Testing

In a man undergoing an evaluation for osteoporosis, laboratory testing is intended to identify correctable causes of bone loss. Appropriate tests are shown in Table 2.

OSTEOPOROSIS PREVENTION IN MEN

The principles of fracture prevention in men are similar to those in women. In early life, excellent nutrition and exercise appear to have positive effects on bone mass. These principles and the avoidance of lifestyle factors known to be associated with bone loss (Table 1) remain important throughout life. Calcium and vitamin D appear to provide beneficial effects on bone mass and fractures in men as in women. Recommendations for both sexes include 1000 mg of calcium for those 30–50 years of age and 1200 mg after age 50, with suggested vitamin D intakes of 1000 IU. In those at risk for falls, attempts to increase strength and balance may be beneficial.

TREATMENT OF OSTEOPOROSIS IN MEN

Ensuring adequate calcium and vitamin D intake and appropriate physical activity are essential foundations for preserving and enhancing bone mass in men who have osteoporosis. Secondary causes of osteoporosis should be identified and treated. In addition, there are pharmacologic therapies that have been shown to enhance BMD, and in some cases reduce fracture risk in men. Although the available data are not as extensive as in women, these therapies appear to be as effective in men as in women. The treatment indications for these drugs are similar in men and women.

- Idiopathic osteoporosis. Alendronate and parathyroid hormone are both effective in improving BMD[18,19] and are effective regardless of age or gonadal function. Alendronate therapy is associated with a reduction in vertebral fracture risk. A summary of the available randomized, controlled trials in men is given in Table 3.
- Glucocorticoid-induced osteoporosis. Bisphosphonate therapy (alendronate, risedronate) is effective in improving BMD, and although the data are not extensive, also probably reduces fracture risk.[20,21]
- Hypogonadal osteoporosis. Testosterone replacement therapy increases BMD in men with established hypogonadism,[2] but whether fracture risk is reduced is unknown. In older men with less severe, age-related reductions in gonadal function, the usefulness of testosterone is unproven. Moreover, the long-term risks of testosterone therapy in older men are unknown. Therefore, testosterone replacement therapy is appropriate for the management of the hypogonadal syndrome, but the treatment of osteoporosis in a man with low testosterone levels should be undertaken with a bisphosphonate or parathyroid hormone.

REFERENCES

1. Seeman E 2001 Sexual dimorphism in skeletal size, density, and strength. J Clin Endocrinol Metab **86:**4576–4584.
2. Orwoll ES, Klein RF 2001 Osteoporosis in men: Epidemiology, pathophysiology, and clinical characterization. In: Marcus R, Feldman D, Kelsey J (eds.) Osteoporosis, 2nd ed. Academic Press, San Diego, CA, USA, pp. 103–149.
3. Seeman E 2002 Pathogenesis of bone fragility in women and men. Lancet **359:**1841–1850.
4. Donaldson LJ, Cook A, Thomson RG 1990 Incidence of fractures in a geographically defined population. J Epidemiol Community Health **44:**241–245.
5. Ismail AA, Pye SR, Cockerill WC, Lunt M, Silman AJ, Reeve J, Banzer D, Benevolenskaya LI, Bhalla A, Armas JB, Cannata JB, Cooper C, Delmas PD, Dequeker J, Dilsen G, Falch JA, Felsch B, Felsenberg D, Finn JD, Gennari C, Hoszowski K, Jajic I, Janott J, Johnell O, Kanis JA, Kragl G, Vaz AL, Lorenc R, Lyritis G, Marchand F, Masaryk P, Matthis C, Miazgowski T, Naves-Diaz M, Pols HAP, Poor G, Rapido A, Raspe HH, Reid DM, Reisinger W, Scheidt-Nave

C, Stepan J, Todd C, Weber K, Woolf AD, O'Neill TW 2002 Incidence of limb fracture across Europe: Results from the European prospective osteoporosis study (EPOS). Osteoporos Int 13:565–571.

6. Group EPOSE 2002 Incidence of vertebral fracture in Europe: Results from the European prospective osteoporosis study (EPOS). J Bone Miner Res 17:716–724.

7. Amin S, Felson DT 2001 Osteoporosis in men. Rheum Dis Clin North Am 27:19–47.

8. Schwartz AV, Kelsey JL, Maggi S, Tuttleman M, Ho SC, Jonsson PV, Poor G, Sisson de Castro JA, Xu L, Matkin CC, Nelson LM, Heyse SP 1999 International variation in the incidence of hip fractures: Cross-national project on osteoporosis for the world health organization program for research aging. Osteoporos Int 9:242–253.

9. Nguyen TV, Eisman JA, Kelly PJ, Sambrook PN 1996 Risk factors for osteoporotic fractures in elderly men. Am J Epidemiol 144:258–261.

10. Vanderschueren D, Boonen S, Bouillon R 2000 Osteoporosis and osteoporotic fractures in men: A clinical perspective. Baillieres Best Pract Res Clin Endocrinol Metab 14:299–315.

11. Khosla S, Melton J III 2002 Estrogen and the male skeleton. J Clin Endocrinol Metab 87:1443–1450.

12. Vanderschueren D, Boonen S, Bouillon R 1998 Action of androgens versus estrogens in male skeletal homeostasis. Bone 23:391–394.

13. Orwoll E 2003 Men, estrogen and bone: Unresolved issues. Osteoporos Int 14:93–98.

14. Leder BZ, Le Blanc KM, Schoenfeld DA, Eastell R, Finkelstein J 2003 Differential effects of androgens and estrogens on bone turnover in normal men. J Clin Endocrinol Metab 88:204–210.

15. Falahati-Nini A, Riggs BL, Atkinson EJ, O'Fallon WM, Eastell E, Khosla S 2000 Relative contributions of testosterone and estrogen in regulating bone resorption and formation in normal elderly men. J Clin Invest 106:1553–1560.

16. Orwoll ES 2001 Androgens: Basic biology and clinical implication. Calcif Tissue Int 69:185–188.

17. Binkley NC, Schmeer P, Wasnich RD, Lenchik L 2002 What are the criteria by which a densitometric diagnosis of osteoporosis can be made in males and non-Caucasians? J Clin Densitom 5(Suppl):19–27.

18. Orwoll E, Ettinger M, Weiss S, Miller P, Kendler D, Graham J, Adami S, Weber K, Lorenc R, Pietschmann P, Vandormael K, Lombardi A 2000 Alendronate for the treatment of osteoporosis in men. N Engl J Med 343:604–610.

19. Orwoll ES, Scheele WH, Paul S, Adami S, Syversen U, Diez-Perez A, Kaufman JM, Clancy AD, Gaich GA 2003 The effect of teriparatide Human Parathyroid Hormone (1–34) therapy on bone density in men with osteoporosis. J Bone Miner Res 18:9–17.

20. Adachi JD, Bensen WG, Brown J, Hanley D, Hodsman A, Josse R, Kendler DL, Lentle B, Olszynski W, Ste-Marie L-G, Tenenhouse A, Chines AA 1997 Intermittent etidronate therapy to prevent corticosteroid-induced osteoporosis. N Engl J Med 337:382–387.

21. Reid DM, Hughes RA, Laan RFJM, Sacco-Gibson NA, Wenderoth DH, Adami S, Eusebio RA, Devogelaer JP 2000 Efficacy and safety of daily residronate in the treatment of corticosteroid-induced osteoporosis in men and women: A randomized trial. J Bone Miner Res 15:1006–1013.

22. Kurland ES, Cosman F, McMahon DJ, Rosen CJ, Lindsay R, Bilezikian JP 2000 Therapy of idiopathic osteoporosis in men with parathyroid hormone: Effects on bone mineral density and bone markers. J Clin Endocrinol Metab 85:3069–3076.

23. Trovas GP, Lyritis GP, Galanos A, Raptou P, Constantelou E 2002 A randomized trial of nasal spray salmon calcitonin in men with idiopathic osteoporosis: Effects on bone mineral density and bone markers. J Bone Miner Res 17:521–527.

Chapter 62.   Glucocorticoid-Induced Osteoporosis

Barbara P. Lukert

Division of Metabolism and Endocrinology, University of Kansas, Kansas City, Kansas

INTRODUCTION

Glucocorticoid-induced osteoporosis (GCOP) has been recognized since Harvey Cushing first described it as a sequela of Cushing's disease.[1] GCOP became a clinical problem of greater significance when cortisone was first used for the treatment of rheumatoid arthritis, and it soon became apparent that patients taking steroids chronically had a high incidence of vertebral fractures.[2] It is now recognized that chronic use of glucocorticoids (GCs) is the most common cause of secondary osteoporosis, and compression fractures of vertebrae are the most devastating consequences of long-term administration.

GC PREPARATIONS

Synthetic derivatives designed in an attempt to diminish the detrimental side effects of cortisol, particularly sodium retention, while augmenting the anti-inflammatory effect of the parent compound, have not succeeded in reducing bone loss. The severity of side effects, other than fluid retention, seem to be proportional to their anti-inflammatory potency. The most frequently prescribed GCs are prednisone, prednisolone, methylprednisolone, betamethasone, dexamethasone, and triamcinolone. Patients prone to adverse side effects of GCs appear to be those with the slowest clearance of the drug.[3] Recent studies suggest that the severity of the effects of GCs on bone may be determined in part by the activity of 11-β hydroxysteroid dehydrogenase (11B-HSD), which controls the interconversion of inactive cortisone to active cortisol.

Route of Administration

The majority of the studies examining the effects of GCs on the skeleton are performed in patients taking oral steroids. Inhaled preparations are highly active topically but weakly active systemically, thus minimizing the risk for suppressing the pituitary-adrenal axis and causing Cushing syndrome. High doses of inhaled steroids may be associated with bone loss. Steroids given by epidural injection are absorbed, and Cushing's syndrome has been reported in patients receiving triamcinolone as paraspinal or epidural injection.[4] The presence of these systemic effects certainly suggests that bone loss may occur.

Clinical Features, and Systemic and Skeletal Manifestations of GC Excess

Patients receiving pharmacologic doses of GCs present with a distinctive clinical picture: centripetal obesity with

---

The author has no conflict of interest.

peripheral subcutaneous fat atrophy, thinning of the skin with increased fragility and ecchymoses, proximal muscle weakness, fluid retention, hyperglycemia, and frequently, vertebral fractures. Fractures caused by bone loss are among the most incapacitating sequela of steroid therapy.

Bone Density

Effect of Oral Steroids. Bone density has been measured in patients taking steroids for a wide variety of diseases. Older retrospective studies reported bone loss varying from 0% to 17% per year.[5] More recent prospective data based on the results derived from the placebo groups in clinical trials show that most people taking GCs lose bone. A meta-analysis on the use of bisphosphonates in GC-induced osteoporosis included 15 studies.[6] The mean change in bone mineral density (BMD) of the spine while taking GCs was −2.97% per year in the placebo group, most of whom were taking calcium and vitamin D. Only 1 in 15 studies failed to observe bone loss. Ten of these studies measured density of the femoral neck also, and they all showed loss of bone in the placebo group with a mean decline of −2.71% per year.

Effect of Inhaled Steroids. A cross-sectional study of bone density and markers of bone remodeling showed that adults taking either inhaled beclomethasone or budesonide in doses of >1500 mg/day for at least 12 months had lower bone density values in the spine and proximal femur.[7,8] Markers of bone formation were decreased, whereas bone resorption markers remained normal.[9] A prospective cohort study of premenopausal women using triamcinolone acetonide showed a dose-related decrease in bone density in the total hip and trochanter but not in the spine or femoral neck.[10] In view of the possibility that inhaled steroids may increase the risk for fracture (see below), adults receiving more than 1000 μg of beclomethasone or budesonide daily and children receiving more than 400 μg daily should be monitored.

Fracture Risk

Oral GCs. The true incidence of osteoporosis-related fractures in patients taking GCs is unknown. Available data were again derived from the control groups of multicenter trials evaluating the efficacy of bisphosphonates and from a retrospective cohort study. In the control groups for bisphosphonate studies in which the placebo group received calcium and vitamin D supplements, the fracture incidence in postmenopausal women ranged from 13% to 21%.[11–13]. No fractures were observed in premenopausal women, and the incidence in men varied from 2.1% to 23.5%. In a retrospective cohort study comparing patients taking oral steroids to those using inhaled steroid, the fracture risk increased within 3 months after the initiation of oral GCs.[14] The risk was dose-dependent, with an increase in risk for vertebral fracture in patients taking as little as 2.5 mg of prednisone daily. The relative risk (RR) for vertebral fracture was 1.55, 2.59, and 5.18 for doses of <2.5, 2.5–7.5, and >7.5, respectively. The hip fracture risk was 0.99 relative to control in patients taking <2.5 mg prednisone daily, rising to 1.77 on daily doses of 2.5–5.0 mg/day and to 2.27 on doses of 7.5 mg or greater.[14]

Although postmenopausal women are at highest risk for fractures, both men and women, old and young, blacks and whites, lose bone, and if they take GCs long enough, it is likely that they will be at risk for fractures.

Inhaled Steroids. The effect of inhaled steroids on fracture risk is less clear. A retrospective cohort study obtained from the General Practice Research Database in the United Kingdom showed that compared with patients using bronchodilators only, inhaled steroid users had an increased relative risk for fractures of the hip and spine of 1.22 and 1.51, respectively.[15] However, there were numerous confounding factors that make it impossible to attribute the increased fracture risk solely to inhaled steroids. For example, the history of the lifetime use of oral steroids was not available, and many of the patients may have been more susceptible to fracture because of previous use of oral steroids.

Histomorphometry

Steroid-induced bone loss occurs primarily in trabecular bone.[16] Bone biopsy specimens taken from the iliac crest of patients taking GCs show a low mineral apposition rate, a reduction of trabecular mean wall thickness, and a decrease in the number of osteoid seams,[16,17] with a consequent decrease in bone volume. The number of apoptotic osteoblasts and osteocytes is increased.[18] The total amount of bone replaced in each remodeling cycle is reduced by 30%. Parameters of bone resorption are elevated, with increases in eroded surface, osteoclast-covered surface, and increased osteoclast number.[18,19]

PATHOGENESIS

Systemic Effects of GCs

Gonadal Hormones. Serum concentrations of estradiol, estrone, dehydroepiandrosterone sulfate, and progesterone are decreased in women taking GCs, and testosterone levels are decreased in men.[20]

Parathyroid Hormone, Vitamin D, and Calcium Absorption

Intestinal Calcium Absorption. Pharmacologic doses of GCs inhibit intestinal absorption of calcium and cause hypercalciuria.[21] In vitro studies show that GCs decrease intestinal mucosal to serosal flux and increase serosal to mucosal flux.[22,23] The effect is at least partially independent of vitamin D.[24] Administration of 1,25(OH)$_2$D improves calcium transport but does not return it to normal.[25] These findings suggest that GC-induced inhibition of calcium absorption is caused by alterations in post-transcriptional events and in mucosal and basolateral membrane transport. Transport is improved by sodium restriction[21] and supplemental calcium.[26]

Effect of Glucocorticoids on Bone

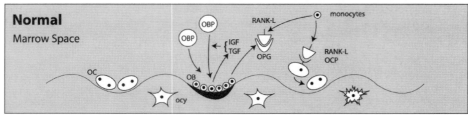

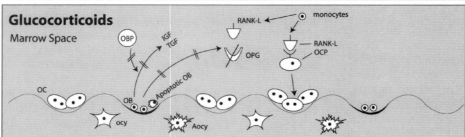

FIG. 1. GC effects. Decreased release of OPG with increased RANKL/OPG ratio causes an increase in osteoclasts and an increased number of sites undergoing remodeling. Decreased differentiation, function, and life span of osteoblasts result in decreased bone formation. An increased number of apoptotic osteocytes cause decreased bone strength. OBP, osteoblast precursor; OCP, osteoclast precursor; OPG, osteoprotegerin; OB, osteoblast; OC, osteoclast; ocy, osteocyte; Aocy, apoptotic osteocyte.

Hyperparathyroidism. Mild hyperparathyroidism has been demonstrated in patients taking long-term GCs in some,[27,28] but not all, studies.[29] A recent review of the role of secondary hyperparathyroidism in the pathogenesis of GC-induced bone loss concluded that the effects of hyperparathyroidism are minor.[30] However, work reported many years ago showing that patients taking steroid had higher parathyroid hormone (PTH) levels and higher levels of urine cyclic adenosine monophosphate (cAMP) suggests that the higher levels of PTH, although within the normal range, were physiologically significant. The importance of hyperparathyroidism is still controversial.

Vitamin D Metabolites. Steroid treated-patients usually have normal serum 25OHD levels, and 1,25(OH)2D concentrations tend to be elevated.[31] When 25OHD levels are low, it is usually because of decreased intake and lack of exposure to sunlight.

Vitamin K. Vitamin K plays an important role in the formation of osteocalcin, a bone matrix protein. Vitamin K is essential for the γ-carboxylation of glutamic acid residues. When menatetrenone, the most potent form of vitamin K, was given to steroid-treated rats, the fall in urine γ-carboxyglutamic acid was prevented, and bone density was preserved.[32]

Direct Effects on Bone Remodeling

Bone Formation. GCs have multiple and complex effects on bone formation (Fig. 1). GCs decrease the number of osteoblasts by decreasing replication and increasing the rate of apoptosis resulting in a short lifespan. The function of osteoblasts is also altered. The synthesis of type I collagen, osteocalcin, mucopolysaccharides, and sulfated glucosaminoglycans is inhibited by glucocorticoids by transcriptional and post-transcriptional mechanisms.[33] In addition to these direct effects, GC action is mediated by changes in skeletal growth factors and their binding proteins. Cortisol suppresses insulin-like growth factor I (IGF-I) gene transcription in osteoblasts. Insulin-like growth factor binding protein-S (IGFBP-5) stimulates bone cell growth, and cortisol decreases the expression of IGFBP-3, -4, and -5 in osteoblasts.

Glucocorticoids decrease the anabolic effects of TGF-β on bone by redistributing the binding of TGF-1 toward extracellular matrix storage sites and away from receptors involved in intracellular signal transduction.[34]

Production of prostaglandin E_2 (PGE$_2$) is inhibited by GCs in tissue culture.[35] GC-induced decrease in cell replication and collagen synthesis is partially reversed when PGE$_2$ is added to GC-treated bones in tissue culture.

GCs enhance the sensitivity of osteoblasts to PTH[36] and potentiate PTH-mediated inhibition of collagen synthesis, alkaline phosphatase activity, and citrate decarboxylation.[37] The renal tubular effects of PTH are also increased by GCs.

GCs decrease the expression of fibroblast growth factor (FGF)-2 and platelet-derived growth factor (PDGF)BB, all factors that are important in fracture healing. The osteoblastic synthesis of hepatocyte growth factor/scatter factor (HGF/SF), a factor that plays a role in tissue regeneration, is inhibited by GCs.[38]

Effects on Bone Resorption. Histomorphometric and calcium kinetic studies suggest that bone resorption is enhanced by GCs.[39,40] The increased bone resorption seems to involve RANKL and osteoprotegerin (OP). RANKL is an osteoblastic signal that binds to an osteoclast receptor, and in association with colony-stimulating factor (CSF)-1, induces osteoclastogenesis. OP is a decoy receptor that binds RANKL, preventing RANKL binding to the osteoclast receptor. TNF-α and interleukin-6 (IL-6) act by inducing RANKL expression. GCs increase the expression of RANKL and CSF-1 and decrease osteoprotegerin expression by human osteoblastic and stromal cells in culture.[41]

Serum levels of OPG are decreased in patients taking GCs for glomerulonephritis. This decrease was accompanied by a significant rise in the markers of bone resorption and a decrease in BMD of the lumbar spine.[42] Low estrogen levels caused by GCs result in higher levels of TNF, which may play a role in bone resorption.

Osteonecrosis

Osteonecrosis (aseptic necrosis or avascular necrosis), a serious complication of GCs, is estimated to occur in 4–25% of patients taking steroids. The hip is most frequently affected, followed by the head of the humerus and the distal femur. Pain is the usual presenting symptom and may be mild in chronic forms of the disease.

The etiology of osteonecrosis remains unclear but may be due to fat emboli, collapse of the epiphysis due to the accumulation of unhealed trabecular microcracks, increased intraosseous pressure caused by fat accumulation leading to mechanical impingement on the sinusoidal vascular bed and decreased blood flow, and/or apoptosis of osteocytes leading to decrease in strength of bone. A review of osteonecrosis is very informative.[43]

Effect on Muscle Strength

Patients taking GCs are prone to myopathy, particularly involving proximal muscles. There is a striking association between the presence of steroid myopathy and osteoporosis. The loss of muscle mass and strength can be attenuated by isokinetic training.[44]

Modulation of Effects of Glucocorticoids

Proinflammatory cytokines in osteoblasts may modulate 11-β hydroxysteroid dehydrogenase isozymes, thus potentiating the effects of GCs. Studies using the G-63 human osteosarcoma cell line and primary cultures of human osteoblasts showed that IL-1β and TNF-α increased cellular sensitivity to physiological concentrations of GCs as shown by induction of serum and GCs-inducible kinase. This effect was associated with inhibition of 11 β-HSD2 activity (conversion of cortisol-cortisone) and mRNA levels in a dose-dependent manner while stimulating reciprocal expression of 11-β-HSD-1 mRNA and activity (conversion of cortisone-cortisol). These results suggest that these cytokines cause an autocrine switch in intracellular corticosteroid metabolism by disabling glucocorticoid inactivation while inducing glucocorticoid activation.[45]

ASSESSMENT OF PATIENTS TREATED WITH GCs

It is important to assess patients when GC therapy is instituted to identify those with hypogonadism, vitamin D deficiency, hypercalciuria, or other conditions that adversely affect bone metabolism.

Bone Density

Trabecular bone (spine, hip, distal radius, pelvis, and ribs) and the cortical rim of the vertebrae are lost more rapidly than cortical bone from the extremities. Earliest changes can be detected in the spine and femoral neck using DXA or quantitative computerized tomography. Evaluation at 6-month intervals for the first 2 years will identify patients who are losing bone rapidly.

PREVENTION AND TREATMENT

Planning GC Therapy

It is prudent to prescribe the lowest effective dose and to use topical preparations whenever possible because the magnitude of bone loss may be related to dose. Alternate day therapy preserves normal function of the pituitary-adrenal axis but does not prevent bone loss.[46]

General Measures

Maintenance of good nutritional status is of obvious importance. The diet should not only provide adequate intakes of calcium and vitamin D but should also be well balanced, with adequate intake of calories to achieve ideal body weight. Sodium restriction is generally desirable because high doses of GCs cause salt and water retention, reduce gastrointestinal absorption, and increase urinary excretion of calcium. If sodium restriction alone does not control hypercalciuria, a thiazide diuretic along with a potassium-sparing diuretic such as amiloride should be added.[21] If this is required, serum potassium levels must be carefully monitored.

An active lifestyle with weight bearing exercise has a positive effect on bone mass and maintains muscle strength, which in turn, decreases falls and their resultant fractures. Every patient should be assessed for signs of myopathy, and appropriate exercises should be prescribed.

Calcium supplements alone reduce bone turnover and may be effective in preventing bone loss in patients receiving long-term, low-dose treatment. Vitamin D plus calcium does not prevent bone loss during the first few months of taking GCs. A recent meta-analysis showed that both vitamin D and its metabolites were more effective in preserving BMD than no therapy or calcium alone.[47] Moreover, the efficacy of bisphosphonates was significantly greater when used in combination with vitamin D. Calcitriol and alfacalcidol may have direct antiresorptive and anabolic effects on bone. However, the meta-analysis just mentioned found no statistical difference between estimates of effect for vitamin D and calcitriol. Calcitriol and other potent metabolites of vitamin D should not be used routinely in the management of GC-induced bone loss until matters of dosage and toxicity are better understood.

Hormone Replacement

Bone density increases in the spine when postmenopausal women taking long-term steroids are given hormone replacement therapy (HRT).[48,49] There is no consistent data on the effect on the hip, and there are no trials large enough to assess the effect of HRT on fracture risk in patients taking GCs. Despite evidence for beneficial effects, it is unlikely that HRT will be used routinely for the prevention or treatment of GC-induced bone loss in view of the recent report from the Women's Health Initiative, showing an increase in the risk for breast cancer and cardiovascular disease in women taking long-term HRT.[50]

BMD of the spine increases when hypogonadal men receiving GCs are treated with testosterone for 1 year. No hip or fracture data are available.

Antiresorptive Drugs

Drugs that limits the depth of the resorption cavity at each remodeling site should minimize the amount of bone loss despite inhibition of bone formation. Calcitonin and the bisphosphonates, alendronate, risedronate, etidronate, and pamidronate, are the antiresorptive drugs (other than estrogen) currently available in the United States.

A meta-regression analysis comparing the efficacy of drug therapies for the management of GC-induced osteoporosis showed that calcitonin given with vitamin D was more effective than no therapy or calcium only, but significantly less effective than bisphosphonates.[47] Etidronate given cyclically and with calcium and vitamin D supplementation (1000 IU/day) improved bone density in preliminary studies.[51] No fracture data are available.

Pamidronate given continuously by the oral route, intravenously every 3 months for 1 year, or as a larger dose once a year prevents bone loss in patients taking prednisone.[52,53]

Alendronate and risedronate preserve bone mass in the spine and hip in patients who start GC therapy within 4 months and in those who have taken GC chronically. Compression fractures of the spine are prevented in postmenopausal women and in men. The studies were not powered to evaluate hip fractures.[12,13,54–56]

A meta-analysis on the use of bisphosphonates in GC-induced osteoporosis included six primary prevention and seven secondary prevention studies involving 842 participants.[6] All 13 studies reported data on bone loss from the lumbar spine, while 8 reported changes at the femoral neck. Twelve studies reported significant improvement in lumbar BMD in the treatment group compared with controls. On average, the treatment and placebo groups had a percentage change in bone density that differed by 4%. Four studies reported a significant improvement in femoral neck BMD, whereas the other four reported no significant difference from the control groups. The mean average change in femoral neck BMD differed by 2.1% between the treated and placebo groups.

Four studies reporting the incidence of new vertebral fractures were included in the meta-analysis. Three found a decreased number of fractures, whereas one study found an increased number in the treatment group. In this analysis, the odds ratio of new fracture did not reach statistical significance (0.8). The author concluded that longer follow-up is required to ascertain the efficacy of bisphosphonates in fracture prevention. This analysis did not include large recent trials using risedronate.[55,56] A 4% increase in BMD would be expected to decrease fracture risk reported in these studies.

Drugs That Stimulate Bone Formation

The most promising anabolic hormone for treating GC-induced bone loss is PTH. PTH causes exuberant increases in BMD in postmenopausal women who are taking GCs and estrogen. Women receiving PTH plus estrogen experienced an 11% increase in BMD of the spine measured by DXA compared with a 1.7% increase in those taking estrogen alone. There were no differences between groups in the density of the hip or forearm. One year after PTH was discontinued, lumbar spine BD increased by another 15%.[57,58]

THERAPY OF THE FUTURE

Recombinant human GH (hGH) prevents protein catabolism and improves protein balance in GC-treated patients.[59] However, the effect on bone loss seems less promising. Attempts to stimulate the local production of growth factors in bone that are altered by GCs, such as IGF-I or TGF-β, may be useful. The search continues for new agents that stimulate replication, differentiation, and function of osteoblasts. The administration of osteoprotegerin, antibodies to RANKL, or agents that alter the secretion of either may be useful in altering the balance between formation and resorption.

There are continuing efforts to develop GCs that retain anti-inflammatory properties but have less effect on calcium metabolism and bone remodeling. There is hope for dissociating the anti-inflammatory effects from effects on bone with the discovery of compounds that dissociate transactivation and transexpression.[60]

Despite the fact that GC-induced osteoporosis has been recognized for over 60 years, it remains a neglected problem. GCs are the mainstay of treatment for a variety of illnesses, and we must be aggressive in our efforts to prevent and treat bone loss, a potentially devastating effect of this very useful class of drugs. GC-induced bone loss is partially reversible. Attempts to prevent the adverse effects of GCs, based on an understanding of the mechanisms involved, should minimize this devastating complication of GC therapy.

REFERENCES

1. Cushing H 1932 Basophile adenomas. J Nerv Ment Dis **76:**50–59.
2. Curtiss PH, Clark WS, Herndon CH 1954 Vertebral fractures resulting from prolonged cortisone and corticotrophin therapy. JAMA **156:**467–469.
3. Kozower M, Veatch L, Kaplan MM 1974 Decreased clearance of prednisolone, a factor in the development of corticosteroid side effects. J Clin Endocrinol Metab **38:**407–412.
4. Edmonds LCVML, Hugher JM 1991 Morbidity from paraspinal depocorticosteroid injections for analgesia: Cushing's syndrome and adrenal suppression. Anesth Analg **72:**820–822.
5. Ruegesegger P, Medici TC, Anlinker M 1983 Corticosteroid-induced bone loss. A longitudinal study of alternate day therapy in patients with bronchial asthma using quantitative computed tomography. Eur J Clin Pharmacol **25:**615–620.
6. Homik JE, Cranney A, Shea B, Tugwell P, Wells G, Adachi J 1999 A metaanalysis on the use of bisphosphonates in corticosteroid induced osteoporosis. J Rheumatol **26:**1148–1157.
7. Wong CA, Walsh LJ, Smith CJP, Wisniewski AF, Lewis SA 2000 Inhaled corticosteroid use and bone-mineral density in patients with asthma. Lancet **355:**1399–1403.

8. Hauache OM, Amarante ECJ, Vieira JGH, Faresin SM, Fernandes ALG, Jardim JR 1999 Evaluation of bone metabolism after the use of an inhaled glucocorticoid (flunisolide) in patients with moderate asthma. Clin Endocrinol (Oxf) **51**:35–39.

9. Ebeling PR, Erbas B, Hopper JL, Wark JD, Rubinfeld AR 1998 Bone mineral density and bone turnover in asthmatics treated with long-term inhaled or oral glucocorticoids. J Bone Miner Res **13**:1283–1289.

10. Israel E, Banerjee TR, Fitzmaurice GM, Kotlov TV, LaHive K, LeBoff MS 2001 Effects of inhaled glucocorticoids on bone density in premenopausal. N Engl J Med **345**:941–947.

11. Adachi J, Bensen W, Hodsman AB 1993 Corticosteroid-induced osteoporosis. Semin Arthritis Rheum **22**:375–384.

12. Saag KG, Emkey R, Schnitzer TJ, Brown JP, Hawkins F 1998 Alendronate for the prevention and treatment of glucocorticoid-induced osteoporosis. N Engl J Med **339**:292–299.

13. Cohen S, Levy RM, Keller M, Boling E, Emkey RD, Greenwald M 1999 Risedronate therapy prevents corticosteroid-induced bone loss: A twelve-month, multicenter, randomized, double-bind, placebo-controlled, parallel-group study. Arthritis Rheum **42**:2309–2318.

14. Van Staa TP, Leufkens HGM, Abenhaim L 2000 Use of oral corticosteroids and risk of fractures. J Bone Miner Res **15**:993–999.

15. Van Staa TP, Leufkens HGM, Cooper C 2001 Use of inhaled corticosteroids and risk of fractures. J Bone Miner Res **16**:581–588.

16. Dempster DW 1989 Bone histomorphometry in glucocorticoid-induced osteoporosis. J Bone Miner Res **4**:137–141.

17. Chavassieux P, Pastoureau P, Chapuy MC, Delmas PD, Meunier PJ 1993 Glucocorticoid-induced inhibition of osteoblastic bone formation in ewes: A biochemical and histomorphometric study. Osteoporos Int **3**:97–102.

18. Weinstein RS, Jilka RL, Parfitt AM, Manolagas SC 1998 Inhibition of osteoblastogenesis and promotion of apoptosis of osteoblasts and osteocytes by glucocorticoids: Potential mechanisms of their deleterious effects on bone. J Clin Invest **102**:274–282.

19. Carbonare LD, Arlot ME, Chavassieux PM, Roux JP, Portero NR 2001 Comparison of trabecular bone microarchitecture and remodeling in glucocorticoid-induced and postmenopausal osteoporosis. J Bone Miner Res **16**:97–103.

20. Montecucco C, Caporali R, Caprotti P, Caprotti M, Notario A 1992 Sex hormones and bone metabolism in postmenopausal rheumatoid arthritis treated with two different glucocorticoids. J Rheumatol **19**:1895–1899.

21. Adams JS, Wahl TO, Lukert BP 1981 Effects of hydrochlorothiazide and dietary sodium restriction on calcium metabolism in corticosteroid treated patients. Metabolism **30**:217–221.

22. Favus MJ, Walling MW, Kimberg DV 1973 Effects of 1,25-dihydroxy-cholecalciferol in intestinal calcium transport in cortisone-treated rats. J Clin Invest **52**:1680–1685.

23. Adams JS, Lukert BP 1980 Effects of sodium restriction on 45-Ca and 22-Na transduodenal flux in corticosteroid-treated rats. Miner Electrolyte Metab **4**:216–226.

24. Shultz TD, Kumar R 1987 Effect of cortisol on [3H] 1,25-dihydroxyvitamin D3 uptake and 1, 25-dihydroxyvitamin D3-induced DNA-dependent RNA polymerase activity in chick intestinal cells. Calcif Tissue Int **40**:224–230.

25. Colette C, Monnier L, Pares Herbute N, Blotman F, Mirouze J 1987 Calcium absorption in corticoid treated subjects–effects of a single oral dose of calcitriol. Horm Metab Res **19**:335–338.

26. Reid IR, Ibbertson HK 1986 Calcium supplements in the prevention of steroid-induced osteoporosis. Am J Clin Nutr **44**:287–290.

27. Lukert BP, Adams JS 1976 Calcium and phosphorus homeostasis in man. Arch Intern Med **136**:1249–1253.

28. Suzuki Y, Ichikawa Y, Saito E, Homma M 1983 Importance of increased urinary calcium excretion in the development of secondary hyperparathyroidism of patients under glucocorticoid therapy. Metabolism **32**:151–156.

29. Lund B, Storm TL, Lund B 1985 Bone mineral loss, bone histomorphometry and vitamin D metabolism in patients with rheumatoid arthritis on long-term glucocorticoid treatment. Clin Rheumatol **4**:143–149.

30. Rubin MR, Bilezikian JP 2002 The role of parathyroid hormone in the pathogenesis of glucocorticoid-induced osteoporosis—A re-examination of the evidence. J Clin Endocrinol Metab **87**:4033–4041.

31. Bikle DD, Halloran BP, Fong L, Steinbach L, Shellito J 1993 Elevated 1,25-dihydroxyvitamin D levels in patients with chronic obstructive pulmonary disease treated with prednisone. J Clin Endocrinol Metab **76**:456–461.

32. Hara K, Akiyama Y, Ohkawa I, Tajima T 1993 Effects of menatetrenone on prednisolone-induced bone loss in rats. Bone **14**:813–818.

33. Canalis EM, Delaney AM 2002 Mechanisms of glucocorticoid action in bone. Ann NY Acad Sci **966**:73–81.

34. Centrella M, McCarthy TL, Canalis EM 1991 Glucocorticoid regulation of transforming growth factor B1 activity and binding in osteoblast-enriched cultures from fetal rat bone. Mol Cell Biol **11**:4490–4496.

35. Raisz LG, Simmons HA 1985 Effects of parathyroid hormone and cortisol on prostaglandin production by neonatal rat calvaria in vitro. Endocr Res **11**:59–74.

36. Chen TL, Feldman D 1978 Glucocorticoid potentiation of the adenosine 3′, 5′-monophosphate response to parathyroid hormone in cultured rat bone cells. Endocrinology **102**:589–596.

37. Wong GL 1979 Basal activities and hormone responsiveness of osteoclast-like and osteoblast-like bone cells are regulated by glucocorticoids. J Biol Chem **254**:6337–6340.

38. Blanquaert F, Pereira RC, Canalis E 2000 Cortisol inhibits hepatocyte growth factor/scatter factor expression and induces c-met transcripts in osteoblasts. Am J Physiol **278**:509–515.

39. Dempster DW, Arlot MA, Meunier PJ 1983 Mean wall thickness and formation periods of trabecular bone packets in corticosteroid-induced osteoporosis. Calcif Tissue Int **35**:410–417.

40. Meunier PJ, Dempster DW, Edouard C, Chapuy MC, Arlot M, Charhon S 1984 Bone histomorphometry in corticoidsteroid-induced osteoporosis and Cushing's syndrome. Adv Exp Med Biol **171**:191–200.

41. Hofbauer LC, Gori FRBL, Lacey DL, Dunstan CR, Spelsberg TC, Khosla S 1999 Stimulation of osteoprotegerin ligand and inhibition of osteoprotegerin production by glucocorticoids in human osteoblastic lineage cells: Potential paracrine mechanisms of glucocorticoid-induced osteoporosis. Endocrinology **140**:4382–4389.

42. Sasaki N, Kusano E, Ando Y, Nemoto J, Iimura O, Ito C 2002 Changes in osteoprotegerin and markers of bone metabolism during glucocorticoid treatment in patients with chronic glomerulonephritis. Bone **30**:853–858.

43. Mankin HJ 1992 Nontraumatic necrosis of bone (osteonecrosis). N Engl J Med **326**:1473–1478.

44. Horber FF, Scheidegger JR, Grunig BE, Frey FJ 1985 Thigh muscle mass and function in patients treated with glucocorticoids. Eur J Clin Invest **15**:302–307.

45. Cooper MS, Bujalska I, Rabbit EH, Walker EA, Bland R, Sheppard MC 2001 Modulation of 11 beta-hydroxysteroid dehydrogenase isozymes by proinflammatory cytokines in osteoblasts: An autocrine switch from glucocorticoid inactivation to activation. J Bone Miner Res **16**:1037–1044.

46. Gluck OS, Murphy WA, Hahn TJ, Hahn BH 1985 Bone loss in adults receiving alternate day glucocorticoid therapy. A comparison with daily therapy. Arthritis Rheum **24**:892–898.

47. Amin S, Lin JM, Simms RW, Felson DT 2002 The comparative efficacy of drug therapies used for the management of corticosteroid-induced osteoporosis: A meta-regression. J Bone Miner Res **17**:1512–1526.

48. Lukert BP, Johnson BE, Robinson RG 1992 Estrogen and progesterone replacement therapy reduces glucocorticoid-induced bone loss. J Bone Miner Res **7**:1063–1069.

49. Hall GM, Daniels M, Doyle DV, Spector TD 1994 Effect of hormone replacement therapy on bone mass in rheumatoid arthritis patients treated with and without steroids. Arthritis Rheum **37**:1499–1505.

50. Writing Group for the Women's Health Initiative Investigators 2002 Risks and benefits of estrogen plus progestin in healthy postmenopausal women. JAMA **288**:321–333.

51. Mulder H, Smelder HA 1992 Effect of cyclical etidronate regimen on prophylaxis of bone loss of glucocorticoid (prednisone) therapy in postmenopausal women. J Bone Miner Res **7**:S331.

52. Reid IR, King AR, Alexander CJ, Ibbertson HK 1988 Prevention of steroid-induced osteoporosis with (3-amino-1-hydroxypropylidene)-1, 1-bisphosphonate (APD). Lancet **1**:143–146.

53. Boutsen Y, Jamart J, Esselinckx W, Devogelaer JP 2001 Primary prevention of glucocorticoid-induced osteoporosis with intravenous pamidronate and calcium: A prospective controlled 1-year study comparing a single infusion, and infusion given once every 3 months, and calcium alone. J Bone Miner Res **16**:104–112.

54. Adachi J, Saag KG, Delmas PD, Liberman UA, Emkey RD, Seeman E 2001 Two-year effects of alendronate on bone mineral density and vertebral fracture in patients receiving glucocorticoids. Arthritis Rheum **44**:202–211.

55. Reid DM, Hughes RA, Laan R, Sacco-Gibson NA, Wenderoth DH 2000 Efficacy and safety of daily risedronate in the treatment of corticosteroid-induced osteoporosis in men and women: A randomized trial. J Bone Miner Res **15**:1006–1012.

56. Wallach S, Reid DM, Hughes RA, Hosking DJ, Laan RF, Doherty SM 2000 Effects of risedronate treatment on bone density and vertebral fracture in patients on corticosteroid therapy. Calcif Tissue Int **67**:277–285.
57. Lane NE, Sanchez S, Modin GW, Genant HK, Pierini E, Arnaud CD 1998 Parathyroid hormone treatment can reverse corticosteroid-induced osteoporosis. J Clin Invest **102**:1627–1633.
58. Lane NE, Sanchez S, Modin GW, Genant HK, Pierini E, Arnaud CD 2000 Bone mass continues to increase at the hip after parathyroid hormone treatment is discontinued in glucocorticoid-induced osteoporosis: Results of a randomized controlled clinical trial. J Bone Miner Res **27**:944–951.
59. Horber FF, Haymond MW 1990 Human growth hormone prevents the protein catabolic side effects of prednisone in humans. J Clin Invest **86**:265–272.
60. Vayssiere BM, Dupont S, Choquart A, Petit F, Garcia T, Marchandeau C 1997 Synthetic glucocorticoids that dissociate transactivation and AP-1 transrepression exhibit antiinflammatory activity in vivo. Mol Endocrinol **11**:1245–1253.

Chapter 63. Transplantation Osteoporosis

Adi Cohen,[1] Peter Ebeling,[2] Stuart Sprague,[3] and Elizabeth Shane[1]

[1]College of Physicians and Surgeons, Columbia University, New York, New York; [2]The Royal Melbourne Hospital, The University of Melbourne, Victoria, Australia; and [3]Evanston Northwestern Healthcare, Feinberg School of Medicine, Northwestern University, Evanston, Illinois

INTRODUCTION

Transplantation is an established therapy for end-stage diseases of the kidney, heart, liver, and lung, and for certain hematologic conditions. Survival has improved dramatically and increased survival has been accompanied by greater awareness of complications such as osteoporosis. In this chapter, we discuss the clinical features of bone disease particular to different types of organ failure, the various immunosuppressive medications that contribute to the pathophysiology of transplantation bone disease, the clinical features of osteoporosis specific to different types of organ transplantation, and the prevention and treatment of osteoporosis in transplant recipients.

This subject topic has been addressed in several recent chapters and reviews[1–5] that contain detailed references.

BONE DISEASE IN CANDIDATES FOR ORGAN TRANSPLANTATION

Chronic Kidney Disease

Some form of renal osteodystrophy is universal in patients with chronic kidney disease (CKD). A complete discussion of renal osteodystrophy is beyond the scope of this chapter. Suffice it to say that patients with kidney failure have the most complex form of pretransplant bone disease. Several different pathogenetic mechanisms may be involved that may ultimately lead to one or more types of bone disease including osteitis fibrosa cystica as a result of secondary hyperparathyroidism (SHPT), some form of low turnover bone disease (osteomalacia, adynamic bone disease, aluminum bone disease), osteoporosis, osteosclerosis, and β_2-microglobulin amyloidosis. In addition, hypogonadism, metabolic acidosis, and certain medications (loop diuretics, heparin, glucocorticoids, or cyclosporine) may also affect bone health before transplantation

In dialysis patients, the prevalence of low bone mineral density (BMD) is increased at the spine, hip, and distal radius. Risk factors for low BMD include female gender, white race, amenorrhea, lower weight or body mass index (BMI), elevated parathyroid hormone (PTH), duration of hemodialysis, and previous kidney transplantation. Vertebral fracture prevalence is as high as 21% and the relative risk of hip fracture is increased 2- to 14-fold. Fracture risk is increased with older age, female gender, white race,[6] duration of dialysis,[7] diabetic nephropathy,[8] peripheral vascular disease,[6] low spine BMD, and lower PTH levels.

Congestive Heart Failure

Low BMD is also common in patients with severe congestive heart failure (CHF). In one study of patients awaiting heart transplantation, lumbar spine (LS) osteopenia was found in 43%, and osteoporosis in 7%, of these patients.[9] Mild renal insufficiency, vitamin D deficiency, SHPT, and increased bone resorption markers were also common.

End-Stage Liver Disease

Osteoporosis, fractures, and abnormal mineral metabolism are associated with virtually all forms of chronic liver disease. Osteoporosis at the spine or hip (T-score < −2.5 or Z-score < −2) has been reported in 11–52% of patients awaiting liver transplantation.[2,5,10] In a recent study of 243 liver transplant candidates,[11] low BMD was associated with older age, lower body weight, and the presence of cholestatic liver disease. Serum concentrations of 25OHD, PTH, osteocalcin, and testosterone are lower than in healthy controls.[10]

Chronic Respiratory Failure

Osteoporosis may be most common in patients awaiting lung transplantation. Hypoxia, hypercapnia, tobacco, and glucocorticoids may all contribute. Cystic fibrosis (CF) is associated with additional risk factors (pancreatic insufficiency, vitamin D deficiency, calcium malabsorption, hypogonadism, inactivity). Densitometric osteoporosis has been reported in 29–61% of patients with end-stage pulmonary

The authors have no conflict of interest.

disease. A recent study of 74 patients found that chronic glucocorticoid (GC) use, low BMI, and pulmonary function were associated with low BMD.[12] In patients with CF, vertebral and rib fractures were 10- to 100-fold more common than expected among the general population.

CANDIDATES FOR BONE MARROW TRANSPLANTATION

Bone loss in bone marrow transplantation (BMT) recipients is related both to the underlying diseases and to the agents used to treat them. These include GC-induced decreases in bone formation and serum $1,25(OH)_2D_3$, as well as hypogonadism secondary to the effects of high-dose chemotherapy, total body irradiation (TBI), and GCs. Women are particularly sensitive to the adverse effects of TBI and chemotherapy on gonadal function. Ovarian insufficiency occurs in the majority,[13,14] although young, premenarchal women may recover ovarian function. Testosterone levels decline acutely after BMT and then return to normal in most men.[15] There may be long-term impairment of spermatogenesis with elevated follicle-stimulating hormone (FSH) occurring in 47% of men.[13,14] Growth hormone deficiency has been documented in children after BMT[16] and may contribute to low BMD. In patients studied after chemotherapy but before BMT, osteopenia was present in 24% and osteoporosis was present in 4%.[17]

SKELETAL EFFECTS OF IMMUNOSUPPRESSIVE DRUGS

Glucocorticoids

GCs in high doses (e.g., ≥50 mg/day of prednisone or prednisolone) are commonly prescribed immediately after transplantation, with subsequent dose reduction over several weeks and transient increases during rejection episodes. Exposure varies with the organ transplanted, the number and management of rejection episodes, and the practice of transplantation programs. The introduction of cyclosporine A, tacrolimus, and more recently, rapamycin and daclizumab have reduced GC requirements. However, there is still sufficient exposure, particularly during the first few months after transplantation, to cause substantial bone loss.

The skeletal effects of GCs are discussed in detail elsewhere and will be reviewed only briefly here. GCs reduce BMD predominantly at trabecular sites, and even small doses are associated with markedly increased fracture risk. GCs cause direct and profound reductions in bone formation by decreasing osteoblast replication, differentiation, and lifespan, and by inhibiting genes for type I collagen, osteocalcin, insulin-like growth factors, bone morphogenetic proteins and other bone matrix proteins, transforming growth factor β (TGFβ), and RANKL. Direct effects of GCs on bone resorption are minor relative to formation. However, GCs may increase bone resorption indirectly by inhibiting synthesis of gonadal steroids and inducing SHPT from reduced intestinal and renal calcium absorption, although hyperparathyroidism (HPT) is thought to be of minor importance in the pathogenesis of steroid-induced bone loss.[18]

Calcineurin Inhibitors: Cyclosporine A and Tacrolimus

The introduction of cyclosporine (CsA) to transplantation regimens was associated with a marked reduction in rejection episodes and improved survival. CsA inhibits calcineurin, a T-cell phosphatase, and reduces T-cell function through suppression of regulatory genes expressing products such as interleukin (IL)-2, interleukin receptors, and the proto-oncogenes H-ras and c-myc.[19] Although in vitro studies demonstrated that CsA inhibits bone resorption in cultured bone, in vivo rodent studies suggest that CsA has independent adverse effects on bone and mineral metabolism that could contribute to bone loss after organ transplantation.[19] In the rat, CsA administration caused severe bone loss particularly in trabecular bone, which was associated with marked increases in resorption and formation, and with increased levels of osteocalcin and $1,25(OH)_2D_3$.[19] The CsA-mediated bone loss was associated with testosterone deficiency,[20] independent of renal function,[19] and attenuated by parathyroidectomy.[21] Antiresorptive agents such as estrogen, raloxifene, calcitonin, and alendronate prevented CsA-induced bone loss.[19] CsA may cause bone loss by direct effects on calcineurin genes expressed in osteoclasts[22] or indirectly through alterations in T-cell function.[23] These animal studies suggest that CsA could be responsible for the high-turnover aspects of posttransplantation bone disease. However, the effects of CsA on the human skeleton are still unclear, particularly in view of reports that kidney transplant patients receiving CsA in a steroid-free regimen[24-26] do not lose bone.

Tacrolimus (FK506), another calcineurin inhibitor (CI) that inhibits cytokine gene expression, T-cell activation, and T-cell proliferation, also causes trabecular bone loss in the rat.[19] Fewer studies have evaluated the skeletal effects of FK506 in humans. Both cardiac[27] and liver[28] transplant recipients sustained rapid bone loss with FK506. However, FK506 may cause less bone loss in humans than CsA.[29,30] Liver transplant recipients taking FK506 were exposed to less prednisone and had significantly higher femoral neck (FN) BMD 2 years after transplantation than those receiving CsA.[30] Thus, FK506-based regimens may benefit the skeleton by allowing for the use of lower GC doses.

Other Immunosuppressive Agents

Limited information is available regarding the effects of other immunosuppressive drugs on BMD and bone metabolism. Azathioprine, sirolimus (rapamycin), and mycophenolate mofetil do not cause bone loss in the rat model. The skeletal effects of newer agents, such as Daclizumab, have not been studied. However, by reducing GC requirements, they may be relatively beneficial to the skeleton.

CLINICAL FEATURES OF TRANSPLANTATION OSTEOPOROSIS

Kidney Transplantation

In general, renal osteodystrophy improves after transplantation, with at least partial resolution of HPT during the

Table 1. Osteoporosis After Solid Organ Transplantation

Type of transplant	Prevalence after transplantation		Bone loss: first post-transplant year	Fracture incidence
	Osteoporosis*	Fractures		
Kidney[†]	11–56%	Vertebral: 3–29% Peripheral: 11–43%	Spine: 4–9% Hip: 8%	Vertebral: 3–10% Peripheral: 10–50%
Heart	25–50%	Vertebral: 22–35%	Spine: 3–8% Hip: 6–11%	10–36%
Liver	30–46%	Vertebral: 29–47%	Spine: 0–24% Hip: 2–4%	Vertebral: 24–65%
Lung	57–73%	42%	Spine: 1–5% Hip: 2–5%	18–37%

* Accepted definitions included BMD of spine and/or hip (by DXA) ≥2 SD below age- and sex-matched controls or ≥2.5 SD below young normal controls.
† Definition of osteoporosis also included BMD of predominantly cortical sites such as the femoral shaft or proximal radius that are adversely affected by excessive PTH secretion.

first year. However, bone resorption remains elevated in a substantial proportion of kidney transplant recipients and histomorphometric studies show osteoblast dysfunction and decreased mineral apposition rate, consistent with GC effect.[31,32] Persistent hyperphosphaturia with resultant hypophosphatemia may also predispose to bone loss. In some patients, this is the result of persistent or residual HPT. However, in many patients, it occurs in the absence of HPT and may persist for many years.

Cross-sectional studies of patients evaluated several years after kidney transplantation have reported osteoporosis (defined as a BMD Z-score ≤ −2 or a T-score ≤ −2.5) in 17–49% at the spine (LS), 11–56% at the FN, and 22–52% at the radius.[1–5] Several studies have shown a correlation between cumulative GC dose and BMD.

The majority of bone loss occurs in the first 6–18 months after transplantation and ranges from 4% to 9% at the LS and 5% to 8% at the hip. Some studies report gender differences in the site of bone loss, with men losing more bone at the hip.[33,34] One study documented significantly less bone loss over the first year in patients receiving alternate day prednisone.[35] Bone loss has not been consistently related to gender, patient age, cumulative GC dose, rejection episodes, activity level, or PTH levels.

Longitudinal studies also document ongoing, although less rapid, bone loss several years after kidney transplantation. In a recent study of patients evaluated approximately 7

Table 2. Changes in LS and FN BMD and Total Body Bone Mineral Content (TBBMC) 12 Months After BMT

Study	n	LS-BMD	FN-BMD	TBBMC
Stern JM et al. 1996	9	−9.5%	—	—
Ebeling PR et al. 1999	39	−3.9%	−11.7%	−3.5%
Valimaki MJ et al. 1999	22	−5.7%	−8.0	—
Kashyap A et al. 2000	21	−3.0%	−11.6%	—
Schulte C et al. 2000	81	−7.2%	−11.9%	−3.8%
Kang MI et al. 2000	31	−2.2%*	−6.2%	—
Buchs N et al. 2001[†]	23	0	−5.6%	−3.1%
Lee WL et al. 2002	67	−3.3%	−8.9% (Total hip)	—

* Not significant.
† 75% treated with intravenous pamidronate.

years after transplantation, those with elevated bone turnover markers lost more bone at the spine and the hip than those with normal bone turnover.[36] In kidney transplant patients studied approximately 10 years after transplantation, GC withdrawal was associated with a significant increase in LS and FN BMD, an increase in markers of bone formation, and little change in markers of bone resorption.[37]

Although increasing time since transplantation is considered to be a risk factor for low BMD, studies examining BMD after the first few years do not consistently show ongoing bone loss. One study noted declines in LS BMD,[38] whereas others have noted improved BMD or no significant decline.[39–42] One noted slight improvement at the LS accompanied by a small decline at the FN,[43] and two found that while some patients improve, others worsen.[36,44] Allograft recipients with progressively worsening BMD had elevated bone turnover markers in one study[36] but not another.[44] Despite the improvements in BMD after the first post-transplant year noted in some reports, most studies show that BMD remains low up to 20 years after transplantation.

In kidney transplant patients, fractures affect appendicular sites (hips, long bones, ankles, feet) more commonly than axial sites (spine and ribs).[45] Women and patients transplanted for diabetic nephropathy are at particularly increased risk of fractures. A recent cohort study of 101,039 patients with end-stage renal disease (ESRD) found that kidney transplantation was associated with a 34% greater risk of hip fracture compared with patients continuing on dialysis.[8] The majority of fractures occur within the first 3 years after transplantation.

Kidney-Pancreas Transplantation

Particularly severe osteoporosis has been documented in transplant recipients with type 1 diabetes. In patients evaluated a mean of 40 ± 23 months after transplantation, 23% had osteoporosis at the LS and 58% had osteoporosis at the FN.[46] Vertebral or nonvertebral fractures were documented in 45%, and fractures were more prevalent in patients with osteoporosis at the LS ($p = 0.05$).[46] Other retrospective studies have documented a fracture prevalence of 26–49% several years after kidney-pancreas transplantation.[5,47]

Cardiac Transplantation

The prevalence of densitometric osteoporosis in long-term cardiac transplant recipients has been reported to be 28% at the LS and 20% at the FN. Observational studies[1–5] have demonstrated that the most rapid rate of bone loss occurs in the first year. LS BMD declines by 6–10% during the first 6 months, with little decrease thereafter. In some studies, there has been partial recovery of LS BMD in later years. FN BMD falls by 6–11% in the first year and stabilizes thereafter in most cases. BMD declines at the largely cortical proximal radius site over the second and third years, perhaps reflecting post-transplant SHPT. Vitamin D deficiency and testosterone deficiency (in men) are associated with more severe bone loss during the first year. Some studies have found correlations between GC dose and bone loss.

Vertebral fracture prevalence rates range between 22% and 35% in long-term cardiac transplant recipients. Vertebral fracture incidence was 36% during the first year after cardiac transplantation.[48] The majority of fractures involved the spine and occurred within the first 6 months. Similarly, a European study of 105 patients[49] reported that one-third of patients sustained a vertebral fracture by the end of the third year. An LS T-score below −1.0 conferred a greater risk (hazard ratio, 3.1) of vertebral fracture.[49]

With respect to the biochemical correlates of bone loss, there are transient increases in markers of bone resorption and decreases in markers of bone formation (osteocalcin) soon after transplantation that return to the upper end of the normal range by 6–12 months after transplantation. Others have observed sustained high bone turnover that differs from the low-turnover state and decreased osteocalcin levels found in patients on GCs alone. SHPT, perhaps related to CsA-induced renal insufficiency, has been documented in some studies.

Liver Transplantation

The progression of osteoporosis after liver transplantation resembles that following cardiac transplantation.[49] Bone loss and fracture rates are highest in the first 6–12 months. Spine BMD declined by 2–24% during the first year in earlier studies. In contrast to these, a more recent study documented bone loss of only 2.3% at the femoral neck, with preservation of spinal BMD during the first year after liver transplantation,[50] and another documented increases in BMD at 1 year.[51] Fracture rates range from 24% to 65%, and as with cardiac transplantation, ribs and vertebrae are the most common sites. Women with primary biliary cirrhosis seem to be at greatest risk. Recovery of BMD at the spine and hip has been documented during the second and third years after transplantation in patients receiving no treatment for bone disease. Type of liver disease, GC exposure, and markers of bone turnover do not reliably predict bone loss or fracture risk. However, older age and pretransplant BMD at the LS and FN predicted post-transplantation fractures in one recent prospective study,[10] and pretrans-

plant vertebral fractures predicted post-transplant vertebral fractures in two recent prospective studies.[49,52]

The high turnover state documented after liver transplantation contrasts with decreased bone formation and low turnover seen before transplantation. This change from low to high bone turnover may be because of resolution of cholestasis or hypogonadism, increased PTH secretion, CsA or FK506, or a combination of factors. Although PTH is generally normal after liver transplantation, significant increases in PTH have been observed during the first 3–6 months.[10,51] As in cardiac transplant patients, it is possible that a decline in renal function caused by renal effects of CsA or FK506 may lead to the development of SHPT.

Lung Transplantation

The prevalence of osteoporosis is very high in lung transplant recipients, with rates as high as 73%. During the first year after lung transplantation, rates of bone loss at the LS and FN range from 2% to 5%.[1–5] Fracture rates are also high during the first year, ranging from 18% to 37%, even in patients who received antiresorptive therapy to prevent bone loss. Some,[53] but not all,[54] studies have found that bone loss correlates with GC dose. Bone turnover markers are consistent with increased resorption and formation.[54] A post-transplantation bone biopsy study of patients with CF showed increased osteoclastic and decreased osteoblastic activity.[55]

BMT

BMT is the treatment of choice for patients with certain hematological malignancies, the majority of whom will survive many years thereafter. Osteoporosis after allogeneic BMT has a complex pathogenesis that is related to effects of treatment and effects on the stromal cell compartment of the bone marrow.[2,56,57] Similar to solid organ transplantation, bone resorption increases while bone formation decreases,[15,57,58] resulting in early, rapid bone loss that is most severe at the proximal femur. Other differences relate to patients being younger, a short interval between diagnosis and BMT, and pre-transplantation factors. In addition to osteoporosis, osteomalacia and avascular necrosis occur.

Small cross-sectional studies have shown decreased FN and LS BMD in adults and children after allogeneic (allo) BMT. Up to 29% and 52% of survivors have T-scores < −1.0 at the LS and FN, respectively.[59] Osteoporosis is more common at proximal femur sites than at the spine. Patients who are younger than 18 years of age at the time of BMT may fail to acquire adequate bone mass, and low BMD in this population may also be related to smaller bone size.[60] Longitudinal studies[15,57,58,61] have shown rapid bone loss in the first 6–12 months after BMT that is greater at the proximal femur than the spine and total body (Table 2) and is highly variable (Fig. 1). Most studies suggest that little additional bone loss occurs after this time. Studies of long-term survivors of BMT have shown that losses from the proximal femur are not regained.[62]

The pathogenesis of BMT-related bone loss is quite complex. Contributing factors include cumulative GC exposure, whether given before BMT or for treatment of graft-versus

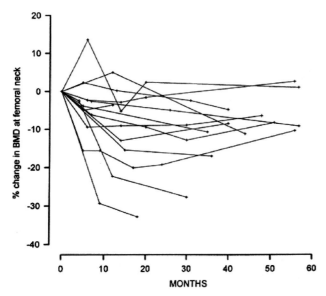

FIG. 1. Cumulative percentage changes in FN BMD in patients with three or more BMD measurements after allogeneic BMT.

host disease (GVHD). Bone loss has been related to duration of CsA exposure[61] and may also be a direct effect of GVHD itself on bone cells. Abnormal cellular or cytokine-mediated bone marrow function may affect bone turnover and BMD after BMT.[63] Both myeloablative treatment and BMT stimulate the early release of cytokines.[63] BMT also has adverse effects on bone marrow osteoprogenitors. Osteocyte viability is decreased after BMT,[64] and osteocytes are replaced by differentiation of host stromal cells.[65] Bone marrow stromal cells are damaged by high-dose chemotherapy, TBI, GCs, and CsA, reducing osteoblastic differentiation from osteoprogenitor cells. Colony forming units-fibroblasts are reduced for up to 12 years after BMT.[56,59] In this regard, high-dose chemotherapy is an important factor, irrespective of gonadal status.[56] Vitamin D deficiency is relatively common after BMT. Treatment with vitamin D improves BMD in patients with vitamin D deficiency and intestinal GVHD.[66,67] Avascular necrosis develops in 10–20% of allo-BMT survivors, a median of 12 months after BMT.[59,61] GC treatment of chronic GVHD is the most important risk factor.

MECHANISMS OF POST-TRANSPLANTATION BONE LOSS

The body of research published over the past decade into the natural history and pathogenesis of transplantation osteoporosis has yielded fairly consistent data that now enable us to develop a unifying hypothesis of the mechanisms of post-transplantation bone loss and fracture. It seems very clear that the mechanisms differ according to the amount of time that has elapsed since transplantation. There seem to be two main phases of bone loss (Fig. 2) that can best be differentiated by the presence (Fig. 2A) or absence (Fig. 2B) of high-dose GCs in the immunosuppressive regimen.

During the first 6 months after transplantation, GC doses are generally high enough to profoundly suppress bone

formation. Virtually every published study has found serum markers of bone formation, particularly osteocalcin, to be suppressed in the early post-transplant period. There are also consistent reports of increased urinary markers of bone resorption during the same time frame. This increase is probably caused by suppressive effects of GCs on osteoblast synthesis of OPG, on the hypothalamic-pituitary-gonadal axis, and on calcium transport across the intestinal, renal tubular, and parathyroid cell membranes. In addition, the well-known nephrotoxic effects of CsA and FK506 result in measurable declines in renal function and decreased synthesis of $1,25(OH)_2D_3$ that also inhibits calcium transport in the gut. Thus, both CIs and GCs have the potential to cause secondary increases in PTH secretion, which in turn increases osteoclast-mediated bone resorption. In addition, both CsA and FK506 may increase bone resorption directly. The concomitant administration of high dose GCs and CsA (or FK506) is therefore associated with uncoupling of resorption and formation. During this phase of the post-transplant period, there is rapid bone loss and high fracture rates.

As prednisone doses are tapered below 5 mg/day, osteoblast function recovers, and the suppressive effects on bone

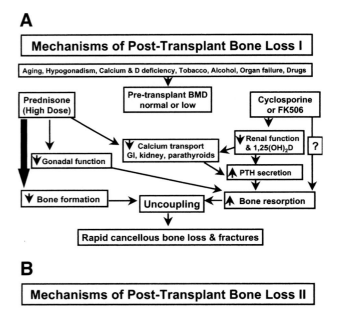

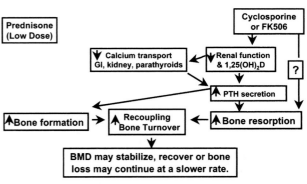

FIG. 2. (A) Mechanisms of bone loss in the early post-transplantation period. (B) Mechanisms of bone loss in the later post-transplantation period, after GC doses are tapered.

formation are reversed (Fig. 2B). However, adverse effects of CsA and FK506 remain—both direct effects on the skeleton and indirect effects mediated by renal toxicity of these drugs that result in SHPT. Thus, resorption remains elevated. With tapering of GCs, bone formation increases also, resulting in "recoupling" of bone turnover. Rates of bone loss slow, and there may even be some recovery, particularly at the spine. Whenever steroid doses are increased for treatment of rejection or stress, the pathophysiologic picture resembles the first phase.

PREVENTION AND MANAGEMENT OF OSTEOPOROSIS

Before Transplantation

Because of the high prevalence of osteoporosis, osteopenia, and abnormal bone and mineral metabolism in patients awaiting transplantation and the morbidity caused by osteoporosis after transplantation, it is our position that all candidates for organ transplantation would benefit from an evaluation of bone health. BMD of the hip and spine should be measured before transplantation, preferably at the time of acceptance to the waiting list. Spine radiographs should be performed to detect prevalent fractures. If BMD is low, an evaluation for secondary causes of osteoporosis should be undertaken, and if detected, should be treated specifically. All patients should receive the recommended daily allowance for calcium and vitamin D (1000–1500 mg of calcium and 400–800 IU of vitamin D). Patients with kidney failure should be evaluated and treated for renal osteodystrophy according to currently accepted standards.

Whether therapy for osteoporosis before transplantation reduces fracture risk after transplantation is presently unclear. Bisphosphonates, in particular, suppress bone resorption for up to 12 months after discontinuation of therapy. Transplantation with bisphosphonates already "on board," may prevent the increase in resorption that develops immediately after grafting and could theoretically mitigate post-transplant bone loss. Moreover, antiresorptive therapy clearly increases BMD and reduces fractures in other populations. Therefore, individuals awaiting lung, liver, and heart transplantation with osteoporosis or osteopenia should be evaluated and treated similarly to others with these conditions. The pretransplant waiting period is often long enough (1–2 years) to achieve significant improvements in BMD. The situation is clearly different and more complex in patients awaiting kidney transplantation. Because there are few published data on the use of antiresorptive drugs in patients with CKD, it is not possible to make general recommendations for these individuals. Furthermore, the use of bisphosphonates in patients with kidney disease may increase the incidence of low bone turnover and adynamic bone disease.

After Organ Transplantation

Virtually all studies have shown that bone loss is most rapid immediately after transplantation. Fractures may occur very early and affect patients with both low and normal pretransplant BMD. Therefore, we believe that most patients (even those with normal BMD) should have preven-

tive therapy instituted immediately after transplantation. In addition, there is an ever-enlarging population transplanted months or years before that have never been evaluated or treated for osteoporosis.

The majority of therapeutic trials have focused on the use of vitamin D metabolites and antiresorptive drugs, particularly bisphosphonates. In the discussions to follow, we will distinguish where possible between studies that focus on the early post-transplant period (prevention trials) and those that include mainly patients with established bone loss who are more than 6–12 months distant from transplantation and have thus passed the phase of most rapid demineralization (treatment trials).

Vitamin D and Analogs

Vitamin D metabolites may reduce post-transplantation bone loss by reversing GC-induced decreases in intestinal calcium absorption and by mitigating secondary HPT.[68] Theoretically, they could reduce GC exposure by virtue of their immunomodulatory effects.[68]

Parent vitamin D, in doses of 400-1000 IU, does not prevent significant post-transplantation bone loss. However, 25OHD (calcidiol) has been associated with significant increases in LS BMD during the 18 months after cardiac transplantation.[69,70] Calcidiol has also been shown to prevent ongoing bone loss in long-term cardiac transplant recipients.[69] $1,25(OH)_2D_3$ (calcitriol) has been studied in heart, lung, liver, and kidney transplant recipients. The results of these trials have been contradictory.

Sambrook et al. published a double-blind study of heart or lung transplant recipients randomly assigned to receive either placebo or calcitriol (0.5–0.75 μg/day) for either 12 or 24 months after transplantation.[71] LS bone loss at 2 years did not differ between groups, averaging 3.0% for those treated with calcium alone, 2.9% for those treated with calcitriol for 2 years, and 5.6% for those treated with calcitriol for the first year followed by calcium alone for the second year. FN bone loss at 24 months averaged 8.3% for those treated with calcium alone, 5.0% for those treated with calcitriol for 2 years, and 7.4% for those treated with calcitriol for the first year followed by calcium alone for the second year. Although fracture rates were lower in the calcitriol-treated subjects, this study lacked sufficient statistical power to be certain. A second study from this group compared rates of bone loss in patients randomized to receive calcitriol (0.5 μg/day) or two cycles of etidronate during the first 6 months after heart or lung transplantation and then followed for an additional 12 months.[72] The results were compared with historical controls transplanted approximately 5 years before. Significant and comparable bone loss (3–8%) occurred at the LS and FN in both treated groups. Although LS bone loss was less pronounced than in the reference group, lack of a concurrently transplanted population, although unavoidable, limits the ability to ascribe this to the intervention. Both studies suggest that rapid bone loss resumes in heart and lung transplant recipients after cessation of calcitriol.[71,72] Moreover, their results are in agreement with others who observed that cardiac transplant recipients randomized to either alphacalcidol or cyclic etidronate sustained considerable bone loss at the LS (alphacalcidol, 7.0%; etidronate, 10.3%) and FN (alphacalcidol, 5.6%; etidronate, 8.9%) during the first year after transplantation.[73] Other studies of calcitriol in long-term kidney[42] and heart transplant recipients,[74] have found no benefit of calcitriol for protection from early post-transplant bone loss. Hypercalcemia and hypercalciuria, common side effects of vitamin D metabolites, may develop at any point during treatment. Frequent monitoring of urine and serum is required. In our opinion, active vitamin D metabolites should not be selected as first-line treatment because of their limited effectiveness and narrow therapeutic window.

Bisphosphonates

Several studies[75–82] suggest that intravenous bisphosphonates prevent bone loss and fractures after transplantation. An open-label study of a single intravenous dose of pamidronate (60 mg) followed by four cycles of etidronate (400 mg every 3 months) and daily low-dose calcitriol (0.25 μg) prevented LS and FN bone loss and reduced fracture rates in heart transplant recipients compared with historical controls.[79] Repeated doses of intravenous pamidronate in heart,[76,83] kidney,[77] and lung[75,84] transplant recipients have been shown to prevent LS and FN bone loss. Bianda et al. reported LS and FN bone loss at 12 months after cardiac transplantation of only 1.9% and 1.4%, respectively, in patients who received a small dose of pamidronate (0.5 mg/kg every 3 months), while in patients randomized to nasal calcitonin (200 IU/day) plus calcitriol (0.25–0.5 μg/day), LS BMD fell by 7.4% and FN BMD by 6.3%.[76] Some have reported fracture reduction while others[75] have not. Recent randomized trials of the more potent intravenous bisphosphonate, ibandronate, in liver[80] and kidney[85] transplant recipients have also found a significant protective effect on BMD at 1 year. However, in a recent trial in which patients were randomized to receive either a single dose of intravenous pamidronate administered 1–3 months before liver transplantation or no treatment, LS BMD did not decline significantly in either group during the first post-transplant year, whereas FN BMD fell comparably and the incidence of new fractures was the same.[50]

Studies evaluating early prophylaxis with cyclic etidronate in heart and liver transplant recipients found no benefit. A more recent study found a protective effect of etidronate in lung and heart recipients compared with historical, untreated controls (although significant bone loss occurred in both groups).[72]

Alendronate has also been compared with calcitriol. In a small study ($N = 20$) of kidney transplant recipients, a regimen of alendronate (10 mg/day), calcium carbonate (2 g/day), and calcitriol (0.25 μg/day) was associated with a 6.3% increase in LS BMD in the first 6 months after transplantation compared with a decrease of 5.8% with calcium and calcitriol alone.[78] A 1-year trial comparing alendronate, calcitriol, and calcium to calcitriol and calcium treatment alone in 40 kidney transplant recipients in whom therapy was begun an average of 5 years after transplantation reported an increase of 5% at the LS and 4.5% at the FN in the alendronate-treated group[86]; BMD remained stable in the patients treated with calcitriol alone. In a 1-year trial, in which patients were randomized immediately after cardiac transplantation to receive either alendronate (10 mg/day) or calcitriol (0.25 μg bid), bone loss at the LS and hip was prevented by both regimens compared with control subjects who received only calcium and vitamin D.[81]

In our opinion, bisphosphonates are the most promising approach for the management of transplantation osteoporosis. However, controversies remain regarding optimal administration of bisphosphonates. These include whether continuous or intermittent therapy should be used, duration of therapy, the level of renal impairment at which bisphosphonates should be avoided, whether they are safe in kidney transplant recipients with adynamic bone disease, and their use after pediatric transplantation.

Calcitonin

Calcitonin is relatively ineffective in preventing bone loss after transplantation.

Hormone Replacement Therapy

Hormone replacement therapy (HRT) protects the skeleton in women treated with GCs, as well as in women receiving liver, lung, and bone marrow transplantation. Because amenorrhea is a common sequela of BMT in women, they should receive HRT whenever possible. In light of recent data suggesting increased rates of coronary events and stroke in postmenopausal women treated with estrogen and progesterone, the risks of this therapy would likely outweigh the benefits in most other types of organ transplantation.

In cardiac transplant recipients, testosterone falls immediately after transplantation and normalizes 6–12 months later. In a recent study evaluating male cardiac transplant recipients treated with intravenous ibandronate, hypogonadal men who received testosterone supplementation showed an improved BMD response at 1 year compared with hypogonadal men who did not receive testosterone.[87] It is not known whether treatment with testosterone in men prevents bone loss after BMT. In general, testosterone replacement should be reserved for men with true hypogonadism. Potential risks of testosterone therapy, such as prostatic hypertrophy, hyperlipidemia, and abnormal liver enzymes, may have particular relevance for this population.

SUMMARY AND CONCLUSIONS

Pre-transplantation bone disease and post-transplantation immunosuppressive regimens combining high doses of GCs (e.g., prednisone at >10 mg/day) and CIs (CsA or FK506) interact to produce a particularly severe form of osteoporosis characterized by rapid bone loss and increased fracture rates. Early rapid bone loss occurs in the setting of uncoupled bone turnover with many studies documenting increased bone resorption and decreased bone formation. Management of these patients should combine assessment and treatment of pre-transplantation bone disease with preventive therapy in the immediate post-transplantation period, because most bone loss occurs in the first months after grafting. In addition, bone mass measurement and therapy of osteoporosis in the long-term organ transplant recipient should be addressed. There are no pre-transplantation variables that reliably predict post-transplantation bone loss and fracture in the individual patient. Therefore, all organ transplant recipients should be considered at risk for post-transplantation bone loss and fractures. Although newer studies suggest that rates of bone loss and fracture may be lower in more recently transplanted patients, morbidity from transplantation osteoporosis remains unacceptably high. Data from clinical trials suggest that bisphosphonates are the safest and most promising agents for the prevention and treatment of post-transplantation osteoporosis.

REFERENCES

1. Shane E 2003 Transplantation osteoporosis. In: Orwoll E, Bliziotes M (eds.) Osteoporosis: Pathophysiology and Clinical Management. Humana Press, Totowa, NJ, USA, pp. 537–567.
2. Shane E, Epstein S 2001 Transplantation osteoporosis. Transplant Rev (Orlando) 15:11–32.
3. Epstein S, Shane E 2001 Transplantation osteoporosis. In: Marcus R, Feldman D, Kelsey J (eds.) Osteoporosis, vol. 2. Academic Press, San Diego, CA, USA, pp. 327–340.
4. Cohen A, Shane E 2001 Transplantation osteoporosis. Curr Opin Endocrinol Diabetes 8:283–290.
5. Cohen A, Shane E 2003 Osteoporosis after solid organ and bone marrow transplantation. Osteoporos Int (in press).
6. Stehman-Breen CO, Sherrard DJ, Alem AM, Gillen DL, Heckbert SR, Wong CS, Ball A, Weiss NS 2000 Risk factors for hip fracture among patients with end-stage renal disease. Kidney Int 58:2200–2205.
7. Alem AM, Sherrard DJ, Gillen DL, Weiss NS, Beresford SA, Heckbert SR, Wong C, Stehman-Breen C 2000 Increased risk of hip fracture among patients with end-stage renal disease. Kidney Int 58:396–399.
8. Ball AM, Gillen DL, Sherrard D, Weiss NS, Emerson SS, Seliger SL, Kestenbaum BR, Stehman-Breen C 2002 Risk of hip fracture among dialysis and renal transplant recipients. JAMA 288:3014–3018.
9. Shane E, Mancini D, Aaronson K, Silverberg SJ, Seibel MJ, Addesso V, McMahon DJ 1997 Bone mass, vitamin D deficiency and hyperparathyroidism in congestive heart failure. Am J Med 103:197–207.
10. Monegal A, Navasa M, Guanabens N, Peris P, Pons F, Martinez de Osaba MJ, Ordi J, Rimola A, Rodes J, Munoz-Gomez J 2001 Bone disease after liver transplantation: A long-term prospective study of bone mass changes, hormonal status and histomorphometric characteristics. Osteoporos Int 12:484–492.
11. Ninkovic M, Love SA, Tom B, Alexander GJ, Compston JE 2001 High prevalence of osteoporosis in patients with chronic liver disease prior to liver transplantation. Calcif Tissue Int 69:321–326.
12. Tschopp O, Boehler A, Speich R, Weder W, Seifert B, Russi EW, Schmid C 2002 Osteoporosis before lung transplantation: Association with low body mass index, but not with underlying disease. Am J Transplant 2:167–172.
13. Keilholz U, Max R, Scheibenbogen C, Wuster C, Korbling M, Haas R 1997 Endocrine function and bone metabolism 5 years after autologous bone marrow/blood-derived progenitor cell transplantation. Cancer 79:1617–1622.
14. Tauchmanova L, Selleri C, Rosa GD, Pagano L, Orio F, Lombardi G, Rotoli B, Colao A 2002 High prevalence of endocrine dysfunction in long-term survivors after allogeneic bone marrow transplantation for hematologic diseases. Cancer 95:1076–1084.
15. Valimaki M, Kinnunen K, Volin L, Tahtela R, Loyttniemi E, Laitinen K, Makela P, Keto P, Ruutu T 1999 A prospective study of bone loss and turnover after allogeneic bone marrow transplantation: Effect of calcium supplementation with or without calcitonin. Bone Marrow Transplant 23:355–361.
16. Couto-Silva AC, Trivin C, Esperou H, Michon J, Fischer A, Brauner R 2000 Changes in height, weight and plasma leptin after bone marrow transplantation. Bone Marrow Transplant 26:1205–1210.
17. Schulte C, Beelen D, Schaefer U, Mann K 2000 Bone loss in long-term survivors after transplantation of hematopoietic stem cells: A prospective study. Osteoporos Int 11:344–353.
18. Rubin MR, Bilezikian JP 2002 Clinical review 151: The role of parathyroid hormone in the pathogenesis of glucocorticoid-induced osteoporosis. A re-examination of the evidence. J Clin Endocrinol Metab 87:4033–4041.
19. Epstein S 1996 Post-transplantation bone disease: The role of immunosuppressive agents on the skeleton. J Bone Miner Res 11:1–7.
20. Bowman AR, Sass DA, Dissanayake IR, Ma YF, Liang H, Yuan Z, Jee WS, Epstein S 1997 The role of testosterone in cyclosporine-induced osteopenia. J Bone Miner Res 12:607–615.
21. Epstein S, Dissanayake A, Goodman GR, Bowman A, Zhou H, Ma Y, Jee WS 2001 Effect of the interaction of parathyroid hormone and cyclosporine A on bone mineral metabolism in the rat. Calcif Tissue Int 68:240–247.
22. Awumey E, Moonga B, Sodam B, Koval A, Adebanjo O, Kumegawa M, Zaide M, Epstein S 1999 Molecular and functional evidence for calcineurin alpha and beta isoforms in the osteoclasts. Novel insights into the mode of action of cyclosporine A. Biochem Biophys Res Commun 254:148–252.
23. Buchinsky F, Ma Y, Mann G, Rucinski B, Bryer H, Romero D, Jee W, Epstein S 1996 T lymphocytes play a critical role in the development of cyclosporine induced osteopenia. Endocrinology 137:2278–2285.
24. Ponticelli C, Aroldi A 2001 Osteoporosis after organ transplantation. Lancet 357:1623.
25. Grotz W, Mundinger A, Gugel B, Exner V, Reichelt A, Schollmeyer P 1994 Missing impact of cyclosporine on osteoporosis in renal transplant recipients. Transplant Proc 26:2652–2653.
26. McIntyre HD, Menzies B, Rigby R, Perry-Keene DA, Hawley CM, Hardie IR 1995 Long-term bone loss after renal transplantation: Comparison of immunosuppressive regimens. Clin Transpl 9:20–24.
27. Stempfle HU, Werner C, Echtler S, Assum T, Meiser B, Angermann CE, Theisen K, Gartner R 1998 Rapid trabecular bone loss after cardiac transplantation using FK506 (tacrolimus)-based immunosuppression. Transplant Proc 30:1132–1133.
28. Park KM, Hay JE, Lee SG, Lee YJ, Wiesner RH, Porayko MK, Krom RA 1996 Bone loss after orthotopic liver transplantation: FK 506 versus cyclosporine. Transplant Proc 28:1738–1740.
29. Goffin E, Devogelaer JP, Depresseux G, Squifflet JP, Pirson Y 2001 Osteoporosis after organ transplantation. Lancet 357:1623.
30. Monegal A, Navasa M, Guanabens N, Peris P, Pons F, Martinez de Osaba MJ, Rimola A, Rodes J, Munoz-Gomez J 2001 Bone mass and mineral metabolism in liver transplant patients treated with FK506 or cyclosporine A. Calcif Tissue Int 68:83–86.
31. Julian BA, Laskow DA, Dubovsky J, Dubovsky EV, Curtis JJ, Quarles LD 1991 Rapid loss of vertebral bone density after renal transplantation. N Engl J Med 325:544–550.
32. Monier-Faugere M, Mawad H, Qi Q, Friedler R, Malluche HH 2000 High prevalence of low bone turnover and occurrence of osteomalacia after kidney transplantation. J Am Soc Nephrol 11:1093–1099.
33. Horber FF, Casez JP, Steiger U, Czerniack A, Montandon A, Jaeger PH 1994 Changes in bone mass early after kidney transplantation. J Bone Miner Res 9:1–9.
34. Almond MK, Kwan JTC, Evans K, Cunningham J 1994 Loss of regional bone mineral density in the first 12 months following renal transplantation. Nephron 66:52–57.
35. Masse M, Girardin C, Ouimet D, Dandavino R, Boucher A, Madore F, Hebert MJ, Leblanc M, Pichette V 2001 Initial bone loss in kidney transplant recipients: A prospective study. Transplant Proc 33:1211.
36. Cruz DN, Wysolmerski JJ, Brickel HM, Gundberg CG, Simpson CA, Mitnick MA, Kliger AS, Lorber MI, Basadonna GP, Friedman AL, Insogna KL, Bia MJ 2001 Parameters of high bone-turnover predict bone loss in renal transplant patients: A longitudinal study. Transplantation 72:83–88.
37. Farmer CKT, Hampson G, Vaja S, Abbs IC, Hilton RM, Koffman G, Watkins J, Sacks SH, Fogelman I 2002 Late low dose steroid withdrawal in renal transplant recipients increases bone formation and bone mineral density without altering renal function: A randomized controlled trial. J Bone Miner Res 17:S1;S158.
38. Pichette V, Bonnardeaux A, Prudhomme L, Gagne M, Cardinal J, Ouimet D 1996 Long-term bone loss in kidney transplant recipients: A cross-sectional and longitudinal study. Am J Kidney Dis 28:105–114.
39. Hurst G, Alloway R, Hathaway D, Somerville T, Hughes T, Gaber A 1998 Stabilization of bone mass after renal transplant with preemptive care. Transplant Proc 30:1327–1328.
40. Moreno A, Torregrosa JV, Pons F, Campistol JM, Martinez de Osaba MJ, Oppenheimer F 1999 Bone mineral density after renal transplantation: Long-term follow-up. Transplant Proc 31:2322–2323.
41. Nowacka-Cieciura E, Durlik M, Cieciura T, Lewandowska D, Baczkowska T, Kukula K, Lao M, Szmidt J, Rowinski W 2002 Steroid withdrawal after renal transplantation–risks and benefits. Transplant Proc 34:560–563.
42. Cueto-Manzano AM, Konel S, Freemont AJ, Adams JE, Mawer B, Gokal R, Hutchison AJ 2000 Effect of 1,25-dihydroxyvitamin D3 and calcium carbonate on bone loss associated with long-term renal transplantation. Am J Kidney Dis 35:227–236.

43. Grotz W, Rump AL, Niessen H, Schmidt-Gayt A, Reichelt G, Kirste G, Olchewski G, Schollmeyer P 1998 Treatment of osteopenia and osteoporosis after kidney transplantation. Transplantation **66**:1004–1008.

44. Brandenburg VM, Ketteler M, Fassbender WJ, Heussen N, Freuding T, Floege J, Ittel TH 2002 Development of lumbar bone mineral density in the late course after kidney transplantation. Am J Kidney Dis **40**:1066–1074.

45. Ramsey-Goldman R, Dunn JE, Dunlop DD, Stuart FP, Abecassis MM, Kaufman DB, Langman CB, Salinger MH, Sprague SM 1999 Increased risk of fracture in patients receiving solid organ transplants. J Bone Miner Res **14**:456–463.

46. Smets YF, van der Pijl JW, de Fijter JW, Ringers J, Lemkes HH, Hamdy NA 1998 Low bone mass and high incidence of fractures after successful simultaneous pancreas-kidney transplantation. Nephrol Dial Transplant **13**:1250–1255.

47. Chiu MY, Sprague SM, Bruce DS, Woodle ES, Thistlethwaite JR Jr, Josephson MA 1998 Analysis of fracture prevalence in kidney-pancreas allograft recipients. J Am Soc Nephrol **9**:677–683.

48. Shane E, Rivas M, Staron RB, Silverberg SJ, Seibel M, Kuiper J, Mancini D, Addesso V, Michler RE, Factor-Litvak P 1996 Fracture after cardiac transplantation: A prospective longitudinal study. J Clin Endocrinol Metab **81**:1740–1746.

49. Leidig-Bruckner G, Hosch S, Dodidou P, Ritchel D, Conradt C, Klose C, Otto G, Lange R, Theilmann L, Zimmerman H, Pritsch M, Zeigler R 2001 Frequency and predictors of osteoporotic fractures after cardiac or liver transplantation: A follow-up study. Lancet **357**:342–347.

50. Ninkovic M, Love S, Tom BD, Bearcroft PW, Alexander GJ, Compston JE 2002 Lack of effect of intravenous pamidronate on fracture incidence and bone mineral density after orthotopic liver transplantation. J Hepatol **37**:93–100.

51. Floreani A, Mega A, Tizian L, Burra P, Boccagni P, Baldo V, Fagiuoli S, Naccarato R, Luisetto G 2001 Bone metabolism and gonad function in male patients undergoing liver transplantation: A two-year longitudinal study. Osteoporos Int **12**:749–754.

52. Ninkovic M, Skingle SJ, Bearcroft PW, Bishop N, Alexander GJ, Compston JE 2000 Incidence of vertebral fractures in the first three months after orthotopic liver transplantation. Eur J Gastroenterol Hepatol **12**:931–935.

53. Spira A, Gutierrez C, Chaparro C, Hutcheon MA, Chan CK 2000 Osteoporosis and lung transplantation: A prospective study. Chest **117**:476–481.

54. Shane E, Papadopoulos A, Staron RB, Addesso V, Donovan D, McGregor C, Schulman LL 1999 Bone loss and fracture after lung transplantation. Transplantation **68**:220–227.

55. Haworth CS, Webb AK, Egan JJ, Selby PL, Hasleton PS, Bishop PW, Freemont TJ 2000 Bone histomorphometry in adult patients with cystic fibrosis. Chest **118**:434–439.

56. Banfi A, Podesta M, Fazzuoli L, Sertoli MR, Venturini M, Santini G, Cancedda R, Quarto R 2001 High-dose chemotherapy shows a dose-dependent toxicity to bone marrow osteoprogenitors: A mechanism for post-bone marrow transplantation osteopenia. Cancer **92**:2419–2428.

57. Lee WY, Cho SW, Oh ES, Oh KW, Lee JM, Yoon KH, Kang MI, Cha BY, Lee KW, Son HY, Kang SK, Kim CC 2002 The effect of bone marrow transplantation on the osteoblastic differentiation of human bone marrow stromal cells. J Clin Endocrinol Metab **87**:329–335.

58. Kang MI, Lee WY, Oh KW, Han JH, Song KH, Cha BY, Lee KW, Son HY, Kang SK, Kim CC 2000 The short-term changes of bone mineral metabolism following bone marrow transplantation. Bone **26**:275–279.

59. Tauchmanova L, Serio B, Del Puente A, Risitano AM, Esposito A, De Rosa G, Lombardi G, Colao A, Rotoli B, Selleri C 2002 Long-lasting bone damage detected by dual-energy x-ray absorptiometry, phalangeal osteosonogrammetry, and in vitro growth of marrow stromal cells after allogeneic stem cell transplantation. J Clin Endocrinol Metab **87**:5058–5065.

60. Nysom K, Holm K, Michaelsen KF, Hertz H, Jacobsen N, Muller J, Molgaard C 2000 Bone mass after allogeneic BMT for childhood leukaemia or lymphoma. Bone Marrow Transplant **25**:191–196.

61. Ebeling P, Thomas D, Erbas B, Hopper L, Szer J, Grigg A 1999 Mechanism of bone loss following allogeneic and autologous hematopoeitic stem cell transplantation. J Bone Miner Res **14**:342–350.

62. Lee WY, Kang MI, Baek KH, Oh ES, Oh KW, Lee KW, Kim SW, Kim CC 2002 The skeletal site-differential changes in bone mineral density following bone marrow transplantation: 3-year prospective study. J Korean Med Sci **17**:749–754.

63. Lee WY, Kang MI, Oh ES, Oh KW, Han JH, Cha BY, Lee KW, Son HY, Kang SK, Kim CC 2002 The role of cytokines in the changes in bone turnover following bone marrow transplantation. Osteoporos Int **13**:62–68.

64. Michelson JD, Gornet M, Codd T, Torres J, Lanighan K, Jones R 1993 Bone morphology after bone marrow transplantation for Hodgkin's and non- Hodgkin's lymphoma. Exp Hematol **21**:475–482.

65. Athanasou NA, Quinn J, Brenner MK, Prentice HG, Graham A, Taylor S, Flannery D, McGee JO 1990 Origin of marrow stromal cells and haemopoietic chimaerism following bone marrow transplantation determined by in situ hybridisation. Br J Cancer **61**:385–389.

66. Arekat MR, And G, Lemke S, Moses AM 2002 Dramatic improvement of BMD following vitamin D therapy in a bone marrow transplant recipient. J Clin Densitom **5**:267–271.

67. Hattori M, Morita N, Tsujino Y, Yamamoto M, Tanizawa T 2001 Vitamins D and K in the treatment of osteoporosis secondary to graft-versus-host disease following bone-marrow transplantation. J Intern Med Res **29**:381–384.

68. Sambrook P 1999 Alfacalcidol and calcitriol in the prevention of bone loss after organ transplantation. Calcif Tissue Int **65**:341–343.

69. Meys E, Terreaux-Duvert F, Beaume-Six T, Dureau G, Meunier PJ 1993 Effects of calcium, calcidiol, and monofluorophosphate on lumbar bone mass and parathyroid function in patients after cardiac transplantation. Osteoporos Int **3**:329–332.

70. Garcia-Delgado I, Prieto S, Fragnas LG, Robles E, Rufilanchas T, Hawkins F 1997 Calcitonin, editronate and calcidiol treatment in bone loss after cardiac transplantation. Calcif Tissue Int **60**:155–159.

71. Sambrook P, Henderson NK, Keogh A, MacDonald P, Glanville A, Spratt P, Bergin P, Ebeling P, Eisman J 2000 Effect of calcitriol on bone loss after cardiac or lung transplantation. J Bone Miner Res **15**:1818–1824.

72. Henderson K, Eisman J, Keogh A, MacDonald P, Glanville A, Spratt P, Sambrook P 2001 Protective effect of short-tem calcitriol or cyclical etidronate on bone loss after cardiac or lung transplantation. J Bone Miner Res **16**:565–571.

73. Van Cleemput J, Daenen W, Geusens P, Dequeker P, Van De Werf F, VanHaecke J 1996 Prevention of bone loss in cardiac transplant recipients. A comparison of biphosphonates and vitamin D. Transplantation **61**:1495–1499.

74. Stempfle HU, Werner C, Echtler S, Wehr U, Rambeck WA, Siebert U, Uberfuhr P, Angermann CE, Theisen K, Gartner R 1999 Prevention of osteoporosis after cardiac transplantation: A prospective, longitudinal, randomized, double-blind trial with calcitriol. Transplantation **68**:523–530.

75. Aris RM, Lester GE, Renner JB, Winders A, Blackwood AD, Lark RK, Ontjes DA 2000 Efficacy of pamidronate for osteoporosis in cystic fibrosis patients following lung transplantation. Am J Respir Crit Care Med **162**:941–946.

76. Bianda T, Linka A, Junga G, Brunner H, Steinert H, Kiowski W, Schmid C 2000 Prevention of osteoporosis in heart transplant recipients: A comparison of calcitriol with calcitonin and pamidronate. Calcif Tissue Int **67**:116–121.

77. Fan S, Almond MK, Ball E, Evans K, Cunningham J 2000 Pamidronate therapy as prevention of bone loss following renal transplantation. Kidney Int **57**:684–690.

78. Kovac D, Lindic J, Kandus A, Bren AF 2001 Prevention of bone loss in kidney graft recipients. Transplant Proc **33**:1144–1145.

79. Shane E, Rodino MA, McMahon DJ, Addesso V, Staron RB, Seibel MJ, Mancini D, Michler RE, Lo SH 1998 Prevention of bone loss after heart transplantation with antiresorptive therapy: A pilot study. J Heart Lung Transplant **17**:1089–1096.

80. Hommann M, Abendroth K, Lehmann G, Patzer N, Kornberg A, Voigt R, Seifert S, Hein G, Scheele J 2002 Effect of transplantation on bone: Osteoporosis after liver and multivisceral transplantation. Transplant Proc **34**:2296–2298.

81. Shane E, Addesso V, Namerow P, Maybaum S, Staron R, Lo S, Zucker M, Pardi S, Mancini D 2002 Prevention of bone loss after cardiac transplantation with alendronate or calcitriol: Efficacy and safety. J Bone Miner Res **17**:S1;S135.

82. Arlen DJ, Lambert K, Ioannidis G, Adachi JD 2001 Treatment of established bone loss after renal transplantation with etidronate. Transplantation **71**:669–673.

83. Krieg M, Seydoux C, Sandini L, Goy JJ, Berguer DG, Thiebaud D, Bruckhardt P 2001 Intravenous pamidronate as a treatment for osteoporosis after heart transplantation: A prospective study. Osteoporos Int **12**:112–116.

84. Trombetti A, Gerbase MW, Spiliopoulos A, Slosman DO, Nicod LP, Rizzoli R 2000 Bone mineral density in lung-transplant recipients before and after graft: Prevention of lumbar spine post-transplantation-

accelerated bone loss by pamidronate. J Heart Lung Transplant **19:** 736–743.

85. Grotz W, Nagel C, Poeschel D, Cybulla M, Petersen KG, Uhl M, Strey C, Kirste G, Olschewski M, Reichelt A, Rump LC 2001 Effect of ibandronate on bone loss and renal function after kidney transplantation. J Am Soc Nephrol **12:**1530–1537.

86. Giannini S, Dangel A, Carraro G, Nobile M, Rigotti P, Bonfante L, Marchini F, Zaninotto M, Dalle Carbonare L, Sartori L, Crepaldi G

2001 Alendronate prevents further bone loss in renal transplant recipients. J Bone Miner Res **16:**2111–2117.

87. Fahrleitner A, Prenner G, Tscheliessnigg KH, Leb G, Piswanger-Solkner CJ, Obermayer-Pietsch B, Dimai HP, Dobnig H 2002 Testosterone supplementation has additional benefits on bone metabolism in cardiac transplant recipients receiving intravenous bisphosphonate treatment: A prospective study. J Bone Miner Res **17:**S1;S388.

Chapter 64. Osteoporosis and Rheumatic Diseases

Steven R. Goldring

Department of Medicine, Beth Israel Deaconess Medical Center, Harvard Medical School and New England Baptist Bone and Joint Institute, Harvard Institutes of Medicine, Boston, Massachusetts

INTRODUCTION

The rheumatic diseases include a diverse group of disorders that share in common their propensity to affect articular structures. The most commonly involved joints are the so-called diarthrodial joints that consist of two articulating surfaces lined by hyaline cartilage. Arthritic processes most often affect the cartilage surfaces and the synovial lining but may also involve the subchondral bone and joint capsule. Amphiarthroses that are characterized by fibrocartilaginous union (e.g., the intervertebral discs) are also frequently affected in rheumatic disorders.

Osteoarthritis is a prototypical example of a rheumatic disease in which the pathological events are restricted almost entirely to the joint structures. Many of the rheumatic diseases, however, may affect extra-articular organ systems, and these conditions are often accompanied by significant systemic symptoms that may dominate the clinical picture. These illnesses, which include, for example, conditions such as rheumatoid arthritis (RA), systemic lupus erythematosus (SLE), and the spondyloarthropathies, are believed to be initiated by disturbances in immune regulation that involve complex interactions between unique host genetic susceptibility and specific environmental factor(s). In these disorders, skeletal tissues may be involved not only at juxta-articular and subchondral sites, but in addition, there is evidence that many of these conditions may produce generalized effects on bone remodeling that affect the entire skeleton.

Among the rheumatic disorders, RA represents an excellent model for gaining insights into the effects of local as well as systemic consequences of inflammatory processes on skeletal tissue remodeling. Three principal forms of bone disease have been described in RA. The first is characterized by a focal process that affects the bone at the joint margins adjacent to the inflammatory synovial lesion. In RA, the synovial lining of diarthrodial joints is the target of an intense immunologic and inflammatory process that is associated with the proliferation of the synovial lining cells and infiltration of the tissue by inflammatory cells, including lymphocytes, plasma cells, and activated macrophages. The proliferative synovial tissue (pannus) attaches to the immediately adjacent bone at the joint margins and induces a progressive focal osteolytic process that gives rise to the characteristic cystic bone "erosions," which can be detected radiographically.[1,2] Recent studies employing magnetic resonance imaging have shown that these erosions occur very early in the course of the disease and progress throughout the illness unless therapeutic interventions are used.[3,4]

Examination of the interface between the pannus and bone at the sites of erosions reveals the presence of resorption lacunae populated by multinucleated cells expressing the full repertoire of authentic osteoclasts, including the expression of TRACP, cathepsin K, and the calcitonin receptor.[5-11] Several groups have demonstrated that cells cultured from synovial tissues from RA patients or animal models of inflammatory arthritis can be induced to form osteoclasts, suggesting that the osteoclast-like cells at the bone-pannus interface are derived from precursors present within the inflamed synovial tissues.[9-14] Further evidence implicating osteoclasts in the pathogenesis of focal joint erosions is provided by two recent studies in which inflammatory arthritis was induced in animals lacking the ability to form osteoclasts. In the studies by Pettit et al.,[15] receptor activator of NF-$\kappa\beta$ ligand knock-out mice were used, and in the studies by Redlich et al., animals lacking the c-*fos* gene were used.[16] In both models, there was minimal evidence of focal bone erosions despite extensive pannus formation and cartilage destruction. These observations provide further evidence that osteoclasts represent the final common cellular pathway for bone resorption in inflammatory joint disease.

The unique propensity of the inflamed synovium in RA to induce bone resorption is likely related to its capacity to produce a variety of factors with potent osteoclast differentiation and activation activity, including RANKL, interleukin (IL)-1α and -β, IL-6, IL-11, IL-15, IL-17, monocyte colony-stimulating factor, TNF-α, and parathyroid hormone–related peptide, the factor implicated in the pathogenesis of humoral hypercalcemia of malignancy.[10,17-26] Particular attention has focused on RANKL because of its potent osteoclastogenic activity. In several different animal models of inflammatory arthritis, treatment with osteopro-

The author has no conflict of interest.

tegerin (the soluble receptor that inhibits its activity) results in marked suppression of bone erosions.[16,22,27]

A second form of bone disease observed in patients with RA is the presence of juxtaarticular osteopenia adjacent to inflamed joints. Histological examination of this bone tissue reveals the presence of frequent osteoclasts and increased osteoid and resorptive surfaces consistent with increased bone turnover.[5,28] Local aggregates of inflammatory cells, including macrophages and lymphocytes, are often detected in the marrow space. It has been suggested that these cells are derived from the synovial lining and that they migrate into the marrow where they release local products that affect bone remodeling.[5] Decreased joint motion and immobilization in response to the joint inflammation likely represent additional contributing factors to this local bone loss.

The third form of bone disease associated with RA is the presence of generalized axial and appendicular osteopenia at sites that are distant from inflamed joints.[29-31] Although there are conflicting data concerning the effects of RA on skeletal mass, the presence of a generalized reduction in bone mass has been confirmed using multiple different techniques, and there is compelling evidence that this reduction is associated with an increased risk of hip and vertebral fracture.[32-36] The conflicting data are in part related to the fact that most observations have been based on cross-sectional studies and have focused on patients late in the evolution of their disease when factors such as disability, corticosteroid, and other treatments may confound the analyses. Histomorphometric analysis of bone biopsy specimens from patients with RA indicate that, in the absence of corticosteroid use, the cellular basis of the generalized reduction in bone mass is related to a decrease in bone formation rather than an increase in bone resorption.[37-39] However, these conclusions differ from the results of more recent studies in which biochemical markers of bone turnover have been used to evaluate patients with RA, and these studies indicate that there is increased bone-resorbing activity. Higher rates of bone resorption were associated with more severe disease activity, especially in patients receiving chronic corticosteroids.[40-44]

Several factors have emerged as important determinants of bone mass in patients with RA, and these include age and menopausal status, reduced mobility, disease activity, the influence of antirheumatic therapy (especially corticosteroids), and disease duration.[42,45-53] A large longitudinal prospective study by Gough et al.[45] concluded that significant amounts of generalized skeletal bone was lost early in RA and that this loss was associated with disease activity. These findings support the previous observations of Als et al.,[54] who also noted a significant decrease in bone mass during the early phases of RA.

There is still considerable controversy regarding the effects of corticosteroids in affecting the progression of bone loss in RA. In part, this is related to the tendency to use these medications in patients with more severe disease. Some authors suggest that if steroids satisfactorily suppress inflammation and maintain mobility, their deleterious effects may be outweighed.[45,46] Results from the recent COBRA trial, in which high-dose prednisolone was used as a component of an induction therapy protocol associated with disease-modifying agents, indicate that glucocorticoids

may contribute to a reduced tendency to develop focal bone erosions.[44,55] Interestingly, patients enrolled in this protocol developed transient bone loss in the lumbar spine that may have been related to the effects of glucocorticoids on reducing bone formation. Presently, it is premature, however, to generally advocate the use of corticosteroids in patients with RA because there is considerable evidence that their chronic use is associated with many potentially serious extraskeletal complications.[56] This cautionary note is supported by the findings of Saag et al.,[32] who noted that low-dose long-term prednisone use, equal to or greater than 5 g/day, was correlated in a dose-dependent fashion with the development of several adverse reactions, including fracture.

Although not associated with focal bone erosions, generalized bone loss is also a significant clinical problem in patients with SLE. Reductions in both cortical as well as trabecular bone mass have been reported, even in the absence of corticosteroid treatment.[57-60] As in patients with RA, the effects of systemic inflammation, decreased physical activity, nutritional factors, sex steroid influences, and drug treatments all likely contribute to the adverse effects on generalized bone mass. Similar factors contribute to the reduced bone mass, delayed skeletal linear growth, and increased incidence of fractures in patients with a history of juvenile chronic (rheumatoid) arthritis.[61-63]

Ankylosing spondylitis is characterized by inflammation at the entheses in the spine and peripheral skeleton. Although local bone erosions may be detected early in the course of the disease, new bone formation and ankylosis of the spine eventually develop in many patients. Several studies have documented an increased incidence of spinal compression fractures in patients with this disorder.[64-67] Because of the chronic back pain experienced by many patients with ankylosing spondylitis and the high incidence of paraspinal calcifications and syndesmophytes, many of these fractures are not detected. The decrease in axial bone density has been attributed to the effects of immobilization of the spine associated with the progressive ankylosis, although systemic inflammation, as in RA, may also be a contributing factor.[68,69]

In contrast to the observations in individuals with inflammatory arthropathies, several authors have suggested that there is a reduced frequency of osteoporosis in patients with osteoarthritis.[70-75] Hart et al.[76] examined the relationship between osteoarthritis of the hand, knee, and spine and bone density using DXA of the spine and femoral neck. Their results suggest that the two conditions are inversely related. Adjustments for age, physical activity, and obesity, as well as smoking and hormone replacement therapy, did not affect results. The mechanisms that account for this observed relationship are not clearly defined.

REFERENCES

1. Goldring SR, Gravallese EM 2000 Mechanisms of bone loss in inflammatory arthritis: Diagnosis and therapeutic implications. Arthritis Res **2**:33–37.
2. Gravallese EM, Goldring SR 2000 Cellular mechanisms and the role of cytokines in bone erosions in rheumatoid arthritis. Arthritis Rheum **43**:2143–2151.
3. McGonagle D, Conaghan PG, O'Connor P, Gibbon W, Green M,

Wakefield R, Ridgway J, Emery P 1999 The relationship between synovitis and bone changes in early untreated rheumatoid arthritis; a controlled magnetic resonance imaging study. Arthritis Rheum **42:** 1706–1711.

4. Conaghan PG, O'Connor P, McGonagle D, Astin P, Wakefield RJ, Gibbon WW, Quinn M, Karim Z, Green MJ, Proudman S, Issacs J, Emery P 2003 Elucidation of the relationship between synovitis and bone damage: A randomized magnetic resonance imaging study of individual patients with early rheumatoid arthritis. Arthritis Rheum **48:**64–71.

5. Bromley M, Woolley DE 1984 Histopathology of the rheumatoid lesion: Identification of cell types at sites of cartilage erosion. Arthritis Rheum **27:**857–863.

6. Gravallese EM, Harada Y, Wang JT, Gorn AH, Thornhill TS, Goldring SR 1998 Identification of cell types responsible for bone resorption in rheumatoid arthritis and juvenile rheumatoid arthritis. Am J Pathol **152:**943–951.

7. Haynes DR, Crotti TN, Loric M, Bain GI, Atkins GJ, Findlay DM 2001 Osteoprotegerin and receptor activator of nuclear factor kappaB ligand (RANKL) regulate osteoclast formation by cells in the human rheumatoid arthritic joint. Rheumatology (Oxford) **40:**623–630.

8. Leisen JCC, Duncan H, Riddle JM, Pitchford WC 1988 The erosive front: A topographic study of the junction between the pannus and the subchondral plate in the macerated rheumatoid metacarpal head. J Rheumatol **15:**17–22.

9. Kuratani T, Nagata K, Kukita T, Hotokebuchi T, Nakasima A, Iijima T 1998 Induction of abundant osteoclast-like multinucleated giant cells in adjuvant arthritic rats with accompanying disordered high bone turnover. Histol Histopathol **13:**751–759.

10. Romas E, Bakharevski O, Hards DK, Kartsogiannis V, Quinn JMW, Ryan PFJ, Martin J, Gillespie MT 2000 Expression of osteoclast differentiation factor at sites of bone erosion in collagen-induced arthritis. Arthritis Rheum **43:**821–826.

11. Suzuki Y, Nishikaku F, Nakatuka M, Koga Y 1998 Osteoclast-like cells in murine collagen induced arthritis. J Rheumatol **25:**1154–1160.

12. Suzuki Y, Tsutsumi Y, Nakagawa M, Suzuki H, Matsushita K, Beppu M, Aoki H, Ichikawa Y, Mizushima Y 2001 Osteoclast-like cells in an in vitro model of bone destruction by rheumatoid synovium. Rheumatology (Oxford) **40:**673–682.

13. Chang JS, Quinn JM, Demaziere A, Bulstrode CJ, Francis MJ, Duthie RB, Athanasou NA 1992 Bone resorption by cells isolated from rheumatoid synovium. Ann Rheum Dis **51:**1223–1229.

14. Fujikawa Y, Shingu M, Torisu T, Itonaga I, Masumi S 1996 Bone resorption by tartrate-resistant acid phosphatase-positive multinuclear cells isolated from rheumatoid synovium. Br J Rheumatol **35:**213–217.

15. Pettit AR, Ji H, von Stechow D, Muller R, Goldring SR, Choi Y, Benoist C, Gravallese EM 2001 TRANCE/RANKL knockout mice are protected from bone erosion in a serum transfer model of arthritis. Am J Pathol **159:**1689–1699.

16. Redlich K, Hayer S, Maier A, Dunstan C, Tohidast-Akrad M, Lang S, Turk B, Pietschmann P, Woloszczuk W, Haralambous S, Kollias G, Steiner G, Smolen J, Schett G 2002 Tumor necrosis factor-α–mediated joint destruction is inhibited by targeting osteoclasts with osteoprotegerin. Arthritis Rheum **46:**785–792.

17. Feldman M, Brennan FM, Chantry D, Haworth C, Turner M, Abney E, Buchan G, Barrett K, Barkley D, Chu A, Field M, Maini RN 1990 Cytokine production in the rhumatoid joint: Implications for treatment. Ann Rheum Dis **49:**480–486.

18. Funk JL, Cordaro LA, Wei H, Benjamin JB, Yocum DE 1998 Synovium as a source of increased amino-terminal parathyroid hormone-related protein expression in rheumatoid arthritis: A possible role for locally produced parathyroid hormone-related protein in the pathogenesis of rheumatoid arthritis. J Clin Invest **101:**1362–1371.

19. Chabaud M, Lubberts E, Joosten L, van Den Berg W, Miossec P 2001 IL-17 derived from juxta-articular bone and synovium contributes to joint degradation in rheumatoid arthritis. Arthritis Res **3:**168–177.

20. Gravallese EM, Manning C, Tsay A, Naito A, Pan C, Amento E, Goldring SR 2000 Synovial tissue in rheumatoid arthritis is a source of osteoclast differentiation factor. Arthritis Rheum **43:**250–258.

21. Horwood NJ, Kartsogiannis V, Quinn JMW, Romas E, Martin TJ, Gillespie MT 1999 Activated T lymphocytes support osteoclast formation in vitro. Biochem Biophys Res Commun **265:**144–150.

22. Kong YY, Feige U, Sarosi I, Bolon B, Tafuri A, Morony S, Capparelli C, Li J, Elliott R, McCabe S, Wong T, Campagnuolo G, Moran E, Bogoch ER, Van G, Nguyen LT, Ohashi PS, Lacey DL, Fish E, Boyle WJ, Penninger JM 1999 Activated T cells regulate bone loss and joint destruction in adjuvant arthritis through osteoprotegerin ligand. Nature **402:**304–309.

23. Okano K, Tsukazaki T, Ohtsuru A, Namba H, Osaki M, Iwasaki K, Yamashita S 1996 Parathyroid hormone-related peptide in synovial fluid and disease activity of rheumatoid arthritis. Br J Rheumatol **35:**1056–1062.

24. Ogata Y, Kukita A, Kukita T, Komine M, Miyahara A, Miyazaki S, Kohashi O 1999 A novel role of IL-15 in the development of osteoclasts: Inability to replace its activity with IL-2. J Immunol **162:**2754–2760.

25. Romas E, Gillespie M, Martin T 2002 Involvement of receptor activator of NF-κβ ligand and tumor necrosis factor-α in bone destruction in rheumatoid arthritis. Bone **30:**340–346.

26. Romas E, Martin TJ 1997 Cytokines in the pathogenesis of osteoporosis. Osteoporos Int **7:**S47–S53.

27. Romas E, Sims N, Hards D, Lindsay M, Quinn J, Ryan P, Dunstan C, Martin T, Gillespie M 2002 Osteoprotegerin reduces osteoclast numbers and prevents bone erosion in collagen-induced arthritis. Am J Pathol **161:**1419–1427.

28. Shimizu S, Shiozawa S, Shiozawa K, Imura S, Fujita T 1985 Quantitative histologic studies on the pathogenesis of periarticular osteoporosis in rheumatoid arthritis. Arthritis Rheum **28:**25–31.

29. Joffe I, Epstein S 1991 Osteoporosis associated with rheumatoid arthritis: Pathogenesis and management. Semin Arthritis Rheum **20:**256–272.

30. Peel NF, Eastell R, Russell RGG 1991 Osteoporosis in rheumatoid arthritis–the laboratory perspective. Br J Rheumatol **30:**84–85.

31. Woolf AD 1991 Osteoporosis in rheumatoid arthritis–the clinical viewpoint. Br J Rheumatol **30:**82–84.

32. Saag K, Rochelle K, Caldwell J, Brasington R, Burmeister L, Zimmerman B, Kohler J, Furst D 1994 Low dose long-term corticosteroid therapy in rheumatoid arthritis; an analysis of serious adverse events. Am J Med **96:**115–123.

33. Spector TD, Hall GM, McCloskey EV, Kanis JA 1993 Risk of vertebral fracture in women with rheumatoid arthritis. BMJ **306:**558.

34. Verstraeten A, Dequeker J 1986 Vertebral and peripheral bone density content and fracture incidence in postmenopausal patients with rheumatoid arthritis: Effects of low-dose corticosteroids. Ann Rheum Dis **45:**852–857.

35. Hooyman JR, Melton LJ, Nelson AM, O'Fallon WM, Riggs BL 1984 Fractures after rheumatoid arthritis; a population based study. Arthritis Rheum **27:**1353–1361.

36. Beat AM, Bloch DA, Fries JF 1991 Predictors of fractures in early rheumatoid arthritis. J Rheumatol **18:**804–808.

37. Compston JE, Vedi S, Croucher PI, Garrahan NJ, O'Sullivan MM 1994 Bone turnover in non-steroid treated rheumatoid arthritis. Ann Rheum Dis **53:**163–166.

38. Kroger H, Arnala I, Alhava EM 1991 Bone remodeling in osteoporosis associated with rheumatoid arthritis. Calcif Tissue Int **49:**S90.

39. Mellish RWE, O'Sullivan MM, Garrahan NJ, Compston JE 1987 Iliac crest trabecular bone mass and structure in patients with non-steroid treated rheumatoid arthritis. Ann Rheum Dis **46:**830–836.

40. Hall GM, Spector TD, Delmas PD 1995 Markers of bone metabolism in postmenopausal women with rheumatoid arthritis. Effects of corticosteroids and hormone replacement therapy. Arthritis Rheum **38:**902–906.

41. Gough AK, Peel NF, Eastell R, Holder RL, Lilley J, Emery P 1994 Excretion of pyridinium crosslinks correlates with disease activity and appendicular bone loss in early rheumatoid arthritis. Ann Rheum Dis **53:**14–17.

42. Gough A, Sambrook P, Devlin J, Huissoon A, Njeh C, Robbins S, Nguyen T, Emery P 1998 Osteoclastic activation is the principal mechanism leading to secondary osteoporosis in rheumatoid arthritis. J Rheumatol **7:**1282–1289.

43. Iwamoto J, Takeda T, Ichimura S 2003 Urinary cross-linked N-telopeptides of type I collagen levels in patients with rheumatoid arthritis. Calcif Tissue Int **72:**491–497.

44. Garnero P, Landewe R, Boers M, Verhoeven A, Van Der Linden S, Christgau S, van der Heijde DM, Boonen A, Geusens P 2002 Association of baseline levels of markers of bone and cartilage degradation with long-term progression of joint damage in patients with early rheumatoid arthritis: The COBRA study. Arthritis Rheum **46:**2847–2856.

45. Gough AK, Lilley J, Eyre S, Holdin R, Emery P 1994 Generalized bone loss in patients with rheumatoid arthritis. Lancet **344:**23–27.

46. Kirwan JR 1995 The effects of glucocorticoids on joint destruction in rheumatoid arthritis. N Engl J Med **333:**142–146.

47. Kroger H, Honkanen R, Saarikoski S, Alhava E 1994 Decreased axial

bone mineral density in perimenopausal women with rheumatoid arthritis. Ann Rheum Dis **53:**18–23.

48. Laan R, van Riel P, van Erning L, Lemmens JA, Ruijs SH, van-de-Putte LB 1992 Vertebral osteoporosis in rheumatoid arthritis arthritis patients: Effects of low-dose prednisone therapy. Br J Rheumatol **31:**91–96.

49. Laan RF, van-Riel PL, van-de-Putte LB 1992 Bone mass in patients with rheumatoid arthritis. Ann Rheum Dis **51:**826–832.

50. Sambrook PN, Eisman A, Champion G, Yeates MG, Pocock NA, Eberl S 1987 Determinants of axial bone loss in rheumatoid arthritis. Arthritis Rheum **30:**721–728.

51. Sambrook P, Nguyen T 1992 Vertebral osteoporosis in rheumatoid arthritis. Br J Rheum **31:**573–574.

52. Sambrook P, Birmingham J, Champion D, Kelly P, Kempler S, Freund J, Eisman J 1992 Postmenopausal bone loss in rheumatoid arthritis: Effect of estrogens and androgens. J Rheumatol **19:**357–361.

53. Sambrook P, Spector T, Seeman E, Bellamy N, Russel R, Buchanan RR, Martin NG, Prince R, Owen E, Silman A, Eisman J 1995 Osteoporosis in rheumatoid arthritis: A monozygotic co-twin control study. Arthritis Rheum **38:**806–809.

54. Als OS, Gotfredsen A, Riis BJ, Christisnsen C 1985 Are disease duration and degree of functional impairment determinants of bone loss in rheumatoid arthritis? Ann Rheum Dis **44:**406–411.

55. Verhoeven AC, Boers M, Te Koppele JM, van der Laan WH, Markusse HM, Geusens P, Van Der Linden S 2001 Bone turnover, joint damage, and bone mineral density in early rheumatoid arthritis treated with combination therapy including high-dose prednisolone. Rheumatology (Oxford) **40:**1231–1237.

56. Fries JF, Williams CA, Ramsey DR, Bloch DA 1993 The relative toxicity of disease-modifying antirheumatic drugs. Arthritis Rheum **44:**406–411.

57. Becker A, Fischer R, Scherbaum WA, Schneider M 2001 Osteoporosis in systemic lupus erythematosus: Impact of disease duration and organ damage. Lupus **10:**809–814.

58. Dykman TR, Gluck OS, Murphy WA, Hahn TJ, Hahn BH 1985 Evaluation of factors associated with glucocorticoid-induced osteopenia in patient with rheumatic diseases. Arthritis Rheum **28:**361–368.

59. Dhillon VB, Davies MC, Hall ML, Round JM, Ell PJ, Jacobs HS, Snaith ML, Isenberg DA 1990 Assessment of the effect of oral corticosteroids on bone mineral density in systemic lupus erythematosus: A preliminary study with dual energy xray absorptiometry. Ann Rheum Dis **49:**624–626.

60. Kalla AA, Fataar AB, Jessop SJ, Bewerunge L 1993 Loss of trabecular bone mineral density in systemic lupus erythematosus. Arthritis Rheum **36:**1726–1734.

61. Loftus J, Allen R, Hesp R, David J, Reid DM, Wright DJ, Green JR, Reeve J, Ansell BM, Woo PM 1991 Randomized, double-blind trial of deflazacort versus prednisone in juvenile chronic (or rheumatoid)

62. Varonos S, Ansell BM, Reeve J 1987 Vertebral collapse in juvenile chronic arthritis: Its relationship with glucocorticoid therapy. Calcif Tissue Int **41:**75–78.

63. French AR, Mason T, Nelson AM, Crowson CS, O'Fallon WM, Khosla S, Gabriel SE 2002 Osteopenia in adults with a history of juvenile rheumatoid arthritis. A population based study. J Rheumatol **29:**1065–1070.

64. Hanson CA, Shagrim JW, Duncan H 1971 Vertebral osteoporosis in ankylosing spondylitis. Clin Orthop **74:**59–64.

65. Ralston SH, Urquhart GD, Brzeski M, Sturrock RD 1990 Prevalence of vertebral compression fractures due to osteoporosis in ankylosing spondylitis. BMJ **300:**563–565.

66. Will R, Bhalla A, Palmer R, Ring F, Calin A 1989 Osteoporosis in early ankylosing spondylitis: A primary pathological event? Lancet **23:**1483–1485.

67. Hitchons PW, From AM, Brenton MD, Glaser JA, Torner JC 2002 Fractures of the thoracolumbar spine complicating ankylosing spondylitis. J Neurosurg **97:**218–222.

68. Dos Santos FP, Constantin A, Laroche M, Destombes F, Bernard J, Mazieres B, Cantagrel A 2001 Whole body and regional bone mineral density in ankylosing spondylitis. J Rheumatol **28:**547–549.

69. Maillefert JF, Aho LS, Maghraoui A, Dougados M, Roux CR 2001 Changes in bone density in patients with ankylosing spondylitis: A two year follow-up study. Osteoporos Int **12:**605–609.

70. Cooper C, Cook PL, Osmond C, Fisher L, Cawley MID 1991 Osteoarthritis of the hip and osteoporosis of the proximal femur. Ann Rheum Dis **50:**540–542.

71. Dequeker J 1985 The relationship between osteoporosis and osteoarthritis. Clin Rheum Dis **11:**271–296.

72. Nevitt MC, Lane NE, Scott JC, Hochberg MC, Pressman AR, Genant HK, Cummings SR 1995 Radiographic osteoarthritis of the hip and bone mineral density. Arthritis Rheum **38:**560–562.

73. Price T, Hesp R, Mitchell R 1987 Bone density in generalized osteoarthritis. J Rheumatol **14:**560–562.

74. Felson DT, Lawrence RC, Dieppe PA, Hirsch R, Helmick CG, Jordan JM, Kington RS, Lane NE, Nevitt MC, Zhang Y, Sowers M, McAlindon T, Spector TD, Poole AR, Yanovski SZ, Ateshian G, Sharma L, Buckwalter JA, Brandt KD, Fries JF 2000 Osteoarthritis: New insights. Part 1: The disease and its risk factors. Ann Intern Med **133:**635–646.

75. Lane NE, Nevitt MC 2002 Osteoarthritis, bone mass, and fractures: How are they related? Arthritis Rheum **46:**1–4.

76. Hart DJ, Mootoosamy I, Doyle DV, Spector TD 1994 The relationship between osteoarthritis and osteoporosis in the general population: The Clingford Study. Ann Rheum Dis **53:**158–162.

Chapter 65.   Juvenile Osteoporosis

Michael E. Norman

INTRODUCTION

The diagnosis of osteoporosis in children is usually made when skeletal radiographs reveal either fractures primarily in the axial skeleton (e.g., spine) and/or a generalized decrease in mineralized bone (e.g., osteopenia) in the absence of rickets or excessive bone resorption (e.g., osteitis fibrosa). Juvenile osteoporosis occurs typically before the onset of puberty, but it also may be seen in younger children, especially when they are growing rapidly. It may be caused by an inherited condition that is clinically evident from birth or early infancy, or it may be acquired during childhood. There are primary and idiopathic forms and a number of secondary forms of juvenile osteoporosis. The condition is uncommon; as of 1997, ~150 cases of idiopathic juvenile osteoporosis (IJO) had been reported in the literature.[1] However, the onset of osteoporosis just before or after the onset of puberty can have far-reaching effects, because one-half of skeletal mass is acquired during the adolescent years.

PATHOPHYSIOLOGY

True osteoporosis is defined histomorphometrically by a decreased total amount of normally formed bone. During bone formation (modeling) and bone remodeling, two fun-

The author has no conflict of interest.

damental defects may occur, singly or in combination: (1) a defect in bone-forming cells leading to decreased or defective matrix formation or (2) abnormalities in the coupling of bone formation and resorption, in which an imbalance develops between matrix formation (mineralization) and bone resorption, with the latter predominating. An inherited group of disorders known as osteogenesis imperfecta (OI) usually represents defects in bone-forming cells in which mutations in one of the two genes encoding type I procollagen produce defective matrix. IJO and the secondary causes of osteoporosis were initially thought to represent examples of bone resorption exceeding bone formation.[2] More recently, however, Rauch et al. have suggested that the primary defect in IJO may actually be diminished bone formation, secondary to impaired osteoblast function, seen primarily on cancellous bone surfaces.[3] IJO and chronic corticosteroid therapy are the most important forms of acquired juvenile osteoporosis. Early reports of calcium balance suggested that IJO changes, with initially negative or inappropriately neutral balances,[4,5] progressing to positive balance during the healing phase,[5,6] and in response to vitamin D administration. Pre-existing calcium deficiency for any reason, but particularly in adolescence and in pregnancy, may lead to especially severe forms of IJO.[7] Jowsey and Johnson[8] and Hoekman et al.[9] presented histological evidence of increased bone resorption, whereas Smith[10] and Reed et al.[11] found decreased bone formation as the major pathophysiologic event in IJO, a finding recently confirmed by Rauch et al.[3] Evans et al.[12] and Marder et al.[13] suggested a role for 1,25-dihydroxyvitamin D [1,25(OH)$_2$D] deficiency in the pathogenesis of IJO. Several reports also suggested a role for calcitonin deficiency in some patients.[14,15] The bone loss noted in astronauts undergoing prolonged periods of weightlessness in space may be analogous to IO, with rapid resorption of weight-bearing bones and suppressed bone formation. Both weightlessness and IJO seem to be reversible.[10] Some have speculated that IJO, like weightlessness, consists of some fundamental disturbance in the mechanical forces that stimulate new bone formation in the growing and young adult skeleton. Recent data in adult osteoporotic patients suggest impaired bone formation related in part to reduced insulin-like growth factor I secretion.[11] Dawson et al. recently extended the relationship between the clinical phenotypes of OI and corresponding mutations in the genes encoding type I collagen to include two siblings with features of IJO.[16] In so doing, they identified the first genetic abnormality in IJO; a mismatch in type I collagen α2 (e.g., COL1A2) mRNA, defined as a single base mutation (e.g., 1715G-A).

CLINICAL FEATURES

The typical child with IJO is immediately prepubertal and healthy. A recent series of 21 children with IJO indicated a mean age at onset of 7 years with a range of 1–13 years and no gender differences.[17] Symptoms begin with an insidious onset of pain in the lower back, hips, and feet, and difficulty walking. Knee and ankle pain and fractures of the lower extremities may be present, as well as diffuse muscle weakness. IJO affects both sexes equally; family and dietary

TABLE 1. DIFFERENTIAL DIAGNOSIS OF JUVENILE OSTEOPOROSIS

Primary
  Calcium deficiency
  Idiopathic juvenile osteoporosis
  Osteogenesis imperfecta
    Multiple subtypes
Secondary
  Endocrine
    Cushing syndrome
    Diabetes mellitus
    Glucocorticoid therapy
    Thyrotoxicosis
    Gonadal dysgenesis
  Gastrointestinal
    Biliary atresia
    Glycogen storage disease, type I
    Hepatitis
    Malabsorption
  Inborn errors of metabolism
    Homocystinuria
    Lysinuric protein intolerance
  Miscellaneous
    Acute lymphoblastic leukemia
    Anticonvulsant therapy
    Cyanotic congenital heart disease
    Immobilization
    Anorexia nervosa

histories are negative. Physical examination may be entirely normal or may reveal thoracolumbar kyphosis or kyphoscoliosis, pigeon-chest deformity, crown/pubis to pubis/heel ratio of less than 1.0, loss of height, deformities of the long bones, and limp. Generally, these physical abnormalities are reversible, and spontaneous recovery is noted in most patients,[2,16] although several of the original patients subsequently developed crippling deformities that left them wheelchair bound with cardiorespiratory abnormalities.[4] The history and physical examination of children with secondary forms of osteoporosis reflect the primary disease more than the osteoporosis (Table 1). There is usually a family history of osteoporosis or of the primary disease, evidence of failure to thrive, immobilization, or administration of corticosteroid or anticonvulsant drugs.

BIOCHEMICAL FEATURES

No proven biochemical abnormalities are characteristic of IJO, and no known endocrine disorder has been identified. In some children,[4,5,9] calcium balance is markedly negative or inappropriately neutral, and serum calcium levels are normal. Urine calcium excretion may be normal or elevated. Serum phosphorus, bicarbonate, magnesium, and alkaline phosphatase levels also are normal. The disease eventually resolves with time and the onset of puberty and can be detected by improvement in calcium balance. Increased urinary hydroxyproline excretion, an indirect indicator of increased bone resorption, as well as hypercalcemia and suppressed parathyroid hormone (PTH) secretion have been observed in some patients. Suppression of PTH secretion reduces 1,25(OH)$_2$D synthesis and decreases intestinal

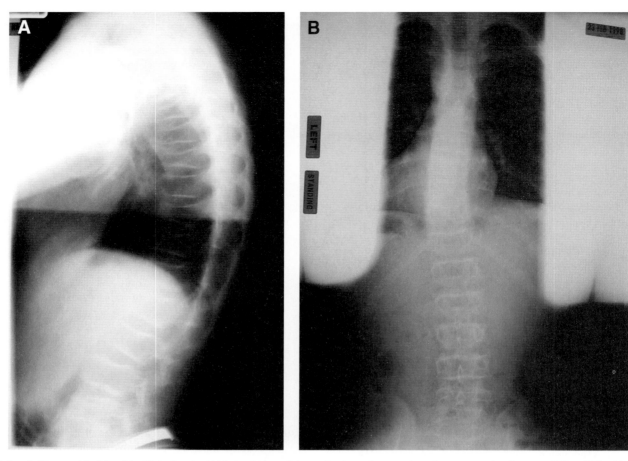

FIG. 1. A 10-year-old white girl with back pain. (A) Lateral view of thoracolumbar spine reveals wedge compression fracture of T8 and T9 with patchy sclerosis of T7. There was generalized osteopenia of the skeleton, confirmed by computed tomography. (B) Anterior view of the same patient reveals loss of height of T8 on the right side. The vertebral bodies are osteopenic.

calcium absorption, contributing to the negative calcium balance.[9] An abnormality in one of the collagen-linked markers of bone and connective tissue disorders, carboxy-terminal propeptide of type I procollagen, was reduced in the serum of IJO patients compared with disease controls with OI and Ehlers-Danlos syndrome.[18] However, these findings occurred only in prepubertal children and have not as yet been confirmed. In secondary forms of osteoporosis, biochemical and clinical clues to diagnosis depend on the underlying primary disease.[5,13]

RADIOLOGIC FEATURES

Conventional radiography is a relatively insensitive method for detecting bone loss; ~30% of skeletal mineral must be lost before osteopenia can be appreciated. In the absence of fractures or rickets, osteomalacia may be difficult to distinguish from osteoporosis as the cause of osteopenia. Looser lines or changes of secondary hyperparathyroidism favor rickets or osteomalacia, whereas biconcave vertebral deformities favor osteoporosis. Children with fully expressed IJO present with generalized osteopenia, fractures of the weight-bearing bones, and collapsed or misshapen vertebrae. Disc spaces may be widened asymmetrically because of wedging of the vertebral bodies (Fig. 1). Sclerosis may be noted. Long bones are usually normal in length and cortical width, unlike the thin, gracile bones of children with osteogenesis imperfecta. The pathognomonic radiographic finding of IJO is neo-osseous osteoporosis, an impaction-type fracture occurring at sites of newly formed weight-bearing metaphyseal bone. Typically such fractures are seen at the distal tibiae, adjacent to the ankle joint and adjacent to the knee and hip joints.[5,10] By using photon absorptiometry and computed tomography for detection of decreased bone mineral density (BMD), childhood osteoporosis may be diagnosed much earlier.

BONE BIOPSY

Few qualitative or quantitative studies of bone tissue have been performed in childhood osteoporosis. From microradiographs of bone, Cloutier et al.[6] and Jowsey and Johnson[8] reported increased bone resorption in IJO. They speculated that excessive dietary phosphorus intake may have stimulated parathyroid-mediated bone resorption. In contrast, Smith,[10] by using quantitative static histology of iliac bone, found indirect evidence of decreased bone formation, which was later confirmed by Rauch et al.[3] employing double tetracycline-labeled iliac bone biopsy specimens to assess changes by dynamic bone histomorphometry.

TABLE 2. DIFFERENTIAL DIAGNOSIS: OSTEOGENESIS IMPERFECTA (OI) VS. IDIOPATHIC JUVENILE OSTEOPOROSIS (IJO)

Characteristic	OI	IJO
Family history	Often positive	Negative
Age at onset	Birth	2–3 years before puberty
Duration of signs/symptoms	Lifelong (intermittent)	1–4 years
Physical findings	Thin gracile bones, short stature	Upper-lower segment ratio < 1.0
	Multiple deformities and contractures	Dorsal kyphoscoliosis
		Pectus carinatum
		Abnormal gait
	Extraskeletal features—	
	blue sclerae, deafness*	
	lax joints, hernias	
	abnormal dentition	
Calcium balance	Positive	Negative (in acute phase)
Radiologic findings	Pathologic fractures seen primarily in the appendicular skeleton but rarely in the metaphyseal regions of long bones	Pathologic fractures seen primarily in the axial skeleton but also in the metaphyseal regions of long bones
	Narrow long bones	Long bones with thin cortices
	Thin ribs	Wedge compression fractures of spine
	Wormian skull bones	
Molecular studies (dermal fibroblasts)	Abnormal collagen	? normal collagen

* Classic, dominantly inherited form.

DIFFERENTIAL DIAGNOSIS

OI is the most important entity to consider in the differential diagnosis of IJO.[19] Comparisons with IJO are listed in Table 2. OI can usually be differentiated from IJO by clinical characteristics, radiologic findings, and a positive family history. Diseases resulting in osteoporosis in childhood that must be differentiated from IJO are outlined in Table 1. Secondary causes of osteoporosis must be excluded in those children without the typical features of IJO. As a result, the diagnosis of IJO is reached by excluding secondary causes of osteoporosis and OI.

THERAPY

Because IJO is almost always a self-limited disease centered around the peripubertal years, prompt and definitive diagnosis is key to preventing progressive deformities of the spine and preserving bone mass, the latter to forestall the development of progressive osteoporosis during the adult years. A number of specific medical therapies have been tried in IJO,[2] the most promising of which are the bisphosphonates, which act by blocking bone resorption. In the initial 1985 report, bisphosphonate treatment in a single case of IJO resulted in a dramatic clinical, biochemical, and radiological response.[9] More recent studies involving groups of children have shown similar beneficial responses without significant adverse effects when treatment has been extended out to as much as 8 years.[20,21] Glorieux et al. reported significant increases in BMD and reductions in the fracture rate of 30 children with OI, treated from 1.5 to 3.0 years with cyclical oral doses of pamidronate, a second generation bisphosphonate.[21] There were no significant adverse effects on fracture healing, growth rates, or the appearance of growth plates on X-ray noted in any of the children. Shaw et al. administered intravenous pamidronate to five children with osteoporosis of diverse causes,[22] with the rapid resolution of bone pain and a marked increase in general activity and mobility in all. As noted in the Glorieux study, there was a corresponding increase in BMD and a fall in the fracture rate in every patient. One patient sustained a transient allergic-type reaction to the initial infusion of pamidronate, which did not recur. As a result of these preliminary but encouraging findings, the National Institute of Child Health and Human Development has initiated a randomized, double-blind, placebo-controlled trial of alendronate (Fosamax; Merck and Co., Inc., West Point, PA, USA), a third generation aminobisphosphonate in the treatment of childhood osteoporosis.[23] Endpoints will be changes in BMD and the rate of pathological fractures. While a number of other bone building agents such as calcitriol, growth hormone, insulin-like growth factor (IGF)-1, and PTH have shown some promise in the management of IJO, most reports are anecdotal, and these therapies remain unproven.[2] Sodium fluoride increases bone mass and has been reported to reduce fracture rates in primary vertebral osteoporosis.[24] However, fluoride treatment has been associated with a number of toxicity symptoms and musculoskeletal complaints in adults, and it remains unclear whether the hyperosteoidosis associated with this therapy produces increased bone strength. Notwithstanding, these reports of the potential beneficial effects of various medical therapies, the prompt institution of supportive care such as non-weight bearing, crutch walking, and physical therapy is crucial to avoiding long-term sequelae, in anticipation of spontaneous recovery at the onset of puberty. Secondary osteoporosis in most children is reversible when treatment of the underlying disease proves to be successful.

PROGNOSIS

With the exception of a few patients who develop progressive lower extremity, spine, and chest-wall deformities and require confinement to wheelchairs or bed, the prognosis of IJO is generally excellent. Distinguishing features have been recognized that identify the subgroup of children with poor prognosis. The prognosis of OI is dependent on the inherited subtype. The most effective treatment of secondary osteoporosis is successful therapy of the underlying disease. Failing this, supportive care should be provided as with IJO.

REFERENCES

1. Villaverde V, Inocencio JD, Merino R, Garcia-Consuegra J 1998 Difficulty walking. A presentation of idiopathic juvenile osteoporosis. J Rheumatol 25:173–176.
2. Kaufmann RP, Overton TH, Shifflet M, Jennings JC 2001 Osteoporosis in children and adolescent girls: Case report of idiopathic juvenile osteoporosis and review of the literature. Obstet Gynecol Surv 56:492–504.
3. Rauch F, Travers R, Norman ME, Taylor A, Parfitt AM, Glorieux FH 2002 The bone formation defect in idiopathic juvenile osteoporosis is surface-specific. Bone 31:85–89.
4. Dent CE, Friedman M 1965 Idiopathic juvenile osteoporosis. Q J Med 34:177–210.
5. Brenton DP, Dent CE 1976 Idiopathic juvenile osteoporosis. In: Bickel JH, Stern J (eds.) Inborn Errors of Calcium and Bone Metabolism. University Park Press, Baltimore, MD, USA, pp. 223–238.
6. Cloutier MD, Hayles AB, Riggs BL, Jowsey J, Bickel WH 1967 Juvenile osteoporosis: Report of a case including a description of some metabolic and microradiographic studies. Pediatrics 40:649–655.
7. Koo WW, Chesney RW, Mitchel N 1995 Case report: Effect of pregnancy on idiopathic juvenile osteoporosis. Am J Med Sci 309:223–225.
8. Jowsey J, Johnson KA 1972 Juvenile osteoporosis: Bone findings in seven patients. J Pediatr 81:511–517.
9. Hoekman K, Papapoulos SE, Peters ACB, Bijvoet OL 1985 Charac-
teristics and bisphosphonate treatment of a patient with juvenile osteoporosis. J Clin Endocrinol Metab 61:952–956.
10. Smith R 1980 Idiopathic osteoporosis in the young. J Bone Joint Surg Br 62:417–427.
11. Reed BY, Zeswekh JE, Sakhaee K, Breslau N, Gottschalk F, Pak CYC 1995 Serum IGF-I is low and correlated with osteoblastic surface in idiopathic osteoporosis. J Bone Miner Res 10:1218–1224.
12. Evans RA, Dunstan CR, Hills E 1983 Bone metabolism in idiopathic juvenile osteoporosis: A case report. Calcif Tissue Int 35:58.
13. Marder HK, Tsang RC, Hug G, Crawford AC 1982 Calcitriol deficiency in idiopathic juvenile osteoporosis. Am J Dis Child 136:914–917.
14. Saggese G, Bertelloni S, Baroncelli GI, Perri G, Calderazzi A 1991 Mineral metabolism and calcitriol therapy in idiopathic juvenile osteoporosis. Am J Dis Child 145:457–461.
15. Jackson EC, Strife CF, Tsang RC, Marder HK 1988 Effect of calcitonin replacement therapy in idiopathic juvenile osteoporosis. Am J Dis Child 142:1237–1239.
16. Dawson PA, Kelly TE, Marini J 1999 Extension of phenotype associated with structural mutations in type I collagen: Siblings with juvenile osteoporosis have an alpha2(I)Gly436-arg substitution. J Bone Miner Res 14:449–455.
17. Smith R 1995 Idiopathic juvenile osteoporosis: Experience of twenty-one patients. Br J Rheumatol 34:68–77.
18. Proszyska K, Wieczorek E, Olszaniecka M, Lorenc RS 1996 Collagen peptides in osteogenesis imperfecta, idiopathic juvenile osteoporosis and Ehlers-Danlos syndrome. Acta Paediatr 85:688–691.
19. Teotia M, Teotia SPS, Singh RK 1979 Idiopathic juvenile osteoporosis. Am J Dis Child 133:894–900.
20. Brumsen C, Hamdy NAT, Papapoulos SE 1997 Long term effects of bisphosphonates on the growing skeleton. Medicine (Baltimore) 76:266–283.
21. Glorieux FH, Bishop NJ, Plotkin H, Chabot G, Lanoue G, Travers RT 1998 Cyclic administration of pamidronate in children with severe osteogenesis imperfecta. N Engl J Med 339:947–952.
22. Shaw NJ, Boivin CM, Crabtree NJ 2000 Intravenous pamidronate in juvenile osteoporosis. Arch Dis Child 83:143–145.
23. National Institute of Child Health and Human Development 1998 Treatment of childhood osteoporosis with alendronate (Fosamax). Available online at http://clinicaltrials.gov/ct/guishow/NCT00001-20:jsessionid=B32103B4D5S8E8251E021.
24. Harrison JE 1990 Fluoride treatment for osteoporosis. Calcif Tissue Int 46:287–288.

Chapter 66. Secondary Causes of Osteoporosis: Thyrotoxicosis and Lack of Weight Bearing

Daniel T. Baran

Regional Medical Director, Merck & Co., Inc., Westwood, Massachusetts; and Department of Orthopedics and Medicine, UMASS Memorial Health Care, Worcester, Massachusetts

THYROTOXICOSOS

Thyroid hormone increases bone remodeling.[1] Although both osteoblast and osteoclast activities are increased by elevated levels of thyroid hormone, osteoclast activity predominates, with a resultant loss of bone mass. It appears that thyroid hormones stimulate osteoclastic bone resorption by an indirect effect mediated by osteoblasts. The presence of osteoblasts is required for thyroid hormones to increase bone resorption.[2,3]

Thyroid hormone directly stimulates osteoblast production of alkaline phosphatase,[4] osteocalcin,[5] and insulin like-growth factor.[6] Thyrotoxicosis is associated with increased serum levels of osteocalcin[7] and alkaline phosphatase.[8] Despite increased osteoblastic activity, the enhanced bone formation cannot compensate for thyroid hormone-induced increments in bone resorption. The increased bone resorption is detected by increased urinary levels of hydroxyproline and collagen cross-links in thyrotoxic patients.[1,9,10] The levels of these biochemical markers of bone turnover appear to correlate with circulating levels of thyroid hormone.

In thyrotoxicosis, the surface area of unmineralized ma-

Dr. Baran is an employee of Merck & Co., Inc.

trix (osteoid) is increased. In contrast to osteomalacia, mineralization rates are increased. The increased bone turnover in the presence of excessive levels of thyroid hormone is characterized by an increase in the number of osteoclasts, the number of resorption sites, and the ratio of resorptive to formative surfaces. In contrast to the normal bone-remodeling cycle, which lasts about 200 days, in thyrotoxic patients, the cycle is shortened, primarily because of a decrease in the length of the formation period, with failure to replace resorbed bone completely.[1] The changes in cortical bone in thyrotoxicosis are characterized by increased porosity[1] and alterations in the gene-expression markers.

In summary, thyroid hormone effects on osteoblasts and osteoclasts result in alterations in mineral metabolism and in the remodeling cycle, manifested by histological and molecular changes in bone. These changes appear to be reflected in altered bone mineral density (BMD).

Bone mass is reduced in patients with thyrotoxicosis.[11,12] The detrimental effects of elevated thyroid hormone levels on the skeleton appear to occur more frequently in female patients and at cortical bone sites.[13] As a result of the decrease in BMD, individuals with a history of thyrotoxicosis have an increased risk of fracture[14] and sustain fractures at an earlier age than individuals who have never been thyrotoxic.[15]

The decreased BMD noted in thyrotoxic patients is reversible after effective treatment. Normalization of the thyroid function test results in significant increases in axial and appendicular BMD compared with pretreatment values.[11,12] If the detrimental skeletal effects of supraphysiologic levels of thyroid hormone were restricted to individuals with thyrotoxicosis, therapy would be expected to prevent any further skeletal damage, and in fact, restore at least a portion of the bone mass that was lost before effective treatment.

Administration of high doses of thyroid hormone to suppress thyroid-stimulating hormone (TSH) secretion in patients with differentiated thyroid carcinoma and nontoxic goiter is considered appropriate therapy for those conditions. In patients prone to osteoporosis, however, this therapy may aggravate fracture risk. TSH-suppressive therapy has been reported to increase[16] and to have no effect[17] on biochemical markers of bone turnover. Likewise, TSH-suppressive doses of thyroid hormone have been reported to decrease or to have no effect on BMD in women. Meta-analyses of the reports in which BMD was assessed in women receiving TSH-suppressive doses of thyroxine concluded that treatment led to a 1% increase in annual bone loss in postmenopausal women.[18,19] Exogenous hyperthyroidism has been identified as a secondary contributor to osteoporosis in otherwise healthy women with osteoporosis.[20] Thyroid hormone replacement therapy in the absence of TSH suppression has been reported to have variable effects on BMD.[19,21]

LACK OF WEIGHT BEARING

Numerous studies have documented the beneficial effects of weight-bearing forces on the skeleton. Increased physical activity is associated with increased bone mass in individuals of all ages.[22] Conversely, lack of weight bearing, whether caused by paralysis,[23] space flight,[24] immobilization,[25] or stress shielding adjacent to prosthetic implants,[26,27] is associated with a decrease in bone mass. Immobilization of the upper extremity after surgery is attended by a decrease in BMD. Interestingly, while one extremity is immobilized, there is an increase in BMD in the contralateral extremity, perhaps the result of greater forces placed on the non-immobilized extremity.[28] The rapidity and extent of bone loss in the absence of normal weight-bearing forces is exemplified by stress shielding adjacent to femoral prostheses and the natural history of bone loss after paralysis. Within 2 months of surgery, there is a 12% decrease in BMD adjacent to the prosthesis, and by 24 months, there is a 25% decrease.[26] This bone loss, which can be prevented by bisphosphonates,[29] can be a serious problem in revision surgery because bone deficiencies may limit reconstructive options.[30] Similarly, much of the decrease in bone mass after paralysis occurs within the first year,[31] with increases in biochemical markers of bone resorption being the earliest indicators of bone loss.[32] These observational studies indicate the importance of limiting inactivity and immobilization when possible. The potential use of pharmacologic agents in the maintenance of BMD in the absence of normal mechanical forces has yet to be fully determined.

REFERENCES

1. Mosekilde L, Eriksen EF, Charles P 1990 Effects of thyroid hormone on bone and mineral metabolism. Endocrinol Metab Clin North Am 19:35–63.
2. Allain TJ, Chambers TJ, Flanagan AM, McGregor AM 1992 Triiodothyronine stimulates rat osteoclastic bone resorption by an indirect effect. J Endocrinol 133:327–331.
3. Britto JM, Fenton AJ, Holloway WR, Nicholson GC 1994 Osteoblasts mediate thyroid hormone stimulation of osteoclastic bone resorption. Endocrinology 134:169–176.
4. Sato K, Han DC, Fujii Y, Tsushima T, Shizume K 1987 Thyroid hormone stimulates alkaline phosphatase activity in cultured rat osteoblastic cells (ROS 17/2.8) through 3, 5, 3-triiodo-L-thyronine nuclear receptors. Endocrinology 120:1873–1881.
5. Rizzoli R, Poser J, Burgi U 1986 Nuclear thyroid hormone receptors in cultured bone cells. Metabolism 35:71–74.
6. Milne M, Kang M-I, Quail JM, Baran DT 1998 Thyroid hormone excess increases insulin-like growth factor 1 transcripts in bone marrow cell cultures: Divergent effects on vertebral and femoral cell cultures. Endocrinology 139:2527–2534.
7. Garrel DR, Delmas PD, Malaval L, Tournaire J 1986 Serum bone Gla protein: A marker of bone turnover in hyperthyroidism. J Clin Endocrinol Metab 62:1052–1055.
8. Cooper DS, Kaplan MM, Ridgway EC, Maloof F, Daniels GH 1979 Alkaline phosphatase isoenzyme patterns in hyperthyroidism. Ann Intern Med 90:164–168.
9. Harvey RD, McHardy KC, Reid IW, Paterson F, Bewsher PD, Duncan A, Robins SP 1991 Measurement of bone collagen degradation in hyperthyroidism and during thyroxine replacement therapy using pyridinium cross-links as specific urinary markers. J Clin Endocrinol Metab 72:1189–1194.
10. Krakerauer JC, Kleerekoper M 1992 Borderline low serum thyrotropin level is correlated with increased fasting urinary hydroxyproline excretion. Arch Intern Med 152:360–364.
11. Rosen CJ, Adler RA 1992 Longitudinal changes in lumbar bone density among thyrotoxic patients after attainment of euthyroidism. J Clin Endocrinol Metab 75:1531–1534.
12. Diamond T, Vine J, Smart R, Butler P 1994 Thyrotoxic bone disease in women: A potentially reversible disorder. Ann Intern Med 120:8–11.

13. Ben-Shlomo A, Hagag P, Evans S, Weiss M 2001 Early postmenopausal bone loss in hyperthyroidism. Maturitas **39:**19–27.
14. Cummings SR, Nevitt MC, Browner WS, Stone K, Fox KM, Ensrud KE, Cauley J, Black D, Vogt TM 1995 Risk factors for hip fracture in white women: Study of osteopenic fractures research group. N Engl J Med **332:**767–773.
15. Solomon BL, Wartofsky L, Burman KD 1993 Prevalence of fractures in postmenopausal women with thyroid disease. Thyroid **3:**17–23.
16. Toivonen J, Tahtela R, Laitinen K, Risteli J, Valimaki MJ 1998 Markers of bone turnover in patients with differentiated thyroid cancer with and following withdrawal of thyroxine suppressive therapy. Eur J Endocrinol **138:**667–673.
17. Mikosch P, Jauk B, Gallowitsch HJ, Pipam W, Kresnik E, Lind P 2001 Suppressive levothyroxine therapy has no significant influence on bone degradation in women with thyroid carcinoma: A comparison with other disorders affecting bone metabolism. Thyroid **11:**257–263.
18. Faber J, Galloe AM 1994 Changes in bone mass during prolonged subclinical hyperthyroidism due to L-thyroxine treatment: A meta-analysis. Eur J Endocrinol **130:**350–356.
19. Uzzan B, Campos J, Cucherat M, NonyP, Boissel JP, Perret GY 1996 Effects on bone mass of long term treatment with thyroid hormones: A meta-analysis. J Clin Endocrinol Metab **81:**4278–4289.
20. Tannebaum C, Clark J, Schwartzman K, Wallenstein S, Lapinski R, Meier D, Luckey M 2002 Yield of laboratory testing to identify secondary contributors to osteoporosis in otherwise healthy women. J Clin Endocrinol Metab **87:**4431–4437.
21. Duncan WE, Chung A, Solomon B, Wartofsky L 1994 Influence of clinical characteristics and parameters associated with thyroid hormone therapy on the bone mineral density of women treated with thyroid hormone. Thyroid **4:**183–190.
22. Snow CM, Shaw JM, Matkin CC 1996 Physical activity and risk for osteoporosis. In: Marcus R, Feldman D, Kelsey J (eds.) Osteoporosis. Academic Press, San Diego, CA, USA, pp. 511–528.
23. Elias AN, Gwinup G 1992 Immobilization osteoporosis in paraplegia. J Am Paraplegia Soc **15:**163–170.
24. Bikle DD, Halloran BP, Morey-Holton E 1997 Spaceflight and the skeleton: Lessons learned for the earthbound. Endocrinologist **7:**10–22.
25. Marchetti ME, Houde JP, Steinberg GG, Crane GK, Goss TP, Baran DT 1996 Humeral bone density losses after shoulder surgery and immobilization. J Shoulder Elbow Surg **5:**471–476.
26. Marchetti ME, Steinberg GG, Greene JM, Jenis LG, Baran DT 1996 A prospective study of proximal femur bone mass following cemented and uncemented hip arthroplasty. J Bone Miner Res **11:**1033–1039.
27. Kroger H, Miettinen H, Arnala I, Koski E, Rushton N, Suomalainen O 1996 Evaluation of periprosthetic bone using dual energy x ray absorptiometry: Precision of the method and effect of operation on bone mineral density. J Bone Miner Res **11:**1526–1530.
28. Houde JP, Schulz LA, Morgan WJ, Breen T, Warhold L, Crane GK, Baran DT 1995 Bone mineral density changes in the forearm after immobilization. Clin Orthop **317:**199–205.
29. Wilkinson JM, Stockley I, Peel NF, Hamer AJ, Elson RA, Barrington NA, Eastell R 2001 Effect of pamidronate in preventing bone loss after total hip arthroplasty: A randomized, double-blind, controlled trial. J Bone Miner Res **16:**556–564.
30. Rubash HE, Sinha RK, Shanbhag AS, Kim SY 1998 Pathogenesis of bone loss after total hip arthroplasty. Orthop Clin North Am **29:**173–186.
31. Biering-Sorensen F, Bohr H, Schaadt O 1990 Longitudinal study of bone mineral content in the lumbar spine, the forearm, and the lower extremities after spinal cord injury. Eur J Clin Invest **20:**330–335.
32. Maimoun L, Couret I, Micallef JP, Peruchon E, Mariano-Goulart D, Rossi M, Lerowx JL, Ohanna F 2002 Use of bone biochemical markers with dual-energy x-ray absorptiometry for early determination of bone loss in persons with spinal cord injury. Metabolism **51:**958–963.

Chapter 67.   Orthopaedic Complications of Osteoporosis

Christopher M. Bono and Thomas A. Einhorn

Department of Orthopaedic Surgery, Boston University Medical Center, Boston, Massachusetts

INTRODUCTION

The ability of bone to perform as the supporting structure of the body lies within its mechanical properties. Normal bone easily withstands the demands of everyday function. However, osteoporotic bone can fail under normal, subcatastrophic loads. Advances in pharmacologic treatment of osteoporosis could dramatically decrease the incidence of fragility fractures. Importantly, the effectiveness of such therapeutics is potentiated by early treatment. Unfortunately, fracture is commonly the seminal event of long-standing irreversible bone loss.

The occurrence of a fragility fracture is an insensitive way for physicians to identify patients with osteoporosis, although its specificity is very high. Despite this, the vast majority of patients who present with fractures are not appropriately diagnosed with osteoporosis. Freedman et al.[1] found that only 2.8% of woman over 55 years of age underwent bone mineral density (BMD) testing after being diagnosed and treated for a distal radius fracture. Notwithstanding, only 23% were treated with an anti-osteoporosis medication. Similarly, Gardner et al.[2] found between 11%

and 29% of patients with hip fractures were given a prescription for an anti-osteoporosis agent at the time of hospital discharge. In both studies, the chances that osteoporosis would go untreated increased with age.

The link between decreased BMD and increased fracture risk has been well established. It has been demonstrated in various skeletal regions, most notably the hip, wrist, and spine. Fractures can lead to pain and dysfunction that may potentiate medical comorbidities.[3–7] The focus of orthopedic intervention is to minimize these sequelae through stabilization, enhancement of fracture healing, and aggressive rehabilitation. Fracture fixation is challenging, because the weakened bone may not be amenable to conventional methods of treatment.

A large percentage of surgical candidates for osteoporotic fracture fixation are elderly. This consideration, in addition to the poor capacity of osteoporotic bone to engage standard fixation devices used in fracture management, results in unique challenges when planning stabilization procedures. Moreover, the ability of osteoporotic bone to support joint arthroplasty implants or rigid spinal instrumentation is diminished; thus, prudent preoperative planning and careful intraoperative technique is crucial to minimizing failures and optimizing results.

The authors have no conflict of interest.

PRINCIPLES OF OSTEOPOROTIC FRACTURE TREATMENT

Fractures are the most common orthopedic manifestation of osteoporosis. While each fracture must be considered individually, management is guided by common principles of skeletal trauma care including timely fixation, achievement of mechanical stability, and biological optimization of the bone healing environment.

1. Timely Fixation. The timing of fracture fixation is influenced by the anatomical region involved. Hip fractures directly and immediately affect patients' ability to ambulate. Left untreated, the patient is recumbent and at risk for decubitus ulcers, thromboembolic events, and pulmonary decompensation. Mortality risk is higher in patients treated nonoperatively.[8] Surgery should not be routinely delayed for medical optimization.[9] Usually, the patient is in the best medical condition at the time of initial admission, with further deterioration more likely with greater time elapsed. For these reasons, hip fractures are preferably surgically treated within the first 24–48 h after injury. Zuckerman et al.[9] found that delay in hip fracture fixation of more than 2 calendar days significantly increased the 1-year mortality rate in cognitively intact, ambulatory individuals. Others have observed that surgery performed within 24 h significantly reduced mortality rates.[10] Vertebral fractures can have detrimental effects on pulmonary function, quality of life, and the ability to perform activities of daily living. In contrast to hip fractures, these effects occur gradually and can be cumulative as subsequent fractures are sustained. Vertebral augmentation techniques (i.e., vertebroplasty and kyphoplasty) have introduced a new and useful tool for minimally invasive treatment of painful fractures.[11,12] The optimal time to stabilize osteoporotic vertebral compression fractures, however, remains to be defined. Current recommendations call for a period of at least 4–6 weeks of conservative treatment, including bracing, physical therapy, and pharmacologic pain management, which ameliorates symptoms in some patients. In addition, because chronically painful fractures can lead to physical deconditioning as well as emotional and psychological distress, patients who have pain that persists beyond this interval may also be effectively treated by vertebral augmentation.

2. Mechanical Stability. Stable fixation is a fundamental component of fracture treatment. This is usually achieved with some type of metallic device or implant, whether a plate, intramedullary rod, or prosthesis. In normal bone, it is preferable to use a very rigid implant because it provides maximal stability. This is achieved through a relatively unyielding interface between the bone and metal. This may not be possible in osteoporotic bone. Therefore, the surgeon may choose devices that do not derive their stability wholly from the bone-metal interface. An example of this is an intramedullary nail. In comparison to a plate, which lies on the outside surface of a bone, a nail is inserted into the medullary canal. Mechanically this achieves two important goals. First, the device is centered within the bone so that stresses are more evenly dispersed throughout the implant. Second, it allows more of the bone at the fracture site to share the loads borne by the extremity. Sliding hip screws rely on a similar principle, enabling the broad cancellous surfaces of an intertrochanteric fracture to bear the majority of the load, while the primary function of the implant is to keep the fragments aligned. One of the purposes of stable fixation is to allow early range of motion, weight bearing, and ambulation. In addition, it minimizes further pain and soft tissue injury by decreasing motion at the fracture site. Early failure of fracture fixation in osteoporotic bone is most influenced by the severity of BMD loss.[13,14] While no independent risk factor exists to the authors' knowledge, meticulous surgical technique, such as optimal lag screw placement into the femoral head/neck for treatment of hip fractures, is important to the durability of fixation.[15]

3. Fracture and Bone Healing. Modern principles of fracture fixation include delicate handling of the surrounding soft tissues. Whereas early techniques of fracture surgery involved extensive periosteal stripping and wide exposure of the fracture, this lead to devitalization of the bone's blood supply and intrinsic healing potential. By preserving the soft-tissue envelope surrounding the fracture site, healing is optimized. This is achieved using methods of indirect reduction and stabilization. Devices such as an intramedullary nail or a sliding hip screw are inserted into the bone at a distance from the site of the fracture and facilitate fracture reduction and stabilization without exposing the fracture itself. Active methods of promoting bone healing have recently been developed. These include substances that are introduced in or around a fracture to promote bone healing. The active components are select human proteins that have been replicated by recombinant DNA technology. These *bone morphogenetic proteins* (BMPs), namely BMP-7 (OP-1) and BMP-2, have led to higher union rates in nonunions as well as open tibia fractures, respectively.[16,17] These substances may also be useful in promoting the healing of osteoporotic fractures; however, the ability of recombinant proteins to enhance the healing of osteoporotic fractures has not specifically been established. Spinal fusion is also disadvantaged in osteoporotic bone.[18] The efficacy of BMP delivered in a collagen sponge has been investigated in human spinal fusion.[19] These materials show remarkable promise, resulting in fusion rates of nearly 100% in some trials. This represents a dramatic improvement over the approximate 60–85% success rate with autograft alone.[20] Currently, BMP-2 is approved as an alternative for autogenous bone graft for anterior interbody fusions performed to treat painful degenerative disc disease. While use of BMP-7 with posterior spinal fusion is being investigated, it is currently not Food and Drug Administration (FDA)-approved for use in this manner. As the majority of fusion procedures in the elderly are posterior, further data are required to define the role of these substances in spinal fusion in osteoporotic bone. Agents to treat osteoporosis may also have a positive effect on fracture healing. High doses of

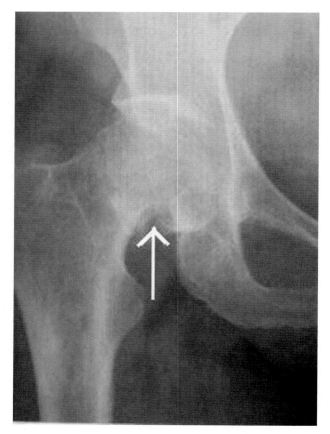

FIG. 1. Displaced femoral neck fractures (arrow) have a high nonunion rate and frequently progress to avascular necrosis of the femoral head.

parathyroid hormone (PTH) administered to rats seem to enhance fracture healing.[21] Although further clinical investigation is warranted, it must be recognized that the effects of comparably high levels of PTH in people may not be achievable without collateral deleterious effects. While these preliminary findings are encouraging, the role of PTH on bone healing in humans has yet to be determined.[22,23]

TREATMENT OF SPECIFIC FRACTURES

Hip

Hip fracture types can be classified according to anatomic region. Femoral neck fractures occur within the confines of the hip capsule. The blood vessels that supply the femoral head and neck are also intracapsular and lie directly on the bone. Fracture displacement can easily disrupt these vessels. Small displacements usually do not cause a vascular insult, and these fractures have a good chance of healing with appropriate internal fixation. Grossly displaced fractures have a risk of nonunion as the blood vessels are usually disrupted leading to an insufficient blood supply to the fracture site. Furthermore, disruption of the vessels can lead to avascular necrosis of the femoral head. In elderly patients in particular, it may be preferable to replace the injured bone rather than attempt to fix it, because this treatment usually

leads to a more favorable outcome with a better chance for early mobilization and rehabilitation of the patient.

Nondisplaced or impacted fractures are treated with stable internal fixation. This is best achieved using multiple screws placed parallel to and within the femoral neck, crossing the fracture site. The lag-type screw design creates compression at the bone ends that increases stability and promotes union. This procedure is minimally invasive because the screws can be placed through percutaneous, stabwound incisions incurring little blood loss and preserving the soft tissue envelope surrounding the fracture site. High rates of union have been achieved using internal fixation of non- or minimally displaced femoral neck fractures.

The treatment of displaced femoral neck fractures is more controversial (Fig. 1). Options include reduction and internal fixation or prosthetic replacement. The advantage of reduction and internal fixation is that it can be performed through a limited incision with minimal blood loss. The major disadvantage is that, despite an anatomic reduction and stable fixation, the fracture may not heal. This can lead to significant pain, morbidity, and the necessity of additional surgery. Prosthetic replacement eliminates these concerns. However, it is a more extensive procedure, with its own set of complications such as dislocation, loosening, and infection.

The current literature suggests that prosthetic replacement may have advantages in the treatment of displaced femoral neck fractures in the elderly (Fig. 2). It seems to result in a lower reoperation rate and better long-term hip function.[24,25] These advantages must be considered in light of the preoperative mental and functional level of the patient as fewer complications have been observed with internal

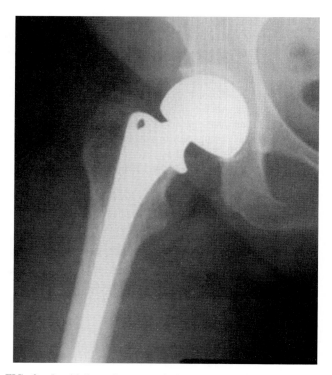

FIG. 2. In elderly patients, prosthetic replacement is preferred. This procedure provides excellent pain relief and enables early weight bearing. In this case, a bipolar hemiarthroplasty was performed.

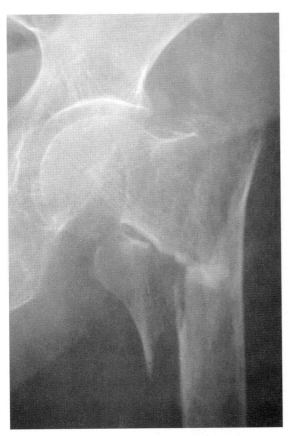

FIG. 3. Intertrochanteric fractures heal much more reliably than femoral neck fractures. For this reason, they are treated with some form of reduction and internal fixation. (Radiographs provided courtesy of Paul Tornetta III, MD, Boston University Medical Center, Boston, MA, USA.)

fixation versus hemiarthroplasty in nonambulatory patients who have severe mental disorders.[24,25]

Intertrochanteric fractures occur within the broad cancellous region between the greater trochanter and the lesser trochanter (Fig. 3). They are extracapsular and have an excellent blood supply that is not compromised by the displacement of the fracture, and therefore, have a much higher rate of healing than femoral neck fractures. However, they are more prone to deformity, such as varus angulation and shortening. The treatment of intertrochanteric fractures is much less controversial, with most authors agreeing that early internal fixation is optimal. Stable fixation is crucial. Various methods of internal fixation are available including dynamic sliding hip screws and intramedullary hips devices (Fig. 4). Some believe intramedullary devices may have a mechanical advantage in osteoporotic bone because of better load-sharing properties. However, a clear advantage of one device versus another has not been demonstrated.

Distal Femur/Proximal Tibia

Fractures around the knee, either supracondylar femur or proximal tibia fractures, are common in the elderly. Supracondylar fractures occur at the transitional region between the dense cortical bone of the distal femoral shaft and the softer metaphyseal bone of the femoral condyles. They often occur by low-energy mechanisms in severely osteopenic patients. In some cases, the fracture can extend into the joint. This predisposes to arthrosis, especially if the fracture is displaced. Proximal tibia fractures can occur from abnormal bending forces applied to the knee. While the knee naturally bends in the sagittal plane (flexion and extension), it does not normally move in the coronal plane (varus and valgus), and thus, forces delivered to the side of a knee, such as that imparted by the bumper of a car, can result in a tibial plateau fracture.

Treatment of supracondylar femur fractures is dependent on a number of factors. Fractures that involve the joint surface should be reduced under direct vision by the surgeon and internally fixed. This is most commonly performed with lag screws. Anatomic reduction of the articular surface decreases the chances of arthrosis and probably the likelihood of painful arthritis. Many times, intra-articular fractures occur in combination with supracondylar fractures. This presents a particular treatment challenge in that the screws placed to stabilize the condylar fragments can obstruct the placement of implant needed to fix the condyles to the femoral shaft. Careful preoperative planning of the placement of all components of the fixation system is necessary to avoid these difficulties.

Supracondylar fractures also present unique challenges.

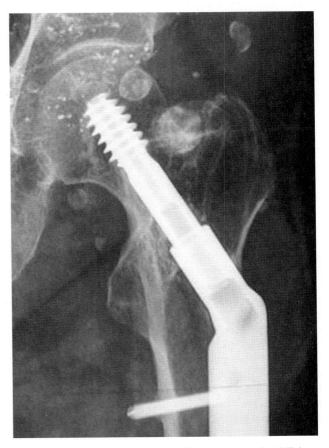

FIG. 4. A dynamic hip screw is an effective method of stabilizing an intertrochanteric fracture. The implant design allows compression across the fracture site with weightbearing.

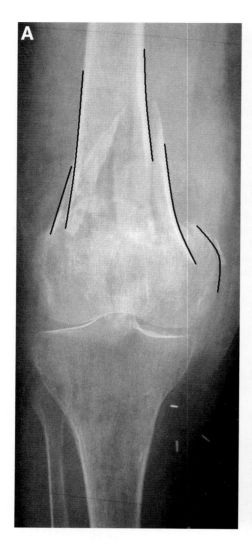

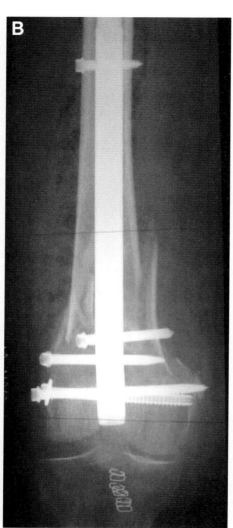

FIG. 5. (A) The black lines delineate the cortical disruption of a complex supracondylar femur fracture. (B) Intramedullary nails are an effective method of stabilizing supracondylar fractures. One advantage of this technique is that the implant can be inserted through a small incision in the knee, leaving the soft tissues around the fracture site intact. (Radiographs provided courtesy of Paul Tornetta III, MD, Boston University Medical Center, Boston, MA, USA.)

The location of the fracture determines the implant choice. Fractures that occur just above the intercondylar notch (located between the two femoral condyles) are generally fixed with a device known as a blade plate. The advantage of the blade plate is that excellent rotational control is achieved in the sagittal plane without the aid of additional screws. The main disadvantage is that it is more technically demanding to insert than other devices.

A dynamic condylar screw and plate can be used to treat more proximal fractures. This device is easier to use than the blade plate. However, stable fixation requires that the distal fragment be long enough to accept an additional screw. As with the blade plate, multiple screws are used to fix a long plate to the lateral cortex of the femoral shaft.

Intramedullary nails can also be used to stabilize supracondylar fractures (Figs. 5A and 5B). The advantage of using a nail is that it can be placed through a small incision within the knee joint. Furthermore, incisions around the fracture site are avoided, which maintains the soft tissue envelope, maximizing the blood supply to the fractured fragments. Intramedullary devices are centered within the bone, allowing more concentric load bearing. The main disadvantage of a nail is that distal fixation relies on only

two to three locking screws. In severely osteoporotic bone, these screws have poor purchase and a tendency to "back out." Newer screw designs have a nut that is placed from the opposite side that threads over the screw tip to lock it in place.

Proximal tibia fractures in bone supporting the knee, often referred to as fractures of the tibial plateau, frequently involve the articular surface. In some patterns, one or more large fragments are produced. In osteoporotic patients, a more common pattern is for an isolated portion of the articular surface to be pushed down (i.e., depressed) into the soft cancellous metaphysis of the proximal tibia. This creates an incongruent articular surface that can later lead to painful arthritis.

Fixation of tibial plateau fractures relies on restoration of the joint surface. With large fragments, open reduction and screw fixation is preferred. When only a portion of the joint surface is depressed, the reduction can be performed through less invasive maneuvers. A small window can be made in the cortex along the proximal shaft. A bone tamp can then be inserted underneath the articular fragment to push it back into place. Bone graft can be packed to support

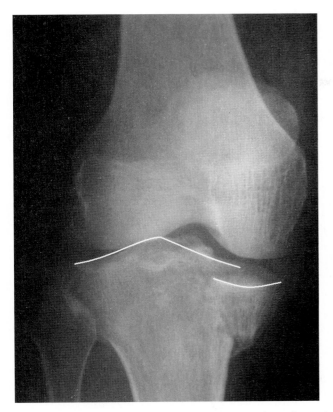

FIG. 6. Tibial plateau fractures occur in the elderly from abnormal bending forces across knee. Pieces of the articular surface are pushed into the soft cancellous bone of the proximal tibia. The white line delineates the articular surface, accentuating the incongruity of the medial joint. Optimally, the articular surface is reduced, and the fracture is stabilized with screws and plates. (Radiographs provided courtesy of Paul Tornetta III, MD, Boston University Medical Center, Boston, MA, USA.)

the reduction, and screws introduced using a percutaneous approach may be inserted to strengthen the repair (Fig. 6).

In the proximal tibia and to a lesser degree the distal femur, compression of the osteoporotic cancellous bone can lead to large voids or gaps. Despite anatomic or near anatomic reduction of the main fragments, these gaps can persist. They may be filled with bone graft or bone cement, known as polymethylmethacrylate (PMMA). PMMA can be inserted as a viscous liquid so that it assumes the exact shape of the void or gap. It quickly hardens to provide stable support to the surrounding bone. The disadvantage of PMMA is its nonresorbability, which can result in a rim of tissue reaction or lysis around its borders. This can compromise fixation and may increase the risk for infection. PMMA can also be used to improve the fixation of screws in osteopenic bone. Similarly, it is injected in a liquid state into the screw hole. The screw is then inserted, and the cement is allowed to harden around it, creating a strong bond between the bone and metal. A new material, recently approved for augmentation of fractures of the long bones by the Food and Drug Administration, may be an effective alternative to PMMA. Norian SRS (Norian Corp., Cupertino, CA, USA), a resorbable calcium- and phosphate-based cement, has been shown in limited clinical trails to provide support to the proximal tibia in plateau fractures in which

such voids are likely to jeopardize stability.[26] Its use as a means of enhancing screw fixation in osteoporotic bone has not been determined.

A newer plate device, the Less Invasive Stabilization System (LISS), has been recently developed. It enables better fixation in osteoporotic bone using a minimally invasive approach. Plates are inserted through a small slit-like incision along the lateral and distal part of the knee. The plate is then guided along the cortex without actually opening the skin or dissecting the muscle overlying the bone. Using a special guide, screws are inserted into the plate through stab-wound incisions. In contrast to standard plates in which the screw is able to toggle within its hole, the screws of the LISS plate have threads around their heads that lock them into the plate. Thus, every screw derives its stability not only from purchase within the bone but also from its fixation to the plate. Promising results using this device in osteoporotic bone have been reported.[27]

Wrist

Distal radius fractures are the most common fractures encountered by orthopedic surgeons, accounting for approximately 15% of emergency room visits for fractures.[28] They are particularly common in the elderly who are subject to frequent falls because as the upper extremity is outstretched in an attempt to break the fall, the soft metaphyseal bone of the distal radius fails under the impact of this

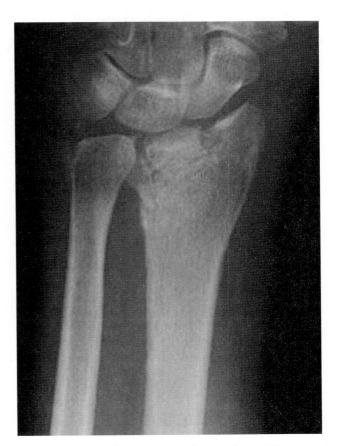

FIG. 7. Distal radius fractures commonly occur from a fall on an outstretched hand.

© 2003 American Society for Bone and Mineral Research

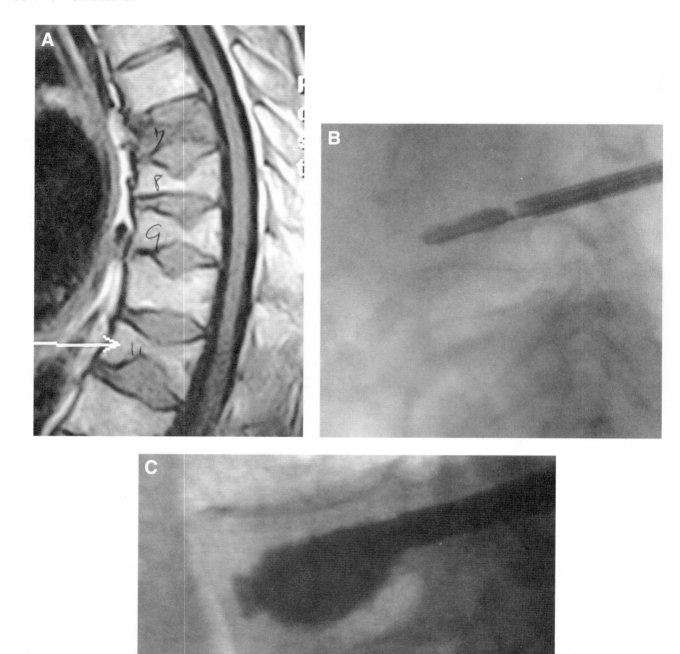

FIG. 8. (A) Osteoporotic compression fractures are best detected by magnetic resonance imaging (MRI). On T1 images, decreased signal indicates an acute fracture. On T2 images, increased signal is suggestive of a recent injury. (B) Persistently painful fractures can be stabilized using kyphoplasty. This technique involves insertion of an inflatable balloon tamp to reduce the fracture and restore vertebral body height. (C) Methacrylate cement is injected to maintain fracture reduction.

load. Fractures of the distal radius usually occur earlier in life than hip fractures and should be interpreted as an indicator of significant bone loss. In fact, patients who have sustained an osteoporotic distal radius fracture are at about twice the risk for a subsequent hip fracture compared with the general population.[29]

As with the other fractures discussed, various treatments exist. Management is influenced by the fracture pattern and

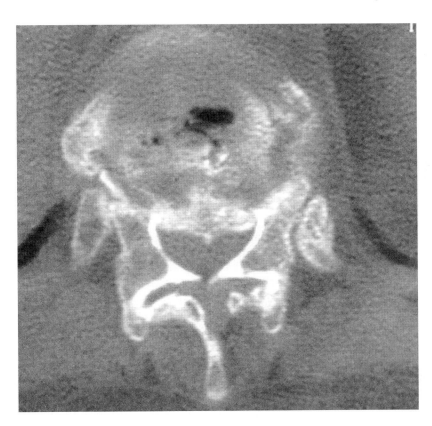

FIG. 9. Burst fractures are less common than osteoporotic compression fractures. However, they frequently result in canal compromise, which is best detected by computerized tomography (CT) images.

location, as well as the relative functional demands of the patient. Regardless of the pattern, nondisplaced fractures should be treated in a well-molded cast for approximately 6 weeks. Longer periods of immobilization can lead to worsened osteopenia and wrist stiffness.

Fractures of the metaphysis of the distal radius are common. Typically, the distal fragment tilts into extension. Small amounts of angulation may be acceptable. However, greater degrees of tilt are indications for closed reduction. Closed reduction relies on forces placed on the bone through the skin. As the skin in elderly patients can be quite fragile, care must be taken not to create degloving injuries. Gentle reduction also decreases the likelihood of further comminution at the fracture site. With small amounts of comminution, the fracture can be held in an acceptable position using a cast. With more comminution, a cast may allow redisplacement. In these injuries, it is preferable to maintain the alignment using a fixation device. Traditionally, this is accomplished with either an external fixator or plate (Fig. 7). These devices derive their stability from screw-thread purchase. In osteoporotic bone, this can be suboptimal, which may lead to construct failure. Surgery is reserved for patients who have substantially displaced fractures and for active patients in whom wrist function is vital to maintain their independence.

Much like the LISS plate, low profile plates with fixed angle capabilities have been developed for the distal radius specifically to address poor fixation in osteoporotic bone. Conceptually, the plates act as a mini-blade plate that supports the fracture through the dense bone directly underneath the articular surface. Variations of these devices have been developed for both the dorsal and volar surface of the

radius. While they can be quite effective, proper use is technically demanding. It requires gentle technique to avoid further bony comminution. Stable fixation, however, can allow early range of motion and avoid the detrimental immobilization effects of a cast. The exact indications for these procedures remains to be defined.

Injectable bone cements such as Norian SRS have been developed to aid in the treatment of osteoporotic distal radius fractures because they may offer mechanical support to stably reduced fractures. While not a replacement for surgery, this technique can be used as an adjunct to cast treatment. In one randomized prospective series, better wrist function was noted using Norian SRS bone cement compared with cast treatment alone.[30] Importantly, use of the bone cement reduces the time in the cast to 2 versus 6 weeks. It does not appear to affect maintenance of the initial reduction.

Spine

The most common vertebral injury in patients with osteoporosis is a compression fracture. This injury can occur with very low energy mechanisms, such as picking up a bag of groceries or a forceful cough or sneeze. Pain can be acute in onset and may persist for long periods of time. The thoracolumbar spine is the most commonly involved region, and the thoracolumbar junction (T12–L1) is the most commonly involved segment. Fractures can lead to pain, deformity (such as kyphosis or kyphoscoliosis), pulmonary compromise, and eating disorders, such as early satiety.[5,6] Osteoporotic compression fractures can significantly diminish a patient's overall quality of life and ability to perform activities of daily living.

In the mid-1980s, a procedure known as vertebroplasty was developed in Europe.[11] It involved the percutaneous injection of PMMA into a fractured vertebral body. With its introduction to the United States in the mid 1990s, a variation of vertebroplasty was developed known as kyphoplasty.[12] While similar to vertebroplasty, kyphoplasty involves the insertion of various tools, including an inflatable bone tamp, which is used to restore the height of the compressed vertebra, before insertion of cement (Figs. 8A–8C). This step seems to have two main advantages: First, it offers the possibility of reversing vertebral compression height loss and kyphosis in affected patients. Second, as the higher pressure injections used during vertebroplasty have led to high rates of cement extrusion (between 20% and 70%), creating a cavity for the PMMA with kyphoplasty has resulted in lower rates of cement extrusion (averaging about 9%).[4,12] Because cement extrusion has been associated with pulmonary emboli, respiratory distress, and neural injury, concerns regarding these complications have led many to prefer kyphoplasty over vertebroplasty for those patients in whom this procedure is indicated. Fortunately, the vast majority of cases of cement extrusion are clinically asymptomatic.

As noted above, there is still a lack of consensus regarding the optimal time to stabilize osteoporotic vertebral compression fractures. Current recommendations call for a period of at least 4–6 weeks of conservative treatment after the injury is sustained. This treatment includes bracing, physical therapy, and pharmacologic pain management. The main indication for vertebral augmentation is the treatment of persistently painful acute or chronic osteoporotic compression fractures. In the authors' experience, patients with fractures as old as 1–2 years can have dramatic pain relief. Progressive painless collapse, documented radiographically, may be an indication for kyphoplasty because of its unique ability to restore vertebral height. Local spine infection (i.e., active osteomyelitis) and uncorrectable coagulopathy are relative contraindications to the procedures.

The rates of pain relief with vertebroplasty and kyphoplasty are between 90% and 100%. From a recent study of patients undergoing kyphoplasty, stabilization of the fractures led to significant functional improvements.[4] In a large multicenter study, kyphoplasty enabled reliable restoration of vertebral body height if performed within 3 months of the injury.[12] Other reports have been more modest, documenting between 50% and 60% height restoration.[4] Vertebroplasty, while providing lasting pain relief, has not demonstrated this ability.

Burst fractures can also occur in the osteoporotic spine. They are most common in the T12 and L1 vertebrae (Fig. 9).[31] In contradistinction to simple compression fractures, they, by definition, involve the posterior aspect of the vertebral body. This can result in compromise of the spinal canal and neurologic impairment.[32–34] Treatment with vertebroplasty or kyphoplasty is usually contraindicated in such situations. Open surgical treatment includes anterior decompression by removing the offending bony fragments. After this subtotal vertebrectomy, the missing bone is replaced with structural autograft, allograft, or a cylindrical titanium mesh cage filled with morcellized graft. The graft or cage should have as broad a surface as possible to evenly disperse forces to the intact, but osteopenic, vertebral endplates above and below the engrafted site. The vertebral bodies are stabilized by anterior instrumentation, such as fixation with a plate and screws. Posterior instrumentation and fusion is performed in a staged fashion to provide additional stability. Such operations should be reserved for patients with neurologic compromise or progressive deformity that may risk injury to the neural elements.

CONSIDERATIONS FOR RECONSTRUCTIVE OPERATIONS

Elderly patients are prone to degenerative joint processes throughout the skeleton. Hip and knee arthritis can be debilitating, making even short walks difficult to negotiate. While medical treatment can be effective early in the course of the disease, patients with more severe disease can benefit from joint replacement. Hip arthroplasty is widely successful and has been ranked the number one most satisfying elective procedure of all operations. As with fracture fixation, the durability of joint reconstruction is dependent on the quality of the bone.

Degenerative changes in the spine can lead to significant problems as well. Arthritis of the disc spaces and facet joints can lead to bony overgrowth. These prominences can eventually impinge on the cauda equina and nerve roots. Furthermore, degeneration can lead to deformities such as kyphosis and scoliosis. Reconstruction of the spine often involves fusion for unstable segments. The strength of screws placed into the vertebral bodies is dependent on the BMD. Reconstruction of the osteoporotic spine must be carefully biomechanically planned.

Total Joint Arthroplasty

The techniques and principles of total joint arthroplasty remain the same in osteoporotic patients as they do for patients with normal skeletons. However, extreme care must be taken when preparing the bones for acceptance of the implants. Preparation of the femoral canal, for example, for a total hip prosthesis involves insertion of sequentially increasing sized reamers that can place large expanding (hoop) stresses on the cortical bone. This step must be carefully performed in the osteoporotic bone to avoid cortical blow out.

Most surgeons advocate the use of PMMA to augment fixation of total joint prostheses in osteoporotic bone. Thus, uncemented, so-called *press-fit* implants are usually reserved for normal bone. Some newly developed press-fit implants have a hydroxyapatite coating that may increase osteoconductivity. Such implants have demonstrated promising results with total hip replacements in osteoporotic patients.[35] The hydroxyapatite coating seems to decrease the rate of loosening. Such alternatives may avoid cement-related intraoperative complications such as transient hypotension.

Spinal Reconstruction

Elderly osteoporotic patients frequently present with spinal deformities and spinal stenosis. These conditions are usually secondary to a degenerative disorder of the spine. Scoliosis or kyphosis can lead to walking imbalance and intractable pain. In select cases, spinal reconstruction may be indicated. These extensive procedures involve combined anterior and posterior procedures.[36] Anterior surgery involves multilevel discectomies followed by fusion. This releases the main deforming forces of the curve, but also creates an iatrogenically unstable spine. It is followed by posterior instrumentation and fusion. In younger patients with adolescent idiopathic deformities, an anterior or posterior procedure can be performed alone. These methods rely on large corrective forces imparted by the instrumentation and would lead to unacceptably early construct failure in weak bone. To decrease the loads borne at each level, multilevel segmental fixation with devices such as pedicle screws or hooks are needed. These measures substantially increase the morbidity of the operation. Procedures for correcting spinal deformity in osteoporotic patients should be performed by experienced surgeons in well-equipped centers in conjunction with a multi-disciplinary team for medical optimization.

Spinal stenosis most commonly occurs in the lumbar spine. It may cause neurogenic claudication with ambulation, characterized by burning pain or a feeling of fatigue in the legs. In some patients with spinal stenosis, decompression with laminectomy is indicated.[37] This is often accompanied by spinal fusion in cases of instability. While the use of instrumentation has demonstrated increased fusion rates, osteopenic bone may be too soft to hold screws or hooks.[38] Longer operative times, greater blood loss, and device-related complications are additional drawbacks.

SUMMARY

Osteoporosis presents a number of challenges to orthopedic surgeons. These are related to complications of the disorder itself, such as fragility fractures, or to the treatment of other conditions, such as large joint arthritis or degenerative spinal disease. Orthopedic surgeons must maintain a greater awareness of the significance of fragility fractures. They must also take a more active role in prompting definitive diagnosis and treatment of the underlying metabolic disorder in addition to appropriate treatment of the fractures. The use of BMPs offers a bright future for improving the rate of fracture healing and spinal fusion in osteoporotic individuals. Continued advancements in the development of bioresorbable cements may obviate the use of nonresorbable materials such as PMMA in the percutaneous stabilization of extremity and spinal fractures.

REFERENCES

1. Freedman KB, Kaplan FS, Bilker WB, Strom BL, Lowe RA 2000 Treatment of osteoporosis: Are physicians missing an opportunity? J Bone Joint Surg Am **82:**1063–1070.
2. Gardner JJ, Flik KR, Mooar P, Lane JM 2002 Improvement in the undertreatment of osteoporosis following hip fracture. J Bone Joint Surg Am **84:**1342–1348.
3. Dzupa V, Bartonicek J, Skala-Rasenbaum J, Prikazsky V 2002 Mortality in patients with proximal femoral fractures during the first year after the injury. Acta Chir Orthop Traumatol Cech **69:**39–44.
4. Lieberman IH, Dudeney S, Reinhardt MK, Bell G 2001 Initial out-
come and efficacy of "kyphoplasty" in the treatment of painful osteoporotic vertebral compression fractures. Spine **26:**1631–1638.
5. Leidig-Bruckner G, Minne HW, Schlaich C, Wagner G, Scheidt-Nave C, Bruckner T, Gebest HJ, Ziegler R 1997 Clinical grading of spinal osteoporosis: Quality of life components and spinal deformity in women with chronic low back pain and women with vertebral osteoporosis. J Bone Miner Res **12:**663–675.
6. Schlaich C, Minne HW, Bruckner T, Wagner G, Gebest HJ, Grunze M, Ziegler R, Leidig-Bruckner G 1998 Reduced pulmonary function in patients with spinal osteoporotic fractures. Osteoporos Int **8:**261–267.
7. Walker N, Norton R, Vander Hoorn S, Rodgers A, MacMahon S, Clark T, Gray H 1999 Mortality after hip fracture: Regional variation in New Zealand. N Z Med J **112:**269–271.
8. Hoerer D, Volpin G, Stein H 1993 Results of early and delayed surgical fixation of hip fractures in the elderly: A comparative retrospective study. Bull Hosp Jt Dis **53:**29–33.
9. Zuckerman JD, Skovron ML, Koval KJ, Aharonoff G, Frankel VH 1995 Postoperative complications and mortality associated with operative delay in older patients who have a fracture of the hip. J Bone Joint Surg Am **77:**1551–1556.
10. Hamlet WP, Lieberman JR, Freedman EL, Dorey FJ, Fletcher A, Johnson EE 1997 Influence of health status and the timing of surgery on mortality in hip fracture. Am J Orthop **26:**621–627.
11. Deramond H, Depriester C, Galibert P, Le Gars D 1998 Percutaneous vertebroplasty with polymethylmethacrylate. Technique, indications, and results. Radiol Clin North Am **36:**533–546.
12. Garfin SR, Yuan H, Lieberman IH 2000 Early outcomes in the minimally-invasive reductions and fixation of compression fractures. Proceedings of the North American Spine Society, New Orleans, LA, USA, pp. 184–185.
13. Goh JC, Shah KM, Bose K 1995 Biomechanical study on femoral neck fracture fixation in relation to bone mineral density. Clin Biomech (Bristol, Avon) **10:**304–308.
14. Spangler L, Cummings P, Tencer AF, Mueller BA, Mock C 2001 Biomechanical factors and failure of transcervical hip fracture repair. Injury **32:**223–228.
15. Baumgaertner MR, Curtin SL, Lindskog DM, Keggi JM 1995 The value of the tip-apex distance in predicting failure of fixation of peritrochanteric fractures of the hip. J Bone Joint Surg Am **77:**1058–1064.
16. Friedlander GE, Perry CR, Cole JD, Cook SD, Cierny G, Muschler GF, Zych GA, Calhoun JH, LaForte AJ, Yin S 2001 Osteogenic protein-1 (bone morphogenetic protein-7) in the treatment of tibial nonunions. J Bone Joint Surg Am **83:**S151–S158.
17. Govender S, Csimma C, Genant HK, Valentin-Opran A 2002 Recombinant human bone morphogenetic protein-2 for treatment of open tibial fractures. J Bone Joint Surg Am **84:**2123–2134.
18. Simmons E, Kuhele J, Lee J, Lee L, Grynpas M 2002 Evaluation of metabolic bone disease as a risk factor for lumbar fusion. Spine J **2:**99S.
19. Boden SD, Zdebick TA, Sandhu HS, Heim SE 2000 The use of rhBMP-2 in Interbody fusion cages. Spine **25:**376–381.
20. Bono C, Lee C 2002 Critical analysis of trends in fusion for degenerative disc disease over the last twenty-years: Influence of technique on fusion rate and clinical outcome. Spine J **2:**47S–48S.
21. Nakajima A, Shimoji N, Shiomi K, Shimizu S, Moriya H, Einhorn TA, Yamazaki M 2002 Mechanisms for the enhancement of fracture healing in rats treated with intermittent low-dose human parathyroid hormone (1–34). J Bone Miner Res **17:**2038–2047.
22. Morley P, Whitfield JF, Willick GE 2001 Parathyroid hormone: An anabolic treatment for osteoporosis. Curr Pharm Des **7:**671–687.
23. Hardy JR, Conlan D, Haty S, Gregg PJ 1993 Serum ionized calcium and its relationship to parathyroid hormone after tibial fracture. J Bone Joint Surg Br **75:**645–649.
24. Johansson T, Jacobsson SA, Ivarsson I, Knutsson A, Wahlstrom O. 2000 Internal fixation versus total hip arthroplasty in the treatment of displaced femoral neck fractures: A prospective randomized study of 100 hips. Acta Orthop Scand 597–602.
25. Ravikumar KJ, Marsh G 2000 Internal fixation versus hemiarthroplasty versus total hip arthroplasty for displaced subcapital fractures of femur-13 year results of a prospective randomised study. Injury **31:**793–797.
26. Lobenhoffer P, Gerich T, Witte F, Tscherne H 2002 Use of an injectable calcium phosphate bone cement in the treatment of tibial plateau fractures: A prospective study of twenty-six cases with twenty-month mean follow-up. J Orthop Trauma **16:**143–149.
27. Schandelmaier P, Stephan C, Krettek C, Tscherne H 2000 Distal fractures of the femur. Unfallchirurg **103:**428–436.

28. Mallmin H, Ljunghall S 1992 Incidence of Colle's fracture in Upssala. A prospective study of a quarter million population. Acta Orthop Scand **63:**213–215.

29. Kannus P, Parkkari J, Sievanen H, Heinonen A, Vuori L, Jarvinen M 1996 Epidemiology of hip fractures. Bone **18**(Suppl):57S–63S.

30. Sanchez-Sotelo J, Munuera L, Madero R 2000 Treatment of fractures of the distal radius with a remodellable bone cement: A prospective, randomised study using Norian SRS. J Bone Joint Surg Br **82:**856–863.

31. Chavda DV, Brantigan JW 1994 Burst fractures of the twelfth thoracic vertebra in a middle aged man with osteoporosis. Nebr Med J **79:**193–199.

32. Nguyen HV, Ludwig S, Gelb D 2003 Osteoporotic vertebral burst fractures with neurologic compromise. J Spinal Disord Tech **16:**10–19.

33. Korovessis P, Marziotis T, Piperos G, Spyropoulos P 1994 Spontaneous burst fracture of the thoracolumbar spine in osteoporosis associated with neurological impairment: A report of seven cases and review of the literature. Eur Spine J **3:**286–288.

34. Tanaka S, Kubota M, Fujimoto Y, Hayashi J, Nishikawa K 1993 Conus medullaris syndrome secondary to an L1 burst fracture in osteoporosis. A case report. Spine **8:**2131–2134.

35. Kligman M, Kirsh G 2000 Hydroxyapatite-coated total hip arthroplasty in osteoporotic patients. Bull Hosp Jt Dis **59:**136–139.

36. Kostuik JP 1990 Anterior Kostuik-Harrington distraction systems for the treatment of kyphotic deformities. Spine **15:**169–180.

37. Grob D, Humke T, Dvorak J 1995 Degenerative lumbar spinal stenosis. Decompression with and without arthrodesis. J Bone Joint Surg Am **77:**1036–1041.

38. Fischgrund J, Mackay M, Herkowitz H, Brower R, Montgomery DM, Kurz LT 1997 Volvo award winner in clinical studies: Degenerative lumbar spondylolisthesis with spinal stenosis. A prospective, randomized study comparing decompressive laminectomy and arthrodesis with and without spinal instrumentation. Spine **22:**2807–2812.

Metabolic Bone Diseases or Osteomalacia

Chapter 68.   Nutritional and Drug-Induced Rickets and Osteomalacia

John M. Pettifor

MRC Mineral Metabolism Research Unit and the Department of Paediatrics, Chris Hani Baragwanath Hospital and the University of the Witwatersrand, Johannesburg, South Africa

INTRODUCTION

Once a scourge for people living in cities of northern Europe and North America, nutritional rickets and osteomalacia were considered by the latter half of the 20th century to have been all but eradicated from a number of countries except in a few at-risk groups such as preterm infants, the elderly, and the infirm. This was made possible through health education, the availability of vitamin D supplements, and the fortification of foods such as milk. However, over the past two decades, attention has been drawn to an apparent resurgence of the problem not only in the United States but also in a number of developing countries.

Rickets is a disorder associated with a failure of or delay in the mineralization of endochondral new bone formation at the growth plates, while osteomalacia is characterized by a failure of mineralization of newly formed osteoid at sites of bone turnover or periosteal and endosteal apposition. Thus, in children, whose growth plates (physes) are not closed, rickets and osteomalacia are found together, while in adults with fused growth plates, only osteomalacia will be noted. Although distinguishing between the two conditions might seem arbitrary, it is possible that the two conditions might respond differently to treatment, as has been suggested in children with X-linked hypophosphatemic rickets.

The causes of rickets and osteomalacia are numerous, and many of the causes will be discussed here and elsewhere. In this chapter, nutritional and drug-induced causes will be described.

NUTRITIONAL CAUSES OF RICKETS/ OSTEOMALACIA

Nutritional rickets/osteomalacia may be caused by deficiencies of vitamin D, calcium, or phosphorus. While each of these causes will be considered separately, each may contribute to a greater or lesser degree to the disease in an individual patient.

Vitamin D Deficiency

Although considered to be a nutrient, vitamin D is found in only small quantities in the majority of natural foods, and these supplies are generally insufficient to meet the vitamin D requirements of humans. Vitamin D sufficiency is maintained in most populations through its formation in the skin from 7-dehydrocholesterol under the influence of ultraviolet-B (UVB) irradiation from sunlight. In situations of impaired dermal synthesis, as may occur in countries of extreme latitude (e.g., in northern Europe, northern China and northern North America), because of extensive clothing coverage of the skin (in the Middle Eastern region),[1] in darkly pigmented persons living in countries with limited UVB irradiation, in the elderly (because of decreased substrate being available for dermal synthesis of vitamin D), or because of the use of sunscreens, food fortification (of milk in the United States), or vitamin D supplementation may be necessary to maintain an adequate vitamin D status.

Despite vitamin D fortification of foods in some countries and the recommendation of vitamin D supplementation in at-risk populations (particularly breastfed infants, the elderly, and the infirm), vitamin D deficiency rickets/ osteomalacia continues to be public health problem in a number of countries: in the United States, increasing numbers of reports are highlighting rickets in infants of black parents, especially in those who have been breastfed for prolonged periods.[2] It is possible that in these toddlers low dietary calcium intakes during the weaning period may exacerbate the problem. In the United Kingdom and other northern European countries, Asian and immigrant populations (from Turkey and African countries) appear to be particularly at risk, where the disease affects not only breastfed infants but also occurs in adolescents and women. In the Middle East, a high prevalence of rickets and osteomalacia has been described in Muslim women and their infants.[3] In Tibet and Mongolia, clinical rickets has been described in over 60% of young infants.[4] Other groups particularly at risk are those individuals living in areas of poor UVB irradiation, who are vegan or vegetarian, or who have other extreme dietary restrictions such as macrobiotic

---

diets. With the improvement in health care in many developed countries, life expectancy has increased dramatically resulting in large numbers of elderly and infirm, often living in retirement villages or old-age homes, where there are limited opportunities of receiving adequate sunlight exposure. In such situations vitamin D deficiency may develop insidiously, resulting in impaired muscle function, bone pain, and an increased risk of fractures.

Pathogenesis. Vitamin D, or more specifically the active metabolite $1,25(OH)_2D$, is essential for maintaining normocalcemia through ensuring adequate intestinal calcium absorption. Inadequate intestinal calcium absorption, particularly in the growing child, leads to a fall in blood ionized calcium concentrations and secondary hyperparathyroidism. Low $1,25(OH)_2D$ levels may contribute to the secondary hyperparathyroidism through the reduction of the suppressive effects of $1,25(OH)_2D$ on parathyroid hormone (PTH) gene transcription. Secondary hyperparathyroidism has a number of effects, which produce the typical biochemical changes seen in vitamin D deficiency. Through its actions on the kidney, urinary calcium excretion is decreased, and renal tubular phosphate loss is increased, reducing the tubular reabsorption of phosphate (TRP) and TmP/GFR. As a consequence of the increased phosphate loss, serum phosphate levels are typically reduced, despite an increase in phosphate release from bone. Increased bone resorption, which occurs through the indirect effect of PTH to increase both osteoclast numbers and activity, leads to osteopenia. Although $1,25(OH)_2D$ has effects on osteoblast differentiation and osteoclast precursors, it is thought that the major osseous features of vitamin D deficiency rickets and osteomalacia are as a result of the effects of hypocalcemia and hypophosphatemia on bone mineralization and of the effects of secondary hyperparathyroidism on bone turnover.

Clinical Features. The clinical features of rickets are more rapid in onset and generally of a more severe nature than those of osteomalacia, which may take several years to manifest. Although the features of rickets characteristically manifest as deformities of the skeletal system, other organ systems, such as the muscular and immune systems, are involved as well. In the young infant, symptoms and signs of hypocalcemia (tetany, apneic episodes, stridor, or convulsions) may be the only features.

The skeletal features in the infant and young child include skull abnormalities, such as a delay in closure of the anterior fontanelle, softening of the skull bones leading to craniotabes, and parietal and frontal bossing giving the hot-cross bun appearance. Chest deformities include enlargement of the costochondral junctions leading to the rachitic rosary, indrawing of the lower ribs at the sites of attachment of the diaphragm resulting in the Harrison's sulcus, and narrowing of the lateral diameter of the chest (violin case deformity). The softening of the ribs and enlargement of the costochondral junctions in association with muscular hypotonia and the inability to clear secretions may lead to severe respiratory distress and an increase in the severity and frequency of lower respiratory tract infections.[5] Weight bearing leads to deformities of the long bones and the characteristic enlargement of the growth plates, especially palpable at the wrist and knee. Deformities of the long bones depend on the stresses placed on the bones, such that in the young infant bowing of the distal radius and ulna and anterior bowing of the tibia may occur. In the toddler, exaggeration of the normal bow-legs (varus deformity) is frequent, while in the older child, knock-knees (valgus deformity) or mixed valgus and varus deformities of the legs (windswept deformity) may occur. Long standing rickets may result in deformities of the pelvis with narrowing of the pelvic outlet with resultant increased risk of obstructed labor in females later in life. Minimal trauma fractures of the long bones may occur, particularly in the young infant and in the elderly with osteomalacia. Bone pain is often a feature in severe rickets/osteomalacia, which in the older patient may be confused with arthritis. Delay in the eruption of permanent dentition, and enamel hypoplasia of both primary and secondary teeth may occur.

Muscular hypotonia may be pronounced, resulting in a delay in gross motor milestones, while in older children and adults with osteomalacia, proximal muscle weakness may result in difficulties in getting out of chairs and climbing stairs. A waddling gait may also be present.

Although in vitro studies clearly show a role for $1,25(OH)_2D$ in immune modulation,[6] there are few studies which have documented impaired immunity in subjects with vitamin D deficiency.[7]

Laboratory Investigations. The typical biochemical features of vitamin D deficiency rickets/osteomalacia are hypocalcemia, hypophosphatemia, and elevated PTH and alkaline phosphatase values. Although serum calcium and phosphorus values may occasionally be within the normal reference range for age before treatment, once treatment has commenced, values tend to rise. Serum 25-hydroxyvitamin D (25OHD) levels are typically lower than normal, with the majority of patients having values below 5 ng/ml (12.5 nM). These low levels of 25OHD are a hallmark of vitamin D deficiency and help to differentiate the latter from other causes of rickets/osteomalacia. The measurement of serum $1,25(OH)_2D$ levels is not particularly helpful in differentiating the various causes of nutritional rickets/osteomalacia because values may be low, normal, or elevated. Markers of bone turnover reflect the increased activity associated with secondary hyperparathyroidism. Urine calcium excretion is typically low, while the TRP and TmP/GFR are decreased. A generalized aminoaciduria and/or bicarbonaturia is also present.

Radiological Findings. The radiographic changes associated with rickets can develop very rapidly, which is different from those of osteomalacia, which may take years to become radiographically apparent. The classical features of rickets occur at the growth plates of long bones and are best seen at the distal end of the radius and ulna or at the tibial and femoral growth plates around the knee. The features at the growth plate include widening of the physis with fraying, cupping and splaying of the metaphyses (Fig. 1), and

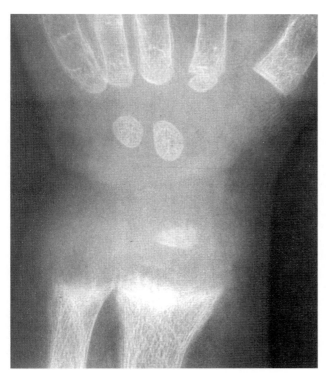

FIG. 1. X-ray of the wrist of an infant with vitamin D deficiency rickets. Note the widened growth plate, the fraying and splaying of the distal metaphyses of the radius and ulna, the poor developed ulna epiphysis, and the coarsening and sparseness of the metaphyseal trabeculae.

underdevelopment of the epiphysis. The earliest sign at the wrist is considered to be a loss of the clear demarcation between the growth plate and the metaphysis with loss of the provisional zone of calcification. The diaphyses of the long bones appear osteopenic and may show thinning of the cortices with periosteal new bone formation. Looser zones, which manifest as short radiolucent lines through the cortex perpendicular to the shaft, are typical of osteomalacia, although they may be seen rarely in other metabolic bone diseases. They are most frequently noted in the medial cortices of the femurs and in the pelvis and ribs. Because of the secondary hyperparathyroidism, the trabecular pattern of the metaphyses becomes coarse and sparse.

In adults with osteomalacia, the most common feature is that of osteopenia, which may be confused with osteoporosis. Only rarely may Looser zones be noted to suggest the diagnosis of osteomalacia. Thus, unlike the typical picture of rickets in children, osteomalacia in adults is difficult to diagnose radiographically and requires biochemical, and often, histological confirmation.[8]

Treatment. The mainstay of treatment is the provision of vitamin D (D_2 or D_3) to correct the vitamin deficiency. In infants and young children, vitamin D drops, 5000–15,000 IU/day (125–375 μg) for 1–2 months, effectively raise 25OHD levels to normal and correct serum calcium, phosphorus, and PTH values usually within 2–3 weeks, although the elevated alkaline phosphatase values and radiological abnormalities take longer to return to normal. An early radiographic sign of healing is the appearance of the provi-

sional zone of calcification at the boundary between the physis and metaphysis, which appears as a well-defined sclerotic line. Older children and adults may be treated on a similar regimen, but compliance is probably better if a weekly dose of vitamin D 50,000 IU (1.25 mg) is taken orally for several months. In some countries, a single oral or intramuscular dose of vitamin D 600,000 IU (15 mg) is preferred. There is no indication for or advantage in using one of the vitamin D metabolites, 25OHD or 1,25(OH)$_2$D, or the vitamin D analog, 1α-hydroxycholecalciferol, for the treatment of simple nutritional vitamin D deficiency. However, the metabolites may be more effective in the management of vitamin D deficiency resulting from intestinal malabsorption syndromes.[9] In this situation, ultraviolet irradiation of the skin may also be effective.

Calcium supplements may also be recommended in the initial stages of management especially if dietary calcium intakes are poor, and advice on ensuring a dietary calcium intake near to the adequate intake or RDA for age should be given. Initially symptomatic hypocalcemia may require parenteral calcium administration to correct the symptoms.

Prevention. Despite the availability of cheap and effective means of preventing vitamin D deficiency, it remains a public health problem in a number of countries in specific age or cultural groups. It is these groups that need to be targeted with educational messages, and possibly, vitamin D supplementation. Table 1 lists the recommended dietary intakes for vitamin D in the United Kingdom and North America. It should be noted that in both countries, higher intakes are recommended in the elderly to compensate for possible decreased sun exposure, decreased dermal synthesis of vitamin D, and decreased responsiveness of the small intestine to vitamin D. In the United Kingdom, infants under 6 months of age also have higher dietary recommendations, because it is assumed that sunlight exposure is limited and that exclusively breastfed infants receive little vitamin D from breast milk.[10] The United Kingdom also recommends that all breastfed infants should receive vitamin D supplements, while the American Academy of Pediatrics suggests only that at-risk infants should be considered for supplementation. In countries, such as in the Middle East and Turkey, where vitamin D deficiency is prevalent among mothers, it makes sense to supplement the mother during

TABLE 1. RECOMMENDED VITAMIN D INTAKES IN THE UNITED KINGDOM AND NORTH AMERICA

Age	UK recommended nutrient intake (μg/d)[44]	U.S./Canadian adequate intake (μg/d)[45]
0–6 months	8.5	5
7 months–3 years	7	5
4–50 years	0*	5
50+ years	10 (61+ years)	10 (51–70 years)
		15 (71+ years)
Pregnancy and lactation	10	5

* The United Kingdom believes that healthy ambulatory persons should be able to obtain their vitamin D requirement from sunlight exposure.

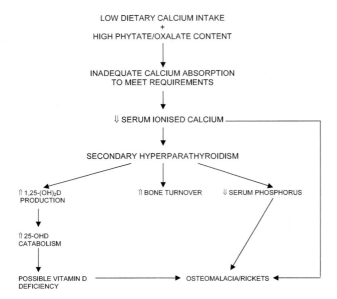

LOW DIETARY CALCIUM INTAKE
+
HIGH PHYTATE/OXALATE CONTENT
↓
INADEQUATE CALCIUM ABSORPTION
TO MEET REQUIREMENTS
↓
⇓ SERUM IONISED CALCIUM
↓
SECONDARY HYPERPARATHYROIDISM

⇑ 1,25-(OH)₂D PRODUCTION   ⇑ BONE TURNOVER   ⇓ SERUM PHOSPHORUS

⇑ 25-OHD CATABOLISM

POSSIBLE VITAMIN D DEFICIENCY   OSTEOMALACIA/RICKETS

FIG. 2. The pathogenesis of rickets/osteomalacia caused by dietary calcium deficiency.

pregnancy to provide the breastfed newborn with stores of vitamin D and to reduce the incidence of neonatal hypocalcemia.[1] Although a daily supplement of 400 IU (10 µg) vitamin D is highly effective in preventing rickets in infants and young children, in situations where compliance may be a problem, intermittent high doses of vitamin D (100,000 IU [2.5 mg] every 3 months) have been shown to be successful.[11] Vitamin D supplementation should also be considered in the infirm and elderly because normal food sources and the limited sun exposure are generally insufficient to meet the vitamin D requirements of these groups.

Dietary Calcium Deficiency

Over the past 20 or so years, growing interest has been shown in the role of low dietary calcium intakes in the pathogenesis of rickets in children. In the 1970s, a few isolated reports appeared of sick infants on highly modified low-calcium diets developing rickets that responded to calcium supplements.[12] More recently, studies from South Africa,[13] Nigeria,[14] and Bangladesh[15] have suggested that dietary calcium deficiency may be a major cause of rickets in children outside the infant age group living in developing countries. Characteristically, the children live in tropical or subtropical climates and are thus exposed to adequate amounts of sunshine. They consume a diet that is very low in calcium (estimated at ≈200 mg calcium daily, or about 20% of the recommended dietary allowance), is relatively monotonous, contains almost no dairy products, and is high in phytates and oxalates.

Pathogenesis. It is suggested that the low dietary calcium intake, often exacerbated by a high oxalate and phytate content that impairs intestinal calcium absorption, is unable to meet the demands of the growing skeleton. This results in a fall in serum ionized calcium concentration, which in turn, stimulates secondary hyperparathyroidism and a cascade of

biochemical changes similar to those described in vitamin D deficiency (Fig. 2). Dietary calcium deficiency may also affect vitamin D metabolism through stimulation of 1,25(OH)₂D production, which itself, in turn, leads to an increase in the catabolism of 25OHD. In situations of relative vitamin D insufficiency, this increased catabolism of 25OHD may precipitate vitamin D deficiency. Such increased catabolism of 25OHD has been proposed as the pathogenesis of the high prevalence of rickets in the Asian community in the United Kingdom.[16] There is some evidence that a similar mechanism may be important in the pathogenesis of rickets in black infants and toddlers. It is important to point out that isolated dietary calcium deficiency and vitamin D deficiency are at the two ends of the pole as far as the pathogenesis of nutritional rickets is concerned; in between these two poles are combinations of the two causes, such that vitamin D sufficiency may be converted to vitamin D deficiency by low dietary calcium intakes, and vitamin D insufficiency may precipitate dietary calcium deficiency by preventing optimal calcium absorption.[17] It is likely that many cases of nutritional rickets have a combination of these two deficiencies to varying degrees in their pathogenesis.

Clinical Presentation. Although calcium deficiency rickets has been described in young infants, this is the exception, as the majority of young infants are fed breast milk or milk formulas, which are good calcium sources. Calcium deficiency rickets typically occurs after the weaning period, when calcium intakes fall as a result of the low calcium content of traditional diets of many communities in developing countries. In Nigeria, the mean age of presentation is around 4 years, although the onset of symptoms may have occurred several years earlier.[18] In South Africa, the mean age of presentation is older, around 8 years. The typical presentation is that of progressive lower limb deformities (bow-legs, knock-knees, or windswept deformities; Fig. 3). The other features of rickets tend to be less pronounced than in vitamin D deficiency, although rachitic rosaries and enlarged wrists are useful clinical signs.[19] In the Nigerian study, delayed motor milestones were noted by the parents.[18] In the South African children, one of the striking differences between vitamin D deficiency and dietary calcium deficiency was noted to be the absence of muscle weakness in the calcium deficiency group.[20]

Laboratory Investigations and Radiological Features. The biochemical features of dietary calcium deficiency are very similar to those of vitamin D deficiency (i.e., hypocalcemia, variable hypophosphatemia, and elevated alkaline phosphatase and PTH values). However, the distinguishing features relate to differences in vitamin D status. In typical dietary calcium deficiency, serum 25OHD values are within the normal range (>10 ng/ml [>25 nM]), and 1,25-(OH)₂D values are elevated, as would be expected in response to hypocalcemia.

The radiographic features of dietary calcium deficiency rickets are similar to those described for vitamin D deficiency with growth plate changes, osteomalacia, and features of secondary hyperparathyroidism (Fig. 4).

the affected communities. However, the use of locally available foods, such as ground dried fish with its bones, or the addition of limestone to the food, might be beneficial.

Phosphate Deficiency

Isolated nutritional phosphate deficiency is an uncommon cause of rickets/osteomalacia because phosphorus is ubiquitous in foods, and the usual dietary intake of phosphate meets the recommended dietary allowances in most situations. However, such mineral deficiency may occur in the breastfed, very low birth weight (VLBW) infant,[21] during prolonged parenteral nutrition in sick patients,[22] and in patients on prolonged antacid therapy.[23] It should be noted that low serum phosphate levels may be a major contributing factor to the pathogenesis of rickets/osteomalacia caused by vitamin D deficiency. However, in that situation, phosphate depletion is dependent on secondary hyperparathyroidism that arises in response to impaired intestinal calcium absorption.

Pathogenesis. Phosphate deficiency induced by either dietary insufficiency or reduced intestinal absorption results in a fall in serum phosphate levels in association with increased renal reabsorption of phosphate (increased TRP or

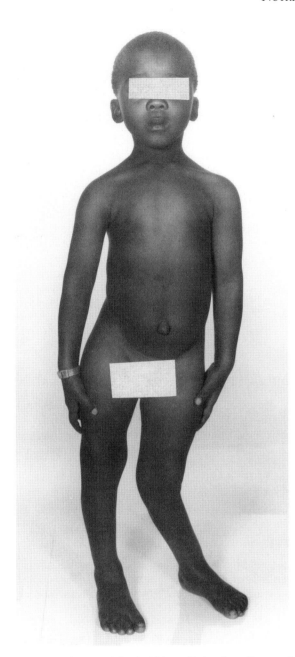

FIG. 3. A girl from rural South Africa suffering from dietary calcium deficiency rickets with windswept deformities of the legs.

Treatment. A number of studies have documented the effectiveness of oral calcium supplements (1000 mg/day for 6 months) without supplemental need for vitamin D in the treatment of dietary calcium deficiency rickets.[14] However, in communities in which it is unclear whether vitamin D insufficiency is playing a role or not, it is prudent to add vitamin D supplements to the regimen.

Prevention. In developing countries, where dietary calcium deficiency is prevalent, prevention of the disease by increase in the consumption of calcium rich foods may be problematic, because dairy products are often scarce and too expensive for

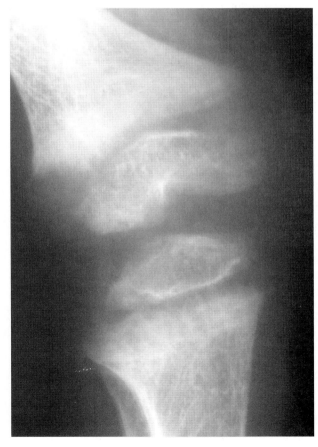

FIG. 4. X-rays of the knee of a child with dietary calcium deficiency. The changes are similar to those described in vitamin D deficiency with widening of the growth plates and splaying and fraying of the metaphyses.

© 2003 American Society for Bone and Mineral Research

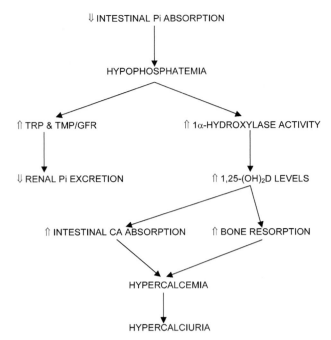

⇓ INTESTINAL Pi ABSORPTION

↓

HYPOPHOSPHATEMIA

⇑ TRP & TMP/GFR   ⇑ 1α-HYDROXYLASE ACTIVITY

⇓ RENAL Pi EXCRETION   ⇑ 1,25-(OH)₂D LEVELS

⇑ INTESTINAL CA ABSORPTION   ⇑ BONE RESORPTION

HYPERCALCEMIA

HYPERCALCIURIA

FIG. 5. The pathogenesis of the biochemical abnormalities in phosphate deficiency rickets/osteomalacia.

TmP/GFR). Hypophosphatemia stimulates renal 1α-hydroxylase with a consequent increase in serum 1,25(OH)$_2$D levels, which lead to increased bone resorption and intestinal calcium absorption and hypercalciuria (Fig. 5). Unlike vitamin D deficiency, PTH levels and vitamin D status are normal in phosphate depletion syndromes. Hypophosphatemia results in impaired bone mineralization and the development of rickets and osteomalacia.

Clinical Presentation and Laboratory Investigations. Metabolic bone disease is a common problem in very low birth weight preterm infants. It typically manifests between 6 and 12 weeks postnatally and has been estimated to occur radiologically in over 50% of infants with birth weights <1000 g, and in over 20% of those weighing <1500 g. The disease is most common in those infants who are breast milk or soy formula fed, or in those who have had prolonged illnesses requiring periods of parenteral nutrition, corticosteroid, or diuretic administration. The clinical manifestations vary from a picture of mildly undermineralized bones to severe rickets with multiple fractures and deformities, which, if involving the ribs, may be severe enough to lead to respiratory distress. The biochemical changes associated with the development of the disease include a rise in alkaline phosphatase levels and the development of hypophosphatemia (<1.8 mM). It is difficult to give a cut-off value for alkaline phosphatase because different assays are used by various laboratories, but a value greater than 7-fold that of the adult normal is highly suggestive of rickets in the preterm infant. Urine phosphate excretion is reduced, whereas urine calcium excretion is increased.

The clinical picture and biochemical abnormalities in prolonged parenteral nutrition are very similar to those described above. The reasons for the development of metabolic bone disease relate to the difficulty in providing adequate amounts of calcium and phosphorus in TPN solutions. These problems have been largely overcome in the newer parenteral nutrition solutions.

Treatment. Although the pathogenesis of metabolic bone disease in very low birth weight infants is multifactorial, the major factor seems to be an inadequate intake of phosphate.

Soy-based formulas should be avoided, because their phosphorus content is generally less readily available, and if VLBW infants are fed breast milk, then breast milk fortifiers, which increase the Ca and Pi content of the intake (among other nutrients) should be provided until the infant is ready for discharge from hospital. An oral Pi intake of ≈120 mg/kg/day should be achieved. An adequate vitamin D intake of 200 IU/kg/day should also be ensured.[24]

Metabolic bone disease as a consequence of total parenteral nutrition should be treated by providing adequate amounts of Ca and Pi in the intravenous solutions. Furthermore, vitamin D sufficiency should also be maintained.

DRUG-INDUCED RICKETS/OSTEOMALACIA

The causes of drug-induced rickets/osteomalacia may be divided into three large groups: those that primarily result in hypocalcemia, those that primarily cause hypophosphatemia, and those that have a direct effect on the mineralization process. Drugs or medications may cause rickets/osteomalacia through each of the three mechanisms described above (Table 2).

Drugs Resulting in Hypocalcemia

Drugs that inhibit the production or intestinal absorption of vitamin D or interfere with its metabolism or action on its target organs may all produce hypocalcemia and consequent rickets/osteomalacia.

TABLE 2. CAUSES OF DRUG-INDUCED RICKETS/OSTEOMALACIA

Drugs resulting in hypocalcemia
  Inhibitors of vitamin D formation or intestinal absorption
    Sunscreens
    Cholestyramine
  Increased catabolism of vitamin D or its metabolites
    Anticonvulsants
Drugs resulting in hypophosphatemia
  Inhibitors of intestinal phosphate absorption
    Aluminum-containing antacids
  Impaired renal phosphate reabsorption
    Cadmium
    Ifosfamide
    Saccharated ferric oxide
Direct impairment of mineralization
  Parenteral aluminum
  Fluoride
  Etidronate

Sunscreens. With the increasing concern about the adverse effects of sunlight and particularly UV irradiation on the skin among the general public, sunscreen usage has become more prevalent. The extensive use of these products may impair vitamin D_3 formation in the skin, resulting in vitamin D deficiency rickets/osteomalacia, particularly in those subjects whose vitamin D status might normally be marginal. Recently rickets in children has been reported to be as a consequence of the use of sunscreens in the United Kingdom.[25]

Cholestyramine. Similarly, impairment of vitamin D absorption from the gastrointestinal tract may also lead to osteomalacia as has been reported with the prolonged use of cholestyramine, an anion exchange resin used to bind bile salts in the gut in post-ileectomy diarrhea.[26]

Anticonvulsants. A number of drugs have been described to interfere with the normal metabolism of vitamin D to 25OHD and $1,25(OH)_2D$, leading to alterations in calcium homeostasis and rickets/osteomalacia by increasing the catabolism of vitamin D and its metabolites through inducing hepatic cytochrome P450 enzymes. These include a number of anticonvulsants (phenobarbitone, phenytoin, and carbamazepine).[27] Phenytoin has been shown to have direct effects on decreasing calcium absorption and increasing bone resorption as well. The development of rickets/osteomalacia is more common in those subjects on anticonvulsant therapy who have limited exposure to sunlight, such as those who are institutionalized[28] or handicapped, where the prevalence has been reported to be as high as 60%. Severe convulsions or spastic cerebral palsy may result in frequent long-bone fractures in such situations.

Typically, the biochemical abnormalities include hypocalcemia, low 25OHD levels, and elevated alkaline phosphatase and PTH values. It is unclear what the prevalence of anticonvulsant associated bone disease is in ambulatory patients, because some studies have shown little effect of anticonvulsants on calcium homeostasis.[29] The disturbances in calcium homeostasis can be prevented or rapidly corrected by the use of vitamin D supplements (up to 4000 IU [100 μg] per day), although alkaline phosphatase levels may remain elevated, especially in phenobarbitone-treated subjects through induction of hepatic enzymes.

Drugs Resulting in Hypophosphatemia

Drugs may induce hypophosphatemia by either impairing phosphate absorption from the gastrointestinal tract or by increasing phosphate loss from the kidney.

Inhibitors of Intestinal Phosphate Absorption. As has been discussed earlier in this chapter, phosphate deficiency through an inadequate dietary intake is very unlikely to occur as phosphate is found ubiquitously in the diet. An important exception to this is found in the breastfed VLBW infant, because breast milk contains inadequate phosphate, and possibly calcium, to meet the demands of the very rapidly growing infant during the first several months of life.

Aluminum-Containing Antacids. Inadequate intestinal phosphate absorption may occur through the inhibition of its absorption through the long-term use of aluminum-containing antacids, which bind phosphate, thereby making it unavailable for absorption. The milk-alkali syndrome is characterized by clinical features of hypophosphatemia (muscle weakness and rickets/osteomalacia) and by hypercalcemia, elevated alkaline phosphatase levels, and normal PTH values but elevated $1,25(OH)_2D$ levels. Typically, such patients have a history of consuming large quantities of aluminum-containing antacids, often with the consumption of milk to manage chronic dyspeptic symptoms. Aluminum given parenterally over a prolonged period of time also causes osteomalacia, but the mechanism is thought to be different from that of oral aluminum administration (see Impaired Mineralization). Phosphate depletion as a result of antacid ingestion can be effectively treated by removing the aluminum-containing antacids. Provision of oral Pi supplements may also be considered until the bone disease responds (clinical improvement in bone pain and muscle weakness, elevation of serum phosphorus values, and a fall in alkaline phosphatase concentrations).

Impaired Renal Phosphate Reabsorption. A number of heavy metals, such as cadmium,[30] and drugs, such as ifosfamide[31,32] and saccharated ferric oxide,[33] have been implicated in causing rickets/osteomalacia through damage to renal tubular function.

Cadmium. Cadmium exposure leads to Itai-Itai disease, which was first described in Japan.[34] The pathogenesis of the osteoporosis and osteomalacia in the disease is not completely elucidated, but cadmium exposure has been shown to lead to permanent damage to glomerular and tubular function, leading to low molecular proteinuria with the excretion of β_2-microglobulin, phosphaturia, and progressive renal failure. Hypophosphatemia and reduced levels of $1,25(OH)_2D$ are characteristic of the disease. Whether cadmium's direct effects on osteoclast and osteoblast function are important in the pathogenesis of the disease are unclear.

Ifosfamide. Ifosfamide, a chemotherapeutic agent used in the treatment of solid tumors, has been reported to produce a renal Fanconi syndrome and hypophosphatemic rickets/osteomalacia, particularly in children, although the complication has also been noted in adults.[31,32]

Saccharated Ferric Oxide. Prolonged intravenous use of saccharated ferric oxide (SFO) for the treatment of iron deficiency anemia causes reversible proximal renal tubular damage, hypophosphatemia, and depressed $1,25(OH)_2D$ levels, leading to osteomalacia.[33] SFO is also thought to inhibit mineralization directly. Cessation of therapy and the use of oral phosphate supplements correct the biochemical and histological abnormalities.

Impairment of Mineralization

A number of agents are known to produce rickets/osteomalacia through direct inhibition of mineralization at the mineralization front in bone and in the growth plate cartilage. These include aluminum,[35] fluoride,[36] and etidronate, a first generation bisphosphonate.[37]

Aluminum. The mechanism by which parenterally acquired aluminum causes rickets/osteomalacia is different from that associated with the oral use of aluminum containing antacids in subjects with normal renal function (see earlier section). The two major conditions, in which aluminum accumulation may occur, are total parenteral nutrition and hemodialysis. In both situations, the aluminum is acquired through contamination of the total parenteral nutrition or hemodialysis fluids. Aluminum may also accumulate through the use of aluminum phosphate binders in patients with impaired renal function. Aluminum inhibits PTH release and 1α-hydroxylase activity. Furthermore, it seems to have direct effects on bone, inhibiting osteoblastic activity and preventing mineralization of preformed osteoid. The net result of all these effects is the production of an adynamic bone disease, or a low bone turnover osteomalacia/rickets.[38] The severity of the bone disease correlates with the extent of stainable aluminum at the bone surfaces. With the increased awareness of the importance of aluminum contamination as a cause of bone disease in patients receiving total parenteral nutrition or hemodialysis, regulations have been introduced to reduce the contamination.[35] This has been assisted by the removal of casein hydrolysates as the protein source in total parenteral nutrition solutions. Furthermore, aluminum-based phosphate binding agents have been replaced by the use of calcium based oral medications, or other resins, in renal failure patients. Aluminum bone disease may respond to the use of deferoxamine, a chelating agent.

Fluoride. The attention of researchers in the developed world has been focused on the toxic effects of fluoride on bone since the introduction of oral fluoride as an experimental drug for the treatment of osteoporosis.[39] However, in a number of developing countries, such as India, South Africa, and Kenya, which have areas of endemic fluorosis, the harmful effects of the excessive ingestion of fluoride have been known for many years.[40] Fluoride is incorporated in the newly formed hydroxyapatite crystal at the mineralization front, where it stabilizes the crystal and prevents its dissolution; furthermore, it stimulates osteoblastic activity but also inhibits mineralization. The mineralization defect is aggravated by low dietary calcium intakes. Although there is good evidence that fluoride therapy increases vertebral bone density, there is no good evidence that it reduces fracture rates in osteoporosis.[39]

Endemic fluorosis, following the long-term ingestion of water with fluoride contents of between 3 and 16 ppm, is associated with the insidious onset of generalized bone pain, stiffness, rigidity, and limitation of movement at the spine and the development of crippling deformities.[41] In children, endemic genu valgum and clinical features of rickets

have been described.[42,43] Radiographically, osteosclerosis and irregular osteophyte formation are noted in the spine with calcification of the intervertebral ligaments. The pelvis also shows osteosclerotic changes with calcification of the sacrotuberous and sacroiliac ligaments. Similarly, interosseous membrane calcification is noted in the forearms and lower limbs. In children, features of rickets at the growth plate and osteomalacia with Looser zones may be noted. Histologically, widened osteoid seams, mineralization defects, poorly mineralized new bone formation, and features of increased bone turnover have been described together with areas of hypermineralization.

Etidronate. The bisphosphonates have become established therapeutic agents in the management of osteoporosis, Paget's disease, and hypercalcemia of malignancy, among other generalized bone conditions. However, they are all analogs of pyrophosphate, an endogenous inhibitor of mineralization. Etidronate, the first bisphosphonate to be approved for clinical use, has been shown to induce impaired mineralization at high doses (20 mg/kg).[37] At lower doses, the incidence of osteomalacia was reduced markedly but was still evident in biopsy specimens. The newer generations of bisphosphonates do not appear to have the same side effects and have been used extensively in the management of osteoporosis without evidence of impairing mineralization.

REFERENCES

1. Andiran N, Yordam N, Ozon A 2002 Risk factors for vitamin D deficiency in breast-fed newborns and their mothers. Nutrition **18:**47–50.
2. Kreiter SR, Schwartz RP, Kirkman HN Jr, Charlton PA, Calikoglu AS, Davenport ML 2000 Nutritional rickets in African American breast-fed infants. J Pediatr **137:**153–157.
3. Sedrani SH 1986 Are Saudis at risk of developing vitamin D deficiency? Saudi Med J **7:**427–433.
4. Harris NS, Crawford PB, Yangzom Y, Pinzo L, Gyaltsen P, Hudes M 2001 Nutritional and health status of Tibetan children living at high altitudes. N Engl J Med **344:**341–347.
5. Muhe L, Luiseged S, Mason KE, Simoes EAF 1997 Case-control study of the role of nutritional rickets in the risk of developing pneumonia in Ethiopian children. Lancet **349:**1801–1804.
6. DeLuca HF, Cantorna MT 2001 Vitamin D: Its role and uses in immunology. FASEB J **15:**2579–2585.
7. Lorente F, Fontan G, Jara P, Casas C, Garcia-Rodriguez MC, Ojeda JA 1976 Defective neutrophil motility in hypovitaminosis D rickets. Acta Paediatr Scand **65:**695–699.
8. Parfitt AM 1997 Vitamin D and the pathogenesis of rickets and osteomalacia. In: Feldman D, Glorieux FH, Pike JW (eds.) Vitamin D. Academic Press, San Diego, CA, USA, pp. 645–662.
9. Basha B, Rao DS, Han ZH, Parfitt AM 2000 Osteomalacia due to vitamin D depletion: A neglected consequence of intestinal malabsorption. Am J Med **108:**296–300.
10. Specker BL, Tsang RC, Hollis BW 1985 Effect of race and diet on human-milk vitamin D and 25-hydroxyvitamin D. Am J Dis Child **139:**1134–1137.
11. Zeghoud F, Ben-Mekhbi H, Djeghri N, Garabedian M 1994 Vitamin D prophylaxis during infancy: Comparison of the long-term effects of three intermittent doses (15, 5, or 2.5 mg) on 25-hydroxyvitamin D concentrations. Am J Clin Nutr **60:**393–396.
12. Kooh SW, Fraser D, Reilly BJ, Hamilton JR, Gall D, Bell L 1977 Rickets due to calcium deficiency. N Engl J Med **297:**1264–1266.
13. Marie PJ, Pettifor JM, Ross FP, Glorieux FH 1982 Histological osteomalacia due to dietary calcium deficiency in children. N Engl J Med **307:**584–588.
14. Thacher TD, Fischer PR, Pettifor JM, Lawson JO, Isichei CO, Reading

JC, Chan GM 1999 A comparison of calcium, vitamin D, or both for nutritional rickets in Nigerian children. N Engl J Med 341:563–568.

15. Fischer PR, Rahman A, Cimma JP, Kyaw-Myint TO, Kabir AR, Talukder K, Hassan N, Manaster BJ, Staab DB, Duxbury JM, Welch RM, Meisner CA, Haque S, Combs GF Jr 1999 Nutritional rickets without vitamin D deficiency in Bangladesh. J Trop Pediatr 45:291–293.

16. Clements MR 1989 The problem of rickets in UK Asians. J Hum Nutr Diet 2:105–116.

17. Pettifor JM 1994 Privational rickets: A modern perspective. J Roy Soc Med 87:723–725.

18. Thacher TD, Fischer PR, Pettifor JM, Lawson JO, Isichei C, Chan GM 2000 Case-control study of factors associated with nutritional rickets in Nigerian children. J Pediatr 137:367–373.

19. Thacher TD, Fischer PR, Pettifor JM 2002 The usefulness of clinical features to identify active rickets. Ann Trop Paediatr 22:229–237.

20. Pettifor JM 1991 Dietary calcium deficiency. In: Glorieux FH (ed.) Rickets. Raven Press, New York, NY, USA, pp. 123–143.

21. Backstrom MC, Kuusela AL, Maki R 1996 Metabolic bone disease of prematurity. Ann Med 28:275–282.

22. Klein GL, Chesney RW 1986 Metabolic bone disease associated with total parenteral nutrition. In: Lebenthal E (ed.) Total Parenteral Nutrition: Indication, Utilization, Complications, and Pathophysiological Considerations. Raven Press, New York, NY, USA, pp. 431–443.

23. Pivnick EK, Kerr NC, Kaufman RA, Jones DP, Chesney RW 1995 Rickets secondary to phosphate depletion. A sequela of antacid use in infancy. Clin Pediatr (Phila) 34:73–78.

24. Backstrom MC, Maki R, Kuusela AL, Sievanen H, Koivisto AM, Ikonen RS, Kouri T, Maki M 1999 Randomised controlled trial of vitamin D supplementation on bone density and biochemical indices in preterm infants. Arch Dis Child 80:F161–F166.

25. Zlotkin S 1999 Vitamin D concentrations in Asian children living in England. Limited vitamin D intake and use of sunscreens may lead to rickets. BMJ 318:1417.

26. Compston JE, Horton LW 1978 Oral 25-hydroxyvitamin D_3 in the treatment of osteomalacia associated with ileal resection and cholestyramine therapy. Gastroenterology 74:900–902.

27. Hahn TJ, Hendin BA, Scharp CR, Haddad JG 1972 Effect of chronic anticonvulsant therapy on serum 25-hydroxycalciferol levels in adults. N Engl J Med 287:900–904.

28. Bischof F, Basu D, Pettifor JM 2002 Pathological long-bone fractures in residents with cerebral palsy in a long-term care facility in South Africa. Dev Med Child Neurol 44:119–122.

29. Ala-Houhala M, Korpela R, Koivikko M, Koskinen T, Koskinen M,

Koivula T 1986 Long-term anticonvulsant therapy and vitamin D metabolism in ambulatory pubertal children. Neuropediatrics 17:212–216.

30. Berglund M, Akesson A, Bjellerup P, Vahter M 2000 Metal-bone interactions. Toxicol Lett 112–113:219–225.

31. Kintzel PE 2001 Anticancer drug-induced kidney disorders. Drug Saf 24:19–38.

32. Garcia AA 1995 Ifosfamide-induced Fanconi syndrome. Ann Pharmacother 29:590–591.

33. Sato K, Shiraki M 1998 Saccharated ferric oxide-induced osteomalacia in Japan: Iron-induced osteopathy due to nephropathy. Endocr J 45:431–439.

34. Jarup L 2002 Cadmium overload and toxicity. Nephrol Dial Transplant 17:35–39.

35. Klein GL 1995 Aluminum in parenteral solutions revisited–again. Am J Clin Nutr 61:449–456.

36. Kleerekoper M 1996 Fluoride and the skeleton. Crit Rev Clin Lab Sci 33:139–161.

37. Silverman SL, Hurvitz EA, Nelson VS, Chiodo A 1994 Rachitic syndrome after disodium etidronate therapy in an adolescent. Arch Phys Med Rehabil 75:118–120.

38. Tannirandorn P, Epstein S 2000 Drug-induced bone loss. Osteoporos Int 11:637–659.

39. Haguenauer D, Welch V, Shea B, Tugwell P, Adachi JD, Wells G 2000 Fluoride for the treatment of postmenopausal osteoporotic fractures: A meta-analysis. Osteoporos Int 11:727–738.

40. Mithal A, Trivedi N, Gupta SK, Kumar S, Gupta RK 1993 Radiological spectrum of endemic fluorosis: Relationship with calcium intake. Skeletal Radiol 22:257–261.

41. Teotia SPS, Teotia M 1984 Endemic fluorosis in India: A challenging national health problem. J Assoc Physicians India 32:347–352.

42. Krishnamachari KAVR, Sivakumar B 1976 Endemic genu valgum: A new dimension to the fluorosis in India. Fluoride 9:185–200.

43. Pettifor JM, Schnitzler CM, Ross FP, Moodley GP 1989 Endemic skeletal fluorosis in children: Hypocalcemia and the presence of renal resistance to parathyroid hormone. Bone Miner 7:275–288.

44. Department of Health 1998 Nutrition and Bone Health, Report on Health and Social Subjects, vol. 49. The Stationary Office, London, UK, pp. 114–115.

45. Standing Committee on the Scientific Evaluation of Dietary Reference Intakes, Food and Nutrition Board, Institute of Medicine 1997 Vitamin D. In: Dietary Reference Intakes for Calcium, Phosphorus, Magnesium, Vitamin D, and Fluoride. National Academy Press, Washington, DC, USA, pp. 250–281.

Chapter 69.   Vitamin D–Dependent Rickets

Uri A. Liberman[1] and Stephen J. Marx[2]

[1]Felsenstein Medical Research Center, Department of Physiology and Pharmacology, Sackler School of Medicine, Tel Aviv University, Tel Aviv, Israel; and [2]Metabolic Diseases Branch, National Institute of Diabetes and Digestive and Kidney Diseases, National Institutes of Health, Bethesda, Maryland

INTRODUCTION

Vitamin D–dependent rickets (VDDR) types I and II are rare inborn errors of vitamin D metabolism, characterized by all of the classical clinical, radiologic, biochemical, and histological features of vitamin D deficiency, despite adequate vitamin D intake and without a therapeutic response to an accepted vitamin D–replacement therapy. The two syndromes differ (Table 1) in the circulating concentration of 1,25-dihydroxyvitamin D [1,25(OH)$_2$D], the therapeutic response to 1α-hydroxylated active vitamin D metabolites,

and obviously, in the primary defect in vitamin D metabolism.

VDDR TYPE I

Prader et al.[1] in 1961 were the first to report two young children with VDDR-I and coin the phrase "pseudovitamin D deficiency" to describe this syndrome. The disease manifests itself before 2 years of age and often during the first 6 months of life. Complete remission could be obtained but was dependent on continuous therapy with high doses of vitamin D. Family studies revealed this to be a genetic disorder with autosomal recessive inheritance,[2] and link-

The authors have no conflict of interest.

TABLE 1. VITAMIN D–DEPENDENT RICKETS

| | Serum concentrations | | | | |
	Calcium	25(OH)D	1,25(OH)$_2$D	IPTH	Presumed defect
VDDR-I	↓	N- ↓	↓↓	↑	Renal 25(OH)D-1-hydroxylase
VDDR-II	↓	N- ↓	N- ↑	↑	Intracellular 1,25(OH)$_2$D receptor

age analysis assigned the gene responsible for the disease to chromosome 12q13.[3]

The gene encoding the 25(OH)D-1α-hydroxylase of mouse kidney, human keratinocyte, and peripheral mononuclear cells was localized on chromosome 12q 13.1–13.3, which maps to the disease locus of VDDR-I.[4–9] There are no direct measures of the renal enzyme proving defective 1α-hydroxylase activity. There are several indirect observations to support this etiology. First, circulating levels of 25(OH)D are normal or elevated, depending on previous vitamin D treatment. Second, serum concentrations of 1,25(OH)$_2$D are very low. Third, while massive doses (100–300 times the daily recommended dose) of vitamin D or 25(OH)D are required to maintain remission of rickets, physiological replacement doses of calcitriol are sufficient to achieve the same effect. Fourth, it was reported that cells isolated from the placenta of two women with this disease had deficient activity of the decidual enzyme 25(OH)D-1α-hydroxylase.[10] Finally, the 1α-hydroxylase gene from more than 25 families with VDDR-I and some of their first degree healthy relatives were analyzed by direct sequencing, site-directed mutagenesis, and cDNA expression in transfected cells.[4–9,11] All patients had homozygous mutations, while parents or other healthy siblings were heterozygous for the mutation. Most patients of French-Canadian origin had the same mutation, causing a frameshifting and a premature stop codon in the putative heme-binding domain.[6] The same mutation was observed in additional families of diverse origin.[11] All other patients had either a base-pair deletion causing premature termination codon upstream from the putative ferredoxin and heme-binding domains or missense mutations.[3,6–9,11] No 1α-hydroxylase activity was detected when the mutant enzyme was expressed in various cells. The sequence of the human 1α-hydroxylase gene from keratinocytes and peripheral blood mononuclear cells has recently been shown to be identical with the renal gene,[3,6–9,11] thus supporting the use of these accessible cells as a proxy to study the renal tubular enzymatic defect. Taken together, these observations support the notion that the etiology of this hereditary disease is a defect in the renal tubular 25(OH)D-1α-hydroxylase activity.

The beneficial therapeutic effect of high circulating levels of 25(OH)D in patients with VDDR-I treated with vitamin D or 25(OH)D$_3$ where 1,25(OH)$_2$D concentrations remain low has several possible explanations. First, 25(OH)D at high concentrations may activate the specific intracellular receptor for 1,25(OH)$_2$D, whose affinity with 25(OH)D is about two orders of magnitude lower than for the active hormone. Second, high concentrations of the substrate 25(OH)D may drive the local production of 1,25(OH)$_2$D in some tissues in a paracrine or autocrine manner. Finally, a metabolite of 25(OH)D may act directly on target tissues.

VDDR TYPE II

In 1978, Brooks et al.[12] described a patient with hypocalcemia, osteomalacia, and elevated circulating levels of 1,25(OH)$_2$D. Treatment with vitamin D$_3$ resulted in a further increase in serum 1,25(OH)$_2$D levels and corrected the hypocalcemia of the patient. The term "vitamin D–dependent rickets type II" was suggested to describe this disorder. Based on additional case reports, in which about one-half of the patients with this disorder did not respond to any form of vitamin D therapy and therefore were not dependent on the vitamin, and some in vivo and in vitro studies to be discussed, the term VDDR-II seems to be a misnomer. We therefore suggest the term "hereditary resistance to 1,25(OH)$_2$D" as more appropriate to describe this syndrome. However, because of convention and convenience, the term VDDR-II will be retained in this chapter.

Clinical Manifestations

The clinical, radiologic, histological, and biochemical characteristics common to all patients with VDDR-II are rickets and/or osteomalacia of varying severity; no history or biochemical evidence of vitamin D or calcium deficiency; hypocalcemia and/or secondary hyperparathyroidism; no remission with physiologic doses of vitamin D or its active metabolites; and increased serum levels of 1,25(OH)$_2$D before or during treatment with calciferol preparations.[13]

Patients with VDDR-II show the highest serum levels of 1,25(OH)$_2$D found in any living system. These levels could represent the end result of synergistic action of three potential stimulators of the 25(OH)D-1-hydroxylase, namely, hypocalcemia, secondary hyperparathyroidism, and hypophosphatemia; they might also reflect an additional defect in regulation of the renal hydroxylase.

There are about 60 known kindreds with this syndrome.[12–51] Contrary to the homogeneity of the clinical and biochemical presentation of VDDR-I, a marked heterogeneity exists in VDDR-II.

Affected children appear normal at birth, and the metabolic bone disease presents early, usually before 2 years of age. However, late onset of the disease was reported in several sporadic cases, presenting in some patients in their teens[12]; in one patient, the onset of osteomalacia was at 45 years of age.[16] All cases with late presentation have been normocalcemic, and they represent the mildest form of the disease.

A peculiar feature of the syndrome that appears in about two-thirds of the kindreds is alopecia that varies from sparse hair to total alopecia without eyelashes. In some patients, additional ectodermal anomalies, such as multiple milia, epidermal cysts, and oligodontia, appear as well.[15] The alopecia may be obvious at birth but usually develops during the first months of life. Alopecia seems to be a marker of a more severe form of the disease as judged by the earlier age of the presentation of the disease, the marked clinical aberrations, the number of patients who did not respond to treatment with high doses of vitamin D and metabolites (in contrast to the complete remission achieved in almost all patients with normal hair), and the high levels of serum $1,25(OH)_2D$ recorded during successful and unsuccessful therapy.[29,52] Although some patients with alopecia have a satisfactory calcemic response to high doses of vitamin D and metabolites, none have shown improvement of hair growth.

The notion that total alopecia is probably a direct consequence of resistance to $1,25(OH)_2D$ is supported by the following observations: (1) alopecia is present in kindreds with different biochemical and molecular defects in the $1,25(OH)_2D$ receptor-effector system; (2) high-affinity uptake of $[^3H]1,25(OH)_2D_3$ occurred in the nucleus of the outer root sheath cells of the hair follicle of rodents; and (3) the epidermis and hair follicles contain a calcium-binding protein that is at least partially vitamin D dependent. Alopecia has been observed only with end-organ resistance to $1,25(OH)_2D$ and has not been noted with hereditary or acquired states associated with low-circulating levels of $1,25(OH)_2D$. Thus, either the deficiency in vitamin D action is more severe in VDDR-II, or alternatively, $1,25(OH)_2D$ may have an effect on differentiation of the hair follicle in the fetus that is unrelated to mineral homeostasis.

Parental consanguinity and multiple siblings with the same defect occur in about one-half of the reported kindreds with VDDR-II, suggesting an autosomal recessive mode of inheritance in these and perhaps all kindreds. Parents of patients appear phenotypically normal. However, in vitro studies of cultured cells from parents of some kindreds with VDDR-II revealed heterogeneity of their $1,25(OH)_2D_3$ receptor (VDR), that is, expression of both a normal and an abnormal VDR allele. The affected children expressed only the abnormal allele.[53,54] There is a striking clustering of patients close to the Mediterranean, and most of the patients reported from Europe and North America are descendants of families originating from around the Mediterranean as well. Notable exceptions are several kindreds reported from Japan.[16,18,34]

Classification by Cellular Defect

Studies on the nature of the intracellular defect in the $1,25(OH)_2D$ receptor-effector system of patients with VDDR-II became possible with demonstration that cells originating from tissues easily accessible for biopsy contain receptors for the hormone that are similar if not identical to those of classical target tissues. The cells used are mainly dermal fibroblasts, but keratinocytes, cells derived from bone, and peripheral blood mononuclear (PBM) cells (mitogen-stimulated T-lymphocytes and Epstein–Barr [EB] virus–transformed lymphocytes) have been used as well.[20–23,25,29,33,54–56] These cells are used to assess most of the steps in $1,25(OH)_2D$ action from cellular uptake to bioresponse and to elucidate the molecular aberrations in the hormone receptor protein and the nuclear DNA that encodes for it.[53,54] The latter became feasible with the cloning and sequencing of the human VDR chromosomal gene.

Several methods have been used to characterize the hormone–receptor interaction, including binding capacity and affinity of $[^3H]1,25(OH)_2D_3$ to intact cells, nuclei, or high-salt-soluble extract (cytosol)[57–60]; measurements of receptor content by monoclonal antibodies with radiological immunoassay or Western blot analysis[53,61,62]; and characterization of the hormone–receptor complex on continuous sucrose gradient and heterologous DNA-cellulose columns.[21,29,30,63] For studies on the molecular defects, isolation, amplification, and sequencing of genomic VDR DNA, as well as cloning and sequencing of VDR cDNA and recreation of the mutant VDR in vitro, have been used. In vitro bioeffects of $1,25(OH)_2D$ on the various cells have been assayed by induction of the 25(OH)D-24-hydroxylase in skin- and bone-derived cells,[24,27,64,65] osteocalcin synthesis in cells derived from bone,[65] inhibition of cell proliferation in PBM cells[33,56] and dermal fibroblasts,[23,66] a mitogenic effect on dermal fibroblasts,[66] and stimulation of cyclic cGMP production in cultured skin fibroblasts.[67]

Heterogeneity of the cellular and molecular defects of the vitamin D receptor-effector system had been revealed in studies of different kindreds with VDDR-II. However, based on the hormone–receptor–nuclear interaction, three different classes of intracellular defects have been identified.

1. Hormone binding defects. These include the following. (1) Markedly decreased capacity (number of binding sites was about 10% of controls) in one patient, who did not respond to prolonged treatment with high doses of active calciferol metabolites.[24] (2) Decreased hormone binding affinity. $[^3H]1,25(OH)_2D_3$ binding affinity is reduced 20- to 30-fold with normal binding capacity of soluble (cytosolic) dermal fibroblasts extract. A complete remission of the disease in these patients could be achieved by high doses of vitamin D or its active metabolites.[31,45] An additional patient had a modest decrease of the affinity of the receptor for $1,25(OH)_2D_3$ when measured at 0°C and a substantial decrease in affinity of approximately 8-fold when the binding was measured at 24°C. A missense point mutation in the VDR gene encoding the hormone binding domceine was elucidated.[45] (3). No hormone binding. Immeasurable specific binding of $[^3H]1,25(OH)_2D_3$ to either high-salt-soluble cell extract and/or intact cells or nuclei. Studies in several kindreds with this defect (including an extended kindred with eight patients studied) revealed undetectable levels of VDR by immunoblots on an immunoradiometric assay in most kindreds.[49,57,61,62,68] This is the most common abnormality observed. In the majority of these patients, high concentrations of $1,25(OH)_2D$ in serum or culture medium did not evoke a biological or biochemical re-

sponse in vivo or in vitro. Different point mutations in the DNA region transcribing the hormone binding domain of VDR were described.[57,61,62] In five affected kindreds, the nucleotide substitution resulted in a stop codon in the coding sequence (which was different for each kindred), thus causing a truncated receptor having no or only a nonfunctional part of the hormone binding site of the VDR. In an additional patient a missense mutation resulted in the substitution of arginine by leucine.[57] It is of interest that in a cotransfection assay, normal transcription could be induced in the presence of 1000-fold higher levels of the hormone than were needed for the wild-type VDR. This may indicate that the mutation caused an extreme decrease in the affinity of the receptor to $1,25(OH)_2D_3$. Recently, two siblings without alopecia and no response to any dose of $1,25(OH)_2D$ in vivo and in vitro were described.[49] These patients had a missense mutation that caused a substitution of tryptophan by arginine at amino acid 286 of the VDR. This substitution in a normal size VDR abolished completely the binding of $1,25(OH)_2D$ to its receptor. The tryptophan in this position is critical for the positioning of calcitriol in the VDR; this was unveiled recently by the three-dimensional arrangement of the VDR and its ligand based on its crystal structure.[58]

2. Deficient nuclear localization. Normal or near-normal binding affinity and capacity of $[^3H]1,25(OH)_2D_3$ binding to soluble cell extract. Normal binding to heterologous DNA but immeasurable localization of $[^3H]1,25(OH)_2D_3$ to nuclei in intact cells.[20,25,38,41] An identical defect was demonstrated with cells cultured from a bone biopsy of one patient[20] and in mitogen-stimulated PBM cells from several kindreds.[34] These patients were treated successfully with high doses of vitamin D and its active metabolites.[13,20,38,41] No mutation was found on sequencing VDR cDNA of some of these patients.[62] However, recently, two DDII unrelated patients were described with a lowered $1,25(OH)_2D_3$ retention in intact cell incubated at 37°C. Two different point mutations leading to impaired heterodimerization with a retinoid X receptor (RXR) were demonstrated. The magnitude of the defect, the response in vivo to the hormone, and in vitro to $1,25(OH)_2D_3$ and RXR were different between these two missense mutations.[41] The fact that no mutation in the VDR coding region was observed in three additional kindreds with the same phenotypical defect may suggest that the genetic defect affects another component of the receptor effector system that is essential for the VDR function as a nuclear transcription factor. It has been recently shown that coactivation complexes are essential for the ligand induced transactivation of VDR.[69] Very recently, a patient with hereditary resistance to $1,25(OH)_2D$ without alopecia was described in abstract form. Sequencing of the VDR DNA revealed a missense mutation in the ligand-binding domain that caused a substitution of glutamic acid to lysine at amino acid 120. This receptor exhibits many normal properties including calcitriol binding, dimerization, and binding to vitamin D response elements in the DNA. However, a marked impairment in binding coactivators

that are essential for the transactivation of the hormone receptor complex and the initiation of the physiological response was observed.[51]

3. There is normal or near-normal $[^3H]1,25(OH)_2D_3$ binding to soluble cell extract and to nuclei of intact cells, but decreased affinity of the hormone–receptor complex to heterologous DNA.[30,54,63] No biological response to high doses of vitamin D or its active metabolites either in vivo or in vitro was documented in almost all patients with this type of defect.[15,30,63] A single nucleotide missense mutation within exon 2 or 3 encoding the DNA binding domain of the VDR was demonstrated in genomic DNA isolated from fibroblasts and/or EB virus-transformed lymphocytes from members from eight unrelated kindreds with this defect.[36,54,55,70] Different single-nucleotide mutations were found with the exception of two unrelated patients that share the same defect. All mutations caused a single amino acid substitution localized to the region of the two zinc fingers of the vitamin D receptor protein. This region is essential for DNA binding of the hormone–receptor complex. It is worthwhile mentioning that the DNA binding domain of the VDR is evolutionarily highly conserved throughout all members of the v-ERB-A–related proteins that include the receptors for steroid hormones, thyroid hormones, and retinoic acid. A mouse model of the disease was created by targeted ablation of the second zinc finger of the VDR-DNA binding domain. Homozygous mice who were phenotypically normal at birth, developed hypocalcemia, secondary hyperparathyroidism, rickets, osteomalacia, and alopecia, with normal survival to at least 6 months.[71] Supplementation with a calcium-enriched diet can prevent or treat most of the disturbances in mineral and bone metabolism in these animal models except alopecia.[59] It is of interest that targeting expression of the human VDR to keratinocytes of VDR null mice prevented alopecia.[72]

IN VITRO POST-TRANSCRIPTIONAL AND TRANSCRIPTIONAL EFFECT OF $1,25(OH)_2D_3$

In vitro bioeffects of the hormone on various cells in patients with hereditary resistance to $1,25(OH)_2D$ have been assayed mainly by two procedures: induction of 25(OH)D-24-hydroxylase and inhibition of mitogen-stimulated PBM cells. $1,25(OH)_2D_3$ induces 25(OH)D-24 hydroxylase activity in skin-derived fibroblasts,[21–24,27,30–32,38,40,47–51,54,55,59,65,68,70] mitogen-stimulated lymphocytes,[73] and cells originating from bone[74] in a dose-dependent manner. In cells from normal subjects, maximal and half-maximal induction of the enzyme was achieved by 10^{-8} and 10^{-9} M concentrations of $1,25(OH)_2D_3$, respectively. Dermal fibroblast or PBM cells from patients with no calcemic response to maximal doses of vitamin D or its metabolites in vivo did not show any 25(OH)D-24-hydroxylase response to very high concentrations of $1,25(OH)_2D_3$ in vitro, whereas dermal fibroblasts from patients with a calcemic response to high doses of vitamin D or its metabolites in vivo showed inducible 24-hydroxylase with supraphysiological concentrations of $1,25(OH)_2D_3$ in vitro. Physiological concentrations of $1,25(OH)_2D_3$ partially inhibit mitogen-induced DNA synthesis in peripheral lymphocytes with a half-maximal inhibition achieved at 10^{-10} M of the hormone.[33,56] Mitogen-stimulated lymphocytes from several kindreds with defects characterized as no hormone binding or deficient binding to DNA, with no calcemic response to high doses of vitamin D and its metabolites in vivo, showed no inhibition of lymphocyte proliferation in vitro with concentrations of up to 10^{-6} M $1,25(OH)_2D_3$. Additional methods to measure bioeffects of $1,25(OH)_2D_3$ on various cells in vitro were carried out only in few patients and included inhibition of dermal fibroblasts proliferation,[24] induction of osteocalcin synthesis in cells derived from bone,[65] a mitogenic effect on dermal fibroblasts,[66] and stimulation of cGMP production in cultured skin fibroblasts.[67] It is noteworthy that, in all assays mentioned without exception, each patient's cell showed severely deficient responses.

Cellular Defects and Clinical Features

Normal hair was described with most phenotypes of the cellular defects the exception being patients with deficient hormone binding capacity and affinity, but this could be because of the fact that only one or two kindreds were described per subgroup. Normal hair is usually associated with a milder form of the disease, as judged by the age of onset, severity of the clinical features, and usually the complete clinical and biochemical remission on high doses of vitamin D or its metabolites. Notable exceptions are three kindreds (four patients), two of them described only recently, without alopecia that displayed resistance both in vivo (no clinical remission on circulating calcitriol level up to 100 times the mean normal adult values) and in vitro [no induction of 25(OH)D-24-hydroxylase activity in dermal fibroblasts by up to 10^{-8} M $1,25(OH)_2D_3$].[32,49,51] Only approximately one-half of the patients with alopecia have shown satisfactory clinical and biochemical remission to high doses of vitamin D or its active 1α-hydroxylated metabolites, but the dose requirement is ~10-fold higher than in patients with normal hair.[52]

It seems that patients' defects characterized as deficient hormone binding affinity and deficient nuclear uptake achieve complete clinical and biochemical remission on high doses of vitamin D or its active 1α-hydroxylated metabolites. Most of the patients with other types of defects could not be cured with high doses of vitamin D or its metabolites. However, it should be emphasized that not all of the patients received treatment for a long enough period of time and with sufficiently high doses (see Treatment).

Diagnosis

Clinical features of early onset rickets with no history of vitamin D deficiency, total alopecia, parental consanguinity, additional siblings with the same disease, serum biochemistry of hypocalcemic rickets, elevated circulating levels of $1,25(OH)_2D$, and normal to high levels of 25(OH)D (Table 1) support the diagnosis of hereditary resistance to $1,25(OH)_2D$. The issue becomes more complicated when the clinical features are atypical (i.e., late onset of the disease, sporadic cases, and normal hair). Failure of a therapeutic trial with calcium and/or physiological replacement doses of vitamin D or its metabolites may support the diagnosis, but the final direct proof requires the demonstration of a cellular, molecular, and functional defect in the VDR-effector system.

Treatment

In about one-half of the kindreds with VDDR-II [hereditary resistance to $1,25(OH)_2D$], the bioeffects of $1,25(OH)_2D_3$ were measured in vitro. An invariable correlation (with one exception) was documented between the in vitro effect and the therapeutic response in vivo—that is, patients with no calcemic response to high levels of serum calcitriol showed no effects of $1,25(OH)_2D_3$ on their cells in vitro [either induction of 25(OH)D-24-hydroxylase or inhibition of lymphocyte proliferation] and vice versa. If the predictive therapeutic value of the in vitro cellular response to $1,25(OH)_2D_3$ could be substantiated convincingly, it may eliminate the need for time-consuming and expensive therapeutic trials with massive doses of vitamin D or its active metabolites. In the meantime, it is mandatory to treat every patient with this disease irrespective of the type of receptor defect.

An adequate therapeutic trial must include vitamin D at a dose that is sufficient to maintain high serum concentrations of $1,25(OH)_2D_3$ because the patients can produce high hormone levels if supplied with enough substrate. If high serum calcitriol levels are not achieved, it is advisable to treat with 1α-hydroxylated vitamin D metabolites in daily doses of up to 6 μg/kg weight, or a total of 30–60 μg, and calcium supplementation of up to 3 g of elemental calcium daily; therapy must be maintained for a period sufficient to mineralize the abundant osteoid (usually 3–5 months). Therapy may be considered a failure if no change in the clinical, radiological, or biochemical parameters occurs during continuous and frequent follow-up while serum $1,25(OH)_2D$ concentrations are maintained at ~100 times the mean normal range.

In some patients with no response to adequate therapeutic trials with vitamin D or its metabolites, a remarkable clinical and biochemical remission of their bone disease, including catch-up growth, was obtained by treatment with large amounts of calcium. This was achieved by long-term (months) intracaval infusions of up to 1000 mg of calcium daily.[39,49,60,65,75] Another way to increase calcium input into the extracellular compartment is to increase net gut absorption, independent of vitamin D, by increasing calcium intake.[76] This approach is limited by dose and patient tolerability and was actually used successfully in only one patient.

CONCLUSION

In summary, two inborn errors in vitamin D metabolism are presented and discussed. The important message is not just the description of a rare curiosity of nature but rather the finding that rare aberrations of natural metabolic processes are important to unveil basic physiologic, biochemical, and molecular mechanisms in general and in humans in particular.

© 2003 American Society for Bone and Mineral Research

REFERENCES

1. Prader A, Illig R, Heierli E 1961 Eline besondere Form der primaren vitamin D-resistenten Rachitis mit Hypocalcemie und autosomal-dominanten Erbgang: Die hereditare Psuedo-Mangelrachi tis. Helv Paediatr Acta **16:**452–468.
2. Fraser D, Kooh SW, Kind P, Tanaka Y, DeLuca HF 1973 Pathogenesis of hereditary vitamin D-dependent rickets: An inborn error of metabolism involving defective conversion of 25-hydroxyvitamin D to 1α, 25-dihydroxy-vitamin D. N Engl J Med **289:**817–822.
3. Labuda M, Morgan K, Glorieux FH 1990 Mapping autosomal recessive vitamin D-dependency Type I to chromosome 12q14 by linkage analysis. Am J Hum Genet **46:**28–36.
4. Fu GK, Lin D, Zhang MY, Bikle DD, Shackleton CH, Miller WL, Portale AA 1997 Cloning of human 25-hydroxyvitamin D1α-hydroxylase and mutations causing vitamin D-dependent rickets type 1. Endocrinology **11:**1961–1970.
5. St. Arnaud R, Messerlian S, Moir JM, Omdahl JL, Glorieux FH 1997 The 25-hydroxyvitamin D₃-1α-hydroxylase gene maps to the pseudovitamin D deficiency rickets (PDDR) disease locus. J Bone Miner Res **12:**1552–1559.
6. Wang JT, Lin CJ, Burridge SM, Fu GK, Labuda M, Portale AA, Miller WL 1998 Genetics of vitamin D 1α-hydroxylase deficiency in 17 families. Am J Hum Genet **63:**1694–1702.
7. Yoshida T, Monkawa T, Tenenhouse HS, Goodyear P, Shinki T, Suda T, Wakino S, Hayashi M, Saruta T 1998 Two novel 1α-hydroxylase in French-Canadians with vitamin D dependency rickets type II. Kidney Int **54:**1437–1443.
8. Kitanaka S, Takeyama K, Murayama A, Sato T, Okumura K, Nogami M, Hasegawa Y, Niimi H, Yanagisawa J, Tanaka T, Kato S 1998 Inactivating mutations in the 25-hydroxyvitamin D₃ 1α-hydroxylase gene in patients with pseudovitamin D-deficiency rickets. N Engl J Med **338:**653–661.
9. Kitanaka S, Murayama A, Sakaki T, Inoue K, Seino Y, Fukumoto S, Shima M, Yukizane S, Takayanagi M, Niimi H, Takeyama K, Kato S 1999 No enzyme activity of 25-hydroxyvitamin D₃ 1α-hydroxylase gene product in pseudovitamin D-deficiency rickets with mild clinical manifestation. J Clin Endocrinol Metab **84:**4111–4117.
10. Glorieux FH, Arabian A, Delvin EE 1995 Pseudo-vitamin D deficiency: Absence of 25-hydroxyvitamin D 1α-hydroxylase activity in human placenta decidua cells. J Clin Endocrinol Metab **80:**2255–2258.
11. Smith SJ, Rucka AK, Berry JL, Davies M, Mylchreest S, Paterson CR, Heath DA, Tassabehji M, Read AP, Mee AP, Mawer EB 1999 Novel mutations in the 1α-hydroxylase (P450c1) gene in three families with pseudovitamin D-deficiency rickets resulting in loss of functional enzyme activity in blood derived macrophages. J Bone Miner Res **14:**730–739.
12. Brooks MH, Bell NH, Love L, Stern PH, Ordei E, Queener SJ 1978 Vitamin D dependent rickets type II resistance of target organs to 1,25-dihydroxyvitamin D. N Engl J Med **293:**996–999.
13. Marx SJ, Spiegel AM, Brown EM, Gardner DG, Downs RW Jr, Attie M, Hamstra AJ, DeLuca HF 1978 A familial syndrome of decrease in sensitivity of 1,25-dihydroxyvitamin D. J Clin Endocrinol Metab **47:**1303–1310.
14. Rosen JF, Fleischman AR, Fineberg L, Hamstra A, DeLuca HF 1979 Rickets with alopecia: An inborn error of vitamin D metabolism. J Pediatr **94:**729–735.
15. Liberman UA, Samuel R, Halabe A, Kauli R, Edelstein S, Weisman Y, Papapoulos SE, Clemens TL, Fraher LJ, O'Riordan JLH 1980 End-organ resistance to 1,25-dihydroxy cholecalciferol. Lancet **1:**504–506.
16. Fujita T, Nomura M, Okajima S, Suzuya H 1980 Adult-onset vitamin D-resistant osteomalacia with unresponsiveness to parathyroid hormone. J Clin Endocrinol Metab **50:**927–931.
17. Sockalsosky JJ, Westrom RA, DeLuca HF, Brown DM 1980 Vitamin D-resistant rickets: End-organ unresponsiveness to 1,25(OH)₂D₃. J Pediatr **96:**701–703.
18. Tauchiya Y, Matsuo N, Cho H, Kumagai M, Yasaka A, Suda T, Orimo H, Shiraki M 1980 An unusual form of vitamin-D-dependent rickets in a child: Alopecia and marked end-organ hyposensitivity to biological active vitamin D. J Clin Endocrinol Metab **51:**685–690.
19. Bear S, Tieder M, Kohelet D, Liberman UA, Vine E, Bar-Joseph G, Gabizon D, Borochowitz ZU, Varon M, Modai D 1981 Vitamin D resistant rickets with alopecia: A form of end-organ resistance to 1,25-dihydroxyvitamin D. Clin Endocrinol (Oxf) **14:**395–402.
20. Eil C, Liberman UA, Rosen JF, Marx SJ 1981 A cellular defect in hereditary vitamin D-dependent rickets type II: Defective nuclear uptake of 1,25-dihydroxyvitamin D in cultured skin fibroblasts. N Engl J Med **304:**1588–1591.
21. Feldman D, Chen T, Cone C, Hirst M, Shari S, Benderli A, Hochberg Z 1982 Vitamin D resistant rickets with alopecia: Cultured skin fibroblasts exhibit defective cytoplasmic receptors and unresponsiveness to 1,25(OH)₂D₃. J Clin Endocrinol Metab **55:**1020–1025.
22. Balsan A, Garabedian M, Liberman UA, Eil C, Bourdeau A, Guillozo H, Grimberg R, DeDeunff MJ, Lieberherr M, Guimbaud P, Broyer M, Marx SJ 1983 Rickets and alopecia with resistance to 1,25-dihydroxyvitamin D: Two different clinical courses with two different cellular defects. J Clin Endocrinol Metab **57:**824–830.
23. Clemens TL, Adams JC, Horiuchi N, Gilchrist BA, Cho H, Ysuchiya Y, Matsuo N, Suda T, Holick MJ 1983 Interaction of 1,25-dihydroxyvitamin D3 with keratinocytes and fibroblasts from skin of a subject with vitamin D-dependent rickets type II: A model for the study of action of 1,25-dihydroxyvitamin D3. J Clin Endocrinol Metab **56:**824–830.
24. Griffin JE, Zerwekh JE 1983 Impaired stimulation of 25-hydroxyvitamin D-24-hydroxylase in fibroblasts from a patient with vitamin D-dependent rickets, type II. J Clin Invest **72:**1190–1199.
25. Liberman UA, Eil C, Marx SJ 1983 Resistance to 1,25-dihydroxyvitamin D: Association with heterogeneous defects in cultured skin fibroblasts. J Clin Invest **71:**192–200.
26. Malloy PJ, Weisman Y, Feldman D 1994 Hereditary 1 alpha, 25-dihydroxyviamin D-resistant rickets resulting from a mutation in the vitamin D receptor deoxyribonucleic acid-binding domain. J Clin Endocrinol Metab **78:**313–316.
27. Chen TL, Hirst MA, Cone CM, Hochberg Z, Tietze HU, Feldman D 1984 1,25-Dihydroxyvitamin D resistance, rickets and alopecia: Analysis of receptors and bioresponse in cultured skin fibroblasts from patients and parents. J Clin Endocrinol Metab **59:**383–388.
28. Hochberg Z, Benderli Z, Levy J, Weisman Y, Chen T, Feldman D 1984 1,25-Dihydroxyvitamin D resistance, rickets and alopecia. Am J Med **77:**805–811.
29. Marx SJ, Liberman UA, Eil C, Gamblin GT, DeGrange DA, Balsan S 1984 Hereditary resistance to 1,25-dihydroxyvitamin D. Recent Prog Horm Res **40:**589–620.
30. Hirst MA, Hochman HI, Feldman D 1985 Vitamin D resistance and alopecia: A kindred with normal 1,25-dihydroxy-vitamin D3 binding but decreased receptor affinity for deoxyribonucleic acid. J Clin Endocrinol Metab **60:**490–495.
31. Castells S, Greig F, Fusi MA, Finberg L, Yasumura S, Liberman UA, Eil C, Marx SJ 1986 Severely deficient binding of 1,25-dihydroxyvitamin D to its receptor in a patient responsive to high doses of this hormone. J Clin Endocrinol Metab **63:**252–256.
32. Fraher LJ, Karmali R, Hinde FRJ, Hendy GN, Jani H, Nicholson L, Grant D, O'Riordan JLH 1986 Vitamin D-dependent rickets type II: Extreme end organ resistance to 1,25-dihydroxyvitamin D3 in a patient without alopecia. Eur J Pediatr **145:**389–395.
33. Takeda E, Kuzoda T, Saijo T, Toshima K, Naito E, Kobashi H, Iwakuni Y, Miyao M 1986 Rapid diagnosis of vitamin D-dependent rickets type II by use of phyto-hemagglutinin-stimulated lymphocytes. Clin Chim Acta **155:**245–250.
34. Takeda E, Kuroda Y, Saijo T, Naito E, Kobashi H, Yokota I, Miyao M 1987 1 alpha-hydroxyvitamin D3 treatment of three patients with 1,25-dihydroxyvitamin D-receptor-defect rickets and alopecia. Pediatrics **80:**97–101.
35. Takeda E, Yokota I, Kawakami I, Hashimoto TT, Kuroda Y, Arase S 1989 Two siblings with vitamin D-dependent rickets type II: No recurrence of rickets for 14 years after cessation of therapy. Eur J Pediatr **149:**54–57.
36. Saijo T, Ito M, Takeda E, Mahbubul Huq AHM, Naito E, Yokota I, Sine T, Pike JW, Kuroda Y 1991 A unique mutation in the vitamin D receptor gene in three Japanese patients with vitamin D-dependent rickets type II: Utility of single-strand conformation polymorphism analysis for heterozygous carrier detection. Am J Hum Genet **49:**668–673.
37. Simonin G, Chabrol B, Moulene E, Bollini G, Strouc S, Mattei JF, Giraud F 1992 Vitamin D resistant rickets type II: Apropos of 2 cases. Pediatrics **47:**817–820.
38. Hewison M, Rut AR, Kristjansson K, Walker RE, Dillon MJ, Hughes MR, O'Riordan JLH 1993 Tissue resistance to 1,25-dihydroxyvitamin D without a mutation of the vitamin D receptor gene. Clin Endocrinol (Oxf) **39:**663–670.
39. Lin JP, Uttley WE 1993 Intraatrial calcium infusions, growth and development in end-organ resistance to vitamin D. Arch Dis Child **69:**689–692.
40. Yagi H, Ozono K, Miyake H, Nagashima K, Kuroume T, Pike JW 1993 A new point mutation in the deoxyribonucleic acid-binding domain of the vitamin D receptor in a kindred with hereditary 1,25-

dihydroxyvitamin D resistant rickets. J Clin Endocrinol Metab **76:** 509–512.

41. Whitfield GK, Selznick SH, Haussler CA, Hsieh JC, Galligan MA, Jurutka PW, Thompson PD, Lee SM, Zerwekh JE, Haussler MR 1996 Vitamin D receptors from patients with resistance to 1,25-dihydroxyvitamin D_3: Point mutations confer reduced transactivation in response to ligand and impaired intereaction with the retinoid X receptor heterodimeric partner. Mol Endocrinol **10:**1617–1631.
42. Lin Nu-T, Malloy PJ, Sakati N, Al-Ashwal A, Feldman D 1996 A novel mutation in the deoxyribonucleic acid-binding domain of the vitamin D receptor causes hereditary 1,25-dihydroxyvitamin D resistant rickets. J Clin Endocrinol Metab **81:**2564–2569.
43. Hawa NS, Cockerill FJ, Vadher S, Hewison M, Rut AR, Pike JW, O'Riordan JLH, Farrow SM 1996 Identification of a novel mutation in hereditary vitamin D resistant rickets causing exon skipping. Clin Endocrinol (Oxf) **45:**85–92.
44. Mechica JB, Leite MOR, Mendoca BB, Frazzatto EST, Borelli A, Latronico AC 1997 A novel nonsense mutation in the first zinc finger of the vitamin D receptor causing hereditary 1,25-dihydroxyvitamin D resistant rickets. J Clin Endocrinol Metab **82:**3892–3894.
45. Malloy PJ, Eccleshall TR, Gross C, van Maldergem L, Bouillion R, Feldman D 1997 Hereditary vitamin D resistant rickets caused by a novel mutation in the vitamin D receptor that results in decreased affinity for hormone and cellular hyporesponsiveness. J Clin Invest **99:**297–304.
46. Cockerill FJ, Hawa NS, Yousaf N, Hewison M, O'Riordan JFL, Farrow SM 1997 Mutations in the vitamin D receptor gene in three kindreds associated with hereditary vitamin D resistant rickets. J Clin Endocrinol Metab **82:**3156–3160.
47. Zhu WJ, Malloy PJ, Delvin E, Chabot G, Feldman D 1998 Hereditary 1,25-dihydroxyvitamin D-resistant rickets due to an opal mutation causing premature termination of the vitamin D receptor. J Bone Miner Res **13:**259–264.
48. Malloy PJ, Zhu W, Zhao XY, Pehling GB, Feldman D 2001 A novel inborn error in the ligand-binding domain of the vitamin D receptor causes hereditary vitamin D-resistant rickets. Mol Genet Metab **73:**138–148.
49. Nguyen TM, Adiceam P, Kottler ML, Guillozo M, Rizk-Rabin F, Brouillard F, Lagier P, Palix C, Garnier JM, Garabedian M 2002 Tryptophan missense mutation in the ligand-binding domain of the vitamin D receptor causes severe resistance to 1,25-dihyroxyvitamin D. J Bone Miner Res **17:**1728–1737.
50. Malloy PJ, Pike JW, Feldman D 1999 The vitamin D receptor and the syndrome of hereditary 1,25-dihydroxyvitamin D-resistant rickets. Endocr Rev **20:**156–188.
51. Malloy DJ, Xu R, Peng L, Clark PA, Feldman D 2002 A novel mutation in helix 12 of the VDR impairs coactivator interaction and causes hereditary 1,25-dihydroxyvitamin D-resistant rickets without alopecia. J Bone Miner Res **17:**S1;S216.
52. Marx SJ, Bliziotes MM, Nanes M 1986 Analysis of the relation between alopecia and resistance to 1,25-dihydroxyvitamin D. Clin Endocrinol (Oxf) **25:**373–381.
53. Malloy PJ, Hochberg Z, Pike JW, Feldman D 1989 Abnormal binding of vitamin D receptors to deoxyribonucleic acid in a kindred with vitamin D dependent rickets type II. J Clin Endocrinol Metab **68:**263–269.
54. Hughes MR, Malloy PJ, Kieback DG, Kesterson RA, Pike JW, Feldman D, O'Malley BW 1988 Point mutations in the human vitamin D receptor gene associated with hypocalcemic rickets. Science **242:**1702–1705.
55. Sone T, Marx SJ, Liberman UA, Pike JW 1990 A unique point mutation in the human vitamin D receptor chromosomal gene confers hereditary resistance to 1,25-dihydroxyvitamin D3. Mol Endocrinol **4:**623–631.
56. Koren R, Ravid A, Liberman UA, Hochberg Z, Weisman J, Novogrodsky A 1985 Defective binding and functions of 1,25-dihydroxyvitamin D3 receptors in peripheral mononuclear cells of patients with end-organ resistance to 1,25-dihydroxyvitamin D. J Clin Invest **76:**2012–2015.
57. Kristjansson K, Rut AR, Hewison M, O'Riordan JLH, Hughes MR 1993 Two mutations in the hormone binding domain of the vitamin D receptor causes tissue resistance to 1,25-dihydroxyvitamin D_3. J Clin Invest **92:**12–16.
58. Rochel N, Wurtz JM, Mitschler A, Klaholz B, Moras D 2000 The crystal structure of the nuclear receptor for vitamin D bound to its natural ligand. Mol Cell **5:**173–179.
59. Delling G, Demay MB 1998 Normalization of mineral ion homeostasis by dietary means prevents hyperparathyroidism, rickets, and osteomalacia, but not alopecia in vitamin D receptor-ablated mice. Endocrinology **139:**4391–4396.
60. Weisman Y, Bab I, Gazit D, Spirer Z, Jaffe M, Hochberg Z 1987 Long-term intracaval calcium infusion therapy in end-organ resistance to 1,25-dihydroxyvitamin D. Am J Med **83:**984–990.
61. Malloy PJ, Hochberg Z, Tiosano D, Pike JW, Hughes MR, Feldman D 1990 The molecular basis of hereditary 1,25-dihydroxyvitamin D3 resistant rickets in seven related families. J Clin Invest **86:**2017–2079.
62. Weise RJ, Goto H, Prahl JM, Marx SJ, Thomas M, Al-Aqeel A, DeLuca HF 1993 Vitamin D-dependency rickets type II: Truncated vitamin D receptor in three kindreds. Mol Cell.Endocrinol **90:**197–201.
63. Liberman UA, Eil C, Marx SJ 1986 Receptor positive hereditary resistance to 1,25-dihydroxyvitamin D. Chromatography of hormone-receptor complexes on DNA-cellulose shows two classes of mutations. J Clin Endocrinol Metab **62:**122–126.
64. Gamblin GT, Liberman UA, Eil C, Downs RW Jr, DeGrange DA, Marx SJ 1985 Vitamin D-dependent rickets type II, defective induction of 25-hydroxyvitamin D3–24-hydroxylase by 1,25-dihydroxyvitamin D3 in cultured skin fibroblasts. J Clin Invest **75:**954–960.
65. Balsan S, Garabedian M, Larchet M, Gorski AM, Cournot G, Tau C, Bourdeau A, Silve C, Ricour C 1986 Long term nocturnal calcium infusions can cure rickets and promote normal mineralization in hereditary resistance to 1,25-dihydroxyvitamin D. J Clin Invest **77:**1661–1667.
66. Barsony J, McKoy W, DeGrange DA, Liberman UA, Marx SJ 1989 Selective expression of a normal action of 1,25-dihydroxyvitamin D3 receptor in human skin fibroblasts with hereditary severe defects in multiple action of this receptor. J Clin Invest **83:**2093–2101.
67. Barsony J, Marx SJ 1988 A receptor-mediated rapid action of 1α, 25-dihydroxycholecalciferol: Increase of intracellular cyclic GMP in human skin fibroblasts. Proc Natl Acad Sci USA **85:**1223–1226.
68. Ritchie HH, Hughes MR, Thompson ET, Hochberg Z, Feldman D, Pike JW, O'Mally BW 1989 An ochre mutation in the vitamin D receptor gene causes hereditary 1,25-dihydroxyvitamin D3 resistant rickets in three families. Proc Natl Acad Sci USA **86:**9783–9787.
69. Freedman LP 1999 Increasing the complexity of coactivation in nuclear receptor signaling. Cell **97:**5–8.
70. Rut AR, Hewison K, Kristjansson K, Luisi B, Hughes M, O'Riordan JLH 1994 Two mutations causing vitamin D resistant rickets: Modeling on the basis of steroid hormone receptor DNA-binding domain crystal structures. Clin Endocrinol (Oxf) **41:**581–590.
71. Li YC, Piroo AE, Amling M, Delling G, Baron R, Bronson R, Demay MB 1997 Targeted ablation of the vitamin D receptor: An animal model of vitamin D-dependent rickets type II with alopecia. Proc Natl Acad Sci USA **94:**9831–9835.
72. Chen CH, Sakai Y, Demay MB 2001 Targeting expression of the human vitamin D receptor to the keratinocytes of vitamin D receptor null mice prevents alopecia. Endocrinology **142:**5386–5389.
73. Takeda E, Yokota I, Ito M, Kobashi I, Saijo T, Kuroda Y 1990 25-hydroxyvitamin D-24-hydroxylase in phyto-hemagglutinin-stimulated lymphocytes: Intermediate bioresponse to 1,25-dihydroxyvitamin D_3 of cells from parents of patients with vitamin D dependent rickets type II. J Clin Endocrinol Metab **70:**1068–1074.
74. Liberman UA, Eil C, Holst P, Rosen JF, Marx JS 1983 Hereditary resistance to 1,25-dihydroxyvitamin D: Defective function of receptors for 1,25-dihydroxyvitamin D in cells cultured from bone. J Clin Endocrinol Metab **57:**958–962.
75. Bliziotes M, Yergey AL, Nanes MS, Muenzer J, Begley MG, Vieira NE, Kher KK, Brandi ML, Marx SJ 1988 Absent intestinal response to calciferols in hereditary resistance to 1,25-dihydroxyvitamin D: Documentation and effective therapy with high dose intravenous calcium infusions. J Clin Endocrinol Metab **66:**294–300.
76. Sakati N, Woodhouse NTY, Niles N, Harji H, DeGrange DA, Marx SJ 1986 Hereditary resistance to 1,25-dihydroxyvitamin D: Clinical and radiological improvement during high-dose oral calcium therapy. Horm Res **24:**280–287.

Chapter 70. Hypophosphatemic Vitamin D–Resistant Rickets

Francis H. Glorieux

Departments of Surgery, Pediatrics and Human Genetics, McGill University, and Shriners Hospital for Children, Montreal, Quebec, Canada

INTRODUCTION

Bone growth and mineralization require adequate availability of calcium and phosphate, the two major constituents of hydroxyapatite, which is the crystalline part of bone tissue. Defective supply of either calcium or phosphate will result in impaired mineralization, which causes rickets at the growth-plate level and osteomalacia at the corticoendosteal level. Thus, in growing individuals, both lesions will be present, whereas by definition, only osteomalacia can possibly develop in adults.

Deficiency in calcium, as a consequence of insufficient intake,[1] vitamin D simple deficiency, or abnormal metabolism,[2] will induce hypocalcemia, rickets, and osteomalacia. The latter will be characterized by osteopenia as a consequence of the increased resorption induced by hyperparathyroidism secondary to hypocalcemia.

In chronic hypophosphatemia, although clinical and radiologic manifestations of rickets are similar to those seen in calcium deficiency, osteomalacia is characterized by an accumulation of unmineralized osteoid along the trabeculae. Because calcemia is normal, there is no secondary hyperparathyroidism and therefore no increased osteoclast activity or excessive resorption. Consequently, bone mass is not decreased. It is, in fact, often measured above normal values for age.

CLASSIFICATION OF HYPOPHOSPHATEMIC SYNDROMES

There are acquired and congenital forms of hypophosphatemia. In most instances, the acquired forms can be controlled by acting on the underlying causes (insufficient phosphate intake, increased renal loss secondary to a mesenchymal tumor, or an altered tubular function). However, the inherited syndromes present a challenge sometimes for diagnosis and always for management. The most frequent of the hypophosphatemic syndromes was described more than 50 years ago by Albright et al.,[3] who coined the term "hypophosphatemic vitamin D–resistant rickets." It is inherited as an X-linked dominant trait,[4] with the mutant gene being located in the distal part of the short arm of the X chromosome[5]; thus, it is often referred to as X-linked hypophosphatemia (XLH). In 1976, a homologous mutation was discovered in the mouse (hyp).[6] The high degree of conservatism of the mammalian X chromosome and comparative mapping of the human and mouse gonosomes[7] support the contention of a close analogy between the human and murine mutations. Active studies have thus been pursued in parallel in the two species to better understand the phenotypic expression of the abnormal genes. A rarer form of hypophosphatemic rickets, inherited as an autosomal dominant trait (ADHR),[8] has attracted attention lately because of the implication in its pathophysiology of the newly identified fibroblast growth factor (FGF)23.

CLINICAL EXPRESSION

In XLH, the classic triad, fully expressed in hemizygous male patients, consists of (1) hypophosphatemia, (2) lower limb deformities, and (3) stunted growth rate. Although low serum phosphate (Pi) is evident early after birth, it is only at the time of weight bearing that leg deformities and progressive departure from normal growth rate become sufficiently striking to attract attention and make parents seek medical opinion. An often overlooked clinical sign is the appearance of the teeth. There is no enamel hypoplasia in XLH as opposed to what is seen in hypocalcemic rickets. Hypophosphatemic rickets rather presents with dentin defects that are not apparent on examination but that may cause dental abscesses and early decay in the young adult. In several families, isolated hypophosphatemia can be found in some heterozygous female subjects. Thus, this trait is considered the marker for the mutation.[4] These healthy trait carriers provide evidence that hypophosphatemia, and renal Pi waste cannot solely explain the abnormal phenotype. ADHR patients present with isolated renal phosphate waste and a variable degree of clinical severity (incomplete penetrance).[8]

BASIC DEFECT

Several studies based on genetic linkage and multilocus analysis have allowed fine mapping of the *HYP* gene to the Xp22.1–22.2 region of the X chromosome between markers DXS41 and DXS43. Subsequently, a candidate gene was identified.[9] This gene, first called *PEX* and subsequently *PHEX*, codes for a membrane-bound endopeptidase. Further characterization of its full sequence and tissue expression will be needed to dissect its role in phosphate homeostasis. *PHEX* mutations have been identified in a large number of XLH kindreds as well as in patients with no family history.[9,10] The latter point indicates that familial and sporadic cases share a similar etiology. A regularly updated list of *PHEX* mutations can be found on the World Wide Web (www.phexdb.mcgill.ca).

The most intriguing question regarding XLH concerns the primary lesion causing the disease. It has long been accepted that hypophosphatemia is the consequence of a primary inborn error of phosphate transport, probably located in the proximal nephron. It is noteworthy that the defect is less severe in female heterozygotes than it is in

The author has no conflict of interest.

male hemizygotes.[11] This gene-dose effect indicates that the observed defect is close to the abnormal gene product. The abnormality in the *Hyp* mouse has been localized to the brush border of the proximal tubular cells.[12] The possibility that it would be secondary to the presence of a humoral hypophosphatemic factor[13] has received experimental support from kidney cross-transplantation studies in the mouse model.[14]

Because of the close link between the phosphate-repletion status and 1,25-dihydroxyvitamin D [1,25(OH)$_2$D] synthesis, the metabolism of this hormone has been extensively studied in mutant individuals. It is important to point out that there is no simple 1,25(OH)$_2$D deficiency (as seen in vitamin D pseudodeficiency) and that there is no close correlation between extracellular Pi concentration and 1,25(OH)$_2$D synthesis. Rather the reported inappropriate response of 1,25(OH)$_2$D synthesis to a low phosphate challenge,[15] although there is no abnormality in the response to a low calcium challenge,[16] points to the vitamin D metabolism abnormality being secondary to the primary Pi transport defect and its consequences on intracellular Pi economy.

Studies both in humans and mice indicate that defective bone formation in XLH is linked to an intrinsic osteoblast defect. The hypomineralized periosteocytic lesions (HPLs), which are a hallmark of XLH, never completely disappear, even after active mineralization has been restored at the endosteal surfaces. After more than 2 years of efficient therapy, HPLs are still present around 20% of the osteocytes in the newly formed osteons.[17] Because HPLs are never present in other chronic hypophosphatemic states, this observation gives substance to the early proposal that there may be an osteoblast primary metabolic defect in XLH.[18] The lesions are also present in the *Hyp* mouse,[19] in which an abnormal osteoblast response to 1,25(OH)$_2$D has been demonstrated.[20] Studies conducted with osteoblasts isolated from mouse calvaria have provided morphologic evidence that Hyp osteoblasts, even when transplanted in a normal environment, are unable to produce adequate amounts of mineralized matrix.[21] Deletions in the *Phex* gene have been reported in the *Hyp* mouse, which confirms definitely its validity as a model for XLH.[22] It is interesting that *Phex* is predominantly expressed in normal osteoblasts, whereas the transcript is not detectable in Hyp osteoblasts.[23] This suggests that a bone gene product may be part of a pathway that regulates phosphate homeostasis and underscores the central role of an osteoblast defect in the etiology of XLH. Unraveling this mechanism must await the identification of the putative circulating factor, which may be a natural substrate for the PHEX protein. One step into that direction was made by the identification of the molecular basis of ADHR. Econs et al. have demonstrated that the affected individuals carry a mutation in the gene encoding FGF23, a new member of the FGF family.[24] Interestingly, FGF23 was found to be overexpressed in cells cultured from mesenchymal tumors causing severe hypophosphatemic osteomalacia.[25] The recent observations that serum concentrations of FGF23 are elevated in patients with oncogenic osteomalacia (OHO) and in most patients with XLH,[26] allow us to postulate a unifying hypothesis to explain the etiology of the hypophosphatemia in XLH,

ADHR, and OHO.[27] In XLH, the inactivating *PHEX* mutations fail to degrade FGF23, whereas in ADHR, the mutant FGF23 protein is not cleared by *PHEX* because the mutation has abolished a presumptive cleavage site, leading to an excess of FGF23 in the circulation. In contrast, in OHO, overproduction of FGF23 exceeds the capacity of the normal PHEX activity. Thus, in the three syndromes, different mechanisms lead to increased serum concentration of FGF23, supporting the contention that FGF23 is a substrate for PHEX and a major hyperphosphaturic factor. As attractive as it is, this hypothesis has not been proven yet. For instance, when osteoblast specific transgene Phex expression was crossed into the *Hyp* background (in the mouse), it improved the defective mineralization of bone and teeth but did not correct the hypophosphatemia and altered vitamin D metabolism associated with the disorder.[28] Thus, additional factors are likely at play to control the latter two functions.

RESPONSE TO TREATMENT

Based on the established renal Pi waste, therapy has centered on often aggressive Pi replacement (1–3 g elemental Pi/day in four or five doses). To offset the hypocalcemic effect of Pi supplementation, which has sometimes caused severe secondary hyperparathyroidism, large (20,000–75,000 IU/day) amounts of vitamin D were added to the regimen. With adequate compliance to such a combined treatment, growth rate improved markedly, and there was radiologic evidence of healed rickets.[29,30] The early observation that heterozygous girls responded better to treatment than hemizygous boys[29] was substantiated, supporting the concept of a gene-dose effect in this X-linked dominant disorder.[31] However, histological studies of iliac crest bone biopsy specimens showed that the osteomalacic component of the bone disease was hardly improved.[32] It was only by substituting 1,25(OH)$_2$D for vitamin D at the dose of 30–70 ng/kg/day that improvement and sometimes healing of the mineralization defect was observed on the trabecular surfaces.[33–36]

LONG-TERM EFFECTS OF TREATMENT

Except for occasional osmotic diarrhea, Pi supplementation has not caused any harmful effects. Coated tablets are preferred to liquid forms because they provide a slower rate of absorption. Tablets are also made of a mixture of sodium and potassium salts, avoiding the high sodium load so frequent with the solutions.

Before 1978, large amounts of vitamin D were administered to offset the hypocalcemic effect of Pi supplementation and the ensuing iatrogenic hyperparathyroidism. This was often difficult to control, and several cases of autonomous hyperparathyroidism were encountered that could only be treated surgically.[29] The substitution of 1,25(OH)$_2$D for vitamin D has now allowed a more precise control of parathyroid hormone (PTH) secretion throughout the treatment period. It thus appears that 1,25(OH)$_2$D, through its direct effect on PTH release, is able to maintain PTH levels within acceptable limits, together with ensuring adequate bone modeling and remodeling.[35–37] Interestingly, this may also be the case for $24,25(OH)_2D_3$. A placebo-controlled trial based on the addition of the metabolite (10 μg/day) to the standard protocol [$1,25(OH)_2D$ and phosphate] showed that better control of the therapy-induced hyperparathyroidism was achieved over a 2-year period.[38]

One major concern with the long-term administration of $1,25(OH)_2D$ is a possible deterioration of renal function through interstitial nephrocalcinosis. Frequent ultrasound observations of echodense renal pyramids have been reported.[39] Histological studies confirmed that they correspond to mineral deposits exclusively made of calcium phosphate.[40] Whether the induction of such deposits is primarily related to the phosphate load or to the long-term use of $1,25(OH)_2D$ is not clear. Such findings are, however, not directly related to evidence of decreased renal function. Our experience with 18 patients treated for an average of 8 years indicates that two-thirds of them present with profiles of increased echogenicity of the renal pyramids (too quickly labeled nephrocalcinosis), but no alteration of renal function (FH Glorieux, unpublished data, 1998). Thus, long-term use of $1,25(OH)_2D$ associated with supplemental Pi and with frequent monitoring of urinary calcium excretion to avoid episodes of hypercalciuria should be considered a safe and efficient way to control the clinical expression of the *PHEX* mutation. When hypercalciuria develops, adjustment of the $1,25(OH)_2D$ dosage is necessary.

Because stunted growth is a major consequence of the XLH phenotype, the use of recombinant human growth hormone (rhGH), as a third therapeutic component, was also advocated.[41] The hormone increased serum Pi levels, and over a 24-week period, appeared to positively affect growth rate, in 11 XLH children. These results have been substantiated by long-term (2–3 years) studies showing that adding rhGH to phosphate and $1,25(OH)_2D$ had a significant positive effect on growth in young XLH patients.[42,43] These studies have not been extended through the completion of the growth process (closure of the epiphyses), so it is premature to conclude that the basic treatment protocol should be uniformly modified.

TREATMENT OF ADULT PATIENTS

With early initiation of therapy and good compliance throughout the growing period, clinical results are usually satisfactory in terms of stature achieved and prevention of lower-limb deformities. An important question is whether one should maintain the demanding treatment schedule combining $1,25(OH)_2D$ and phosphate, after fusion of the epiphyseal plates. Because growth has ceased and bone turnover is reduced, the appropriateness of maintaining a high phosphate intake can rightly be questioned. The demonstration that, in 18 symptomatic XLH adult patients who received Pi + $1,25(OH)_2D$ for 4 years, the treatment resulted in significant clinical and histomorphometric improvement[44] suggests that such an approach is worthwhile. Its optimal duration, however, remains unresolved. Because strict compliance to Pi supplements on a five-dose per day schedule is difficult, one may envisage that continuing

$1,25(OH)_2D$ alone, through its stimulation of bone turnover and intestinal phosphate absorption, would retain the good results obtained with the combined therapy. Preliminary observations in six XLH patients indicated that $1,25(OH)_2D$ alone (at a dose of 1–2 μg/day) positively influenced the parameters of bone mineralization over an 11- to 17-month period (FH Glorieux, unpublished data, 1992). Such studies should allow better definition of a long-term strategy for metabolic and clinical control of adult XLH patients.

CONCLUSION

Despite the persistent questions about the pathogenesis of hypophosphatemic vitamin D–resistant rickets, medical control of its clinical expression has greatly improved over the last 15 years. The combination of large amounts of phosphate salts and supraphysiological doses of $1,25(OH)_2D$ has allowed normal growth and adequate bone-matrix mineralization. With close and careful follow-up, the regimen is safe, and no deleterious effects on renal function are to be expected. Uncertainty continues with regard to the treatment of asymptomatic adult subjects.

REFERENCES

1. Marie PJ, Pettifor JM, Ross FP, Glorieux H 1982 Histologic osteomalacia due to dietary calcium deficiency in children. N Engl J Med **307:**584–588.
2. Glorieux FH, Pettifor JM 1984 Metabolic bone disease. In: Kelly VC (ed.) Practice of Pediatrics, vol. 7. Harper & Row, New York, NY, USA, pp. 1–17.
3. Albright F, Butler AM, Bloomberg E 1937 Rickets resistant to vitamin D therapy. Am J Dis Child **54:**529–547.
4. Winters RW, Graham JB, Williams TF, McFalls VW, Burnett CH 1958 A genetic study of familial hypophosphatemia and vitamin D resistant rickets with a review of the literature. Medicine (Baltimore) **37:**97–142.
5. Thakker RV, Read AP, Davies KE, Whyte MP, Weksberg R, Glorieux F, Davies M, Mountford RC, Harris R, King A 1987 Bridging markers defining the map position of X-linked hypophosphatemic rickets. J Med Genet **24:**756–760.
6. Eicher EM, Southard JL, Scriver CR, Glorieux FH 1976 Hypophosphatemic mouse model for human familial hypophosphatemic (vitamin D resistant) rickets. Proc Natl Acad Sci USA **73:**4667–4671.
7. Davisson MT 1987 X-linked genetic homologies between mouse and man. Genomics **1:**213–227.
8. Bianchine JW, Stambles AA, Harrison HE 1971 Familial hypophosphatemic rickets showing autosomal dominant inheritance. Birth Defects **7:**287–294.
9. The HYP Consortium 1995 A gene (PEX) with homologies to endopeptidases is mutated in patients with X-linked hypophosphatemic rickets. Nat Genet **11:**130–136.
10. Dixon PH, Christie PT, Wooding C, Trump D, Grieff M, Holm I, Gertner JM, Schmidtke J, Shah B, Shaw N, Smith C, Tau C, Schlessinger D, Whyte MP, Thakker RV 1998 Mutational analysis of the PHEX gene in X-linked hypophosphatemia. J Clin Endocrinol Metab **33:**3615–3623.
11. Glorieux F, Scriver CR 1972 Loss of a PTH sensitive component of phosphate transport in X-linked hypophosphatemia. Science **147:**997–1000.
12. Tenenhouse HS, Scriver CR, McInnes RR, Glorieux FH 1978 Renal handling of phosphate in vivo and in vitro by the X-linked hypophosphatemic male mouse (Hyp/Y): Evidence for a defect in the brush border membrane. Kidney Int **14:**236–244.
13. Bonjour J-P, Caverzasio J, Muhlbauer R, Trechsel U, Troehler U 1982 Are 1,25(OH)2D production and tubular phosphate transport regulated by one common mechanism which would be defective in X-linked hypophosphatemic rickets? In: Norman AW, Schaefer K, Herrath D, Grigoleit H-G (eds.) Vitamin D: Chemical, Biochemical

and Clinical Endocrinology of Calcium Metabolism. Walter de Gruyter, New York, NY, USA, pp. 427–433.

14. Nesbitt T, Coffman TM, Griffiths R, Drezner MK 1992 Cross-transplantation of kidneys in normal and Hyp mice: Evidence that the Hyp mouse phenotype is unrelated to an intrinsic renal defect. J Clin Invest **89:**1453–1459.

15. Lobaugh B, Drezner MK 1983 Abnormal regulation of renal 25-dihydroxyvitamin D-1-α-hydroxylase in the X-linked hypophosphatemic mouse. J Clin Invest **71:**400–403.

16. Meyer RA Jr, Gray RW, Ross BA, Kiebzak GM 1982 Increased plasma 1,25-dihydroxyvitamin D after low calcium challenge in X-linked hypophosphatemic mice. Endocrinology **111:**174–177.

17. Marie PJ, Glorieux FH 1983 Relations between hypomineralized periosteocytic lesions and bone mineralization in vitamin D resistant rickets. Calcif Tissue Int **35:**443–448.

18. Frost HM 1958 Some observations on bone mineral in a case of vitamin D resistant rickets. Henry Ford Hosp Med Bull **6:**300–302.

19. Glorieux FH, Ecarot-Charrier B 1987 X-linked vitamin D-resistant rickets: Is osteoblast activity defective? In: Cohn DV, Martin TJ, Meunier PJ (eds.) Calcium Regulation and Bone Metabolism, vol 9. Excerpta Medica, Amsterdam, The Netherlands, pp. 227–231.

20. Yamamoto T, Ecarot B, Glorieux FH 1992 Abnormal response of osteoblasts from Hyp mice to 1,25-dihydroxyvitamin D3. Bone **13:**209–215.

21. Ecarot-Charrier E, Glorieux FH, Travers R, Desbarats M, Bouchard F, Hinek A 1988 Defective bone formation by transplanted Hyp mouse bone cells into normal mice. Endocrinology **123:**768–773.

22. Strom TM, Francis F, Lorenz B, Boddrich A, Econs MJ, Lehrach H, Meitinger T 1997 Pex gene deletions in Gy and Hyp mice provide mouse models for X-linked hypophosphatemia. Hum Mol Genet **6:**165–171.

23. Du L, Desbarats M, Viel J, Glorieux FH, Cawthorn C, Ecarot B 1996 cDNA cloning of the murine pex gene implicated in X-linked hypophosphatemia and evidence for expression in bone. Genomics **36:**22–28.

24. The ADHR Consortium 2000 Autosomal dominant hypophosphataemic rickets is associated with mutations in FGF23. Nat Genet **26:**345–348.

25. White KE, Jonsson KB, Carn G, Hampson G, Spector TD, Mannstadt M, Lorenz-Depiereux B, Miyauchi A, Yang IM, Ljunggren O, Meitinger T, Strom TM, Juppner H, Econs MJ 2001 The Autosomal Dominant Hypophosphatemic Rickets (ADHR) gene is a secreted polypeptide overexpressed by tumours that cause phosphate wasting. J Clin Endocrinol Metab **86:**497–500.

26. Jonsson KB, Zahradnik R, Larsson T, White KE, Sugimoto T, Imanishi Y, Yamamoto T, Hampson G, Koshiyama H, Ljunggren O, Oba K, Yang IM, Miyauchi A, Econs MJ, Lavigne J, Juppner H 2003 Fibroblast growth factor 23 in oncogenic osteomalacia and X-linked hypophosphatemia. N Engl J Med **348:**1656–1663.

27. Thakker R Hereditary hypophosphatemic rickets: Role for a fibroblast growth factor, FGF23. Available online at http://www.bonekey_IBMS.org. pp. 2001027–0.

28. Bai X, Miao D, Panda D, Grady S, McKee MD, Goltzman D, Karaplis AC 2002 Partial rescue of the hyp phenotype by osteoblast-targeted PHEX (Phosphate-regulating gene with Homologies to Endopeptidases on the X Chromosome) expression. Mol Endocrinol **16:**2913–2925.

29. Glorieux FH, Scriver CR, Reade TM, Goldman H, Roseborough A 1972 Use of phosphate and vitamin D to prevent dwarfism and rickets in X-linked hypophosphatemia. N Engl J Med **281:**481–487.

30. Verge CF, Lam A, Simpson JM, Cowell CR, Howard NJ, Silink M 1991 Effects of therapy in X-linked hypophosphatemic rickets. N Engl J Med **325:**1843–1848.

31. Petersen DJ, Boniface AM, Schranck FW, Rupich RC, Whyte MP 1992 X-linked hypophosphatemic rickets: A study (with literature review) of linear growth response to calcitriol and phosphate therapy. J Bone Miner Res **7:**583–597.

32. Glorieux FH, Bordier PJ, Marie P, Delvin EE, Travers R 1980 Inadequate bone response to phosphate and vitamin D in familial hypophosphatemic rickets. In: Massry S, Ritz E, Rapada A (eds.) Homeostasis of Phosphate and Other Minerals. Plenum Press, New York, NY, USA, pp. 227–232.

33. Glorieux FH, Marie PJ, Pettifor JM, Delvin EE 1980 Bone response to phosphate salts, ergocalciferol and calcitriol in hypophosphatemic vitamin D-resistant rickets. N Engl J Med **303:**1023–1031.

34. Costa T, Marie PJ, Scriver CR, Cole DE, Reade TM, Nogrady B, Glorieux FH, Delvin EE 1981 X-linked hypophosphatemia: Effect of calcitriol on renal handling of phosphate, serum phosphate, and bone mineralization. J Clin Endocrinol Metab **52:**463–472.

35. Drezner MK, Lyles KW, Haussler MR, Harrelson JM 1980 Evaluation of a role for 1,25-dihydroxyvitamin D in the pathogenesis and treatment of X-linked hypophosphatemic rickets and osteomalacia. J Clin Invest **66:**1020–1032.

36. Harrell RM, Lyles KW, Harrelson JM, Friedman NE, Drezner MK 1985 Healing of bone disease in X-linked hypophosphatemic rickets/osteomalacia: Induction and maintenance with phosphorus and calcitriol. J Clin Invest **75:**1858–1868.

37. Bettinelli A, Bianchi ML, Mazazucchi E, Gandolini G, Appliani AC 1991 Acute effects of calcitriol and phosphate salts on mineral metabolism in children with hypophosphatemic rickets. J Pediatr **118:**373–376.

38. Carpenter TO, Keller M, Schwarts D, Mitnick M, Smith C, Ellison A, Carey D, Comite F, Horst R, Travers R, Glorieux FH, Gundberg CM, Poole AR, Insogna KL 1996 24, 25-Dihydroxyvitamin D supplementation corrects hyperparathyroidism and improves skeletal abnormalities in X-linked hypophosphatemic rickets: A clinical research center study. J Clin Endocrinol Metab **81:**2381–2388.

39. Goodyear PR, Kronick JB, Jequier S, Reade TM, Scriver CR 1987 Nephrocalcinosis and its relationship to treatment of hereditary rickets. J Pediatr **111:**700–704.

40. Alon U, Donaldson DL, Hellerstein S, Warady BA, Harris DJ 1992 Metabolic and histologic investigation of the nature of nephrocalcinosis in children with hypophosphatemic rickets and in the Hyp mouse. J Pediatr **120:**899–905.

41. Wilson DM, Lee PDK, Morris AH, Reiter EO, Gertner JM, Narcus R, Quarmby VE, Rosenfeld RG 1991 Growth hormone therapy in hypophosphatemic rickets. Am J Dis Child **145:**1165–1170.

42. Saggese G, Baroncelli GI, Bertolloni S, Perri G 1995 Long-term growth hormone treatment in children with renal hypophosphatemic rickets: Effects on growth, mineral metabolism and bone density. J Pediatr **127:**395–402.

43. Seikaly MG, Brown R, Baum M 1997 The effect of recombinant human growth hormone in children with X-linked hypophosphatemia. Pediatrics **100:**879–884.

44. Sullivan W, Carpenter T, Glorieux FH, Travers R, Insogna K 1992 A prospective trial of phosphate and 1,25-dihydroxyvitamin D3 therapy in symptomatic adults with X-linked hypophosphatemic rickets. J Clin Endocrinol Metab **75:**879–885.

Chapter 71.   Tumor-Induced Osteomalacia

Suzanne M. Jan de Beur

Department of Medicine, The Johns Hopkins University School of Medicine, Baltimore, Maryland

INTRODUCTION

Tumor induced osteomalacia (TIO), or oncogenic osteomalacia, is an acquired, paraneoplastic syndrome of renal phosphate-wasting that resembles genetic forms of hypophosphatemic rickets. Although first described in 1947 by McCrance,[1] the tumor was not identified as the underlying cause of syndrome until 1959.[2] Since this initial observation, clinical and experimental studies implicate the humoral factor(s) that tumors produce in the profound biochemical and skeletal alterations that characterize TIO. TIO is a rare disorder, with approximately 120 cases reported in the literature[3]; however, progress in understanding its pathogenesis is contributing to our understanding of hypophosphatemic disorders and of normal phosphate homeostatic mechanisms.

CLINICAL AND BIOCHEMICAL MANIFESTATIONS

Although the preponderance of TIO patients is adults (usually diagnosed in the sixth decade), this syndrome may present at any age. In the clinical setting, these patients report long-standing, progressive muscle and bone pain, weakness, and fatigue. These symptoms often predate the recurrent fractures that complicate TIO. Children with TIO display rachitic features including gait disturbances, growth retardation, and skeletal deformities. The occult nature of this metabolic syndrome delays its recognition, and the average time from onset of symptoms to a correct diagnosis often exceeds 2.5 years.[3] An average of 5 years elapses from the time of diagnosis to the identification of the underlying tumor.[4] Until this time, the diagnosis is uncertain, and other renal phosphate wasting syndromes must be considered. Therefore, it is important to note that in patients with TIO, a family history of hypophosphatemia and bone disorders is absent. Extensive and serial physical examination in combination with imaging is frequently required to successfully detect the causal tumor.

The biochemical hallmarks of TIO are low serum concentrations of phosphate, phosphaturia secondary to reduced proximal renal tubular phosphate reabsorption, and frankly low or inappropriate normal levels of serum calcitriol [$1,25(OH)_2D$] that are expected to be elevated in the face of hypophosphatemia. The degree of hypophosphatemia is usually profound and can range from 0.7 to 2.4 mg/dl.[3] However, serum calcium and 25-hydroxyvitamin D are invariably normal, and serum concentrations of intact parathyroid hormone (PTH) are only occasionally elevated. Alkaline phosphatase is typically elevated. A more global proximal tubular defect that results in glucosuria, and amino aciduria occasionally accompanies phosphaturia. Bone histomorphometry reveals severe osteomalacia with clear evidence of a mineralization defect. The dual defect of renal phosphate wasting in concert with impaired calcitriol synthesis results in poor bone mineralization and fractures.[3,5] If untreated, severe osteomalacia leads to fractures of the long bones as well as vertebra and ribs with resultant chest wall deformity and respiratory compromise.

DIAGNOSTIC EVALUATION

Laboratory Studies

When evaluating a patient with suspected TIO, the work-up includes fasting serum phosphorus, a chemistry panel with serum calcium, alkaline phosphatase, and creatinine, an intact PTH level, and serum $1,25(OH)_2D$. In addition, 24-h urine phosphate, creatinine, calcium, amino acids, and glucose are measured. As an indication of renal tubular phosphate clearance, the threshold for the renal tubular reabsorption of phosphate (TRP) is calculated. In some instances when confirmation of the diagnosis is warranted, a tetracycline-labeled, iliac crest bone biopsy is obtained for bone histomorphometric studies. Markedly increased osteoid surface with an increased mineralization lag time indicative of osteomalacia is observed in TIO.

Imaging

General. Plain radiographs exhibit characteristics of osteomalacia including generalized osteopenia, pseudofractures, and coarsened trabeculae. Radiographs of children with TIO show widened epiphyses and other features of rickets. Diffuse skeletal uptake, referred to as a "superscan," and focal uptake at sites of fractures are characteristic features on [99]Technecium bone scintigraphy. In general, plain films show features of osteomalacia; however, it is impossible to differentiate the underlying etiology of the osteomalacia with these modalities.

Tumor Localization. Detection and localization of the culprit tumor in TIO is imperative because complete surgical resection is curative. However, the mesenchymal tumors that cause this syndrome are often small, slow growing, and frequently situated in unusual anatomical sites; therefore, conventional imaging techniques often fail to localize them. Because in vitro studies show that many mesenchymal tumors express somatostatin receptors (SSTR),[6] ^{111}In-pentetreotide scintigraphy (octreotide scan), a scanning technique that employs a radiolabeled somatostatin analog, has been used to successfully detect and localize these tumors in some patients with TIO.[4,7] The mesenchymal tumors that express SSTR are not limited to those associated with TIO, thus careful biochemical confirmation of the syndrome is necessary before embarking on exhaustive imaging efforts.[6]

With conventional imaging such as magnetic resonance scanning or computed tomography, special attention di-

---

Dr. Jan de Beur serves as a co-investigator with Genzyme Corporation.

rected to craniofacial locations and the extremities is indicated because these are more common locations for tumors in TIO, although tumors have been found distributed through out the body.

DIFFERENTIAL DIAGNOSIS

In contrast to more common forms of osteomalacia that share clinical features with TIO, TIO patients have normal serum calcium, serum 25-hydroxyvitamin D, intact PTH, and phosphaturia (reduced TRP). However, TIO is biochemically indistinguishable from several inherited forms of hypophosphatemic rickets; X linked hypophosphatemic rickets (XLH), and autosomal dominant hypophosphatemic rickets (ADHR).[8] Because patients with XLH and ADHR exhibit a variable age of onset, it is critical to take a careful family history in patients with hypophosphatemia. The clinical consequences of TIO are typically present for many years before the causal tumor is identified; this further obscures the clinical distinction between TIO and inherited forms of hypophosphatemic, vitamin D–resistant rickets. Serum fibroblast growth factor (FGF)-23 levels are generally elevated in patients with TIO but are also elevated in some patients with XLH. Normal serum FGF-23 levels do not eliminate the diagnosis of TIO.[9,10] The diagnosis of TIO is dependent on the identification of the culprit tumor and remission of the syndrome after complete tumor resection. In cases where complete resection is not possible, the diagnosis remains presumptive. Genetic testing of the *PHEX* and *FGF-23* genes, which are defective in XLH and ADHR, respectively, is commercially available and may be indicated when a definitive diagnosis is necessary.[11]

Another inherited renal phosphate-wasting syndrome, hereditary hypophosphatemic rickets with hypercalciuria (HHRH), is clinically similar to TIO with bone pain, osteomalacia, and muscle weakness as prominent features, yet the distinction is easily made with biochemical testing. Both syndromes are characterized by hypophosphatemia owing to decreased renal phosphorus reabsorption; however, patients with HHRH exhibit elevated levels of calcitriol and hypercalciuria that distinguish it from TIO, XLH, and ADHR.[8,12]

Recently, heterozygous, dominant-negative, mutations in the renal type IIa sodium-phosphate co-transporter gene (*NPT-2*) were identified in two patients with hypophosphatemia secondary to renal phosphate wasting and osteopenia or nephrolithiasis. The prominent symptoms of bone pain and muscle weakness seen in TIO are absent in those with *NPT-2* mutations. Furthermore, the presence of hypercalciuria and elevated calcitriol make these patients easily distinguishable from patients with TIO.[13]

TUMORS

The mesenchymal tumors that are associated with TIO are characteristically slow-growing, complex, polymorphous neoplasms that have been subdivided into four groups based on their histological features: (1) phosphaturic mesenchymal tumor, mixed connective tissue type (PMTMCT); (2) osteoblastoma-like tumors; (3) ossifying fibrous-like tumors; and (4) nonossifying fibrous-like tumors.[14] The PMTMCT subtype is the most common and comprises approximately 70–80% of the mesenchymal tumors associated with TIO.[14,15] Characterized by an admixture of spindle cells, osteoclast-like giant cells, prominent blood vessels, cartilage-like matrix, and metaplastic bone, these tumors occur equally in soft tissue and bone. Although typically benign, malignant variants of PMTMCT have been described.

FGF-23 message is abundantly expressed in these tumors,[16–18] and FGF-23 protein is detectable by immunoblot[18] and immunohistochemistry.[15,19] In one series, 17 of 21 PMTMCT tumors had detectable FGF-23 protein expression.[15] The granular cytoplasm within the spindle cells exhibits the most consistent staining and seems to be the source of FGF-23.

These mesenchymal tumors are small, indolent and remotely located. Although found in a variety of anatomical locations, including the long bones, the nasopharynx, the sinuses, and the groin,[4] these tumors are most commonly located in the extremities and appendicular skeleton.[15] While tumor localization is frequently a prolonged and arduous task, once detected, the anatomical inaccessibility of the tumors make complete resection difficult. Successful tumor detection requires careful physical examination, diligent follow-up, and periodic imaging.

Although TIO is typically caused by benign mesenchymal tumors, the syndrome has also been associated with a variety carcinomas,[20,21] neurofibromatosis,[22] linear nevus syndrome, and fibrous dysplasia of bone.[23] Because the multiplicity of lesions and resultant inability to completely resect the entire tumor burden, demonstration of biochemical and radiographic improvement with surgery has been lacking save for a few cases.[22,24]

PATHOPHYSIOLOGY

With the identification of the genetic defects in X-linked and autosomal dominant forms of hypophosphatemic rickets and the discovery of novel phosphate-regulatory genes in tumors associated with TIO, the past several years have brought dramatic advances in our understanding of the molecular and biochemical bases of inherited and acquired hypophosphatemic disorders.

Dual Defect: Renal Phosphate Wasting and Abnormal Vitamin D Metabolism

The basic pathophysiology of TIO is hypophosphatemia secondary to inhibition of renal phosphate reabsorption compounded by a vitamin D synthetic defect that blunts the compensatory rise in calcitriol in response to hypophosphatemia. Profound hypophosphatemia results in muscle pain and weakness, osteomalacia, and fractures. Experimental evidence suggests that the biochemical and skeletal defects in TIO are caused by a humoral factor (or factors), coined "phosphatonin," produced by mesenchymal tumors. Tumor extracts can inhibit phosphate transport in vitro[25–29] and produce phosphaturia and hypophosphatemia in vivo.[30] Extracts from a heterotransplanted tumor inhibits renal 25-hydroxyvitamin D-1-α-hydroxylase activity in cultured kidney cells.[31] Furthermore, complete surgical resection of tumor tissue results in normalization of serum phosphate and calcitriol, reversal of renal phosphate loss, and eventually, remineralization of bone.[3,5]

Identifying "Phosphatonin": FGF-23

Although several groups have reported tumor cultures or tumor extracts inhibit phosphate transport, slow growth of cultured tumor cells and the frequent loss of phosphate-inhibitory activity in culture hampered the identification of the phosphaturic substance produced by these tumors. By examining highly expressed genes in TIO tumors, several investigators[17,32,33] have identified several candidate genes for the phosphaturic substance produced by these tumors. Included among these genes is *FGF-23*, a novel FGF, which was contemporaneously identified by positional cloning as the defective gene in autosomal dominant hypophosphatemic rickets.[34] FGF-23 is highly expressed in TIO tumors[17,18,33] but only low levels in normal tissue.[34]

Conditioned media and purified FGF-23 can inhibit phosphate transport in opossum kidney cells (OK), a model of renal proximal tubular epithelium.[16,35] When injected into mice, FGF-23 reduces serum phosphate and increases fractional excretion of phosphorus.[33,36] Mice chronically exposed to FGF-23–transfected Chinese hamster ovary (CHO) cell xenografts become hypophosphatemic with increased renal phosphate clearance, show reduced bone mineralization, and have reduced expression of renal 25-hydroxyvitaminD-1-α-hydroxylase with decreased circulating levels of calcitriol.[33] The biochemical and skeletal abnormalities of transgenic mice that overexpress FGF-23 mimic human TIO.[37] Conversely, FGF-23–deficient mice exhibit growth retardation and early death, with biochemical abnormalities that include hyperphosphatemia, elevated calcitriol, and hypercalcemia.[37]

Circulating FGF-23 is detectable in human serum.[9,10] Individuals with TIO exhibit elevated serum levels of FGF-23 that plummet after complete tumor resection. However, some individuals with TIO have normal levels or only mildly elevated levels—underscoring the heterogeneous composition of "phosphatonin." Elevated serum FGF-23 levels are also observed in XLH, albeit to a more modest degree.[9,10]

FGF-23 is also central in the pathogenesis of ADHR. Missense mutations in one of two arginine residues at positions 176 or 179 have been identified in affected members of four unrelated ADHR families.[34] This clustering of missense mutations suggests that they are activating mutations. Furthermore, the mutated arginine residues, located in the consensus proprotein convertase cleavage RXXR motif, prevent the degradation of FGF-23 and thus may result in prolonged or enhanced FGF-23 action.[16,36,38] Moreover, FGF-23 exhibits more potent biological action than the native FGF-23,[39,40] in its ability to reduce *Npt-2* gene expression and 25-dihydroxyvitamin D-1-α-hydroxylase protein.[39]

Amassing evidence suggests that FGF-23 may be key in the pathogenesis of XLH. XLH is caused by mutations in the *PHEX* gene,[41] which encodes an M13 metalloprotease.

Speculation about the function of *PHEX* paired with data that implicate both an intrinsic osteoblast defect[42] and a humoral factor in the pathogenesis of XLH[43–45] lead to the hypothesis that the substrate for PHEX is the humoral factor responsible for TIO. The endogenous substrate for PHEX remains unknown. However, the preponderance of experimental evidence suggests that FGF-23 is cleaved by PHEX,[16,46] although not all investigators are in agreement.[47]

It is clear that FGF-23 plays a central role in three distinct disorders of renal phosphate wasting. In TIO, tumors produce FGF-23 that then exerts its activity at the proximal renal tubule to inhibit tubular reabsorption of phosphate and downregulate the 25-hydroxyvitaminD-1-α-hydroxylase, resulting in hypophosphatemia and osteomalacia. In ADHR, FGF-23 bears mutations that enhance it biological activity and render it resistant to proteolytic cleavage, and again, the result is hypophosphatemia, phosphaturia, bone deformity, and rickets. In XLH, mutated PHEX is not able to cleave FGF-23, its presumed substrate, and FGF-23 accumulates in the circulation and exerts its phosphaturic activity at the renal proximal tubule. Whether FGF-23 is only important in these rare disorders of renal phosphate wasting or is a key regulator of physiologic phosphate homeostasis remains to be demonstrated.

Other "Phosphatonin" Candidates

Frizzled Related Protein 4. Gene expression profiles of mesenchymal tumors associated with TIO[17] demonstrated several genes that encoded secreted proteins that were highly and differentially expressed. This analysis revealed a second "phosphatonin" candidate, secreted frizzled related protein 4 (sFRP4).[48] FRPs are a class of molecules that inhibit Wnt signaling by acting as a decoy receptor. Wnt signaling is important in development especially of the skeleton and kidney. Recently, two disorders of bone mass accrual have been linked to activation or inhibition of Wnt signaling through it co-receptor, LRP5. Activating mutations in LRP5 result in autosomal dominant high bone mass trait,[49,50] whereas a number of inactivating mutations in LRP5 have been identified in osteoporosis pseudoglioma syndrome.[51] Thus, it is possible that modulation of Wnt signaling may be important in regulating determinants of bone mass including some aspects of mineral ion homeostasis. Several lines of evidence suggest sFRP4 has phosphaturic properties. sFRP4 inhibits phosphate transport in cultured renal epithelial cells,[52] it reduces fractional excretion of phosphorus when infused into mice and rats, and with longer-term exposure, sFRP4 produces hypophosphatemia with blunting of the compensatory increase in 25-hydroxyvitamin D-1-α-hydroxylase expression induced by hypophosphatemia.[53] Whether sFRP4 is elevated in the serum of patient with TIO in currently unknown.

Matrix Extracellular Phosphoglycoprotein. Matrix extracellular phosphoglycoprotein (MEPE)/osteoregulin is a recently identified secreted protein that displays structural features of an extracellular matrix protein and is highly expressed in bone marrow and differentiated osteoblasts.[32]

Three independent investigators demonstrated MEPE is highly expressed in mesenchymal tumors associated with TIO.[17,32,33] MEPE-deficient mice exhibit increased bone density caused by enhanced bone mineralization,[54] whereas overexpression of MEPE in TIO is associated with impaired bone mineralization, suggesting that MEPE is an important negative regulator of bone mineralization. Currently, there is no evidence that MEPE directly inhibits phosphate transport, but intriguing data are emerging that MEPE may be a substrate for PHEX.[46]

TREATMENT

The definitive treatment for TIO is complete resection of the tumor that results in rapid correction of the biochemical derangements and remineralization of bone.[55] However, even after the diagnosis of TIO is made, the tumor often remains obscure or incompletely resected. In the case of malignant tumors associated with TIO, such as prostate cancer, complete resection may not be possible. Therefore, many times medical management of this disorder is necessary.

The current practice is to treat TIO with phosphorus supplementation in combination with calcitriol. The phosphorus supplementation serves to replace ongoing renal phosphorus loss and the calcitriol supplements replace insufficient renal production of 1,25 dihydroxyvitamin D and enhance renal and gastrointestinal phosphate reabsorption. Generally, patients are treated with phosphorus (2 g/day), in divided doses, and calcitriol (1–3 μg/day).[3] In some cases, administration of calcitriol alone may improve the biochemical abnormalities seen in TIO and heal the osteomalacia.[56] Therapy and dosing should be tailored to improve symptoms, maintain fasting phosphorus in the low normal range, normalize alkaline phosphatase, and control secondary hyperparathyroidism, without inducing hypercalcemia or hypercalciuria. With appropriate treatment, muscle and bone pain will improve, and healing of the osteomalacia will ensue.

Monitoring for therapeutic complications of high doses of calcitriol and phosphorus is important to prevent unintended hypercalcemia, nephrocalcinosis, and nephrolithiasis. Although parathyroid autonomy has been reported in only a few cases of TIO, the true incidence is likely higher with prolonged treatment with phosphorus (alone or in combination with vitamin D) because it stimulates parathyroid function that can eventually lead to autonomy. To assess safety and efficacy of therapy, monitoring of serum and urine calcium, renal function, and parathyroid status is recommended every 3–6 months.

Octreotide in vitro and in vivo has been shown to inhibit secretion of hormones by many neuroendocrine tumors. The expression of SSTRs that bind octreotide by some mesenchymal tumors provided the rationale for a therapeutic trial of octreotide in several patients with TIO and residual tumor. In one case, treatment with subcutaneous octreotide 50–100 μg three times a day resulted in correction of hypophosphatemia, improvement in phosphaturia, and reduction in alkaline phosphatase.[7] However, in two other patients, despite 8 weeks of treatment with subcutaneous octreotide up to 200 μg three times daily, serum levels of phosphorus and calcitriol failed to increase, and the tubular reabsorption of phosphate remained depressed.[4] Given the limited and mixed experience with octreotide treatment in TIO, this therapy should be reserved for the most severe cases that are refractory to current medical therapy.

As we understand the pathophysiology of this disorder more fully, specific therapies directed at attenuating the effect of excess FGF-23 and the other humoral factors elaborated in TIO no doubt will be developed.

REFERENCES

1. McCrance RA 1947 Osteomalacia with Looser's nodes (milkman's syndrome) due to a raised resistance to vitamin D acquired about the age of 15 years. Q J Med 16:33–46.
2. Prader A, Illig R, Uehlinger RE, Stalder G 1959 Rachitis infolge knochentumors (Rickets caused by bone tumors). Helv Pediatr Acta 14:554–565.
3. Drezner MK 1999 Tumor-induced osteomalacia. In: Favus MJ (ed.) Primer on Metabolic Bone Diseases and Disorders of Mineral Metabolism, 4th ed. Lippincott-Raven, Philadelphia, PA, USA, pp. 331–337.
4. Jan de Beur SM, Streeten EA, Civelek AC, McCarthy EF, Uribe L, Watts N, Marx S, Sharon M, Levine MA 2002 Localization of mesenchymal tumors causing oncogenic osteomalacia with somatostatin receptor imaging. Lancet 359:761–763.
5. Kumar R 2000 Tumor-induced osteomalacia and the regulation of phosphate homeostasis. Bone 27:333–338.
6. Reubi JC, Waser B, Laissue JA, Gebbers JO 1996 Somatostatin and vasoactive intestinal peptide receptors in human mesenchymal tumors: in vitro identification. Cancer Res 56:1922–1931.
7. Seufert J, Ebert K, Muller J, Eulert J, Hendrich C, Werner E, Schuuze N, Schulz G, Kenn W, Richtmann H, Palitzsch KD, Jakob F 2001 Octreotide therapy for tumor-induced osteomalacia. N Engl J Med 345:1883–1888.
8. Jan de Beur SM, Levine MA 2002 Molecular pathogenesis of hypophosphatemic rickets. J Clin Endocrinol Metab 87:2467–2473.
9. Yamazaki Y, Okazaki R, Shibata M, Hasegawa Y, Satoh K, Tajima T, Takeuchi Y, Fujita T, Nakahara K, Yamashita T, Fukumoto S 2002 Increased circulatory level of biologically active full-length FGF-23 in patients with hypophosphatemic rickets/osteomalacia. J Clin Endocrinol Metab 87:4957–4960.
10. Jonsson KB, Zahradnik R, Larsson T, White KE, Sugimoto T, Imanishi Y, Yamamoto T, Hampson G, Koshiyama H, Ljunggren O, Oba K, Yang IM, Miyauchi A, Econs MJ, Lavigne J, Juppner H 2003 Fibroblast growth factor 23 in oncogenic osteomalacia and X-linked hypophosphatemia. N Engl J Med 348:1656–1663.
11. Gene Testing for XLH (PHEX) and ADHR (FGF-23) are Commercially Available. Available online at www.genedx.com and www.medichecks.com. Accessed on June 17 2003.
12. Teider M, Modai D, Samuel R 1985 Hereditary hypophosphatemic rickets with hypercalciuria. N Engl J Med 312:611–617.
13. Prie D, Huart V, Bakouh N, Planelles G, Dellis O, Gerard B, Hulin P, Benque-Blanchet F, Silve C, Grandchamp B, Friedlander G 2002 Nephrolithiasis and osteoporosis associated with hypophosphatemia caused by mutations in the type 2a sodium-phosphate cotransporter. N Engl J Med 347:983–991.
14. Weidner N, Santa CD 1987 Phosphaturic mesenchymal tumors. A polymorphous group causing osteomalacia or rickets. Cancer 59:1442–1454.
15. Folpe AL, Fanburg-Smith JC, Weiss SW, the Phosphaturic Mesenchymal Tumor Study Group 2003 Most phosphaturic mesenchymal tumors are a single entity: An analysis of 31 cases. Mod Pathol 16:12A.
16. Bowe A, Finnegan R, Jan de Beur SM, Vassiliadis J, Cho J, Levine MA, Kumar R, Schiavi SC 2001 FGF-23 Inhibits phosphate transport in vitro and is a substrate for the PHEX endopeptidase. Biochem Biophys Res Commun 284:977–981.
17. Jan de Beur SM, Finnegan RB, Vassiliadis J, Cook B, Barberio D, Estes S, Manavalon P, Petroziello J, Madden S, Cho JY, Kumar R, Levine MA, Schiavi SC 2002 Tumors associated with oncogenic osteomalacia express markers of bone and mineral metabolism. J Bone Miner Res 17:1102–1110.
18. White KE, Jonsson KB, Carn G, Hampson G, Spector TD, Mannstadt M, Lorenz-Depiereux B, Miyauchi A, Yang IM, Ljunggren O,

Meitinger T, Strom TM, Juppner H, Econs MJ 2001 The autosomal dominant hypophosphatemic rickets (ADHR) gene is a secreted polypeptide overexpressed by tumors that cause phosphate wasting. J Clin Endocrinol Metab **86**:497–500.

19. Larsson T, Zahradnik R, Lavigne J, Ljunggren O, Juppner H, Jonsson KB 2003 Immunohistochemical detection of FGF-23 protein in tumors that cause oncogenic osteomalacia. Eur J Endocrinol **148**:269–276.

20. Lyles KW, Berry WR, Haussler M, Harrelson JM, Drezner MK 1980 Hypophosphatemic osteomalacia: Association with prostatic carcinoma. Ann Intern Med **93**:275–278.

21. Shaker JL, Brickner RC, Divgi AB, Raff H, Findling JW 1995 Case report: Renal phosphate wasting, syndrome of inappropriate antidiuretic hormone, and ectopic corticotropin production in small cell carcinoma. Am J Med Sci **310**:38–41.

22. Saville PD, Nassim JR, Stevenson FH 1955 Osteomalacia in von Recklinghausen's neurofibromatosis: Metabolic study of a case. Br Med J **1**:1311–1313.

23. Dent CE, Gertner JM 1976 Hypophosphataemic osteomalacia in fibrous dysplasia. Q J Med **45**:411–420.

24. Ivker R, Resnick SD, Skidmore R 1997 Hypophosphatemic vitamin D-resistant rickets, precocious puberty, and the epidermal nevus syndrome. Arch Dermatol **133**:1557–1561.

25. Cai Q, Hodgson SF, Kao PC, Lennon VA, Klee GG, Zinsmiester AR, Kumar R 1994 Brief report: Inhibition of renal phosphate transport by a tumor product in a patient with oncogenic osteomalacia. N Engl J Med **330**:1645–1649.

26. Wilkins GE, Granleese S, Hegele RG, Holden J, Anderson DW, Bondy GP 1995 Oncogenic osteomalacia: Evidence for a humoral phosphaturic factor. J Clin Endocrinol Metab **80**:1628–1634.

27. Nelson AE, Namkung HJ, Patava J, Wilkinson MR, Chang AC, Reddel RR Robinson BG, Mason R 1996 Characteristics of tumor cell bioactivity in oncogenic osteomalacia. Mol Cell Endocrinol **124**:17–23.

28. Rowe PS, Ong AC, Cockerill FJ, Goulding JN, Hewison M 1996 Candidate 56 and 58 kDa protein(s) responsible for mediating the renal defects in oncogenic hypophosphatemic osteomalacia. Bone **18**:159–169.

29. Jonsson K, Mannstadt M, Miyauchi A, Yang IM, Stein G, Ljunggren O, Juppner H 2001 Extracts from tumors causing oncogenic osteomalacia inhibit phosphate uptake in opossum kidney cells. J Endocrinol **169**:613–620.

30. Popovtzer MM 1981 Tumor-induced hypophosphatemic osteomalacia (TIO): Evidence for a phosphaturic cyclic AMP-independent action of tumor extract. Clin Res **29**:418A.

31. Miyauchi A, Fukase M, Tsutsumi M, Fujita T 1998 Hemangiopericytoma-induced osteomalacia: Tumor transplantation in nude mice causes hypophosphatemia and tumor extracts inhibit renal 25-hydroxyvitamin D-1-hydroxylase activity. J Clin Endocrinol Metab **67**:46–53.

32. Rowe PS, de Zoysa PA, Dong R, Wang HR, White KE, Econs MJ, Oudet CL 2000 MEPE, a new gene expressed in bone marrow and tumors causing osteomalacia. Genomics **67**:54–68.

33. Shimada T, Mizutani S, Muto T, Yoneya T, Hino R, Takeda S, Takeuchi Y, Fujita T, Fukumoto S, Yamashita T 2001 Cloning and characterization of FGF23 as a causative factor of tumor-induced osteomalacia. Proc Natl Acad Sci USA **98**:6500–6505.

34. The ADHR Consortium 2000 Autosomal dominant hypophosphataemic rickets is associated with mutations in FGF 23. Nat Genet **26**:45–348.

35. Yamashita T, Konishi M, Miyake A, Inui Ki, Itoh N 2002 Fibroblast Growth Factor (FGF)-23 inhibits renal phosphate reabsorption by activation of themitogen-activated protein kinase pathway. J Biol Chem **27**:28265–28270.

36. Shimada T, Muto T, Urakawa I, Yoneya I, Yamazaki Y, Okawa K, Takeuchi Y, Fujita T, Fukumoto S, Yamashita T 2002 Mutant FGF-23 responsible for autosomal dominant hypophosphatemic rickets is resistant to proteolytic cleavage and causes hypophophatemia in vivo. Endocrinology **143**:3179–3182.

37. Shimada T, Mizutani S, Kakitani M, Hasegawa H, Yamazaki Y, Ohguma A, Takeuchi Y, Fujita T, Fukumoto S, Tomizuka K, Yamashita T 2002 Targeted ablation of FGF-23 causes hyperphophatemia, increased 1, 25-dihydroxyvitamin D level and severe growth retardation. J Bone Miner Res **17**:S168.

38. White KE, Carn G, Lorenz-Depiereux B, Benet-Pages A, Strom TM, Econs MJ 2001 Autosomal dominant hypophosphatemic rickets mutations stabilize FGF-23. Kidney Int **60**:2079–2086.

39. Bai XY, Miao D, Goltzman D, Karaplis AC 2003 The autosomal dominant hypophosphatemic rickets R176Q mutation in fibroblast growth factor 23 resists proteolytic cleavage and enhances in vivo biological potency. J Biol Chem **278**:9843–9849.

40. Saito H, Kusano K, Kinosaki M, Ito H, Hirata M, Segawa H, Miyamoto K, Fukushima N 2003 Human fibroblast growth factor-23 mutants suppress Na+-dependent phosphate co-transport activity and 1alpha, 25-dihydroxyvitamin D3 production. J Biol Chem **278**:2206–2211.

41. The HYP Consortium 1995 A gene (PEX) with homologies to endopeptidases is mutated in patients with X-linked hypophosphatemic rickets. Nat Genet **11**:130–136.

42. Ecarot-Charrier B, Glorieux FH, Travers R, Desbarats M, Bouchard F, Hinek A 1988 Defective bone formation by transplanted *Hyp* mouse bone cells into normal mice. Endocrinology **123**:768–773.

43. Meyer RA Jr, Meyer MH, Gray RW 1989 Parabiosis suggests a humoral factor is involved in X-linked hypophosphatemia in mice. J Bone Miner Res **4**:493–500.

44. Nesbitt T, Coffman TM, Griffiths R, Drezner MK 1992 Cross transplantation of kidneys in normal and *Hyp* mice: Evidence that the *Hyp* phenotype is unrelated to an intrinsic renal defect. J Clin Invest **89**:1453–1459.

45. Lajeunesse D, Meyer RA, Hamel L 1996 Direct demonstration of a humorally mediated inhibition of of renal phosphate transport in the *Hyp* mouse. Kidney Int **50**:1531–1538.

46. Campos M, Couture C, Hirata IY, Juliano MA, Loisel TP, Crine P, Juliano L, Boileau G, Carmona AK 2003 Human recombinant PHEX has a strict S1′ specificity for acidic residues and cleaves peptides derived from FGF-23 and MEPE. Biochem J (in press).

47. Guo R, Lui S, Spurney RF, Quarles LD 2001 Analysis of recombinant Phex: An endopeptidase in search of a substrate. Am J Physiol Endocrinol Metab **281**:E837–E847.

48. Schiavi SC, Moe OW 2002 Phosphatonins: A new class of phosphate-regulating proteins. Curr Opin Nephrol Hypertens **11**:423–430.

49. Boyden LM, Mao J, Belsky J, Mitzner L, Farhi A, Mitnick MA, Wu D, Insogna K, Lifton RP 2002 High bone density due to a mutation in LDL receptor related protein 5. N Engl J Med **346**:1513–1521.

50. Little RD, Carulli JP, Del Mastro RG, Dupuis J, Osborne M, Folz C, Manning SP, Swain PM, Zhao SC, Eustace B, Lappe MM, Spitzer L, Zweier S, Braunschweiger K, Benchekroun Y, Hu X, Adair R, Chee L, FitzGerald MG, Tulig C, Caruso A, Tzellas N, Bawa A, Franklin B, McGuire S, Nogues X, Gong G, Allen KM, Anisowicz A, Morales AJ, Lomedico PT, Recker SM, Van Eerdewegh P, Recker RR, Johnson ML 2002 A mutation in the LDL receptor related protein 5 gene results in the autosomal dominant high bone mass trait. Am J Hum Genet **70**:11–19.

51. Gong Y, Slee RB, Fukai N, Rawadi G, Roman-Roman S, Reginato AM, Wang H, Cundy T, Glorieux FH, Lev D, Zacharin M, Oexle K, Marcelino J, Suwairi W, Heeger S, Sabatakos G, Apte S, Adkins WN, Allgrove J, Arslan-Kirchner M, Batch JA, Beighton P, Black GC, Boles RG, Boon LM, Borrone C, Brunner HG, Carle GF, Dallapiccola B, De Paepe A, Floege B, Halfhide ML, Hall B, Hennekam RC, Hirose T, Jans A, Juppner H, Kim CA, Keppler-Noreuil K, Kohlschuetter A, LaCombe D, Lambert M, Lemyre E, Letteboer T, Peltonen L, Ramesar RS, Romanengo M, Somer H, Steichen-Gersdorf E, Steinmann B, Sullivan B, Superti-Furga A, Swoboda W, van den Boogaard MJ, Van Hul W, Vikkula M, Votruba M, Zabel B, Garcia T, Baron R, Olsen BR, Warman ML, Osteoporosis-Pseudoglioma Syndrome Collaborative Group 2001 LDL receptor related protein 5 (LRP-5) affects bone accrual and eye development. Cell **107**:513–523.

52. Vassiliadis J, Jan de Beur SM, Bowe AE, Finnegan R, Levine MA, Kumar R, Schiavi SC 2001 Frizzled Related Protein 4 expression is elevated in tumors associated with oncogenic osteomalacia and inhibits phosphate transport *in vitro*. J Bone Miner Res **16**:S11.

53. Berndt TJ, Vassiliadis J, Reczek D, Schiavi SC, Kumar R 2002 Effect of the acute infusion of Fizzed Related Protein 4 (FRP-4), a protein highly expressed in tumors associated with osteomalacia, on phosphate excretion in vivo. J Bone Miner Res **17**:S158.

54. Gowen LC, Petersen DN, Mansolf AL, Qi H, Stock JL, Tkalcevic GT, Simmons HA, Crawford DT, Chidsey-Frink KL, Ke HZ, McNeish JD, Brown TA 2003 Targeted disruption of the osteoblast/osteocyte factor 45 gene (OF45) results in increased bone formation and bone mass. J Biol Chem **278**:1998–2007.

55. Shane E, Parisien M, Henderson JE, Dempster DW, Feldman F, Hardy MA, Tohme JF, Karaplis AC, Clemens TL 1997 Tumor-induced osteomalacia: Clinical and basic studies. J Bone Miner Res **12**:1502–1511.

56. Drezner MK, Feinglos MN 1977 Osteomalacia due to 1alpha, 25-dihydroxycholecalciferol deficiency. Association with a giant cell tumor of bone. J Clin Invest **60**:1046–1053.

Chapter 72. Hypophosphatasia

Michael P. Whyte

Division of Bone and Mineral Diseases, Washington University School of Medicine at Barnes-Jewish Hospital and Center for Metabolic Bone Disease and Molecular Research, Shriners Hospitals for Children, St. Louis, Missouri

INTRODUCTION

Hypophosphatasia (OMIM 146300, 241500, 241510) is a rare, heritable type of rickets or osteomalacia that occurs in all races (although especially uncommon in blacks). The incidence for the severe forms is approximately 1 per 100,000 births; mild forms are more prevalent.[1,2] Approximately 300 cases have been reported. This inborn error of metabolism is characterized biochemically by subnormal activity of the tissue-nonspecific (bone/liver/kidney) isoenzyme of alkaline phosphatase (TNSALP). Activity of the tissue-specific intestinal, placental, and germ-cell ALP isoenzymes is not diminished.[3]

Although there is considerable overlap in severity among them, four principal clinical forms of hypophosphatasia are reported depending on the age at which skeletal lesions are discovered: perinatal, infantile, childhood, and adult. When dental manifestations alone are present, the condition is called *odontohypophosphatasia*. Generally, the earlier the onset of skeletal problems, the more severe the clinical course.[1,2]

CLINICAL PRESENTATION

Although some TNSALP is normally present in all tissues, hypophosphatasia affects predominantly the skeleton and teeth. Severity of clinical expression is, however, remarkably variable (e.g., death may occur in utero or mild symptoms may go undiagnosed in adults).[1,2]

Perinatal hypophosphatasia manifests during gestation. Pregnancies may be complicated by polyhydramnios. Typically, extreme skeletal hypomineralization causes caput membranaceum and short and deformed limbs apparent at birth. Rarely, an unusual bony spur protrudes from a major long bone.[4] Most affected newborns survive only briefly while suffering increasing respiratory compromise and sometimes unexplained fever, anemia (perhaps from encroachment on the marrow space by excessive osteoid), failure to gain weight, irritability, periodic apnea with cyanosis and bradycardia, intracranial hemorrhage, and pyridoxine-dependent seizures. Survival is very rare.[1,2]

Infantile hypophosphatasia becomes clinically apparent before 6 months of age. Developmental milestones often seem normal until poor feeding, inadequate weight gain, hypotonia, and wide fontanels are noted. Rachitic deformities then manifest. Hypercalcemia and hypercalciuria can cause recurrent vomiting, nephrocalcinosis and, occasionally, renal compromise. Despite widely "open" fontanels (actually hypomineralized areas of calvarium), functional craniosynostosis can occur. Raised intracranial pressure may be associated with bulging of the anterior fontanel, proptosis, and papilledema. Mild hypertelorism and brachycephaly can appear. A flail chest predisposes to pneumonia. During the months after diagnosis, there may be spontaneous improvement or progressive skeletal deterioration. About 50% of patients die within 1 year. Prognosis seems to improve if there is survival beyond infancy.[1,2]

Childhood hypophosphatasia varies greatly in severity. Premature loss of deciduous teeth (<5 years of age) from hypoplasia or aplasia of dental cementum is a major clinical hallmark. Odontohypophosphatasia is diagnosed when radiographs show no evidence of skeletal disease. The lower incisors are typically lost first, but in severe cases. the entire dentition can be affected. Exfoliation occurs without root resorption; teeth slide intact from sockets. Dental radiographs often show enlarged pulp chambers and root canals forming "shell teeth." The prognosis for the permanent dentition is more favorable. When rickets is present, delayed walking with a waddling gait, short stature, and a dolichocephalic skull with frontal bossing are often apparent. Static myopathy is a poorly understood complication. Childhood hypophosphatasia may improve spontaneously during puberty, but recurrence of skeletal symptoms is likely during adult life.[1,2]

Adult hypophosphatasia usually presents during middle age, often with painful and poorly healing, recurrent, metatarsal stress fractures. Pain in the thighs or hips can reflect femoral pseudofractures. About 50% of patients give histories consistent with rickets and/or premature loss of deciduous teeth during childhood.[5] Chondrocalcinosis occurs frequently and calcium pyrophosphate dihydrate crystal deposition disease and calcific periarthritis trouble some patients.[6] Femoral pseudofractures generally mend after intramedullary rodding.[7]

LABORATORY FINDINGS

Hypophosphatasia is diagnosed from a consistent clinical history and physical findings, radiographic or histopathological evidence of rickets or osteomalacia, and the presence of low serum ALP activity (hypophosphatasemia).[1] Diagnosticians must appreciate changes in the normal range for serum ALP activity with age, and understand that rarely other conditions (including severe cases of osteogenesis imperfecta and cleidocranial dysplasia) and treatments can cause hypophosphatasemia.[1]

Rickets/osteomalacia in hypophosphatasia is distinctly unusual because serum levels of calcium and inorganic phosphate (Pi) are not reduced. In fact, hypercalcemia and hypercalciuria occur frequently in perinatal and infantile hypophosphatasia, apparently because of dyssynergy between gut absorption of calcium and defective skeletal growth and mineralization (severely affected patients may also show progressive skeletal demineralization).[8] Affected children and adults have serum Pi levels that are above mean levels for age-matched controls, and about 50%

The author has no conflict of interest.

are hyperphosphatemic. Enhanced renal reclamation of Pi (increased TmP/GFR) accounts for this abnormality.[1] In serum, vitamin D metabolite concentrations are typically normal.[1] Parathyroid hormone levels may be suppressed.

At least three phosphocompounds accumulate endogenously in hypophosphatasia[1,3]: phosphoethanolamine (PEA), inorganic pyrophosphate (PPi), and pyridoxal 5'-phosphate (PLP). Demonstration of phosphoethanolaminuria supports the diagnosis but is not specific because PEA can be modestly increased in a variety of other disorders, and normal levels can occur in mild cases. Assay of PPi in plasma and urine is a research technique. If vitamin B_6 supplements are not taken, an elevated plasma level of PLP seems to be the most sensitive and specific test for hypophosphatasia among these markers. In general, the lower the serum level of ALP activity for age and the greater the plasma PLP level, the more severe the clinical manifestations.[1,3]

RADIOLOGIC FINDINGS

Perinatal hypophosphatasia manifests pathognomonic features.[9] In extreme cases, the skeleton may be so poorly calcified that only the base of the skull is visualized. In less remarkable patients, the calvarium may be ossified at central portions of individual membranous bones and give the illusion that the sutures are open and widely separated. Marked skeletal undermineralization occurs with severe rachitic changes. Segments of the spinal column may appear missing. Fractures are also common.

Infantile hypophosphatasia causes characteristic but less severe changes.[9] Abrupt transition from relatively normal appearing diaphyses to hypomineralized metaphyses can suggest a sudden metabolic deterioration. Worsening rickets with progressive skeletal demineralization and fracture heralds a lethal outcome. Skeletal scintigraphy may identify closed sutures that appear widened radiographically.

Childhood hypophosphatasia often features characteristic "tongues" of radiolucency that project from rachitic growth plates into metaphyses (Fig. 1). True, premature fusion of cranial sutures can cause a "beaten-copper" appearance of the skull.

Adult hypophosphatasia is associated with osteopenia, metatarsal stress fractures, chondrocalcinosis, and proximal femoral pseudofractures.

HISTOPATHOLOGIC FINDINGS

Nondecalcified sections of bone reveal histological features of rickets or osteomalacia (without secondary hyperparathyroidism) in all clinical forms of hypophosphatasia except odontohypophosphatasia.[1] However, biochemical or histochemical detection of low ALP activity in osseous tissue distinguishes hypophosphatasia from other disorders. Open cranial "sutures" are actually uncalcified osteoid. Dental histopathology shows aplasia or hypoplasia of cementum. Enlarged pulp chambers indicate impaired dentinogenesis. Changes vary from tooth to tooth.

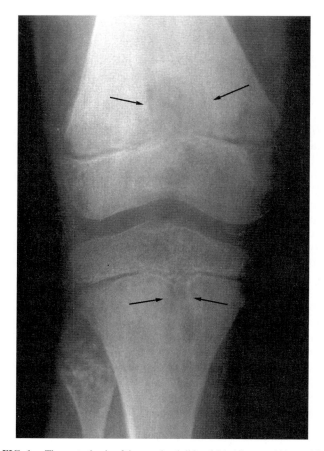

FIG. 1. The metaphysis of the proximal tibia of this 10-year-old boy with mild childhood hypophosphatasia shows a subtle but characteristic "tongue" of radiolucency (arrows). Note, however, that his rickets does not manifest with widening of the growth plate.

INHERITANCE

Perinatal and infantile hypophosphatasia are inherited as autosomal recessive traits. Parents of these severely affected patients usually have low or low-normal serum ALP activity and sometimes mildly elevated plasma PLP levels and modest phosphoethanolaminuria. Challenge with vitamin B_6 (pyridoxine) orally is followed by a distinctly abnormal increment in plasma PLP levels in patients, and perhaps in most carriers.[1]

The mode of inheritance for the milder forms of hypophosphatasia, odontohypophosphatasia, and adult-onset disease can be autosomal dominant or recessive.[1,10,11]

BIOCHEMICAL GENETIC DEFECT

In keeping with an inborn error of metabolism that selectively compromises the TNSALP isoenzyme, autopsy studies of perinatal and infantile hypophosphatasia show profound deficiency of ALP activity in bone, liver, and kidney, but not in the intestine or placenta. More than 100 different mutations have been identified worldwide in the *TNSALP* gene.[10,11]

PATHOGENESIS

Studies of vitamin B_6 metabolism in hypophosphatasia indicate that TNSALP regulates the extracellular concentration of a variety of phosphocompounds.[3] Accumulation of PPi, an inhibitor of hydroxyapatite crystal formation and growth, is increasingly incriminated in the impaired skeletal mineralization.[2,3,12] The *TNSALP* knockout mouse model, which recapitulates infantile hypophosphatasia,[13] is helping to clarify the physiological role of TNSALP.

TREATMENT

There is no established medical therapy for hypophosphatasia. Marrow cell transplantation seemed to rescue and improve a patient with the infantile form.[8] Dietary Pi restriction to correct hyperphosphatemia and thereby reduce inhibition of TNSALP by Pi is being tested in milder cases.[14]

Unless there is documented deficiency, it seems important to avoid traditional treatments for rickets or osteomalacia (e.g., vitamin D sterols and mineral supplementation) because circulating levels of calcium, Pi, 25(OH)D, and $1,25(OH)_2D$ are usually not reduced.[1] Furthermore, traditional regimens may exacerbate any predisposition to hypercalcemia or hypercalciuria.

The hypercalcemia of perinatal or infantile hypophosphatasia may respond to restriction of dietary calcium and to salmon calcitonin and/or glucocorticoid therapy.[15] Fractures in children and adults do mend; however, healing may be delayed, including after osteotomy. Placement of load-sharing intramedullary rods, rather than load-sparing plates, seems best for the acute or prophylactic treatment of fractures and pseudofractures in adults.[7] Expert dental care is important. Dentures may be necessary even for pediatric patients.

PRENATAL DIAGNOSIS

Perinatal hypophosphatasia can be detected in utero. Combined use of serial sonography (with attention to the limbs as well as to the skull) and radiologic study of the fetus have been successful in the second trimester.[16] First-trimester diagnosis is now DNA-based.[16] Importantly, however, some cases of childhood hypophosphatasia may manifest bowing in utero that does not reflect a lethal skeletal dysplasia and corrects postnatally.[4]

REFERENCES

1. Whyte MP 2001 Hypophosphatasia. In: Scriver CR, Beaudet AL, Sly WS, Valle D, Childs B, Vogelstein B (eds.) The Metabolic and Molecular Bases of Inherited Disease, 8th ed. McGraw-Hill, New York, NY, USA, pp. 5313–5329.
2. Caswell AM, Whyte MP, Russell RGG 1992 Hypophosphatasia and the extracellular metabolism of inorganic pyrophosphate: Clinical and laboratory aspects. Crit Rev Clin Lab Sci 28:175–232.
3. Whyte MP 2002 Hypophosphatasia: Nature's window on alkaline phosphatase function in man. In: Bilezikian J, Raisz L, Rodan G (eds.) Principles of Bone Biology, 2nd ed. Academic Press, San Diego, CA, pp. 1229–1248.
4. Pauli RM, Modaff P, Sipes SL, Whyte MP 1999 Mild hypophosphatasia mimicking severe osteogenesis imperfecta in utero: Bent but not broken. Am J Med Genet 86:434–438.
5. Weinstein RS, Whyte MP 1981 Heterogeneity of adult hypophosphatasia: Report of severe and mild cases. Arch Intern Med 141:727–731.
6. Chuck AJ, Pattrick MG, Hamilton E, Wilson R, Doherty M 1989 Crystal deposition in hypophosphatasia: A reappraisal. Ann Rheum Dis 48:571–576.
7. Coe JD, Murphy WA, Whyte MP 1986 Management of femoral fractures and pseudofractures in adult hypophosphatasia. J Bone Joint Surg Am 68:981–990.
8. Whyte MP, Kurtzburg J, McAlister WH, Podgornik MN, Mumm SR, Coburn SP, Ryan LM, Miller CR, Gottesman GS, Martin PL 2003 Marrow cell transplantation for infantile hypophosphatasia. J Bone Miner Res 18:624–636.
9. Shohat M, Rimoin DL, Gerber HE, Lachman RS 1991 Perinatal hypophosphatasia: Clinical, radiologic, and morphologic findings. Pediatr Radiol 21:421–427.
10. Henthorn PS, Raducha M, Fedde KN, Lafferty MA, Whyte MP 1992 Different missense mutations at the tissue-nonspecific alkaline phosphatase gene locus in autosomal recessively inherited forms of mild and severe hypophosphatasia. Proc Natl Acad Sci USA 89:9924–9928.
11. Mornet E 2000 Hypophosphatasia: The mutations in the tissue-nonspecific alkaline phosphatase gene. Hum Mutat 15:309–315.
12. Hessle L, Johnson KA, Anderson HC, Narisawa S, Sali A, Goding JW, Terkeltaub R, Millan JL 2002 Tissue-nonspecific alkaline phosphatase and plasma cell membrane glycoprotein-1 are central antagonistic regulators of bone mineralization. Proc Natl Acad Sci USA 99:9445–9449.
13. Fedde KN, Blair L, Silverstein J, Coburn SP, Ryan LM, Weinstein RS, Waymire K, Narisawa S, Millan JL, MacGregor GR, Whyte MP 1999 Alkaline phosphatase knock-out mice recapitulate the metabolic and skeletal defects of infantile hypophosphatasia. J Bone Miner Res 14:2015–2026.
14. Wenkert D, Podgornik MN, Coburn SP, Ryan LM, Mumm S, Whyte MP 2002 Dietary phosphate restriction therapy for hypophosphatasia: Preliminary observations. J Bone Miner Res 17:S384.
15. Barcia JP, Strife CF, Langman CB 1997 Infantile hypophosphatasia: Treatment options to control hypercalcemia, hypercalciuria, and chronic bone demineralization. J Pediatr 130:825–828.
16. Henthorn PS, Whyte MP 1995 Infantile hypophosphatasia: Successful prenatal assessment by testing for tissue-nonspecific alkaline phosphatase gene mutations. Prenat Diagn 15:1001–1006.

Chapter 73. Fanconi Syndrome and Renal Tubular Acidosis

Peter J. Tebben[1,3] and Rajiv Kumar[1–5]

[1]Division of Endocrinology, Diabetes, Metabolism and Nutrition; [2]Division of Nephrology; [3]Department of Internal Medicine; [4]Mayo Proteomic Research Center; and [5]Department of Biochemistry and Molecular Biology, Mayo Clinic, Rochester, Minnesota

DEFINITION AND PRESENTATION

Fanconi syndrome is a disorder of renal proximal tubules characterized by decreased reabsorption of phosphorus, glucose, and amino acids. These findings are often accompanied by metabolic acidosis secondary to proximal tubular bicarbonate wasting (type II RTA). Impaired handling of potassium, calcium, uric acid, sodium, water, and low molecular weight proteins have also been described.[1–6] Laboratory findings include hypophosphatemia, hyperphosphaturia, and a low tubular maximum for inorganic phosphate; hypobicarbonatemia, excessive bicarbonate excretion in the urine, and a low tubular maximum for bicarbonate; glycosuria and aminoaciduria; elevated serum alkaline phosphatase, and normal serum calcium, normal parathyroid hormone (PTH), normal serum 25-hydroxyvitamin D [25(OH)D$_3$], and inappropriately normal serum 1α, 25-dihydroxyvitamin D [1α,25(OH)$_2$D$_3$] concentrations. Radiological studies reveal osteomalacia or rickets.

Children with Fanconi syndrome present clinically with growth failure and rickets. Fanconi syndrome has been associated with many diseases (Table 1), including the lysosomal storage disease, cystinosis, which is the most common inherited cause in the pediatric population. Adults present with osteomalacia, which manifests as bone pain, proximal muscle weakness, and spontaneous fractures. Multiple myeloma is the most common cause of Fanconi syndrome in adults. The diagnosis can be established by showing the biochemical abnormalities noted above: a reduced tubular maximum for phosphate, glycosuria with normal plasma glucose concentrations, and generalized aminoaciduria. Because some patients will have phosphorus values that fall in the low normal range, it is useful to calculate the fractional excretion of phosphorus, which will be elevated in Fanconi syndrome.

PHYSIOLOGY OF SOLUTE TRANSPORT IN THE PROXIMAL TUBULE

The transport of filtered solute across the proximal tubular membrane requires multiple specialized transport proteins that are present in the luminal brush border. Amino acids are almost entirely reabsorbed in the proximal tubule by a variety of sodium-dependent transporters.[7,8] Transporters for acidic, basic, and neutral amino acids have been identified, as well as carriers that are specific to single amino acids.[8] In Fanconi syndrome, all amino acids are lost in excess in the urine; however, urinary amino acid losses do not seem to be of clinical consequence. Glucose normally is reabsorbed with great efficiency primarily by

the proximal tubule. This is accomplished by sodium-dependent secondary active transport. Two separate transporters have been identified: a high capacity low affinity transporter (SGLT2) in the S1 segment and a low capacity high affinity transporter (SGLT1) in the S3 segment.[8–10] Glucose is transported out of the epithelial cells through the basolateral membrane by the sodium-glucose transporter GLUT2.[10] Under normal conditions, very little glucose passes from the proximal tubule into the final urine. Glycosuria may contribute to polyuria and polydipsia often seen in Fanconi syndrome but is otherwise clinically insignificant. Reabsorption of inorganic phosphorus (Pi) occurs pri-

TABLE 1. DISORDERS ASSOCIATED WITH THE FANCONI SYNDROME

Acquired	Heritable
Multiple myeloma	Cystinosis
Lymphoma	Lowe syndrome
Light chain nephropathy	Hereditary fructose intolerance
Amyloidosis	Tyrosinemia
Sjögren's syndrome	Galactosemia
Nephrotic syndrome	Glycogen storage disease
Renal transplantation	Wilson's disease
Balkan nephropathy	Cytochrome oxidase deficiency
Paroxysmal nocturnal	Subacute necrotizing encephalomyelopathy
hemoglobinuria	Alport syndrome
Vitamin D deficiency	Medullary cystic disease
Interstitial nephritis/	Idiopathic (AD, AR, XLR)
uveitis syndrome	Fanconi-Bickel syndrome
Renal vein thrombosis	Dent's disease
	GRACILE syndrome
Drugs	Rod-cone dystrophy, sensorineural
Outdated tetracycline	deafness, and renal dysfunction
Methyl-3-chromone	
6-Mercaptopurine	
Gentamicin	
Valproic acid	
Streptozocin	
Isophthalanilide	
Ifosphamide	
Cephalothin	
Heavy Metals	
Lead	
Cadmium	
Mercury	
Uranium	
Platinum	
Copper	
Bismuth	
Other	
Parquat	
Lysol	
Toluene inhalation	

The authors have no conflict of interest.

marily in the proximal tubule by a sodium-phosphate co-transporter system.[11–13] The sodium-phosphate type II (NaPi-2) co-transporter is located in the brush border of renal tubular epithelial cells and is influenced by dietary phosphorus intake and PTH.[14,15]

MECHANISMS OF ACIDIFICATION OF THE URINE

The two main mechanisms the kidney uses to maintain acid-base balance include proximal tubule HCO_3^- reabsorption and distal tubule H^+ excretion.[16–21] Under physiologic conditions, 80–90% of filtered HCO_3^- is reabsorbed in the proximal tubule principally by a Na^+-H^+ exchange mechanism. The distal tubule excretes H^+ and thus regenerates bicarbonate. In addition, NH_3 generation by the kidney facilitates the secretion of H^+ ion. Renal tubular acidosis results from a failure to reabsorb bicarbonate in the proximal tubule or a failure to generate or secrete H^+ in the distal tubule.

Type II renal tubular acidosis (RTA), which is often associated with Fanconi syndrome, results from excessive losses of bicarbonate from the proximal tubule. The urine pH in type II RTA can be variable, in contrast to type I in which it is consistently greater than 5.5. This is because of the ability of the proximal tubule to reabsorb the filtered load of HCO_3^- once the serum level falls below a given threshold. If untreated, the serum HCO_3^- will usually remain greater than 12, and the urine pH may fall below 5.5. Shortly after HCO_3^- is administered for treatment or for diagnostic purposes, the transport maximum for HCO_3^- will be exceeded, and the urine pH will rise significantly. A urine pH greater than 6.5 with a serum HCO_3^- 22 or less will establish the diagnosis.[22] An elevated fractional excretion of HCO_3^- in response to a bicarbonate load can also differentiate type II from type I RTA.

In type I RTA, the distal tubule is unable to excrete hydrogen ions appropriately. As a result, the serum bicarbonate level can drop less than 10, and the urine pH is inappropriately elevated (greater than 5.5).[23] Hypokalemia and nephrolithiasis are common clinical findings. These characteristics can help distinguish type I from type II RTA. Type I RTA can occur in Fanconi syndrome if there is damage to the distal tubule as well as the proximal tubule by the causal agent (e.g., drug or metal).

PATHOGENESIS OF HYPOPHOSPHATEMIA AND BONE DISEASE IN FANCONI SYNDROME

Phosphaturia and hypophosphatemia are hallmarks of Fanconi syndrome. Pi plays a vital role in bone mineralization and normally is incorporated into osteoid that has been deposited by osteoblasts. When Pi is not available in sufficient quantity, osteomalacia will result with thickened osteoid seams that are readily apparent on bone biopsy.[24] The extracellular pool of phosphorus is regulated by dietary intake as well as the influence $1\alpha,25(OH)_2D_3$ and PTH.[25–30] $25(OH)D_3$ conversion to the more active metabolite, $1\alpha,25(OH)_2D_3$, can be stimulated by low serum Pi through a PTH-independent mechanism.[31] $1\alpha,25(OH)_2D_3$ in-

creases Pi absorption in the intestine and Pi reabsorption in the kidney.[32,33]

Renal proximal tubule epithelial cells have a high metabolic requirement. Generalized cellular toxicity seems more likely to account for the syndrome than multiple transport defects, because so many filtered solutes are affected. Fanconi syndrome probably results from disrupted mitochondrial ATP production and/or Na^+/K^+-ATPase activity.[34–37] Either of these mechanisms can lead to a diminished sodium electrochemical gradient that drives the majority of solute transport across the luminal membrane. It is likely that multiple toxic proteins, drugs, insoluble metabolic products, or metals alter proximal tubule cell function in a global manner by diverse pathways. The end result is reduced solute reabsorption. PTH, which is elevated in some patients with Fanconi syndrome, acts to reduce the number of NaPi-2 co-transporters in the luminal membrane, thereby reducing the tubular transport maximum for phosphorus and inducing phosphaturia. In the nondiseased state, a low phosphorus diet will increase the number of co-transporters in the brush border in an attempt to maintain normal extracellular Pi levels.[15,38] A maleic acid–induced model of Fanconi syndrome in rats results in downregulation of the NaPi-2 co-transporter,[39] offering another possible explanation for phosphaturia and hypophosphatemia see in human Fanconi syndrome.

The expected elevation of $1\alpha,25(OH)_2D_3$ concentrations in the face of hypophosphatemia are not seen in Fanconi syndrome. The result is a relative or absolute vitamin D deficiency. The $25(OH)_2D_3$ 1α-hydroxylase is a multi-component mitochondrial enzyme located in the renal cortex, the activity of which is reduced in an experimental model of the Fanconi syndrome.[40] Significant hepatic damage or reduced renal mass associated with many of the diseases listed in Table 1 may also account for some of vitamin D deficiency. However, vitamin D deficiency has been described in Fanconi syndrome patients without significant liver disease and with normal or minimally reduced glomerular filtration rates (GFR).[24,41,42]

The bone disease in Fanconi syndrome could be worsened by the presence of acidosis. RTA is commonly seen in patients with Fanconi syndrome. It is generally a type II RTA, although defects in H^+ ion excretion may also be present.

The pathogenesis of bone disease in chronic metabolic acidosis is multifactorial. As previously discussed, Fanconi syndrome manifests as rickets and linear growth failure in children and osteomalacia in adults. It is assumed that phosphaturia and hypophosphatemia play a major role in the development of rickets/osteomalacia. However, acidosis can cause bone disease independent of phosphate wasting. Bone serves as a large reservoir of buffer for the excess H^+.[43] Acute and chronic acidosis induces demineralization of bone and increased urinary losses of calcium.[43,44] Patients with RTA have lower bone mineral density (BMD) and increased osteoid volume compared with reference values.[45,46] Osteoblast-like cells cultured in an acidic environment show an increased response to PTH and increased mRNA for the PTH/PTHrP receptor.[47] This would presumably increase bone turnover in favor of resorption. Cultured mouse calvaria exposed to an acidic environment

TABLE 2. SERUM CALCIUM, PHOSPHORUS, PTH, 25(OH)$_2$D, AND 1,25(OH)$_2$D$_3$ CONCENTRATIONS AND URINE SOLUTE CONCENTRATIONS IN VARIOUS HYPOPHOSPHATEMIC CONDITIONS

Condition	sPi	sCa	sPTH	s25(OH)D	s1,25(OH)$_2$D	U_{Pi}	FE_{Pi}	U_{Ca}	FE_{Ca}	U_{HCO_3}	FE_{HCO_3}	U_{Glu}	FE_{Glu}	U_{AA}
Fanconi syndrome	D	N	N or I	N	D or N	I	I	N	N	I	I	I	I	I
Nutritional vitamin D deficiency, malabsorption	D	D	I	D	V	I	I	D	D	N or I	N or I	N	N	N or I
Impaired intestinal Pi absorption (use of binders)	D	N or I	D or N	N	I	D	D	I	I	N	N	N	N	N
X-linked hypophosphatemic rickets (XLH)	D	N	N	N	D or N	I	I	N	N	N	N	N	N	N
Autosomal dominant hypophosphatemic rickets (ADHR)	D	N	N	N	D or N	I	I	N	N	N	N	N	N	N
Tumor-induced osteomalacia	D	N	N	N	D or N	I	I	N	N	N	N	N	N	N
Vitamin D–dependent rickets (type 1)	D or low N	D	I	N	D	I	I	D	D	N or I	N or I	N	N	N or I
Vitamin D–dependent rickets (type 2)	D	D	I	N	I	I	I	D	D	N or I	N or I	N	N	N or I
Primary hyperparathyroidism	D or low N	I	I	N	N or I	I	I	I	D	N or I	N or I	N	N	N or I
Humoral hypercalcemia of malignancy	D or low N	I	D or N	N	D or N	I	I	I	D	N or I	N or I	N	N	N or I
Hereditary hypophosphatemic rickets with hypercalciuria	D	N	D or N	N	I	I	I	I	I	N	N	N	N	N

D, decreased; I, increased; N, normal; V, variable.

show increased osteoclastic and decreased osteoblastic activity as determined by measurements of collagen synthesis, alkaline phosphatase activity, and β-glucuronidase activity compared with controls.[43,48] Vitamin D metabolism is likely also affected as evidenced by impaired conversion of 25(OH)D$_3$ in the rat kidney exposed to a low pH.[49,50] There are many pathways by which chronic acidosis seems to be inhibiting bone formation and enhancing demineralization.

DIFFERENTIAL DIAGNOSIS

Hypophosphatemia is seen in several metabolic bone disorders that should be distinguished from Fanconi syndrome. This can usually be accomplished by determining serum phosphorus, calcium, PTH, 25-hydroxyvitamin D, and 1,25-dihydroxyvitamin D concentrations, as well as urine studies to measure excretion rates of several filtered solutes. Other disorders mimicking Fanconi syndrome are listed in Table 2.

TABLE 3. VITAMIN D ANALOGS

Vitamin D	Potency relative to D$_3$	Duration of toxicity with renal failure (days)
D$_3$ (cholecalciferol)	1	17–30
Dihydrotachysterol	100	17–30
25(OH)D$_3$	500	15–30
1α(OH)D$_3$	5000	5–15
1,25(OH)$_2$D$_3$	5000	2–7

Adapted with permission from Johnson WJ 1984 Vitamin D: Basic and Clinical Aspects. Kluwer, Hague, Netherlands, p. 651.

TREATMENT

Treatment of Fanconi syndrome–induced bone disease should be based on its underlying cause. If the associated disease can be treated or offending agent removed (Table 1), Fanconi syndrome may resolve and the metabolic bone disease remit. The relative contribution of disordered phosphorus, bicarbonate, vitamin D$_3$, and calcium metabolism may vary in individual patients. Phosphate and calcium replacement have been reported to improve osteomalacia and rickets in Fanconi syndrome.[46,51–55] Neutral phosphate (1–4 g/day) in divided doses are commonly required to maintain phosphorus levels. Vitamin D replacement with vitamin D$_2$ or D$_3$ [25(OH)$_2$D$_3$ and 1,25(OH)$_2$D$_3$] have been successfully used.[24,46,51,52] Many diseases associated with Fanconi syndrome are also characterized by renal failure. The relative potency and duration of toxicity varies with

TABLE 4. BICARBONATE REPLACEMENT

Potassium citrate (Urocit-K)	
540-mg tablet	5 mEq per tablet
1080-mg tablet	10 mEq per tablet
Potassium citrate + citric acid	
Oral solution (Polycitra-K)	2 mEq/1 ml
Crystals (Polycitra-K)	30 mEq per packet
Sodium citrate + citric acid (Bicitra or Shohl's solution)	1 mEq/1 ml
Potassium citrate + sodium citrate + citric acid (Polycitra)	2 mEq/1 ml
Sodium bicarbonate	
325-mg tablet	3.87 mEq per tablet
650-mg tablet	7.74 mEq per tablet
Baking soda	60 mEq/teaspoon

vitamin D analogs and should be taken into account when choosing which form to use (Table 3).

Alkali therapy alone can improve RTA-associated osteomalacia.[56] Oral bicarbonate in doses of 10–20 mEq/kg/day are typically required to correct the acidosis caused by proximal RTA with or without Fanconi syndrome. Generally, distal RTA bicarbonate requirements are considerably less (1–2 mEq/kg/day in divided doses). However, infants and children with distal RTA may require substantially higher doses to maintain normal growth.[57] Many forms of alkali replacement are available (Table 4) and can be tailored to the individual patient needs. In type I RTA, it is often necessary to replace potassium before initiating alkali replacement, because correction of the acidosis will worsen hypokalemia. Treatment of type IV RTA includes a low potassium diet, alkali replacement, and occasionally, a loop diuretic.

REFERENCES

1. Sebastian A, McSherry E, Morris RC Jr 1971 On the mechanism of renal potassium wasting in renal tubular acidosis associated with the Fanconi syndrome (type 2 RTA). J Clin Invest 50:231–243.
2. Rodriguez Soriano J, Houston IB, Boichis H, Edelmann CM Jr 1968 Calcium and phosphorus metabolism in the fanconi syndrome. J Clin Endocrinol Metab 28:1555–1563.
3. Rodriquez-Soriano J, Vallo A, Castillo G, Oliveros R 1980 Renal handling of water and sodium in children with proximal and distal renal tabular acidosis. Nephron 25:193–198.
4. Houston IB, Boichis H, Edelmann CM Jr 1968 Fanconi syndrome with renal sodium wasting and metabolic alkalosis. Am J Med 44:638–646.
5. Dillard MG, Pesce AJ, Pollak VE, Boreisha I 1971 Proteinuria and renal protein clearances in patients with renal tubular disorders. J Lab Clin Med 78:203–215.
6. Lee DB, Drinkard JP, Rosen VJ, Gonick HC 1972 The adult Fanconi syndrome: Observations on etiology, morphology, renal function and mineral metabolism in three patients. Medicine (Baltimore) 51:107–138.
7. Murer H 1982 Renal transport of amino acids: Membrane mechanisms. Contrib Nephrol 33:14–28.
8. Moe OW, Berry CA, Rector FC Jr 2000 Renal transport of glucose, amino acids, sodium, chloride, and water. In: Brenner BM (ed.) The Kidney, vol. 1. Saunders, Philadelphia, PA, USA, pp. 375–415.
9. Kanai Y, Lee WS, You G, Brown D, Hediger MA 1994 The human kidney low affinity Na+/glucose cotransporter SGLT2. Delineation of the major renal reabsorptive mechanism for D-glucose. J Clin Invest 93:397–404.
10. Brown GK 2000 Glucose transporters: Structure, function and consequences of deficiency. J Inherit Metab Dis 23:237–246.
11. Murer H, Kohler K, Lambert G, Stange G, Biber J, Forster I 2002 The renal type IIa Na/Pi cotransporter: Structure-function relationships. Cell Biochem Biophys 36:215–220.
12. Biber J, Murer H, Forster I 1998 The renal type II Na+/phosphate cotransporter. J Bioenerg Biomembr 30:187–194.
13. Biber J, Custer M, Magagnin S, Hayes G, Werner A, Lotscher M, Kaissling B, Murer H 1996 Renal Na/Pi-cotransporters. Kidney Int 49:981–985.
14. Murer H, Lotscher M, Kaissling B, Levi M, Kempson SA, Biber J 1996 Renal brush border membrane Na/Pi-cotransport: Molecular aspects in PTH-dependent and dietary regulation. Kidney Int 49:1769–1773.
15. Murer H, Hernando N, Forster I, Biber J 2001 Molecular aspects in the regulation of renal inorganic phosphate reabsorption: The type IIa sodium/inorganic phosphate co-transporter as the key player. Curr Opin Nephrol Hypertens 10:555–561.
16. Kurtzman NA 2000 Renal tubular acidosis syndromes. South Med J 93:1042–1052.
17. Kurtzman NA 1990 Disorders of distal acidification. Kidney Int 38:720–727.
18. Batlle D, Kurtzman NA 1982 Distal renal tubular acidosis: Pathogenesis and classification. Am J Kidney Dis 1:328–344.
19. Arruda JA, Kurtzman NA 1980 Mechanisms and classification of deranged distal urinary acidification. Am J Physiol 239:F515–F523.
20. Gluck SL, Iyori M, Holliday LS, Kostrominova T, Lee BS 1996 Distal urinary acidification from Homer Smith to the present. Kidney Int 49:1660–1664.
21. Bastani B, Gluck SL 1996 New insights into the pathogenesis of distal renal tubular acidosis. Miner Electrolyte Metab 22:396–409.
22. Gluck SL 1998 Acid-base. Lancet 352:474–479.
23. Rodriguez-Soriano J 2000 New insights into the pathogenesis of renal tubular acidosis–from functional to molecular studies. Pediatr Nephrol 14:1121–1136.
24. Clarke BL, Wynne AG, Wilson DM, Fitzpatrick LA 1995 Osteomalacia associated with adult Fanconi's syndrome: Clinical and diagnostic features. Clin Endocrinol (Oxf) 43:479–490.
25. Berndt T, Knox FG 1992 Renal regulation of phosphate excretion. In: Seldin DW Giebisch G (eds.) The Kidney: Physiology and Pathophysiology, 2nd ed. Raven Press, LTD, New York, NY, USA, pp. 2511–2532.
26. Kumar R 1988 Osteomalacia. In: Bardin CW (ed.) Current Therapy in Endocrinology and Metabolism, 3rd ed. B.C. Decker, Inc, Philadelphia, PA, USA, pp.361–365.
27. Kumar R 1990 Vitamin D metabolism and mechanisms of calcium transport. J Am Soc Nephrol 1:30–42.
28. Kumar R 2002 New insights into phosphate homeostasis: Fibroblast growth factor 23 and frizzled-related protein-4 are phosphaturic factors derived from tumors associated with osteomalacia. Curr Opin Nephrol Hypertens 11:547–553.
29. Kumar R 1997 Phosphatonin–a new phosphaturetic hormone? (Lessons from tumour-induced osteomalacia and X-linked hypophosphatasemia). Nephrol Dial Transplant 12:11–13.
30. Kumar R 2000 Tumor-induced osteomalacia and the regulation of phosphate homeostasis. Bone 27:333–338.
31. Tanaka Y, Deluca HF 1973 The control of 25-hydroxyvitamin D metabolism by inorganic phosphorus. Arch Biochem Biophys 154:566–574.
32. Steele TH, Engle JE, Tanaka Y, Lorenc RS, Dudgeon KL, DeLuca HF 1975 Phosphatemic action of 1,25-dihydroxyvitamin D3. Am J Physiol 229:489–495.
33. Tanaka Y, Deluca HF 1974 Role of 1,25-dihydroxyvitamin D3 in maintaining serum phosphorus and curing rickets. Proc Natl Acad Sci USA 71:1040–1044.
34. Guan S, el-Dahr S, Dipp S, Batuman V 1999 Inhibition of Na-K-ATPase activity and gene expression by a myeloma light chain in proximal tubule cells. J Investig Med 47:496–501.
35. Batuman V, Guan S, O'Donovan R, Puschett JB 1994 Effect of myeloma light chains on phosphate and glucose transport in renal proximal tubule cells. Ren Physiol Biochem 17:294–300.
36. Coor C, Salmon RF, Quigley R, Marver D, Baum M 1991 Role of adenosine triphosphate (ATP) and NaK ATPase in the inhibition of proximal tubule transport with intracellular cystine loading. J Clin Invest 87:955–961.
37. Castano E, Marzabal P, Casado FJ, Felipe A, Pastor-Anglada M 1997 Na+, K(+)-ATPase expression in maleic-acid-induced Fanconi syndrome in rats. Clin Sci (Lond) 92:247–253.
38. Hoag HM, Martel J, Gauthier C, Tenenhouse HS 1999 Effects of Npt2 gene ablation and low-phosphate diet on renal Na(+)/phosphate cotransport and cotransporter gene expression. J Clin Invest 104:679–686.
39. Haviv YS, Wald H, Levi M, Dranitzki-Elhalel M, Popovtzer MM 2001 Late-onset downregulation of NaPi-2 in experimental Fanconi syndrome. Pediatr Nephrol 16:412–416.
40. Brewer ED, Tsai HC, Szeto KS, Morris RC Jr 1977 Maleic acid-induced impaired conversion of 25(OH)D3 to 1,25(OH)2D3: Implications for Fanconi's syndrome. Kidney Int 12:244–252.
41. Baran DT, Marcy TW 1984 Evidence for a defect in vitamin D metabolism in a patient with incomplete Fanconi syndrome. J Clin Endocrinol Metab 59:998–1001.
42. Colussi G, De Ferrari ME, Surian M, Malberti F, Rombola G, Pontoriero G, Galvanini G, Minetti L 1985 Vitamin D metabolites and osteomalacia in the human Fanconi syndrome. Proc Eur Dial Transplant Assoc Eur Ren Assoc 21:756–760.
43. Bushinsky DA, Frick KK 2000 The effects of acid on bone. Curr Opin Nephrol Hypertens 9:369–379.
44. Eiam-ong S, Kurtzman NA 1994 Metabolic acidosis and bone disease. Miner Electrolyte Metab 20:72–80.
45. Domrongkitchaiporn S, Pongsakul C, Stitchantrakul W, Sirikulchayanonta V, Ongphiphadhanakul B, Radinahamed P, Karnsombut P, Kunkitti N, Ruang-raksa C, Rajatanavin R 2001 Bone mineral density and histology in distal renal tubular acidosis. Kidney Int 59:1086–1093.

46. Dalmak S, Erek E, Serdengecti K, Okar I, Ulku U, Basaran M 1996 A case study of adult-onset hypophosphatemic osteomalacia with idiopathic fanconi syndrome. Nephron 72:121–122.
47. Disthabanchong S, Martin KJ, McConkey CL, Gonzalez EA 2002 Metabolic acidosis up-regulates PTH/PTHrP receptors in UMR 106–01 osteoblast-like cells. Kidney Int 62:1171–1177.
48. Krieger NS, Sessler NE, Bushinsky DA 1992 Acidosis inhibits osteoblastic and stimulates osteoclastic activity in vitro. Am J Physiol 262:F442–F448.
49. Reddy GS, Jones G, Kooh SW, Fraser D 1982 Inhibition of 25-hydroxyvitamin D3–1-hydroxylase by chronic metabolic acidosis. Am J Physiol 243:E265–E271.
50. Kawashima H, Kraut JA, Kurokawa K 1982 Metabolic acidosis suppresses 25-hydroxyvitamin in D3–1alpha-hydroxylase in the rat kidney. Distinct site and mechanism of action. J Clin Invest 70:135–140.
51. Zeier M, Ritz E 2000 The bedridden osteomalacic patient with Fanconi syndrome in pre-terminal renal failure. Nephrol Dial Transplant 15:1880–1882.
52. Lambert J, Lips P 1989 Adult hypophosphataemic osteomalacia with Fanconi syndrome presenting in a patient with neurofibromatosis. Neth J Med 35:309–316.
53. Long WS, Seashore MR, Siegel NJ, Bia MJ 1990 Idiopathic Fanconi syndrome with progressive renal failure: A case report and discussion. Yale J Biol Med 63:15–28.
54. Smith R, Lindenbaum RH, Walton RJ 1976 Hypophosphataemic osteomalacia and Fanconi syndrome of adult onset with dominant inheritance. Possible relationship with diabetes mellitus. Q J Med 45:387–400.
55. Harrison NA, Bateman JM, Ledingham JG, Smith R 1991 Renal failure in adult onset hypophosphatemic osteomalacia with Fanconi syndrome: A family study and review of the literature. Clin Nephrol 35:148–150.
56. Richards P, Chamberlain MJ, Wrong OM 1972 Treatment of osteomalacia of renal tubular acidosis by sodium bicarbonate alone. Lancet 2:994–997.
57. McSherry E, Morris RC Jr 1978 Attainment and maintenance of normal stature with alkali therapy in infants and children with classic renal tubular acidosis. J Clin Invest 61:509–527.

Chapter 74.   Renal Osteodystrophy in Adults and Children

William G. Goodman,[1] Jack W. Coburn,[1] Eduardo Slatopolsky,[3] Isidro B. Salusky,[2] and L. Darryl Quarles[4]

[1]Department of Medicine and [2]Department of Pediatrics, David Geffen School of Medicine at UCLA, Los Angeles, California; [3]Renal Division, Washington University, St. Louis, Missouri; and [4]Center for Bone and Mineral Disorders, Duke University, Durham, North Carolina

INTRODUCTION

Mineral metabolism is a closely integrated process involving the kidneys, intestine, parathyroid glands, and bone. When renal function declines, mineral homeostasis is disrupted, resulting in diverse manifestations in bone and other tissues. In its broadest sense, the term renal osteodystrophy encompasses all the disorders of bone and mineral metabolism associated with chronic kidney disease.

Both the excretory and the metabolic components of renal function participate in regulating mineral metabolism. The total body balances for calcium, phosphorus, magnesium, and other minerals are modulated by adjusting amounts excreted in the urine. Reductions in net acid excretion by the kidney lead to systemic acidosis, affecting both the mineral content of bone and bone cell metabolism. Substances such as aluminum and β-2-microglobulin may be retained in patients with impaired renal function, leading to specific disorders of the bones and joints.[1,2]

In regard to renal metabolism, the kidney is a major target organ for parathyroid hormone (PTH), and it also serves as an important site for the degradation of PTH. Calcitriol, or 1,25-dihydroxyvitamin D, is the biologically most active form of vitamin D, and it is synthesized predominantly by epithelial cells of the proximal nephron. Calcitriol has diverse hormonal actions in a variety of tissues, serving as a key determinant of intestinal calcium absorption and as an important regulator of pre-pro-PTH gene transcription. Calcitriol also modifies cell proliferation and differentiated cellular functions in bone, cartilage, and the parathyroid glands. Because even modest reductions in kidney function substantially alter renal excretory and metabolic capacity, mineral homeostasis is progressively compromised in patients with chronic renal failure.[3]

Disturbances in the regulation of PTH synthesis and secretion, parathyroid gland hyperplasia, and alterations in calcium and vitamin D metabolism are key contributors to the pathogenesis of renal bone disease. Together with other factors such as systemic acidosis and the retention of aluminum or β-2-microglobulin, the skeletal lesions that develop in patients with renal failure reflect complex interactions among several pathogenic components.

RENAL BONE DISEASES

The renal bone diseases represent a spectrum of skeletal disorders ranging from high-turnover lesions arising predominantly from excess PTH secretion to low-turnover lesions of diverse etiology that are typically associated with normal or reduced plasma PTH levels (Fig. 1).[4] Transitions among histological subtypes are determined by one or more dominant pathogenic factors. Such changes can be documented by bone biopsy and quantitative bone histology, which represents the definitive method for the diagnosis of renal osteodystrophy. Because plasma PTH levels represent the major determinant of bone formation and turnover in patients with chronic kidney disease, alterations in parathyroid gland function associated with renal failure play a pivotal role in the pathogenesis and evolution of renal osteodystrophy.[5,6]

Regulation of PTH Synthesis and Secretion

PTH is synthesized in parathyroid cells and stored in secretory granules, providing a reservoir of hormone that is

---

The authors have no conflict of interest.

Spectrum of Renal Osteodystrophy

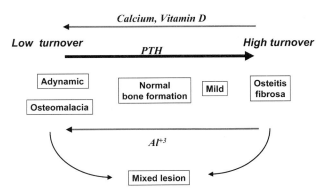

FIG. 1. The spectrum of renal osteodystrophy. (Reproduced from Salusky IB, Goodman WG, Growth hormone and calcitriol as modifiers of bone formation in renal osteodystrophy, Kidney Int 1995:**48:**657–665 with permission from Blackwell Publishing.)

available for release into the peripheral circulation. Pre-pro-PTH gene transcription is negatively regulated by interactions between 1,25-dihydroxyvitamin D bound to the vitamin D receptor (VDR) and a response element located 100–125 bp upstream from the transcriptional start site.[7] A calcium response element located approximately 3.6 kb upstream from the gene for pre-pro-PTH confers additional negative regulatory transcriptional control by calcium.[8] As such, pre-pro-PTH gene transcription is enhanced by reductions in the availability of either 1,25-dihydroxyvitamin D or calcium, whereas gene transcription and PTH synthesis are reduced when 1,25-dihydroxyvitamin D and calcium are abundant.

It is now known that the minute-to-minute release of PTH from parathyroid cells is regulated by a G-protein–coupled receptor that is located in the cell membrane.[9] The calcium-sensing receptor (CaSR) contains 1078 amino acids that form seven membrane spanning segments and a long extracellular domain containing clusters of acidic amino acids that probably interact with calcium and other extracellular cations.[10] The CaSR is expressed abundantly in parathyroid tissue.[11] Increases in blood ionized calcium concentration activate the CaSR and inhibit PTH release, whereas decreases in extracellular calcium concentration inactivate the CaSR and trigger PTH secretion.[11–13]

Although minute-to-minute variations in PTH secretion are regulated by the CaSR, there is a non-suppressible component of PTH secretion that persists even at high blood ionized calcium concentrations. Basal amounts of hormone are thus discharged into the circulation even when serum calcium levels are markedly elevated (Fig. 2).[14] The peptides released from the parathyroid cell vary according to the prevailing concentration of ionized calcium in blood, probably reflecting changes in intracellular hormone degradation.[15,16] When serum calcium levels are reduced, secretion of the full-length, biologically active hormone comprised of 84 amino acids, or PTH(1-84), predominates. In contrast, the secretion of PTH(1--84) decreases when blood ionized calcium levels rise, whereas the release of aminoterminally truncated PTH fragments increases.[16]

Pathogenesis of High-Turnover Bone Disease (Secondary Hyperparathyroidism)

Several factors contribute to sustained increases in plasma PTH levels, and ultimately, to the development of high-turnover skeletal lesions in patients with chronic renal failure (Fig. 3). Among these are hypocalcemia, impaired renal calcitriol production, skeletal resistance to the calcemic actions of PTH, alterations in the regulation of pre-pro-PTH gene transcription, reductions in VDR and CaSR expression in the parathyroids, and hyperphosphatemia caused by diminished renal phosphorus excretion.[3]

Because blood ionized calcium levels represent the most immediate stimulus for PTH secretion, disturbances that lead to hypocalcemia in patients with kidney disease promote excess PTH secretion. Renal 1,25-dihydroxyvitamin D production serves to maintain serum calcium levels by promoting active intestinal calcium absorption, by facilitating calcium release from bone, and by enhancing renal tubular calcium reabsorption. Serum 1,25-dihydroxyvitamin D levels decline progressively, however, as renal function diminishes, with wide-ranging effects on mineral homeostasis.[17] Although serum 1,25-dihydroxyvitamin D levels vary considerably at any given level of renal function, the proportion of patients with subnormal values increases as renal failure worsens. Such changes account, at least in part, for impaired intestinal calcium absorption and for moderate reductions in serum calcium concentration in patients with moderate to advanced renal failure.[18] Diminished VDR expression in intestinal epithelial cells may also contribute.[19,20]

Skeletal resistance to the calcemic actions of PTH further compromises the ability to maintain serum calcium levels in those with advanced renal disease. During infusions of parathyroid extract, increases in serum calcium concentration are less in patients with moderate to advanced renal failure than in normal subjects, and the correction of hypocalcemia occurs more slowly.[21] Thus, higher serum PTH levels are required to elicit equivalent biological responses in patients with chronic renal failure.[22,23] Abnormalities in vitamin D metabolism have been reported to account for these changes, but alterations in VDR expression could also contribute. In addition, expression of the receptor for PTH/

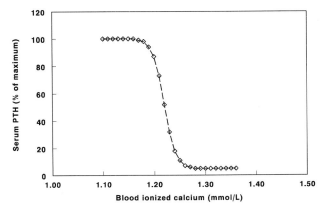

FIG. 2. The inverse sigmoidal relationship between blood ionized calcium concentrations and serum PTH levels in normal subjects.

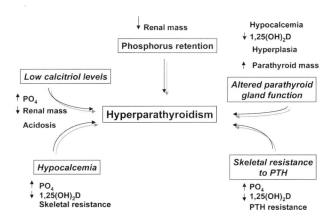

FIG. 3. Factors that contribute to the pathogenesis of secondary hyperparathyroidism.

PTHrP is reduced in renal failure. This change is probably attributable to renal failure per se rather than to PTH-mediated downregulation of its own receptor because receptor expression is low in uremic animals regardless of the prevailing serum level of PTH.[24] Decreases in PTH/PTHrP receptor expression may contribute, therefore, to tissue resistance to the actions of PTH in renal failure.

VDR expression is also reduced in parathyroid tissue from humans and experimental animals with secondary hyperparathyroidism caused by renal failure.[25] This disturbance may disrupt the normal feedback inhibition of pre-pro-PTH gene transcription by 1,25-dihydroxyvitamin D. Abnormalities in binding of the VDR to vitamin D-response elements within DNA may further interfere with the regulation of pre-pro-PTH gene transcription.[26] Because calcitriol upregulates its own receptor,[27] reductions in VDR expression in renal failure may simply reflect the low serum levels that characterize the disorder. Nevertheless, differences in gene expression in hyperplastic tissues and metabolic changes caused by uremia per se represent additional mechanisms by which VDR expression in the parathyroid glands may be altered in renal failure.

Because 1,25-dihydroxyvitamin D is a potent inhibitor of cell proliferation, disturbances in renal calcitriol production and/or reductions in VDR expression may contribute to the development of parathyroid hyperplasia in chronic kidney disease.[28] Vitamin D receptor expression is markedly reduced in parathyroid tissues that exhibit a nodular pattern of

tissue hyperplasia, whereas lesser reductions occur in glands with a diffuse histological pattern.[29] Interestingly, the extent of glandular enlargement is generally greater in nodular parathyroid hyperplasia.[30] The clonal expansion of subpopulations of parathyroid cells and selected chromosomal deletions represent additional mechanisms that may influence parathyroid gland enlargement.[31]

The development and progression of parathyroid gland hyperplasia is an important component of renal secondary hyperparathyroidism.[32] Once established, parathyroid enlargement is difficult to reverse because rates of apoptosis in parathyroid tissue are quite low, and the half-life of parathyroid cells is estimated to be approximately 30 years.[33] Clinical assessments of parathyroid gland function show that differences in functional parathyroid gland size largely account for wide variations in basal plasma PTH levels in patients with chronic renal failure.[34] The secretion of PTH from massively enlarged parathyroid glands may ultimately become uncontrolled because of the ongoing non-suppressible component of PTH release leading to hypercalcemia and progressive bone disease in patients with end-stage renal disease (ESRD).

Expression of the CaSR is reduced by 30–70% as judged by immunohistochemical methods in hyperplastic parathyroid tissues obtained from human subjects with renal failure.[35] Such changes may thus render parathyroid cells less sensitive to the inhibitory effect of calcium on PTH secretion. Because 1,25-dihydroxyvitamin D upregulates CaSR expression, disturbances in vitamin D metabolism may be involved.[36,37]

The relationship between the duration and/or the severity of renal failure and decreases in parathyroid CaSR expression has yet to be determined. In vivo studies of parathyroid gland function in patients with ESRD indicate that calcium-sensing by the parathyroid glands is altered in advanced but not in mild to moderate secondary hyperparathyroidism (Table 1). [38,39] Such findings are consistent with in vitro assessments that show that calcium-regulated PTH release is altered in parathyroid cells obtained from hyperplastic tissues removed from patients undergoing parathyroidectomy for severe secondary hyperparathyroidism.[40] In contrast, evidence of a calcium-sensing defect is not found in patients with moderate renal insufficiency who do not require dialysis.[41] These in vivo findings in mild to moderate secondary hyperparathyroidism have yet to be confirmed by in vitro assessments of calcium-regulated PTH release or

TABLE 1. BIOCHEMICAL FEATURES AND SETPOINT ESTIMATES IN NORMAL SUBJECTS, PATIENTS WITH MODERATE SECONDARY HYPERPARATHYROIDISM (2°HPT) DOCUMENTED BY BONE BIOPSY, PATIENTS WITH ADVANCED SECONDARY HYPERPARATHYROIDISM STUDIED SEVERAL DAYS BEFORE UNDERGOING SUBTOTAL PARATHYROIDECTOMY (PRE-PTX), AND PATIENTS WITH PRIMARY HYPERPARATHYROIDISM (1°HPT)

	Normal (n = 20)	2°HPT (n = 31)	Pre-PTX (n = 8)	1°HPT (n = 3)
Blood ionized calcium (mmol/l)	1.22 ± 0.04	1.22 ± 0.07	1.27 ± 0.08*†	1.38 ± 0.08*†‡
Basal serum PTH level (pg/ml)	26 ± 6	536 ± 395*	1026 ± 324*†	88 ± 25*
Set point for calcium-regulated PTH release (mmol/l)	1.21 ± 0.04	1.22 ± 0.05	1.28 ± 0.08*†	1.35 ± 0.06*†‡

Values are means ± SD.
* $p < 0.05$ vs. Normal.
† $p < 0.01$ vs. 2°HPT.
‡ $p < 0.001$ vs. Pre-PTX.

CaSR expression because parathyroid tissues from such individuals are not readily available. It remains uncertain, therefore, whether alterations in CaSR expression contribute substantially to alterations in parathyroid gland function in early stages of chronic renal failure.

Phosphorus retention and hyperphosphatemia have been recognized for many years as important factors in the pathogenesis of secondary hyperparathyroidism. The disorder can be prevented in experimental animals with chronic renal failure when dietary phosphorus intake is reduced in proportion to glomerular filtration rate (GFR).[42] Dietary phosphate restriction also lowers plasma PTH levels in patients with moderate renal failure.[43,44] Phosphorus retention and hyperphosphatemia seem to aggravate secondary hyperparathyroidism in several ways. Extreme elevations in serum phosphorus concentration may lead to the formation of soluble complexes of calcium and phosphorus in plasma, thereby lowering blood ionized calcium concentrations and stimulating PTH secretion. Phosphorus impairs renal 1α-hydroxylase activity directly and reduces 1,25-dihydroxyvitamin D synthesis.[44] In addition, either phosphorus abundance or renal failure per se may affect post-transcriptional events that influence PTH mRNA stability and hormone synthesis.[45,46] Finally, phosphorus retention may aggravate parathyroid gland hyperplasia by altering the expression of factors involved in cell cycle regulation and cell proliferation.[47]

In summary, the causes of secondary hyperparathyroidism caused by chronic renal failure are numerous and diverse. As plasma PTH levels becomes persistently elevated, osteoblastic and osteoclastic activity in bone increases, leading to high rates of bone formation and turnover. Overall, plasma PTH values generally predict the histological severity of secondary hyperparathyroidism as assessed by bone biopsy and quantitative bone histology in patients with ESRD who are not being treated with active vitamin D sterols and in those given small daily oral doses of calcitriol. Less in known about this relationship in patients given large intermittent doses of vitamin D sterols to manage secondary hyperparathyroidism.

The osseous changes of renal secondary hyperparathyroidism are often much more pronounced than those of primary hyperparathyroidism, probably because of the higher plasma levels of PTH. Values are typically 5- to 10-fold above the upper limit of normal in patients with secondary hyperparathyroidism caused by ESRD, and they may reach levels that are 20–40 times higher than normal. By comparison, plasma PTH levels in most patients with primary hyperparathyroidism are only 2- to 3-fold above the upper limit of normal.

In contrast to those with ESRD, patients with moderate renal failure who do not require dialysis often have overt histological evidence of secondary hyperparathyroidism when PTH levels are only modestly elevated.[48] The discrepancy in disease severity between these two groups with markedly different plasma PTH levels is probably because of differences in tissue resistance to the biological actions of PTH or in the extent to which vitamin D metabolism has been disrupted.

Pathogenesis of Low-Turnover Bone Disease (Adynamic Bone and Osteomalacia)

Secondary hyperparathyroidism develops almost invariably in untreated patients with progressive kidney disease. An increasing proportion of patients do not, however, have markedly elevated plasma PTH levels at the time regular dialysis is begun. Many have bone biopsy evidence of adynamic renal osteodystrophy, which is characterized by subnormal rates of bone formation and turnover. The prevalence of adynamic skeletal lesions has also increased in adult patients undergoing regular dialysis. Approximately 40% of those treated with hemodialysis and more than one-half of those receiving peritoneal dialysis have plasma PTH levels that are only minimally elevated or fall within the normal range, values typically associated with normal or reduced rates of bone formation and turnover in patients with ESRD.[49]

Adynamic renal osteodystrophy currently accounts for most cases of low-turnover bone disease in patients with ESRD. Osteomalacia is seen much less often. Bone formation and turnover are reduced in both disorders, but osteomalacia is characterized by an additional defect in skeletal mineralization.

In the 1970s and 1980s, aluminum intoxication accounted for most cases of adynamic bone and osteomalacia in patients with chronic renal failure. Two distinct patterns of aluminum exposure were identified: one from inadequate water purification during the preparation of dialysis solutions and the other from the long-term ingestion of aluminum-containing, phosphate-binding agents.[50] Bone aluminum deposition was a prominent finding in patients with either adynamic lesions or osteomalacia. Both disorders were associated with bone and muscle pain, proximal myopathy, and skeletal fracture.[50] Bone histology improved and bone formation increased when aluminum overload was treated effectively.

Aluminum has diverse effects on bone and mineral metabolism.[51] It inhibits the proliferation and the differentiated function of osteoblasts, reduces collagen synthesis, and suppresses PTH secretion.[52-54] As such, adynamic bone from aluminum toxicity may arise both from direct inhibitory actions on osteoblasts and from indirect effects mediated by low plasma PTH levels.[51] Aluminum also interferes directly with skeletal mineralization, leading to changes of osteomalacia.[55,56]

Risk factors for aluminum-related bone disease included previous parathyroidectomy, a history of renal transplantation and graft failure, bilateral nephrectomy, and diabetes mellitus. By promoting the formation of soluble complexes with aluminum, citrate markedly enhances intestinal aluminum absorption, and its use in patients with renal failure who are also ingesting aluminum-containing medications must be avoided.[57,58] High plasma PTH levels seem to partially offset the adverse skeletal effects of aluminum. This may account for the somewhat greater risk of aluminum-related bone disease in diabetic patients and those who have undergone parathyroidectomy, conditions associated with low plasma PTH values.[59,60]

Fortunately, aluminum-related bone disease is now uncommon. Diabetes, corticosteroid therapy, and increasing

Adynamic / Aplastic Bone
Etiology

- **Aluminum toxicity**
- **Diabetes**
- **Corticosteroid therapy**
- **Hypoparathyroidism**
  - Surgical
  - Medical
- **Immobilization**
- **Malnutrition**

- **Advanced age - Osteoporosis**
- **Excess doses of vitamin D sterols**
- **Calcium supplementation**
  - **Oral calcium salts**
  - **Dialysate**

FIG. 4. Pathogenic considerations in adynamic renal osteodystrophy.

age account for adynamic lesions in many patients (Fig. 4). In this regard, the proportion of diabetic and elderly patients with ESRD continues to increase. The histological features of adynamic renal osteodystrophy without evidence of bone aluminum deposition are indistinguishable from those caused by osteoporosis from any of a variety of causes unless trabecular bone volume is also reduced. Decreases in bone mass and histological evidence of trabecular bone loss are not integral components of the adynamic lesion of renal osteodystrophy, and their presence suggests a component of osteoporosis.

The widespread use of large doses of oral calcium as a phosphate-binding agent and the use of large doses of active vitamin D sterols to treat secondary hyperparathyroidism probably account for recent increases in the prevalence of adynamic bone in patients with ESRD.[49] Both interventions can lead to sustained reductions in plasma PTH levels. Calcitriol may also suppress osteoblastic activity directly when given in large intermittent doses to patients undergoing regular dialysis.[61]

The long-term consequences of adynamic renal osteodystrophy, when not caused by aluminum toxicity, remain uncertain. Some studies suggest that the risk of skeletal fracture may be greater.[62,63] Soft tissue and vascular calcification might be aggravated by frequent episodes of hypercalcemia, but this has not yet been documented. In prepubertal children, adynamic renal osteodystrophy has been associated with reductions in linear growth.[64]

For patients with osteomalacia, aluminum toxicity must be excluded if there is a history of sustained aluminum ingestion or if there are concerns about the adequacy of water purification procedures in dialysis facilities. Evidence of inadequate vitamin D nutrition, which is not uncommon, should be sought by measuring serum 25-hydroxyvitamin D levels.[65,66] Long-term treatment with phenytoin and/or phenobarbital has been associated with osteomalacia in nonuremic persons, and a higher incidence of symptomatic bone disease has been reported in dialysis patients receiving these drugs.[67] Persistent hypocalcemia and/or hypophosphatemia can lead to osteomalacia in some patients. In infants and small children, excess dietary phosphorus restriction should be avoided because serum phosphorus levels are higher normally in this age group and the skeletal requirements for phosphorus are greater than in older children or adults. Overall, improvements in the management of

mineral metabolism and decreases in the use of aluminum-containing medications have markedly lowered the prevalence of osteomalacia in patients with ESRD.

HISTOLOGICAL FEATURES OF RENAL OSTEODYSTROPHY

The use of bone biopsy has contributed substantially to our understanding of renal bone disease. Quantitative histomorphometry of bone provides information about the status of skeletal mineralization, the structural characteristics of cancellous and cortical bone, the levels of osteoblastic and osteoclastic activity, and the presence or absence of marrow fibrosis. Measurements of bone formation can also be obtained using the technique of double tetracycline labeling, and such information is often needed for correct diagnostic interpretation.

Methods for achieving double tetracycline labeling of bone differ among laboratories, but the following approach is suitable for patients with renal failure. Patients are given either demeclocycline, 300 mg orally bid, or tetracycline HCl, 500 mg orally bid, for 2 days, followed by a 10- to 20-day interval during which no tetracycline is given. A second course of oral tetracycline HCl, 500 mg bid, is then given for another 2 days. Bone biopsy should be obtained 3–7 days after finishing the second course of oral tetracycline. For pediatric patients, doses of tetracycline should not exceed 10 mg/kg/day.

Histochemical staining procedures are done to show deposits of aluminum, iron, and amyloid in bone, and the aluminum content of bone can be measured by atomic absorption spectroscopy in separate samples obtained at the time of biopsy. Iliac crest bone biopsy can be done safely as an outpatient procedure with little morbidity both in adults and in children.[68]

High-Turnover Bone Disease

Osteitis fibrosa is the most common high-turnover lesion of renal osteodystrophy both in adults and in children.[4,69] The disorder represents the response of bone to persistently high plasma PTH levels. There is histological evidence of active bone resorption with increases in the number and size of osteoclasts and in the number of resorption bays, or Howship's lacunae, within cancellous bone (Table 2). Fibrous tissue is found immediately adjacent to bony trabeculae, or it may accumulate more extensively within the marrow space (Fig. 6). Partial or complete fibrous replacement of bony trabeculae can occur in more advanced cases.

Osteoblastic activity is increased in patients with osteitis fibrosa,[4,69] and the combined increase in osteoblastic and osteoclastic activity accounts for high rates of bone remodeling and turnover in secondary hyperparathyroidism. Bone formation is elevated, and values are often two to four times greater than normal (Table 2). The number of osteoblasts is substantially increased, and a greater proportion of cancellous bone surface is covered with newly formed osteoid. Overall, the amount of osteoid is moderately elevated, and many osteoid seams have a woven or hatched appearance, similar to that of a straw basket. This is a characteristic

TABLE 2. HISTOLOGICAL FEATURES OF HIGH-TURNOVER RENAL OSTEODYSTROPHY

	Mild lesion of 2°HPT	Osteitis fibrosa
Bone formation		
Trabecular bone volume	Normal	Normal–high
Osteoid volume	Normal–high	Normal–high
Osteoid seam thickness	Normal	Normal–high
Number of osteoblasts	High	Very high
Bone formation rate	High	Very high
Mineralization lag time	Normal	Normal
Bone resorption		
Eroded bone perimeter	High	Very high
Number of osteoclasts	High	Very high
Marrow fibrosis	Absent	Present

feature of skeletal disorders where collagen synthesis and deposition rates are markedly increased, and it reflects the disordered arrangement of collagen fibrils within osteoid seams when bone formation proceeds rapidly.

Patients with moderate increases in osteoclastic activity and bone formation and in whom there is little or no evidence of peritrabecular fibrosis are classified as mild lesions of renal osteodystrophy (Table 2). The disorder is a less severe manifestation of hyperparathyroid bone disease.[4,69] Plasma PTH levels are elevated, but values are substantially lower than in patients with overt osteitis fibrosa.[70,71] Other biochemical and radiographic manifestations of secondary hyperparathyroidism may be present. Because the histological changes of the mild lesion are less striking than those of overt osteitis fibrosa, tetracycline-based measurements of bone formation are useful for distinguishing this subgroup of patients from those with either normal rates of bone formation or adynamic lesions (Table 2).[4,69]

Low-Turnover Bone Disease

Osteomalacia is the most striking histological manifestation of low-turnover renal bone disease. Excess osteoid, or unmineralized bone collagen, accumulates in bone because of a primary defect in mineralization. Osteoid seams are wide, and they have multiple lamellae (Table 3); the extent of trabecular bone surface covered with osteoid is also increased. In contrast, osteoblastic activity is markedly reduced, and bone formation often cannot be measured because of the lack of tetracycline uptake (Table 3). In patients with aluminum-related osteomalacia, the bone aluminum content is elevated. Deposits of aluminum can be seen along trabecular bone surfaces using histochemical staining methods,[4,69,72] and the histological severity of osteomalacia in such cases corresponds to the amount of surface stainable aluminum in trabecular bone.[73]

Bone biopsy specimens from patients with the adynamic lesion of renal osteodystrophy exhibit normal or reduced amounts of osteoid, no tissue fibrosis, diminished numbers of osteoblasts and osteoclasts, and low or unmeasurable rates of bone formation (Table 3; Fig. 6).[4,69,74] The disorder was originally described in patients with aluminum toxicity, and aluminum deposition along trabecular bone surfaces was a prominent finding.[74] In vivo studies in experimental animals suggest the disorder is a forerunner of overt histological osteomalacia when bone aluminum deposition is the underlying cause.[52] Thus, bone aluminum levels are not as high in this subgroup of patients compared with those with aluminum-related osteomalacia.

Currently, most adult and pediatric dialysis patients with adynamic renal osteodystrophy do not have evidence of bone aluminum deposition. Other factors are now more common causes of adynamic bone (Fig. 4).

Mixed Lesion of Renal Osteodystrophy

Some patients have histological features of both osteitis fibrosa and osteomalacia. This combination of findings is called the mixed lesion of renal osteodystrophy.[75] Patients have biochemical evidence of secondary hyperparathyroidism, but other factors account for defects in skeletal mineralization. Persistent hypocalcemia and/or hypophosphatemia are found in some patients,[75] and nutritional vitamin D deficiency is present in others. Mixed lesions of

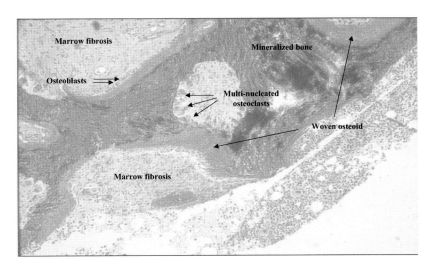

FIG. 5. Goldner-stained section of undecalcified bone from a patient with osteitis fibrosa caused by end-stage renal disease. Magnification ×50. Mineralized bone stains dark, and osteoid appears light. Fibrous tissue has accumulated within the marrow space immediately adjacent to bone, and the serrated margins along the bone surface represent sites of osteoclastic bone resorption.

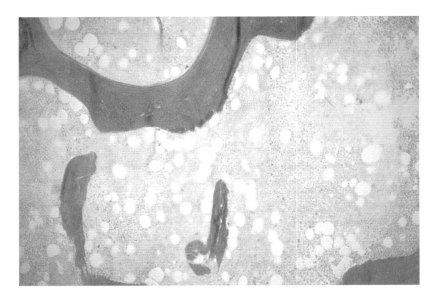

FIG. 6. Goldner-stained section of undecalcified bone from a patient with adynamic renal osteodystrophy. Magnification ×50. Mineralized bone stains dark, and osteoid appears light. There is little osteoid, osteoid seams are very narrow, and there is an overall paucity of both osteoclasts and osteoblasts.

renal osteodystrophy can be seen in patients with osteitis fibrosa who are in the process of developing aluminum-related bone disease or in those with aluminum-related osteomalacia who are responding favorably to treatment with deferoxamine with increases in bone formation.[76] Mixed renal osteodystrophy can thus represent a transitional state between the high-turnover lesions of secondary hyperparathyroidism and the low-turnover disorders of osteomalacia or adynamic bone.[51]

CLINICAL MANIFESTATIONS

The signs and symptoms of renal osteodystrophy are rather nonspecific, and the extent of various laboratory and radiographic abnormalities often fail to correspond with the severity of clinical manifestations.[3] Common features include bone pain, muscle weakness, skeletal deformities, and extraskeletal calcifications. In children, growth retardation is a prominent feature.

Bone Pain

Bone pain is often present in patients with renal osteodystrophy; its onset is insidious, and symptoms progress gradually over many months. Pain is diffuse and nonspecific, but it is often aggravated by weight bearing or by changes in posture. When localized, the lower back, hips, and legs are most often affected. Pain in the heels or ankles may be a presenting complaint.[3] Occasionally, the initial manifestation is an acute arthritis or peri-arthritis that is not relieved by massage or by the application of heat locally. Severe bone pain is more common in patients with aluminum-related bone disease than in those with osteitis fibrosa, and it is a prominent clinical feature of this disorder.[77] There is marked variation among patients, however, and some with advanced secondary hyperparathyroidism are severely incapacitated. The physical examination is generally unremarkable unless fractures or skeletal deformities are present.

Muscle Weakness

Proximal myopathy develops in some patients with advanced renal failure. Symptoms appear slowly, and weakness and aching are the most common manifestations both in adults and in children.[3] The physiological basis of this disorder is not understood. Favorable clinical responses have been noted in some patients after treatment with calcitriol or 25-hydroxyvitamin D, after parathyroidectomy, after successful renal transplantation, or during treatment of aluminum-related bone disease with deferoxamine.[3] The role of abnormal vitamin D metabolism in the pathogenesis of uremic myopathy remains uncertain, but a careful evaluation must be done to exclude severe secondary hyperpara-

TABLE 3. HISTOLOGICAL FEATURES OF LOW-TURNOVER RENAL OSTEODYSTROPHY

	Adynamic	Osteomalacia
Bone formation		
Trabecular bone volume	Normal, low	Variable Low, normal, or high
Osteoid volume	Normal, low	High–very high
Osteoid seam thickness	Normal, low	High–very high
Number of osteoblasts	Low	Low
Bone formation rate	Low–very low	Low–very low
Mineralization lag time	Normal*	Prolonged
Bone resorption		
Eroded bone perimeter	Normal, low	
Number of osteoclasts	Low	Low; may be normal or high
Marrow fibrosis	Absent	Absent

* As measured by conventional histomorphometric methods, the mineralization lag time (Mlt), which reflects the average value for all osteoid seams, may be prolonged in adynamic renal osteodystrophy. In contrast, the osteoid maturation time (O.mt), which represents values for osteoid seams that are undergoing active mineralization as judged by the uptake of tetracycline into bone, is normal in the adynamic lesion. The disparity between values for Mlt and O.mt is attributable to the lower proportion of osteoid seams undergoing active mineralization at any given point in time.

thyroidism or bone aluminum toxicity. In those with prominent symptoms of muscle pain and weakness, an empiric therapeutic trial of calcitriol or 25-hydroxyvitamin D is warranted.

Skeletal Deformities

Bone deformities are a prominent manifestation of renal osteodystrophy, particularly in children with long-standing renal failure. The frequency of skeletal deformity in pediatric patients is probably related to high rates of linear bone growth and skeletal modeling during endochondral bone formation in the immature skeleton. Bone deformities can affect both the axial and appendicular skeleton.

The pattern of deformity varies with age in children with chronic kidney disease. In patients younger than 4 years old, changes of secondary hyperparathyroidism most often resemble those of vitamin D–deficient rickets; characteristic features include rachitic rosary, Harrison's grooves, and enlargement of the wrists and ankles caused by widening of the metaphysis beneath the growth plate of long bones. Craniotabes and frontal bossing of the skull occur in children who develop renal failure in the first 2 years of life.[78]

The onset of overt renal failure before the age of 10 years is often associated with deformities of long bones; bowing is the most frequent change. Genu valgum is a common manifestation at any age, and ulnar deviation of hands, pes varus, "swelling" of the wrists, ankles, or medial ends of clavicles caused by metaphyseal widening and pseudo-clubbing are frequently observed. Despite regular treatment with vitamin D sterols, 20–25% of pediatric patients undergoing long-term dialysis require orthopedic procedures to correct skeletal deformities.[79]

Slipped epiphyses are another serious complication of renal bone disease in pediatric patients. The disorder typically occurs in those with severe secondary hyperparathyroidism,[78] and the femoral epiphysis is affected most often. Dental abnormalities, including enamel defects and malformations of the teeth, occur in children with congenital renal disease because mineral metabolism is disturbed early in life.[78]

In adults with aluminum-related bone disease, skeletal deformities are confined predominantly to the axial skeleton; changes include lumbar scoliosis, kyphosis, and distortion of the thoracic cage. Adult patients with severe osteitis fibrosa may develop rib deformities and pseudo-clubbing.

Growth Retardation

Children with chronic renal failure almost invariably exhibit growth retardation; contributing factors include metabolic acidosis, malnutrition, renal bone disease, and disturbances in the growth hormone-insulin-like growth factor I (IGF-I) axis.[80] Treatment with calcitriol has been reported to improve linear growth in children with advanced secondary hyperparathyroidism,[81] but increases in growth during treatment with vitamin D, 25-hydroxyvitamin D, or calcitriol have not been found consistently in children undergoing maintenance dialysis. Indeed, linear growth may be less in prepubertal children with adynamic renal osteodystrophy.[64]

Extraskeletal Manifestations

Several types of soft tissue calcification can be detected by radiographic examination. Most frequent are tumoral or periarticular calcifications. These are due mostly to amorphous deposits containing both calcium and phosphorus that are sometimes associated with acute periarticular inflammation, and the clinical presentation may suggest acute arthritis. Such calcifications commonly develop when serum phosphorus levels are greater than 8–9 mg/dl or when the calcium-phosphorus ion product in serum exceeds a value of $70–75 \text{ mg}^2/\text{dl}^2$.[82] They can resolve almost completely if reductions in serum phosphorus can be achieved and maintained. Although extraskeletal calcifications are more common with advancing age, they can also occur in children with ESRD.

Visceral calcifications are rather infrequent, and their chemical composition may differ. The lungs, heart, kidneys, skeletal muscle, and stomach are involved most often. Pulmonary calcification can cause restrictive lung disease that may be progressive, and the disorder persists even after successful kidney transplantation or parathyroidectomy.

Vascular calcification is common in patients with chronic renal failure, and it involves the medial layer of small and medium-sized arteries predominantly, a lesion known as Monckerberg's sclerosis. Calcifications occur diffusely and continuously within the arterial wall. Medial calcification is common in diabetic patients, and the radiographic appearance differs from the irregular pattern of calcified intimal plaques. It is best detected by lateral views of the ankle or anterior-posterior views of the hands or feet using magnification techniques with macroradioscopy.[83] Imaging techniques such as electron beam computed tomography may be useful for detecting calcification in the coronary arteries or cardiac valves.[84] Medial wall calcification is usually asymptomatic, but the palpation of peripheral pulses and blood pressure measurements may be difficult in affected limbs. Reductions in vascular compliance caused by medial wall calcification adversely affect cardiovascular hemodynamics by raising systolic blood pressure, widening pulse pressure, and increasing pulse wave velocity.[85–87]

It is now apparent that vascular calcification in patients with ESRD is associated with serious adverse clinical outcomes including cardiovascular disease and high mortality rates from cardiovascular causes.[88] In part, vascular calcification in such patients is related to disturbances in mineral metabolism such as phosphorus retention and hyperphosphatemia. Indeed, high serum phosphorus levels have been identified as an independent risk factor for death in adults undergoing regular hemodialysis.[89] Episodes of hypercalcemia and calcium retention caused by the use of large amounts of calcium as a phosphate-binding agent and from the administration of large doses of vitamin D sterols may also contribute.

Although soft-tissue and vascular calcification in ESRD has traditionally been thought to represent dystrophic calcification due predominantly to passive, physical-chemical processes, there is now considerable evidence that vascular calcification is a regulated process that may be modulated by various genes and proteins normally involved in bone and mineral metabolism.[90] Some of these such as matrix-

Gla-protein and osteopontin act as localized tissue specific inhibitors of vascular calcification, whereas others such as fetuin are circulating inhibitors of soft-tissue calcification.[91–93] Although beyond the scope of the current discussion, the role of renal failure as a potential modifier of selected regulators of soft-tissue and vascular calcification is a subject of considerable interest for future investigation.

In some patients with extensive vascular calcification, ischemic necrosis of the skin, muscle, and/or subcutaneous tissues can develop. The condition is variously known as calcific uremic arteriolopathy (CUA) or "calciphylaxis."[94] Its pathogenesis is not understood, but the disorder has been described in patients with chronic kidney disease, in those receiving regular dialysis, and in transplant recipients.[94] Most cases in early studies had advanced secondary hyperparathyroidism with markedly elevated PTH levels. Reports of clinical improvement after parathyroidectomy suggested that very high PTH levels played a pathogenic role. It is now evident, however, that CUA can occur in patients with adynamic renal osteodystrophy when plasma PTH levels are not substantially elevated. Morbidity is severe and mortality rates are extremely high. Risk factors identified in various studies include female gender, increasing age, obesity, large doses of calcium-containing medications, and the use of the anti-coagulant warfarin. It is quite possible that disturbances in the regulation of tissue-specific inhibitors of vascular calcification play a role in the pathogenesis of CUA.[95]

AMYLOIDOSIS IN PATIENTS WITH CHRONIC RENAL FAILURE

Most adult patients with ESRD who are treated with dialysis for more than 7–10 years develop amyloid deposits with a unique amyloid fibril protein that is derived from β_2-microglobulin (β_2M), a normal plasma constituent. Patients present with multiple bone cysts, pathological fractures, carpal tunnel syndrome, scapulohumeral arthritis, and spondyloarthropathy. [2,96–98] Involvement of the musculoskeletal system with bone pain and articular symptoms makes it difficult to separate dialysis-related amyloidosis from other forms of renal osteodystrophy.

β_2-microglobulin is a low molecular weight protein of approximately 12,000 Da that is produced by many cells, particularly lymphoid cells and other cells with high rates of turnover. In cells of this type, β_2M stabilizes the structure of the MHC class I antigen on the cell surface, but β_2M is released when the complexes are shed from the cell membrane. Approximately 180–250 mg of β_2M is normally generated each day. Almost all available β_2M is filtered at the glomerulus and is then catabolized by renal tubular epithelial cells.[97,99] With advanced renal failure, β_2M accumulates in plasma, and levels increase to values 50 times greater than normal in anuric dialysis patients.[100]

Histologically, β_2M amyloid fibrils are similar in appearance to amyloid AA; however, β_2M amyloid deposits are predominantly osteoarticular, leading to musculoskeletal manifestations.[97,99] Both the slow rate of appearance and the predilection for bone and articular structures suggest that elevated serum β_2M levels do not fully account for the clinical syndrome observed in patients with chronic renal failure. Increased age-related glycosylation products,[101] certain specific proteases[102] and inhibitors of other proteases[103] have each been suggested as factors that lead to the deposition of β_2M amyloid in bony structures and in synovial tissues. In rare cases, systemic deposits occur, and these may be fatal.[104]

The clinical features of amyloid deposition rarely appear before 5 years of dialysis therapy, and the disorder is more common in patients who start regular dialysis after the age of 50 years.[105] Carpal tunnel syndrome is the most frequent clinical feature, but shoulder pain, other arthritic complaints, and cystic bone lesions are common. Deposits of β_2M are found in periarticular structures, joints, bone (Fig. 4), and tendon sheaths. Far less commonly, the liver, spleen, rectal mucosa, or blood vessels are involved.

Skeletal manifestations include generalized arthritis, erosive arthritis, and joint effusions. Scapulohumeral involvement with shoulder pain is a common clinical presentation. Generalized arthritis can lead to pain and stiffness, decreased joint mobility, joint effusions, and deformities. Characteristically, pain is worse at night or when the patient must sit quietly for several hours during dialysis sessions; joint motion or activity can provide temporary relief. Erosive arthritis can involve the metacarpophalangeal joints, the interphalangeal joints, shoulders, wrists, and knees; effusions sometimes occur at these sites. The cervical spine is the most common site of destructive spondyloarthropathy.[106]

By radiography, bone cysts are most common at the ends of long bones, particularly the femoral head and proximal humerus, and they may also be found in the metacarpal and carpal bones. Multiple cystic lesions are common, and serial radiographs often show cyst enlargement with time. Cystic deposits of β_2M may resemble brown tumors of osteitis fibrosa; however, their location and the presence of multiple rather than solitary cysts suggest that amyloid deposition is responsible. Cystic changes most commonly occur at sites of tendonous insertions, and pathologically these may represent "amyloidomas" that have replaced trabecular bone. Fractures sometimes occur at these sites, and hip fractures in dialysis patients commonly arise at sites of β_2M deposition.[107]. Ultrasound examinations of the shoulder are a simple noninvasive method to assess progressive tendonous involvement with β_2M amyloid deposits.[108]

The fraction of patients afflicted with amyloidosis increases progressively with the duration of dialysis therapy; thus, 70–80% of adult patients treated with hemodialysis for 10 or more years will have clinical features of β_2M amyloidosis.[98,99] The distinction between this disorder and either severe secondary hyperparathyroidism or aluminum-related bone disease can be difficult, and thorough clinical, biochemical, and radiographic evaluations are required; β_2M amyloidosis can coexist with either high-turnover or low-turnover lesions of renal osteodystrophy.[107]

The overall clinical management of amyloidosis in patients with ESRD has thus far proven unsatisfactory. The carpal tunnel syndrome may respond to surgical correction, but it often recurs. The use of highly permeable dialysis membranes can slightly lower serum levels of β_2M, but there is no evidence that this intervention alters disease progression.[97,99] There is some evidence that patients treated from the onset of long-term dialysis with poly-acrilonitrile (PAN) membranes have a delayed appearance of certain clinical features of dialysis amyloidosis compared with those treated with conventional cellulosic dialyzers.[105] Successful renal transplantation is followed by symptomatic relief in most patients, but there is no evidence that bony or soft tissue lesions actually regress after renal transplantation.[109]

BIOCHEMICAL FEATURES OF RENAL OSTEODYSTROPHY

Serum calcium levels are often within the lower range of normal or modestly reduced in untreated patients with moderate to advanced renal failure. After treatment with dialysis is begun, values usually rise and may return to normal. The magnitude of the increase in serum calcium levels is partly related to the calcium concentration in dialysis solutions. In patients treated with CAPD who are not receiving vitamin D supplements, serum calcium levels can often be maintained within the normal range.

Calcium tablets and aluminum-containing phosphate binders have been replaced with agents that are safer and are associated with less frequent hypocalcemia in patients with progressive kidney disease. Indeed, normal or high serum calcium levels are found not infrequently, even in patients who are not receiving vitamin D sterols. Such findings underscore the importance of the passive, vitamin D–independent component of intestinal calcium transport as a determinant of net calcium absorption when sufficiently large amounts of calcium are given to patients with renal failure.

The development of hypercalcemia in patients undergoing regular dialysis warrants prompt and thorough investigation. Common causes include marked hyperplasia of the parathyroid glands caused by severe secondary hyperparathyroidism, adynamic renal osteodystrophy, treatment with calcitriol or other active vitamin D sterols, and the administration of large oral doses of calcium. Less frequent causes are aluminum-related bone disease, immobilization, malignancy, and granulomatous disorders such as sarcoidosis or tuberculosis that lead to extrarenal 1,25-dihydroxyvitamin D production.[3] Basal serum calcium levels are generally higher in patients with adynamic bone than in subjects with other skeletal lesions of renal osteodystrophy, and episodes of hypercalcemia occur more often.[70] Because skeletal calcium uptake is limited in the adynamic lesion, calcium entering the extracellular fluid from dialysate or after intestinal absorption cannot adequately be buffered in bone, and serum calcium levels rise.[110] Lowering the doses of calcium-containing, phosphate-binding agents and decreasing dialysate calcium concentrations temporarily usually corrects the hypercalcemia.

When the GFR falls below 20–25% of normal, hyperphosphatemia may develop. Thus, phosphate-binding agents and dietary phosphorus restriction may be required to avoid phosphate retention. Because the efficiency of phosphorus removal is rather limited with both hemodialysis and peritoneal dialysis, these additional measures are needed to adequately control weekly total body phosphorus balance in patients with ESRD who ingest adequate amounts of dietary protein.

In advanced renal failure, serum magnesium levels rise because of diminished renal magnesium excretion. Values are normal or slightly elevated when the concentration of magnesium in dialysate is kept between 0.5 and 0.8 mEq/liter.[111] The use of magnesium-containing laxatives or antacids can abruptly raise serum magnesium levels in patients with renal failure,[112] and these medications should be avoided. Serum magnesium levels should be measured frequently and regularly if magnesium-containing medications are used.

Serum alkaline phosphatase values are fair markers of the severity of secondary hyperparathyroidism in patients with renal failure. Osteoblasts express large amounts of the bone isoenzyme of alkaline phosphatase, and serum levels are usually elevated when osteoblastic activity and bone formation rates are increased. High levels generally correspond to the extent of histological change in patients with high-turnover lesions of renal osteodystrophy, and values frequently correlate with plasma PTH levels.[113] Serum total alkaline phosphatase measurements may also be useful for monitoring the skeletal response to treatment with vitamin D sterols in patients with osteitis fibrosa. Values that decrease progressively over several months usually indicate histological improvement.

New assays for bone-specific alkaline phosphatase may provide useful information about the level of osteoblastic activity in patients with renal osteodystrophy.[114] Measurements of the serum levels of osteocalcin and other biochemical markers of bone metabolism have generally not proven to be reliable indices of bone formation and turnover in patients with chronic kidney disease.[115,116]

Plasma aluminum levels are usually markedly elevated in patients with renal failure who have ongoing exposure to aluminum-containing medications or to inadequately purified dialysate.[117–119] As such, plasma aluminum levels should be monitored at regular intervals in patients undergoing maintenance dialysis, particularly in those who continue to use aluminum-containing, phosphate-binding medications. Plasma aluminum levels do not, however, serve as a reliable indicator of the extent of aluminum retention in tissues.[120] Serum levels can fall substantially after aluminum-containing medications have been discontinued despite persistent aluminum retention in tissues. For these reasons, deferoxamine (DFO) infusions have been used as a noninvasive diagnostic test for aluminum loading and may provide useful information about the extent of tissue aluminum accumulation in patients with chronic renal failure.[121]

Plasma PTH levels vary widely in patients with advanced renal failure, but double antibody immunometric assays generally provide reliable and reproducible results in patients with renal failure. Indeed, plasma PTH measurements using first-generation immunometric assays (vide infra) are used extensively for the initial diagnosis of renal osteodystrophy and to monitor therapy. The reference range of normal for these assays is 10–65 pg/ml (1–6 pM). Plasma PTH values are better than other biochemical indices for distinguishing between patients with secondary hyperparathyroidism and those with adynamic lesions of bone.[22,70,122] In untreated patients and in those receiving small daily oral doses of calcitriol, bone biopsy evidence of secondary hyperparathyroidism is found when plasma PTH

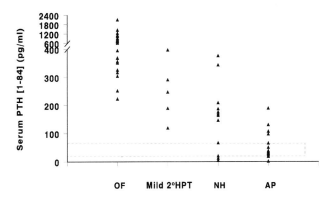

FIG. 7. Serum PTH levels as determined using a first-generation immunometric assay in dialysis patients with various histological subtypes of renal osteodystrophy. OF, osteitis fibrosa; mild 2HPT, mild lesion of secondary hyperparathyroidism;

levels are above 250–300 pg/ml (25–30 pM; Fig. 7). In contrast, values in patients with adynamic lesions are usually below 150 pg/ml (15 pM) and are often below 100 pg/ml (10 pM; Fig. 7). Both in children and in adults with ESRD, plasma PTH levels 2- to 3-fold above the upper limit of normal generally correspond to normal rates of bone formation as documented by bone biopsy.[22,122]

In contrast to the findings in patients with ESRD, plasma PTH levels that exceed the upper limit of normal in patients with chronic kidney disease who do not yet require dialysis are often associated with histological evidence of secondary hyperparathyroidism.

Until recently, the first-generation immunometric PTH assays that have been used widely for the past 12–15 years were thought to detect either predominantly or exclusively full length PTH(1-84). It is now apparent, however, that these assays cross-react with other large amino-terminally truncated PTH fragments.[123] In contrast, recently introduced second-generation immunometric PTH assays detect PTH(1-84) exclusively.[123,124] When measured by second-generation assays, plasma PTH concentrations are on average 40–45% lower than values obtained using first-generation assays both in subjects with normal renal function and in those with ESRD. Several studies indicate, however, that values obtained with each assay are highly correlated.

The proper interpretation of PTH measurements in patients with renal failure depends largely on the extent to which values reflect bone histology as documented by bone biopsy. These relationships have been established for first-generation immunometric PTH assays, but only limited information is available using second-generation assays. It remains to be determined, therefore, whether second-generation immunometric PTH will serve as better predictors of bone histology in patients with chronic kidney disease.

RADIOGRAPHIC FEATURES OF RENAL OSTEODYSTROPHY

Osteitis Fibrosa

Subperiosteal erosions are one of the most consistent radiographic findings in patients with secondary hyperpara-thyroidism and their extent corresponds to plasma PTH and alkaline phosphatase levels.[125] Patchy osteosclerosis is also common accounting for the classic "rugger jersey" appearance of the spine on lateral views of the thoracic vertebrae and for the "salt and pepper" appearance of the skull on radiographs. Skeletal roentgenographs may be normal, however, in patients with mild to moderate secondary hyperparathyroidism. Subperiosteal erosions may be seen in patients with aluminum-related osteomalacia,[126] emphasizing the need for independent biochemical or histological confirmation of secondary hyperparathyroidism.

Subperiosteal erosions are detected at the margins of the digital phalanges, at the distal ends of the clavicles, beneath the surfaces of the ischium and pubis, at the sacroiliac joints, and at the junction of the metaphysis and diaphysis of long bones. Fine grain films and a hand lens of 6–7× magnification can help to detect erosions in radiographs of the hands.[127] In pediatric patients, metaphyseal changes, or growth zone lesions, are common, and these have been described as "rickets-like lesions." This radiographic finding of secondary hyperparathyroidism differs from that of true vitamin D deficiency.[78] Both subperiosteal erosions of the digits and growth zone lesions are best demonstrated by examining X-ray films of the hands. In children, the presence of growth zone changes is a reliable indicator of the severity of secondary hyperparathyroidism as judged by the serum levels of PTH and alkaline phosphatase.[125]

Slipped epiphyses are among the most striking clinical and radiographic manifestations of renal osteodystrophy in children, and they are usually a consequence of advanced osteitis fibrosa in uremic children.[78] The age of patients often determines the site affected. In preschool children, epiphyseal slippage occurs in either the upper or lower femoral region or in the distal tibial epiphysis, but not in the distal radius or distal ulna. In contrast, the upper femoral epiphysis and the distal epiphyses of the forearm are affected most often in older children. Severe epiphyseal slippage can lead to gross deformities of the skeleton with ulnar deviation of the hands and abnormalities in gait.

Osteomalacia

The radiographic features of osteomalacia are less specific than for secondary hyperparathyroidism. Indeed, pseudofractures are the only pathognomonic finding in adults. These are straight, wide radiolucent bands in cortical bone oriented perpendicular to the long axis. Fractures of the ribs and hips and compression fractures of the vertebral bodies are more common in dialysis patients with osteomalacia than in those with osteitis fibrosa.[77]

Rickets-like lesions have been described in pediatric patients with aluminum-related osteomalacia, and these changes can resolve after treatment with deferoxamine.[128] Rachitic changes in children are not specific, however, and bone biopsy is usually required to determine the specific type of bone disease in pediatric patients with end-stage renal failure.

Amyloidosis

Cystic changes in bone, particularly if they are large, suggest amyloid deposits. Cysts most commonly involve the metacarpals and regions immediately adjacent to large joints near the site of tendon insertions; the hip, wrist, proximal humerus, pubic ramus, and proximal tibia are affected most often, but the carpal and tarsal bones may also be involved. Radiographs may reveal fractures at the site of cyst formation. Multiple bone cysts suggest amyloidosis, whereas brown tumors occur more often as isolated cystic lesions, usually in the ribs, mandible, or maxillae.

Bone Scan

The compounds used most frequently for skeletal scintigraphy are technetium-labeled bisphosphonates, mainly ^{99}Tc-methylene diphosphonate. Bone scintigraphy may reveal fractures, pseudofractures, or extraskeletal calcifications, and local increases in tracer uptake can occur in areas of amyloid deposition. Patients with osteitis fibrosa often exhibit symmetrical increases in isotope activity in the skull, mandible, sternum, shoulders, vertebral bodies, and distal portions of the femur and tibia. Collectively, these findings have been termed the "super scan." In contrast, the skeletal uptake of isotopic tracers is less in patients with aluminum-related osteomalacia than in those with osteitis fibrosa.[129] Despite such general trends, findings on bone scans often do not agree with data obtained by bone biopsy.[130] As such, bone scans provide supportive information, but they are of limited diagnostic value in the assessment of patients with renal bone disease.

MANAGEMENT OF RENAL OSTEODYSTROPHY

The successful clinical management of patients with renal osteodystrophy includes measures to counteract or correct several important pathogenic factors. Key objectives include (1) maintenance of normal serum calcium and phosphorus levels; (2) prevention of extraskeletal calcifications; (3) avoidance of exposure to toxic agents such as aluminum and excess iron; (4) judicious use of vitamin D sterols and phosphate-binding agents; and (5) selective use of chelating agents such as deferoxamine to manage aluminum intoxication.

Dietary Management

Adequate control of serum phosphorus levels is important for preventing soft-tissue calcification and for managing secondary hyperparathyroidism in patients with advanced renal failure. The intake of phosphorus in the diet ranges normally from 1.0 to 1.3 g per day in adults, but it must be lowered to 400–800 mg/day to prevent hyperphosphatemia in patients with renal failure. Such diets are generally unpalatable, and long-term compliance is difficult to achieve.[131] Consequently, phosphate-binding antacids are often required to adequately control hyperphosphatemia when glomerular filtration rates decrease to 20–25% of normal.

To substantially reduce dietary phosphorus content, the intake use of dairy products must be sharply curtailed. Phosphorus-restricted diets contain only limited amounts of calcium, often in the range of 500–600 mg. Patients with chronic kidney disease who abide by current recommendations thus commonly have a dietary calcium intake that is insufficient to meet nutritional requirements. Modest dietary calcium supplementation will be needed in most patients to achieve a total daily calcium intake approaching 1500 mg as recommended by the World Health Organization. The impact of concurrent therapy with calcium-containing or calcium-free phosphate-binding agents must be considered when assessing overall calcium nutrition in patients with chronic kidney disease.

Phosphate-Binding Agents

Phosphate-binding agents diminish intestinal phosphate absorption by forming poorly soluble complexes with phosphorus in the intestinal lumen. In the past, aluminum-containing medications were used widely, but these should be used sparingly, if at all, to avoid aluminum loading and aluminum toxicity. If they are used, the duration of treatment should be limited, and doses must be kept as low as possible. The concurrent administration of citrate-containing compounds must be avoided, and plasma aluminum levels should be monitored regularly.

Calcium carbonate and calcium acetate are the two most widely used phosphate-binding medications. They have similar efficacy. Calcium citrate can also be used as a phosphate-binding agent, but citrate can enhance intestinal aluminum absorption in patients receiving aluminum-containing medications and should thus be used with caution.[57,132] Calcium-containing agents should be ingested with meals to maximize the efficiency of phosphorus binding and to limit net intestinal calcium absorption. Although reasonably effective for controlling serum phosphorus levels in patients with ESRD, very large doses of calcium are required. Total daily calcium intake usually far exceeds 1500–2000 mg of elemental calcium and may be as great as 4 g or more. Episodes of hypercalcemia thus represent a major treatment-related side effect.[133,134]

The use of very large doses of calcium as a phosphate-binding agent has been associated with evidence of soft-tissue and vascular calcification in patients with ESRD.[135,136] As a result, alternative phosphate-binding strategies that limit cumulative calcium intake to 1500–2000 mg per day from both dietary and medicinal sources have been proposed.[137] These rely on the availability of calcium-free, phosphate-binding agents.

Sevelamer hydrochloride, or hydrogel of cross-linked poly-allylamine hydrochloride (RenaGel), is an ion exchange polymer that was designed specifically as a phosphate-binding agent.[138] It does not contain calcium or aluminum. In short-term clinical trials, sevelamer has been shown to be as effective as calcium acetate for controlling serum phosphorus levels with a substantially lower incidence of episodes of hypercalcemia.[139] In longer-term studies, total daily doses averaging 5 g were sufficient to maintain serum phosphorus levels at approximately 5.8–6.0 mg/dl, (1.8–2.0 mM) in patients undergoing regular hemodialysis. Interestingly, the serum levels of total cholesterol and low-density lipoprotein cholesterol decrease by 20–30% during treatment, whereas high-density lipoprotein cholesterol levels rise.[138,140,141] In patients with chronic renal failure who do not require dialysis, modest reductions in serum carbon dioxide levels, reflecting decreases in plasma bicarbonate concentrations, may occur during treatment with sevelamer. This change is probably because of the release of protons from the resin during the phosphate binding.

Lanthanum carbonate has been evaluated in large clinical trials and has been shown to be an effective phosphate-binding agent.[142] It is not yet available for clinical use. Magnesium carbonate was reported to be an effective phosphate-binder when used together with magnesium-free dialysate in patients undergoing regular hemodialysis,[143] but gastrointestinal side effects often complicate sustained treatment with magnesium-containing compounds.

Vitamin D Sterols

Despite dietary phosphate restriction and maintenance of an adequate dietary calcium intake, the use of appropriate levels of calcium in dialysate, and the regular ingestion of phosphate-binding agents, a substantial proportion of patients with ESRD develop secondary hyperparathyroidism. Treatment with active vitamin D sterols is thus required in many patients. Although calcifediol, or 25-hydroxyvitamin D_3, 1α-hydroxyvitamin D_3, and dihydrotachysterol have all been shown to be effective in managing secondary hyperparathyroidism, calcitriol and other recently introduced vitamin D sterols such as paricalcitol and doxercalciferol are used much more widely.

Daily oral doses of calcitriol are effective in patients with symptomatic renal osteodystrophy.[144,145] Treatment is started using small doses, and these are periodically adjusted upward if serum calcium and phosphorus levels remain within acceptable bounds. Bone pain diminishes, muscle strength, and gait-posture improve, and osteitis fibrosa frequently resolves either partially or completely.[146] When measured using reliable assays, PTH levels decrease in those who respond favorably to treatment. Similar findings have been reported in patients given daily oral doses of 1α-hydroxyvitamin D_3, which undergoes 25-hydroxylation in the liver to form calcitriol.[147,148]

Doses of oral calcitriol in most clinical trials have ranged from 0.25 to 1.5 μg/day. Hypercalcemia is the most common side effect, but most adult patients tolerate daily doses of 0.25–0.50 μg without marked increases in serum calcium levels. Pediatric patients may require somewhat larger daily oral doses of calcitriol. Growth velocity has been reported to increase during calcitriol therapy in some children with severe bone disease.[81]

Oral calcitriol therapy is now used relatively infrequently in patients treated with regular hemodialysis because vitamin D sterols can be given conveniently by the intravenous route during dialysis sessions. Parenteral dosing strategies assure patient compliance and achieve high plasma sterol levels that may enhance the suppressive actions of vitamin D on PTH synthesis. It is also possible that this therapeutic approach lessens the effect of vitamin D administration to promote intestinal calcium transport. Calcitriol, paricalcitol,

and doxercalciferol are each available as parenteral preparations.

Large intermittent oral doses of calcitriol can be used to treat secondary hyperparathyroidism in patients undergoing peritoneal dialysis in whom parenteral therapy is not practical.[149,150] When given two or three times per week, the cumulative weekly dose of calcitriol is somewhat greater than with daily therapy. Dosage regimens have ranged from 0.5–1.0 to 3.5–4.0 μg thrice weekly or from 2.0 to 5.0 μg twice weekly. Low doses should be used initially, but upward adjustments to the dose can be made if serum calcium and phosphorus levels are adequately controlled.

The development of hypercalcemia during calcitriol therapy may predict the underlying skeletal lesion of renal osteodystrophy. When hypercalcemia occurs after several months of treatment and previously elevated serum PTH and alkaline phosphatase levels have returned toward normal, it is likely that osteitis fibrosa has substantially resolved. In contrast, hypercalcemia that occurs within the first several weeks of treatment suggests the presence of either low-turnover bone disease, which in some cases is due to bone aluminum deposition, or severe secondary hyperparathyroidism.[146] Bone biopsy and measurements of bone aluminum content may be needed to exclude aluminum-related bone disease. If there is evidence of autonomous hyperparathyroidism, parathyroidectomy is required.

In adult hemodialysis patients, the intravenous administration of calcitriol thrice weekly effectively lowers serum PTH levels.[151] A portion of this response seems to be independent of changes in serum ionized calcium.[151] As mentioned previously in regard to intermittent oral calcitriol therapy, somewhat larger cumulative weekly doses of calcitriol are achievable using an intermittent dosage regimen.

Increases in serum calcium and phosphorus levels often limit the doses of calcitriol that can be given safely to patients with ESRD, particularly in patients who are also ingesting large oral doses of calcium as a phosphate-binding agent. Concerns have also grown in recent years about the potential for aggravating soft-tissue and vascular calcification during the medical management of secondary hyperparathyroidism. The use of intravenous calcitriol has thus been largely replaced by treatment with new analogs of vitamin D such as paricalcitol and doxercalciferol. Both are vitamin D2 derivatives. Each has been shown to effectively lower plasma PTH levels by 50–60% over 12–16 weeks of treatment in hemodialysis patients with secondary hyperparathyroidism in association with only modest increases in serum calcium and phosphorus concentrations.[152] As such, paricalcitol and doxercalciferol may provide a wider margin of safety for managing calcium and phosphorus metabolism during the treatment of secondary hyperparathyroidism.

Reductions in plasma PTH levels are used most often to assess the efficacy of treatment for secondary hyperparathyroidism with active vitamin D sterols. Although serum PTH levels generally reflect the severity of bone disease in untreated patients with secondary hyperparathyroidism and in those receiving small daily oral doses of calcitriol, similar relationships may not apply during treatment with larger intermittent doses of vitamin D sterols given twice or thrice weekly.[61] Bone formation and turnover may fall dramatically during intermittent calcitriol therapy, and a substantial fraction of patients develop adynamic renal osteodystrophy.[61] In some, adynamic lesions are seen after marked reductions in plasma PTH levels, but PTH values may remain elevated in others despite substantial decreases in bone formation.[61] Such findings suggest that large intermittent doses of calcitriol diminish osteoblastic activity and lower bone formation rates directly by PTH-independent mechanisms. Accordingly, plasma PTH levels should be monitored regularly during intermittent calcitriol therapy, and the dose of calcitriol should be lowered when serum PTH levels fall to values four to five times the upper limit of normal to reduce the risk of developing adynamic bone. Whether new vitamin D analogs also diminish osteoblastic activity and lower bone formation in a manner similar to that observed during intermittent calcitriol therapy remains to be determined.

Calcimimetic agents are small organic molecules that act as allosteric activators of the CaSR.[153] In parathyroid cells, they lower the threshold for receptor activation by extracellular calcium ions and diminish PTH secretion. When given to patients with secondary hyperparathyroidism, serum PTH levels fall within 1–2 h after drug administration.[154,155] Calcimimetic compounds thus represent a novel way of controlling excess PTH secretion in patients with secondary hyperparathyroidism.

Clinical trials have documented that the calcimimetic agents effectively lower plasma PTH levels during long-term treatment without increasing serum calcium or phosphorus concentrations in adult hemodialysis patients with secondary hyperparathyroidism. Serum phosphorus levels and values for the calcium-phosphorus ion product in serum often decline as plasma PTH levels fall during treatment. Experimental evidence suggests that calcimimetic agents may also impede the development of parathyroid gland hyperplasia, an integral component of secondary hyperparathyroidism caused by chronic renal failure. Calcimimetics agents thus have considerable potential for the treatment of with secondary hyperparathyroidism.

Parathyroidectomy

Certain events indicate the need to consider parathyroid surgery in patients with advanced secondary hyperparathyroidism. In all instances, the diagnosis of aluminum-related bone disease must be considered and excluded before parathyroidectomy, and evidence of severe secondary hyperparathyroidism should be thoroughly documented by biochemical, radiographic, and if necessary, bone histological criteria.[3] Specific indications for parathyroidectomy include (1) persistent hypercalcemia with serum calcium levels above 11.0–11.5 mg/dl; (2) intractable pruritus that does not respond to intensive dialysis or to other medical interventions; (3) progressive extraskeletal calcifications and/or persistent hyperphosphatemia despite the continued use of dietary phosphorus restriction and phosphate-binding agents; (4) severe bone pain or fractures; and (5) the development of calciphylaxis.[156] Other causes of hypercalcemia such as sarcoidosis, malignancy, or the intake of excess amounts of calcium or vitamin D must be considered and excluded.

There is ongoing disagreement about the use of subtotal versus total parathyroidectomy in patients with chronic renal failure.[157,158] The 15–30% incidence of recurrent secondary hyperparathyroidism in patients undergoing subtotal parathyroidectomy is a legitimate concern, and the availability of calcitriol and other active vitamin D sterols greatly facilitates the management of hypocalcemia after total parathyroidectomy. For patients who may subsequently undergo renal transplantation, the preservation of residual parathyroid tissue after subtotal parathyroidectomy helps to maintain calcium homeostasis when renal function is restored.

It is generally not advisable to implant remnants of parathyroid tissue removed at parathyroidectomy into the forearm or other sites in an effort to preserve parathyroid function after surgery. Such grafts may exhibit autonomous secretory behavior, and they occasionally spread locally into surrounding tissues leading to recurrent hyperparathyroidism. Adequate surgical resection may be difficult.

Management of Aluminum Intoxication

The clinical manifestations and histological features of aluminum-related bone disease improve during deferoxamine (DFO) therapy in patients undergoing regular dialysis,[159,160] and aluminum removal during hemodialysis and peritoneal dialysis increases substantially after intravenous or subcutaneous doses of DFO.[161,162] After 4–10 months of therapy, clinical benefit was observed in a large proportion of patients with severe bone disease.[50,160]

Biochemical changes during DFO treatment include reductions in serum calcium levels and increases in serum alkaline phosphatase values, findings consistent with improvements in skeletal mineralization and osteoblastic activity. Plasma PTH levels rise modestly in most patients, but it is not known whether this change is caused by aluminum removal from the parathyroid glands or to a fall in serum calcium concentrations. Serial bone biopsy specimens generally show increases in bone formation and improvements in mineralization.[160] The amount of surface stainable aluminum in bone decreases in most patients who improve with treatment, but patients who have undergone previous parathyroidectomy respond less well or not at all.[160]

Serious and often lethal infections with *Rhizipus* and *Yersinia* species can develop in dialysis patients given DFO.[163–167] The chelation of iron by DFO enhances iron delivery to certain organisms, increasing their pathogenic potential.[168–170] Such findings emphasize the need to use DFO judiciously in the treatment of aluminum intoxication in patients undergoing regular dialysis.

DFO should be given only to patients with symptomatic aluminum intoxication, and evidence of tissue toxicity should be fully documented before therapy is begun. Doses of DFO should not exceed 0.5–1.0 g/week, and plasma aluminum levels should be measured regularly. Subcutaneous administration avoids the high serum levels of ferrioxamine that can occur after intravenous doses, an approach that may limit the risk of opportunistic infection. In asymptomatic patients with aluminum deposition in bone, bone histology and bone formation can improve solely by withdrawing aluminum-containing medications and using calcium carbonate to control serum phosphorus levels.[171]

REFERENCES

1. Goodman WG 1990 Aluminum metabolism and the uremic patient. In: Simpson DJ (ed.) Nutrition and Bone Development. Oxford University Press, New York, NY, USA, pp. 269–294.
2. Kleinman KS, Coburn JW 1989 Amyloid syndromes associated with hemodialysis. Kidney Int 35:567–575.
3. Coburn JW, Slatopolsky E 1990 Vitamin D, parathyroid hormone, and the renal osteodystrophies. In: Brenner B, Rector F (eds.) The Kidney. W. B. Saunders, Co., Philadelphia, PA, USA, pp. 2036–2120.
4. Sherrard DJ, Ott SM, Maloney NA, Andress DL, Coburn JW 1983 Uremic osteodystrophy: Classification, cause and treatment. In: Frame B, Potts J (eds.) Clinical Disorders of Bone Mineral Metabolism. Excerpta Medica, Amsterdam, The Netherlands, pp. 254–259.
5. Salusky IB, Goodman WG 1995 Growth hormone and calcitriol as modifiers of bone formation in renal osteodystrophy. Kidney Int 48:657–665.
6. Goodman WG, Belin TR, Salusky IB 1996 In vivo assessments of calcium-regulated parathyroid hormone release in secondary hyperparathyroidism. Kidney Int 50:1834–1844.
7. Okazaki T, Zajac JD, Igarashi T, Ogata E, Kronenberg HM 1991 Negative regulatory elements in the human parathyroid hormone gene. J Biol Chem 266:21903–21910.
8. Okazaki T, Ando K, Igarashi T, Ogata E, Fujita T 1992 Conserved mechanism of negative gene regulation by extracellular calcium. Parathyroid hormone gene versus atrial natriuretic polypeptide gene. J Clin Invest 89:1268–1273.
9. Brown EM, Pollak M, Seidman CE, Seidman JG, Chou YH, Riccardi D, Hebert SC 1995 Calcium-ion-sensing cell-surface receptors. N Engl J Med 333:234–240.
10. Garrett JE, Capuano IV, Hammerland LG, Hung BC, Brown EM, Hebert SC, Nemeth EF, Fuller F 1995 Molecular cloning and functional expression of human parathyroid calcium receptor cDNAs. J Biol Chem 270:12919–12925.
11. Brown EM, Gamba G, Riccardi D, Lombardi M, Butters R, Kifor O, Sun A, Hediger MA, Lytton J, Hebert SC 1993 Cloning and characterization of an extracellular Ca(2+)-sensing receptor from bovine parathyroid. Nature 366:575–580.
12. Brown EM 1991 Extracellular Ca^{2+} sensing, regulation of parathyroid cell function, and the role of Ca^{2+} and other ions as extracellular (first) messengers. Physiol Rev 71:371–411.
13. Brown EM 1993 Mechanisms underlying the regulation of parathyroid hormone secretion in vivo and in vitro. Curr Opin Nephrol Hypertens 2:541–551.
14. Mayer GP, Habener JF, Potts JT Jr 1976 Parathyroid hormone secretion in vivo. Demonstration of a calcium-independent nonsuppressible component of secretion. J Clin Invest 57:678–683.
15. Mayer GP, Keaton JA, Hurst JC, Habener JF 1979 Effects of plasma calcium concentration on the relative proportion of hormone and carboxyl fragments in parathyroid venous blood. Endocrinology 104:1778–1784.
16. D'Amour P, Rousseau L, Rocheleau B, Pomier-Layrargues G, Huet PM 1996 Influence of Ca2+ concentration on the clearance and circulating levels of intact and carboxy-terminal iPTH in pentobarbital-anesthetized dogs. J Bone Miner Res 11:1075–1085.
17. Brandstrom H, Jonsson KB, Ohlsson C, Vidal O, Ljunghall S, Ljunggren O 1998 Regulation of osteoprotegerin mRNA levels by prostaglandin E2 in human bone marrow stroma cells. Biochem Biophys Res Commun 247:338–341.
18. Coburn JW, Kopple JD, Brickman AS 1973 Study of intestinal absorption of calcium in patients with renal failure. Kidney Int 3:264–272.
19. Szabo A, Ritz E, Schmidt-Gayk H, Reichel H 1996 Abnormal expression and regulation of vitamin D receptor in experimental uremia. Nephron 73:619–628.
20. Patel SR, Ke HQ, Hsu CH 1994 Regulation of calcitriol receptor and its mRNA in normal and renal failure rats. Kidney Int 45:1020–1027.
21. Massry SG, Coburn JW, Lee DBN, Jowsey J, Kleeman CR 1973 Skeletal resistance to parathyroid hormone in renal failure. Ann Intern Med 78:357–364.
22. Quarles LD, Lobaugh B, Murphy G 1992 Intact parathyroid hormone overestimates the presence and severity of parathyroid-mediated osseous abnormalities in uremia. J Clin Endocrinol Metab 75:145–150.
23. Cohen-Solal ME, Sebert JL, Boudaillez B, Marie A, Moriniere PH, Gueris J, Bouillon R, Fournier A 1991 Comparison of intact, midregion, and carboxy-terminal assays of parathyroid hormone for the diagnosis of bone disease in hemodialyzed patients. J Clin Endocrinol Metab 73:516–524.
24. Linkhart TA, Mohan S 1989 Parathyroid hormone stimulated release of insulin-like growth factor I (IGF-I) and IGF-II from neonatal mouse calvaria in organ culture. Endocrinology 125:1484–1491.
25. Korkor AB 1987 Reduced binding of ^{3}H-1,25-dihydroxyvitamin D in the parathyroid glands of patients with renal failure. N Engl J Med 316:1573–1577.
26. Sawaya BP, Koszewski NJ, Qi Q, Langub MC, Monier-Faugere MC, Malluche HH 1997 Secondary hyperparathyroidism and vitamin D receptor binding to vitamin D response elements in rats with incipient renal failure. J Am Soc Nephrol 8:271–278.
27. Strom M, Sandgren ME, Brown TA, DeLuca HF 1989 1,25-Dihydroxyvitamin D_3 up-regulates the 1,25-dihydroxyvitamin D_3 receptor in vivo. Proc Natl Acad Sci USA 86:9770–9773.
28. Szabo A, Merke J, Beier E, Mall G, Ritz E 1989 1,25($OH)_2$ vitamin D_3 inhibits parathyroid cell proliferation in experimental uremia. Kidney Int 35:1049–1056.
29. Fukuda N, Tanaka H, Tominaga Y, Fukagawa M, Kurokawa K, Seino Y 1993 Decreased 1,25-dihydroxyvitamin D_3 receptor density is associated with a more severe form of parathyroid hyperplasia in chronic uremic patients. J Clin Invest 92:1436–1443.
30. DeFrancisco AM, Ellis HA, Owen JP, Cassidy MJD, Farndon JR, Ward MK, Kerr DNS 1985 Parathyroidectomy in chronic renal failure. Q J Med 55:289–315.
31. Arnold A, Brown MF, Ureña P, Gaz RD, Sarfati E, Drüeke TB 1995 Monoclonality of parathyroid tumors in chronic renal failure and in primary parathyroid hyperplasia. J Clin Invest 95:2047–2053.
32. Parfitt AM 1997 The hyperparathyroidism of chronic renal failure: A disorder of growth. Kidney Int 52:3–9.
33. Lloyd HM, Parfitt AM, Jacobi JM, Willgoss DA, Craswell PW, Petrie JJB, Boyle PD 1989 The parathyroid glands in chronic renal failure: A study of their growth and other properties made on the basis of findings in patients with hypercalcemia. J Lab Clin Med 114:358–367.
34. Sanchez CP, Goodman WG, Ramirez JA, Belin TR, Segre GV, Salusky IB 1995 Calcium-regulated parathyroid hormone secretion in adynamic renal osteodystrophy. Kidney Int 48:838–843.
35. Kifor O, Moore FD Jr, Wang P, Goldstein M, Vassilev P, Kifor I, Hebert SC, Brown EM 1996 Reduced immunostaining for the extracellular Ca^{+2}-sensing receptor in primary and uremic secondary hyperparathyroidism. J Clin Endocrinol Metab 81:1598–1606.
36. Canaff L, Hendy GN 2002 Human calcium-sensing receptor gene. Vitamin D response elements in promoters p1 and p2 confer transcriptional responsiveness to 1,25-dihydroxyvitamin d. J Biol Chem 277:30337–30350.
37. Brown AJ, Zhong M, Finch J, Ritter C, McCracken R, Morrissey J, Slatopolsky E 1996 Rat calcium-sensing receptor is regulated by vitamin D but not by calcium. Am J Physiol 270:F454–F460.
38. Goodman WG, Veldhuis JD, Belin TR, Van Herle AJ, Jüppner H, Salusky IB 1998 Calcium-sensing by parathyroid glands in secondary hyperparathyroidism. J Clin Endocrinol Metab 83:2765–2772.
39. Ramirez JA, Goodman WG, Gornbein J, Menezes C, Moulton L, Segre GV, Salusky IB 1993 Direct in vivo comparison of calcium-regulated parathyroid hormone secretion in normal volunteers and patients with secondary hyperparathyroidism. J Clin Endocrinol Metab 76:1489–1494.
40. Brown EM, Wilson RE, Eastman RC, Pallotta J, Marynick S 1982 Abnormal regulation of parathyroid hormone release by calcium in secondary hyperparathyroidism due to chronic renal failure. J Clin Endocrinol Metab 54:172–179.
41. Messa P, Vallone C, Mioni G, Geatti O, Turrin D, Passoni N, Cruciatti A 1994 Direct in vivo assessment of parathyroid hormone-calcium relationship curve in renal patients. Kidney Int 46:1713–1720.
42. Slatopolsky E, Caglar S, Pennell JP, Taggart DB, Canterbury JM, Reiss E, Bricker NS 1971 On the pathogenesis of hyperparathyroidism in chronic experimental renal insufficiency in the dog. J Clin Invest 50:492–499.
43. Llach F, Massry SG 1985 On the mechanism of secondary hyperparathyroidism in moderate renal insufficiency. J Clin Endocrinol Metab 61:601–606.
44. Portale AA, Booth BE, Halloran BP, Morris RC Jr 1984 Effect of dietary phosphorus on circulating concentrations of 1,25-dihydroxyvitamin D and immunoreactive parathyroid hormone in

children with moderate renal insufficiency. J Clin Invest **73**:1580–1589.

45. Denda M, Finch J, Slatopolsky E 1996 Phosphorus accelerates the development of parathyroid hyperplasia and secondary hyperparathyroidism in rats with renal failure. Am J Kidney Dis **28**:596–602.

46. Yalcindag C, Silver J, Naveh-Many T 1999 Mechanism of increased parathyroid hormone mRNA in experimental uremia: Roles of protein RNA binding and RNA degradation. J Am Soc Nephrol **10**:2562–2568.

47. Dusso AS, Pavlopoulos T, Naumovich L, Lu Y, Finch J, Brown AJ, Morrissey J, Slatopolsky E 2001 p21(WAF1) and transforming growth factor-alpha mediate dietary phosphate regulation of parathyroid cell growth. Kidney Int **59**:855–865.

48. Hamdy NA, Kanis JA, Beneton MNC, Brown CB, Juttmann JR, Jordans JGM, Josse S, Meyrier A, Lins RL, Fairey IT 1995 Effect of alfacalcidol on natural course of renal bone disease in mild to moderate renal failure. Br Med J **310**:358–363.

49. Pei Y, Hercz G, Greenwood C, Sherrard DJ, Segre G, Manuel A, Saiphoo C, Fenton S 1992 Non-invasive prediction of aluminum bone disease in hemo- and peritoneal dialysis patients. Kidney Int **41**:1374–1382.

50. Coburn JW, Norris KC, Nebeker HG 1986 Osteomalacia and bone disease arising from aluminum. Semin Nephrol **6**:68–89.

51. Goodman WG, Leite Duarte ME 1991 Aluminum: Effects on bone and role in the pathogenesis of renal osteodystrophy. Miner Electrolyte Metab **17**:221–232.

52. Goodman WG 1984 Short-term aluminum administration in the rat: Reductions in bone formation without osteomalacia. J Lab Clin Med **103**:749–757.

53. Sedman AB, Alfrey AC, Miller NL, Goodman WG 1987 Tissue and cellular basis for impaired bone formation in aluminum-related osteomalacia in the pig. J Clin Invest **79**:86–92.

54. Morrissey J, Rothstein M, Mayor G 1983 Suppression of parathyroid hormone secretion by aluminum. Kidney Int **23**:699–704.

55. Blumenthal NC, Posner AS 1984 *In vitro* model of aluminum-induced osteomalacia: Inhibition of hydroxyapatite formation and growth. Calcif Tissue Int **36**:439–441.

56. Klein GL, Vaccaro ML, Lee TC, Bishop JE, Jongen M, Kurokawa K, Coburn JW, Norman AW 1986 Aluminum loading is associated with reduced serum levels of 1,25(OH)$_2$-vitamin D in rats following parathyroid hormone administration. Biochem Med Metab Biol **36**:363–368.

57. Molitoris BA, Froment DH, Mackenzie TA, Huffer WH, Alfrey AC 1989 Citrate: A major factor in the toxicity of orally administered aluminum compounds. Kidney Int **36**:949–953.

58. Froment DPH, Molitoris BA, Buddington B, Miller N, Alfrey AC 1989 Site and mechanism of enhanced gastrointestinal absorption of aluminum by citrate. Kidney Int **36**:978–984.

59. de Vernejoul MC, Marchais S, London G, Morieux C, Bielakoff J, Miravet L 1985 Increased bone aluminum deposition after subtotal parathyroidectomy in dialyzed patients. Kidney Int **27**:785–791.

60. Felsenfeld AJ, Harrelson JM, Gutman RA, Wells SA, Drezner MK 1982 Osteomalacia after parathyroidectomy in patients with uremia. Ann Intern Med **960**:34–39.

61. Goodman WG, Ramirez JA, Belin TR, Chon Y, Gales B, Segre GV, Salusky IB 1994 Development of adynamic bone in patients with secondary hyperparathyroidism after intermittent calcitriol therapy. Kidney Int **46**:1160–1166.

62. Atsumi K, Kushida K, Yamazaki K, Shimizu S, Ohmura A, Inoue T 1999 Risk factors for vertebral fractures in renal osteodystrophy. Am J Kidney Dis **33**:287–293.

63. Coco M, Rush H 2000 Increased incidence of hip fractures in dialysis patients with low serum parathyroid hormone. Am J Kidney Dis **36**:1115–1121.

64. Kuizon BD, Goodman WG, Jüppner H, Boechat I, Nelson P, Gales B, Salusky IB 1998 Diminished linear growth during treatment with intermittent calcitriol and dialysis in children with chronic renal failure. Kidney Int **53**:205–211.

65. Eastwood JB, Harris E, Stamp TCB, de Wardener HE 1976 Vitamin D deficiency in the osteomalacia of chronic renal failure. Lancet **2**:1209–1211.

66. Thomas MK, Lloyd-Jones DM, Thadhani RI, Shaw AC, Deraska DJ, Kitch BT, Vamvakas EC, Dick IM, Prince RL, Finkelstein JS 1998 Hypovitaminosis D in medical inpatients. N Engl J Med **338**:777–783.

67. Pierides AM, Ellis HA, Ward M, Simpson W, Peart KM, Alvarez-Ude F, Uldall PR, Kerr DNS 1976 Barbiturate and anticonvulsant treatment in relation to osteomalacia with haemodialysis and renal transplantation. Br Med J **1**:190–193.

68. Rao SD 1983 Practical approach to bone biopsy. In: Recker RR (ed.) Bone Histomorphometry: Techniques and Interpretation. CRC Press, Boca Raton, FL, USA, pp. 3–11.

69. Salusky IB, Coburn JW, Brill J, Foley J, Slatopolsky E, Fine RN, Goodman WG 1988 Bone disease in pediatric patients undergoing dialysis with CAPD or CCPD. Kidney Int **33**:975–982.

70. Salusky IB, Ramirez JA, Oppenheim WL, Gales B, Segre GV, Goodman WG 1994 Biochemical markers of renal osteodystrophy in pediatric patients undergoing CAPD/CCPD. Kidney Int **45**:253–258.

71. Sherrard DJ, Hercz G, Pei Y, Maloney N, Greenwood C, Manuel A, Saiphoo C, Fenton SS, Segre GV 1993 The spectrum of bone disease in end-stage renal failure: An evolving disorder. Kidney Int **43**:436–442.

72. Llach F, Felsenfeld AJ, Coleman MD, Pederson JA 1984 Prevalence of various types of bone disease in dialysis patients. In: Robinson RR (ed.) Nephrology, Proceedings of the Ninth International Congress of Nephrology, vol 2. Springer-Verlag, New York, NY, USA, pp. 1375–1382.

73. Hodsman AB, Sherrard DJ, Alfrey AC, Ott SM, Brickman AS, Miller NL, Maloney NA, Coburn JW 1982 Bone aluminum and histomorphometric features of renal osteodystrophy. J Clin Endocrinol Metab **54**:539–546.

74. Andress DL, Maloney NA, Endres DB, Sherrard DJ 1986 Aluminum-associated bone disease in chronic renal failure: High prevalence in a long-term dialysis population. J Bone Miner Res **1**:391–398.

75. Sherrard DJ, Baylink DJ, Wergedal JE, Maloney NA 1974 Quantitative histological studies on the pathogenesis of uremic bone disease. J Clin Endocrinol Metab **39**:119–135.

76. Sherrard DJ 1986 Renal osteodystrophy. Semin Nephrol **6**:56–67.

77. Llach F, Felsenfeld AJ, Coleman MD, Keveney JJ Jr, Pederson JA, Medlock TR 1986 The natural course of dialysis osteomalacia. Kidney Int **29**:S74–S79.

78. Mehls O 1984 Renal osteodystrophy in children: Etiology and clinical aspects. In: Fine RN, Gruskin AB (eds.) Endstage Renal Disease in Children. W. B. Saunders, Philadelphia, PA, USA, pp. 227–250.

79. Salusky IB, Brill J, Oppenheim W, Goodman WG 1989 Features of renal osteodystrophy in pediatric patients receiving regular peritoneal dialysis. Semin Nephrol **9**:37–42.

80. Stickler GB, Bergen BJ 1973 A review: Short stature in renal disease. Pediatr Res **7**:978–982.

81. Chesney RW, Moorthy AV, Eisman JA, Tax DK, Mazess RB, DeLuca HF 1978 Increased growth after long-term oral 1,25-vitamin D$_3$ in childhood renal osteodystrophy. N Engl J Med **298**:238–242.

82. Ibels LS, Alfrey AC, Huffer WE, Craswell PW, Anderson JT, Weil R3 1979 Arterial calcification and pathology in uremic patients undergoing dialysis. Am J Med **66**:790–796.

83. Meema HE, Oreopoulos DG, Rapoport A 1987 Serum magnesium and arterial calcification in end-stage renal disease. Kidney Int **32**:388–394.

84. Braun J, Oldendorf M, Moshage W, Heidler R, Zeitler E, Luft FC 1996 Electron beam computed tomography in the evaluation of cardiac calcifications in chronic dialysis patients. Am J Kidney Dis **27**:394–401.

85. Marchais SJ, Metivier F, Guerin AP, London GM 1999 Association of hyperphosphataemia with haemodynamic disturbances in end-stage renal disease. Nephrol Dial Transplant **14**:2178–2183.

86. Blacher J, Guerin AP, Pannier B, Marchais SJ, London GM 2001 Arterial calcifications, arterial stiffness, and cardiovascular risk in end-stage renal disease. Hypertension **38**:938–942.

87. Blacher J, Safar ME, Guerin AP, Pannier B, Marchais SJ, London GM 2003 Aortic pulse wave velocity index and mortality in end-stage renal disease. Kidney Int **63**:1852–1860.

88. Ganesh SK, Stack AG, Levin NW, Hulbert-Shearon T, Port FK 2001 Association of elevated serum PO(4), Ca x PO(4) product, and parathyroid hormone with cardiac mortality risk in chronic hemodialysis patients. J Am Soc Nephrol **12**:2131–2138.

89. Block GA, Hulbert-Shearon TE, Levin NW, Port FK 1998 Association of serum phosphorus and calcium x phosphorus product with mortality risk in chronic hemodialysis patients: A national study. Am J Kidney Dis **31**:607–617.

90. Schinke T, Karsenty G 2000 Vascular calcification: A passive process in need of inhibitors. Nephrol Dial Transplant **15**:1272–1274.

91. Shanahan CM, Proudfoot D, Farzaneh-Far A, Weissberg PL 1998 The role of Gla proteins in vascular calcification. Crit Rev Eukaryot Gene Expr **8**:357–375.

92. Speer MY, McKee MD, Guldberg RE, Liaw L, Yang HY, Tung E,

Karsenty G, Giachelli CM 2002 Inactivation of the osteopontin gene enhances vascular calcification of matrix Gla protein-deficient mice: Evidence for osteopontin as an inducible inhibitor of vascular calcification in vivo. J Exp Med **196**:1047–1055.

93. Ketteler M, Bongartz P, Westenfeld R, Wildberger JE, Mahnken AH, Bohm R, Metzger T, Wanner C, Jahnen-Dechent W, Floege J 2003 Association of low fetuin-A (AHSG) concentrations in serum with cardiovascular mortality in patients on dialysis: A cross-sectional study. Lancet **361**:827–833.

94. Gipstein RM, Coburn JW, Adams JA, Lee DBN, Parsa KP, Sellars A, Suki WN, Massry SG 1976 Calciphylaxis in man: A syndrome of tissue necrosis and vascular calcification in 11 patients with chronic renal failure. Arch Intern Med **136**:1273–1280.

95. Goodman WG 2001 Vascular calcification in chronic renal failure. Lancet **358**:1115–1116.

96. Bardin T, Kuntz D, Zingraff J, Voisin MC, Zelmar A, Lansaman J 1985 Synovial amyloidosis in patients undergoing long-term hemodialysis. Arthritis Rheum **28**:1052–1058.

97. Koch KM 1992 Dialysis-related amyloidosis. Kidney Int **41**:1416–1429.

98. Bazzi C, Arrigo G, Luciani L, Casazza F, Saviotti M, Malaspina D, Bonucci E, Ballanti P, Amaducci S, Lattuada P, Manna G, Pozzi F, D'Amico G 1995 Clinical features of 24 patients on regular hemodialysis treatment (RDT) for 16–23 years in a single unit. Clin Nephrol **44**:96–107.

99. Zingraff J, Drüeke T 1991 Can the nephrologist prevent dialysis-related amyloidosis? Am J Kidney Dis **18**:1–11.

100. Gejyo F, Homma N, Suzuki M, Arakawa KM 1986 Serum levels of B-2-microglobulin as a new form of amyloid protein in patients undergoing long-term hemodialysis. N Engl J Med **314**:585–586.

101. Miyata T, Inagi R, Iida Y, Sato M, Yamada N, Oda O, Maeda K, Seo H 1994 Involvement of β_2-microglobulin modified with advanced glycation end products in the pathogenesis of hemodialysis-associated amyloidosis. Induction of human monoctye chemotaxis and macrophage secretion of tumor necrosis factor-α and interleukin-1. J Clin Invest **93**:521–528.

102. Linke RP, Hampl H, Lobeck H, Ritz E, Bommer J, Waldherr R, Eulitz M 1989 Lysine-specific cleavage of β_2-microglobulin in amyloid deposits associated with hemodialysis. Kidney Int **36**:675–681.

103. Campistol JM, Shirahama T, Abraham CR, Rodgers OG, Solé M, Cohen AS, Skinner M 1992 Demonstration of plasma proteinase inhibitors in β_2-microglobulin amyloid deposits. Kidney Int **42**:915–923.

104. Campistol JM, Cases A, Torras A, Soler M, Munoz-Gomez J, Montoliu J, Lopez-Pedret J, Revert L 1987 Visceral involvement of dialysis amyloidosis. Am J Nephrol **7**:390–393.

105. van Ypersele de Strihou CA, Jadoul M, Malghem J, Maldague B, Jamart J, The Working Party on Dialysis Amyloidosis 1991 Effect of dialysis membrane and patient's age on signs of dialysis-related amyloidosis. Kidney Int **41**:1012–1019.

106. Ohashi K, Hara M, Kawai R, Ogura Y, Honda K, Nihei H, Mimura N 1992 Cervical discs are most susceptible to beta2-microglobulin amyloid deposition in the vertebral column. Kidney Int **41**:1646–1654.

107. Onishi S, Andress DL, Maloney NA, Coburn JW, Sherrard DJ 1991 Bone deposition of beta-2-microglobulin in hemodialysis patients. Kidney Int **39**:990–995.

108. McMahon LP, Radford J, Dawborn JK 1991 Shoulder ultrasound in dialysis-related amyloidosis. Clin Nephrol **35**:227–232.

109. Jadoul M, Malgehm J, Pirson Y, Maldague B, van Ypersele de Strihou CA 1989 Effect of renal transplantation on the radiological signs of dialysis amyloid osteoarthropathy. Clin Nephrol **32**:194–197.

110. Kurz P, Monier-Faugere MC, Bognar B, Werner E, Roth P, Vlachojannis J, Malluche HH 1994 Evidence for abnormal calcium homeostasis in patients with adynamic bone disease. Kidney Int **46**:855–861.

111. Stewart WK, Fleming LW 1973 The effects of dialysate magnesium on plasma and erythocyte magnesium and potassium concentrations during maintenance haemodialysis. Nephron **10**:221–231.

112. Guillot AP, Hood VL, Runge CF, Gennari FJ 1982 The use of magnesium-containing phosphate binders in patients with end-stage renal disease on maintenance hemodialysis. Nephron **30**:114–117.

113. Hruska KA, Teitelbaum SL, Kopelman R, Richardson CA, Miller P, Debman J, Martin K, Slatopolsky E 1978 The predictability of the histological features if uremic bone disease by non-invasive techniques. Metab Bone Dis Relat Res **1**:39–44.

114. Couttenye MM, D'Haese P, Van Hoof VO, Lemoniatou E, Goodman

115. Charhon SA, Delmas PD, Malaval L, Chavassieux PM, Arlot M, Chapuy MC, Meunier PJ 1986 Serum bone Gla-protein in renal osteodystrophy: Comparison with bone histomorphometry. J Clin Endocrinol Metab **63**:892–897.

116. Ureña P, de Vernejoul MC 1999 Circulating biochemical markers of bone remodeling in uremic patients. Kidney Int **55**:2141–2156.

117. Pierides AM, Edwards WG Jr, Cullu US Jr, McCall JT, Ellis HA 1980 Hemodialysis encephalopathy with osteomalacic fractures and muscle weakness. Kidney Int **18**:115–124.

118. Felsenfeld AJ, Gutman RA, Llach F, Harrelson JM 1982 Osteomalacia in chronic renal failure: A syndrome previously reported only with maintenance dialysis. Am J Nephrol **2**:147–154.

119. Coburn JW, Nebeker HG, Hercz G, Milliner DS, Ott SM, Andress DL, Sherrard DJ, Alfrey AC 1984 Role of aluminum accumulation in the pathogenesis of renal osteodystrophy. In: Robinson RR (ed.) Nephrology, vol. 2. Springer-Verlag, New York, NY, USA, pp. 1383–1395.

120. Alfrey AC 1986 Aluminum metabolism. Kidney Int **29**(Suppl 18):S8–S11.

121. Milliner DS, Nebeker HG, Ott SM, Andress DL, Sherrard DJ, Alfrey AC, Slatopolsky EA, Coburn JW 1984 Use of the deferoxamine infusion test in the diagnosis of aluminum-related osteodystrophy. Ann Intern Med **101**:775–779.

122. Broman GE, Trotter M, Peterson RR 1958 The density of selected bones of the human skeleton. Am J Physiol Anthropology **16**:197–211.

123. John MR, Goodman WG, Gao P, Cantor TL, Salusky IB, Jüppner H 1999 A novel immunoradiometric assay detects full-length human PTH but not amino-terminally truncated fragments: Implications for PTH measurements in renal failure. J Clin Endocrinol Metab **84**:4287–4290.

124. Gao P, Scheibel S, D'Amour P, John MR, Rao DS, Schmidt-Gayk H, Cantor TL 2001 Development of a novel immunoradiometric assay exclusively for biologically active whole parathyroid hormone 1–84: Implications for improvement of accurate assessment of parathyroid function. J Bone Miner Res **16**:605–614.

125. Salusky IB, Fine RN, Kangarloo H, Gold R, Paunier L, Goodman WG, Brill JE, Gilli G, Slatopolsky E, Coburn JW 1987 "High-dose" calcitriol for control of renal osteodystrophy in children on CAPD. Kidney Int **32**:89–95.

126. Shimada H, Nakamura M, Marumo F 1983 Influence of aluminium on the effect of 1-alpha-(OH)D$_3$ on renal osteodystrophy. Nephron **35**:163–170.

127. Meema HE, Schatz DL 1970 Simple radiologic demonstration of cortical bone loss in thyrotoxicosis. Radiology **97**:9–15.

128. Andreoli SP, Smith JA, Bergstein JM 1985 Aluminum bone disease in children: Radiographic features from diagnosis to resolution. Radiology **156**:663–667.

129. Karsenty G, Vigneron N, Jorgetti V, Fauchet M, Zingraff J, Drüeke T, Cournot-Witmer G 1986 Value of the 99-mTc-methylene diphosphonate bone scan in renal osteodystrophy. Kidney Int **29**:1058–1065.

130. Hodson EM, Howman-Gilles RB, Evans RB, Banutonich G, Hills EE, Sherbon K, Back BD, Horvath SS, Tiller DJ 1981 The diagnosis of renal osteodystrophy: A comparison of technitium99 pyrophosphate bone scintography with other techniques. Clin Nephrol **16**:24–28.

131. Barsotti G, Guiducci A, Ceardella G, Giovannetti S 1981 Effects on renal function of a low-nitrogen diet supplemented with essential amino acids and ketoanalogues and of hemodialysis and free protein supply in patients with chronic renal failure. Nephron **27**:113–117.

132. Bakir AA, Hryhorczuk DO, Berman E, Dunea G 1986 Acute fatal hyperaluminemic encephalopathy in undialyzed and recently dialyzed uremic patients. Trans Am Soc Artif Intern Organs **32**:171–176.

133. Salusky IB, Coburn JW, Foley J, Nelson P, Fine RN 1986 Effects of oral calcium carbonate on control of serum phosphorus and changes in plasma aluminum levels after discontinuation of aluminum-containing gels in children receiving dialysis. J Pediatr **108**:767–770.

134. Slatopolsky E, Weerts C, Lopez-Hilker S, Norwood K, Zink M, Windus M, Delmez J 1986 Calcium carbonate is an effective phosphate binder in patients with chronic renal failure undergoing dialysis. N Engl J Med **315**:157–161.

135. Goodman WG, Goldin J, Kuizon BD, Yoon C, Gales B, Sider D, Wang Y, Chung J, Emerick A, Greaser L, Elashoff RM, Salusky IB

2000 Coronary artery calcification in young adults with end-stage renal disease who are undergoing dialysis. N Engl J Med **342:**1478–1483.

136. Guérin AP, London GM, Marchais SJ, Metivier F 2000 Arterial stiffening and vascular calcifications in end-stage renal disease. Nephrol Dial Transplant **15:**1014–1021.

137. Block GA, Port FK 2000 Re-evaluation of risks associated with hyperphosphatemia and hyperparathyroidism in dialysis patients: Recommendations for a change in management. Am J Kidney Dis **35:**1226–1237.

138. Chertow GM, Burke SK, Lazarus JM, Stenzel K, Wombolt D, Goldberg DI, Bonventre JV, Slatopolsky E 1997 Poly[allylamine hydrochloride] (RenaGel): A noncalcemic phosphate binder for the treatment of hyperphosphemia in chronic renal failure. Am J Kidney Dis **29:**66–71.

139. Chertow GM, Dillon M, Burke SK, Steg M, Bleyer AJ, Garrett BN, Domoto DT, Wilkes BM, Wombolt DG, Slatopolsky EA 1999 A randomized trial of sevelamer hydrochloride (RenaGel) with and without supplemental calcium. Strategies for the control of hyperphosphatemia and hyperparathyroidism in hemodialysis patients. Clin Nephrol **51:**18–26.

140. Wilkes BM, Reiner D, Kern M, Burke S 1998 Simultaneous lowering of serum phosphate and LDL-cholesterol by sevelamer hydrochloride (RenaGel) in dialysis patients. Clin Nephrol **50:**381–386.

141. Chertow GM, Burke SK, Dillon MA, Slatopolsky E 1999 Long-term effects of sevelamer hydrochloride on the calcium x phosphate product and lipid profile of haemodialysis patients. Nephrol Dial Transplant **14:**2709–2714.

142. Hutchison AJ 1999 Calcitriol, lanthanum carbonate, and other new phosphate binders in the management of renal osteodystrophy. Perit Dial Int **19**(Suppl 2)**:**S408–S412.

143. O'Donovan R, Baldwin D, Hammer M, Moniz C, Parsons V 1986 Substitution of aluminum salts by magnesium salts in control of dialysis hyperphosphatemia. Lancet **1:**880–882.

144. Baker LR, Muir JW, Sharman VL, Abrams SM, Greenwood RN, Cattell WR, Goodwin FJ, Marsh FP, Adami S, Hately W, Hattersly LA, Morgan AG, Papapoulos SE, Revell PA, Tucker AK, Chaput de Saintonge DM, O'Riordan JLH 1986 Controlled trial of calcitriol in hemodialysis patients. Clin Nephrol **26:**185–191.

145. Berl T, Berns AS, Huffer WE, Hammill K, Alfrey AC, Arnaud CD, Schrier RW 1978 1,25-dihydroxycholecalciferol effects in chronic dialysis. A double-blind controlled study. Ann Intern Med **88:**774–780.

146. Ott SM, Maloney NA, Coburn JW, Alfrey AC, Sherrard DJ 1982 The prevalence of bone aluminum deposition in renal osteodystrophy and its relation to the response to calcitriol therapy. New Engl J Med **307:**709–713.

147. Pierides AM, Simpson W, Ward MK, Ellis HA, Dewar JH, Kerr DNS 1976 Variable response to long-term 1α-hydroxycholecalciferol in hemodialysis osteodystrophy. Lancet **1:**1092–1095.

148. Kanis JA, Henderson RG, Heynen G, Ledingham JGG, Russell RGG, Smith R, Walton RJ 1977 Renal osteodystrophy in nondialysed adolescents: Long-term treatment with 1α-hydroxycholecalciferol. Arch Dis Child **52:**473–481.

149. Fukagawa M, Kitaoka M, Kaname S, Okazaki R, Matsumoto T, Ogata E, Hoshino M, Inada T, Sekine T, Kurokawa K 1990 Suppression of parathyroid gland hyperplasia by 1,25(OH)$_2$D$_3$ pulse therapy. N Engl J Med **315:**421–422.

150. Martin KJ, Bullal HS, Domoto DT, Blalock S, Weindel M 1992 Pulse oral calcitriol for the treatment of hyperparathyroidism in patients on continuous ambulatory peritoneal dialysis: Preliminary observations. Am J Kidney Dis **19:**540–545.

151. Slatopolsky E, Weerts C, Thielan J, Horst RL, Harter H, Martin KJ 1984 Marked suppression of secondary hyperparathyroidism by intravenous administration of 1,25-dihydroxycholecalciferol in uremic patients. J Clin Invest **74:**2136–2143.

152. Tan AU Jr, Levine BS, Mazess RB, Kyllo DM, Bishop CW, Knutson JC, Kleinman KS, Coburn JW 1997 Effective suppression of parathyroid hormone by 1 alpha-hydroxy-vitamin D$_2$ in hemodialysis patients with moderate to severe secondary hyperparathyroidism. Kidney Int **51:**317–323.

153. Nemeth EF 1996 Calcium receptors as novel drug targets. In: Bilezikian JP, Raisz LG, Rodan GA (eds.) Principles in Bone Biology. Academic Press, Inc., San Diego, CA, USA, pp. 1019–1035.

154. Silverberg SJ, Bone HG III, Marriott TB, Locker FG, Thys-Jacobs S, Dziem G, Kaatz S, Sanguinetti EL, Bilezikian JP 1997 Short-term inhibition of parathyroid hormone secretion by a calcium-receptor agonist in patients with primary hyperparathyroidism. N Engl J Med **337:**1506–1510.

155. Antonsen JE, Sherrard DJ, Andress DL 1998 A calcimimetic agent acutely suppresses parathyroid hormone levels in patients with chronic renal failure. Rapid communication. Kidney Int **53:**223–227.

156. Llach F 1990 Parathyroidectomy in chronic renal failure: Indications, surgical approach, and the use of calcitriol. Kidney Int **38**(Suppl 29)**:**S62–S68.

157. Kaye M, D'Amour P, Henderson J 1989 Elective total parathyroidectomy without autotransplant in end-stage renal disease. Kidney Int **35:**1390–1399.

158. Kaye M 1989 Parathyroidectomy in end-stage renal disease. J Lab Clin Med **114:**334–335.

159. Malluche HH, Smith AJ, Abreo K, Faugere MC 1984 The use of deferoxamine in the management of aluminium accumulation in bone in patients with renal failure. N Engl J Med **311:**140–144.

160. Ott SM, Andress DL, Nebeker HG, Milliner DS, Maloney NA, Coburn JW, Sherrard DJ 1986 Changes in bone histology after treatment with desferrioxamine. Kidney Int **29**(Suppl 18)**:**S108–S113.

161. Hercz G, Salusky IB, Norris KC, Fine RN, Coburn JW 1986 Aluminum removal by peritoneal dialysis: Intravenous vs. intraperitoneal deferioxamine. Kidney Int **30:**944–948.

162. Milliner DS, Hercz G, Miller JH, Shinaberger JH, Nissenson AR, Coburn JW 1986 Clearance of aluminum by hemodialysis: Effect of deferoxamine. Kidney Int **29**(Suppl 18)**:**S100–S103.

163. Windus DW, Stokes TJ, Julian BA, Fenves AZ 1987 Fatal rhizopus infections in hemodialysis patients receiving deferoxamine. Ann Intern Med **107:**678–680.

164. Boelaert JR, Valcke YL, Vanderbroucke DH 1985 Yersinia enterocolitica bacteraemia in hemodialysis. Proc Euro Dial Transplant Assoc **22:**283.

165. Gallant T, Freedman MH, Vellend H, Francombe WH 1986 Yersinia sepsis in patients with iron overload treated with deferoxamine. N Engl J Med **314:**1643.

166. Hoen B, Renoult E, Jonon B, Kessler M 1988 Septicemia due to Yersinia enterocolitica in a long-term hemodialysis patient after a single desferrioxamine administration. Nephron **50:**378–379.

167. Segal R, Zoller KA, Sherrard DJ, Coburn JW Mucormycosis: A life-threatening complication of deferoxamine therapy in long-term dialysis patients. Kidney Int **33:**238.

168. Abe F, Inaba H, Katoh T, Hotchi M 1990 Effects of iron and desferrioxamine of Rhizopus infection. Mycopathologica **110:**81–91.

169. Van Cutsem J, Boelaert JR 1989 Effects of deferoxamine, feroxamine and iron on experimental mucormycosis (zygomycosis). Kidney Int **36:**1061–1068.

170. Robins-Browne RM, Prpic JK 1985 Effects of iron and desferrioxamine on infections with Yersinia enterocolitica. Infect Immun **47:**774–779.

171. Hercz G, Andress DL, Nebeker HG, Shinaberger JH, Sherrard DJ, Coburn JW 1988 Reversal of aluminum-related bone disease after substituting calcium carbonate for aluminum hydroxide. Am J Kidney Dis **11:**70–75.

Genetic, Developmental, and Dysplastic Skeletal Disorders

Introduction

Michael P. Whyte

Division of Bone and Mineral Diseases, Washington University School of Medicine at Barnes-Jewish Hospital and Center for Metabolic Bone Disease and Molecular Research, Shriners Hospitals for Children, St. Louis, Missouri

Physicians can encounter a great diversity of rare genetic, developmental, and dysplastic skeletal disorders.[1–5] Some are simply radiographic curiosities; some are lethal. Some cause focal bony abnormalities; some feature generalized disturbances of skeletal growth, modeling, or remodeling, leading to osteosclerosis, hyperostosis, or osteoporosis. A few are associated with overt derangements in mineral homeostasis. Most are important because they are heritable and harbor clues concerning factors and pathways that regulate mineral metabolism and skeletal homeostasis. Cumulatively, the number of such patients is substantial.[1–5]

This section provides a concise overview of several of the more common or more revealing of the genetic, developmental, and dysplastic skeletal disorders beginning with those traditionally grouped as sclerosing bone dysplasias.[2–4] Sub-

sequently, one finds descriptions of a few additional important heritable or sporadic developmental and dysplastic conditions.

REFERENCES

1. McKusick VA 1998 Mendelian Inheritance in Man. A Catalog of Human Genes and Genetic Disorders, 12th ed. The Johns Hopkins University Press, Baltimore, MD, USA.
2. Royce PM, Steinmann B (eds.) 2002 Connective Tissue and Its Heritable Disorders, 2nd ed. Wiley-Liss, Inc., New York, NY, USA.
3. Scriver CR, Beaudet AL, Sly WS, Valle D, Childs B, Vogelstein B (eds.) 2001 The Metabolic and Molecular Bases of Inherited Disease, 8th ed. McGraw-Hill, New York, NY, USA.
4. Whyte MP 1997 Skeletal disorders characterized by osteosclerosis or hyperostosis. In: Avioli LV, Krane SM (eds.) Metabolic Bone Disease, 2nd ed. Academic Press, San Diego, CA, USA, pp. 697–738.
5. Beighton P (ed.) 1993 McKusick's Heritable Disorders of Connective Tissue. Mosby Year Book, St. Louis, MO, USA.

Chapter 75.   Sclerosing Bone Disorders

Michael P. Whyte

Division of Bone and Mineral Diseases, Washington University School of Medicine at Barnes-Jewish Hospital and Center for Metabolic Bone Disease and Molecular Research, Shriners Hospitals for Children, St. Louis, Missouri

INTRODUCTION

Osteosclerosis and hyperostosis refer to trabecular and cortical bone thickening, respectively.[1] Increased skeletal mass is caused by many rare (often hereditary) dysplastic conditions,[2] as well as by a variety of dietary, metabolic, endocrine, hematologic, infectious, and neoplastic problems (Table 1).[1] The following sections describe the principal disorders among the bone dysplasias and other unusual conditions associated with localized or generalized osteosclerosis and hyperostosis.

OSTEOPETROSIS

Osteopetrosis (marble bone disease) was first described in 1904 by Albers-Schönberg.[3] More than 300 cases have been reported.[4] Two major clinical forms are well delineated: the autosomal dominant adult (benign) type that is associated with relatively few symptoms[5] and the autosomal recessive infantile (malignant) type that is typically fatal during infancy or early childhood if untreated.[6] A rarer autosomal recessive "intermediate" form presents during childhood with some of the difficulties and signs of malignant osteopetrosis, but its impact on life expectancy is not known.[7] A fourth clinical type, also inherited as an autosomal recessive trait, was initially called the syndrome of *osteopetrosis with renal tubular acidosis and cerebral calcification*, but represents an inborn error of metabolism,

---

The author has no conflict of interest.

TABLE 1. DISORDERS THAT CAUSE HIGH BONE MASS

Dysplasias and Dysostoses
    Autosomal dominant osteosclerosis
    Central osteosclerosis with ectodermal dysplasia
    Craniodiaphyseal dysplasia
    Craniometaphyseal dysplasia
    Dysosteosclerosis
    Endosteal hyperostosis (van Buchem disease and
    sclerosteosis)
    Frontometaphyseal dysplasia
    Infantile cortical hyperostosis (Caffey disease)
    Juvenile Paget disease (osteoectasia with hyperphosphatasia or
    hyperostosis corticalis)
    Melorheostosis
    Metaphyseal dysplasia (Pyle disease)
    Mixed sclerosing bone dystrophy
    Oculodento-osseous dysplasia
    Osteodysplasia of Melnick and Needles
    Osteopathia striata
    Osteopetrosis
    Osteopoikilosis
    Progressive diaphyseal dysplasia (Engelmann disease)
    Pycnodysostosis
    Tubular stenosis (Kenny-Caffey syndrome)
Metabolic
    Carbonic anhydrase II deficiency
    Fluorosis
    Heavy metal poisoning
    Hepatitis C–associated osteosclerosis
    Hypervitaminosis A,D
    Hyper-, hypo-, and pseudohypoparathyroidism
    Hypophosphatemic osteomalacia
    Milk-alkali syndrome
    Renal osteodystrophy
    X-linked hypophosphatemia
Other
    Axial osteomalacia
    Diffuse idiopathic skeletal hyperostosis (DISH)
    Erdheim-Chester disease
    Fibrogenesis imperfecta ossium
    High bone mass phenotype
    Hypertrophic osteoarthropathy
    Ionizing radiation
    Leukemia
    Lymphomas
    Mastocytosis
    Multiple myeloma
    Myelofibrosis
    Osteomyelitis
    Osteonecrosis
    Paget disease
    Sarcoidosis
    Sickle cell disease
    Skeletal metastases
    Tuberous sclerosis

(Reprinted from Dynamics of Bone and Cartilage Metabolism: Principles and Clinical Applications, Seibel MJ, Robins SP, Bilezikian JP, Rare bone diseases, pp. 605–621, 1999 with permission of Elsevier.)

carbonic anhydrase II deficiency.[4] Neuronal storage disease with malignant osteopetrosis has been reported in several patients and seems to reflect a distinct entity.[8] There also appear to be especially rare forms of osteopetrosis called "lethal," "transient infantile," and "postinfec-

tious."[4] A new syndrome of *osteopetrosis, lymphedema, anhydrotic ectodermal dysplasia, and immunodeficiency* (OL-EDA-ID) was characterized as an X-linked trait affecting boys.[9] Recently, the first report of drug-induced osteopetrosis concerned a boy treated with high doses of pamidronate.[10]

Although a diversity of clinical and hereditary types of osteopetrosis makes it apparent that defects in several different genes and a variety of biological disturbances cause this disorder in humans, the pathogenesis of all true forms involves failure of osteoclast-mediated resorption of the skeleton.[4] Consequently, primary spongiosa (calcified cartilage deposited during endochondral bone formation) persists as a histopathological marker.[11] Understandably, the term "osteopetrosis" has been used generically for some other conditions with radiodense skeletons but lacking this hallmark, but we should now be precise. In fact, it is crucial to recognize that therapeutic approaches for true forms of osteopetrosis, for which the pathogenesis is partly elucidated, may be hazardous for other sclerosing bone disorders.[4]

Clinical Presentation

Infantile osteopetrosis manifests during the first year of life.[6] Recurrence within sibships and an increased incidence of parental consanguinity implicate transmission as an autosomal recessive trait. Nasal stuffiness caused by malformation of the mastoid and paranasal sinuses is an early symptom. Cranial foramina do not widen fully, and this can gradually paralyze optic, oculomotor, and facial nerves. There is also failure to thrive. Eruption of the dentition is delayed. Bones may appear dense on radiographic study but are fragile. Some patients develop hydrocephalus or sleep apnea. Blindness can also be caused by retinal degeneration or raised intracranial pressure.[12] Recurrent infection and spontaneous bruising and bleeding are common problems from myelophthisis because of excessive bone, abundant osteoclasts, and fibrous tissue crowding the marrow spaces. Hypersplenism and hemolysis may exacerbate severe anemia. Physical examination shows short stature, a large head, frontal bossing, an "adenoid" appearance, nystagmus, hepatosplenomegaly, and *genu valgum*. Untreated children usually die during the first decade of life from hemorrhage, pneumonia, severe anemia, or sepsis.[6]

Intermediate osteopetrosis causes short stature. Some patients develop cranial nerve deficits, macrocephaly, ankylosed teeth that predispose to osteomyelitis of the jaw, recurrent fractures, and mild or occasionally moderately severe anemia.[7] A variant, CA II deficiency, is described in the next section.

Adult osteopetrosis is a developmental disorder where radiographic abnormalities appear during childhood. In some kindreds, generations are skipped, and carriers show no X-ray disturbances. Although affected individuals can be asymptomatic,[5] the long bones are brittle and fractures do occur. Facial palsy, deafness, osteomyelitis of the mandible, compromised vision or hearing, psychomotor delay, carpal tunnel syndrome, slipped capital femoral epiphysis, and

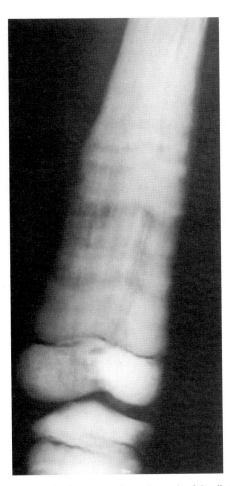

FIG. 1. Osteopetrosis. Anteroposterior radiograph of the distal femur of a 10-year-old boy shows a widened metadiaphyseal region with characteristic alternating dense and lucent bands. (Reprinted from Metabolic Bone Disease, Whyte MP, Murphy WA, Osteopetrosis and other sclerosing bone disorders, 1990 with permission of Elsevier.)

osteoarthritis can be additional problems.[13] Two principal types of adult osteopetrosis have been proposed.[14]

Neuronal storage disease with osteopetrosis features severe skeletal manifestations and is characterized by the additional complications of epilepsy and neurodegenerative disease.[8] *Lethal osteopetrosis* manifests in utero and results in stillbirth.[4] *Transient infantile osteopetrosis* inexplicably resolves during the first few months of life.[4]

Radiological Features

Generalized, symmetrical increase in bone mass is the major radiographic finding in osteopetrosis.[15] Trabecular and cortical bone appear thickened. In the severe forms, all three principal components of skeletal development are disturbed; bone growth, modeling, and remodeling. Most of the skeleton is uniformly dense, but alternating sclerotic and lucent bands are commonly noted in the iliac wings and near the ends of the long bones. Metaphyses are typically broadened and may have a club-shape or "Erlenmeyer flask" deformity (Fig. 1). Rarely, the distal phalanges in the hands are eroded (more common in pyknodysostosis). Pathologi-

cal fracture of long bones is not rare. Rachitic-like changes in growth plates may occur,[16] perhaps reflecting secondary hyperparathyroidism. In the axial skeleton, the skull is usually thickened and dense, especially at the base, and the paranasal and mastoid sinuses are underpneumatized (Fig. 2). Vertebrae may show, on lateral view, a "bone-in-bone" (endobone) configuration.

Albers-Schönberg disease, the adult form of osteopetrosis, manifests with progressive osteosclerosis beginning in childhood, with selective thickening of the base of the skull together with typical vertebral end-plate accentuation that causes an endobone or "rugger jersey" appearance of the spine.[13,14] In the various forms of osteopetrosis, skeletal scintigraphy can reveal fractures and osteomyelitis.[17] Magnetic resonance imaging (MRI) may help to monitor patients with severe disease who undergo bone marrow transplantation, because successful engraftment will enlarge medullary spaces.[18] Computed tomography (CT) and MRI findings concerning the heads of affected infants and children have been detailed.[19]

Laboratory Findings

In infantile osteopetrosis, serum calcium levels generally reflect the dietary intake.[20] Hypocalcemia can occur and may be severe enough to engender rachitic changes in growth plates. Secondary hyperparathyroidism with elevated serum levels of calcitriol is commonly present.[21] Acid phosphatase (ACP) activity is often increased in serum. Presence of the brain isoenzyme of creatine kinase (BB-CK) in serum is a biochemical marker for genuine forms of osteopetrosis.[22] Apparently, the ACP and BB-CK originate from patient osteoclasts.[22] In adult osteopetrosis,

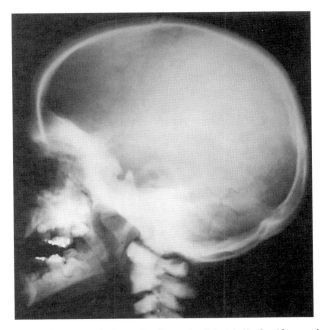

FIG. 2. Osteopetrosis. Lateral radiograph of the skull of a 13-year-old boy shows osteosclerosis, especially apparent at the base. (Reprinted from Metabolic Bone Disease, Whyte MP, Murphy WA, Osteopetrosis and other sclerosing bone disorders, 1990 with permission of Elsevier.)

© 2003 American Society for Bone and Mineral Research

standard biochemical indices of mineral homeostasis are usually unremarkable. However, parathyroid hormone (PTH) levels can be increased in serum.[14]

Histopathological Findings

The radiographic features of the osteopetroses can be diagnostic.[15] Nevertheless, failure of osteoclasts to resorb skeletal tissue provides a histological finding that is pathognomonic[23]: that is, remnants of mineralized primary spongiosa persist as "islands" or "bars" of calcified cartilage within mature bone (Fig. 3).

Human osteopetroses may feature increased, normal, or decreased numbers of osteoclasts. In the infantile form, these cells are usually, but not always, abundant and are found at bone surfaces.[24] Their nuclei are especially numerous, yet the ruffled borders or clear zones that characterize healthy osteoclasts are absent.[25] Fibrous tissue often crowds the marrow spaces.[25] Adult osteopetrosis may show increased amounts of osteoid and osteoclasts can be few and lack ruffled borders, or they can be especially numerous and large.[26] A common histological finding is "woven" bone.[23]

Etiology and Pathogenesis

The pathogenesis of all true forms of osteopetrosis involves diminished osteoclast-mediated skeletal resorption.[27,28] However, the potential causes of osteoclast failure are many and complex.[4,28] Abnormalities could occur in the osteoclast stem cell, its microenvironment, osteoclast precursor cells, the mature heterokaryon, or the bone matrix could be at fault.[4,11] In 1996, an osteoblast defect was reported in two severely affected patients.[29] Cases of osteopetrosis with neuronal storage disease (characterized by accumulation of ceroid lipofuscin) may involve a defect centered in lysosomes.[8] Virus-like inclusions have been found in the osteoclasts of a few sporadic cases of benign osteopetrosis, but their significance is uncertain.[30] Synthesis of an abnormal PTH,[31] or defective production of interleukin (IL)-2[32] or superoxide[33]—factors necessary for bone resorption—may also be pathogenetic defects. In fact, leukocyte function studies in the infantile form have revealed abnormalities in circulating monocytes and granulocytes.[33,34] Ultimately, impaired skeletal resorption causes fragility because fewer collagen fibrils properly connect osteons, and there is defective remodeling of woven bone to compact bone.[11]

Most forms of human osteopetrosis seem to be heritable and transmitted as autosomal traits. The molecular bases are now being discovered.[4] Loss of the chloride channel 7 as a result of mutations in the *CLCN7* gene on chromosome 16p13.3 has been reported rarely in patients with autosomal recessive malignant osteopetrosis but worldwide in adult osteopetrosis, type II (Albers-Schönberg disease).[4] Autosomal recessive infantile osteopetrosis had been found in a small number of patients to reflect mutations in *ATP6I* (TC1RG1) encoding the α3 subunit of the vacuolar proton pump.[35] Hence, deactivating mutations of three genes are currently recognized and compromise CA II, the α_3 subunit of the vacuolar H^+ pump, and chloride channel 7 in osteoclasts.[15] Of interest, together they enable H^+ formation

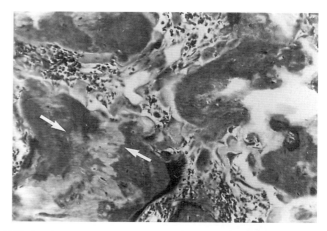

FIG. 3. Osteopetrosis. A characteristic area of lightly stained calcified primary spongiosa (arrows) is found within darkly stained mineralized bone.

and secretion by osteoclasts.[4] Hence, the majority of the human osteopetroses reflect defects in osteoclast-mediated acidification. *OL-EDA-ID* is caused by a mutation in an essential modulator of NF-κB.[9]

Treatment

Because the etiology, pattern of inheritance, and prognosis for the various forms of osteopetrosis can differ, a correct diagnosis is crucial before therapy is attempted. Infants or young children with CA II deficiency may have radiographic features consistent with malignant osteopetrosis, yet subsequent X-ray studies can show spontaneous gradual resolution of their bony sclerosis.[4] Intermediate osteopetrosis is relatively benign compared with the infantile type. A precise diagnosis from among the various forms of osteopetrosis may require investigation of the family, careful evaluation of the patient's disease severity and progression, and gene studies.[4]

Bone Marrow Transplantation

Bone marrow transplantation (BMT) has remarkably improved some patients with infantile osteopetrosis.[36,37] In 1980, transplanted osteoclasts, but not osteoblasts, were shown to be of donor origin.[38] Such observations bolstered the hypothesis that osteopetrosis is caused by defective osteoclast-mediated bone resorption and that osteoclast progenitor cells derive from marrow.[38] However, patients with severely crowded medullary spaces appear less likely to engraft after BMT. Hence, early intervention with BMT seems to be more successful. Accordingly, histomorphometric studies of bone may help to assess the outcome of this procedure. Use of marrow from HLA-nonidentical donors warrants continued study.[30] Recently, purified blood progenitor cells from HLA-haploidentical parents has been effective.[39] It is understandable that BMT may not benefit all patients,[4] because a variety of defects (not all of which are intrinsic to marrow) could theoretically cause osteopetrosis. Successful BMT can engender hypercalcemia as osteoclast function begins.[40]

Hormonal and Dietary Therapy

Some success in treating osteopetrosis has been reported with a calcium-deficient diet. Conversely, supplementation of dietary calcium may be necessary for symptomatic hypocalcemia in severely affected infants or children.[16] Large oral doses of calcitriol (1,25-dihydroxyvitamin D_3), together with limited dietary calcium intake (to prevent hypercalciuria/hypercalcemia), seems to occasionally improve infantile osteopetrosis.[41] Calcitriol may help by stimulating dormant osteoclasts. Nevertheless, some patients seem to become resistant to this treatment.[27,33] Long-term infusion of PTH helped one infant,[31] perhaps by enhancing calcitriol synthesis. The observation that leukocytes from severely affected individuals have diminished production of superoxide led to administration of recombinant human interferon γ-1b and clinical, laboratory, and histopathological evidence of benefit.[27,33] In 2000, interferon γ-1b received Food and Drug Administration (FDA) approval in the United States for severe osteopetrosis.

High-dose glucocorticoid treatment stabilizes pediatric patients with pancytopenia and hepatomegaly. Prednisone and a low-calcium/high-phosphate diet may be an alternative to BMT.[42] A recent case report describes apparent cure of the malignant form using prednisone therapy.[43]

Supportive

Hyperbaric oxygenation can be an important adjunctive treatment for osteomyelitis of the jaw. Surgical decompression of the optic and facial nerves may benefit some patients.

Early prenatal diagnosis of osteopetrosis by ultrasound has generally been unsuccessful. Conventional radiographic studies occasionally diagnose malignant osteopetrosis late in pregnancy.[44] However, mutation detection is rapidly becoming increasingly useful.[4]

CARBONIC ANHYDRASE II DEFICIENCY

In 1983, the autosomal recessive syndrome of *osteopetrosis with renal tubular acidosis (RTA) and cerebral calcification* was discovered to be an inborn error of metabolism caused by deficiency of the *carbonic anhydrase II (CA II)* isoenzyme.[45]

Clinical Presentation

Description of more than 50 cases of CA II deficiency has revealed considerable clinical variability among affected families.[46,47] The perinatal history is typically unremarkable, but in infancy or early childhood, patients may sustain a fracture or manifest failure to thrive, developmental delay, or short stature. Mental subnormality is common, but not invariable. Compression of the optic nerves and dental malocclusion are additional complications. Renal tubular acidosis (RTA) may explain the hypotonia, apathy, and muscle weakness that trouble some patients. Periodic hypokalemic paralysis has been reported. Although fracture is unusual, recurrent breaks in long bones can cause significant morbidity.[46] Life expectancy does not seem to be short-ened, but to date the oldest published cases have been young adults.[48,49]

Radiological Features

CA II deficiency resembles other forms of osteopetrosis on radiographic study, except that cerebral calcification develops during childhood and the osteosclerosis and defects in skeletal modeling diminish spontaneously (rather than increase) over years.[50] Skeletal radiographs are typically abnormal at diagnosis, although findings can be subtle at birth. CT has demonstrated that the cerebral calcification appears between 2 and 5 years of age, increases during childhood, affects gray matter of the cortex and basal ganglia, and is similar if not identical to that of idiopathic hypoparathyroidism or pseudohypoparathyroidism.

Laboratory Findings

Bone marrow examination is unremarkable. If anemia is present, it is generally mild and of nutritional origin. Metabolic acidosis occurs as early as the neonatal period. Both proximal and distal RTA have been described[51]; distal (type I) RTA seems to be better documented. Additional understanding, however, is required.[51] Aminoaciduria and glycosuria are absent.[48]

Autopsy studies have not been reported.[48] Histopathological examination of bone from four individuals, who represented two affected families, revealed characteristic areas of unresorbed calcified primary spongiosa.[50]

Etiology and Pathogenesis

The CA isoenzymes accelerate the first step in the reaction $CO_2 + H_2O \leftrightarrows H_2CO_3 \leftrightarrows H^+ + HCO_3^-$. Accordingly, they function importantly in acid-base regulation. CA II is present in many tissues, such as brain, kidney, erythrocytes, cartilage, lung, and gastric mucosa.[52] The other CA isoenzymes have a more limited distribution.

All of 21 patients from 12 unrelated kindreds of diverse ethnic and geographic origin were shown to have selective deficiency of CA II in erythrocytes.[48] Red cell CA II levels are approximately one-half normal in carriers.[48,49] Although deficiency of CA II remains to be shown in tissues other than erythrocytes, the presence of osteopetrosis, RTA, and cerebral calcification in patients predicted a global deficiency of CA II and important function in bone, kidney, and perhaps brain.[49] In fact, a variety of deactivating mutations in the *CA II* gene have now been documented in patients worldwide.[49,52] Further insight concerning CA II is provided from a knockout mouse model.[49]

Treatment

Transfusion of CA II-replete erythrocytes in one patient did not correct the systemic acidosis.[53] RTA in CA II deficiency has been treated with HCO_3^- supplementation, but the long-term impact is unknown. Recently, BMT corrected the osteopetrosis, slowed the cerebral calcification, but did not alter the RTA.[54]

PYCNODYSOSTOSIS

Pycnodysostosis may have afflicted the French impressionist painter Henri de Toulouse-Lautrec (1864–1901).[55] More than 100 cases from 50 families have been described since the disorder was delineated in 1962.[56] Pycnodysostosis is transmitted as an autosomal recessive trait; parental consanguinity has been reported for about 30% of patients. Most case descriptions have come from Europe or the United States, but the dysplasia has been found in Israelis, Indonesians, Asian Indians, and Africans. Pycnodysostosis seems to be especially common in the Japanese.[57] In 1996, the genetic defect, compromising cathepsin K, was discovered.[58]

Clinical Presentation

Pycnodysostosis is generally diagnosed during infancy or early childhood because of disproportionate short stature associated with a relatively large cranium and dysmorphic features that include fronto-occipital prominence, obtuse mandibular angle, small facies and chin, high-arched palate, dental malocclusion with retained deciduous teeth, proptosis, bluish sclerae, and a beaked and pointed nose.[59] The anterior fontanel and other cranial sutures are usually open. Fingers are short and clubbed from acro-osteolysis or aplasia of terminal phalanges, fingernails are hypoplastic, and hands are small and square. The thorax is narrow and there may be pectus excavatum, kyphoscoliosis, and increased lumbar lordosis. Recurrent fractures typically involve the lower limbs and cause *genu valgum* deformity. Patients are, however, usually able to walk independently. Visceral manifestations and rickets have been described. Mental retardation affects about 10% of cases.[59] Adult height ranges from 4 ft 3 in to 4 ft 11 in. Recurrent respiratory infections and right heart failure, from chronic upper airway obstruction caused by micrognathia, trouble some patients.

Radiographic Features

Pycnodysostosis shares many radiographic features with osteopetrosis. For example, both conditions cause generalized osteosclerosis and are associated with recurrent fractures. Furthermore, the osteosclerosis is developmental, uniform, first becomes apparent in childhood, and increases with age. However, the marked modeling defects of the severe forms of osteopetrosis do not occur in pycnodysostosis, although long bones manifest hyperostosis and narrow medullary canals. Additional findings that help to differentiate pycnodysostosis include delayed closure of cranial sutures and fontanels (prominently the anterior) (Fig. 4), obtuse mandibular angle, wormian bones, gracile clavicles that are hypoplastic at their lateral segments, hypoplasia or aplasia of the distal phalanges and ribs, and partial absence of the hyoid bone.[60] Endobones and radiodense striations are absent.[15] However, the calvarium and base of the skull are sclerotic, and the orbital ridges are radiodense. Hypoplasia of facial bones, sinuses, and terminal phalanges are characteristic. Vertebrae are dense, yet their transverse processes are uninvolved; anterior and posterior concavities occur. Lumbosacral spondylolisthesis is not uncommon,

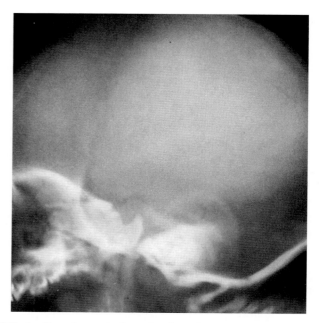

FIG. 4. Pycnodysostosis. Lateral radiograph of the skull of an infant shows that the cranial sutures are markedly widened. The base is sclerotic. (Reprinted from Metabolic Bone Disease, Whyte MP, Murphy WA, Osteopetrosis and other sclerosing bone disorders, 1990 with permission of Elsevier.)

and lack of segmentation of the atlas and axis may be present. Madelung deformity can affect the forearms.

Laboratory Findings

Serum calcium and inorganic phosphate levels and alkaline phosphatase activity are usually unremarkable. Anemia is not a problem. Histopathological study shows cortical bone structure that seems normal despite the appearance of diminished osteoclastic and osteoblastic activity.[61] Electron microscopy of bone from two patients suggested that degradation of collagen might be defective, perhaps from an abnormality in the bone matrix or in the osteoclast.[61] In chondrocytes, abnormal inclusions have been described.

Etiology and Pathogenesis

Early studies of pycnodysostosis indicated that absorption of dietary calcium may be increased. Both the rate of bone accretion and the size of the exchangeable calcium pool seemed reduced.[62] Accordingly, diminished rates of bone resorption potentially explained the osteosclerosis. Also, virus-like inclusions were found in the osteoclasts of two affected brothers.[63]

In 1993, the killing activity and IL-1 secretion of circulating monocytes were found to be low.[64] In 1996, defective growth hormone secretion and low serum insulin-like growth factor (IGF)-1 levels were reported in five of six affected children.[65] Discovery of the molecular basis for pycnodysostosis occurred in 1996 with identification of deactivating mutation of the gene encoding cathepsin K.[58] Cathepsin K, a lysosomal cysteine protease, is highly expressed in osteoclasts. Impaired collagen degradation seems to be a fundamental pathogenetic defect.[58]

Treatment

There is no effective medical therapy for pycnodysostosis. Bone marrow transplantation has not been reported. Fractures of the long bones are typically transverse. They usually heal at a satisfactory rate, although delayed union and massive callus formation have been described. Internal fixation of long bones is formidable because of their hardness. Extraction of teeth is similarly difficult; fracture of the jaw has occurred.[59] Osteomyelitis of the mandible may require treatment with a combined antibiotic and surgical approach. The orthopedic problems have been briefly reviewed.[66]

PROGRESSIVE DIAPHYSEAL DYSPLASIA (CAMURATI-ENGELMANN DISEASE)

Progressive diaphyseal dysplasia (PDD) was characterized by Cockayne in 1920.[67] Camurati found that the condition is heritable. Engelmann described the severe typical form in 1929.[68] In 2000, mutations were identified in the *TGFβ1* gene.[69] PDD is transmitted as an autosomal dominant trait. All races are affected. Descriptions of more than 100 cases show that the clinical and radiological penetrance is quite variable.[70] The characteristic feature is hyperostosis that occurs gradually on both the periosteal and endosteal surfaces of long bones. In severe cases, the skull and axial skeleton are also involved, and osteosclerosis is widespread. Some carriers have no radiographic changes, but bone scintigraphy is abnormal.

Clinical Presentation

PDD typically presents during childhood with limping or a broad-based and waddling gait, leg pain, muscle wasting, and decreased subcutaneous fat in the extremities. Understandably, these features can be mistaken for muscular dystrophy.[71] Severely affected patients also have a characteristic body habitus that includes an enlarged head with prominent forehead, proptosis, and thin limbs with thickened bones and little muscle mass. Cranial nerve palsies may develop when the skull is affected. Puberty is sometimes delayed. Raised intracranial pressure can occur. Physical findings include palpable bony thickening and skeletal tenderness. Some patients have hepatosplenomegaly, Raynaud's phenomenon, and other findings suggestive of vasculitis.[72] Although radiological studies typically show progressive disease, the clinical course is variable, and remission of symptoms seems to occur in some patients during adult life.[73]

Radiological Features

The principal radiographic feature of PDD is hyperostosis of major long bone diaphyses caused by proliferation of new bone on both the periosteal and the endosteal surfaces.[15] The sclerosis is fairly symmetrical and gradually spreads to

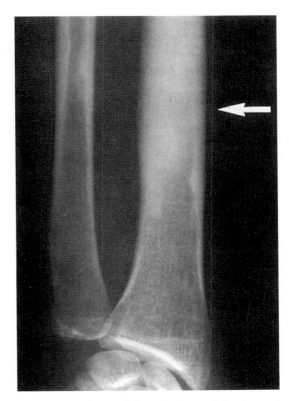

FIG. 5. Progressive diaphyseal dysplasia (Camurati-Engelmann disease). The distal radius of this 20-year-old woman has a characteristic area of patchy thickening (arrow) of the periosteal and endosteal surfaces of the diaphysis.

involve metaphyses. However, the epiphyses are characteristically spared (Fig. 5). The tibias and femora are most commonly involved; less frequently, the radii, ulnae, humeri and, occasionally, the short tubular bones are affected. The scapulae, clavicles, and pelvis may also become thickened. Typically, the shafts of long bones gradually widen and develop irregular surfaces. The age-of-onset, rate of progression, and degree of bony involvement are highly variable. With relatively mild disease, especially in adolescents or young adults, radiographic and scintigraphic abnormalities may be confined to the long bones of the lower limbs. Maturation of the new bone increases the degree of hyperostosis. However, in severely affected children, some areas of the skeleton can appear osteopenic.

Bone scanning typically reveals focally increased radionuclide accumulation in affected areas of the skeleton.[74] Clinical, radiographic, and scintigraphic findings are generally concordant. In some patients, however, bone scans are unremarkable despite considerable radiographic abnormality. This mismatch seems to reflect advanced but quiescent disease.[74] Markedly increased radioisotope accumulation with minimal radiographic findings can disclose active but early skeletal disease.[74] MRI and CT findings delineating cranial involvement have been reported.[75]

Laboratory Findings

Routine biochemical parameters of bone and mineral metabolism are typically normal in PDD, although serum alkaline phosphatase activity and urinary hydroxyproline levels are elevated in some patients. Modest hypocalcemia and significant hypocalciuria occur in some affected individuals who have severe disease and appear to reflect positive calcium balance.[73] Mild anemia and leukopenia and elevated erythrocyte sedimentation rate may also be present.[72]

Histopathology shows new bone formation along diaphyses. Peripheral to the original bony cortex, there is disorganized, newly-formed, woven bone undergoing centripetal maturation and then incorporation into the cortex.[70] Electron microscopy of muscle has shown myopathic changes and vascular abnormalities.[71]

Etiology and Pathogenesis

The clinical and laboratory features of severe PDD and its responsiveness to glucocorticoid treatment have led some investigators to suggest that this disorder is a systemic condition (i.e., an inflammatory connective tissue disease).[72] Some especially mild cases were believed to represent a separate autosomal recessive condition called Ribbing's disease.[76] However, sporadic cases of PDD do occur, and mild clinical forms can be transmitted as an autosomal dominant trait with variable penetrance.[77]

Aberrant differentiation of monocytes/macrophages to fibroblasts, and hence to osteoblasts, has been discussed as a fundamental pathogenetic feature.[78]

Just before identification of its genetic basis, PDD was thought to be more severe in ensuing generations ("anticipation").[77] PDD is now known to reflect mutations in the gene that encodes transforming growth factor B_1 ($TGF\beta1$). A "latency-associated peptide" encoded by this gene is mutated and remains bound to $TGF\beta1$ keeping it constitutively active in skeletal matrix.[69,79] Severity is variable among kindred members. However, there seems to some locus heterogeneity.[80,81]

Treatment

PDD is a chronic and somewhat unpredictable condition.[82] Symptoms may remit during adolescence or adult life. After initial use in 1967 for this disorder, glucocorticoid therapy (typically prednisone given in small doses on an alternate day schedule) has become a well-documented, effective treatment that can relieve bone pain and apparently correct histological abnormalities in affected bone.[83] Complete relief of localized pain has followed surgical removal of diseased diaphyseal bone, forming a "cortical window."[84] Bisphosphonate therapy may increase bone pain.[85]

ENDOSTEAL HYPEROSTOSIS

In 1955, van Buchem et al. first described the condition *hyperostosis corticalis generalisata*.[86] Their report led to characterization of the disorders that are considered endosteal hyperostoses.

Van Buchem Disease

Van Buchem disease is an autosomal recessive, clinically severe condition[86] that is differentiated from an autosomal dominant, more benign form of endosteal hyperostosis (Worth type)[86,87] and an autosomal recessive, severe disorder called *sclerosteosis*. The entity is considerably less common than the cumulative number of case reports might suggest.[88]

Clinical Presentation. *Van Buchem disease* has been described in children and adults; sex distribution seems to be equal. Progressive asymmetrical enlargement of the jaw occurs during puberty. The adult mandible is markedly thickened with a wide angle, but there is no prognathism, and dental malocclusion is uncommon. Patients may be symptom free; however, recurrent facial nerve palsy, deafness, and optic atrophy from narrowing of cranial foramina are common and can begin as early as infancy. Long bones may become painful with applied pressure, but they are not fragile, and joint range-of-motion is generally normal. Sclerosteosis has been differentiated clinically from van Buchem disease because sclerosteosis patients are excessively tall and have syndactyly.[89]

Radiological Features. Endosteal cortical thickening that produces a dense and homogeneous diaphyseal cortex that narrows the medullary canal is the major radiographic feature of van Buchem disease. The hyperostosis is selectively endosteal; long bones are properly modeled. However, generalized osteosclerosis affects the base of the skull, facial bones, vertebrae, pelvis, and ribs. The mandible becomes enlarged (Fig. 6). Cranial CT features have been characterized.[90]

Laboratory Findings. Alkaline phosphatase activity in serum is primarily of skeletal origin and may be increased; calcium and inorganic phosphate levels are unremarkable. Van Buchem and colleagues suggested that the excessive bone was essentially of normal quality.

Etiology and Pathogenesis. Van Buchem disease and sclerosteosis were once predicated to be allelic disorders—their clinical/radiographic differences likely reflecting epistatic effects of modifying genes.[89] Now, we know that deactivating mutations in the *SOST* gene cause sclerosteosis,[91] whereas van Buchem disease involves a 52-kb deletion downstream of *SOST*.[92]

Treatment. There is no specific medical therapy. Surgical decompression of narrowed foramina may help cranial nerve palsies.[93] Surgery has also been used to recontour the mandible.[94]

Sclerosteosis

Sclerosteosis (cortical hyperostosis with syndactyly), like van Buchem disease, is an autosomal recessive form of

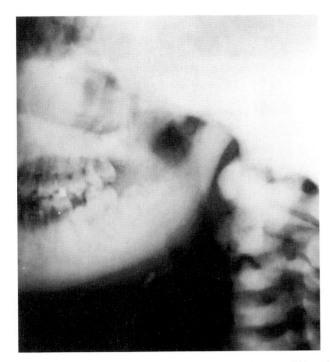

FIG. 6. Endosteal hyperostosis. Lateral radiograph of the mandible and facial bones of a 9-year-old boy with van Buchem disease shows dense sclerosis of all osseous structures. (Reprinted from Metabolic Bone Disease, Whyte MP, Murphy WA, Osteopetrosis and other sclerosing bone disorders, 1990 with permission of Elsevier.)

endosteal hyperostosis. It occurs primarily in Afrikaners or others of Dutch ancestry.[89] Initially, sclerosteosis was distinguished from van Buchem disease by some radiographic differences and the presence of syndactyly. Subsequent clinical studies predicted both disorders were "allelic" and involved defects in the same gene.[89] We now know that the genetic defects are different.[91,92]

Clinical Presentation. At birth, only syndactyly may be noted.[95] During early childhood, overgrowth and sclerosis of the skeleton involves especially the skull and causes facial disfigurement. Patients are tall and heavy beginning in childhood. Understandably, the term "gigantism" has been used. However, deafness and facial palsy caused by nerve entrapment are also prominent problems. The mandible has a rather square configuration. Raised intracranial pressure and headache may be sequelae of a small cranial cavity. The brainstem can become compressed. Syndactyly from either cutaneous or bony fusion of the middle and index fingers is typical, but of variable severity. The fingernails are dysplastic. Patients are not prone to fracture, and their intelligence is normal. Life expectancy may be shortened.[96]

Radiological Features. Except when bony syndactyly is present, the skeleton is normal in early childhood. The principal radiographic feature is progressive bone thickening that causes widening of the skull and prognathism.[97] In the long bones, modeling defects occur and the cortices are thickened. The vertebral pedicles, ribs, pelvis, and tubular

bones may also become somewhat dense. CT has shown fusion of the ossicles and narrowing of the internal auditory canals and cochlear aqueducts.[89]

Histopathological Findings. In an American kindred with sclerosteosis, dynamic histomorphometry of the skull of one patient showed thickened trabeculae and osteoidosis where the rate of bone formation was increased; osteoclastic bone resorption appeared to be quiescent.[97]

Etiology and Pathogenesis. Enhanced osteoblast activity with failure of osteoclasts to compensate for increased bone formation seems to explain the dense bone of sclerosteosis.[98] No abnormality of calcium homeostasis or of pituitary gland function has been documented.[99] The pathogenesis of the neurological defects has been described in detail.[98]

In 1998, van Buchem disease was mapped to chromosome 17q12-q21.[100] In 2000, deactivating mutations in a gene called *SOST* within this region were discovered in sclerosteosis patients of Afrikaner descent.[91]

Treatment. There is no specific medical treatment for sclerosteosis. Surgical correction of syndactyly is especially difficult if there is bony fusion. Prognathism cosmesis is complicated by dense mandibular bone. Management of associated neurological dysfunction has been reviewed.[98]

OSTEOPOIKILOSIS

Osteopoikilosis literally translated means spotted bones. This condition, usually a radiographic curiosity, is transmitted as an autosomal dominant trait with a high degree of penetrance.[101] Affected individuals may also have a form of connective tissue nevus called *dermatofibrosis lenticularis disseminata*; the disorder is then called the *Buschke-Ollendorff syndrome*.[102] The bony lesions are asymptomatic, but if not recognized, can precipitate studies for other important conditions, including metastatic disease to the skeleton.[103] Hence, family members at risk should be screened with a radiograph of the hand/wrist and knee after childhood.

Clinical Presentation

Osteopoikilosis is typically an incidental finding. Musculoskeletal pain, recorded in many cases, is probably coincidental. The nevi usually involve the lower trunk or extremities and occur before puberty, sometimes congenitally. This dermatosis characteristically appears as small asymptomatic papules; however, they are sometimes yellow or white discs or plaques, deep nodules, or streaks.[102]

Radiological Features

The characteristic radiographic finding is numerous small foci of osteosclerosis of variable shape (usually round or oval).[15] Commonly affected sites are the ends of the short tubular bones, the metaepiphyseal regions of the long bones,

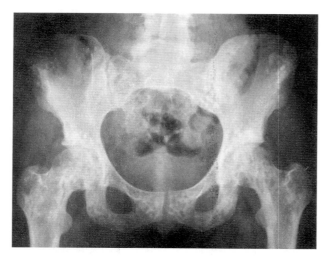

FIG. 7. Osteopoikilosis. Characteristic features shown here include the spotted appearance of the pelvis and metaepiphyseal regions of the femora. (Reproduced with permission from Whyte MP 1995 Rare disorders of skeletal formation and homeostasis. In: Becker KN, ed., Principles and Practice of Endocrinology and Metabolism, 2nd ed. Lippincott-Raven Publishers, Philadelphia, PA, USA.)

and the tarsal, carpal, and pelvic bones (Fig. 7). These foci do not change shape and size for decades, but they may mimic metastatic lesions. However, radionuclide accumulation is not increased on bone scanning.[103]

Histopathological Studies

Dermatofibrosis lenticularis disseminata is characterized by excessive amounts of unusually broad, markedly branched, interlacing elastin fibers in the dermis; the epidermis is normal.[103] The foci of osteosclerosis are thickened trabeculae that merge with surrounding normal bone or islands of cortical bone that include Haversian systems. Mature lesions seem to be remodeling slowly.[104]

OSTEOPATHIA STRIATA

Osteopathia striata is characterized by linear striations at the ends of long bones and in the ileum.[15] Like osteopoikilosis, it is a radiographic curiosity when the skeletal findings occur alone. However, osteopathia striata is also a feature of a variety of clinically important syndromes, including *osteopathia striata with cranial sclerosis*[105] and *osteopathia striata with focal dermal hypoplasia*.[106]

Clinical Presentation

Isolated osteopathia striata is transmitted as an autosomal dominant trait. The musculoskeletal symptoms that may have led to the radiographic studies are probably unrelated. However, when there is also sclerosis of the skull, cranial nerve palsies are common.[105] Until recently, this condition was considered an autosomal dominant trait, but now perhaps an X-linked dominant disorder.[107] Osteopathia striata with focal dermal hypoplasia (*Goltz syndrome*) is a serious X-linked recessive problem in which affected boys have

widespread linear areas of dermal hypoplasia through which adipose tissue can herniate. They also have a variety of additional bony defects in their limbs.[106] Histopathological studies of bone have not been described.

Radiological Features

Gracile linear striations in the cancellous regions of the skeleton, particularly in the metaepiphyses of major long bones and in the periphery of the iliac bones, are the characteristic radiographic findings (Fig. 8).[15] The carpal, tarsal, and tubular bones of the hands and feet are less commonly and more subtly affected. The striations appear unchanged for years. Radionuclide accumulation is not increased during bone scanning.[103]

Treatment

The bone lesions are benign. Although unlikely to be misdiagnosed, radiographic screening after childhood of family members at risk would seem prudent. In one family with osteopathia striata and cranial sclerosis, the diagnosis was reportedly made prenatally by ultrasound examination.[108]

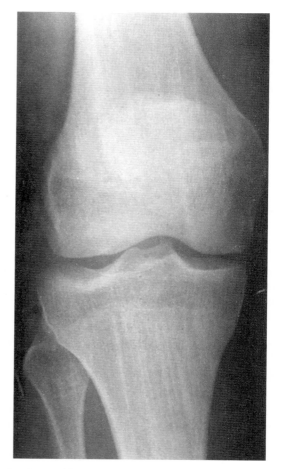

FIG. 8. Osteopathia striata. Characteristic longitudinal striations are present in the femur and tibia of this 17-year-old girl.

MELORHEOSTOSIS

Melorheostosis, from the Greek, refers to flowing hyperostosis of the limbs. The skeletal radiographic findings have been likened to wax that has dripped down the side of a candle. After its initial description in 1922,[109] about 200 cases have been reported.[110,111] No Mendelian pattern of inheritance has been found; the disorder occurs sporadically.

Clinical Presentation

Melorheostosis typically manifests during childhood. Usually there is monomelic involvement; bilateral disease, when it occurs, is generally asymmetrical. Cutaneous changes that overlie affected skeletal sites are not uncommon. Of 131 patients reported in one investigation, 17% had linear scleroderma-like patches and hypertrichosis. Fibromas, fibrolipomas, capillary hemangiomas, lymphangiectasia, and arterial aneurysms also occur.[112,113] Soft-tissue abnormalities are often noted before the hyperostosis is discovered. Pain and stiffness are the major symptoms. Affected joints can contract and deform. In affected children, leg length inequality occurs because of soft tissue contractures and premature fusion of epiphyses. The skeletal lesions seem to progress most rapidly during childhood. During the adult years, melorheostosis may or may not gradually extend.[114] Nevertheless, pain is a more frequent symptom in adults because of subperiosteal new bone formation.

Radiological Features

Dense, irregular, and eccentric hyperostosis of both the cortex and the adjacent medullary canal of a single bone, or several adjacent bones, is the characteristic radiographic finding in melorheostosis (Fig. 9).[15,111] Any anatomical region or bone may be affected, but the lower extremities are most commonly involved. Bone can also develop in soft tissues near affected skeletal areas, particularly near joints. Melorheostotic bone has increased blood flow and avidly accumulates radionuclide during bone scanning.[115]

Laboratory Findings

Routine laboratory studies (e.g., serum calcium and inorganic phosphate levels and alkaline phosphatase activity) are normal.

Histopathological Findings

The skeletal lesion in melorheostosis features endosteal thickening during infancy and childhood and then periosteal new bone formation during adult life.[111] Bony lesions are sclerotic with thickened irregular lamellae that may occlude Haversian systems. Marrow fibrosis may also be present.[111] Unlike in true scleroderma, the collagen of the scleroderma-like lesions of melorheostosis appears normal. Thus, this dermatosis has been called *linear melorheostotic scleroderma*.[112,116]

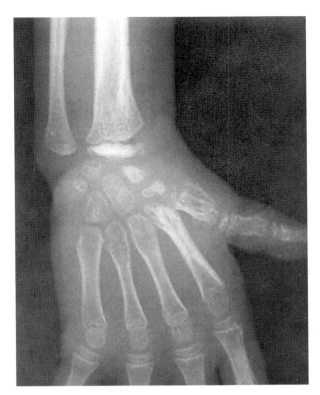

FIG. 9. Melorheostosis. Characteristic patchy osteosclerosis is most apparent in the radius and second metacarpal of this 8-year-old girl.

Etiology and Pathogenesis

The distribution of melorheostosis and its associated soft-tissue lesions in sclerotomes, myotomes, and dermatomes suggests that a segmentary, embryogenetic defect explains this sporadic condition.[112,116] Linear scleroderma may reflect the primary abnormality that extends deep into the skeleton. Recent studies of affected skin suggest altered expression of several adhesion proteins.[117]

Treatment

Surgical correction of contractures can be difficult; recurrent deformity is common. Distraction techniques, however, have reportedly had promising outcomes.[118]

MIXED SCLEROSING BONE DYSTROPHY

Mixed sclerosing bone dystrophy is a rare skeletal dysplasia in which features of osteopoikilosis, osteopathia striata, melorheostosis, cranial sclerosis, or additional osseous defects occur together in various combinations in one individual.[119]

Clinical Presentation

Patients may experience the problems typically associated with the individual patterns of osteosclerosis; for example, cranial sclerosis may result in cranial nerve palsy, and melorheostosis can cause localized bone pain.[119]

Radiological Features

Two or more dense bone patterns are noted (osteopoiki-losis, osteopathia striata, melorheostosis, cranial sclerosis, generalized cortical hyperostosis, focal osteosclerosis, or progressive diaphyseal dysplasia). However, just one region of the skeleton may be affected.

Bone scanning shows increased radionuclide uptake in the areas of greatest skeletal sclerosis.[119,120]

Histopathological Findings

Although the term "osteopetrosis" has been applied to the generalized osteosclerosis that occurs in some patients, his-topathology has failed to show remnants of calcified primary spongiosa (see osteopetrosis).[119,120]

Etiology and Pathogenesis

Delineation of mixed sclerosing bone dystrophy suggests a common etiology and pathogenesis for its individual osteosclerotic patterns. However, osteopoikilosis and most forms of osteopathia striata are heritable, whereas mixed sclerosing bone dystrophy, like melorheostosis, seems to be a sporadic disorder.[119,120]

Treatment

There is no medical treatment. Contractures or neurovascular compression by osteosclerotic lesions can require surgical intervention.

AXIAL OSTEOMALACIA

Axial osteomalacia is characterized radiographically by coarsening of the trabecular pattern of the axial but not the appendicular skeleton.[121] Fewer than 20 patients have been described. Most affected individuals have been sporadic cases, but dominant transmission has been reported[118]; thus, further understanding is needed.

Clinical Presentation

Most patients with axial osteomalacia have been middle-aged or elderly men; a few middle-aged women have been described. However, radiographic manifestations are likely to be detectable earlier.[122] The majority of cases have presented with dull, vague, and chronic axial bone pain (often in the cervical region) that prompted radiographic study. Family histories are usually negative for skeletal disease.

Radiological Features

Abnormalities are essentially confined to the spine and pelvis, where trabeculae are coarsened and form a pattern resembling other types of osteomalacia.[123] However, Looser zones (a radiologic hallmark of osteomalacia) have not been reported. The cervical spine and ribs seem to be the most severely affected; the lumbar spine is abnormal to a lesser degree. Several patients have also had features of

ankylosing spondylitis.[124,125] Radiographic survey of the appendicular skeleton is unremarkable.

Laboratory Studies

In a few patients, serum inorganic phosphate levels tended to be low.[124,125] In others, osteomalacia occurred despite normal serum levels of calcium, inorganic phosphate, 25-hydroxyvitamin D and 1,25-dihydroxyvitamin D. Serum alkaline phosphatase activity (bone isoenzyme) may be increased.

Histopathological Findings

Iliac crest specimens have distinct corticomedullary junctions, but the cortices can be especially wide and porous. Trabeculae are of variable thickness; total bone volume may be increased. Collagen has a normal lamellar pattern on polarized-light microscopy. Increased width and extent of osteoid seams involves trabecular bone surfaces and cortical bone spaces. Tetracycline labeling confirms the defective skeletal mineralization and results in fluorescent "labels" that are single, irregular, and wide.[122] Osteoblasts are flat and inactive-appearing "lining" cells, with reduced Golgi zones and rough endoplasmic reticulum and increased amounts of cytoplasmic glycogen, but these cells do stain intensely for alkaline phosphatase activity. Changes of secondary hyperparathyroidism are absent.[122]

Etiology and Pathogenesis

Axial osteomalacia possibly results from an osteoblast defect.[126] Electron microscopy of iliac crest bone from one patient[122] revealed osteoblasts that had an inactive appearance but were able to form matrix vesicles within abundant osteoid.

Treatment

Effective medical therapy has not been reported. The natural history for axial osteomalacia, however, seems relatively benign. Methyltestosterone and stilbestrol have been tested without success.[126] Vitamin D_2 (as much as 20,000 U/day for 3 years) was similarly without beneficial effect.[126] Slight improvement in skeletal histology, but not in symptoms, was reported for calcium and vitamin D_2 therapy in a study of four cases.[124] Long-term follow-up of one patient showed that symptoms and radiographic findings did not change.[126]

FIBROGENESIS IMPERFECTA OSSIUM

Fibrogenesis imperfecta ossium was first described in 1950. Approximately 10 cases have been reported.[127,128] Although radiographic studies suggest generalized osteopenia, the coarse and dense appearance of trabecular bone explains why this condition is included among the osteosclerotic disorders. The clinical, biochemical, radiological, and histopathological features of fibrogenesis imperfecta ossium and axial osteomalacia have been carefully contrasted.[1]

Clinical Presentation

Fibrogenesis imperfecta ossium typically presents during middle age or later. Both sexes are affected. Gradual onset of intractable skeletal pain that rapidly progresses is the characteristic symptom. Subsequently, there is a debilitating course with progressive immobility. Spontaneous fractures are also a prominent feature. Patients generally become bedridden. Physical examination shows marked bony tenderness.

Radiological Features

Radiographic changes are noted throughout the skeleton, except in the skull. Initially, there may be only osteopenia and a slightly abnormal appearance of trabecular bone.[128] Subsequently, the changes become more consistent with osteomalacia (i.e., further alterations of the trabecular bone pattern, heterogeneous bone density, and thinning of cortical bone). The corticomedullary junctions become indistinct as cortices are replaced by an abnormal pattern of trabecular bone. Areas of the skeleton may have a mixed lytic and sclerotic appearance.[127,128] The generalized osteopenia causes remaining trabeculae to appear coarse and dense in a "fish-net" pattern. Pseudofractures may develop. Deformities secondary to fractures can be present, although bony contours are typically normal. Some patients have a "rugger jersey" spine. Long bone shafts may show periosteal reaction. In fibrogenesis imperfecta ossium and axial osteomalacia, the distribution of the radiographic abnormalities (generalized versus axial) distinguishes the two conditions. Furthermore, the histopathological features are clearly different.[1]

Laboratory Findings

Serum calcium and inorganic phosphate concentrations are normal, but alkaline phosphatase activity is increased. Hydroxyproline levels in urine may be normal or elevated.[128] Typically, there is no aminoaciduria or other evidence of renal tubular dysfunction. Acute agranulocytosis and macroglobulinemia have been reported.

Histopathological Findings

The osseous lesion is a form of osteomalacia, although the amount of affected bone varies considerably from area to area.[128] Aberrant collagen is found in regions with abnormal mineralization patterns, but this protein is unremarkable in other tissues. Polarized-light microscopy shows that the abnormal collagen fibrils lack birefringence. Electron microscopy reveals that the collagen fibrils are thin and randomly organized in a "tangled" pattern. Cortical bone in the shaft of the femora and tibias may show the least abnormality. Osteoid seams are thick. Osteoblasts and osteoclasts can be abundant. In some regions, peculiar circular

matrix structures of 300–500 nm diameter have been observed.[128] Unless bone specimens are viewed with polarized-light or electron microscopy, fibrogenesis imperfecta ossium can be mistaken for osteoporosis or other forms of osteomalacia.[128]

Etiology and Pathogenesis

The etiology is unknown. Genetic factors have not been implicated for this sporadic condition. It seems to be an acquired disorder of collagen synthesis in lamellar bone. Subperiosteal bone formation and collagen synthesis in nonosseous tissues appears to be normal.

Treatment

There is no recognized medical therapy. Temporary clinical improvement can occur.[128] Treatment with vitamin D (or an active metabolite) together with calcium supplementation has been tried without significant benefit. Indeed, ectopic calcification complicated high-dose vitamin D_2 therapy in one patient. Synthetic salmon calcitonin, sodium fluoride, and $24,25(OH)_2D$ have also been used without apparent benefit.[128] Treatment with melphalan and prednisolone seemed to help one patient.[129]

PACHYDERMOPERIOSTOSIS

Pachydermoperiostosis (hypertrophic osteoarthropathy: primary or idiopathic) causes clubbing of the digits, hyperhidrosis and thickening of the skin on especially the face and forehead (*cutis verticis gyrata*), and periosteal new bone formation that occurs prominently in the distal limbs. Autosomal dominant inheritance with variable expression is established,[130] but autosomal recessive transmission also seems to occur.[131]

Clinical Presentation

Men seem to be more severely affected than women, and blacks more commonly than whites. The age at presentation is variable, but symptoms typically first manifest during adolescence.[130,131] All three principal features (clubbing, periostitis, and pachydermia) trouble some patients; others have just one or two of these findings. Clinical expression emerges over a decade, but the disorder can then become quiescent.[132] Progressive gradual enlargement of the hands and feet may result in a "pawlike" appearance. Some affected individuals are described as "acromegalic." Arthralgias of the elbows, wrists, knees, and ankles are common. Occasionally, the small joints are also painful. Acroosteolysis has been reported. Symptoms of pseudogout can occur. Chondrocalcinosis, with calcium pyrophosphate crystals in synovial fluid, troubled one patient. Stiffness and limited mobility of both the appendicular and the axial skeleton can develop. Compression of cranial or spinal nerves has been described. Cutaneous changes include coarsening, thickening, furrowing, pitting, and oiliness of especially the scalp and face. Fatigue is not uncommon.

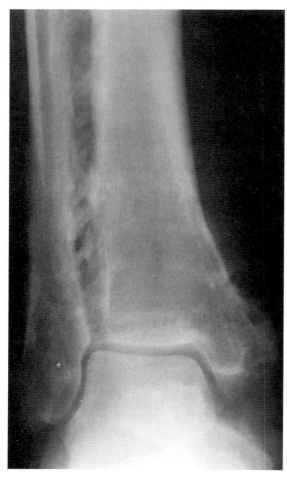

FIG. 10. Pachydermoperiostosis. Anteroposterior radiograph of the ankle shows ragged periosteal reaction along the interosseous membrane between the tibia and fibula (note also the proliferative bone formation along the medial malleolus). (Reproduced with permission from Whyte MP 1995 Rare disorders of skeletal formation and homeostasis. In: Becker KN, ed., Principles and Practice of Endocrinology and Metabolism, 2nd ed. Lippincott-Raven Publishers, Philadelphia, PA, USA.)

Myelophthisic anemia with extramedullary hematopoiesis may occur. Life expectancy is not compromised.[132]

Radiological Features

Severe periostitis that thickens the distal portions of the tubular bones—typically the radius, ulna, tibia, and fibula—is the principal radiographic abnormality (Fig. 10). The metacarpals, tarsals/metatarsals, clavicles, pelvis, base of the skull, and phalanges may also be affected. Clubbing is obvious, and acro-osteolysis can occur. The spine is rarely involved. Ankylosis of joints, especially in the hands and in the feet, may trouble older patients.[15]

The major diagnostic challenge is secondary hypertrophic osteoarthropathy (pulmonary or otherwise). The radiographic features of this condition are, however, somewhat different. In secondary hypertrophic osteoarthropathy, periosteal reaction typically has a smooth, undulating appearance.[133] In pachydermoperiostosis, periosteal proliferation is more exuberant, has an irregular appearance, and often

involves epiphyses. Bone scanning in either condition reveals symmetrical, diffuse, regular uptake along the cortical margins of long bones, especially in the legs. This feature results in a "double stripe" sign.

Laboratory Findings

Periosteal new bone formation roughens the surface of cortical bone.[134] This newly synthesized osseous tissue undergoes cancellous compaction and can accordingly be difficult to distinguish on histopathological examination from the original cortex.[134] There may also be osteopenia of trabecular bone from quiescent formation.[15] Mild cellular hyperplasia and thickening of subsynovial blood vessels is found near synovial membranes.[135] Electron microscopy shows layered basement membranes. Typically, synovial fluid is unremarkable.

Etiology and Pathogenesis

Pachydermoperiostosis has not been mapped within the human genome. A controversial hypothesis suggests that initially some unknown circulating factor acts on vasculature to cause hyperemia and thus alters soft tissues; later, blood flow is reduced.[131] In one patient, skin fibroblasts reportedly synthesized decreased and increased amounts of collagen and decorin, respectively.[136]

Treatment

There is no established medical treatment. Painful synovial effusions may respond to nonsteroidal anti-inflammatory drugs.[137] Colchicine reportedly helped arthralgias, clubbing, folliculitis, and pachyderma in one patient.[138] Contractures or neurovascular compression by osteosclerotic lesions may require surgical intervention.

HEPATITIS C–ASSOCIATED OSTEOSCLEROSIS

In 1992, a new syndrome was delineated that featured acquired, severe, generalized osteosclerosis and hyperostosis in former intravenous drug abusers infected with hepatitis C virus.[139] Approximately a dozen cases have been reported.

Periosteal, endosteal, and trabecular bone thickening occur throughout the skeleton except, apparently, in the cranium (Fig. 11). During active disease, bones in the forearms and legs are painful. Osteodensitometry shows values 200–300% above age- and sex-matched control means. Bone remodeling seems, from biochemical markers, accelerated during active disease and may respond to pamidronate or to calcitonin therapy. Gradual, spontaneous remission of pain and normalization of bone turnover may occur. Exposure to blood contaminated with hepatitis C virus is the historical feature common to all patients.[140] Distinctive abnormalities in the IGF system feature increased circulating levels of IGF binding protein 2[141] and "big" IGF II.[142]

HIGH BONE MASS PHENOTYPE

Some mutations of the *LRP5* gene encoding low density lipoprotein receptor-related protein 5 cause increased skeletal

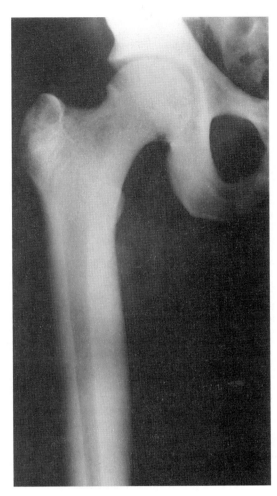

FIG. 11. Hepatitis C–associated osteosclerosis. Anteroposterior view of the proximal right femur of this middle-aged, former intravenous drug abuser shows diffuse bony sclerosis with marked cortical thickening. The medullary cavity is narrow and the periosteal margins of the cortex are mildly convex, suggesting endosteal and periosteal bone apposition, respectively. The cortices of the greater and lesser trochanters are relatively spared. The trabecular pattern in the femoral neck is especially prominent. (Reproduced from J Bone Miner Res 1996;554–558 with permission of the American Society for Bone and Mineral Research.)

mass of good quality.[143] Some patients have *torus palitinus*.[144] Enhanced *wnt* signaling stimulates osteoblasts.[144]

OTHER SCLEROSING BONE DYSPLASIAS

Table 1 lists the relatively large number of conditions that cause focal or generalized increases in skeletal mass.[1,145] Of note, sarcoidosis characteristically causes cysts within coarsely reticulated bone; occasionally, however, sclerotic areas are found in the axial skeleton or in long tubular bones. These skeletal changes may develop well after the pulmonary disease is arrested. Although multiple myeloma typically presents with generalized osteopenia or with discrete osteolytic lesions, widespread osteosclerosis can occur. Lymphoma, myelofibrosis, and mastocytosis are additional hematologic causes of increased bone mass. Metastatic carcinoma, primarily prostatic, commonly causes dense bone. Diffuse osteosclerosis is also relatively frequent in secondary hyperparathyroidism (e.g., renal disease), but occurs rarely in primary hyperparathyroidism. Fluorosis, intoxication with vitamin A or vitamin D, heavy metal poisoning, milk-alkali syndrome, ionizing radiation, osteomyelitis, and osteonecrosis are additional explanations for increased bone mass.[1,145]

REFERENCES

1. Whyte MP 1997 Skeletal disorders characterized by osteosclerosis or hyperostosis. In: Avioli LV, Krane SM (eds.) Metabolic Bone Disease, 2nd ed. Academic Press, San Diego, CA, USA, pp. 697–738.
2. McKusick VA 1998 Mendelian Inheritance in Man: A Catalog of Human Genes and Genetic Disorders, 12th ed. The Johns Hopkins University Press, Baltimore, MD, USA.
3. Albers-Schönberg H 1904 Rontgenbilder einer seltenen, Knochenerkrankung. Meunch Med Wochenschr 51:365.
4. Whyte MP 2002 Osteopetrosis. In: Royce PM, Steinmann B (eds.) Connective Tissue and Its Heritable Disorders. Wiley-Liss, Inc., New York, NY, USA, pp. 789–807.
5. Johnston CC Jr, Lavy N, Lord T, Vellios F, Merritt AD, Deiss WP Jr 1968 Osteopetrosis: A clinical, genetic, metabolic, and morphologic study of the dominantly inherited, benign form. Medicine (Baltimore) 47:149–167.
6. Loria-Cortes R, Quesada-Calvo E, Cordero-Chaverri E 1977 Osteopetrosis in children: A report of 26 cases. J Pediatr 91:43–47.
7. Kahler SG, Burns JA, Aylsworth AS 1984 A mild autosomal recessive form of osteopetrosis. Am J Med Genet 17:451–464.
8. Jagadha V, Halliday WC, Becker LE, Hinton D 1988 The association of infantile osteopetrosis and neuronal storage disease in two brothers. Acta Neuropathol (Berl) 75:233–240.
9. Dupuis-Girod S, Corradini N, Hadj-Rabia S, Fournet JC, Faivre L, Le Deist F, Durand P, Doffinger R, Smahi A, Israel A, Courtois G, Brousse N, Blanche S, Munnich A, Fischer A, Casanova JL, Bodemer C 2002 Osteopetrosis, lymphedema, anhidrotic ectodermal dysplasia, and immunodeficiency in a boy and incontinentia pigmenti in his mother. Pediatrics 109:1–6.
10. Whyte MP, Wenkert D, Clements KL, McAlister WH, Mumm S 2003 Bisphosphonate-induced osteopetrosis. N Engl J Med 394:455–461.
11. Marks SC Jr 1987 Osteopetrosis. Multiple pathways for the interception of osteoclast function. Appl Pathol 5:172–183.
12. Vanier V, Miller R, Carson BS 2000 Bilateral visual improvement after unilateral optic canal decompression and cranial vault expansion in a patient with osteopetrosis, narrowed optic canals, and increased intracranial pressure. J Neurol Neurosurg Psychiatry 69:405–406.
13. Benichou OD, Lareo JD, De Verenjoul MC 2000 Type II autosomal dominant osteopetrosis (Albers-Schönberg disease): Clinical and radiological manifestations in 42 patients. Bone 26:87–83.
14. Bollerslev J 1989 Autosomal dominant osteopetrosis: Bone metabolism and epidemiological, clinical and hormonal aspects. Endocr Rev 10:45–67.
15. Resnick D, Niwayama G 2002 Diagnosis of Bone and Joint Disorders, 4th ed. WB Saunders, Philadelphia, PA, USA.
16. Di Rocco M, Buoncompagni A, Loy A, Dellacqua A 2000 Osteopetrorickets: Case report. Eur J Paediatr Neurol 159:579–581.
17. Park H-M, Lambertus J 1977 Skeletal and reticuloendothelial imaging in osteopetrosis: Case report. J Nucl Med 18:1091–1095.
18. Rao VM, Dalinka MK, Mitchell DG, Spritzer CE, Kaplan F, August CS, Axel L, Kressel HY 1986 Osteopetrosis: MR characteristics at 1.5 T. Radiology 161:217–220.
19. Elster AD, Theros EG, Key LL, Chen MYM 1992 Cranial imaging in autosomal recessive osteopetrosis (parts I & II). Radiology 183:129–144.
20. Key LL, Carnes D, Cole S, Holtrop M, Bar-Shavit Z, Shapiro F, Arceci R, Steinberg J, Gundberg C, Kahn A, Teitelbaum S, Anast C 1984 Treatment of congenital osteopetrosis with high dose calcitriol. N Engl J Med 310:409–415.
21. Cournot G, Trubert-Thil CL, Petrovic M, Boyle A, Cormier C, Girault D, Fischer A, Garabedian M 1992 Mineral metabolism in infants with malignant osteopetrosis: Heterogeneity in plasma 1,25-dihydroxyvitamin D levels and bone histology. J Bone Miner Res 7:1–10.
22. Whyte MP, Chines A, Silva DP Jr, Landt Y, Ladenson JH 1996 Creatine kinase brain isoenzyme (BB-CK) presence in serum distinguishes osteopetrosis among the sclerosing bone disorders. J Bone Miner Res 11:1438–1443.

23. Revell PA 1986 Pathology of Bone. Springer-Verlag, Berlin, Germany.

24. Flanagan AM, Massey HM, Wilson C, Vellodi A, Horton MA, Steward CG 2002 Macrophage colony-stimulating factor and receptor activator NF-κB ligand fail to rescue osteoclast-poor human malignant infantile osteopetrosis in vitro. Bone 30:85–90.

25. Helfrich MH, Aronson DC, Everts V, Mieremet RHP, Gerritsen EJA, Eckhardt PG, Groot CG, Scherft JP 1991 Morphologic features of bone in human osteopetrosis. Bone 12:411–419.

26. Bollerslev J, Steiniche T, Melsen F, Mosekilde L 1986 Structural and histomorphometric studies of iliac crest trabecular and cortical bone in autosomal dominant osteopetrosis: A study of two radiological types. Bone 10:19–24.

27. Whyte MP 1995 Chipping away at marble bone disease. N Engl J Med 332:1639–1640.

28. Teitelbaum SL, Tondravi MM, Ross FP 1996 Osteoclast biology. In: Marcus R, Feldman D, Kelsey J (eds.) Osteoporosis. Academic Press, San Diego, CA, USA, pp. 61–94.

29. Lajeunesse D, Busque L, Mènard P, Brunette MG, Bonny Y 1996 Demonstration of an osteoblast defect in two cases of human malignant osteopetrosis. Correction of the phenotype after bone marrow transplant. Bone 98:1835–1842.

30. Mills BG, Yabe H, Singer FR 1988 Osteoclasts in human osteopetrosis contain viral-nucleocapsid-like nuclear inclusions. J Bone Miner Res 3:101–106.

31. Glorieux FH, Pettifor JM, Marie PJ, Delvin EE, Travers R, Shepard N 1981 Induction of bone resorption by parathyroid hormone in congenital malignant osteopetrosis. Metab Bone Dis Relat Res 3:143–150.

32. Key LL, Ries WL, Schiff R 1987 Osteopetrosis associated with interleukin-2 deficiency. J Bone Miner Res 2:S2;85.

33. Key LL, Rodriguiz RN, Willi SM, Wright NM, Hatcher HC, Eyre DR, Cure JK, Griffin PP, Ries WL 1995 Recombinant human interferon gamma therapy for osteopetrosis. N Engl J Med 332:1594–1599.

34. Beard CJ, Key L, Newburger PE, Ezekowitz RA, Arceci R, Miller B, Proto P, Ryan T, Anast C, Simons ER 1986 Neutrophil defect associated with malignant infantile osteopetrosis. J Lab Clin Med 108:498–505.

35. Sobacchi C, Frattini A, Orchard P, Porras O, Tezcan I, Andolina M, Babul-Hirji R, Baric I, Canham N, Chitayat D, Dupuis-Girod S, Ellis I, Etzioni A, Fasth A, Fisher A, Gerritsen B, Gulino V, Horwitz E, Klamroth V, Lanino E, Mirolo M, Musio A, Matthijs G, Nonomaya S, Notarangelo LD, Ochs HD, Superti Furga A, Valiaho J, van Hove JL, Vihinen M, Vujic D, Vezzoni P, Villa A 2001 The mutational spectrum of human malignant autosomal recessive osteopetrosis. Hum Mol Genet 10:1767–1773.

36. Kaplan FS, August CS, Fallon MD, Dalinka M, Axel L, Haddad JG 1988 Successful treatment of infantile malignant osteopetrosis by bone-marrow transplantation: A case report. J Bone Joint Surg Am 70:617–623.

37. Schulz AS, Classen CF, Mihatsch WA, Sigl-Kraetzig M, Wiesneth M, Debatin KM, Friedrich W, Muller SM 2002 HLA-haploidentical blood progenitor cell transplantation in osteopetrosis. Blood 99:3458–3460.

38. Coccia PF, Krivit W, Cervenka J, Clawson C, Kersey JH, Kim TH, Nesbit ME, Ramsay NK, Warkentin PI, Teitelbaum SL, Kahn AJ, Brown DM 1980 Successful bone-marrow transplantation for infantile malignant osteopetrosis. N Engl J Med 302:701–708.

39. Orchard PJ, Dickerman JD, Mathews CH, Frierdich S, Hong R, Trigg ME, Shahidi NT, Finlay JL, Sondel PM 1987 Haploidentical bone marrow transplantation for osteopetrosis. Am J Pediatr Hematol Oncol 9:335–340.

40. Rawlinson PS, Green RH, Coggins AM, Boyle IT, Gibson BE 1991 Malignant osteopetrosis: Hypercalcaemia after bone marrow transplantation. Arch Dis Child 66:638–639.

41. Key LL Jr 1987 Osteopetrosis: A genetic window into osteoclast function. Cases Metab Bone Dis 2:1–12.

42. Dorantes LM, Mejia AM, Dorantes S 1986 Juvenile osteopetrosis: Effects of blood and bone of prednisone and low calcium, high phosphate diet. Arch Dis Child 61:666–670.

43. Iacobini M, Migliaccio S, Roggini M, Taranta A, Werner B, Panero A, Teti A 2001 Case Report: Apparent cure of a newborn with malignant osteopetrosis using prednisone therapy. J Bone Miner Res 16:2356–2360.

44. Ogur G, Ogur E, Celasun B, Baser I, Imirzalioglu N, Ozturk T, Alemdaroglut A 1995 Prenatal diagnosis of autosomal recessive osteopetrosis, infantile type, by x-ray evaluation. Prenat Diagn 15:477–481.

45. Sly WS, Hewett-Emmett D, Whyte MP, Yu YS, Tashian RE 1983 Carbonic anhydrase II deficiency identified as the primary defect in the autosomal recessive syndrome of osteopetrosis with renal tubular acidosis and cerebral calcification. Proc Natl Acad Sci USA 80:2752–2756.

46. Whyte MP 1993 Carbonic anhydrase II deficiency. Clin Orthop 294:52–63.

47. Sly WS, Whyte MP, Sundaram V, Tashian RE, Hewett-Emmett D, Guibaud P, Vainsel M, Baluarte HJ, Graskin A, Al-Mosawi M 1985 Carbonic anhydrase II deficiency in 12 families with the autosomal recessive syndrome of osteopetrosis with renal tubular acidosis and cerebral calcification. N Engl J Med 313:139–145.

48. Sly WS, Shah GN 2001 The carbonic anhydrase II deficiency syndrome: Osteopetrosis with renal tubular acidosis and cerebral calcification. In: Scriver CR, Beaudet AL, Sly WS, Valle D, Child B, Vogelstein B (eds.) The Metabolic and Molecular Bases of Inherited Disease, 8th ed. McGraw-Hill Book Company, New York, NY, USA, pp. 5331–5343.

49. Whyte MP, Murphy WA, Fallon MD, Sly WS, Teitelbaum SL, McAlister WH, Avioli LV 1980 Osteopetrosis, renal tubular acidosis and basal ganglia calcification in three sisters. Am J Med 69:64–74.

50. Sly WS, Whyte MP, Krupin T, Sundaram V 1985 Positive renal response to acetazolamide in carbonic anhydrase II-deficient patients. Pediatr Res 19:1033–1036.

51. Roth DE, Venta PJ, Tashian RE, Sly WS 1992 Molecular basis of human carbonic anhydrase II deficiency. Proc Natl Acad Sci USA 89:1804–1808.

52. Whyte MP, Hamm LL III, Sly WS 1988 Transfusion of carbonic anhydrase-replete erythrocytes fails to correct the acidification defect in the syndrome of osteopetrosis, renal tubular acidosis, and cerebral calcification (carbonic anhydrase II deficiency). J Bone Miner Res 3:385–388.

53. McMahon C, Will A, Hu P, Shah GN, Sly WS, Smith OP 2001 Bone marrow transplantation corrects osteopetrosis in the carbonic anhydrase II deficiency syndrome. Blood 97:1947–1950.

54. Maroteaux P, Lamy M 1965 The malady of Toulouse-Lautrec. JAMA 191:715–717.

55. Maroteaux P, Lamy M 1962 La pycnodysostose. Presse Med 70:999–1002.

56. Sugiura Y, Yamada Y, Koh J 1974 Pycnodysostosis in Japan: Report of six cases and a review of Japanese literature. Birth Defects 10:78–98.

57. Gelb BD, Brömme D, Desnick RJ 2001 Pycnodysostosis: Cathepsin K deficiency. In: Scriver CR, Beaudet AL, Sly WS, Valle D, Child B, Vogelstein B (eds.) The Metabolic and Molecular Bases of Inherited Disease, 8th ed. McGraw-Hill Book Company, New York, NY, USA, pp. 3453–3468.

58. Elmore SM 1967 Pycnodysostosis: A review. J Bone Joint Surg Am 49:153–162.

59. Wolpowitz A, Matisson A 1974 A comparative study of pycnodysostosis, cleidocranial dysostosis, osteopetrosis and acro-osteolysis. S Afr Med J 48:1011–1118.

60. Soto TJ, Mautalen CA, Hojman D, Codevilla A, Piqué J, Pangaro JA 1969 Pycnodysostosis, metabolic and histologic studies. Birth Defects 5:109–115.

61. Everts V, Aronson DC, Beertsen W 1985 Phagocytosis of bone collagen by osteoclasts in two cases of pycnodysostosis. Calcif Tissue Int 37:25–31.

62. Cabrejas ML, Fromm GA, Roca JF, Mendez MA, Bur GE, Ferreyra ME, Demarchi C, Schurman L 1976 Pycnodysostosis: Some aspects concerning kinetics of calcium metabolism and bone pathology. Am J Med Sci 271:215–220.

63. Beneton MNC, Harris S, Kanis JA 1987 Paramyxovirus-like inclusions in two cases of pycnodysostosis. Bone 8:211–217.

64. Karkabi S, Reis ND, Linn S, Edelson G, Tzehoval E, Zakut V, Dolev E, Bar-Meir E, Ish-Shalom S 1993 Pyknodysostosis: Imaging and laboratory observations. Calcif Tissue Int 53:170–173.

65. Soliman AT, Rajab A, AlSalmi I, Darwish A, Asfour M 1996 Defective growth hormone secretion in children with pycnodysostosis and improved linear growth after growth hormone treatment. Arch Dis Child 75:242–244.

66. Edelson JG, Obad S, Geiger R, On A, Artul HJ 1992 Pycnodysostosis: Orthopedic aspects, with a description of 14 new cases. Clin Orthop 280:263–276.

67. Cockayne EA 1920 A case for diagnosis. Proc R Soc Med 13:132–136.

68. Engelmann G 1929 Ein fall von osteopathia hyperostotica (sclerotisans) multiplex infantilis. Fortschr Geb Roentgen **39:**1101–1106.

69. Saito T, Kinoshita A, Yoshiura Ki, Makita Y, Wakui K, Honke K, Niikawa N, Taniguchi N 2001 Domain-specific mutations of a transforming growth factor (TGF)-β1 latency-associated peptide cause Camurati-Engelmann disease because of the formation of a constitutively active form of TGF-β1. J Biol Chem **276:**11469–11472.

70. Hundley JD, Wilson FC 1973 Progressive diaphyseal dysplasia: Review of the literature and report of seven cases in one family. J Bone Joint Surg Am **55:**461–474.

71. Naveh Y, Ludatshcer R, Alon U, Sharf B 1985 Muscle involvement in progressive diaphyseal dysplasia. Pediatrics **76:**944–949.

72. Crisp AJ, Brenton DP 1982 Engelmann's disease of bone: A systemic disorder? Ann Rheum Dis **41:**183–188.

73. Smith R, Walton RJ, Corner BD, Gordon IR 1977 Clinical and biochemical studies in Engelmann's disease (progressive diaphyseal dysplasia). Q J Med **46:**273–294.

74. Kumar B, Murphy WA, Whyte MP 1981 Progressive diaphyseal dysplasia (Englemann's disease): Scintigraphic-radiologic-clinical correlations. Radiology **140:**87–92.

75. Applegate LJ, Applegate GR, Kemp SS 1991 MR of multiple cranial neuropathies in a patient with Camurati-Engelmann disease: Case report. Am Soc Neuroradiol **12:**557–559.

76. Shier CK, Krasicky GA, Ellis BI, Kottamasu SR 1987 Ribbing's disease: Radiographic-scintigraphic correlation and comparative analysis with Engelmann's disease. J Nucl Med **28:**244–248.

77. Saraiva JM 2000 Anticipation in progressive diaphyseal dysplasia. J Med Genet **37:**394–395.

78. Labat ML, Bringuier AF, Seebold C, Moricard Y, Meyer-Mula C, Laporte P, Talmage RV, Grubb SA, Simmons DJ, Milhaud G 1991 Monocytic origin of fibroblasts: Spontaneous transformation of blood monocytes into neo-fibroblastic structures in osteomyelosclerosis and Engelmann's disease. Biomed Pharmacother **45:**289–299.

79. Janssens K, Gershoni-Baruch R, Guanabens N, Migone N, Ralston S, Bonduelle M, Lissens W, Van Maldergem L, Vanhoenacker F, Verbruggen L, Van Hul W 2000 Mutations in the gene encoding the latency-associated peptide of TGF-β1 cause Camurati-Engelmann disease. Nat Genet **26:**273–275.

80. Hecht JT, Blanton SH, Broussard S, Scott A, Hall CR, Mlunsky JM 2001 Evidence for locus heterogeneity in the Camurati-Engelmann (DPD1) Syndrone. Clin Genet **59:**198–200.

81. Makita Y, Nishimura G, Ikegawa S, Ishii T, Ito Y, Okuno A 2000 Intrafamilial phenotypic variability in Engelmann disease (ED): Are ED and Ribbing disease the same entity? Am J Med Genet **91:**153–156.

82. Kaftori JK, Kleinhaus U, Neveh Y 1987 Progressive diaphyseal dysplasia (Camurati-Engelmann): Radiographic follow-up and CT findings. Radiology **164:**777–782.

83. Naveh Y, Alon U, Kaftori JK, Berant M 1985 Progressive diaphyseal dysplasia: Evaluation of corticosteroid therapy. Pediatrics **75:**321–323.

84. Fallon MD, Whyte MP, Murphy WA 1980 Progressive diaphyseal dysplasia (Engelmann's disease): Report of a sporadic case of the mild form. J Bone Joint Surg Am **62:**465–472.

85. Inaoka T, Shuke N, Sato J, Ishikawa Y, Takahashi K, Aburano T, Makita Y 2001 Scintigraphic evaluation of pamidronate and corticosteroid therapy in a patient with progressive diaphyseal dysplasia (Camurati-Engelmann disease). Clin Nucl Med **26:**680–682.

86. Van Buchem FSP, Prick JJG, Jaspar HHJ 1976 Hyperostosis Corticalis Generalisata Familiaris (Van Buchem's Disease). Excerpta, Amsterdam, The Netherlands.

87. Perez-Vicente JA, Rodriguez de Castro E, Lafuente J, Mateo MM, Gimenez-Roldan S 1987 Autosomal dominant endosteal hyperostosis. Report of a Spanish family with neurological involvement. Clin Genet **31:**161–169.

88. Eastman JR, Bixler D 1977 Generalized cortical hyperostosis (van Buchem disease): Nosologic considerations. Radiology **125:**297–304.

89. Beighton P, Barnard A, Hamersma H, van der Wouden A 1984 The syndromic status of sclerosteosis and van Buchem disease. Clin Genet **25:**175–181.

90. Hill SC, Stein SA, Dwyer A, Altman J, Dorwart R, Doppman J 1986 Cranial CT findings in sclerosteosis. Am J Neuroradiol **7:**505–511.

91. Brunkow ME, Gardner JC, Van Ness J, Paeper BW, Kovacevich BR, Proll S, Skonier JE, Zhao L, Sabo PJ, Fu Y, Alisch RS, Gillett L, Colbert T, Tacconi P, Galas D, Hamersma H, Beighton P, Mulligan J 2001 Bone dysplasia sclerosteosis results from loss of the *SOST* gene product, a novel cystine knot-containing protein. Am J Hum Genet **68:**577–589.

92. Balemans W, Patel N, Ebeling M, Van Hul E, Wuyts W, Lacza C, Dioszegi M, Dikkers FG, Hildering P, Willems PJ, Verheij JB, Lindpaintner K, Vickery B, Foernzler D, Van Hul W 2002 Identification of a 52 kb deletion downstream of the *SOST* gene in patients with van Buchem disease. J Med Gent **39:**91–97.

93. Ruckert EW, Caudill RJ, McCready PJ 1985 Surgical treatment of van Buchem disease. J Oral Maxillofac Surg **43:**801–805.

94. Schendel SA 1988 van Buchem disease: Surgical treatment of the mandible. Ann Plast Surg **20:**462–467.

95. Beighton P, Durr L, Hamersma H 1976 The clinical features of sclerosteosis: A review of the manifestations in twenty-five affected individuals. Ann Intern Med **84:**393–397.

96. Barnard AH, Hamersma H, Kretzmar JH, Beighton P 1980 Sclerosteosis in old age. S Afr Med J **58:**401–403.

97. Beighton P, Cremin BJ, Hamersma H 1976 The radiology of sclerosteosis. Br J Radiol **49:**934–939.

98. Stein SA, Witkop C, Hill S, Fallon MD, Viernstein L, Gucer G, McKeever P, Long D, Altman J, Miller NR, Teitelbaum SL, Schlesinger S 1983 Sclerosteosis, neurogenetic and pathophysiologic analysis of an American kinship. Neurology **33:**267–277.

99. Epstein S, Hamersma H, Beighton P 1979 Endocrine function in sclerosteosis. S Afr Med J **55:**1105–1110.

100. Van Hul W, Balemans W, Van Hul E, Dikkers FG, Obee H, Stokroos RJ, Hildering P, Vanhoenacker F, Van Camp G, Willems PJ 1998 Van Buchem disease (hyperostosis corticalis generalisata) maps to chromosome 17q12–q21. Am J Hum Genet **62:**391–399.

101. Berlin R, Hedensio B, Lilja B, Linder L 1967 Osteopoikilosis: A clinical and genetic study. Acta Med Scand **18:**305–314.

102. Uitto J, Santa Cruz DJ, Starcher BC, Whyte MP, Murphy WA 1981 Biochemical and ultrastructural demonstration of elastin accumulation in the skin of the Buschke-Ollendorff syndrome. J Invest Dermatol **76:**284–287.

103. Whyte MP, Murphy WA, Seigel BA 1978 99m Tc-pyrophosphate bone imaging in osteopoikilosis, osteopathia striata, and melorheostosis. Radiology **127:**439–443.

104. Lagier R, Mbakop A, Bigler A 1984 Osteopoikilosis: A radiological and pathological study. Skeletal Radiol **11:**161–168.

105. Rabinow M, Unger F 1984 Syndrome of osteopathia striata, macrocephaly, and cranial sclerosis. Am J Dis Child **138:**821–823.

106. Happle R, Lenz W 1977 Striation of bones in focal dermal hypoplasia: Manifestation of functional mosaicism? Br J Dermatol **96:**133–138.

107. Viot G, Lacombe D, David A, Mathieu M, de Broca A, Faivre L, Gigarel N, Munnich A, Lyonnet S, Le Merrer M, Cormier-Daire V 2002 Osteopathia striata cranial sclerosis: Non-random X-inactivation suggestive of X-linked dominant inheritance. Am J Med Genet **107:**1–4.

108. Kornreich L, Grunebaum M, Ziv N, Shuper A, Mimouni M 1988 Osteopathia striata, cranial sclerosis with cleft palate and facial nerve palsy. Eur J Paediatr Neurol **147:**101–103.

109. Leri A, Joanny J 1922 Une affection non decrite des os. Hyperostose "en coulee" sur toute la longueur d'un membre ou "melorheostose." Bull Mem Soc Med Hop Paris **46:**1141–1145.

110. Murray RO, McCredie J 1979 Melorheostosis and sclerotomes: A radiological correlation. Skeletal Radiol **4:**57–71.

111. Campbell CJ, Papademetriou T, Bonfiglio M 1968 Melorheostosis: A report of the clinical, roentgenographic, and pathological findings in fourteen cases. J Bone Joint Surg Am **50:**1281–1304.

112. Miyachi Y, Horio T, Yamada A, Ueo T 1979 Linear melorheostotic scleroderma with hypertrichosis. Arch Dermatol **115:**1233–1234.

113. Applebaum RE, Caniano DA, Sun CC, Azizkhan RA, Queral LA 1986 Synchronous left subclavian and axillary artery aneurysms associated with melorheostosis. Surgery **99:**249–253.

114. Colavita N, Nicolais S, Orazi C, Falappa PG 1987 Melorheostosis: Presentation of a case followed up for 24 years. Arch Orthop Trauma Surg **106:**123–125.

115. Davis DC, Syklawer R, Cole RL 1992 Melorheostosis on three-phase bone scintigraphy: Case report. Clin Nucl Med **17:**561–564.

116. Wagers LT, Young AW Jr, Ryan SF 1972 Linear melorheostotic scleroderma. Br J Dermatol **86:**297–30.

117. Kim JE, Kim EH, Han EH, Park RW, Park IH, Jun SH, Kim JC, Young MF, Kim IS 2000 A TGF-β-inducible cell adhesion molecular, Big-h3, is upregulated in melorheostosis and involved in oseogeneis. J Cell Biochem **77:**169–178.

118. Atar D, Lehman WB, Grant AD, Strongwater AM 1992 The Ilizarov apparatus for treatment of melorheostosis: Case report and review of the literature. Clin Orthop **281:**163–167.

119. Whyte MP, Murphy WA, Fallon MD, Hahn TJ 1981 Mixed-sclerosing-bone-dystrophy: Report of a case and review of the literature. Skeletal Radiol **6:**95–102.
120. Pacifici R, Murphy WA, Teitelbaum SL, Whyte MP 1986 Mixed-sclerosing-bone-dystrophy: 42-year follow-up of a case reported as osteopetrosis. Calcif Tissue Int **38:**175–185.
121. Frame B, Frost HM, Ormond RS, Hunter RB 1961 Atypical axial osteomalacia involving the axial skeleton. Ann Intern Med **55:**632–639.
122. Whyte MP, Fallon MD, Murphy WA, Teitelbaum SL 1981 Axial osteomalacia: Clinical, laboratory and genetic investigation of an affected mother and son. Am J Med **71:**1041–1049.
123. Christmann D, Wenger JJ, Dosch JC, Schraub M, Wackenheim A 1981 L'osteomalacie axiale: Analyse compare avec la fibrogenese imparfaite. J Radiol **62:**37–41.
124. Nelson AM, Riggs BL, Jowsey JO 1978 Atypical axial osteomalacia: Report of four cases with two having features of ankylosing spondylitis. Arthritis Rheum **21:**715–722.
125. Cortet B, Berniere L, Solau-Gervais E, Hacene A, Cotton A, Delcambre B 2000 Axial osteomalacia with sacroiliitis and moderate phosphate diabetes: Report of a case. Clin Exp Rheumatol **18:**625–628.
126. Condon JR, Nassim JR 1971 Axial osteomalacia. Postgrad Med **47:**817–820.
127. Swan CH, Shah K, Brewer DB, Cooke WT 1976 Fibrogenesis imperfecta ossium. Q J Med **45:**233–253.
128. Lang R, Vignery AM, Jenson PS 1986 Fibrogenesis imperfecta ossium with early onset: Observations after 20 years of illness. Bone **7:**237–246.
129. Ralphs JR, Stamp TCB, Dopping-Hepenstal PJC, Ali SY 1989 Ultrastructural features of the osteoid of patients with fibrogenesis imperfecta ossium. Bone **10:**243–249.
130. Rimoin DL 1965 Pachydermoperiostosis (idiopathic clubbing and periostosis). Genetic and physiologic considerations. N Engl J Med **272:**923–931.
131. Matucci-Cerinic M, Lott T, Jajic IVO, Pignone A, Bussani C, Cagnoni M 1991 The clinical spectrum of pachydermoperiostosis (primary hypertrophic osteoarthropathy). Medicine **79:**208–214.
132. Herman MA, Massaro D, Katz S 1965 Pachydermoperiostosis: Clinical spectrum. Arch Intern Med **116:**919–923.
133. Ali A, Tetalman M, Fordham EW 1980 Distribution of hypertrophic pulmonary osteoarthropathy. Am J Roentgenol **134:**771–780.
134. Vogl A, Goldfischer S 1962 Pachydermoperiostosis: Primary or idiopathic hypertrophic osteoarthropathy. Am J Med **33:**166–187.
135. Lauter SA, Vasey FB, Huttner I, Osterland CK 1978 Pachydermoperiostosis: Studies on the synovium. J Rheumatol **5:**85–95.
136. Wegrowski Y, Gillery P, Serpier H, Georges N, Combemale P, Kalis B, Maquart FX 1996 Alteration of matrix macromolecule synthesis by fibroblasts from a patient with pachydermoperiostosis. J Invest Dermatol **106:**70–74.
137. Cooper RG, Freemont AJ, Riley M, Holt PJL, Anderson DC, Jayson MIV 1992 Bone abnormalities and severe arthritis in pachydermoperiostosis. Ann Rheum Dis **51:**416–419.
138. Matucci-Cerinic M, Fattorini L, Gerini G, Lombardi A, Pignone A, Petrini N, Lotti T 1988 Cochicine treatment in a case of pachydermoperiostosis with acroosteolysis. Rheumatol Int **8:**185–188.
139. Whyte MP, Teitelbaum SL, Reinus WR 1996 Doubling skeletal mass during adult life: The syndrome of diffuse osteosclerosis after intravenous drug abuse. J Bone Miner Res **11:**554–558.
140. Shaker JL, Reinus WR, Whyte MP 1998 Hepatitis C-associated osteosclerosis: Late onset after blood transfusion in an elderly woman. J Clin Endocrinol Metab **84:**93–98.
141. Khosla S, Hassoun AAK, Baker BK, Liu F, Zien NN, Whyte, MP, Reasner CA, Nippoldt TB, Tiegs RD, Hintz RL, Conover CA 1998 Insulin-like growth factor system abnormalities in hepatitis C-associated osteosclerosis: A means to increase bone mass in adults? J Clin Invest **101:**2165–2173.
142. Khosla S, Ballard FJ, Conover CA 2002 Use of site-specific antibodies to characterize the circulating form of big insulin-like growth factor II in patients with hepatitis C-associated osteosclerosis. J Clin Endocrinol Metab **87:**3867–3870.
143. Little RD, Carulli JP, Del Mastro RG, Dupuis J, Osborne M, Folz C, Manning SP, Swain PM, Zhao SC, Eustace B, Lappe MM, Spitzer L, Zweier S, Braunschweiger K, Benchekroun Y, Hu X, Adair R, Chee L, FitzGerald MG, Tulig C, Caruso A, Tzellas N, Bawa A, Franklin B, McGuire S, Nogues X, Gong G, Allen KM, Anisowicz A, Morales AJ, Lomedico PT, Recker SM, Van Eerdewegh P, Recker RR, Johnson ML 2002 A mutation in the LDL receptor-related protein 5 gene results in the autosomal dominant high-bone-mass trait. Am J Hum Genet **70:**11–19.
144. Boyden LM, Mao J, Belsky J, Mitzner L, Farhi A, Mitnick MA, Wu D, Insogna K, Lifton RP 2002 High bone density due to a mutation in LDL-receptor-related protein 5. N Engl J Med **345:**1513–1521.
145. Frame B, Honasoge M, Kottamasu SR 1987 Osteosclerosis, Hyperostosis, and Related Disorders. Elsevier, New York, NY, USA.

Chapter 76. Fibrous Dysplasia

Michael T. Collins and Paolo Bianco

Craniofacial and Skeletal Diseases Branch, National Institute of Dental and Craniofacial Research, National Institutes of Health, Department of Health and Human Services, Bethesda, Maryland; and Dipartimento di Medicina Sperimentale e Patologia, Universita' La Sapienza, Rome, Italy

INTRODUCTION

Fibrous dysplasia of bone (FD; OMIM#174800) is an uncommon skeletal disorder with a broad spectrum of clinical expressions, ranging from an incidentally discovered asymptomatic radiographic finding, involving a single skeletal site, to a severe disabling disease. The disease may involve one bone (monostotic forms), multiple bones (polyostotic FD), or even the entire skeleton (panostotic FD). In polyostotic forms, lesions of different limb bones are often (but not necessarily) ipsilateral.[1] FD may associate with extraskeletal lesions or dysfunction, most commonly cutaneous pigmentation (Figs. 1A and 1B) and hyperfunctioning endocrinopathies including precocious puberty, hyperthyroidism, growth hormone (GH) excess, and Cushing syndrome (McCune-Albright syndrome [MAS]).[2] A renal tubulopathy, which includes renal phosphate wasting, is one of the most common extraskeletal dysfunctions associated with polyostotic disease.[3] More rarely, FD may be associated with myxomas of skeletal muscle (Mazabraud's syndrome)[4] or dysfunction of heart, liver, pancreas, or other organs in the context of the MAS.[5]

ETIOLOGY AND PATHOGENESIS

All forms of FD are caused by activating, missense mutations of the *GNAS1* gene, encoding the α subunit of the

The authors have no conflict of interest.

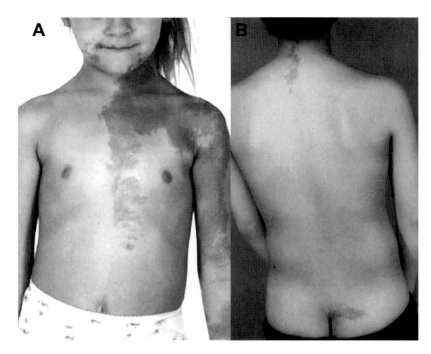

FIG. 1. Café-au-lait skin pigmentation. (A) A typical lesion on the face, chest, and arm of a 5-year-old girl with McCune-Albright syndrome, which shows jagged "coast of Maine" borders and the tendency for the lesions to both respect the midline and follow the developmental lines of Blashko. (B) Typical lesions that are often found on the nape of the neck and crease of the buttocks are shown.

stimulatory G-protein, $G_s\alpha$.[6,7] Mutations occur post-zygotically, are never inherited, and result in a somatic mosaic state. Time of mutation occurrence in development, and size and viability of the mutated clone arising from the single originally mutated cell determine the variable distribution and frequency of the mutated cells in the postnatal organism and the extent and severity of disease.[1] Single base transitions lead to replacement of arginine at position 201 with histidine or cysteine (most commonly) or rarely with other amino acids.[8] As a consequence of the mutation, the catalysis of guanine triphosphate (GTP) to guanine diphosphate (GDP) by $G_s\alpha$ is significantly lowered. Constitutive activation of adenylyl cyclase by the mutated $G_s\alpha$ ensues, and the resulting excess cyclic adenosine monophosphate (cAMP) mediates a number of pathological effects in mutated cells.[1] In bone, mutations impact on cells of the osteogenic lineage, with adverse effects both on osteoprogenitor cells and differentiated osteoblasts.[9,10] Expansion of the osteoprogenitor cell pool leads to their accumulation in marrow spaces, resulting in local loss of hematopoietic tissue and marrow fibrosis. Osteogenic cells derived from mutated skeletal progenitors are functionally and morphologically abnormal and deposit abnormal bone. Bone trabeculae are abnormal in shape (so-called Chinese writing, alphabet soup patterns), collagen orientation, and biochemical composition,[9] and in many cases, are severely undermineralized and abnormally compliant[9,11] (Fig. 2E). The histological pattern may be significantly different at different skeletal sites, and peculiar patterns are seen in craniofacial bones.[12] The hormonal climate influences FD lesions[13] and may significantly alter the local rate of bone remodeling.[11] FD tissue is highly vascularized and therefore prone to bleeding, leading to posthemorrhagic cysts.[14] Arteriovenous shunts are formed, which may, in rare cases, lead to high-output cardiac failure in the presence of extensive skeletal involvement.

CLINICAL FEATURES

Pathological effects of $G_s\alpha$ mutations in osteogenic cells are most pronounced and evident during the phase of rapid bone growth, which translates into the most common clinical presentation during childhood or adolescence.[15] Presentation in infancy is rare and usually heralds severe, widespread disease with multiorgan involvement. Pain, fracture, and deformity are the most common presenting features. In general, children are less likely to complain of pain, per se, and may instead report stiffness or tiredness. In adults, the complaint of pain is common, especially in the ribs, long bones, and craniofacial bones. It is often severe and may require narcotic analgesics. Lesions in the spine and pelvis are usually less painful. Pathological fracture, or stress fracture of weight bearing limb bones, is a prime cause of morbidity. Deformity of limb bones is caused by expansion and abnormal compliance of lesional FD, fracture treatment failure, and local complications such as cyst formation.[1] Deformity of craniofacial bone is solely the result of the overgrowth of lesional bone.

Although any bone may be affected, the skull base and the proximal metaphysis of the femora are the two sites most commonly involved. Femoral disease usually presents in childhood with, limp, fracture, pain, and deformity, ranging from coxa vara to the classical shepherd's crook deformity (Fig. 2A). Radiographically, the lesion may be limited to the metaphysis or extend along the diaphysis for variable length.[14] The picture most commonly observed in children and adolescents consists of an expansile, deforming, medullary lesion, with cortical thinning and an overall "ground glass" density (Fig. 2A). The radiographic picture is significantly affected by the evolution of the lesion over time and by the appearance of superimposed changes, most commonly aneurysmal bone cysts. Hence, lesions observed in

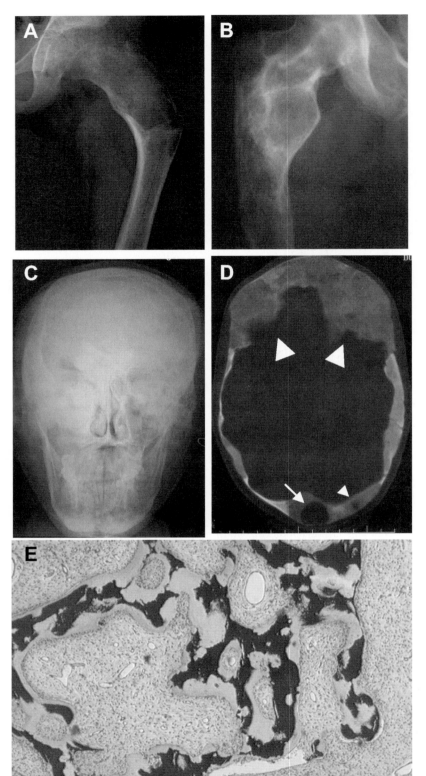

FIG. 2. Radiographic and histological appearance of FD. (A) A proximal femur with typical ground glass appearance and shepherd's crook deformity in a 10-year-old child is shown. (B) The appearance of FD in the femur of an untreated 40-year-old man show the tendency for FD to appear more sclerotic with time. (C) The typical sclerotic appearance of FD in the craniofacial region is shown. (D) A CT image show thickened frontal bone with a mixed solid and cystic appearance (large arrowheads), and lesions in the occipital bone, one with "cystic" changes (small arrowhead) that represents an area of fibrous tissue, as well as a fluid-filled cyst (arrow). (E) Representative histological image of FD. The tissue was processed for undecalcified embedding, which enables to show excess osteoid in the undermineralized fibrous dysplastic bone. The marrow spaces are filled with "fibrous" tissue, consisting of excess, abnormal marrow stromal cells.

adults tend to appear more sclerotic and less homogeneous (Fig. 2B). Sclerosis in FD lesions of the femur and other limb bones, but not in craniofacial lesions, may signify less active disease.

In the skull, FD mostly involves the skull base and facial bones. The typical presentation is in childhood with facial

asymmetry or a "bump" that persists, but symmetric expansion of malar prominences and/or frontal bosses may also be seen. The disease can progress into adulthood and disfiguration may be marked. Abnormal growth and deformity of craniofacial bones may result in encroachment on cranial nerves. Severe adverse consequences are rare,[16] but obvi-

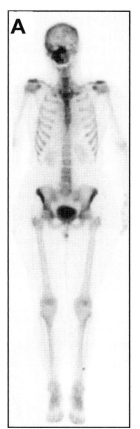
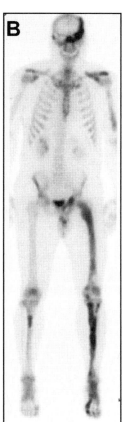
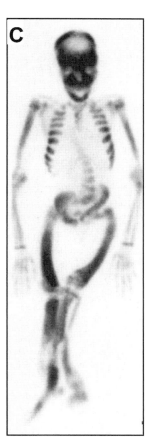

FIG. 3. Bone scintigraphy in FD. Representative ^{99}Tc-MDP bone scans that show tracer uptake at affected skeletal sites are shown. (A) A 50-year-old woman with monostotic FD confined to a single focus involving contiguous bones in the craniofacial region. (B) A 42-year-old man with polyostotic FD shows the tendency for FD to be predominantly (but not exclusively) unilateral and to involve the skull base and proximal femur. (C) A 16-year-old boy with McCune-Albright syndrome and involvement of virtually all skeletal sites (panostotic) is shown.

ously represent one of the most important concerns. FD tissue in craniofacial bones is especially prone to bleeding, herniation through cranial foramina and vascular passages, and formation of posthemorrhagic cysts (Fig. 2D). These events may precipitate blindness when they occur in the vicinities of the optic nerves. Craniofacial FD may have a "ground glass" appearance, but a sclerotic, "pagetoid" appearance is typical (Fig. 2C), and correlates with site-specific, osteosclerotic, histological changes.[12] Lesions in the spine, ribs, and pelvis are common, may be elusive on plain radiographs, and are easily detected by bone scintigraphy, the most sensitive imaging technique for the detection of FD lesions (Fig. 3). Disease in the spine is frequently associated with scoliosis, which may be progressive and require surgery.

Malignancy in FD is rare (<1%).[17] While there is an association with the development of cancer with prior treatment with high dose external beam radiation, it may occur independent of prior exposure to ionizing radiation. Rapid lesion expansion and cortical bone disruption should alert the clinician to the possibility of sarcomatous change. Osteogenic sarcoma is the most common, but not the only type of bone tumor that may complicate FD. The clinical course is usually aggressive, surgery is the primary treatment, and chemotherapeutic regimens do not seem to improve prognosis significantly.

MANAGEMENT AND TREATMENT

Diagnosis of FD must be established based on expert assessment of clinical, radiographic, and histopathological features. Markers of bone turnover are usually elevated.[3] Disease extent is best determined with total body bone scintigraphy, and potential associated metabolic derangements must be accurately screened for and specifically treated. These include not only endocrine dysfunction, but also the occurrence of renal phosphate wasting and hypophosphatemia. Some endocrine dysfunction (e.g., GH excess, Cushing's disease) may significantly affect the course of the skeletal disease.[13] Phosphate wasting impairs the mineralization of FD bone, aggravating deformity and tendency to fracture.[11]

Mutation analysis may be helpful in distinguishing FD from unrelated fibro-osseous lesions of the skeleton, which may mimic FD both clinically and radiographically (osteofibrous dysplasia, ossifying fibromas of jawbones).[1] Multiple nonossifying fibromas, skeletal angiomatosis, and Ollier's disease may sometimes enter the differential diagnosis, which again relies on histology and mutation analysis.

Disease of the proximal femur, in which there is fracture or impending fracture, is often best treated by insertion of intramedullary nails, in an effort to prevent serious deformity and limb length discrepancy.[14,18] Design of specific types of nails is felt to be necessary, and development of such devices is underway.[14] Surgery is not advocated for craniofacial disease unless hearing or vision loss are documented and prophylactic optic nerve decompression appears to be contraindicated.[16] Treatment with bisphosphonates (pamidronate) has been advocated based on observational studies,[19,20] with claims of reduced pain, decreased serum and urine markers of bone metabolism, and improvement in the radiographic appearance of the disease, but the effects of bisphosphonates on the natural history of FD remain to be determined in controlled studies.

REFERENCES

1. Bianco P, Gehron Robey P, Wientroub S 2003 Fibrous dysplasia. In: Glorieux F, Pettifor J, Juppner H (eds.) Pediatric Bone: Biology and Disease. Academic Press, Elsevier, New York, NY, USA, pp. 509–539.
2. Danon M, Crawford JD 1987 The McCune-Albright syndrome. Ergeb Inn Med Kinderheilkd 55:81–115.
3. Collins MT, Chebli C, Jones J, Kushner H, Consugar M, Rinaldo P, Wientroub S, Bianco P, Robey PG 2001 Renal phosphate wasting in fibrous dysplasia of bone is part of a generalized renal tubular dysfunction similar to that seen in tumor- induced osteomalacia. J Bone Miner Res 16:806–813.
4. Cabral CE, Guedes P, Fonseca T, Rezende JF, Cruz Junior LC, Smith J 1998 Polyostotic fibrous dysplasia associated with intramuscular myxomas: Mazabraud's syndrome. Skeletal Radiol 27:278–282.
5. Shenker A, Weinstein LS, Moran A, Pescovitz OH, Charest NJ, Boney CM, Van Wyk JJ, Merino MJ, Feuillan PP, Spiegel AM 1993 Severe endocrine and nonendocrine manifestations of the McCune-Albright syndrome associated with activating mutations of stimulatory G protein GS. J Pediatr 123:509–518.
6. Weinstein LS, Shenker A, Gejman PV, Merino MJ, Friedman E, Spiegel AM 1991 Activating mutations of the stimulatory G protein in the McCune-Albright syndrome. N Engl J Med 325:1688–1695.
7. Bianco P, Riminucci M, Majolagbe A, Kuznetsov SA, Collins MT, Mankani MH, Corsi A, Bone HG, Wientroub S, Spiegel AM, Fisher LW, Robey PG 2000 Mutations of the GNAS1 gene, stromal cell dysfunction, and osteomalacic changes in non-McCune-Albright fibrous dysplasia of bone. J Bone Miner Res 15:120–128.
8. Riminucci M, Fisher LW, Majolagbe A, Corsi A, Lala R, De Sanctis C, Robey PG, Bianco P 1999 A novel GNAS1 mutation R201G, in McCune-Albright syndrome. J Bone Miner Res 14:1987–1989.
9. Riminucci M, Fisher LW, Shenker A, Spiegel AM, Bianco P, Gehron Robey P 1997 Fibrous dysplasia of bone in the McCune-Albright syndrome: Abnormalities in bone formation. Am J Pathol 151:1587–1600.
10. Bianco P, Kuznetsov S, Riminucci M, Fisher LW, Spiegel AM, Gehron Robey P 1998 Reproduction of human fibrous dysplasia of bone in immunocompromised mice by transplanted mosaics of normal and Gs-alpha mutated skeletal progenitor cells. J Clin Invest 101:1737–1744.
11. Corsi A, Collins MT, Riminucci M, Howell PGT, Boyde A, Robey PG, Bianco P 2003 Osteomalacic and hyperparathyroid changes in fibrous dysplasia of bone:core biopsy studies and clinical correlations. J Bone Miner Res (in press).
12. Riminucci M, Liu B, Corsi A, Shenker A, Spiegel AM, Gehron Robey P, Bianco P 1999 The histopathology of fibrous dysplasia of bone in patients with activating mutations of the Gs alpha gene: Site-specific patterns and recurrent histological hallmarks. J Pathol 187:249–258.
13. Akintoye SO, Chebli C, Booher S, Feuillan P, Kushner H, Leroith D, Cherman N, Bianco P, Wientroub S, Robey PG, Collins MT 2002 Characterization of gsp-mediated growth hormone excess in the context of McCune-Albright Syndrome. J Clin Endocrinol Metab 87:5104–5112.
14. Ippolito E, Bray EW, Corsi A, De Maio F, Exner GU, Gehron Robey P, Grill F, Lala R, Massobrio M, Pinggera O, Riminucci M, Snela S, Zambakidis C, Bianco P 2003 Natural history and treatment of Fibrous dysplasia of bone: A multicenter clinico-pathologic study promoted by the European Pediatric Orthopaedic Society. J Pediatr Ortho B 12:155–177.
15. Harris WH, Dudley HR, Barry RJ 1962 The natural history of fibrous dysplasia. An orthopedic, pathological, and roentgenographic study. J Bone Joint Surg Am 44:207–233.
16. Lee JS, FitzGibbon E, Butman JA, Dufresne CR, Kushner H, Wientroub S, Robey PG, Collins MT 2002 Normal vision despite narrowing of the optic canal in fibrous dysplasia. N Engl J Med 347:1670–1676.
17. Ruggieri P, Sim FH, Bond JR, Unni KK 1994 Malignancies in fibrous dysplasia. Cancer 73:1411–1424.
18. Keijser LC, Van Tienen TG, Schreuder HW, Lemmens JA, Pruszczynski M, Veth RP 2001 Fibrous dysplasia of bone: Management and outcome of 20 cases. J Surg Oncol 76:157–168.
19. Liens D, Delmas PD, Meunier PJ 1994 Long-term effects of intravenous pamidronate in fibrous dysplasia of bone. Lancet 343:953–954.
20. Chapurlat RD, Delmas PD, Liens D, Meunier PJ 1997 Long-term effects of intravenous pamidronate in fibrous dysplasia of bone. J Bone Miner Res 12:1746–1752.

Chapter 77.   Osteogenesis Imperfecta

Michael P. Whyte

Division of Bone and Mineral Diseases, Washington University School of Medicine at Barnes-Jewish Hospital and Center for Metabolic Bone Disease and Molecular Research, Shriners Hospitals for Children, St. Louis, Missouri

INTRODUCTION

Osteogenesis imperfecta (OI), sometimes called brittle bone disease, is a heritable disorder of connective tissue involving type I collagen.[1–3] The pathogenesis of all major types (Table 1) centers on a quantitative and often also a qualitative abnormality of this most abundant protein in bone.[1–3] The clinical hallmark of OI is osteopenia causing recurrent fractures and skeletal deformity.[4] However, type I collagen is also present in teeth, sclerae, ligaments, skin, and elsewhere, and many patients with OI have dental disease because of defective formation of dentin (*dentinogenesis imperfecta*).[5] Abnormalities can occur in other tissues that contain this fibrous protein.[1–3] Severity of OI is, however, extremely variable and ranges from stillbirth to perhaps lifelong absence of symptoms. The classification system devised by Sillence,[6] according to clinical features and apparent mode of inheritance, provided a useful framework for prognostication and further biochemical/molecular studies. However, this nosology has limitations, and DNA-based findings have elucidated, especially for the severe forms, the autosomal dominant inheritance pattern.[1–3] The clinical heterogeneity of OI is now understood because a great variety of dominant/negative mutations have been characterized within the two genes that encode the two different, large, protein chains (pro α_1 and pro α_2) that combine to form the type I collagen heterotrimer.[1–3,7]

CLINICAL PRESENTATION

Among the differential diagnosis for OI in infants and children is idiopathic juvenile osteoporosis, Cushing's dis-

The author has no conflict of interest.

TABLE 1. CLINICAL HETEROGENEITY AND BIOCHEMICAL DEFECTS IN OSTEOGENESIS IMPERFECTA (OI)

OI type	Clinical features	Inheritance	Biochemical defects
I	Normal stature, little or no deformity, blue sclerae, hearing loss in about 50% of individuals. Dentinogenesis imperfecta is rare and may distinguish a subset.	AD	Decreased production of type I procollagen. Substitution for residue other than glycine in the triple-helix of the $\alpha_1(1)$
II	Lethal in the perinatal period, minimal calvarial mineralization, beaded ribs, compressed femurs, marked long bone deformity, platyspondyly.	AD (new mutation) AR (rare)	Rearrangements in the COL1A1 and COL1A2 genes Substitutions for glycyl residues in the triple-helical domain of the $\alpha_1(1)$ $\alpha_2(1)$ chain. Small deletion in $\alpha_2(1)$ on the background of a null allele.
III	Progressively deforming bones, usually with moderate deformity at birth. Sclerae variable in hue, often lighten with age. Dentinogenesis imperfecta is common, hearing loss is common. Stature very short.	AD AR	Point mutations in the $\alpha_1(1)$ or $\alpha_2(1)$ chain. Frameshift mutation that prevents incorporation of pro $\alpha_1(1)$ into molecules (noncollagenous defects).
IV	Normal sclerae, mild to moderate bone deformity, and variable short stature. Dentinogenesis imperfecta is common, and hearing loss occurs in some	AD	Point mutations in the $\alpha_2(1)$ chain. Rarely, point mutations in the $\alpha_1(1)$ chain. Small deletions in the $\alpha_2(1)$ chain.

AD, autosomal dominant; AR, autosomal recessive.

Reproduced with permission from Byers PH 2001. Disorders of collagen biosynthesis and structure. In: Scriver CR, Beaudet AL, Sly WA, Valle D, Childs B, Vogelstein B (eds.) The Metabolic and Molecular Bases of Inherited Disease, 8th ed. The McGraw Hill Companies, New York, NY, USA, pp. 5241–5285.

ease, homocystinuria, congenital indifference to pain, and child abuse. However, the disturbances in type I collagen biosynthesis that cause OI usually engender signs and symptoms that readily lead to the correct diagnosis from the patient's medical history, physical features, and radiographic findings.[4] A positive family history is especially helpful, but new mutation is not uncommon.[1] Scleral discoloration ranges from a blue or gray tint that may be startling or subtle. In severe OI, signs and symptoms also include a triangular face, high-pitched voice, short stature, scoliosis, hernias, disproportionately large head compared with body size, and chest deformity. Patients can manifest ligamentous laxity with joint hypermobility, diaphoresis, susceptibility to bruises, fragile and discolored teeth, and hearing loss (occurring in about 50% of patients younger than age 30 years and nearly all who are older).[8] Deafness typically reflects conductive or mixed pathogenesis but sometimes results from sensorineural disturbances.[8] Mitral valve clicks are not uncommon, but primary cardiac disease is unusual. Thoracic distortion predisposes to pneumonia. Patients with even the most deformed skeletons are generally of normal intelligence. Some variability in the severity of OI often occurs among affected individuals in a single family.[1–4]

CLINICAL TYPES

The classification scheme for OI devised in the late 1970s by Silence (Table 1) is based on the disorder's clinical

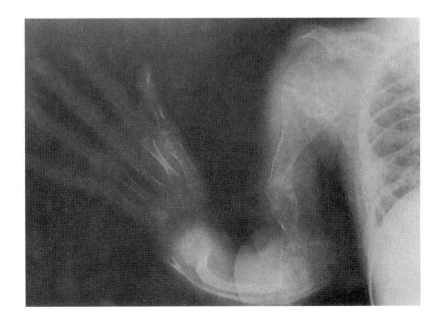

FIG. 1. Osteogenesis imperfecta. Severe changes of OI are apparent in the upper limb of this 14-year-old boy, including marked osteopenia with characteristic thinning of bony cortices, evidence of old fractures, gracile ribs, and limb deformities. (Reprinted from Metabolic Bone and Mineral Disorders, Manolagas SC, Olefsky JM, Hereditary disorders of bone and mineral metabolism, 1988 with permission from Elsevier.)

© 2003 American Society for Bone and Mineral Research

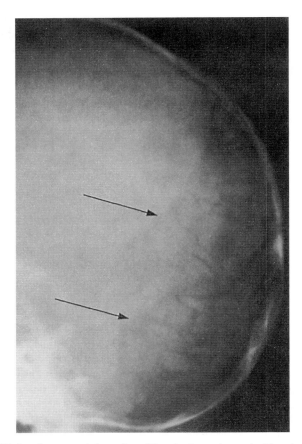

FIG. 2. Osteogenesis imperfecta. Wormian bones (arrows), although not pathognomonic for OI, may be found near the lambdoidal suture of the posterior occiput. (Reproduced with permission from Whyte MP 1995 Rare disorders of skeletal formation and homeostasis. In: Becker KN, ed. Principles and Practice of Endocrinology and Metabolism, 2nd ed. Lippincott-Raven Publishers, Philadelphia, PA, USA.)

manifestations and apparent mode of inheritance.[6] This nosology remains useful, but has been greatly clarified, especially for the more severe types of OI, by revelation of the defects involving type I collagen and their autosomal dominant mode of inheritance.[1–3] Recently, additional clinical types of OI have been proposed,[9] but do not seem to fundamentally involve type I collagen.[2]

Type I OI features sclerae with bluish discoloration (especially apparent during childhood), relatively mild osteopenia with infrequent fractures (deformity is uncommon or slight), and deafness (30% incidence) that first manifests during early adulthood. Typically, patient height is normal. Elderly women with this most mild form of OI can be mistaken as having postmenopausal osteoporosis if they present with fracture during middle age, because radiographic findings may not distinguish between the two disorders. However, more numerous cortical osteocytes may be detected by iliac crest biopsy.[10–12] Type I OI has been subclassified into I-A and I-B disease depending on the absence or (more rarely) the presence, respectively, of dentinogenesis imperfecta. Approximately one-third of cases are new mutations.

Type II OI is usually fatal within the first few weeks or months of life from respiratory complications. Affected newborns are often premature and small for gestational age and have short, bowed limbs, numerous fractures, markedly soft skulls, and small thoraces.

Type III OI features progressive skeletal deformity during childhood from recurrent fractures. Short stature results, in part, from fragmentation of growth plates.[6] Dentinogenesis imperfecta[5] is common.

Type IV OI frequently explains multigeneration disease.[1–3] The sclerae have normal color, but skeletal deformity, dental disease, and hearing loss are usual features.

RADIOGRAPHIC FEATURES

Characteristic findings manifest in severely affected patients.[13] The cardinal features are generalized osteopenia, deformity from recurrent fractures, and modeling (shaping) defects of long bones. The modeling defects are caused by diminished rates of periosteal bone formation that retard circumferential widening of bones. Hence, cortices appear thin and long bones are "gracile." In some severely affected infants, micromelia occurs with major long bones that are short but appear "thick" in external diameter. Multiple and recurrent fractures deform vertebrae as well as long bones (Fig. 1). Wormian bones (Fig. 2) of significant number and size in the skull are a common, but not pathognomonic, feature of OI.[14] Platybasia, which can progress to basilar impression, and excessive pneumatization of the frontal and mastoid sinuses are common in severely affected patients.[14] The pelvis can have a triradiate-shaped appearance. Osteoarthritic changes are common in ambulatory adults with skeletal deformity.

Radiographic abnormalities may worsen markedly during growth—a feature that helps to define progressively deforming (type III) OI. "Popcorn" calcifications are unusual, acquired defects in epiphyses and metaphyses of major long bones (predominantly at the ankles and knees) mainly occurring in type III OI.[15] The finding is believed to result from traumatic fragmentation of growth plate cartilage. The complication severely limits long bone growth and contributes importantly to short stature. It is noted during childhood, but then "resolves" during puberty when endochondral cartilage becomes fully mineralized and replaced by bone. When fractures occur in OI, they are often transverse but heal at normal rates. Occasionally, exuberant callus forms that has been mistaken for skeletal malignancy.

LABORATORY FINDINGS

Routine biochemical parameters of bone and mineral metabolism are typically unremarkable; however, elevations in serum alkaline phosphatase activity, urinary levels of hydroxyproline, or other markers of bone turnover occur in a significant number of patients.[16] Hypercalciuria is common especially in severely affected children, but their renal function is not compromised.[17]

Bone histology reflects the abnormal skeletal matrix, especially in severely affected patients. Polarized-light microscopy often shows an abundance of disorganized (woven) bone or abnormally thin collagen bundles in lamellar osseous tissue.[12] Numerous osteocytes are found in the cortical bone of some patients. This finding seems to reflect decreased amounts of bone produced by individual osteoblasts, yet many cells that are active simultaneously. Subsequently, the overall rate of skeletal turnover can be rapid, as shown by in vivo tetracycline labeling[18] and biochemical markers.[16]

ETIOLOGY AND PATHOGENESIS

Table 1 summarizes the types of molecular/biochemical defects that have been identified in the various clinical forms of OI.[1–3] A hallmark is low levels of type I collagen synthesized in vitro by skin fibroblasts.[1–3] Many specific types of mutation have occurred within the pro-α_1 and pro-α_2 type I collagen genes in patients worldwide.[1–3] The large and complex nature of type I collagen is such that nearly all OI families have unique ("private") mutations in one of these genes. Detailed information appears elsewhere.[1–3,7]

TREATMENT

Promising results are increasingly reported for bisphosphonate treatment in children with OI,[16,19] but the early published trials have not yet been blinded or placebo-controlled, and therapy endpoints remain unclear with drug-induced osteopetrosis a possibility.[20] The response by adults is especially uncertain. Preliminary reports concerning growth hormone injections mention improved linear growth rates and positive changes in bone formation in some affected children.[21] Mouse models for OI provide a new way to test potential therapies.[22,23] Patient treatment requires expert orthopedic, rehabilitative, and dental intervention to care for recurrent fractures, limb deformities, kyphoscoliosis, dental sequelae, etc. Rodding of long bones and bracing of the lower limbs has enabled some affected children to walk. Stapes surgery has been used for hearing loss.[24] The current management of OI has been reviewed.[25]

National support groups (e.g., Osteogenesis Imperfecta Foundation, Inc., USA) are important sources of comfort and lay-language information for patients and their families (www.oif.org).

Genetic counseling should be periodically updated when appropriate, because progress in this area has been considerable. Although rare patients with type II or III OI represent homozygosity for an autosomal recessive trait not understood molecularly, most cases reflect new dominant mutations or germline mosaicism for type I collagen gene defects. Hence, the recurrence risk of this most severe OI phenotype is now estimated to be 5–10%.[1–7] Some mildly affected individuals are mosaics for type I collagen defects and have more severely affected children.[1]

Prenatal diagnosis of severe OI by a variety of techniques, particularly ultrasound examination at 14–18 weeks gestation, has been helpful.[26] Biochemical and genetic studies are proving increasingly successful.[27]

REFERENCES

1. Byers PH 2001 Disorders of collagen biosynthesis and structure. In: Scriver CR, Beaudet AL, Sly WS, Valle D, Childs B, Vogelstein B (eds.) The Metabolic and Molecular Bases of Inherited Disease, 8th ed. McGraw-Hill, New York, NY, USA, pp. 5241–5285.
2. Byers PH, Cole WG 2002 Osteogeneis imperfecta. In: Royce PM, Steinmann B (eds.) Connective Tissue and Its Heritable Disorders. Wiley-Liss Inc., New York, NY, USA, pp. 385–430.
3. Rowe DW, Shapiro JR 1998 Osteogenesis imperfecta. In: Avioli LV, Krane SM (eds.) Metabolic Bone Disease, 2nd ed. Academic Press, San Diego, CA, USA, pp. 651–695.
4. Albright JA, Millar EA 1981 Osteogenesis imperfecta (symposium). Clin Orthop 159:1–156.
5. Krebsbach P, Polverini P 2003 Dental manifestations of disorders of bone and mineral metabolism. In: Favus M (ed.) Primer on the Metabolic Bone Diseases and Disorders of Mineral Metabolism, 5th ed. American Society of Bone and Mineral Research, Washington, DC, USA, pp. 532–536.
6. Silence D 1981 Osteogenesis imperfecta: An expanding panorama of variants. Clin Orthop 159:11–25.
7. Byers PH, Wallis GA, Willing MC 1991 Osteogenesis imperfecta: Translation of mutation to phenotype. Med Genet 28:433–442.
8. Pedersen U 1984 Hearing loss in patients with osteogenesis imperfecta. Scand Audiol Suppl 13:67–74.
9. Glorieux FH, Rauch F, Plotkin H, Ward L, Travers R 2000 Type V osteogenesis imperfecta: A new form of brittle bone disease. J Bone Miner Res 15:1650–1658.
10. Revell PA 1986 Pathology of Bone. Springer-Verlag, Berlin, Germany.
11. Falvo KA, Bullough PG 1973 Osteogenesis imperfecta: A histometric analysis. J Bone Joint Surg Am 55:275–286.
12. Rauch F, Travers R, Parfitt AM, Glorieux FH 2000 Static and dynamic bone histomorphometry in children with osteogenesis imperfecta. Bone 26:581–589.
13. Resnick D, Niwayama G 2002 Diagnosis of Bone and Joint Disorders, 4th ed. WB Saunders, Philadelphia, PA, USA.
14. Cremin B, Goodman H, Prax M, Spranger J, Beighton P 1982 Wormian bones in osteogenesis imperfecta and other disorders. Skeletal Radiol 8:35–38.
15. Goldman AB, Davidson D, Pavlor H, Bullough PG 1980 "Popcorn" calcifications: A prognostic sign in osteogenesis imperfecta. Radiology 136:351–358.
16. Rauch F, Plotkin H, Travers R, Zeitlin L, Glorieux FH 2003 Osteogenesis imperfecta types I, III, and IV: Effect of pamidronate therapy on bone and mineral metabolism. J Clin Endocrinol Metab 88:986–992.
17. Chines A, Boniface A, McAlister W, Whyte M 1995 Hypercalciuria in osteogenesis imperfecta: A follow-up study to assess renal effects. Bone 16:333–339.
18. Baron R, Gertner JM, Lang R, Vighery A 1983 Increased bone turnover with decreased bone formation by osteoblasts in children with osteogenesis imperfecta tarda. Pediatr Res 17:204–207.
19. Glorieux FH, Bishop NJ, Plotkin H, Chabot G, Lanoue G, Travers R 1998 Cyclic administration of pamidronate in children with severe osteogenesis imperfecta. N Engl J Med 339:947–942.
20. Whyte MP, Wenkert D, Clements KL, McAlister WH, Mumm S 2003 Bisphosphonate-induced osteopetrosis. N Engl J Med 349:455–461.
21. Marini JC, Hopkins E, Glorieux FH, Chrousos GP, Reynolds JC, Gundberg CM, Reing CM 2003 Positive linear growth and bone responses to growth hormone treatment in children with types III and IV osteogenesis imperfecta: High predictive value of the carboxyterminal propeptide of type I procollagen. J Bone Miner Res 18:237–243.
22. McBride DJ Jr, Choe V, Shapiro JR, Brodsky B 1997 Altered collagen structure in mouse tail tendon lacking the alpha 2(I) chain. J Mol Biol 170:275–284.
23. Pereira RF, Hume EL, Halford KW, Prockop DJ 1995 Bone fragility in transgenic mice expressing a mutated gene for type I procollagen (COL1A1) parallels the age-dependent phenotype of human osteogenesis imperfecta. J Bone Miner Res 10:1837–1843.
24. Garretsen TJ, Cremers CW 1991 Stapes surgery in osteogenesis imperfecta: Analysis of postoperative hearing loss. Ann Otol Rhinol Laryngol 100:120–130.
25. Binder H, Conway A, Hason S, Gerber LH, Marini J, Weintrob J 1993 Comprehensive rehabilitation of the child with osteogenesis imperfecta. Am J Med Genet 45:265–269.
26. Thompson EM 1993 Non-invasive prenatal diagnosis of osteogenesis imperfecta. Am J Med Genet 45:201–206.
27. Pepin M, Atkinson M, Starman BJ, Byers PH 1997 Strategies and outcomes of prenatal diagnosis for osteogenesis imperfecta: A review of biochemical and molecular studies completed in 129 pregnancies. Prenat Diagn 17:559–570.

Chapter 78. Chondrodystrophies and Mucopolysaccharidoses

Michael P. Whyte

Division of Bone and Mineral Diseases, Washington University School of Medicine at Barnes-Jewish Hospital and Center for Metabolic Bone Disease and Molecular Research, Shriners Hospitals for Children, St. Louis, Missouri

INTRODUCTION

Beginning in the 1960s, concerted efforts to classify the skeletal dysplasias led to recognition of more than 80 such entities.[1] Most seemed to be heritable; however, the nosology at that time was essentially descriptive because the biochemical bases were unknown for nearly all of these disorders, and the molecular/genetic defects were unapproachable. Hence, the early nomenclature is based on the parts of the skeleton that are most involved on radiographic study.[1-4]

Now, as reviewed below, gene mapping, positional cloning, and candidate gene approaches subsequently disclosed the molecular basis of many of these conditions and importantly altered their classification by revealing that many are "allelic" problems involving relatively few genes.[5] Additionally, these recent advances have greatly increased the spectrum of disorders that can now be considered "metabolic bone diseases" (Table 1).[5]

OSTEOCHONDRODYSPLASIAS

The term *osteochondrodysplasia* encompasses a large group of seemingly distinctive entities among the skeletal dysplasias.[6-8] Each is characterized by abnormal growth

The author has no conflict of interest.

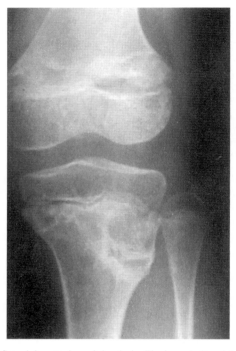

FIG. 2. Spondylometaphyseal dysplasia. The irregularity of the metaphyses in the knees of this 9-year-old girl are sometimes mistaken for rickets.

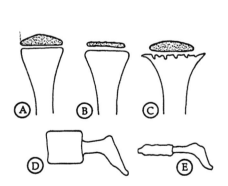

Involvement	Disease Category
A+D	Normal
B+D	Epiphyseal dysplasia
C+D	Metaphyseal dysplasia
B+E	Spondyloepiphyseal dysplasia
C+E	Spondylometaphyseal dysplasia
B+C+E	Spondyloepimetaphyseal dysplasia

FIG. 1. Chondrodysplasias. Classification based on radiographic involvement of long bones and vertebrae.[1] (Reprinted from Emery and Rimoin's Principles and Practice of Medical Genetics, Rimoin DL, Lachman RS, Chondrodysplasias, p. 2796, 1996 with permission from Elsevier.)

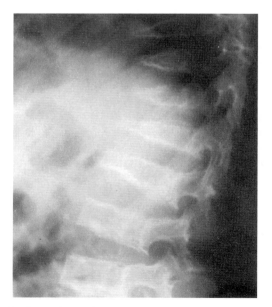

FIG. 3. Spondylometaphyseal dysplasia. Characteristic dysplastic changes at 11 years of age are present in the vertebrae of the patient shown in Fig. 2 and establish a spondylometaphyseal rather than a metaphyseal dysplasia.

TABLE 1. GENE DEFECTS IN OSTEOCHONDRODYSPLASIAS

Disorder	Gene	Protein
1. Achondroplasia group		
Thanatophoric dysplasia, Type I	FGFR3	Fibroblast growth factor
Thanatophoric dysplasia, Type II	"	receptor 3
Achondroplasia	"	"
Hypochondroplasia	"	"
2. Diastrophic dysplasia group		
Diastrophic dysplasia	DTDST	Sulfate transporter
Achondrogenesis I B	"	"
Atelosteogenesis, Type II	"	"
3. Type II collagenopathies		
Achondrogenesis II (Langer-Saldino)	COL2A1	Type II collagen
Hypochondrogenesis	"	"
Kniest dysplasia	"	"
Spondyloepiphyseal dysplasia (SED) congenita	"	"
Spondyloepimetaphyseal dysplasia (SEMD) Strudwick type	"	"
SED with brachydactyly	"	"
Mild SED with premature onset arthrosis	"	"
Stickler dysplasia (heterogeneous, some not linked to COL2A1)	"	"
4. Type XI collagenopathies		
Stickler dysplasia (heterogeneous)	COL11A1	Type XI collagen
Otospondylomegaepiphyseal dysplasia (OSMED)	COL11A2	"
5. Multiple epiphyseal displasias and pseudoachondroplasia		
Pseudoachondroplasia	COMP	Cartilage oligomeric-matrix protein
Multiple epiphyseal dysplasia (MED) (Fairbanks and Ribbing types)	"	"
Other MEDs	COL9A2	Type IX collagen
6. Chondrodysplasia punctata (stippled epiphyses group)		
Rhizomelic type	PEX7	Peroxin-7
Zellweger syndrome	PEX	Peroxin 1,2,5,6
Conradi-Hünermann type	CPXD	
X-linked recessive type	CPXR	
Brachytelephalangic type	ARSE	Arylsulfatase E
7. Metaphyseal dysplasias		
Jansen type	PTHR	PTHR/PTHRP
Schmid type	COL10A1	COL10 α chain
8. Acromelic and acromesomelic dysplasias		
Trichorhinophalangeal dysplasia, type I	TRPS1	
" " , type II (Langer-Giedion)	TRPS1 + EXT1	
Grebe dysplasia	CDMP1	Cartilage-derived morphogenic protein 1
Hunter-Thompson dysplasia	"	"
Brachydactyly type C	"	"
Pseudohypoparathyroidism (Albright Hereditary Osteodystrophy)	GNAS1	Guanine nucleotide binding protein of adenylate cyclase α-subunit
9. Dysplasias with prominant membranous bone involvement		
Cleidocranial dysplasia	CBFA1	Core binding factor α1-subunit
10. Bent-bone dysplasia group		
Campomelic dysplasia	SOX9	SRY-box 9
11. Multiple dislocations with dysplasias		
Larsen syndrome	LAR1	
12. Dysostosis multiplex group		
Mucopolysaccharidosis IH	IDA	α-1-Iduronidase
" IS	"	"
" II	IDS	Iduronidate-2-sulfatase
" IIIA	HSS	Heparan sulfate sulfatase
" IIID	GNS	N-Ac-glucosamine-6-sulfatase
" IVA	GSLNS	Galactose-6-sulfatase
" IVB	GLBI	β-Galactosidase
" VI	ARSB	Arysulfatase B
" VII	GUSB	β-Glucuronidase

Table 1. (Continued)

Disorder	Gene	Protein
Fucosidosis	FUCA	α-Fucosidase
α-Mannosidosis	MAN	α-Mannosidase
β-Mannosidosis	MANB	β-Mannosidase
Aspartyglucosaminuuuria	AgA	Aspartyglucosaminidase
GMI Gangliosidosis, several forms	GLB1	β-Galactosidase
Sialidosis, several forms	NEU	α-Neuraminidase
Sialic acid storage disease	SIASD	
Galactosialidisos, several forms	PPGB	β-Galactosidase protective protein
Multiple sulfatase deficiency		Multiple sulfatases
Mucolipidosis II, III	GNPTA	N-Ac-Glucosamine-phosphotransferase
13. Dysplasias with decreased bone density		
Osteogenesis imperfecta	COL1A1 & A2	Type I procollagen
14. Dysplasias with defective mineralization		
Hypophosphatasia	TNSALP (ALPL)	Alkaline phosphatase
Hypophosphatemic rickets	PHEX	X-linked hypophosphatemia protein
Neonatal hyperparathyroidism	CASR	Calcium sensor
Transient neonatal hyperparathyroidism with hypocalciuric hypercalcemia	"	"
15. Increased bone density without modification of bone shape		
Osteopetrosis with renal tubular acidosis	CA2	Carbonic anhydrase II
Pyknodysostosis	CTSK	Cathespin K
16. Disorganized development of cartilaginous and fibrous components of the skeleton		
Multiple cartilaginous exostoses	EXT1	Exostosin-1
Fibrous dysplasia (McCune-Albright and others)	GNAS1	Guanine nucleotide protein, α-subunit
17. Patella dysplasias		
Nail patella dysplasia	NPS1	

Modified with permission from Springer-Verlag Pediatr Radiol 1998;**28**:737–744.

or development of bone and/or cartilage (see refs. 1, 6, 7, and 8 for a review of the clinical nomenclature). Osteochondrodysplasias are, in turn, subdivided into several groups, some of which feature defects in the growth of tubular bones and/or the spine. These disorders are frequently referred to as chondrodysplasias.[1] The anatomic region of the long bones that is most affected (epiphyses, metaphyses, or diaphyses) is the basis for the subclassification into epiphyseal, metaphyseal, or diaphyseal dysplasia.[1–3] When the vertebrae too are deformed, these conditions are grouped as spondyloepiphyseal dysplasia, and so on (Fig. 1).

Chondrodysplasias that feature primarily metaphyseal defects (metaphyseal dysplasia and spondylometaphyseal dysplasia) may be confused, from their clinical and radiographic appearance, with forms of rickets (Fig. 2). However, biochemical parameters of bone and mineral metabolism are typically normal, and the skeleton is generally well mineralized. [Jansen syndrome, caused by activating mutations in the parathyroid hormone (PTH)/PTH-related peptide (PTHrP) receptor and leading to hypercalcemia, is an interesting exception.[5]] Indeed, the configuration of the metaphyseal defects has led to a useful subclassification scheme devised by experienced radiologists. When abnormalities of the spine are present (Fig. 3), diagnosis of dysplasia and not rickets should be especially evident.

DNA-based technology has mapped and characterized many of the genes and the mutations that cause skeletal dysplasias (Table 1). Our understanding of the molecular/ biochemical bases of these disorders is growing rapidly.[1,5,7,9] Defects in a variety of genes reveal that many proteins are essential for human skeletal development. Abnormalities in type I, II, IX, and X collagen genes cause osteogenesis imperfecta, spondyloepiphyseal dysplasia, multiple epiphyseal dysplasia, and metaphyseal dysplasia (Schmid type), respectively.[1,5,7,8] Cartilage-oligomeric-matrix-protein gene mutations can engender multiple epiphyseal dysplasia and pseudoachondroplasia. Fibroblast growth factor (FGF) receptor-3 gene defects cause achondroplasia.[5,7] The elastin and fibrillin genes are involved in Williams and Marfan syndromes, respectively.[5] Remarkably, however, the majority of skeletal dysplasias are "allelic" disorders involving relatively few genes, but especially those encoding type II collagen and the FGF receptor-3.[8] Nevertheless, the number of "metabolic bone diseases" will continue to grow.

MUCOPOLYSACCHARIDOSES

Mucopolysaccharidoses are inborn errors of metabolism caused by diminished activity of the lysosomal enzymes that degrade glycosaminoglycans (acid mucopolysaccharides) (Table 1).[10,11] Accumulation of these complex carbohydrates within marrow cells leads to skeletal alterations that are generally referred to by radiologists as *dysostosis multiplex*. However, the degree of severity and precise bony manifestations vary according to the specific disorder.[1–5] (See refs. 3 and 4 for detailed radiographic descriptions.)

Patients with dysostosis multiplex share the following radiographic features: osteoporosis with coarsened trabeculae, macrocephaly, dyscephaly, a J-shaped sella turcica, oar-shaped ribs, widened clavicles, oval or hook-shaped vertebral bodies, dysplasia of the capital femoral epiphyses, coxa valga, epiphyseal and metaphyseal dysplasia, proximal tapering of the second and fifth metacarpals, and dysplasia of long tubular bones.[3,4]

REFERENCES

1. Rimoin DL, Lachman RS, Unger S 2002 Chondrodysplasias. In: Rimoin DL, Connor JM, Pyeritz RE (eds.) Emery and Rimoin's Principles and Practice of Medical Genetics, 4th ed. Churchill Livingstone, London, UK, pp. 4071–4115.
2. Wynne-Davies R, Hall CM, Apley AG 1985 Atlas of Skeletal Dysplasias. Churchill Livingstone, Edinburgh, UK.
3. Resnick D, Niwayama G 2002 Diagnosis of Bone and Joint Disorders, 4th ed. WB Saunders, Philadelphia, PA, USA.
4. Taybi H, Lachman RS 1996 Radiology of Syndromes, Metabolic Disorders, and Skeletal Dysplasias, 4th ed. Mosby, St. Louis, USA.
5. McKusick VA 1998 Mendelian Inheritance In Man: A Catalog of Human Genes and Genetic Disorders, 12th ed. Johns Hopkins University Press, Baltimore, MD, USA.
6. Lachman RS 1998 International nomenclature and classification of the osteochondrodysplasias. Pediatr Radiol 28:737–744.
7. Rimoin DL, Lachman RS 1993 Genetic disorders of the osseous skeleton. In: McKusick's Heritable Disorders of Connective Tissue, 5th ed. pp. 557–689.
8. Horton WA, Hecht JT 2001 Chondrodysplasias: Disorders of cartilage matrix proteins. In: Royce PM, Steinmann B (eds.) Connective Tissue and Its Heritable Disorders, 2nd ed. Wiley-Liss, Inc., New York, NY, USA, pp. 909–937.
9. Horton WA 1995 Molecular genetics of the human chondrodysplasias-1995. Eur J Hum Genet 3:357–373.
10. Leroy JG, Wiesmann U 2001 Disorders of lysosomal enzymes. In: Royce PM, Steinmann B (eds.) Connective Tissue and Its Heritable Disorders. Wiley-Liss, Inc., New York, NY, USA, pp. 8494–899.
11. Neufeld EF, Muenzer J 2001 The mucopolysaccharidoses. In: Scriver CR, Beaudet AL, Sly WS, Valle D, Childs B, Vogelstein B (eds.) The Metabolic and Molecular Bases of Inherited Disease, 8th ed. McGraw-Hill, New York, NY, USA, pp. 3421–3452.

SECTION IX

Acquired Disorders of Cartilage and Bone

Introduction

Michael P. Whyte

Division of Bone and Mineral Diseases, Washington University School of Medicine at Barnes-Jewish Hospital and Center for Metabolic Bone Disease and Molecular Research, Shriners Hospitals for Children, St. Louis, Missouri

Physicians who care for patients with metabolic bone diseases encounter a considerable number and variety of acquired skeletal disorders. Among these conditions are neoplasms of cartilage and bone, problems that result from disruption of the vascular supply to the skeleton, and diseases that are characterized by proliferation or infiltration of the marrow space by specific types of cells. In certain "metabolic" bone diseases and some skeletal dysplasias, there is predisposition to neoplastic transformation (e.g., Paget's bone disease, fibrous dysplasia), metabolic disturbances can cause skeletal ischemia (e.g., Cushing syndrome, storage diseases), and infiltrative marrow disorders may be associated with aberrant mineral homeostasis (e.g., sarcoidosis). This section provides an overview of some of the principal acquired disorders of cartilage and bone.

Chapter 79.   Skeletal Neoplasms

Michael P. Whyte

Division of Bone and Mineral Diseases, Washington University School of Medicine at Barnes-Jewish Hospital and Center for Metabolic Bone Disease and Molecular Research, Shriners Hospitals for Children, St. Louis, Missouri

GENERAL CONSIDERATIONS

Among the acquired disorders of cartilage and bone are a variety of neoplasms. Some are malignant and cause considerable morbidity and can metastasize and kill. Others are benign and may even heal spontaneously. Rarely, skeletal tumors behave as though "transitional," with both malignant and benign features. Diagnosis and treatment of bone tumors is a complex and specialized discipline. Only a brief overview is provided here. Additional resources include several comprehensive texts devoted to this topic.[1–7]

Classification of skeletal neoplasms begins with the apparent cell or tissue type of origin (Table 1). The source of the tumor is usually revealed by the kind of tissue that the neoplastic cells make, such as osteoid or cartilage. However, in a few instances (e.g., giant cell tumor of bone), the origin is less clear.[1,6]

Biological behavior of bone tumors importantly influences their classification. Within the two major categories, benign and malignant, there are different degrees of aggressiveness. Biological behavior reflects the capacity of the tumor to exceed its natural barriers. Such barriers may include a tumor capsule (the shell of fibrous tissue or bone around the neoplasm), a reactive zone (composed in part of fibrous tissue or bone that forms between the capsule and

TABLE 1. COMMON SKELETAL NEOPLASMS*

Tissue origin	Benign	Malignant
Osseous		Classic osteosarcoma
		Parosteal osteosarcoma
		Periosteal osteosarcoma
Cartilaginous	Enchondroma	Primary chondrosarcoma
	Exostosis	Secondary chondrosarcoma
Fibrous	Nonossifying fibroma	Fibrosarcoma
		Malignant fibrous histiocytoma
Reticuloendothelial		Ewing's sarcoma
		Multiple myeloma
Unknown	Giant cell tumor in bone	

*See references 1–5 for general reviews.

The author has no conflict of interest.

479

normal tissue), and any adjacent articular cartilage, cortical bone, or periosteum.[1,6,7]

Skeletal neoplasms will be properly managed only when there is a thorough understanding of their clinical presentation and natural history, as well as use of current staging procedures. This often requires histopathological examination.[1,6,8] Proper choice of therapy may include medical and/or surgical approaches.[1–3,5,7,9,10] Optimum patient management can depend on multidisciplinary expertise.[1–7] Improved radiological imaging, histopathological methods, cytogenetic and molecular testing, surgical techniques, and chemotherapeutic regimens have all contributed to better survival and function of patients with skeletal sarcomas. Chemotherapy has improved the treatment of early metastatic deposits.[11–14] Consequently, aggressive limb-salvaging procedures are now possible with survival rates that were previously achieved only by radical amputation.[12,15–18]

BENIGN BONE TUMORS

Benign skeletal tumors, with only rare exceptions, do not metastasize.[19] Nevertheless, as a group, their biological behavior can still be variable and may range from completely inactive to quite aggressive. Fortunately, their behavior can often be predicted by noting the clinical presentation and examining the radiological features of the specific neoplasm[4,20,21]; sometimes, histopathological inspection is also essential.[1,6] Benign tumors can be classified generally as "inactive," "active," or "aggressive."[1,6,19]

Inactive benign bone tumors are sometimes called "latent" or "static." They are encapsulated by mature fibrous tissue or by cortical bone-like material, and do not expand or deform surrounding skeletal tissue. Individual neoplasms will have only a minimal (if any) reactive zone, and their histopathological appearance is that of a benign tumor with a low cell-to-matrix ratio, a well-differentiated matrix, and no cellular hyperchromasia, anaplasia, or pleomorphism. Inactive benign tumors are usually asymptomatic.[1,6,19]

Active benign bone tumors can deform or destroy adjacent cortical bone or joint cartilage as they grow, but they do not metastasize. They are encapsulated within fibrous tissue, although a thin reactive zone can develop. These neoplasms generally cause mild symptoms, but may lead to pathological fractures.[1,6,19]

Aggressive benign bone tumors are not uncommon in children. They show invasive properties resembling low-grade malignancies. The reactive zone forms a capsule or pseudocapsule that prevents the neoplasm itself from extending directly into normal tissue, but the tumor can resorb and destroy adjacent bone and spread to nearby skeletal compartments. Despite their aggressive behavior, the cytological features are benign—including a well-differentiated matrix. These neoplasms cause symptoms and can engender pathological fractures.[1,6,19]

MALIGNANT BONE TUMORS

Malignant skeletal tumors may metastasize. Nevertheless, as a group, their biological behavior also varies considerably.[1–3,5,7] Some grow slowly with a low probability of spreading elsewhere, so that there is typically a long interval between the discovery of the primary neoplasm and the development and recognition of metastases. Others are very aggressive and not only cause rapid and extensive local tissue destruction, but also have a high incidence of metastases so that primary and metastatic lesions are frequently recognized simultaneously. The biological behavior of malignant skeletal tumors can usually be predicted by their clinical, radiological,[4,20,21] and histopathological features.[1,5,6] Assessment of the histopathological type and grade is the best predictor of biological activity and is of paramount importance for successful treatment and accurate prognostication.[1,5,6]

Low-grade sarcomas invade local tissues, but grow slowly and have a low risk of metastasizing. They are usually asymptomatic and manifest as gradually growing masses. Nevertheless, the histopathological features of malignancy are present, such as anaplasia, pleomorphism, and hyperchromasia, together with a few mitotic cells. The tumor capsule can be disrupted in many areas, and there may be an extensive reactive zone that forms a pseudocapsule and contains satellite tumor nodules that slowly erode the various natural barriers. Over time, and after repeatedly unsuccessful surgical excision with tumor recurrences, there is a risk of transformation to a high-grade sarcoma.[1,5,6]

High-grade sarcomas readily extend beyond their reactive zone. They seem to have minimal pseudoencapsulation. Their margins are poorly demarcated. Metastases may appear in seemingly uninvolved areas of the same bone and often in the medullary canal. Extension to nearby tissues destroys cortical bone, articular cartilage, and joint capsules. These tumors show all of the histopathological features that typify malignancy and produce a poorly differentiated (immature) matrix.[1,5,6]

DIAGNOSIS OF BONE TUMORS

A thorough medical history and complete physical examination are the foundation for successful delineation and management of skeletal neoplasms.[22] The patient's age, presence or absence of predisposing conditions (e.g., Paget's bone disease), and anatomical site of the lesion provide important clues to the precise diagnosis.

Radiological studies should be selected both to help establish the tumor type and to provide staging information that will be critical for choosing treatment and for understanding the patient's prognosis.[4,23,24] The tumor "stage" reflects the neoplasm's location and extent, as well as its biological activity or grade, and is based in part on the presence or absence of metastases.[8] Radiographs establish the tumor location, often suggest the underlying histopathological type,[4,20,21] help assess its extent, and guide the selection of additional staging studies. Clinical and radiological examination is completed before biopsy or other surgical procedures.[1,3,7,8,22]

Bone scanning helps to determine if multiple areas of neoplasm are present and if the extent of skeletal involvement exceeds conventional radiographic findings. Avidity for radionuclide uptake generally reflects the tumor's biological activity.[20,21,23,24]

Computed tomography (CT) is especially useful for precisely defining the anatomical extent of the primary lesion, detecting destruction of spongy or cortical bone, assessing compartmental changes, and locating neurovascular structures that may be impinged on by tumor or located near planned surgery.[25] This technique also supplements conventional radiography for detecting pulmonary metastases.

Magnetic resonance imaging (MRI) is particularly helpful for defining tumor soft-tissue extension and for showing any disruption of the marrow space.[24,26,27] Positron emission tomography (PET) is also proving useful.[28]

Angiography can help plan limb-salvage operations, because this procedure may reveal involvement of major neurovascular bundles.[4]

Arthrography assists in showing joint involvement and is therefore useful for assessing whether a cartilaginous tumor is of intra-articular or extra-articular origin.[4]

Biopsy and histopathological study are essential for successful staging and treatment of many skeletal neoplasms.[1,2,29] Open (incisional) biopsy has been the technique of choice if a malignant lesion is suspected, because it secures sufficient tissue for examination.[1,2,29] However, this procedure carries a greater risk of tumor contamination of uninvolved tissues (e.g., by dissecting hematoma) than closed biopsy.[30] Accordingly, open biopsy can potentially compromise a limb-salvage because of added risk of local recurrence. Hence, careful attention must be paid to where the incision for biopsy is made and to the surgical technique.[1–3] Increasingly, fine-needle aspiration biopsy is used.[31] Accessible benign tumors may be removed by incisional biopsy if they are intracapsular or with en bloc marginal incision.[1–3]

INDIVIDUAL TYPES OF SKELETAL NEOPLASIA

Benign and Transitional Bone Tumors

Benign skeletal neoplasms occasionally originate from marrow elements, but most often they arise from cartilage or bone.[32] Typically, these tumors develop before skeletal maturation is complete or during the early adult years, and they are most common in areas of rapid bone growth and cellular metabolism (i.e., epiphyses and metaphyses of major long bones).[33] In some patients or families with specific heritable disorders, benign skeletal tumors (e.g., enchondromas or exostoses) are multiple and have a significantly increased risk of malignant transformation.[34,35] Most benign skeletal tumors, however, are solitary lesions and have a good prognosis.[32] The following paragraphs describe the principal types.

Nonossifying fibroma is the most common bone tumor.[36,37] This lesion is often called a "fibrous cortical defect." It represents a focal, developmental abnormality in periosteal bone formation that results in an area of failed ossification. Nonossifying fibromas most commonly occur in the metaphyses of the distal femur or distal tibia and are located eccentrically in or near the bony cortex.[4,20,21] They are somewhat more prevalent in boys than in girls, develop in the older pediatric population, and are active lesions that enlarge throughout childhood yet typically do not cause symptoms. However, when most of the diameter of a long bone is involved, pathological fracture can occur.[36,37] Ra-

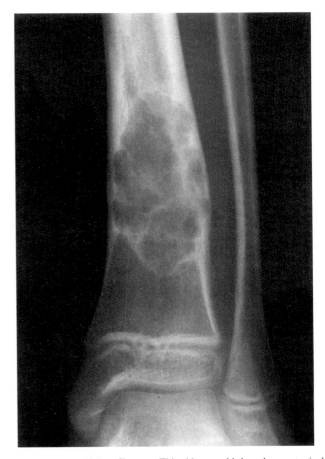

FIG. 1. Nonossifying fibroma. This 11-year-old boy has a typical, benign-appearing lesion of his distal left tibia. It is an ovoid, radiolucent, fibrous tumor located at the metadiaphyseal junction that is slightly expansile and has a multiloculated appearance with regions of cortical scalloping and thinning.

diological study may show a well-demarcated radiolucent zone with apparent trabecularization that results in a multilocular or even in a septated appearance (Fig. 1). Some cortical bone erosion may be present. The radiographic pattern can be considered diagnostic, and further staging is typically unnecessary.[4,21,22] After puberty with skeletal maturation, nonossifying fibromas become inactive or latent and ultimately ossify. Surgical intervention is usually unnecessary unless pathological fracture is a significant risk.[38] Intracapsular curettage is effective, but bone grafting or other stabilizing techniques for fracture prevention or treatment may be required.[36,37] Rarely, nonossifying fibromas cause oncogenic rickets.

Enchondroma is a benign and typically asymptomatic tumor of cartilage caused by focal disruption of endochondral bone formation. It can be considered a dysplasia of the central growth plate.[19,39] Enchondromas seem to arise in metaphyses and may eventually become incorporated into the diaphysis. Solitary lesions are usually noted in adolescence or in early adulthood. They most commonly involve small tubular bones of the hands or feet or the proximal humerus. However, several distinct disorders feature multiple enchondromas (enchondromatosis, Ollier disease, and Maffucci syndrome). A mutant parathyroid hormone

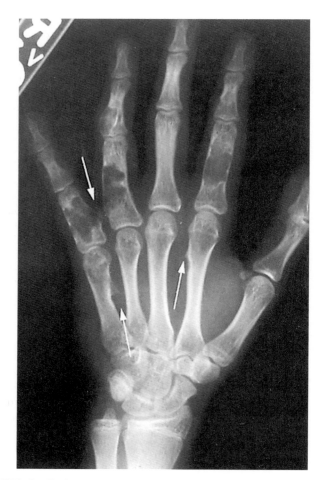

FIG. 2. Enchondromatosis. This 13-year-old girl has multiple, lucent, benign-appearing lesions of the phalanges. Each has produced expansion of the bone as well as cortical scalloping and thinning. Several periosteum-based chondromas are present that show reactive bone formation at their margins (arrows).

Solitary asymptomatic enchondromas are generally benign and require no treatment, although periodic follow-up is indicated. If they become symptomatic and begin to enlarge, careful surveillance is necessary.[39] Imaging techniques may be helpful to search for evidence of malignancy.[4,24,25] Surgical treatment would then be indicated.

Osteochondroma (osteocartilaginous exostosis) is a common dysplasia of cartilage involving the peripheral region of a growth plate.[19,33,39] Mutations within the *EXT1* or *EXT2* genes cause heritable forms of this disorder.[41–43] The lesion can arise in any bone that derives from cartilage, but it usually occurs in a long bone. Typically, either end of a femur, the proximal humerus or tibia, the pelvis, or the scapula is affected. Exostoses present as hard painful masses that are fixed to bone. They enlarge during childhood but become latent in adulthood. These lesions can irritate overlying soft tissues and may form a fluid-filled bursa. A painful and enlarging exostosis during adult life, especially in the pelvis or shoulder girdle, should suggest malignant transformation to a chondrosarcoma.[33,35,39,44] Generally exostoses are solitary, but multiple hereditary exostoses is a well-characterized autosomal dominant entity that can result in significant angular deformity of the lower limbs, clubbing of the radius, and short stature.[34]

Radiographics may show either a flat, sessile, or pedunculated metaphyseal bony lesion of variable density that is typically well defined and covered by a radiolucent carti-

(PTH)/PTH-related peptide (PTHrP) type I receptor has been identified.[40] Fewer than 1% of the solitary asymptomatic tumors undergo malignant transformation, but with enchondromatosis, the risk is estimated to be 10%.[32,37]

Radiographs show a medullary, radiolucent lesion with a well-defined but only slightly thickened bony margin (Fig. 2).[4,20,21] This defect may enlarge slowly during its active phase in adolescence but calcifies when the tumor becomes latent during the adult years. Then it has a diffusely punctate or stippled appearance (Fig. 3). In time, enchondromas become surrounded by dense reactive osseous tissue. Skeletal scintigraphy typically reflects the tumor's biological activity and shows increased radioisotope uptake in the reactive zone (greatly increased uptake suggests malignant transformation). Accordingly, it is prudent to secure for young adults with multiple enchondromas a "baseline" bone scan and radiographs.

Biopsy is often not necessary because the lesion's identity is revealed by characteristic radiography.[4,20,21] Histopathological examination may be required, however, to distinguish benign from low-grade malignant enchondromas. Here, the patient's age is an especially important consideration.[39]

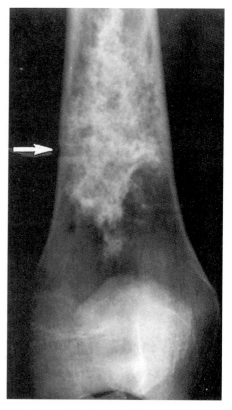

FIG. 3. Enchondroma. This 43-year-old woman has an extensively calcified lesion of the metadiaphyseal region of her distal femur. The calcification is amorphous and dense with little radiolucent component (arrow indicates a biopsy needle track). This lesion is differentiated from a bone infarction, which typically has a dense, linearly marginated periphery.

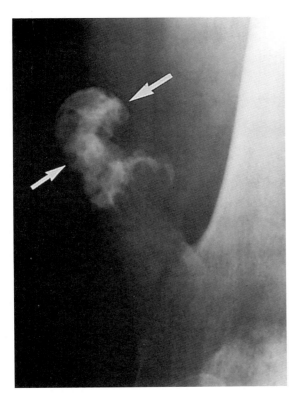

FIG. 4. Osteochondroma (osteocartilagenous exostosis). This 51-year-old woman has a typical pedunculated exostosis of her distal femur. The cortex and trabecular components of the exostosis are continuous with the host bone. Note how the exostosis slants away from the knee joint. The osteocartilagenous cap (arrows) is densely mineralized.

ysis, and they can penetrate into subchondral bone and may even invade articular cartilage. In contrast to other benign skeletal neoplasms, they occasionally metastasize. Accordingly, giant cell tumors of bone are sometimes referred to as "transitional" neoplasms. Overexpression of the c-*myc* oncogene correlates with occurrence of metastasis.[47]

Radiological studies show a relatively large lucent abnormality surrounded by an obvious reactive zone.[4,21,22] The cortex can appear eroded from the endosteal surface (Fig. 5). A trabecular bone pattern may fill in the tumor cavity. Bone scanning can manifest decreased tracer uptake at the center of the lesion (the "doughnut" sign). Histopathological examination shows numerous, scattered, multinucleated giant cells in a proliferative stroma; mitoses are occasionally present.[1,6] The findings differ from the *extraskeletal osteoclastomas* affecting exceptional patients with Paget's bone disease.[48]

Curettage (with bone grafting or use of cement) deals with less advanced lesions. Recurrent or advanced tumors are removed with en bloc wide excision and reconstructive surgery.

Malignant Bone Tumors

Multiple myeloma, a neoplasm of marrow origin, is the most common cancer of the skeleton. However, a considerable variety of malignant tumors arise from bone, cartilage, fibrous tissue, histiocytes, and perhaps endothelial tissue in the skeleton itself.[1,2,5,6]

laginous cap (Fig. 4). Characteristically, there is continuity of tumor and metaphyseal bone.[4,21,22] The diagnosis is rarely difficult. However, following malignant transformation, there may be a soft tissue mass on CT or MRI, and skeletal scintigraphy will show suddenly or considerably increased tracer uptake.

The cartilaginous cap of an exostosis appears histopathologically like a poorly organized growth plate. The trabeculae are not remodeled and thus contain cartilage cores (primary spongiosa).

Excisional treatment of an active exostosis should include the cartilaginous cap and overlying perichondrium to minimize the chance of recurrence.[1,3,7,39] There is about a 5% recurrence rate after marginal excision of a solitary lesion. Malignant degeneration occurs in fewer than 1% of solitary lesions, but the likelihood is almost 10% for multiple hereditary exostoses.[34,35,39]

Giant cell tumor of bone (osteoclastoma) is a common benign bone neoplasm. The cellular origin, however, is unknown.[45–47] Men are more frequently affected than women, typically at 20–40 years of age. These tumors cause chronic and deep pain that mimics an arthropathy. Pathological fracture or effusion into the knee is a common presentation. Frequently, the epiphysis of a distal femur or a proximal tibia is affected. However, the distal radius, proximal humerus, distal tibia, and sacrum are also commonly involved. Often, giant cell tumors enlarge to occupy most of the epiphysis and portions of the adjacent metaph-

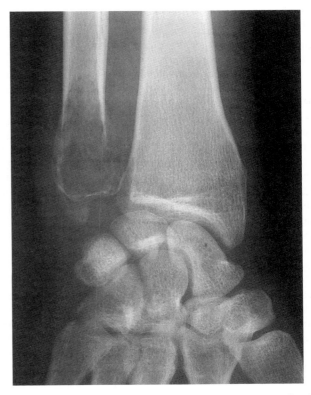

FIG. 5. Giant cell tumor. This 25-year-old man has an expansile, destructive, lucent lesion of the distal ulna. The lesion extends to the end of the bone.

Malignant bone tumors typically cause skeletal pain that is noted particularly at night. Accordingly, this symptom, especially in adolescents or young adults, is reason for evaluation. Treatment of malignant bone tumors is complex and is primarily based on the tumor grade and staging.[1,2,5,6] Only general comments are provided here and concern the principal entities.

Multiple myeloma typically develops during middle age and affects many skeletal sites. Constitutional symptoms can include bone pain, fever, malaise, fatigue, and weight loss. Often there is anemia, thrombocytopenia, and renal failure.[49,50] Hypercalcemia, caused by elaboration of osteoclast-activating factors,[51] occurs in about 20–40% of patients.[52] The diagnosis is made by showing paraproteinemia using serum and urine immunoelectrophoresis and by examining bone marrow for plasmacytosis.[49] Infection with Karposi's sarcoma-associated herpes virus may be involved in the pathogenesis.[53]

Radiographic findings classically include discrete, circular, osteolytic lesions, but generalized osteopenia is actually a more common presentation. Bone scintigraphy can seem unusual because of little tracer uptake in foci of osteolysis.[4,20,21,23]

Myeloma is radiation sensitive and treatable by chemotherapy. Reossification of tumor sites can occur within several months of therapy. Prevention of pathological fractures may require surgical stabilization.[49] The primary mechanism of bone destruction is increased osteoclastic action.[51] Bisphosphonate treatment has helped to decrease fractures and pain.[54]

Osteosarcoma (osteogenic sarcoma) is the most common primary malignancy of the skeleton.[1,7,55,56] There are about 1100–1500 new cases in the United States yearly. This cancer typically develops before age 30 and is somewhat more common in males than in females. Although most of the tumors are the "classic" variety, variants include parosteal, periosteal, and telangiectatic types that have different presentations and prognoses. Cytogenetic aberrations have been characterized.[56,57]

Classic osteosarcoma characteristically arises in the metaphysis of a long bone where there is the most rapid growth. Teenagers are usually affected. In about 50% of cases, these tumors develop near the knee in the distal femur or proximal tibia. Other commonly involved sites are the humerus, proximal femur, and pelvis, but they can begin de novo anywhere in the skeleton. Classic osteosarcomas also derive from malignant transformation of Paget's bone disease.[58]

Typically, an osteosarcoma presents as a tender bony mass. Pain is severe and unremitting. Pathological fracture can occur. They are aggressive neoplasms that readily penetrate metaphyseal cortical bone, and the majority have already infiltrated surrounding soft tissues at the time of diagnosis. At presentation, about 50% of affected adolescents show penetration of their growth plates with epiphyseal involvement, about 20% have metastases elsewhere in the cancerous bone and, in approximately 10%, the tumor has spread to lymph nodes or to lung.[55]

Radiological study shows a destructive lesion that is composed of amorphous osseous tissue with poorly defined margins.[4,20,21,59] Some osteosarcomas are predominantly

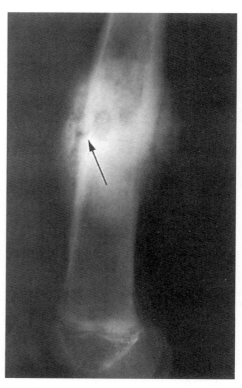

FIG. 6. Central (medullary) osteosarcoma. This 12-year-old boy has a sclerotic diaphyseal lesion that arose in the medullary cavity. It has penetrated the cortex and produced a densely mineralized mass surrounding the femur. Portions of the cortex appear to have been destroyed (arrow), whereas other regions are thickened.

osteoblastic and radiologically dense; others are predominantly osteolytic and radiolucent. Some have a mixed pattern.[20,21] Cortical bone destruction is often apparent (Fig. 6). A characteristic "sunburst" configuration results from spicules of amorphous neoplastic osseous tissue forming perpendicularly to the long axis of the affected bone. This is in contrast to the parallel or "onion skin" appearance of reactive periosteal new bone. Codman's triangle results from reaction and elevation of the periosteum that demarcates a triangular area of cortical bone (see Fig. 8). Bone scintigraphy shows intense uptake of tracer and may disclose more widespread disease than by conventional radiography.[58] CT, MRI, PET, and angiography are helpful, as discussed previously. Microscopic examination typically shows a very malignant stroma that produces an amorphous and immature osteoid in a trabecular pattern.[1–7]

Use of chemotherapy preoperatively[10,14,20,55] has significantly improved the prognosis for this malignancy and has enabled many osteosarcoma patients to be managed by limb-salvage procedures instead of radical amputation.[7,9,17]

Parosteal osteosarcomas are juxtacortical (i.e., they develop between the bony cortex and the soft tissue as a surface neoplasm). Adolescents and young adults are most commonly affected by these slowly growing, low-grade tumors that typically occur as a fixed and painless mass posteriorly on the distal femur or medially on the proximal humerus. They are less aggressive than classic osteosarcomas and can remain separated for a considerable length of

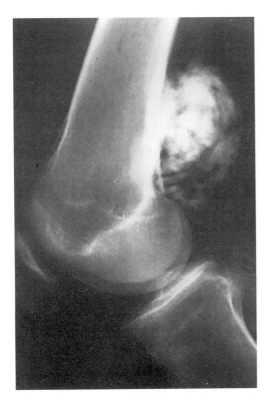

FIG. 7. Parosteal osteosarcoma. This 30-year-old woman has a very densely mineralized mass arising from the periosteal surface of the distal femoral metaphysis posteriorly. This tumor has lobular calcification and is attached to the femur by a broad pedicle.

time from the parent bone by a narrow radiolucent region of soft tissue. Eventually, they may involve the underlying skeleton and degenerate into a high-grade osteosarcoma.[55]

Radiological study typically reveals a densely ossified, broad-based, fusiform mass that seems to encircle the metaphyseal region of a long bone (Fig. 7).[4,20,21,59] Reactive tissue initially separates the neoplasm from the underlying bone that is destroyed once the tumor penetrates the normal cortex into the medullary canal. Parosteal osteosarcomas have mature trabeculae with cement lines resembling Paget's bone disease,[9] however, a low-grade malignant stroma is present. This tumor is often misdiagnosed as benign. Limb-salvage with wide marginal excision is the usual treatment for less advanced disease. The prognosis is good. Chemotherapy is typically not used unless there has been dedifferentiation of the neoplasm.[9,14,55]

Periosteal osteosarcoma often presents as a painless growing mass that extends from the surface of a bone into soft tissue.[55] This uncommon variant of classic osteosarcoma typically affects young adults. Radiological study shows a poorly mineralized mass primarily on a bone surface in an area of cortical erosion. The crater-like lesion has irregular margins with periosteal reaction.[4,20,21] Penetration through cortical bone into the medullary canal occurs more rapidly than with parosteal osteosarcoma. If this complication has occurred, the likelihood of pulmonary metastasis is greater—contributing to its poorer prognosis. Bone scintigraphy shows avid tracer uptake.[59] CT reveals a mass that fills a shallow cortical bone defect but contains minimal

calcification. Malignant mesenchymal stroma with neoplastic osteoid occurs in and around areas of mature cartilage.[4,6,20,21]

Periosteal osteosarcoma is often treated by excision with a wide margin.[51] Adjuvant chemotherapy is used when the tumor has regions of high-grade malignancy.[11,14]

Chondrosarcoma occurs most often between 40 and 60 years of age when this neoplasm develops as a primary tumor.[39,60] About 25% of patients manifest malignant transformation in a pre-existing enchondroma or osteocartilaginous exostosis. Thus, chondrosarcomas usually involve the pelvis, proximal femur, or shoulder girdle. Patients initially experience a persistent dull ache that can mimic arthritis. Variants of the classic form of chondrosarcoma include a high-grade dedifferentiated neoplasm, an intermediate-grade clear cell type, and a low-grade juxtacortical tumor. The particular designation depends on the histopathological pattern and anatomical location.[39,60]

Radiographs show a subtle radiolucent lesion that contains hazy or speckled calcification in a diffuse "salt and pepper" or "popcorn" pattern.[4,20,21] Primary chondrosarcomas can develop either within the medullary canal or on the surface of a bone where they may destroy the cortex and form a mass. On histopathological examination, it can be difficult to show that high-grade tumors are cartilaginous in origin, or that low-grade tumors are actually malignant.[39,45]

Treatment of chondrosarcomas depends on the tumor stage. Limb amputation may be necessary for higher grade tumors. Adjuvant chemotherapy or radiation therapy has been disappointing.[39]

Ewing sarcoma is a highly malignant neoplasm that arises from nonmesenchymal cells in the bone marrow.[61–64] This cancer usually harbors a pathognomonic t(11:12)(q24; q12) translocation[65] and represents a form of primitive neuroectodermal tumor.[59] It typically presents in 10- to 15-year-old children and more commonly affects boys than girls.[1,61–64] Initial manifestations include an enlarging and tender soft tissue swelling together with weight loss, malaise, fever, and lethargy. The erythrocyte sedimentation rate may be elevated, and there can be leukocytosis and anemia. The diaphysis of the femur is most commonly involved; alternatively, an ilium, tibia, fibula, or rib is affected. When this cancer occurs in the pelvis, it is usually found late and has an especially poor prognosis.[1,61–64]

Radiological study typically reveals a diaphyseal lesion of patchy density that destroys cortical bone and frequently causes an "onion skin" appearance of reactive periosteum (Fig. 8).[4,20,21] Bone scanning may show intense tracer uptake that extends considerably beyond the radiographic abnormality.

Chemotherapy can be followed by wide excision or radiation therapy, depending on, among other factors, the anatomical site. Newer therapeutic approaches have reduced the incidence of pulmonary metastases and have markedly improved survival.[1,66] Histological response to preoperative chemotherapy and tumor size are important predictors of event-free survival.[13]

Malignant fibrous histiocytoma occurs more frequently in soft tissues than in the skeleton and is less common than benign fibrous tumors.[1,3,37] This cancer affects adults and

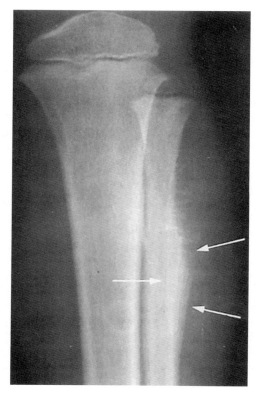

FIG. 8. Ewing sarcoma. This 5-year-old boy has a subtle permeative lesion of the proximal diaphysis of his fibula. The tumor is characterized by layered (onion skin) periosteal reaction forming a Codman's triangle (arrows) and by "sunburst" new bone formation more proximally, which is characteristically perpendicular to the bone's long axis. A large soft tissue mass is associated with the skeletal defects.

often originates in Paget's bone disease or at the site of a skeletal infarct. Typically, this is an aggressive sarcoma that readily spreads within the lymphatics. Bone is infiltrated early on, and pathological fracture is a common presentation.

Radiological study reveals a poorly defined radiolucent lesion that causes cortical bone erosion.[4,19,20] The histopathological pattern is variable from area to area; extremely large and bizarre histiocytic cells are found in some sections, and undifferentiated cells that resemble histiocytic lymphoma are noted in others. Areas that contain fibrous tissue may suggest that the tumor is a fibrosarcoma. Special stains and electron microscopy can be required to establish the diagnosis.[5,6,67] Staging studies direct the therapy, which may require radical resection or amputation and perhaps chemotherapy.[1,39] The prognosis is guarded.[39,67]

Fibrosarcoma causes pain and typically arises in a major long bone of an adolescent or young adult.[1–5,37] Radiological study reveals a poorly defined and destructive lucent lesion in a metaphysis.[4,20,21] Low-grade and high-grade fibrosarcomas have similar radiological and histopathological appearances. Accordingly, electron microscopy may be necessary to reveal the collagenous composition of the matrix of a high-grade tumor.[6,37] Therapy depends on the staging results.[1,3,5]

Metastatic bone tumors are considerably more common than primary skeletal malignancies (with a ratio of about 25

to 1).[1,4,5] Prostate, breast, thyroid, lung, and kidney cancers are the principal neoplasms that metastasize to bone. There is predilection for malignant cells to deposit within blood-forming marrow spaces in the spine, ribs, skull, pelvis, and metaphyses of long bones (particularly the femur and humerus). In children, metastases within the skeleton usually reflect a neuroblastoma, leukemia, or Ewing sarcoma. In teenagers or young adults, lymphomas are the predominant source. After age 30, an adenocarcinoma is the likely primary. Osteoblastic metastases most commonly derive from carcinoma of the prostate or breast. Osteolytic metastases may come from the lung, thyroid, kidney, or gastrointestinal tract.[4,20,22] In a significant number of patients, the origin is not evident, and staging studies with biopsy[31] are performed to explore the possibility of an intrinsic skeletal sarcoma.[1–3,5,6]

REFERENCES

1. Dorfman HD, Czerniak B 1997 Bone Tumors. Mosby-Year Book, Inc., St. Louis, MO, USA.
2. Levesque J 1998 Clinical Guide to Primary Bone Tumors. Williams & Wilkins, Baltimore, MD, USA.
3. Simon M 1997 Surgery for Bone and Soft-Tissue Tumors. Lippincott-Raven Publishers, Philadelphia, PA, USA.
4. Wilner D 1997 Wilner's Radiology of Bone Tumors. W. B. Saunders Company, Philadelphia, PA, USA.
5. Unni K, Dahlin DC 1996 Dahlin's Bone Tumors: General Aspects and Data on 11,087 Cases, 5th ed. Lippincott-Raven, Philadelphia, PA, USA.
6. Greenspan A, Remagen W 1998 Differential Diagnosis Of Tumors And Tumor-Like Lesions Of Bones And Joints. Lippincott-Raven, Philadelphia, PA, USA.
7. Simon MA, Springfield DS 1998 Surgery for Bone and Soft-Tissue Tumors. Lippincott-Raven, Philadelphia, PA, USA.
8. Heare TC, Enneking WF, Heare MM 1989 Staging techniques and biopsy of bone tumors. Orthop Clin North Am 20:273–285.
9. Choong PF, Sim FH 1997 Limb-sparing surgery for bone tumors: New developments. Semin Oncol 13:64–69.
10. Biermann JS, Baker LH 1997 The future of sarcoma treatment. Semin Oncol 24:592–597.
11. Jaffe N 1989 Chemotherapy for malignant bone tumors. Orthop Clin North Am 20:487–503.
12. Sweetnam R 1989 Malignant bone tumor management: 30 years of achievement. Clin Orthop 247:67–73.
13. Wunder JS, Paulian G, Huvos AG, Heller G, Meyers PA, Healey JH 1998 The histologic response to chemotherapy as a predictor of the oncological outcome of operative treatment of Ewing sarcoma. J Bone Joint Surg Am 80:1020–1033.
14. Bramwell VH 1997 The role of chemotherapy in the management of non-metastatic operable extremity osteosarcoma. Semin Oncol 24:561–571.
15. Nichter LS, Menendez LR 1993 Reconstructive considerations for limb salvage surgery. Orthop Clin North Am 24:511–521.
16. McDonald DJ 1994 Limb-salvage surgery for treatment of sarcomas of the extremities. Am J Roentgenol 163:509–513.
17. 1991 In: Langlais F, Tomeno B (eds.) Limb Salvage: Major Reconstruction in Oncologic and Nontumoral Conditions. Springer-Verlag, Berlin, Germany.
18. Weis LD 1999 The success of limb-salvage surgery in the adolescent patient with osteogenic sarcoma. Adolesc Med 10:451–458.
19. Scarborough MT, Moreau G 1996 Benign cartilage tumors. Orthop Clin North Am 27:583–589.
20. Edeiken J, Dalinka M, Karasick D 1990 Edeiken's Roentgen Diagnosis of Diseases of Bone, 4th ed. Williams and Wilkins, Baltimore, MD, USA.
21. Resnick D, Niwayama G 2002 Diagnosis of Bone and Joint Disorders, 4th ed. WB Saunders, Philadelphia, PA, USA.
22. Simon MA 1993 Diagnostic strategy for bone and soft-tissue tumors. J Bone Joint Surg Am 75:622–631.
23. Brown ML 1993 Bone scintigraphy in benign and malignant tumors. Radiol Clin North Am 31:731–738.

24. Murphy WA Jr 1991 Imaging bone tumors in the 1990s. Cancer **67:**1169–1176.
25. Magid D 1993 Two-dimensional and three-dimensional computed tomographic imaging in musculoskeletal tumors. Radiol Clin North Am **31:**426–447.
26. Berquist TM 1993 Magnetic resonance imaging of primary skeletal neoplasms. Radiol Clin North Am **31:**411–424.
27. Redmond OM, Stack JP, Dervan PA, Hurson BJ, Carney DN, Ennis JT 1989 Osteosarcoma: Use of MR imaging and MR spectroscopy in clinical decision making. Radiology **172:**811–815.
28. Cook GJ, Fogelman I 2001 The role of positron emission tomography in skeletal disease. Semin Nucl Med **31:**50–61.
29. Simon MA, Biermann JS 1993 Biopsy of bone and soft-tissue lesions. J Bone Joint Surg Am **75:**616–621.
30. Schwartz HS, Spengler DM 1997 Needle tract recurrences after closed biopsy for sarcoma: Three cases and review of the literature. Ann Surg Oncol **4:**228–236.
31. Wedin R, Bauer HC, Skoog L, Soderlund V, Tani E 2000 Cytological diagnosis of skeletal lesions. Fine-needle aspiration biopsy in 110 tumours. J Bone Joint Surg Br **82:**673–678.
32. Giudici MA, Moser RP Jr, Kransdorf MJ 1993 Cartilaginous bone tumors. Radiol Clin North Am **31:**237–259.
33. Schubiner JM, Simon MA 1987 Primary bone tumors in children. Orthop Clin North Am **18:**577–595.
34. Wicklund CL, Pauli RM, Johnston D, Hecht JT 1995 Natural history study of hereditary multiple exostoses. Am J Med Genet **55:**43–46.
35. Ozaki T, Hillmann A, Blasius S, Link T, Winkelmann W 1998 Multicentric malignant transformation of multiple exostoses. Skeletal Radiol **27:**233–236.
36. Hudson TM, Stiles RG, Monson DK 1993 Fibrous lesions of bone. Radiol Clin North Am **31:**279–297.
37. Marks KE, Bauer TW 1989 Fibrous tumors of bone. Orthop Clin North Am **20:**377–393.
38. Jee WH, Choe BY, Kang HS, Suh KJ, Suh JS, Ryu KN, Lee YS, Ok IY, Kim JM, Choi KH, Shinn KS 1998 Nonossifying fibroma: Characteristics at MR imaging with pathological correlation. Radiology **209:**197–202.
39. Greenspan A 1989 Tumors of cartilage origin. Orthop Clin North Am **20:**347–366.
40. Hopyan S, Gokgoz N, Poor R, Gensure RC, Yu C, Cole WG, Bell RS, Jupper H, Andrulis IL, Wunder JS, Alman BA 2002 A mutant PTH/PTHrP type I receptor in enchondromatosis. Nat Genet **30:**306–310.
41. McCormick C, Leduc Y, Martindale D, Mattison K, Esford LE, Dyer AP, Tufaro F 1998 The putative tumour suppressor EXT1 alters the expression of cell-surface heparan sulfate. Nat Genet **19:**158–161.
42. Bridge JA, Nelson M, Orndal C, Bhatia P, Neff JR 1998 Clonal karyotypic abnormalities of the hereditary multiple exostoses chromosomal loci 8q24.1 (EXT1) and 11p11–12 (EXT2) in patients with sporadic and hereditary osteochondromas. Cancer **82:**1657–1663.
43. McCormick C, Duncan G, Tufaro F 1999 New perspectives on the molecular basis of hereditary bone tumors. Mol Med Today **5:**481–486.
44. Merchan EC, Sanchez-Herrera S, Gonzalez JM 1993 Secondary chondrosarcoma. Four cases and review of the literature. Acta Orthop Belg **59:**76–80.
45. Manaster BJ, Doyle AJ 1993 Giant cell tumors of bone. Radiol Clin North Am **31:**299–323.
46. Richardson MJ, Dickinson IC 1998 Giant cell tumor of bone. Bull Hosp Jt Dis **57:**6–10.
47. Gamberi G, Benassi MS, Bohling T, Ragazzini P, Molendini L, Sollazzo MR, Merli M, Ferrari C, Magagnoli G, Bertoni F, Picci P 1998 Prognostic relevance of C-myc gene expression in giant-cell tumor of bone. J Orthop Res **16:**1–7.
48. Ziambaras K, Totty WA, Teitelbaum SL, Dierkes M, Whyte MP 1997 Extraskeletal osteoclastomas responsive to dexamethasone treatment in Paget bone disease. J Clin Endocrinol Metab **82:**3826–3834.
49. Osserman EF, Merlini G, Butler VP Jr 1987 Multiple myeloma and related plasma cell dyscrasias. JAMA **258:**2930–2937.
50. Lacy MQ, Gertz MA, Hanson CA, Inwards DJ, Kyle RA 1997 Multiple myeloma associated with diffuse osteosclerotic bone lesions: A clinical entity distinct from osteosclerotic myeloma (POEMS syndrome). Am J Hematol **56:**288–293.
51. Roodman GD 1997 Mechanisms of bone lesions in multiple myeloma and lymphoma. Cancer **80:**1557–1563.
52. Mundy GR 1989 Calcium Homeostasis: Hypercalcemia and Hypocalcemia. Martin Dunitz, London, UK.
53. Berenson JR, Vescio RA, Said J 1998 Multiple myeloma: The cells of origin–a two-way street. Leukemia **12:**121–127.
54. Bloomfield DJ 1998 Should bisphosphonates be part of the standard therapy of patients with multiple myeloma or bone metastases from other cancers? An evidence-based review. J Clin Oncol **16:**1218–1225.
55. Meyers PA 1987 Malignant bone tumors in children: Osteosarcoma. Hematol Oncol Clin North Am **1:**655–665.
56. Meyers PA, Gorlick R 1997 Osteosarcoma. Pediatr Clin North Am **44:**973–989.
57. Bridge JA, Nelson M, McComb E, McGuire MH, Rosenthal H, Vergara G, Maale GE, Spanier S, Neff JR 1997 Cytogenetic findings in 73 osteosarcoma specimens and a review of the literature. Cancer Genet Cytogenet **95:**74–87.
58. Hadjipavlou A, Lander P, Srolovitz H, Enker IP 1992 Malignant transformation in Paget disease of bone. Cancer **70:**2802–2808.
59. Fletcher BD 1997 Imaging pediatric bone sarcomas. Diagnosis and treatment-related issues. Radiol Clin North Am **35:**1477–1494.
60. Welkerling H, Dreyer T, Delling G 1991 Morphological typing of chondrosarcoma: A study of 92 cases. Virchows Arch **418:**419–425.
61. Horowitz ME, Tsokos MG, DeLaney TF 1992 Ewing's sarcoma. Cancer J **42:**300–320.
62. Eggli KD, Quiogue T, Moser RP Jr 1993 Ewing's sarcoma. Radiol Clin North Am **31:**325–337.
63. Lawlor ER, Lim JF, Tao W, Poremba C, Chow CJ, Kalousek IV, Kovar H, MacDonald TJ, Sorensen PH 1998 The Ewing tumor family of peripheral primitive neuroectodermal tumors expresses human gastrin-releasing peptide. Cancer Res **58:**2469–2476.
64. Grier HE 1997 The Ewing family of tumors. Ewing's sarcoma and primitive neuroectodermal tumors. Pediatr Clin North Am **44:**991–1004.
65. Maurici D, Perez-Atayde A, Grier HE, Baldini N, Serra M, Fletcher JA 1998 Frequency and implications of chromosome 8 and 12 gains in Ewing sarcoma. Cancer Genet Cytogenet **100:**106–110.
66. Sandoval C, Meyer WH, Parham DM, Kun LE, Hustu HO, Luo X, Pratt CB 1996 Outcome in 43 children presenting with metastatic Ewing sarcoma; the St. Jude Children's Research Hospital experience, 1962 to 1992. Med Pediatr Oncol **26:**180–185.
67. Womer RB 1991 The cellular biology of bone tumors. Clin Orthop **262:**12–21.

Chapter 80. Ischemic Bone Disease

Michael P. Whyte

Division of Bone and Mineral Diseases, Washington University School of Medicine at Barnes-Jewish Hospital and Center for Metabolic Bone Disease and Molecular Research, Shriners Hospitals for Children, St. Louis, Missouri

INTRODUCTION

Regional interruption of blood flow to the skeleton can cause ischemic (aseptic or avascular) necrosis—an important acquired disorder affecting bone and cartilage.[1–4] Ischemia, if sufficiently severe and prolonged, will kill osteoblasts and chondrocytes. Clinical problems arise if subsequent resorption of necrotic tissue during skeletal repair sufficiently compromises bone strength to cause fracture.[1–3]

A change in skeletal density is the principal radiographic feature of ischemic bone disease.[2,3] However, alterations may take several months to appear. Characteristic signs include crescent-shaped subchondral radiolucencies, patchy areas of sclerosis and lucency, bony collapse, and diaphyseal periostitis. Joint space is initially preserved despite the epiphyseal disease.

A variety of conditions cause ischemic bone disease (Table 1) and a great number of clinical presentations occur based primarily on the affected skeletal site. Legg-Calvé-Perthes disease is discussed in some detail here, because it represents an archetypal form. A few additional important clinical presentations are mentioned subsequently.

LEGG-CALVÉ-PERTHES DISEASE

Legg-Calvé-Perthes disease (LCPD) can be defined as idiopathic ischemic necrosis (osteonecrosis) of the capital femoral epiphysis in children.[5–7] It is a common, complex, and controversial problem that affects boys more frequently than girls (4:1 to 5:1). Typically, LCPD presents between 2 and 12 years of age; the mean age at diagnosis is 7 years. When it manifests later in life, the term "adolescent ischemic necrosis" is used to indicate the poorer prognosis compared with when adults suffer ischemic bone disease. Usually, one hip is involved. However, bilateral disease troubles about 20% of patients where our experience suggests that an epiphyseal dysplasia should be considered as a possible explanation for the radiographic findings. Familial incidence varies from 1% to 20%.[5–7]

Although the etiology of LCPD is unknown, the pathogenesis is fairly well understood. Interruption of blood flow to the capital femoral epiphysis is the fundamental skeletal insult. However, ischemia at this site in children can have many causes including raised intracapsular pressure resulting from congenital or developmental abnormalities, episodes of synovitis, venous thrombosis, or perhaps increased blood viscosity.[5–7] Most, if not all, of the capital femoral epiphysis is rendered ischemic. Consequently osteoblasts, osteocytes, and marrow cells may die. Endochondral ossification ceases temporarily because blood flow to chondrocytes in the growth plate is impaired. Articular cartilage, however, remains intact initially because synovial fluid provides nourishment. Revascularization of necrosed areas then follows and proceeds from the periphery to the center of the epiphysis. New bone is deposited on the surface of subchondral cortical or central trabecular osseous debris. Subsequently, the critical process of removal of necrotic bone begins, during which time the rate of bone resorption exceeds the rate of reparative new bone formation. Consequently, subchondral bone is weakened.

If there is no fracture in the area of reparative bone resorption, the child may remain asymptomatic and eventually heal. If, however, fracture occurs, there will be symptoms. Furthermore, trabecular bone collapse can cause a second episode of ischemia.[5–7] Longitudinal growth of the proximal femur can be stunted, because the disrupted blood flow disturbs the physis and metaphysis. Premature closure of the growth plate may occur. As reossification of the epiphysis proceeds, the femoral head will remold its shape according to impacting mechanical forces.[2,3,5–7]

Children with LCPD typically limp, complain of pain in a knee or anterior thigh, and have limited mobility of the hip (especially with abduction or internal rotation). The Trendelenburg sign may be positive. If treatment is not successful, adduction and flexion contractures of the hip can develop, and thigh muscles may atrophy.

Laboratory investigation may show a slightly elevated erythrocyte sedimentation rate. Radiographic examination, which should include anteroposterior and "frog" lateral views for diagnosis and follow-up, often reveals a bone age that is 1–3 years delayed.[2,3] Sequential studies typically show cessation of growth of the capital femoral epiphysis, resorption of necrotic bone, subchondral fracture, reossification, and finally, healing (Fig. 1). Magnetic resonance imaging (MRI) is helpful because signal intensity patterns change with circulatory compromise, soft tissues as well as bone are visualized, and containment of the femoral head can be assessed.[8]

TABLE 1. CAUSES OF ISCHEMIC NECROSIS OF CARTILAGE AND BONE

Endocrine/metabolic
Alcohol abuse
Glucocorticoid therapy
Cushing's syndrome
Gout
Osteomalacia
Storage diseases (e.g., Gaucher disease)
Hemoglobinopathies (e.g., sickle cell disease)
Trauma (e.g., dislocation, fracture)
Dysbaric conditions
Collagen vascular disorders
HIV infection
Irradiation
Pancreatitis
Renal transplantation
Idiopathic, familial

The author has no conflict of interest.

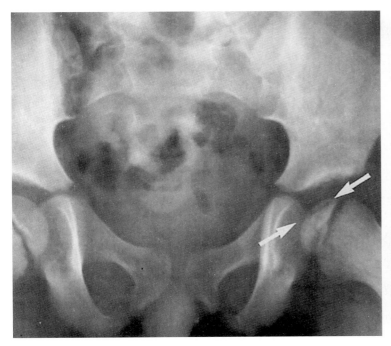
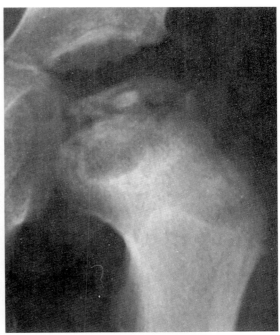

FIG. 1. Legg-Calvé-Perthes disease. (A) The affected left capital femoral epiphysis of this 4-year-old boy is denser and smaller than the contralateral normal side. It shows a radiolucent area that forms the "crescent sign" (arrows) indicative of subchondral bone collapse. (B) Seven months later, there is flattening of the capital femoral epiphysis with widening and irregularity of the femoral neck.

The short-term prognosis for LCPD depends on the severity of femoral head deformity at the completion of the healing phase. The long-term outcome is conditioned by how much secondary degenerative osteoarthritis develops. Generally, the more extensive the involvement of the capital femoral epiphysis, the worse the prognosis. Girls seem to have poorer outcomes than boys, because they tend to have greater involvement of the capital femoral epiphysis and they mature earlier. Sexual maturation means less time for femoral head modeling before closure of the growth plates. Onset at 2–6 years of age causes the least femoral head deformity; onset after 10 years of age has a poor outcome.[5–9]

Treatment for LCPD is directed principally by the orthopedic surgeon.[10] Prevention of femoral head deformity is a major goal. Significant distortion, not mild, predisposes to osteoarthritis. Degenerative joint disease seems to be greatest for children who lose containment of the femoral head by the acetabulum. Hip subluxation and loss of motion from muscle spasm and contractures disproportionately increase mechanical stresses on some regions of the femoral head. Improved coverage of the femoral head by the acetabulum is sought, allowing the acetabulum to act as a mold during reparative reossification.[5–7] Appropriate management may be observation alone, intermittent treatment of symptoms with periodic bed rest, stretching exercises to maintain hip range-of-motion, and early or late surgical prevention or correction of deformity.[10,11] Bed rest does not seem to decrease compressive forces that may stimulate healing and bone modeling if properly distributed.[5–7,10,11] Periodic radiographic follow-up is essential, and arthrography, bone scintigraphy, and especially MRI can be useful.[6,8] The long-term results of

these treatments remain controversial. Whether containment is useful, and how best to achieve it, are clinical questions that are being actively studied.[5–7,10,11]

TABLE 2. COMMON SITES OF OSTEOCHONDROSIS AND
ISCHEMIC NECROSIS OF BONE

Adult skeleton
  Osteochondritis dissecans (König)
  Osteochondrosis of lunate (Kienböck)
  Fractured head of femur (Axhausen, Phemister)
  Proximal fragment of fractured carpal scaphoid
  Fractured head of humerus
  Fractured talus
  Osteonecrosis of the knee (spontaneous or idiopathic ischemic
    necrosis)
  Idiopathic ischemic necrosis of the femoral head
Developing skeleton
  Osteochondrosis of femoral head (Legg-Calvé-Perthes)
  Slipped femoral epiphysis
  Vertebral epiphysitis affecting secondary ossification centers
    (Scheuermann)
  Vertebral osteochondrosis of primary ossification centers (Calvé)
  Osteochondrosis of tibial tuberosity (Osgood-Schlatter)
  Osteochondrosis of tarsal scaphoid (Köhler)
  Osteochondrosis of medial tibial condyle (Blount)
  Osteochondrosis of primary ossification center of patella (Köhler) and
    of secondary ossification center (Sinding Larsen)
  Osteochondrosis of os calcis (Sever)
  Osteochondrosis of head of second metatarsal (Freiberg) and of other
    metatarsals and metacarpals
  Osteochondrosis of the humeral capitellum (Panner)

Reproduced with permission from Edeiken J, Dalinka M, Karasic D (eds). 1990. Edeiken's Roentgen Diagnosis of Diseases of Bone, 4th ed. Williams & Wilkins, Baltimore, MD, USA, p. 937.

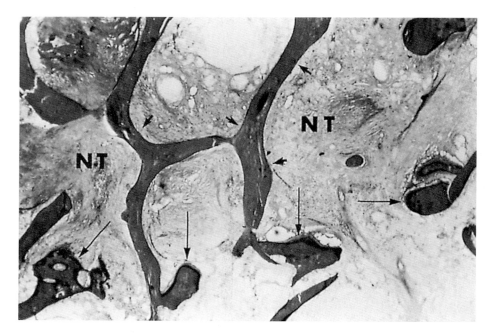

FIG. 2. Ischemic necrosis. This undecalcified section from an affected femoral head shows a typical area of dead bone (arrows) with a smooth acellular surface. A band of necrotic tissue (NT) is visible. Reparative bone formation is occurring in adjacent areas where darkly stained, newly synthesized osteoid is covered by osteoblasts (arrowheads) (Goldner stain, ×160).

OTHER CLINICAL PRESENTATIONS

A considerable variety of conditions can cause ischemic necrosis (Table 1). Recently, HIV infection in adults and children has been added to the list.[12] Numerous clinical presentations manifest in children and adults (Table 2),[1–3] now perhaps including regional migratory osteoporosis.[13] Symptoms result primarily from skeletal disintegration. The specific diagnosis, however, depends on the patient's age, the anatomic site, and the size of the area of bone where blood flow has been interrupted. Legg-Calvé-Perthes disease illustrates particularly well that disruption of the microvasculature of the skeleton predisposes especially subchondral bone to infarction. However, several mechanisms for vascular insufficiency may lead to ischemic bone disease, such as traumatic rupture, internal obstruction, or external pressure compromising blood flow. Arteries, veins, or sinusoids may be involved. The resulting bone disease has been referred to as "ischemic," "avascular," "aseptic," or "idiopathic" necrosis.[1–3]

The pathogenesis of disrupted blood flow in ischemic bone disease is, however, incompletely understood.[1–3] For many types of nontraumatic ischemic necrosis, the predisposed sites within the skeleton seem to recapitulate the physiological conversion of red marrow to fatty marrow with aging.[2] This process occurs from distally to proximally in the appendicular skeleton. As the transition occurs, marrow blood flow decreases. Accordingly, disorders that increase the size and/or number of adipocytes within critical areas of medullary space (e.g., alcohol abuse, Cushing's syndrome) may ultimately compress sinusoids and infarct bone. However, fat embolization, hemorrhage, and abnormalities in the quality of susceptible bone tissue may also be pathogenetic factors in some types of traumatic or nontraumatic ischemic necrosis.[2]

Radiographic features of ischemic bone disease depend on the amount of skeletal revascularization, reossification, and resorption of infarcted bone.[2,3] Revascularization occurs within 6–8 weeks of the ischemic event and may cause trabecular bone resorption (radiolucent bands near necrotic areas). New bone formation then occurs on dead bone surfaces. Over months or years, dead bone may, or may not, be slowly resorbed. Osteosclerosis will occur if new bone encases dead bone and/or if there is bony collapse.

Histopathological study is consistent with the pathogenesis that is suggested radiographically. It shows that these various processes of skeletal death and repair are focal and may be occurring simultaneously (Fig. 2).[4]

After infarction, necrotic bone does not change density for at least 10 days.[2] Currently, MRI is the most sensitive way to detect ischemic necrosis of the skeleton. It is, therefore, particularly useful early on, although occasionally false negatives do occur.[8,14,15] Bone scintigraphy with [99m]technetium diphosphonate, although not specific, can also detect osteonecrosis before radiographic changes are apparent.[16,17] Before the process of revascularization, the infarcted area shows decreased radioisotope uptake. Later, increased tracer accumulation will occur. Computed tomography (CT) is especially helpful for detecting ischemic necrosis of the femoral head, because the bony structure centrally has an "asterisk" shape that is distorted by new bone formation.[18]

The various clinical presentations of ischemic bone disease (Table 2) are sometimes divided into two major anatomic categories: diaphysometaphyseal and epiphysometaphyseal.[2]

Diaphysometaphyseal ischemia can be caused by dysbaric disorders, hemoglobinopathies, collagen vascular diseases, thromboembolic problems, gout, storage disorders (e.g., Gaucher disease), acute or chronic pancreatitis, pheochromocytoma, and other conditions. Typically, large bones (especially the distal femur or proximal tibia) are involved where radiographic changes extend into the metaphysis. Lesions are often symmetrical; however, the size can vary considerably. Small bones may be affected, for example, in

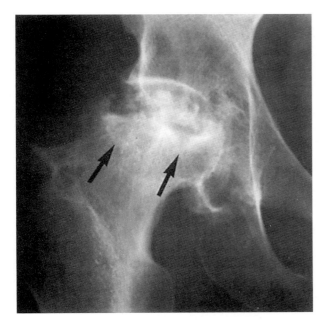

FIG. 3. Ischemic (avascular) necrosis. This 50-year-old man has advanced avascular necrosis of the femoral head. Note that much of the femoral head has been resorbed, causing collapse of the articular surface. The necrotic area is fragmented. A sclerotic zone of reparative tissue (arrows) indicates the interface between viable and necrotic tissues. The acetabular cartilage is focally thin. This finding indicates that he is developing secondary osteoarthritis.

the hands and feet of infants with sickle cell anemia. New bone deposition delineates infarcted bone especially well on radiographic study.

Epiphysometaphyseal infarcts can result from dysbaric conditions, sickle cell disease, Cushing's syndrome, gout, trauma, storage problems, and other disorders. When the lesions are small, they typically affect children or young adults and occur without a history of injury, although occult trauma may actually be important in their pathogenesis. Thrombosis, disease of arterial walls, or abnormalities within adjacent bone, such as those occurring in Gaucher disease or histiocytosis-X, may cause this category of ischemic necrosis.

Osteochondrosis refers to atraumatic ischemic necrosis that typically affects an ossification ("growth") center.[2] *Osteochondritis dissecans* describes a small epiphysometaphyseal infarct that can cause fracture immediately adjacent to a joint space. This lesion appears as a small, dense, button-like area of osseous tissue separated from the intact bone by a radiolucent band. This skeletal fragment can become loose and enter the joint, but it may also heal in place. Larger infarcts are often also idiopathic, occur frequently in adults, and typically involve the hip and the femoral condyles. Large areas of ischemic bone can collapse, thus flattening joint surfaces and destroying articular cartilage. Ultimately, this complication will lead to osteoarthritis (Fig. 3). Very extensive epiphysometaphyseal infarction results from trauma or systemic disease and fre-

quently involves the femoral head (e.g., Legg-Calvé-Perthes disease).[2]

Eponyms for specific presentations of osteochondrosis or ischemic necrosis of the skeleton are numerous and popular (e.g., Blount disease, Scheuermann disease). However, classification according to the involved anatomic site is more informative. Table 2 matches the eponym with the affected skeletal region and helps to illustrate that the patient's age is an important factor for where the skeleton is at risk.[2]

Treatment of ischemic bone disease varies according to the site and size of the lesion and the patient's age, and various aspects remain controversial. Conservative or surgical approaches may be appropriate.[1,19,20]

REFERENCES

1. Pavelka K 2000 Osteonecrosis. Clin Rheumatol **14**:399–414.
2. Edeiken J, Dalinka M, Karasick D 1990 Edeiken's Roentgen Diagnosis of Diseases of Bone, 4th ed. Williams and Wilkins, Baltimore, MD, USA.
3. Resnick D, Niwayama G 2002 Diagnosis of Bone and Joint Disorders, 4th ed. WB Saunders, Philadelphia, PA, USA.
4. Plenk H Jr, Hofmann S, Eschberger J, Gstettner M, Kramer J, Schneider W, Engel A 1997 Histomorphology and bone morphometry of the bone marrow edema syndrome of the hip. Clin Orthop **334**:73–84.
5. Katz JE 1984 Legg-Calvé-Perthes Disease. Praeger, New York, NY, USA.
6. Conway JJ 1993 A scintigraphic classification of Legg-Calvé-Perthes disease. Semin Nucl Med **23**:274–295.
7. Wenger DR, Ward WT, Herring JA 1991 Current concepts review: Legg-Calvé-Perthes disease. J Bone Joint Surg Am **73**:778–788.
8. Lang P, Genant HK, Jergesen HE, Murray WR 1992 Imaging of the hip joint. Computed tomography versus magnetic resonance imaging. Clin Orthop **274**:135–153.
9. Mukherjee A, Fabry G 1990 Evaluation of the prognostic indices in Legg-Calvé-Perthes disease: Statistical analysis of 116 hips. J Pediatr Orthop **10**:153–158.
10. Herring JA 1994 The treatment of Legg-Calvé-Perthes disease. A critical review of the literature. J Bone Joint Surg Am **76**:448–458.
11. Paterson DC, Leitch JM, Foster BK 1991 Results of innominate osteotomy in the treatment of Legg-Calvé-Perthes disease. Clin Orthop **266**:96–103.
12. Gaughan DM, Mofenson LM, Hughes MD, Seage GR III, Ciupak GL, Oleske JM, Pediatric AIDS Clinical Trials Group Protocol 219 Team 2002 Osteonecrosis of the hip (Legg-Calvé-Perthes disease) in human immunodeficiency virus-infected children. Pediatrics **109**:1–8.
13. Trevisan C, Ortolani S, Monteleone M, Mrinoni EC 2002 Case Report: Regional migratory osteoporosis. A pathogenetic hypothesis based on three cases and a review of the literature. Clin Rheumatol **21**:418–425.
14. Mitchell MD, Kundel HL, Steinberg ME, Kressel HY, Alavi A, Axel L 1986 Avascular necrosis of the hip: Comparison of MR, CT, and scintigraphy. Am J Roentgenol **147**:67–71.
15. Mitchell DG, Rao VM, Dalinka MK, Spritzer CE, Alavi A, Steinberg ME, Fallon M, Kressel HY 1987 Femoral head avascular necrosis: Correlation of MR imaging, and clinical findings. Radiology **162**:709–715.
16. Bonnarens F, Hernandez A, D'Ambrosia RD 1985 Bone scintigraphic changes in osteonecrosis of the femoral head. Orthop Clin North Am **16**:697–703.
17. Spencer JD, Maisey M 1985 A prospective scintigraphic study of avascular necrosis of bone in renal transplant patients. Clin Orthop **194**:125–135.
18. Dihlmann W 1982 CT analysis of the upper end of the femur: The asterisk sign and ischemic bone necrosis of the femoral head. Skeletal Radiol **8**:251–258.
19. Canale ST 1998 Campbell's Operative Orthopaedics, 9th ed. CV Mosby, St. Louis, MO, USA.
20. Smith SW, Fehring TK, Griffin WL, Beaver WB 1995 Core decompression of the osteonecrotic femoral head. J Bone Joint Surg Am **77**:674–680.

Chapter 81.   Infiltrative Disorders of Bone

Michael P. Whyte

Division of Bone and Mineral Diseases, Washington University School of Medicine at Barnes-Jewish Hospital and Center for Metabolic Bone Disease and Molecular Research, Shriners Hospitals for Children, St. Louis, Missouri

INTRODUCTION

Several important skeletal disorders feature excessive proliferation or infiltration of specific cell types within marrow spaces. Reviewed briefly here are systemic mastocytosis and histiocytosis-X.

SYSTEMIC MASTOCYTOSIS

Systemic mastocytosis, one of several disorders characterized by increased numbers of mast cells,[1] involves the viscera—principally the liver, spleen, gastrointestinal tract, and lymph nodes.[1-5] Additionally, the skin can contain numerous hyperpigmented macules that reflect dermal mast cell accumulation, a condition called *urticaria pigmentosa* (Fig. 1). Bone marrow is also typically involved and increasingly recognized to cause skeletal pathology. Patients often succumb to a granulocytic neoplasm.[1-3,6]

Symptoms of systemic mastocytosis result primarily from release of mediator substances by the mast cells and include generalized pruritus, urticaria, flushing, episodic hypotension, diarrhea, weight loss, peptic ulcer, and syncope.[1-5] With cutaneous involvement, histamine release occurs from stroking the skin causing urtication (Darier's sign). Skeletal complications develop relatively infrequently but include bone pain or tenderness from deformity resulting from fracture.[1-5,7-10] Serum tryptase elevation is a good, but not disease-specific, marker for systemic mastocytosis.[1] Urinary *N*-methylhistamine increase is an indicator of bone marrow involvement.[11]

Radiographic abnormalities of the skeleton are common in systemic mastocytosis (about 70% of patients). The disturbances have been thoroughly characterized.[12,13] Radiographs classically show diffuse, poorly demarcated, sclerotic, and lucent areas where red marrow is present (i.e., in the axial skeleton) (Fig. 2). However, circumscribed lesions can occur, especially in the skull and in the extremities. These focal findings may be mistaken for metastatic disease. Lytic areas are often small and have a surrounding rim of osteosclerosis; rarely, they are large and can lead to fracture. Progression of the radiographic changes can occur as regional involvement becomes generalized.[12,13] Focal bony changes may be absent despite extensive accumulation of mast cells in the skeleton. Generalized osteopenia (without discrete bony abnormalities) is also a common presentation,[7,8,10] but has a relatively benign prognosis.[14] Bone scintigraphy helps detect involved skeletal areas[15] and can provide information regarding disease activity and prognosis.[16] Reportedly, hip bone density correlates positively with urinary excretion of the histamine metabolite, methylimidazoleacetic acid.[17]

Histopathological correlates of systemic mastocytosis

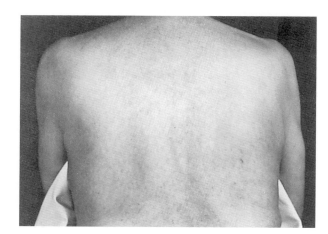

FIG. 1.   Systemic mastocytosis. Numerous characteristic hyperpigmented macules (urticaria pigmentosa) are present on the back of this 61-year-old woman.

within the skeleton are also well characterized.[3,7,18,19] In fact, it is increasingly apparent that examination of undecalcified sections of bone can be an especially effective way to establish the diagnosis. Transiliac crest biopsy may be superior for this purpose to bone marrow aspiration or biopsy.[7,18,19] Undecalcified sections of iliac crest show multiple nodules 150–450 μm in diameter that resemble granulomas (mast cell granulomas). Within the granulomas are characteristic oval or spindle-shaped mast cells, eosinophils, lymphocytes, and plasma cells. The spindle-shaped cells resemble histiocytes or fibroblasts, but they contain granules that stain metachromatically and are actually a type of mast cell (Fig. 3). In addition, the marrow contains increased numbers of these mast cells, individually or in small aggregates.[7,18,19] Tetracycline-based histomorphometry shows rapid skeletal remodeling.[18,19]

The etiology of systemic mastocytosis is unclear.[1-5] Persistence of mast cell disease after bone marrow transplantation (for an additional condition) suggests that a defective myeloid precursor cell is not the cause.[20,21] The disorder seems to be a multi-topic, monoclonal proliferation of cytologically and/or functionally abnormal tissue mast cells.[3] Many patients have a mutation in the *C-KIT* proto-oncogene in abnormal mast cells.[22]

Treatment of systemic mastocytosis is discussed in a number of reviews,[1-5,22-26] and must be "tailored" in individual patients.[1] Severe bone pain from advanced bone disease has been reported to respond to radiotherapy.[27] Bisphosphonates have controlled pain and improved bone density in early trials.[28]

HISTIOCYTOSIS-X

Histiocytosis-X is the term coined in 1953 to unify what had been regarded as three distinct entities: Letterer-Siwe

The author has no conflict of interest.

About 1200 cases of histiocytosis-X are diagnosed yearly in the United States. Sex incidence is equal. Northern Europeans are affected more commonly than Hispanics, and the condition is rare in blacks. Many tissues and organs can be involved, including brain, lung, oropharynx, gastrointestinal tract, skin, and bone marrow. Diabetes insipidus is common because of pituitary infiltration. Prognosis is age-related; infants and the elderly have poorer outcomes. The signs and symptoms of the three principal clinical forms also differ.

Letterer-Siwe disease presents between several weeks and 2 years of age with hepatosplenomegaly, lymphadenopathy, anemia, hemorrhagic tendency, fever, failure to grow, and skeletal lesions. It has ended fatally after just several weeks.[29,30]

Hand-Schüller-Christian disease is a chronic condition that begins in early childhood, although symptoms may not manifest until the third decade.[29,30] The classic triad of findings consists of exophthalmos, diabetes insipidus, and bony lesions. However, this presentation occurs in only 10% of cases. The most common skeletal manifestation is osteolytic lesions in the skull, with overlying soft tissue nodules (Fig. 4).[30,31] Proptosis is associated with destruction of orbital bones. There may be spontaneous remissions and exacerbations. Soft tissue nodules may remit without treatment.

Eosinophilic granuloma occurs most frequently in children between 3 and 10 years of age, and it is rare after the age of 15 years.[28,29] A solitary and painful lesion in a flat bone is the most common finding.[30,31] There may be a soft tissue mass. The calvarium is usually affected, although any bone can be involved. The prognosis is excellent, with monostotic lesions healing spontaneously or responding well to X-ray therapy.

The radiographic findings in the skeleton are similar in the three disorders.[11,12,30,31] Single bony foci are most prevalent. Nevertheless, multiple areas can be affected and show progressive enlargement. Individual lesions are well defined (i.e., "punched-out," osteolytic, and destructive with scalloped edges). They vary from a few millimeters to several centimeters in diameter. Fewer than one-half of these radiolucencies show marginal reactive osteosclerosis. Membranous bones as well as long bones can be affected. In the long bones, defects occur in the medullary canal where there is erosion of the endosteal cortex (commonly in the

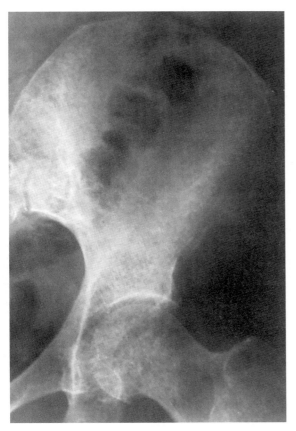

FIG. 2. Systemic mastocytosis. This 81-year-old woman has characteristic diffuse punctuate radiolucencies of her pelvis and hip that indicate a permeative process in the bone marrow.

disease, Hand-Schüller-Christian disease, and eosinophilic granuloma.[29,30] The Langerhans cell is considered the pathognomonic and linking feature, and the condition is now called Langerhans cell histiocytosis.[29,30] Histiocytosis-X seems to result from some poorly understood dysfunction of the immune system.[29] It is an extremely heterogeneous condition. Nevertheless, the tripartite distinction for histiocytosis-X continues to be used because of the generally different clinical courses and prognoses.[29,30]

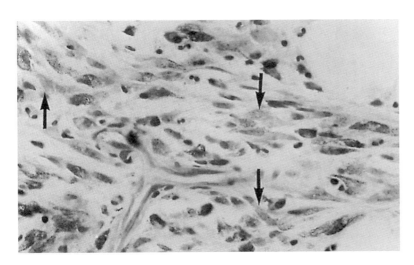

FIG. 3. Mast cell granuloma. A nondecalcified specimen of iliac crest shows a characteristic mast cell granuloma that contains numerous spindle-shaped mast cells (arrows) (Toluidine blue stain ×20).

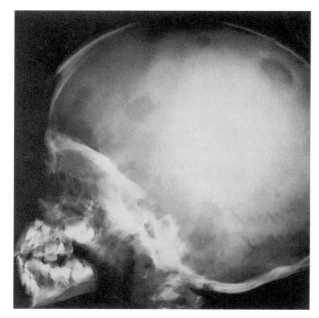

FIG. 4. Hand-Schüller-Christian disease. This 2-year-old boy has multiple, well-defined, beveled-edge, lucent lesions of the skull. Note the extensive destruction of the paranasal sinuses and at the base of the skull.

metaphyseal or epiphyseal regions). Periosteal reaction is frequent and produces a solid layer of new bone. In the skull, the bony tables can be eroded. Destruction of orbital bones may or may not be associated with exophthalmos. *Vertebra plana* (i.e., flattened vertebrae) can result from spinal involvement in young children. Radionuclide accumulation is poor during bone scanning.[11,12] Biochemical parameters of mineral homeostasis are usually normal.

Histiocytosis-X tends to be benign and self-limiting when there is no systemic involvement. Treatment for severe disease includes chemotherapy, radiation therapy, and immunotherapy.[32,33] Methylprednisolone injected into lesions is an effective procedure.[31] Central nervous system involvement is often treated by radiation therapy. Allogeneic bone marrow transplantation was reported to have been successful in a severe case with poor prognosis.[34]

REFERENCES

1. Valent P, Horny HP, Escribano L, Longley BJ, Li CY, Schwartz LB, Marone G, Nunez R, Akin C, Sotlar K, Sperr WR, Wolff K, Brunning RD, Parwaresch RM, Austen KF, Lennert K, Metcalfe DD, Vardiman JW, Bennett JM 2001 Diagnostic criteria and classification of mastocytosis: A consensus proposal. Leuk Res 25:603–625.
2. Valent P 1996 Biology, classification and treatment of human mastocytosis. Wien Klin Wochenschr 108:385–397.
3. Horny HP, Ruck P, Krober S, Kaiserling E 1997 Systemic mast cell disease (mastocytosis). General aspects and histopathological diagnosis. Histol Histopathol 12:1081–1089.
4. Marone G, Spadaro G, Genovese A 1995 Biology, diagnosis and therapy of mastocytosis. Chem Immunol 62:1–21.
5. Genovese A, Spadaro G, Triggiani M, Marone G 1995 Clinical advances in mastocytosis. Int J Clin Lab Res 25:178–188.
6. Lawrence JB, Friedman BS, Travis WD, Chinchilli VM, Metcalfe DD, Gralnick HR 1991 Hematologic manifestations of systemic mast cell disease: A prospective study of laboratory and morphologic features and their relation to prognosis. Am J Med 91:612–624.
7. Fallon MD, Whyte MP, Teitelbaum SL 1981 Systemic mastocytosis associated with generalized osteopenia: Histopathological character-ization of the skeletal lesion using undecalcified bone from two patients. Hum Pathol 12:813–820.
8. Harvey JA, Anderson HC, Borek D, Morris D, Lukert BP 1989 Osteoporosis associated with mastocytosis confined to bone: Report of two cases. Bone 10:237–241.
9. Cook JV, Chandy J 1989 Systemic mastocytosis affecting the skeletal system. J Bone Joint Surg Br 71B:536.
10. Lidor C, Frisch B, Gazit D, Gepstein R, Hallel T, Mekori YA 1990 Osteoporosis as the sole presentation of bone marrow mastocytosis. J Bone Miner Res 5:871–876.
11. Oranje AP, Riezebos P, van Toorenenbergen AW, Mulder PGH, Heide R, Tank B 2002 Urinary N-methylhistamine as an indicator of bone marrow involvement in mastocytosis. Clin Exp Dermatol 27:502–506.
12. Edeiken J, Dalinka M, Karasick D 1990 Edeiken's Roentgen Diagnosis of Diseases of Bone, 4th ed. Williams and Wilkins, Baltimore, MD, USA.
13. Resnick D, Niwayama G 2002 Diagnosis of Bone and Joint Disorders, 4th ed. WB Saunders, Philadelphia, PA, USA.
14. Andrew SM, Freemont AJ 1993 Skeletal mastocytosis. J Clin Pathol 46:1033–1035.
15. Arrington ER, Eisenberg B, Hartshorne MF, Vela S, Dorin RI 1989 Nuclear medicine imaging of systemic mastocytosis. J Nucl Med 30:2046–2048.
16. Chen CC, Andrich MP, Mican JM, Metcalfe DD 1994 A retrospective analysis of bone scan abnormalities in mastocytosis: Correlation with disease category and prognosis. J Nucl Med 35:1471–1475.
17. Johansson C, Roupe G, Lindstedt G, Mellstrom D 1996 Bone density, bone markers and bone radiological features in mastocytosis. Age Ageing 25:1–7.
18. de Gennes C, Kuntz D, de Vernejoul MC 1991 Bone mastocytosis. A report of nine cases with a bone histomorphometric study. Clin Orthop 279:281–291.
19. Chines A, Pacifici R, Avioli LV, Teitelbaum SL, Korenblat PE 1991 Systemic mastocytosis presenting as osteoporosis: A clinical and histomorphometric study. J Clin Endocrinol Metab 72:140–144.
20. Ronnov-Jessen D, Nielsen PL, Horn T 1991 Persistence of systemic mastocytosis after allogeneic bone marrow transplantation in spite of complete remission of the associated myelodysplastic syndrome. Bone Marrow Transplant 8:413–415.
21. Van Hoof A, Criel A, Louwagie A, Vanvuchelen J 1991 Cutaneous mastocytosis after autologous bone marrow transplantation. Bone Marrow Transplant 8:151–153.
22. Fritsche-Polanz R, Jordan JH, Feix Al, Sperr WR, Sunder-Plassmann G, Valent P, Födinger M 2001 Mutation analysis of C-KIT in patients with myelodysplastic syndromes without mastocytosis and cases of systemic mastocytosis. Br J Haematol 113:357–364.
23. Gasior-Chrzan B, Falk ES 1992 Systemic mastocytosis treated with histamine H1 and H2 receptor antagonists. Dermatology 184:149–152.
24. Metcalfe DD 1991 The treatment of mastocytosis: An overview. J Invest Dermatol 96:55S–59S.
25. Póvoa P, Ducla-Soares J, Fernandes A, Palma-Carlos AG 1991 A case of systemic mastocytosis: Therapeutic efficacy of ketotifen. J Intern Med 229:475–477.
26. Kluin-Nelemans HC, Jansen JH, Breukelman H, Wolthers BG, Kluin PM, Kroon HM, Willemze R 1992 Response to interferon α2b in a patient with systemic mastocytosis. N Engl J Med 326:619–623.
27. Johnstone PA, Mican JM, Metcalfe DD, DeLaney TF 1994 Radiotherapy of refractory bone pain due to systemic mast cell disease. Am J Clin Oncol 17:328–330.
28. Brumsen C, Hamady NAT, Papapoulos SE 2002 Osteoporosis and bone marrow mastocytosis: Dissociation of skeletal responses and mast cell activity during long-term bisphosphonate therapy. J Bone Miner Res 17:567–569.
29. Lam KY 1997 Langerhans cell histiocytosis (histiocytosis X). Postgrad Med J 73:391–394.
30. Nezelof C, Basset F 1998 Langerhans cell histiocytosis research. Past, present, and future. Hematol Oncol Clin North Am 12:385–406.
31. Alexander JE, Seibert JJ, Berry DH, Glasier CM, Williamson SL, Murphy J 1988 Prognostic factors for healing of bone lesions in histiocytosis X. Pediatr Radiol 18:326–332.
32. Bollini G, Jouve JL, Gentet JC, Jacquemier M, Bouyala JM 1991 Bone lesions in histiocytosis X. J Pediatr Orthop 11:469–477.
33. Greenberger JS, Crocker AC, Vawter G, Jaffe N, Cassady JR 1981 Results of treatment of 127 patients with systemic histiocytosis (Letterer-Siwe syndrome, Schüller-Christian syndrome and multifocal eosinophilic granuloma). Medicine (Baltimore) 60:311–388.
34. Ringdén O, Aohström L, Lönnqvist B, Boaryd I, Svedmyr E, Gahrton G 1987 Allogeneic bone marrow transplantation in a patient with chemotherapy-resistant progressive histiocytosis X. N Engl J Med 316:733–735.

Chapter 82.   Paget's Disease of Bone

Ethel S. Siris[1] and G. David Roodman[2]

[1]Department of Medicine, Columbia University College of Physicians and Surgeons, New York, New York; and [2]Department of Medicine, University of Pittsburgh School of Medicine, Pittsburgh, Pennsylvania

INTRODUCTION

Paget's disease of bone is a localized disorder of bone remodeling. The process is initiated by increases in osteoclast-mediated bone resorption, with subsequent compensatory increases in new bone formation, resulting in a disorganized mosaic of woven and lamellar bone at affected skeletal sites. This structural change produces bone that is expanded in size, less compact, more vascular, and more susceptible to deformity or fracture than is normal bone.[1] Clinical signs and symptoms will vary from one patient to the next depending on the number and location of affected skeletal sites, as well as on the degree and extent of the abnormal bone turnover. It is believed that most patients are asymptomatic, but a substantial minority may experience a variety of symptoms, including bone pain, secondary arthritic problems, bone deformity, excessive warmth over bone from hypervascularity, and a variety of neurological complications caused in most instances by compression of neural tissues adjacent to pagetic bone.

ETIOLOGY

Although Paget's disease is the second most common bone disease after osteoporosis, little still is known about its pathogenesis—why it is highly localized, the potential role paramyxoviral infection might play, the basis for the unusual geographic distribution, and the contribution of a genetic component to the disease process.

It is abundantly clear that there is a strong genetic predisposition involved in the pathophysiology of Paget's disease. Paget's disease occurs commonly in families and can be transmitted vertically between generations in an affected family. In patients with Paget's disease described in several clinical series, 15–30% have positive family histories of the disorder.[2] An extensive investigation of relatives of 35 patients with Paget's disease in Madrid revealed that 40% of the patients had at least one first-degree relative affected with the disease.[3] Other studies have confirmed an autosomal dominant pattern of inheritance for Paget's disease.[4] Familial aggregation studies in a United States population[5]

suggest that the risk of a first-degree relative of a pagetic subject developing the condition is seven times greater than is the risk for someone who does not have an affected relative.

As yet, no single genetic abnormality has been identified that explains familial Paget's disease. Cody et al.[6] described a predisposition locus on chromosome 18q in a large family with Paget's disease, and other groups have identified different predisposition loci on chromosome 18, and on chromosome 6.[7,8] No specific genes have been identified at these loci, and none are located on chromosome 13, which contains the *RANK ligand* gene. In a Japanese family with atypical Paget's disease, a mutation in the *RANK* gene has been reported,[9] but this mutation is not found in the overwhelming majority of patients with familial Paget's disease.[10]

Recently, Laurin et al.,[11] in Quebec, have mapped a mutation in a gene on 5q35-QTER, which encodes an ubiquitin binding protein, sequestasome-1 ($SQSTM14/p62^{ZIP}$), as a candidate gene for Paget's disease because of its association with the NFκB signaling pathway. This mutation results in a proline to leucine substitution at amino acid-392 of the protein that was not found in 291 controls. The mutation was detected in 11 of 24 French-Canadian families with Paget's disease and 18 unrelated Paget's disease patients. Sequestasome-1 acts as an anchor protein and plays an important role in the NFκB signaling pathway. It binds either TRAF-6 in the interleukin (IL)-1 or RIP-1 in the TNF signaling pathway to activate NFκB. However, the $p62^{ZIP}$ mutation does not completely explain the pagetic phenotype. There is large phenotypic variability in patients with Paget's disease associated with the mutation in $p62^{ZIP}$. For example, one individual who is 77 years old and carried this $p62^{ZIP}$ mutation had no signs of the disease.[12] Moreover, homozygotes and heterozygotes seem to be similarly affected, suggesting that other genetic and/or environmental factors such as a common viral infection may contribute to the variability and the severity of Paget's disease of bone.[12] Hocking et al.[8] have studied a large group of patients with familial Paget's disease and found a mutation in the $p62^{ZIP}$ gene in 19% of the patients. A second mutation in $p62^{ZIP}$, in which a T insertion that introduces a stop code in position 396, was also found in 6% of the families, and a third mutation affecting a splice donor site in intron A was found in 2% of the families. Thus, 30% of patients with familial

Dr. Roodman has served as a consultant and speaker for Novartis. Dr. Siris has served as a consultant for Merck, Novartis, and Procter & Gamble.

Paget's disease have mutations in the $p62^{ZIP}$ gene. These mutations are associated with a variable clinical phenotype, including no evidence of Paget's disease in at least one or two individuals, and they cannot explain the highly localized nature of the disease.

Ethnic and geographic clustering of Paget's disease also has been described, with the intriguing observation that the disorder is quite common in some parts of the world but relatively rare in others. Clinical observations indicate that the disease is most common in Europe, North America, Australia, and New Zealand. Studies surveying radiologists have computed prevalence rates in hospitalized patients older than 55 years in several European cities and found the highest percentages in England (4.6%) and France (2.4%), with other Western European countries reporting slightly lower prevalences (e.g., 0.7–1.7% in Ireland, 1.3% in Spain and West Germany, and 0.5% in Italy and Greece).[13] There is a remarkable focus of Paget's disease in Lancashire, England, where 6.3–8.3% of people older than 55 years in several Lancashire towns had radiographs revealing Paget's disease.[14]

Prevalence rates appear to decrease from north to south in Europe, except for the finding that Norway and Sweden have a particularly low rate (0.3%).[13] Few data are available from Eastern Europe, but Russian colleagues indicate that Paget's disease is not uncommon in that country. The disorder is seen in Australia and in New Zealand at rates of 3–4%.[15] Paget's disease is distinctly rare in Asia, particularly in China, India, and Malaysia, although occasional cases of Indians living in the United States have been documented. Similar radiographic studies have described a prevalence of 0.01–0.02% in several areas of sub-Saharan Africa.[15] In Israel, the disease is seen predominantly in Jews[16] but was recently found to exist in Israeli Arabs as well.[17] In Argentina, the disease seems to be restricted to an area surrounding Buenos Aires and predominantly occurs in patients descended from European immigrants.[18] It is estimated, based on very few studies, that 2–3% of people older than 55 years living in the United States have Paget's disease. It is believed that most Americans with Paget's disease are white and of Anglo-Saxon or European descent. The disorder is described in African-American, and most clinical series from hospitals in major American cities report having African-American patients.[2,19]

Some recent studies have remarked on an apparent decline in the frequency and severity of Paget's disease in both New Zealand and Great Britain.[20,21]

For more than 30 years, studies have suggested that Paget's disease may result from a chronic paramyxoviral infection. This is based on ultrastructural studies by Rebel et al.,[22] who demonstrated that nuclear and cytoplasmic inclusions, which were similar to nucleocapsids from paramyxoviruses, were present in osteoclasts from Paget's disease patients. Mills et al.[23] also reported that the measles virus nucleocapsid antigen was present in osteoclasts from patients with Paget's disease but not from patients with other bone diseases. In some specimens, both measles virus and respiratory syncytial virus nucleocapsid proteins were demonstrated by immunocytochemistry on serial sections. Similarly, Basle et al.[24] have also demonstrated presence of measles virus nucleocapsid protein in patients

with Paget's disease, but also found other paramyxoviral proteins as well.

Recently, Friedrichs et al.[25] have reported the full sequence of the measles virus nucleocapsid protein isolated from a patient with Paget's disease as well as 700 base pairs of measles virus nucleocapsid protein sequence from three other patients. In contrast, Gordon et al.,[26] using in situ hybridization studies, examined specimens from English patients with Paget's disease and found canine distemper virus nucleocapsid protein in 11 of 25 patients. Mee et al.,[27] using highly sensitive in situ polymerase chain reaction (PCR) techniques, found that osteoclasts from 12 of 12 English patients with Paget's disease expressed canine distemper virus nucleocapsid transcripts.

Kurihara et al.[28] have provided evidence for a possible pathophysiologic role for measles virus in the abnormal osteoclast activity in Paget's disease. They transfected the measles virus nucleocapsid gene into normal human osteoclast precursors and demonstrated that the osteoclasts that formed expressed many of the abnormal characteristics of pagetic osteoclasts. However, other workers have been unable to confirm the presence of measles virus or CDV in pagetic osteoclasts[29]; therefore, the role of a chronic paramyxoviral infection in Paget's disease remains controversial.

Among the many questions that need to be explained to understand a putative viral etiology of Paget's disease are (1) since paramyxoviral infections such as measles virus occur worldwide, why does Paget's disease have a very restricted geographic distribution and (2) how does the virus persist in osteoclasts in patients who are immunocompetent for such long periods of time, as measles virus infections generally occur in children rather than adults and Paget's disease is usually diagnosed in patients over the age of 55?

The presence of an acquired or inherited genetic component to explain Paget's disease has its limitations as well. It is very difficult to explain the variable phenotypic presentation of patients with familial Paget's disease, especially that some of these patients who carry the mutated gene do not have Paget's disease although they are over 70 years of age. Furthermore, it is very difficult to explain how a mutation of a specific gene expressed in bone results in a highly focal disease such as Paget's disease. More likely, environmental factors and genetic factors are both required for patients to develop Paget's disease.

PATHOLOGY

Histopathologic Findings in Paget's Disease

The initiating lesion in Paget's disease is an increase in bone resorption. This occurs in association with an abnormality in the osteoclasts found at affected sites. Pagetic osteoclasts are more numerous than normal and contain substantially more nuclei than do normal osteoclasts, with up to 100 nuclei per cell noted by some investigators. In response to the increase in bone resorption, numerous osteoblasts are recruited to pagetic sites where active and rapid new bone formation occurs. It is generally believed that the osteoblasts are intrinsically normal,[30] but this is not proven conclusively.

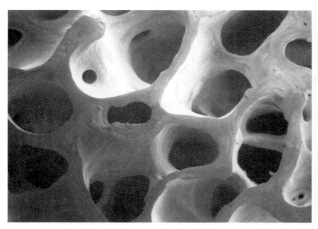 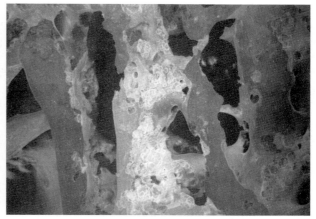

FIG. 1. Scanning electron micrographs with sections of normal bone (left) and pagetic bone (right). Both samples were taken from the iliac crest. The normal bone shows the trabecular plates and marrow spaces to be well preserved, whereas the pagetic bone has completely lost this architectural appearance. Extensive pitting of the pagetic bone is apparent, due to dramatically increased osteoclastic bone resorption. [Photographs courtesy of Dr. David Dempster; reproduced from J Bone Miner Res 1986;**1**:15–21 with permission of the American Society for Bone and Mineral Research (left); and Siris ES, Canfield RE 1995 Paget's disease of bone. In: Becker KL (ed.) Principles and Practice of Endocrinology and Metabolism, 2nd ed. JB Lippincott, Philadelphia, PA, USA, pp. 585–594 (right).]

In the earliest phases of Paget's disease, increased osteoclastic bone resorption dominates, a picture appreciated radiographically by an advancing lytic wedge or "blade-of-grass" lesion in a long bone or by osteoporosis circumscripta, as seen in the skull. At the level of the bone biopsy, the structurally abnormal osteoclasts are abundant. After this, there is a combination of increased resorption and relatively tightly coupled new-bone formation, produced by the large numbers of osteoblasts present at these sites. During this phase, and presumably because of the accelerated nature of the process, the new bone that is made is abnormal. Newly deposited collagen fibers are laid down in a haphazard rather than a linear fashion, creating more primitive woven bone. The woven-bone pattern is not specific for Paget's disease, but it does reflect a high rate of bone turnover. The end product is the so-called mosaic pattern of woven bone plus irregular sections of lamellar bone linked in a disorganized way by numerous cement lines representing the extent of previous areas of bone resorption. The bone marrow becomes infiltrated by excessive fibrous connective tissue and by an increased number of blood vessels, explaining the hypervascular state of the bone. Bone matrix at pagetic sites is usually normally mineralized, and tetracycline labeling shows increased calcification rates. It is not unusual, however, to find areas of pagetic biopsy specimens in which widened osteoid seams are apparent, perhaps reflecting inadequate calcium/phosphorus products in localized areas where rapid bone turnover heightens mineral demands.

In time, the hypercellularity at a locus of affected bone may diminish, leaving the end product of a sclerotic, pagetic mosaic without evidence of active bone turnover. This is so-called burned out Paget's disease. Typically, all phases of the pagetic process can be seen at the same time at different sites in a particular subject. Scanning electron microscopy affords an excellent view of the chaotic architectural changes that occur in pagetic bone and provides the visual imagery that makes comprehensible the loss of structural integrity. Figure 1 compares the appearances of normal and of pagetic bone using this technique. Figure 2 show the mosaic pattern of disorganized bone in Paget's disease in most of the field, contrasted with a normal pattern of new bone deposition after restoration of normal turnover with bisphosphonate therapy.

Biochemical Parameters of Paget's Disease

Increases in the urinary excretion of biomarkers of bone resorption such as collagen cross-links and associated peptides (e.g., NTX, CTX, DPD)[31] reflect the primary lesion in Paget's disease, the increase in bone resorption. Increases in osteoblastic activity are associated with elevated levels of serum alkaline phosphatase. In untreated patients, the values of these two markers rise in proportion to each other, offering a reflection of the preserved coupling between resorption and formation. From the clinical perspective, the

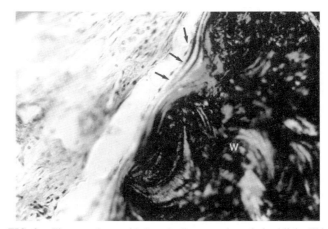

FIG. 2. Iliac crest bone with Paget's disease under polarized light. This patient had been treated with potent bisphosphonate therapy. Older bone is present in a pattern of woven bone (W), but new bone deposition after suppression of increased pagetic turnover shows a normal pattern of bone deposition (arrows).

degree of elevation of these indices offers an approximation of the extent or severity of the abnormal bone turnover, with higher levels reflecting a more active, ongoing localized metabolic process. Interestingly, the patients with the highest alkaline phosphatase elevations (e.g., >10 times the upper limit of normal) typically have involvement of the skull as at least one site of the disorder. Active monostotic disease (other than skull) may have lower biochemical values than polyostotic disease. Lower values (e.g., <3 times the upper limit of normal) may reflect a lesser extent of involvement (i.e., fewer sites on bone scans or radiographs) or a burned-out form of Paget's disease, especially in a very elderly person known to have had extensive polyostotic disease in the past. However, mild elevations in a patient with highly localized disease (e.g., the proximal tibia) may be associated with symptoms and clear progression of disease at the affected site over time. Indeed, a so-called "normal" alkaline phosphatase (e.g., a value a slightly less than the upper limit of normal for the assay) may not truly be normal for the pagetic patient. Today, many would argue that to be confident that the value is normal (and the disease quiescent), a result in the middle of the normal range is required.

In addition to offering some estimate of the degree of abnormal bone turnover, the bone resorption markers and alkaline phosphatase measurements are useful in observing the disorder over time and especially for monitoring the effects of treatment. With the potent new bisphosphonates that are capable of normalizing the biochemical markers (i.e., producing a remission of the bone-remodeling abnormality) in a majority of patients and bringing the markers to near normal in most others, the monitoring role has heightened importance. Urinary resorption markers such as the N-telopeptide of collagen or deoxypyridinoline may become normal in days to a few weeks after bisphosphonate therapy is initiated. It is often most practical and the least expensive, however, to monitor serum alkaline phosphatase as the sole biochemical endpoint, with a baseline measure and subsequent follow-up tests at intervals appropriate for the therapy used. If a patient has concomitant elevations of liver enzymes, a measurement of bone-specific alkaline phosphatase can be especially helpful. Serum osteocalcin, however, is not a useful measurement in Paget's disease.

Serum calcium levels are typically normal in Paget's disease, but they may become elevated in two special situations. First, if a patient with active, usually extensive Paget's disease is immobilized, the loss of the weight-bearing stimulus to new bone formation may transiently uncouple resorption and accretion, so that increasing hypercalciuria and hypercalcemia may occur. This is a relatively infrequent occurrence. Alternatively, when hypercalcemia is discovered in an otherwise healthy, ambulatory patient with Paget's disease, coexistent primary hyperparathyroidism may be the cause. Inasmuch as increased levels of parathyroid hormone (PTH) can drive the intrinsic pagetic remodeling abnormality to even higher levels of activity, correction of primary hyperparathyroidism in such cases is indicated.

Several investigators have commented on the 15–20% prevalence of secondary hyperparathyroidism (associated with normal levels of serum calcium) in Paget's disease, typically seen in patients with very high levels of serum alkaline phosphatase.[32,33] The increase in PTH is believed to reflect the need to increase calcium availability to bone during phases of very active pagetic bone formation, particularly in subjects in whom dietary intake of calcium is inadequate. Secondary hyperparathyroidism and transient decreases in serum calcium also can occur in some patients being treated with potent bisphosphonates such as pamidronate, alendronate, or risedronate. This results from the effective and rapid suppression of bone resorption in the setting of ongoing new-bone formation.[34] Later, as restoration of coupling occurs with time, PTH levels fall. The problem can be largely avoided by being certain that such patients are and remain calcium and vitamin D replete.

Elevations in serum uric acid and serum citrate have been described in Paget's disease and are of unclear clinical significance.[1] Gout has been noted in this disorder, but it is uncertain whether it is more common in pagetic patients than in nonpagetic subjects. Hypercalciuria may occur in some patients with Paget's disease, presumably because of the increased bone resorption, and kidney stones are occasionally found as a consequence of this abnormality.[1]

CLINICAL FEATURES

Paget's disease affects both men and women, with most series describing a slight male predominance. It is rarely observed to occur in individuals younger than age 25 years; it is thought to develop as a clinical entitiy after the age of 40 in most instances, and it is most commonly diagnosed in people over the age of 50. In a survey of over 800 selected patients in the United States, 600 of whom had symptoms, the average age at diagnosis was 58 years.[35] It seems likely that many patients have the disorder for a period of time before any diagnosis is made, especially because it is often an incidental finding.

It is important to emphasize the localized nature of Paget's disease. It may be monostotic, affecting only a single bone or portion of a bone (Fig. 3), or may be polyostotic, involving two or more bones. Sites of disease are often asymmetric. A patient might have a pagetic right femur with a normal left, involvement of only one-half the pelvis, or involvement of several noncontiguous vertebral bodies. Clinical observation suggests that in most instances, sites affected with Paget's disease when the diagnosis is made are the only ones that will show pagetic change over time. Although progression of disease within a given bone may occur (Fig. 4), the sudden appearance of new sites of involvement years after the initial diagnosis is uncommon. This information can be very reassuring for patients who often worry about extension of the disorder to new areas of the skeleton as they age.

The most common sites of involvement include the pelvis, femur, spine, skull, and tibia. The bones of the upper extremity, as well as the clavicles, scapulae, ribs, and facial bones, are less commonly involved, and the hands and feet are only rarely affected. It is generally believed that most patients with Paget's disease are asymptomatic and that the disorder is most often diagnosed when an elevated serum alkaline phosphatase is noted on routine screening or when

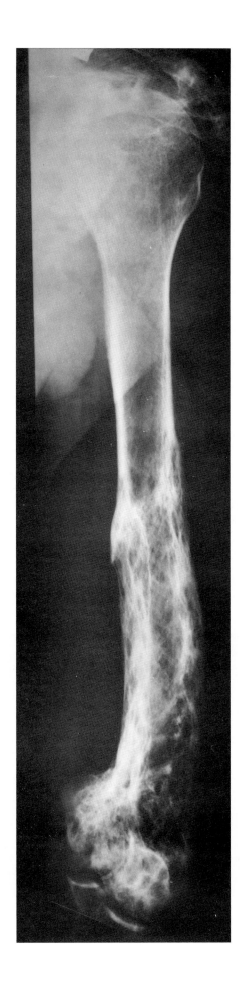

a radiograph taken for an unrelated problem reveals typical skeletal changes. The development of symptoms or complications of Paget's disease is influenced by the particular areas of involvement, the interrelationship between affected bone and adjacent structures, the extent of metabolic activity, and presence or absence of disease progression within an affected site.

Signs and Symptoms

Bone pain from a site of pagetic involvement, experienced either at rest or with motion, is probably the most common symptom. The direct cause of the pain may be difficult to characterize and requires careful evaluation. Pagetic bone has an increased vascularity, leading to a warmth of the bone that some patients perceive as an unpleasant sensation. Small transverse lucencies along the expanded cortices of involved weight-bearing bones or advancing, lytic, blade-of-grass lesions sometimes cause pain. It is postulated that microfractures frequently occur in pagetic bone and can cause discomfort for a period of days to weeks.

A bowing deformity of the femur or tibia can lead to pain for several possible reasons. A bowed limb is typically shortened, resulting in specific gait abnormalities that can lead to abnormal mechanical stresses. Clinically severe secondary arthritis can occur at joints adjacent to pagetic bone (e.g., the hip, knee, or ankle). The secondary gait problems also may lead to arthritic changes on the contralateral nonpagetic side, particularly at the hip.

Back pain in pagetic patients is another difficult symptom to assess. Nonspecific aches and pains may emanate from enlarged pagetic vertebrae in some instances; vertebral compression fractures also may be seen. In the lumbar area, spinal stenosis with neural impingement may arise, producing radicular pain and possibly motor impairment. Degenerative changes in the spine may accompany pagetic changes, and it is useful for the clinician to determine which symptoms arise as a consequence of the pagetic process and which result from degenerative disease of nonpagetic vertebrae. Kyphosis may occur, or there may be a forward tilt of the upper back, particularly when a compression fracture or spinal stenosis is present. Treatment options will differ, depending on the symptoms. When Paget's disease affects the thoracic spine, there may rarely be syndromes of direct spinal cord compression with motor and sensory changes. Several cases of apparent direct cord compression with loss of neural function have now been documented to have resulted from a vascular steal syndrome, whereby hypervascular pagetic bone "steals" blood from the neural tissue.[36]

Paget's disease of the skull, demonstrated radiographically in Fig. 5, may be asymptomatic, but common complaints in up to one-third of patients with skull involvement may include an increase in head size with or without frontal bossing or deformity, or headache, sometimes described as a band-like tightening around the head. Hearing loss may

FIG. 3. Radiograph of a humerus showing typical pagetic change in the distal half, with cortical thickening, expansion, and mixed areas of lucency and sclerosis, contrasted with normal bone in the proximal half.

© 2003 American Society for Bone and Mineral Research

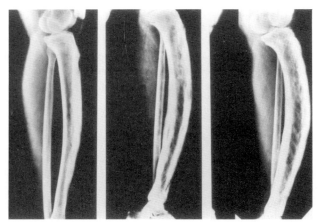

FIG. 4. This series of radiographs of a pagetic tibia show progression of pagetic change and bowing deformity in an untreated patient. This individual's Paget's disease was limited to the tibia and was associated with a serum alkaline phosphatase level that was generally only mildly elevated to about twice the upper limit of normal. Note the distal progression of cortical thickening with time, as well as the worsening of the bowing deformity. (Reproduced from J Bone Miner Res 1997;**12:**691–692 with permission of the American Society for Bone and Mineral Research.)

occur as a result of isolated or combined conductive or neurosensory abnormalities; recent data suggest cochlear damage from pagetic involvement of the temporal bone is an important component.[37] Cranial nerve palsies (such as in nerves II, VI, and VII) occur rarely. With extensive skull involvement, a softening of the base of the skull may produce platybasia, or flattening, with the development of basilar invagination, so that the odontoid process begins to extend upward as the skull sinks downward on it. This feature can be appreciated by various radiographic measures, including skull radiographs and computed tomography (CT) or magnetic resonance imaging (MRI) scans. Although many patients with severe skull changes may have radiographic evidence of basilar invagination, a relatively small number develop a very serious complication, such as direct brainstem compression or an obstructive hydrocephalus and increased intracranial pressure caused by blockage of cerebrospinal fluid flow. Pagetic involvement of the facial bones may cause facial deformity, dental problems, and, rarely, narrowing of the airway. Mechanical changes of these types may lead to a nasal intonation when the patient is speaking.

Fracture through pagetic bone is an occasional and serious complication. These fractures may be either traumatic or pathological, particularly involving long bones with active areas of advancing lytic disease; the most common involve the femoral shaft or subtrochanteric area.[38] The increased vascularity of actively remodeling pagetic bone (i.e., with a moderately increased serum alkaline phosphatase) may lead to substantial blood loss in the presence of fractures caused by trauma. Fractures also may occur in the presence of areas of malignant degeneration, a rare complication of Paget's disease. Far more common are the small fissure fractures along the convex surfaces of bowed lower extremities, which may be asymptomatic, stable, and persistent for years, but sometimes a more extensive transverse lucent area extends medially from the cortex and may lead

to a clinical fracture with time. As described later, there are data indicating that blade-of-grass lytic areas as well as these larger transverse fractures may respond to antipagetic treatment and heal. These types of lesions warrant radiographic follow-up over time. Conversely, the smaller fissure fractures typically do not change with treatment, and in the absence of new pain, rarely require extensive radiographic monitoring. In most cases, fracture through pagetic bone heals normally, although some groups have reported as high as a 10% rate of nonunion.

Neoplastic degeneration of pagetic bone is a relatively rare event, occurring with an incidence of less than 1%. This abnormality has a grave prognosis, typically manifesting itself as new pain at a pagetic site. The most common site of sarcomatous change appears to be the pelvis, with the femur and humerus next in frequency.[39] Typically these lesions are osteolytic. The majority of the tumors are classified as osteogenic sarcomas, although both fibrosarcomas and chondrosarcomas are also seen. Current treatment regimens emphasize maximal resection of tumor mass and chemotherapy and sometimes radiotherapy. Unfortunately, in these typically elderly patients, death from massive local extension of disease or from pulmonary metastases occurs in the majority of cases in 1–3 years.

Benign giant-cell tumors also may occur in bone affected by Paget's disease. These lesions may present as localized masses at the affected site. Radiographic evaluation may disclose lytic changes. Biopsy reveals clusters of large osteoclast-like cells, which some authors believe represent reparative granulomas.[40] These tumors may show a remarkable sensitivity to glucocorticoids, so in many instances, the mass will shrink or even disappear after treatment with prednisone or dexamethasone.[41]

DIAGNOSIS

When Paget's disease is suspected, the diagnostic evaluation should include a careful medical history and physical

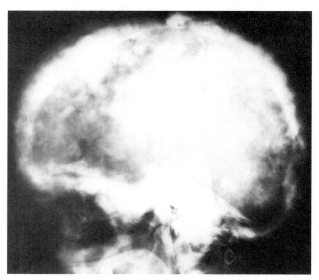

FIG. 5. Typical "cotton-wool" appearance of an enlarged pagetic skull with marked osteoblastic change. The patient had an increase in head size and deafness.

examination. The possibility of a positive family history and a symptom history should be ascertained. Gout, pseudogout, and arthritis are all possible complications of Paget's disease. Rarely, patients with underlying intrinsic heart disease may develop congestive heart failure in the presence of severe Paget's disease. There are also reports suggesting that patients may have an increased incidence of calcific aortic disease.[42] Angioid streaks are seen on funduscopic examination of the eye in some patients with polyostotic Paget's disease. The physical examination also should note the presence or absence of warmth, tenderness, or bone deformity in the skull, spine, pelvis, and extremities, as well as evidence of loss of range of motion at major joints or leg length discrepancy.

Laboratory tests include measurement of serum alkaline phosphatase and in some cases a urinary marker of bone resorption, as described earlier. Radiographic studies (bone scans and conventional radiographs) complete the initial evaluation. Bone biopsy is not usually indicated, because the characteristic radiographic and laboratory findings are diagnostic in most instances.

Bone scans are the most sensitive means of identifying pagetic sites and are most useful for this purpose. Scans are nonspecific, however, and also can be positive in nonpagetic areas that have degenerative changes or, more ominously, may reflect metastatic disease. Plain radiographs of bones noted to be positive on the bone scan provide the most specific information, because the changes noted on the radiograph are usually characteristic to the point of being pathognomonic. Examples of these are shown in Figs. 3–5. Enlargement or expansion of bone, cortical thickening, coarsening of trabecular markings, and typical lytic and sclerotic changes may be found. Radiographs also provide data on the status of the joints adjacent to involved sites, identify fissure fractures, indicate the degree to which lytic or sclerotic lesions predominate, and show the presence or absence of deformity or fracture.

Repeated scans or radiographs are usually unnecessary in observing patients over time, unless new symptoms develop or current symptoms become significantly worse. The possibility of an impending fracture, or rarely, of sarcomatous change should be borne in mind in these situations. Although imaging studies such as CT or MRI scans are not usually required in routine cases, a CT scan may be helpful in the assessment of a fracture where radiographs are not sufficient, and MRI scans are quite useful in assessing the possibility of sarcoma, giant cell tumor, or metastatic disease at a site of Paget's disease, in which case discovery of an accompanying soft tissue mass aids in diagnosis.

The characteristic X-ray and clinical features of Paget's disease usually eliminate problems with differential diagnosis. However, an older patient may occasionally present with severe bone pain, elevations of the serum alkaline phosphatase and urinary N-telopeptide or deoxypyridinoline, a positive bone scan, and less-than-characteristic radiographic areas of lytic or blastic change. Here, the possibility of metastatic disease to bone or some other form of metabolic bone disease (e.g., osteomalacia with secondary hyperparathyroidism) must be considered. Old radiographs and laboratory tests are very helpful in this setting, because normal studies 1 year earlier would make a diagnosis of Paget's disease less likely. A similar dilemma occurs when someone with known and established Paget's disease develops multiple painful new sites; here, too, the likelihood of metastatic disease must be carefully considered, and bone biopsy for a tissue diagnosis may be indicated.

TREATMENT

Antipagetic Therapy

Specific antipagetic therapy consists of those agents capable of suppressing the activity of pagetic osteoclasts. Currently approved agents available by prescription in the United States include five bisphosphonate compounds: orally administered etidronate, tiludronate, alendronate, and risedronate, and intravenously administered pamidronate; and parenterally administered calcitonin. Each of these is discussed later.

Between the mid-1970s when treatments became available for the first time and the mid-1990s, the mainstays of therapy were calcitonin and etidronate. However, these agents should generally be replaced as the first lines of therapy by the newer bisphosphonates, pamidronate, alendronate, and risedronate, all progressively more potent than either etidronate or calcitonin, offering the potential for greater disease suppression and frank remission (i.e., normalization of pagetic indices) for prolonged periods. In addition to the newer bisphosphonates mentioned earlier, clodronate, more potent than etidronate and available in several other countries, has been shown to be effective in Paget's disease.[43] Olpadronate, neridronate, and ibandronate have significant activity as in Paget's disease[44–46]; zoledronate (zoledronic acid) is the most potent bisphosphonate under investigation to date in this disease.[47] Gallium nitrate, approved in the United States for the treatment of cancer hypercalcemia, has been studied for efficacy in Paget's disease.[48] Other symptomatic treatments for Paget's disease, including analgesics, anti-inflammatory drugs, and selected orthopedic and neurosurgical interventions, have important roles in management in many patients.

Two logical indications for treatment of Paget's disease are to relieve symptoms and to prevent future complications. It has been clearly demonstrated that suppression of the pagetic process by any of the available agents can effectively ameliorate certain symptoms in the majority of patients. Symptoms such as bone aches or pain (probably the most common complaints of Paget's disease), excessive warmth over bone, headache caused by skull involvement, low-back pain secondary to pagetic vertebral changes, and some syndromes of neural compression (e.g., radiculopathy and some examples of slowly progressive brainstem or spinal cord compression) are the most likely to be relieved. Pain caused by a secondary arthritis from pagetic bone involving the spine, hip, knee, ankle, or shoulder may or may not respond to antipagetic treatment. Filling in of osteolytic blade-of-grass lesions in weight-bearing bones has been reported in some treated cases with either calcitonin or bisphosphonates. On the other hand, a bowed extremity or other bone deformity will not change after treatment, and deafness is unlikely to improve, although limited studies (with calcitonin) suggest that progression of hearing loss may be slowed.[49]

A second indication for treatment is to prevent the development of late complications in those patients deemed to be at risk, based on their sites of involvement and evidence of active disease, as shown by elevated levels of bone turnover markers. Admittedly, it has not been proved that suppression of pagetic bone turnover will prevent future complications. However, as shown in Fig. 2, there is a restoration of normal patterns of new bone deposition in biopsy specimens after suppression of pagetic activity. It is also clear that active, untreated disease can continue to undergo a persistent degree of abnormal bone turnover for many years, with the possibility of severe bone deformity over time, as shown in Fig. 4. Indeed, substantial (e.g., 50%) but incomplete suppression of elevated indices of bone turnover with older therapies has been associated with disease progression[50]; with bisphosphonates such as pamidronate, alendronate, and risedronate, however, indices become normal after treatment for extended periods in the majority of patients and approach normal in most of the rest.

Thus, in the view of some investigators, the presence of asymptomatic but active disease (i.e., a serum alkaline phosphatase above normal) at sites where the potential for later problems or complications exists (e.g., weight-bearing bones, areas near major joints, vertebral bodies, extensively involved skull) is an indication for treatment.[51] The need for treatment in this setting may be particularly valid in patients who are younger, for whom many years of coexistence with the disorder are likely. However, even in the elderly, one can justify treatment if a degree of bone deformity is present that might create serious problems in the next few years. Others argue that the evidence does not yet support such use, because it has not been shown in clinical trials that disease suppression reduces progression of deformity.[52]

Although controlled studies are not available to prove efficaciousness in this situation, the use of antipagetic therapy before elective surgery on pagetic bone also is recommended.[53] The goal here is to reduce the hypervascularity associated with moderately active disease (e.g., a threefold or more elevation in serum alkaline phosphatase) to reduce the amount of blood loss at operation.

Recently, recommendations for the management of Paget's disease have been published as guideline or management documents by consensus panels in the United States,[51] United Kingdom,[52] and Canada,[54] and the reader is referred to these thoughtful reviews.

Bisphosphonates

The discussion that follows will consider this class of drugs in their ascending order of potency and to some extent in terms of their historical development. It should be emphasized that while any of these medications might be chosen in a specific case, the agents that are considered to be first line at the time of this writing are pamidronate, alendronate, and risedronate.

Etidronate. Etidronate was the first bisphosphonate to have been used clinically in the United States for Paget's dis-

ease[55,56] and was one of the two mainstays of therapy (with salmon calcitonin) for nearly 20 years. It is the least potent of the currently available bisphosphonate drugs. Etidronate is commercially available as Didronel in a 200- or 400-mg tablet. Although only a small percentage of the administered dose is absorbed, 5 mg/kg/day will provide a 50% lowering of biochemical indices and a reduction in symptoms in the majority of patients.

All bisphosphonates have the capacity to impair mineralization of newly forming bone if high enough doses are used. The dose of etidronate is limited by the fact that the doses that most effectively reduce the increased bone resorption can also impair mineralization, compelling the use of lower doses given for no longer than 6 months at a time. Thus, the recommended regimen for the agent is 5 mg/kg/day (i.e., 400 mg in most patients, taken with a small amount of water midway in a 4-h fast any time of day) for a 6-month period, followed by at least 6 months of no treatment. Etidronate is contraindicated in the presence of advancing lytic changes in a weight-bearing bone. Over several years of repeated 6-month-on, 6-month-off cycles, long-term benefit with maintenance of lower levels of pagetic biochemical activity has been observed in many patients, although others have become resistant to it after repeated courses. A failure to adhere to a cyclic low-dose regimen as described can induce bone pain, and occasionally, fracture caused by focal osteomalacia secondary to mineralization problems from excessive etidronate. However, careful cyclic management has been well tolerated by the majority of patients. Occasionally mild transient diarrhea may occur with etidronate, but this does not usually require more than a day or two of withholding the agent, after which it maybe taken again. More severe new pain in patients taking etidronate warrants stopping the drug and evaluating the patient before continuing therapy, to be certain that lytic disease or impending fracture (particularly in a weight-bearing extremity) has not been exacerbated.

In summary, etidronate is well tolerated in most, relatively easy to administer, but affords a less robust suppression of turnover than the newer bisphosphonates and has the associated risk of mineralization problems with over use.

Tiludronate. Tiludronate is about 10 times more potent than etidronate, and its use at effective doses is not associated with mineralization problems. Approved by the Food and Drug Administration (FDA) for Paget's disease in 1997, it is available as Skelid in a 200-mg tablet. The recommended dosage is 400 mg daily for 3 months, with a 3-month post-treatment observation period, after which the serum alkaline phosphatase is likely to have reached its nadir. This approach led to a normal serum alkaline phosphatase at the 6-month point in 24–35% of moderately affected subjects in clinical trials.[57,58] It is generally well tolerated, with a minority of patients experiencing mild upper gastrointestinal upset. It seems to offer the benefits of etidronate without the risk of mineralization problems in patients for whom this might be a concern (e.g., those with lytic disease in lower extremities) and one-half the total number of days of pills in a treatment course. As with etidronate, 400 mg of tiludronate should be taken with some water (in this case 6–8 oz) at least 2 h away from food and the patient should not lie down for the next 30 minutes. Patients also need to be calcium and vitamin D replete, but calcium supplements, like food, should not be taken within 2 h of the tiludronate dose.

Clinical experience with tiludronate is still relatively limited, with few data regarding duration of efficacy. It is a reasonable alternative to etidronate in patients with mild disease because it is well tolerated and requires only 3 months of active treatment. Patients who respond should have serum alkaline phosphatase measured at 3- to 4-month intervals and can be retreated when indices increase above normal or above a nadir level by 25% or more.

Pamidronate. Pamidronate is in the range of 100 times more potent than etidronate. With its availability in the mid-1990s, a new philosophy of and approach to management became available to the clinician. The greater potency of pamidronate (and also of the two newer agents, alendronate and risedronate) allows a majority of patients to experience a normalization of pagetic indices rather than only partial suppression, as is seen with calcitonin, etidronate, and (in most cases) tiludronate. Second, the effects may be longer lasting, so a limited course of treatment may provide up to 1 year or more of disease suppression. Third, all of the potent newer bisphosphonates have a much more favorable ratio of inhibition of bone resorption to inhibition of mineralization, so the threat of focal osteomalacia should be markedly reduced if not eliminated.

With pamidronate, there is an opportunity to individualize the dosing regimen to the needs of the specific patient, and there really is no single best dose. Indeed, the literature is replete with numerous approaches,[59–61] all of which seem to be effective. The package insert for pamidronate, available as Aredia, recommends three daily infusions of 30 mg each, over a period of 4 h each time, in 500 ml of normal saline or 5% dextrose in water. In clinical practice, experience has shown that this is probably not the best mode of administration. This dose is probably not high enough to achieve normalization of indices for many patients, and three daily infusions are highly impractical in most settings. I find that patients with relatively mild disease may experience a substantial reduction of alkaline phosphatase to normal or near normal with a single 60-mg infusion given over a 2-h period in 300–500 ml of 5% dextrose in water. Patients with more moderate to severe disease (e.g., serum alkaline phosphatase levels >3–4 times normal) may require multiple infusions of 60–90 mg infused as described and given on a once weekly or biweekly basis, primarily based on physician and patient convenience. Two to four 60-mg doses or three 90-mg doses may suffice in moderate disease (e.g., serum alkaline phosphatase in the range of 4–5 times normal). Total doses in the range of 300–500 mg may be required in some severe cases (serum alkaline phosphatase ~10–20 times normal), given over a number of weeks.

Suppression of urinary markers can often be noted within a few days after an infusion, but the serum alkaline phosphatase may take up to 2–3 months to reach its nadir. For moderate to severe cases, giving three to four 60-mg doses and then reassessing at 3 months with the possibility of more treatment is a reasonable approach. A successful course of therapy can result in 1 year or more of continued disease suppression, with markers of turnover at normal or near-normal levels. Side effects may include a low-grade fever and flu-like symptoms in the first 24 h after the first ever infusion (decreasing in likelihood with repeated dosing), and the possibility of mild and transient hypocalcemia, hypophosphatemia, and lymphopenia. Venous irritation may arise, especially if an insufficient volume of fluid is used or if the fluid extravasates. It is desirable to provide oral calcium supplements at a dose of 500 mg, two or three times daily, and vitamin D, 400 to 800 U daily, to prevent or ameliorate a reduction in serum calcium and concomitant rise in PTH.

Overall, pamidronate offers the opportunity to titrate the dosage as required in the individual patient, with the possibility of normalization or near normalization of biochemical indices and the potential for substantial and prolonged reduction in disease progression in many patients. In my view, it is most useful in patients with mild disease, in whom a single infusion may afford long-term benefit in a very cost-effective manner, and in severe and refractory cases, in which delivery of drug by vein bypasses problems with oral absorption. It is also the drug of choice for individuals who experience esophageal symptoms from alendronate or risedronate. The need for outpatient intravenous administration of multiple doses may be expensive and inconvenient in some cases. However, the rapid onset of symptomatic improvement and overall potency of the agent make it the drug of choice for cases with neurologic compression syndromes, for severe and painful lytic disease with or without impending fracture, and as a pretreatment of active Paget's disease before elective surgery to shrink the hypervascularity of the pagetic bone and decrease the amount of bleeding at operation. There has been one report of asymptomatic mineralization abnormalities with dosing in the usual clinical range,[62] but this is not the general experience. Recently, there has been a report of patients developing secondary resistance to pamidronate after repeated use.[63]

Alendronate. Approved by the FDA for the treatment of Paget's disease in the fall of 1995, alendronate, sold as Fosamax, is an orally administered aminobisphosphonate that is 700 times more potent than etidronate and is not associated with mineralization problems at therapeutically effective doses. In a study of 89 patients with moderate to severe disease who received 6 months of either alendronate, 40 mg daily, or etidronate, 400 mg/day, alendronate led to a normalized serum alkaline phosphatase in over 63% of subjects compared with 17% for etidronate; overall, alendronate led to a mean fall in alkaline phosphatase of 79% compared with 44% with etidronate.[64] Alendronate seemed to be as well tolerated as etidronate in this study, although symptoms of upper gastrointestinal discomfort or nausea, or the less common but more serious complication of esophageal ulceration, should be watched for at the 40-mg dose. Biopsy specimens from patients treated with alendronate revealed normal patterns of deposition of new bone[64,65] and radiologic improvement.[65] The recommended dose is 40 mg daily for 6 months to be taken with 8 oz of tap water on rising in the morning after an overnight fast. The patient is instructed not to take anything else orally (except more water) and not to lie down for at least 30 minutes after the dose. It is important with alendronate, as with pamidronate and tiludronate, that patients be replete in vitamin D and have a daily calcium intake of 1–1.5 g to avoid hypocalcemia early in the treatment course. Biochemical remissions may persist for 12–18 months after a single course. Retreatment guidelines are incomplete because follow-up data are few, but many physicians have given repeat 6-month courses of alendronate once indices rise above normal with good success in re-establishing complete or partial biochemical remission.

Risedronate. More than 1000 times more potent than etidronate, risedronate is the newest available bisphosphonate, approved by the FDA for use in Paget's disease in 1998. Risedronate is available as Actonel. Studies with risedronate have described the efficacy of a 30-mg dose given for 2[66] or 3[67] months to patients with moderately active disease. These short courses of therapy led to a nearly 80% reduction in serum alkaline phosphatase and normalization of indices of bone turnover in 50–70% of patients. Thus, 30 mg can be given daily for 2 months, with a follow-up measurement of serum alkaline phosphatase 1 month later; if the value is not yet normal or near normal, a third or fourth month could be offered with a good likelihood of normalcy or near normalcy of indices thereafter, with a prolonged period of disease suppression similar to that achieved with pamidronate or alendronate. Once again, adequacy of calcium and vitamin D intake is important to avoid hypocalcemia. The 30-mg risedronate dose is taken with 8 oz of water on arising in the morning after an overnight fast, with no other oral intake (except water) and no lying down for 30 minutes after the dose. In the clinical trials, the main side effects were mild upper gastrointestinal upset in 15% of patients; symptoms of esophageal irritation were not common in these clinical trials with the 30-mg dose but should be kept in mind by the physician until more data are available. A few cases of iritis were seen, something also reported rarely with pamidronate.

Calcitonin

The polypeptide hormone, salmon calcitonin, is available therapeutically as a synthetic formulation for parenteral administration. It, like human and other calcitonins, was first shown to be efficacious in Paget's disease more than 30 years ago.[68,69] At present, the formulation approved for use in Paget's disease in the United States, sold as Miacalcin, must be injected subcutaneously or intramuscularly. A nasal-spray formulation of salmon calcitonin, approved by the FDA for use in postmenopausal osteoporosis, is available, although not specifically approved for treatment of Paget's disease.

The usual starting dose is 100 U (0.5 ml; the drug is available in a 2 ml-vial), generally self-injected subcutane-

ously, initially on a daily basis. Symptomatic benefit may be apparent in a few weeks, and the biochemical benefit (typically about a 50% reduction from baseline in serum alkaline phosphatase) is usually seen after 3–6 months of treatment. After this period, many clinicians reduce the dose to 50–100 U every other day or three times weekly. Often, a dose of 50 U, three times weekly after the first few months of therapy, will maintain the achieved benefit. Patients with moderate to severe disease may require indefinite treatment to maintain a 50% reduction in the biochemical indices and symptomatic relief, but milder or monostotic disease may allow discontinuation of treatment for prolonged periods.

Escape from the efficacy of salmon calcitonin may sometimes occur after a variable period of benefit. In some cases this may be caused by a postulated downregulation of receptors, but in other instances, it may be a consequence of the development of neutralizing antibodies to the salmon polypeptide.[70] The main side effects of parenteral salmon calcitonin include, in a minority of patients, the development of nausea or queasiness, with or without flushing of the skin of the face and ears. These annoying side effects may last from a few minutes to several hours after each injection, although many patients can avoid them by experimenting with taking the agent at bedtime, with food, without food, and so on. Although these side effects are unpleasant, they do not seem to be serious or harmful, and most patients develop tolerance to them. In summary, however, it is apparent that the newer bisphosphonates offer both greater effectiveness and ease of use, suggesting that this agent will be used in the future primarily by patients who do not tolerate oral or intravenous bisphosphonate therapy.

Intranasal calcitonin is available as Miacalcin Nasal Spray. It seems to have a lower incidence of the side effects described earlier. The optimal dose in Paget's disease with the present formulation is not known, but anecdotal evidence suggests that in occasional patients with mild disease, the 200-U single spray dose given daily may lower biochemical indices and relieve mild symptoms, such as increased warmth in a pagetic tibia.

Other Therapies

Analgesics and nonsteroidal anti-inflammatory agents (NSAIDs), as well as newer cox-2 inhibitors, may be tried empirically with or without antipagetic therapy to relieve pain. Pagetic arthritis (i.e., osteoarthritis caused by deformed pagetic bone at a joint space) may cause periods of pain that are often helped by these agents.

Surgery on pagetic bone[53] may be necessary in the setting of established or impending fracture. Elective joint replacement, although more complex with Paget's disease than with typical osteoarthritis, is often very successful in relieving refractory pain. Rarely, osteotomy is performed to alter a bowing deformity in the tibia. Neurosurgical intervention is sometimes required in cases of spinal cord compression, spinal stenosis, or basilar invagination with neural compromise. Although medical management may be beneficial and adequate in some instances, all cases of serious neurological compromise require immediate neurological and neurosurgical consultation to allow the appropriate plan of management to be developed. As improved therapies emerge, long-term suppression of pagetic activity may have a preventive role in Paget's disease and, possibly, may obviate the need for surgical management in many cases.

REFERENCES

1. Kanis JA 1998 Pathophysiology and Treatment of Paget's Disease of Bone, 2nd ed. Martin Dunitz Ltd., London, UK.
2. Siris ES, Canfield RE, Jacobs TP 1980 Paget's disease of bone. Bull NY Acad Med **56:**285–304.
3. Morales-Piga AA, Rey-Rey JS, Corres-Gonzalez J, Garcia-Sagredo IM, Lopez-Abente G 1995 Frequency and characteristics of familial aggregation of Paget's disease of bone. J Bone Miner Res **10:**663–670.
4. McKusick VA 1972 Heritable Disorders of Connective Tissue, 5th ed. CV Mosby, St. Louis, Missouri, USA, pp. 718–723.
5. Siris ES, Ottman R, Flaster E, Kelsey JL 1991 Familial aggregation of Paget's disease of bone. J Bone Miner Res **6:**495–500.
6. Cody JD, Singer FR, Roodman GD, Otterund B, Lewis TB, Leppert M 1997 Genetic linkage of Paget disease of bone to chromosome 18q. Am J Hum Genet **61:**1117–1122.
7. Good DA, Busfield F, Fletcher BH, Duffy DL, Kesting JB, Andersen J, Shaw JT 2002 Linkage of Paget disease of bone to a novel region on human chromosome 18q23. Am J Hum Genet **70:**517–525.
8. Hocking LJ, Herbert CA, Nicholls RK, Williams F, Bennett ST, Cundy T, Nicholson GC, Wuyts W, Van Hul W, Ralston SH 2001 Genomewide search in familial Paget disease of bone shows evidence of genetic heterogeneity with candidate loci on chromosomes 2q36, 10p13, and 5q35. Am J Hum Genet **69:**1055–1061.
9. Sparks AB, Peterson SN, Bell C, Loftus BJ, Hocking L, Cahill DP, Frassica FJ, Streeten EA, Levine MA, Fraser CM, Adams MD, Broder S, Venter JC, Kinzler KW, Vogelstein B, Ralston SH 2001 Mutation screening of the TNFRSF11A gene encoding receptor activator of NF kappa B (RANK) in familial and sporadic Paget's disease of bone and osteosarcoma. Calcif Tissue Int **68:**151–155.
10. Hocking L, Slee F, Haslam SI, Cundy T, Nicholson G, van Hul W, Ralston SH 2000 Familial Paget's disease of bone: Patterns of inheritance and frequency of linkage to chromosome 18q. Bone **26:**577–580.
11. Laurin N, Brown JP, Morissette J, Raymond V 2002 Recurrent mutation of the gene encoding sequestosome 1 (SQSTM1/p62) in Paget disease of bone. Am J Hum Genet 2002 **70:**1582–1588.
12. Laurin N, Morissette J, Raymond V, Brown JP 2002 Large phenotypic variability of Paget disease of bone caused by the P392L sequestasome 1/p62 mutation. J Bone Miner Res **17:**S1:S380.
13. Barker DJ 1984 The epidemiology of Paget's disease of bone. Br Med Bull **40:**396–400.
14. Barker DJP, Chamberlain AT, Guyer PH, Gardner MJ 1980 Paget's disease of bone: The Lancashire focus. BMJ **280:**1105–1107.
15. Barry HC 1969 Paget's Disease of Bone. E & S Livingstone, Edinburgh, Scotland.
16. Dolev E, Samuel R, Foldes J, Brickman M, Assia A, Liberman U 1994 Some epidemiological aspects of Paget's disease in Israel. Semin Arthritis Rheum **23:**228.
17. Lowenthal MN, Alkalay D, Abu Rabbia Y, Liel Y 1995 Paget's disease of bone in Negev Bedouin: Report of two cases. Isr J Med Sci **31:**628–629.
18. Mautalen C, Pumarino H, Blanco MC, Gonzalez D, Ghiringhelli G, Fromm G 1994 Paget's disease: The South American experience. Semin Arthritis Rheum **23:**226–227.
19. Guyer PB, Chamberlain AT 1980 Paget's disease of bone in two American cities. BMJ **280:**985.
20. Cundy T, McAnulty K, Wattie D, Gamble G, Rutland M, Ibbertson HK 1997 Evidence for secular change in Paget's disease. Bone **20:**69–71.
21. Cooper C, Schafheutle K, Dennison E, Kellingray S, Guyer P, Barker D 1999 The epidemiology of Paget's disease in Britain: Is the prevalence decreasing? J Bone Miner Res **14:**192–197.
22. Rebel A, Malkani K, Basle M, Bregeon C 1977 Is Paget's disease of bone a viral infection? Calcif Tissue Res. **22**(Suppl):283–286.
23. Mills BG, Singer FR, Weiner LP, Suffin SC, Stabile E, Holst P 1984 Evidence for both respiratory syncytial virus and measles virus antigens in the osteoclasts of patients with Paget's disease of bone. Clin Orthop **183:**303–311.
24. Basle M, Rebel A, Pouplard A, Kouyoumdjian S, Filmon R, Loepatezour A 1979 Demonstration by immunofluorescence and immuno-

25. peroxidase of an antigen of the measles type in the osteoclasts of Paget's disease of bone. Bull Assoc Anat **63:**263–272.
25. Friedrichs WE, Reddy SV, Bruder JM, Cundy T, Cornish J, Singer FR, Roodman GD 2002 Sequence analysis of measles virus nucleocapsid transcripts in patients with Paget's disease. J Bone Miner Res **17:**145–151.
26. Gordon MT, Mee AP, Sharpe PT 1994 Paramyxoviruses in Paget's disease. Semin Arthritis Rheum **23:**232–234.
27. Mee AP, Dixon JA, Hoyland JA, Davies M, Selby PL, Mawer EB 1998 Detection of canine distemper virus in 100% of Paget's disease samples by in situ-reverse transcriptase-polymerase chain reaction. Bone **23:**171–175.
28. Kurihara N, Reddy SV, Menaa C, Anderson D, Roodman GD 2000 Osteoclasts expressing the measles virus nucleocapsid gene display a pagetic phenotype. J Clin Invest 2000 **105:**607–614.
29. Ooi CG, Walsh CA, Gallagher JA, Fraser WD 2000 Absence of measles virus and canine distemper virus transcripts in long-term bone marrow cultures from patients with Paget's disease of bone. Bone **27:**417–421.
30. Rebel A, Basle M, Pouplard A, Malkani K. Filmon R, Lepatezour A 1980 Bone tissue in Paget's disease of bone: Ultrastructure and immunocytology. Arthritis Rheum 23:1104–1114.
31. Calvo MS, Eyre DR, Gundberg CM 1996 Molecular basis and clinical application of biological markers of bone turnover. Endocr Rev **17:**333–368.
32. Meunier PJ, Coindre JM, Edouard CM, Arlot ME 1980 Bone histomorphometry in Paget's disease: Quantitative and dynamic analysis of pagetic and non-pagetic bone tissue. Arthritis Rheum 23:1095–1103.
33. Siris ES, Clemens TP, McMahon D, Gordon AG, Jacobs TP, Canfield RE 1989 Parathyroid function in Paget's disease of bone. J Bone Miner Res **4:**75–79.
34. Siris ES, Canfield RE 1994 The parathyroids and Paget's disease of bone. In: Bilezikian J, Levine M, Marcus R (eds.) The Parathyroids. Raven Press, New York, NY, USA, pp. 823–828.
35. Siris ES 1991 Indications for medical treatment of Paget's disease of bone. In: Singer FR, Wallach S (eds.) Paget's Disease of Bone: Clinical Assessment. Present and Future Therapy. Elsevier, New York, NY, USA, pp. 44–56.
36. Herzberg L, Bayliss E 1980 Spinal cord syndrome due to non-compressive Paget's disease of bone: A spinal artery steal phenomenon reversible with calcitonin. Lancet **2:**13–15.
37. Monsell EM, Bone HG, Cody DD, Jacobson GP, Newman CW, Patel SG, Divine GW 1995 Hearing loss in Paget's disease of bone: Evidence of auditory nerve integrity. Am J Otol **16:**27–33.
38. Barry HC 1980 Orthopedic aspects of Paget's disease of bone. Arthritis Rheum 23:1128–1130.
39. Wick MR, Siegal GP, Unni KK, McLeod RA, Greditzer HB 1981 Sarcomas of bone complicating osteitis deformans (Paget's disease): 50 years experience. Am J Surg Pathol **5:**47–59.
40. Upchurch KS, Simon LS, Schiller AL, Rosenthal DI, Campion EW, Krane SM 1983 Giant cell reparative granulomas of Paget's disease of bone: A unique clinical entity. Ann Intern Med **98:**35–40.
41. Jacobs TP, Michelsen J, Polay J, D' Adamo AC, Canfield RE 1979 Giant cell tumor in Paget's disease of bone: Familial and geographic clustering. Cancer **44:**742–747.
42. Strickberger SA, Schulman SP, Hutchins GM 1987 Association of Paget's disease of bone with calcific aortic valve disease. Am J Med **82:**953–956.
43. Delmas PD, Chapuy MC, Vignon E, Charhon S, Briancon D, Alexandre C, Edouard C, Meunier PJ 1982 Long-term effects of dichloromethylene diphosphonate in Paget's disease of bone. J Clin Endocrinol Metab **54:**837–844.
44. Gonzalez DC, Mautalen CA 1999 Short term therapy with oral olpadronate in active Paget's disease of bone. J Bone Miner Res **14:**2042–2047.
45. Adami S, Bevilacqua M, Broggini M, Fillipponi P, Ortolani S, Palummeri E, Uliveri F, Nannipieri F, Braga V 2002 2002 Short term intravenous therapy with neridronate in Paget's disease. Clin Exp Rheumatol **20:**55–58.
46. Woitge HW, Oberwittler H, Heichel S, Grauer A, Ziegler R, Seibel MJ 2000 Short- and long-term effects of ibandroante treatment on bone turnover in Paget disease of bone. Clin Chem **46:**684–690.
47. Buckler H, Fraser W, Hosking D, Ryan W, Maricic MJ, Singer F, Davie M, Fogelman I, Birbara CA, Moses AM, Lyles K, Selby P, Richardson P, Seaman J, Zelenakas K, Siris E 1999 Single infusion of zoledronate in Paget's disease of bone: A placebo-controlled, dose ranging study. Bone **24:**81S–85S.
48. Bockman RS, Wilhelm F, Siris E, Singer F, Chausmer A, Bitton R,

Kotler J, Bosco BJ, Eyre DR, Levenson D 1995 A multi-center, trial of low dose gallium nitrate in patients with advanced Paget's disease of bone. J Clin Endocrinol Metab **80:**595–602.

49. EI-Sammaa M, Linthicum FH, House HP, House JW 1986 Calcitonin as treatment for hearing loss in Paget's disease. Am J Otol **7:**241–243.

50. Meunier PJ, Vignot E 1995 Therapeutic strategy in Paget's disease of bone. Bone **17:**489S–49IS.

51. Lyles KW, Siris ES, Singer FR, Meunier PJ 2001 A clinical approach to the diagnosis and management of Paget's disease of bone. J Bone Miner Res **16:**1379–1387.

52. Selby PL, Davie MW, Ralston SH, Stone MD 2002 Guidelines on the management of Paget's disease of bone. Bone **31:**366–373.

53. Kaplan FS 1999 Surgical management of Paget's disease. J Bone Miner Res **2:**34–38.

54. Drake WM, Kendler DL, Brown JP 2001 2001 Consensus statement on the modern therapy of Paget's disease of bone from a Western Osteoporosis Alliance Symposium. Clin Ther **23:**620–626.

55. Altman RD, Johnston CC, Khairi MRA, Wellman H, Serafini AN, Sankey RR 1973 Influence of disodium etidronate on clinical and laboratory manifestations of Paget's disease of bone (osteitis deformans). N Engl J Med **289:**1379–1384.

56. Canfield R, Rosner W, Skinner J, McWhorter J, Resnick L, Feldman F, Kammerman S, Ryan K, Kunigonis M, Bohne W 1977 Diphosphonate therapy of Paget's disease of bone. J Clin Endocrinol Metab **44:**96–106.

57. Roux C, Gennari C, Farrerons J, Devogelaer JP, Mulder H, Kruse HP, Picot C, Titeux L, Reginster JY, Dougados M 1995 Comparative prospective, double-blind, multi-center study of the efficacy of tiludronate and etidronate in the treatment of Paget's disease of bone. Arthritis Rheum **38:**851–858.

58. McClung MR, Tou CK, Goldstein NH, Picot C 1995 Tiludronate therapy for Paget's disease of bone. Bone **17:**493S–496S.

59. Siris ES 1994 Perspectives: A practical guide to the use of pamidronate in the treatment of Paget's disease. J Bone Miner Res **9:**303–304.

60. Harinck HI, Papapoulos SE, Blanksma HJ, Moolenaar AJ, Vermeij P, Bijvoet OL 1987 Paget's disease of bone: Early and late responses to three different modes of treatment with aminohydroxypropylidene bisphosphonate (APD). BMJ **295:**1301–1305.

61. Trombetti A, Arlot M, Thevenon J, Uebelhart B, Meunier PJ 1999 Effects of multiple intravenous pamidronate courses in Paget's disease of bone. Rev Rhum Engl Ed **66:**467–476.

62. Adamson BB, Gallacher SJ, Byars J, Ralston SH, Boyle IT, Boyce BF 1993 Mineralisation defects with pamidronate therapy for Paget's disease. Lancet **342:**1459–1460.

63. Gutteridge DH, Ward LC, Stewart GO, Retallack RW, Will RK, Prince RL, Criddle A, Bhagat CI, Stuckey BG, Price RI, Kent GN, Faulkner DL, Geelhoed E, Gan SK, Vasikaran S 1999 Paget's disease: Acquired resistance to one aminobisphosphonate with retained response to another. J Bone Miner Res **2:**79–84.

64. Siris E, Weinstein RS, Altman R, Conte JM, Favus M, Lombardi A, Lyles K, McIlwain H, Murphy WA Jr., Reda C, Rude R, Seton M, Tiegs R, Thompson D, Tucci JR, Yates AJ, Zimering M 1996 Comparative study of alendronate vs. etidronate for the treatment of Paget's disease of bone. J Clin Endocrinol Metab **81:**961–967.

65. Reid IR, Nicholson GC, Weinstein RS, Hosking DJ, Cundy T, Kotowicz MA, Murphy WA Jr, Yeap S, Dufresne S, Lombardi A, Musliner TA, Thompson DE, Yates AJ 1996 Biochemical and radiologic improvement in Paget's disease of bone treated with alendronate: A randomized, placebo-controlled trial. Am J Med **171:**341–348.

66. Miller PD, Adachi JD, Brown JP, Khairi RA, Lang R, Licata AA, McClung MR, Ryan WG, Singer FR, Siris ES, Tenenhouse A, Wallach S, Bekker PJ, Axelrod DW 1997 Risedronate vs. etidronate: Durable remission with only two months of 30 mg risedronate. J Bone Miner Res **12:**S269.

67. Siris ES, Chines AA, Altman RD, Brown JP, Johnston CC Jr, Lang R, McClung MR, Mallette LE, Miller PD, Ryan WG, Singer FR, Tucci JR, Eusebio RA, Bekker PJ 1998 Risedronate in the treatment of Paget's disease: An open-label, multicenter study. J Bone Miner Res **13:**1032–1038.

68. Woodhouse NJY, Bordier P, Fisher M, Joplin GF, Reiner M, Kalu DN, Foster GV, MacIntyre I 1971 Human calcitonin in the treatment of Paget's bone disease. Lancet **1:**1139–1143.

69. DeRose J, Singer FR, Avramides A, Flores A, Dziadiw R, Baker RK, Wallach S 1974 Response of Paget's disease to porcine and salmon calcitonins: Effects of long term treatment. Am J Med **56:**858–866.

70. Singer FR, Ginger K 1991 Resistance to calcitonin. In: Singer FR, Wallach S (eds.) Paget's Disease of Bone: Clinical Assessment, Present and Future Therapy. Elsevier, New York, NY, USA, pp. 75–85.

Extraskeletal (Ectopic) Calcification and Ossification

Introduction

Michael P. Whyte

Division of Bone and Mineral Diseases, Washington University School of Medicine at Barnes-Jewish Hospital and Center for Metabolic Bone Disease and Molecular Research, Shriners Hospitals for Children, St. Louis, Missouri

A significant number and variety of disorders cause extraskeletal deposition of calcium and phosphate (Table 1). In some, mineral is precipitated as amorphous calcium phosphate or as crystals of hydroxyapatite; in others, osseous tissue is formed. The pathogenesis of the ectopic mineralization is generally ascribed to one of three mechanisms (Table 1). First, a supranormal "calcium-phosphate solubility product" in extracellular fluid can cause metastatic calcification. Second, mineral may be deposited as dystrophic calcification into metabolically impaired or dead tissue despite normal serum levels of calcium and phosphate. Third, ectopic ossification (or true bone formation) occurs in a few disorders for which the pathogenesis is less well understood.

Discussed briefly in this introduction section are these three mechanisms for extraskeletal calcification or ossification. Afterward, there follows a description of three principal disorders that illustrates each pathogenesis.

MECHANISMS FOR EXTRASKELETAL CALCIFICATION AND OSSIFICATION

Calcium and inorganic phosphate are normally present in serum or extracellular fluid at concentrations that form a "metastable" solution. That is, their levels are too low for spontaneous precipitation but sufficiently great to cause hydroxyapatite [$Ca_{10}(PO_4)_6(OH)_2$] formation once crystal nucleation has begun.[1] In health, the presence of a variety of inhibitors of mineralization, such as inorganic pyrophosphate, helps to prevent ectopic calcification.[2]

The pathogenesis of metastatic and dystrophic calcification at the cell level is partially understood. Both processes typically involve mineral accumulation within matrix vesicles and sometimes within mitochondria.[2] Conversely, the mechanisms which initiate ectopic ossification are largely an enigma, but recent studies of progressive osseous heteroplasia (POH) identified deactivating mutations in *GNAS1* (which also causes pseudohypoparathyroidism type IA).[3]

Metastatic calcification can occur from significant hypercalcemia or hyperphosphatemia (especially both) of any etiology (Table 1). In fact, therapy with phosphate supplements during mild hypercalcemia or treatment with vitamin D or calcium during mild hyperphosphatemia may trigger this problem.[4] Mineral deposition can also occur ectopically from hyperphosphatemia despite concomitant hypocalcemia.

Direct precipitation of mineral occurs when the calcium–phosphate solubility product in extracellular fluid is exceeded. A value of 75 (mg/dl × mg/dl) is commonly taken as the limit, which if surpassed, causes mineral precipitation. However, the critical value for renal calcification is not precisely defined and may vary with age.[4] In adults, some consider 70 to be the maximal safe level for the kidney. It is possible that children tolerate a somewhat higher value because they normally have greater serum phosphate concentrations compared with adults. However, this is not well established.[4]

The material that forms in metastatic calcification may be

TABLE 1. DISORDERS ASSOCIATED WITH EXTRASKELETAL CALCIFICATION OR OSSIFICATION

A. Metastatic calcification
  I. Hypercalcemia
    a. Milk-alkali syndrome
    b. Hypervitaminosis D
    c. Sarcoidosis
    d. Hyperparathyroidism
    e. Renal failure
  II. Hyperphosphatemia
    a. Tumoral calcinosis
    b. Hyperparathyroidism
    c. Pseudohypoparathyroidism
    d. Cell lysis after chemotherapy for leukemia
    e. Renal failure
B. Dystrophic calcification
  I. Calcinosis (universalis or circumscripta)
    a. Childhood dermatomyositis
    b. Scleroderma
    c. Systemic lupus erythematosis
  II. Posttraumatic
C. Ectopic ossification
  I. Myositis ossificans (posttraumatic)
    a. Burns
    b. Surgery (joint replacement)
    c. Neurologic injury
  II. Fibrodysplasia (myositis) ossificans progressiva (FOP)
  III. Progressive osseous heteroplasia (POH)
  IV. Osteoma cutis

amorphous calcium phosphate initially, but hydroxyapatite is deposited soon after.[2] The anatomic pattern of deposition varies somewhat between hypercalcemia and hyperphosphatemia, but occurs irrespective of the specific underlying condition or mechanism for the disturbed mineral homeostasis. Additionally, there is a predilection for precipitation into certain tissues.

Hypercalcemia is typically associated with mineral deposits in the kidneys, lungs, and fundus of the stomach. In these "acid-secreting" organs, a local alkaline milieu may account for the calcium deposition. In addition, the media of large arteries, elastic tissue of the endocardium (especially the left atrium), conjunctiva, and periarticular soft tissues are often affected. However, the predisposition for these sites is not well understood. In the kidney, hypercalciuria may cause calcium phosphate casts to form within the tubule lumen, or calculi to develop in the calyces or pelvis. Furthermore, calcium phosphate may precipitate in peritubular tissues. In the lung, calcification affects the alveolar walls and the pulmonary venous system. Well-established causes of metastatic calcification mediated by hypercalcemia include the milk-alkali syndrome, hypervitaminosis D, sarcoidosis, and hyperparathyroidism (Table 1).

Hyperphosphatemia of sufficient severity to cause metastatic calcification occurs in idiopathic hypoparathyroidism or pseudohypoparathyroidism and with the massive cell lysis (release of cellular phosphate) that can follow chemotherapy for leukemia (Table 1). Renal insufficiency is commonly associated with metastatic calcification—the mechanism may involve hyperphosphatemia, hypercalcemia, or both. Of interest (but unexplained), ectopic calcification is more common in pseudohypoparathyroidism (type I) than in idiopathic hypoparathyroidism despite comparable elevations in serum phosphate levels. Furthermore, the location of ectopic calcification in pseudohypoparathyroidism and hypoparathyroidism (e.g., cerebral basal ganglion) is different from observations in hypercalcemia. With hyperphosphatemia, calcification of periarticular subcutaneous tissues is characteristic and may be related to tissue trauma from the movement of joints.

Dystrophic calcification occurs despite a normal serum calcium–phosphate solubility product. Injured tissue of any kind is predisposed to this type of extraskeletal calcification. Apparently, tissues can release material that has nucleating properties. One classic example is the caseous lesion of tuberculosis. However, what local factor predisposes to the precipitation of calcium salts is unknown. Indeed, several mechanisms seem likely. It is clear that mineral precipitation into injured tissue is even more striking and more severe when either the calcium or phosphate level in extracellular fluid is also increased. The deposited mineral, as for metastatic calcification, may be either amorphous calcium phosphate or crystalline hydroxyapatite.

The term "calcinosis" refers to an important type of dystrophic calcification that commonly occurs in (or under) the skin with connective tissue disorders—particularly dermatomyositis, scleroderma, or systemic lupus erythematosus. As the symptoms and the inflammatory process in the subcutaneous tissues from the acute connective tissue disease subside, painful masses of calcium phosphate appear under the skin. Calcinosis may involve a relatively localized area with small deposits in the skin and subcutaneous tissues, especially over the extensor aspects of the joints and the fingertips (calcinosis circumscripta); or, it may be widespread and not only in the skin and subcutaneous tissues, but deeper in periarticular regions as well as areas of trauma (calcinosis universalis). The lesions of calcinosis are small or medium-sized hard nodules that can cause muscle atrophy and contractures. Other etiologies for calcinosis include metastases or trauma that produce necrotic tissue.

Ectopic ossification is associated with two principal etiologies. It occurs sporadically with the fasciitis that follows neurological injury, surgery, burns, or trauma when it is called myositis ossificans. It also occurs as the major feature of a separate, heritable entity—fibrodysplasia (myositis) ossificans progressiva—where the pathogenesis is becoming understood. Some consider the primary reason for the ectopic bone formation in this latter genetic disorder to be a muscle abnormality (myositis ossificans progressiva), whereas others favor a connective tissue defect (fibrodysplasia ossificans progressiva). In all of these conditions, osseous tissue is formed. The bone is lamellar, actively remodeled by osteoblasts and osteoclasts, has haversian systems, and sometimes contains marrow. Apparently, the injured or diseased tissue has the necessary precursor cells and inductive signals to form cartilage and bone.

Described in the following chapters are three disorders—tumoral calcinosis, dermatomyositis, and fibrodysplasia ossificans progressiva (FOP)—that are principal examples of each type of ectopic mineralization.

REFERENCES

1. Fawthrop FW, Russell RGG 1993 Ectopic calcification and ossification. In: Nordin BEC, Need AG, Morris HA, (eds.) Metabolic Bone and Stone Disease, 3rd ed. Churchill Livingstone, Edinburgh, UK, pp. 325–338.
2. Anderson HC 1983 Calcific diseases: A concept. Arch Pathol Lab Med **107**:341–348.
3. Harrison HE, Harrison HC 1979 Disorders of Calcium and Phosphate Metabolism in Childhood and Adolescence. WB Saunders, Philadelphia, PA, USA.
4. Eddy MC, Jan de Beur SM, Yandow SM, McAlister WH, Shore EM, Kaplan FS, Whyte MP, Levine MA 2000 Deficiency of the α-subunit of the stimulatory G protein and severe extraskeletal ossification. J Bone Miner Res **15**:2074–2083.

Chapter 83. Tumoral Calcinosis

Michael P. Whyte

Division of Bone and Mineral Diseases, Washington University School of Medicine at Barnes-Jewish Hospital and Center for Metabolic Bone Disease and Molecular Research, Shriners Hospitals for Children, St. Louis, Missouri

INTRODUCTION

Tumoral calcinosis, first described in 1899, is a heritable disorder that features periarticular metastatic calcification.[1] Hyperphosphatemia is a pathogenetic factor in many patients.[2–4] Mineral deposition manifests as soft tissue masses around the major joints. Typically, the hips and shoulders are affected, although additional joints can be involved.[5] Visceral calcification does not occur, but segments of vasculature may contain deposits.[5] The differential diagnosis includes periarticular metastatic calcification from hypercalcemia associated with renal failure, milk-alkali syndrome, sarcoidosis, and vitamin D intoxication.

CLINICAL PRESENTATION

Most patients in North America with this disorder are black. About one-third of cases are familial. Autosomal recessive inheritance is usually described, although autosomal dominant transmission has also been reported.[1–6] There is no gender preference.

Tumoral calcinosis often presents in childhood, but characteristic masses have been discovered in infancy and in old age. Hyperphosphatemic patients are usually black, have a positive family history, manifest the disease before 20 years of age, and have multiple lesions.[3]

The soft tissue calcifications are typically painless and grow at variable rates.[7] After 1 or 2 years, the masses may be the size of an orange or grapefruit and weigh 1 kg or more. Often they are hard, lobulated, and firmly attached to deep fascia. Occasionally, the swellings infiltrate into muscles and tendons.[3] The major clinical complications are related to the tumors that occur around joints and in skin, marrow, teeth, and blood vessels. Because the deposits are extracapsular, joint range of motion is not impaired unless the tumors are particularly large. There can, however, be compression of adjacent neural structures. The lesions can also ulcerate the skin and form a sinus tract that drains a chalky fluid; this complication may lead to infection. Other potential secondary problems include anemia, low-grade fever, regional lymphadenopathy, splenomegaly, and amyloidosis. Some patients have characteristics of *pseudoxanthoma elasticum* (i.e., skin and vascular calcifications and angioid streaks in the retina). A tooth abnormality, featuring short bulbous roots and calcific deposits that often obliterate pulp chambers, is a dental hallmark.[6,8] Recently, recurrent episodes of bone inflammation have been characterized.[9] This is a lifelong disorder.

RADIOGRAPHIC EXAMINATION

The tumors typically appear as large aggregations of irregular, densely calcified lobules that are confined to soft

The author has no conflict of interest.

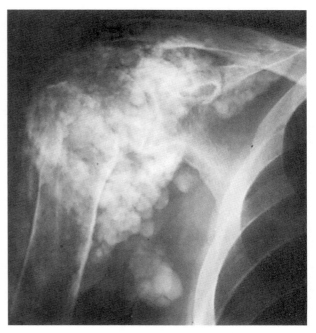

FIG. 1. Tumoral calcinosis. Lobular, periarticular calcifications are present at the right shoulder of this middle-aged man.

tissues (Fig. 1). Radiolucent fibrous septae account for the lobular appearance.[10] Occasionally, fluid layers are seen within the masses. The joints per se are unaffected. Bone texture and density are also unremarkable.

A "diaphysitis" has been recognized using radiographs, computerized tomography (CT), or magnetic resonance imaging (MRI) in some cases of tumoral calcinosis. New bone formation occurs along the endosteal surface of the diaphysis, perhaps from calcific myelitis.[7] This finding may be confused with osteomyelitis or a neoplasm.[11] When only calcific myelitis is present, CT and MRI are excellent tools for diagnosis.[11] Bone scanning, however, is the best method to detect and localize the calcified masses.

Periarticular masses that are radiologically indistinguishable from those of tumoral calcinosis occur in chronic renal failure when mineral homeostasis is poorly controlled.

LABORATORY FINDINGS

Serum calcium levels and alkaline phosphatase activity are usually normal. Hyperphosphatemia and increased serum calcitriol levels occur in some patients.[3,12] The TmP/GFR (phosphate transport maximum/glomerular filtration rate) may be supranormal, but renal function is otherwise unremarkable. Patients are in positive calcium/phosphate balance. Urinary studies reflect both the ongoing calcium and phosphate retention, and some patients are frankly hypocalciuric.

The chalky fluid in lesions is predominantly hydroxyapatite.[13,14]

HISTOPATHOLOGY

The masses of tumoral calcinosis are essentially foreign body granuloma reactions that form multilocular, cystic structures.[15] The early lesion may involve hemorrhage and histiocyte accumulation.[15,16] There are ill-defined, perivascular, reactive-like, solid cell nests admixed with mononuclear and iron-loaded macrophages, or well-organized, variably-sized, fibrohistiocytic nodules embedded in a dense collagenous stroma.[15] The cysts have tough connective tissue capsules, and their fibrous walls contain numerous foreign body giant cells. Mature lesions are filled with calcareous material in a viscous milky fluid. Occasionally, spicules of spongy bone and cartilage are found as well.

ETIOLOGY AND PATHOGENESIS

The genetic basis for tumoral calcinosis is unknown.[1] The precise pathogenesis is poorly understood but may involve the kidney tubule cell. Increased renal reclamation of filtered phosphate seems to be an important pathogenetic factor.[4] In hyperphosphatemic patients, enhanced kidney tubular reabsorption of phosphate occurs independently of suppressed serum parathyroid hormone (PTH) levels.[3,12] Deranged regulation of the renal 25-hydroxyvitamin D, 1-hydroxylase causes increased calcitriol synthesis. Consequently, dietary calcium absorption is enhanced, and serum PTH levels are suppressed.[3,12]

The masses may begin as calcific bursitis but then grow into adjacent fascial planes. Tissue damage with fat necrosis can be a pathogenetic factor.[14]

TREATMENT

Surgical removal of subcutaneous calcified masses may be helpful if they are painful, interfere with function, or are cosmetically unacceptable. When tumor excision is complete, recurrence seems to be unlikely.[17]

Radiation therapy and cortisone treatment have not been effective. Although it might seem that large masses of apatite crystals would be refractory to dissolution, success with aluminum hydroxide therapy (together with dietary phosphate and calcium deprivation) has been reported.[2,18,19] Furthermore, reduction of phosphate levels in extracellular fluid could help to prevent reformation of mineral deposits.[2] Preliminary studies indicate that calcitonin therapy may also be efficacious by enhancing phosphaturia.[20]

Acetazolamide, together with aluminum hydroxide, seemed to be helpful for one patient.[21]

REFERENCES

1. McKusick VA 1998 Mendelian Inheritance in Man: A Catalog of Human Genes and Genetic Disorders, 12th ed. The Johns Hopkins University Press, Baltimore, MD, USA, pp..
2. Mozaffarian G, Lafferty FW, Pearson OH 1972 Treatment of tumoral calcinosis with phosphorus deprivation. Ann Intern Med 77:741–745.
3. Prince MJ, Schaefer PC, Goldsmith RS, Chausmer AB 1982 Hyperphosphatemic tumoral calcinosis. Association with elevation of serum 1,25-dihydroxy-cholecalciferol concentrations. Ann Intern Med 96:586–591.
4. Smack D, Norton SA, Fitzpatrick JE 1996 Proposal for a pathogenesis-based classification of tumoral calcinosis. Int J Dermatol 35:265–271.
5. McGuinness FE 1995 Hyperphosphataemic tumoral calcinosis in Bedouin Arabs–clinical and radiological features. Clin Radiol 50:259–264.
6. Lyles KW, Burkes EJ, Ellis GJ, Lucas KJ, Dolan EA, Drezner MK 1985 Genetic transmission of tumoral calcinosis: Autosomal dominant with variable clinical expressivity. J Clin Endocrinol Metab 60:1093–1096.
7. Narchi H 1997 Hyperostosis with hyperphosphatemia: Evidence of familial occurrence and association with tumoral calcinosis. Pediatrics 99:745–748.
8. Burkes EJ Jr, Lyles KW, Dolan EA, Giammara B, Hanker J 1991 Dental lesions in tumoral calcinosis. J Oral Pathol Med 20:222–227.
9. Blay P, Fernandez-Martinez JM, Diaz-Lopez B 2001 Vertebral involvement in hyperphosphatemic tumoral calcinosis. Bone 28:316–318.
10. Steinbach LS, Johnston JO, Tepper EF, Honda GD, Martel W 1995 Tumoral calcinosis: Radiologic-pathologic correlation. Skeletal Radiol 24:573–578.
11. Martinez S, Vogler JB, Harrelson JM, Lyles KW 1990 Imaging of tumoral calcinosis: New observations. Radiology 174:215–222.
12. Lyles KW, Halsey DL, Friedman NE, Lobaugh B 1988 Correlations of serum concentrations of 1, 25-dihydroxyvitamin D, phosphorus, and parathyroid hormone in tumoral calcinosis. J Clin Endocrinol Metab 67:88–92.
13. Boskey AL, Vigorita VJ, Sencer O, Stuchin SA, Lane JM 1983 Chemical, microscopic and ultrastructural characterization of mineral deposits in tumoral calcinosis. Clin Orthop 178:258–270.
14. Kindbolm L-G, Gunterberg B 1988 Tumoral calcinosis: An ultrastructural analysis and consideration of pathogenesis. APMIS 96:368–376.
15. Pakasa NM, Kalengayi RM 1997 Tumoral calcinosis: A clinicopathological study of 111 cases with emphasis on the earliest changes. Histopathology 31:18–24.
16. Slavin RE, Wen J, Kumar WJ, Evans EB 1993 Familial tumoral calcinosis. A clinical, histopathologic, and ultrastructural study with an analysis of its calcifying process and pathogenesis. Am J Surg Pathol 17:788–802.
17. Noyez JF, Murphree SM, Chen K 1993 Tumoral calcinosis, a clinical report of eleven cases. Acta Orthop Belg 59:249–254.
18. Davies M, Clements MR, Mawer EB, Freemont AJ 1987 Tumoral calcinosis: Clinical and metabolic response to phosphorus deprivation. Q J Med 242:493–503.
19. Gregosiewicz A, Warda E 1989 Tumoral calcinosis: Successful medical treatment. J Bone Joint Surg Am 71A:1244–1249.
20. Salvi A, Cerudelli B, Cimino A, Zuccato F, Giustina G 1983 Phosphaturic action of calcitonin in pseudotumoral calcinosis. Horm Metab Res 15:260.
21. Yamaguchi T, Sugimoto T, Imai Y, Fukase M, Fujita T, Chihara K 1995 Successful treatment of hyperphosphatemic tumoral calcinosis with long-term acetazolamide. Bone 16:247S–250S.

Chapter 84. Dermatomyositis in Children

Michael P. Whyte

Division of Bone and Mineral Diseases, Washington University School of Medicine at Barnes-Jewish Hospital and Center for Metabolic Bone Disease and Molecular Research, Shriners Hospitals for Children, St. Louis, Missouri

INTRODUCTION

Dermatomyositis is a multisystem connective tissue disorder caused by small vessel vasculitis.[1,2] Acute and chronic, non-suppurative inflammation involves especially the skin and striated muscles. Dystrophic calcification often follows episodes of inflammation and can be severely debilitating.[1–6]

CLINICAL PRESENTATION

There are more female than male patients and two peak ages of incidence: childhood (5–15 years) and adulthood (50–60 years). When the disorder manifests before age 16 years, it is called juvenile or childhood dermatomyositis.[1–6] The adult form is associated with malignancy.[7]

In juvenile dermatomyositis, the patient's sex and the age-of-onset of symptoms seem unrelated to the severity of calcinosis, although increased time to diagnosis and treatment worsen this complication.[8] Calcification is generally noted 1–3 years after the disease onset and occurs in 25–50% of patients. However, calcinosis may predate the myopathy.[9] Mineral deposits develop over 1–3 years. In *calcinosis universalis* (see below), calcification occurs throughout the subcutaneous tissues, but primarily in periarticular regions or in areas that are subject to trauma (Fig. 1). In *calcinosis circumscripta*, the deposits are more localized and typically occur around joints. The ectopic mineralization can cause pain, ulcerate the skin, limit mobility, result in contractures, and predispose to abscess formation. Although the dystrophic calcification then typically remains stable, rarely some spontaneous resolution is reported.[1–6] Dystrophic calcification is rare in adults with dermatomyositis.[7]

LABORATORY FINDINGS

Whereas hypercalcemia with hypercalciuria and hyperphosphaturia may occur in juvenile dermatomyositis, parameters of mineral homeostasis are usually normal.[10] Elevated levels of γ-carboxyglutamic acid have been found in the urine of affected children—especially if there is calcinosis.[11] Hydroxyapatite comprises the nucleus of the calcinosis deposits, but other factors (including cytokines and macrophages) are also present.[12]

RADIOGRAPHIC FINDINGS

In juvenile dermatomyositis, four types of dystrophic calcification occur[13]:

1. Superficial masses (small circumscribed nodules or plaques) within the skin
2. Deep, discrete, subcutaneous, nodular masses (Fig. 1) near joints that can impair movement (calcinosis circumscripta)
3. Deep, linear, sheet-like deposits within intramuscular fascial planes (calcinosis universalis)
4. Lacy reticular subcutaneous deposits that encase the torso to form a generalized "exoskeleton"

Children with severe disease refractory to medical therapy seem especially prone to developing exoskeleton-like calcifications. In turn, the exoskeleton is associated with severe calcinosis and poor physical function.

ETIOLOGY AND PATHOGENESIS

Juvenile dermatomyositis seems to be a form of complement-mediated microangiopathy.[14] HLA-DQA1*051 may be a predisposing factor.[15] The precise cause of the dystrophic calcification is unknown. However, immune deficiencies may predispose the patient to this complication.[16] Calcinosis seems to occur in the majority of long-term survivors and may reflect a scarring process. This hypothesis is supported by the observation that mineral deposition appears to occur primarily in the muscles that were most severely affected during the disease's acute phase. Electron microscopy shows that the calcification consists of hydroxyapatite crystals,[17] but other important factors and cells seem to be important constituents.[12]

A variety of mechanisms considered for the dystrophic calcification include release of alkaline phosphatase or free fatty acids from diseased muscle that, in turn, directly precipitate calcium or first bind acid mucopolysaccharides. Increased urinary levels of γ-carboxylated peptides suggest that calcium-binding proteins may be responsible for the mineral deposition.

TREATMENT

High-dose prednisone therapy soon after the onset of symptoms seems to be important for minimizing the risk of calcinosis and for ensuring good, functional recovery.[2,3,18,19] If the response is incomplete, consideration is given to additional immunosuppressive agents,[3,5] including methotrexate and cyclosporine.[20] In a small clinical trial, warfarin treatment to decrease γ-carboxylation was not associated with changes in calcium or phosphorus excretion or in a reduction of calcinosis.[21] Phosphate-binding antacid therapy may reverse the mineral deposition.[22] Remarkable resolution of calcinosis universalis occurred in a young man treated with probenecid to improve renal handling of phosphate.[23] Positive response to alendronate[12] and increasingly positive responses to diltiazem are reported.[24,25] Troublesome calcium deposits can be removed surgically.

The author has no conflict of interest.

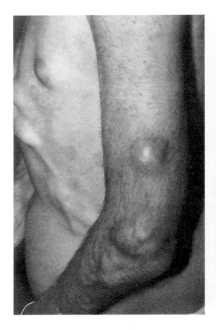 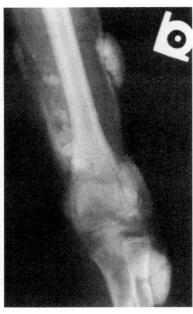

FIG. 1. Calcinosis universalis in childhood dermatomyositis. (A) Characteristic subcutaneous nodules are apparent in the left arm and anterior chest wall of this 15-year-old boy. (B) The nodules in this boy's arm are composed of dense lobular calcifications. In addition, the muscles of the upper arm are encased in a characteristic calcified sheath.

PROGNOSIS

The clinical course of dermatomyositis in children is variable. Some have long-term relapsing or persistent disease, whereas others recover. When recovery is incomplete, there may be severe residual weakness, joint contractures, and calcinosis. The calcinosis may be the principal cause of long-term disability.[1–6,23]

REFERENCES

1. Cassidy JT, Petty RE 2001 Juvenile dermatomyositis. In: Textbook of Pediatric Rheumatology, 4th ed. W. B. Saunders Company, pp. 465–504.
2. Pachman LM 1995 Juvenile dermatomyositis. Pathophysiology and disease expression. Pediatr Clin North Am **42:**1071–1098.
3. Kaye SA, Isenberg DA 1994 Treatment of polymyositis and dermatomyositis. Br J Hosp Med **52:**463–468.
4. Pachman LM 1994 Juvenile dermatomyositis. New clues to diagnosis and pathogenesis. Clin Exp Rheumatol **12:**S69–S73.
5. Ansell BM 1992 Juvenile dermatomyositis. J Rheumatol Suppl **33:**60–62.
6. Olson JC 1992 Juvenile dermatomyositis. Dermatologica **11:**57–64.
7. Jayalakshmi SS, Borgohain R, Mohandas S 2000 Dystrophic calcification in adult dermatomyositis: Neuroimage. Neurol India **48:**407.
8. Pachman LM, Hayford JR, Chung A, Daugherty CA, Pallansch MA, Fink CW, Gewanter HL, Jerath R, Lang BA, Sinacore J, Szer IS, Dyer AR, Hochberg MC 1998 Juvenile dermatomyositis at diagnosis: Clinical characteristics of 79 children. J Rheumatol **25:**1198–1204.
9. Wananukul S, Pongprasit P, Wattanakrai P 1997 Calcinosis cutis presenting years before other clinical manifestations of juvenile dermatomyositis: Report of two cases. Australas J Derm **38:**202–205.
10. Perez MD, Abrams SA, Koenning G, Stuff JE, O'Brien KO, Ellis KJ 1994 Mineral metabolism in children with dermatomyositis. J Rheumatol **21:**2364–2369.
11. Lian JB, Pachman LM, Gundberg CM, Partridge REH, Maryjowski MC 1982 Gamma-carboxyglutamate excretion and calcinosis in juvenile dermatomyositis. Arthritis Rheum **25:**1094–1100.
12. Mukamel M, Horev G, Mimouni M 2001 New insight into calcinosis of juvenile dermatomyositis: A study of composition and treatment. J Pediatr **138:**763–766.
13. Blane CE, White SJ, Braunstein EM, Bowyer SL, Sullivan DB 1984 Patterns of calcification in childhood dermatomyositis. Am J Roentgenol **142:**397–400.
14. Kissel JT, Mendell JR, Rammohan KW 1986 Microvascular deposition of complement membrane attack complex in dermatomyositis. N Engl J Med **314:**329–334.
15. Reed AM, Pachman LM, Hayford J, Ober C 1998 Immunogenetic studies in families of children with juvenile dermatomyositis. J Rheumatol **25:**1000–1002.
16. Moore EC, Cohen F, Douglas SD, Gutta V 1992 Staphylococcal infections in childhood dermatomyositis association with the development of calcinosis, raised IgE concentrations and granulocyte chemotactic defect. Ann Rheum Dis **51:**378–383.
17. Landis WJ 1995 The strength of a calcified tissue depends in part on the molecular structure and organization of its constituent mineral crystals in their organic matrix. Bone **116:**533–544.
18. Bowyer SL, Blane CE, Sullivan DB, Cassidy JT 1983 Childhood dermatomyositis: Factors predicting functional outcome and development of dystrophic calcification. J Pediatr **103:**882–888.
19. DeSilva TN, Kress DW 1998 Management of collagen vascular diseases in childhood. Dermatol Clin **6:**579–592.
20. Reiff A, Rawlings DJ, Shaham B, Franke E, Richardson L, Szer IS, Bernstein BH 1997 Preliminary evidence for cyclosporin A as an alternative in the treatment of recalcitrant juvenile rheumatoid arthritis and juvenile dermatomyositis. J Rheumatol **24:**2436–2443.
21. Moore SE, Jump AA, Smiley JD 1986 Effect of warfarin sodium therapy on excretion of 4-carboxy-l-glutamic acid in scleroderma, dermatomyositis, and myositis ossificans progressiva. Arthritis Rheum **29:**344–351.
22. Wang W-J, Lo W-L, Wong CK 1988 Calcinosis cutis-juvenile dermatomyositis: Remarkable response to aluminum hydroxide therapy (letter). Arch Dermatol **124:**1721–1722.
23. Eddy MC, Leelawattana R, McAlister WH, Whyte MP 1997 Calcinosis universalis complicating juvenile dermatomyositis: Resolution during probenecid therapy. J Clin Endocrinol Metab **82:**3536–3542.
24. Vinen CS, Patel S, Bruckner FE 2000 Regression of calcinosis associated with adult dermatomyositis follow diltiazem therapy. Rheumatology **39:**333–340.
25. Ichiki Y, Akiyama T, Shimozawa N, Suzuki Y, Kondo N, Kitajima Y 2001 An extremely severe case of cutaneous calcinosis with juvenile dermatomyositis, and successful treatment with diltiazem. Br J Dermatol **144:**894–897.

Chapter 85. Fibrodysplasia (Myositis) Ossificans Progressiva

Frederick S. Kaplan, David L. Glaser, and Eileen M. Shore

Division of Molecular Orthopaedics, Department of Orthopaedic Surgery, The University of Pennsylvania School of Medicine, Philadelphia, Pennsylvania

INTRODUCTION

Fibrodysplasia ossificans progressiva (FOP) is a rare heritable disorder of connective tissue disease characterized by (1) congenital malformations of the great toes and (2) recurrent episodes of painful soft-tissue swelling that lead to heterotopic ossification.[1,2]

Post-traumatic myositis ossificans, a different disorder, also features heterotopic bone and cartilage formation within soft tissues. Heterotopic ossification may also follow hip replacement, spinal cord injury, and brain injury.

FOP was first described in 1692; more than 600 cases have been reported.[1,2] This disorder is among the rarest of human afflictions, with an estimated incidence of one per two million live births.[1,2] All races are affected.[2] Autosomal dominant transmission with variable expressivity is established.[3] However, reproductive fitness is low, and most cases are sporadic. Gonadal mosaicism has been described.[4]

CLINICAL PRESENTATION

If the typical congenital skeletal malformations are recognized, FOP can be suspected at birth before soft-tissue lesions occur.[1,2] The characteristic feature is short great toes, caused by malformation (hallux valgus) of the cartilaginous anlage of the first metatarsal and proximal phalanx (Fig. 1). In some cases, the thumbs also are strikingly short. Synostosis and hypoplasia of the phalanges is typical.[1,2] FOP is usually diagnosed when soft-tissue swellings and radiographic evidence of heterotopic ossification are first noted.[1,2]

The severity of FOP differs significantly among patients,[5] although most become immobilized and confined to a wheelchair by the third decade of life.[1,2,6] Typically, episodes of soft-tissue swelling begin during the first decade of life (Fig. 1).[7] Occasionally, the onset occurs as late as early adulthood.

Painful, tender, and rubbery soft-tissue lesions appear spontaneously or may seem to be precipitated by minor trauma including intramuscular injections and influenza-like viral illnesses.[2,8] Swellings develop rapidly during the course of several days. Typically, lesions affect the paraspinal muscles in the back or in the limb girdles and may persist for several months.[9] Aponeuroses, fascia, tendons, ligaments, and connective tissue of voluntary muscles may be affected. Although some swellings may regress spontaneously, most mature through an endochondral pathway, engendering true heterotopic bone.[9] The episodes of induration recur with unpredictable frequency. Some patients seem to have periods of quiescent disease. However, once ossification develops, it is permanent.

Gradually, bony masses immobilize joints and cause contractures and deformity, particularly in the neck and shoulders. Ossification around the hips, typically present by the third decade of life, often prevents ambulation.[6] Involvement of the muscles of mastication (frequently the outcome of injection of local anesthetic or overstretching of the jaw during dental procedures) can severely limit movement of the mandible and ultimately impair nutrition.[10,11] Ankylosis of the spine and rib cage further restricts mobility and may imperil cardiopulmonary function (Fig. 1).[1,2,6,12] Scoliosis is common and associated with heterotopic bone that asymmetrically connects the rib cage to the pelvis.[13] Hypokyphosis results from ossification of the paravertebral musculature. Restrictive lung disease and predisposition to pneumonia may follow. However, the vocal muscles, diaphragm, extraocular muscles, heart, and smooth muscles are characteristically spared.[1] Although secondary amenorrhea may develop, reproduction has occurred.[1–3] Hearing impairment (beginning in late childhood or adolescence) manifests with increased frequency.[14]

RADIOLOGIC FEATURES

Skeletal anomalies and soft-tissue ossification are the characteristic radiologic features of FOP.[15] The principal malformations involve the great toe, although other anomalies of digits in the feet and hands may occur. Exostoses may occur.[9] A remarkable feature of FOP is progressive fusion of cervical vertebrae that may be confused with Klippel-Feil syndrome.[1] The femoral necks may be broad yet short. However, the remainder of the skeleton is generally unremarkable.[15]

Ectopic ossification in FOP progresses in several regular patterns or gradients (proximally before distally, axially before appendicularly, cranially before caudally, and dorsally before ventrally).[7] Paraspinal muscles are involved early in life, with subsequent spread to the shoulders and hips. The ankles, wrists, and jaw may be affected at later stages.[7]

Radiographic and bone scan findings suggest normal modeling and remodeling of heterotopic bone.[16] Fractures are not increased and respond similarly in either the heterotopic or normotopic skeleton.[17]

Bone scans are abnormal before ossification can be demonstrated by conventional radiographs.[16] Computerized tomography and magnetic resonance imaging of early lesions has been described.[18]

LABORATORY FINDINGS

Routine biochemical studies of mineral metabolism are usually normal, although alkaline phosphatase activity in

---

The authors have no conflict of interest.

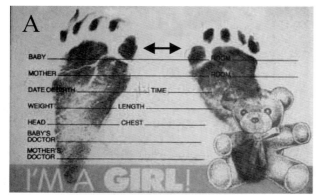

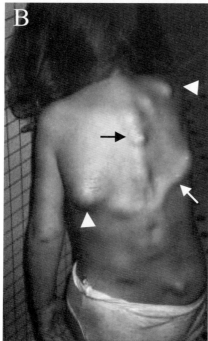

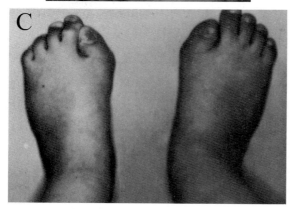

FIG. 1. Fibrodysplasia (myositis) ossificans progressiva. Characteristic features of FOP are seen in early childhood. (A) The presence of short malformed great toes at birth (arrows) heralds (B) the later spontaneous appearance of the preosseous soft tissue lesions on the neck and back (arrowheads) and should provoke suspicion of FOP even before the transformation to heterotopic bone (arrows). (C) An inspection of the toes will confirm the diagnosis and may alleviate the need for a lesional biopsy (trauma) that could exacerbate the condition. (Reprinted from J Bone Miner Res 1997;**12**:855 with permission from the American Society for Bone and Mineral Research.)

serum may be increased, especially during disease "flare-ups".[1,2,19] Urinary basic fibroblast growth factor (FGF) levels may be elevated during disease flare-ups and coincide with the preosseous angiogenic fibroproliferative lesions.[20]

HISTOPATHOLOGY

The earliest stage of FOP lesion formation consists of an intense aggregation of B- and T-lymphocytes in the perivascular spaces of otherwise normal-appearing skeletal muscle.[21] Subsequently, a nearly pure T-cell infiltrate is seen between edematous muscle fibers at the leading edge of an angiogenic fibroproliferative lesion, which is indistinguishable from *aggressive juvenile fibromatosis*.[21,22] Mast cell infiltration is seen at all stages of FOP flare-ups.[23] Misdiagnosis is common but can be avoided by correctly examining the patient's toes. Immunostaining with a monoclonal antibody against bone morphogenetic protein (BMP) 2/4 is intense in FOP lesions, but not in aggressive fibromatosis.[22] Endochondral ossification is the major pathway for heterotopic bone formation.[9] Mature osseous lesions have haversian systems and can contain hematopoietic tissue.

ETIOLOGY AND PATHOGENESIS

The genetic defect causing FOP has been mapped to 4q27–31 based on four small multigenerational families.[24] Dysregulation of *BMP4* gene expression has been reported,[25–27] but mutational screening and linkage exclusion analysis indicate that the molecular defect lies elsewhere.[28] Similarities between FOP and the effects of *Drosophila decapentaplegic* gene (BMP4 homolog) mutations may represent clues to the etiology and pathogenesis.[29] Although mutations in the gene encoding noggin, a BMP antagonist, are not the cause of FOP,[30] FOP cells are unable to appropriately upregulate the expression of multiple BMP antagonists, including noggin and gremlin, in response to a BMP challenge.[31]

TREATMENT

There is no established medical treatment for FOP.[1,2] The disorder's rarity, variable severity, and fluctuating clinical course pose substantial uncertainties when evaluating experimental therapies. Binders of dietary calcium, radiotherapy, and warfarin are ineffective.[1,2,32] Limited benefits have been reported using corticosteroids and disodium etidronate together during flare-ups, or by using isotretinoin to prevent disease activation.[33,34] However, these impressions reflect uncontrolled studies. Accordingly, medical intervention is currently supportive. Nevertheless, physical therapy to maintain joint mobility may be harmful by provoking or exacerbating lesions.[1,2] Surgical release of joint contractures is unsuccessful and risks new, trauma-induced heterotopic ossification.[1,2] Removal of FOP lesions is often followed by significant recurrence. Osteotomy of ectopic bone to mobilize a joint is uniformly counterproductive because additional heterotopic ossification develops at the operative site. Spinal bracing is ineffective, and surgical intervention is associated with numerous complications.[13]

Dental therapy should preclude injection of local anesthetics and stretching of the jaw.[1,2,10,11] In fact, newer dental techniques for focused administration of anesthetic are available. Guidelines for general anesthesia have been reported.[10] Intramuscular injections should be avoided.[8] Prevention of falls is crucial.[35] Measures against recurrent pulmonary infections and onset of cardiopulmonary complications of restrictive lung disease are important.

PROGNOSIS

Despite widespread heterotopic ossification and severe disability, some patients live productive lives into the seventh decade. Most, however, die earlier from pulmonary complications including pneumonia, secondary to restricted ventilation from chest wall involvement.[1,2,12]

PROGRESSIVE OSSEOUS HETEROPLASIA

Research on FOP led to the discovery of progressive osseous heteroplasia (POH), a distinct developmental disorder of heterotopic ossification.[36–38] Like FOP, POH is an autosomal dominant genetic disorder of heterotopic ossification within soft connective tissues. However, unlike in FOP, heterotopic ossification in POH commonly occurs within the dermis and forms by an intramembraneous, rather than an endochondral, pathway.[38] Identification of two patients with POH-like features who also had Albright Hereditary Osteodystrophy suggested the possibility of a genetic link between the two conditions,[38,39] which was confirmed in a third patient with pure POH.[40] These discoveries led to the rapid identification of paternally inherited inactivating mutations of the *GNAS1* gene as the genetic cause of POH.[41]

REFERENCES

1. Connor JM, Evans DAP 1982 Fibrodysplasia ossificans progressiva: The clinical features and natural history of 34 patients. J Bone Joint Surg Br 64:76–83.
2. Kaplan FS, Shore EM, Connor JM 2002 Fibrodysplasia ossificans progressiva. In: Royce PM, Steinmann B (ed.) Connective Tissue and Its Heritable Disorders: Molecular, Genetic, and Medical Aspects, 2nd ed. John Wiley & Sons, New York, NY, USA, pp. 827–840.
3. Delatycki M, Rogers JG 1998 The genetics of fibrodysplasia ossificans progressiva. Clin Orthop 346:15–18.
4. Janoff HB, Muenke M, Johnson LO, Rosenberg A, Shore EM, Okereke E, Zasloff M, Kaplan FS 1996 Fibrodysplasia ossificans progressiva in two half-sisters. Evidence for maternal mosaicism. Am J Med Genet 61:320–324.
5. Janoff HB, Tabas JA, Shore EM, Muenke M, Dalinka MK, Schlesinger S, Zasloff MA, Kaplan FS 1995 Mild expression of fibrodysplasia ossificans progressiva: A report of 3 cases. J Rheumatol 22:976–978.
6. Rocke DM, Zasloff M, Peeper J, Cohen RB, Kaplan FS 1994 Age and joint-specific risk of initial heterotopic ossification in patients who have fibrodysplasia ossificans progressiva. Clin Orthop 301:243–248.
7. Cohen RB, Hahn GV, Tabas JA, Peeper J, Levitz CL, Sando A, Sando N, Zasloff M, Kaplan FS 1993 The natural history of heterotopic ossification in patients who have fibrodysplasia ossificans progressiva. A study of 44 patients. J Bone Joint Surg Am 75:215–219.
8. Lanchoney TF, Cohen RB, Rocke DM, Zasloff MA, Kaplan FS 1995 Permanent heterotopic ossification at the injection site after diphtheria-tetanus-pertussis immunizations in children who have fibrodysplasia ossificans progressiva. J Pediatr 126:762–764.
9. Kaplan FS, Tabas JA, Gannon FH, Finkel G, Hahn GV, Zasloff MA 1993 The histopathology of fibrodysplasia ossificans progressiva: An endochondral process. J Bone Joint Surg Am 75:220–230.
10. Luchetti W, Cohen RB, Hahn GV, Rocke DM, Helpin M, Zasloff M, Kaplan FS 1996 Severe restriction in jaw movement after routine injection of local anesthetic in patients who have progressiva. Oral Surg Oral Med Oral Pathol Oral Radiol Endod 81:21–25.
11. Janoff HB, Zasloff M, Kaplan FS 1996 Submandibular swelling in patients with fibrodysplasia ossificans progressiva. Otolaryngol Head Neck Surg 114:599–604.
12. Kussmaul WG, Esmail AN, Sagar Y, Ross J, Gregory S, Kaplan FS 1998 Pulmonary and cardiac function in advanced fibrodysplasia ossificans progressiva. Clin Orthop 346:104–109.
13. Shah PB, Zasloff MA, Drummond D, Kaplan FS 1994 Spinal deformity in patients who have fibrodysplasia ossificans progressiva. J Bone Joint Surg Am 76:1442–1450.
14. Levy CE, Lash AT, Janoff HB, Kaplan FS 1999 Conductive hearing loss in individuals with fibrodysplasia ossificans progressiva. Am J Audiol 8:29–33.
15. Mahboubi S, Glaser DL, Shore EM, Kaplan FS 2001 Fibrodysplasia ossificans progressiva (FOP). Pediatr Radiol 31:307–314.
16. Kaplan FS, Strear CM, Zasloff MA 1994 Radiographic and scintigraphic features of modeling and remodeling in the heterotopic skeleton of patients who have fibrodysplasia ossificans progressiva. Clin Orthop 304:238–247.
17. Einhorn TA, Kaplan FS 1994 Traumatic fractures of heterotopic bone in patients who have fibrodysplasia ossificans progressiva. Clin Orthop 308:173–177.
18. Shirkhoda A, Armin A-R, Bis KG, Makris J, Irwin RB, Shetty AN 1995 MR imaging of myositis ossificans: Variable patterns at different stages. J Magn Reson Imaging 65:287–292.
19. Lutwak L 1964 Myositis ossificans progressiva: Mineral, metabolic, and radioactive calcium studies of the effects of hormones. Am J Med 37:269–293.
20. Kaplan F, Sawyer J, Connors S, Keough K, Shore E, Gannon F, Glaser D, Rocke D, Zasloff M, Folkman J 1998 Urinary basic fibroblast growth factor: A biochemical marker for preosseous fibroproliferative lesions in patients with FOP. Clin Orthop 346:59–65.
21. Gannon FH, Valentine BA, Shore EM, Zasloff MA, Kaplan FS 1998 Acute lymphocytic infiltration in an extremely early lesion of fibrodysplasia ossificans progressiva. Clin Orthop 346:19–25.
22. Gannon F, Kaplan FS, Olmsted E, Finkel G, Zasloff M, Shore E 1997 Differential immunostaining with bone morphogenetic protein (BMP) 2/4 in early fibromatous lesions of fibrodysplasia ossificans progressiva and aggressive juvenile fibromatosis. Hum Pathol 28:339–343.
23. Gannon FH, Glaser D, Caron R, Thompson LD, Shore EM, Kaplan FS 2001 Mast cell involvement in fibrodysplasia ossificans progressiva. Hum Pathol 32:842–848.
24. Feldman G, Li M, Martin S, Urbanek M, Urtizberea JA, Fardeau M, LeMerrer M, Connor JM, Triffitt J, Smith R, Muenke M, Kaplan FS, Shore EM 2000 Fibrodysplasia ossificans progressiva (FOP), a heritable disorder of severe heterotopic ossification, maps to human chromosome 4q27–31. Am J Hum Genet 66:128–135.
25. Shafritz AB, Shore EM, Gannon FH, Zasloff MA, Taub R, Muenke M, Kaplan FS 1996 Dysregulation of bone morphogenetic protein 4 (BMP4) gene expression in fibrodysplasia ossificans progressiva. N Engl J Med 335:555–561.
26. Lanchoney TF, Olmsted EA, Shore EM, Gannon FA, Rosen V, Zasloff MA, Kaplan FS 1998 Characterization of bone morphogenetic protein 4 receptors in fibrodysplasia ossificans progressiva. Clin Orthop 346:38–45.
27. Olmsted EA, Kaplan FS, Shore EM 2003 Bone morphogenetic protein-4 regulation in fibrodysplasia ossificans progressiva. Clin Orthop 408:331–343.
28. Xu M, Shore EM 1998 Mutational screening of the bone morphogenetic protein 4 gene in a family with fibrodysplasia ossificans progressiva. Clin Orthop 346:53–58.
29. Kaplan F, Tabas JA, Zasloff MA 1990 Fibrodysplasia ossificans progressiva: A clue from the fly? Calcif Tissue Int 47:117–125.
30. Xu MQ, Feldman G, Le Merrer M, Shugart YY, Glaser DL, Urtizberea JA, Fardeau M, Connor JM, Triffitt J, Smith R, Shore EM, Kaplan FS 2000 Linkage exclusion and mutational analysis of the noggin gene in patients with fibrodysplasia ossificans progressiva. Clin Genet 58:291–298.
31. Ahn J, Serrano de La Peña L, Shore EM, Kaplan FS 2003 Paresis of a bone morphogenetic protein antagonist response in a genetic disorder of heterotopic skeletogenesis. J Bone Joint Surg Am 85:667–674.
32. Moore SE, Jump AA, Smiley JD 1986 Effect of warfarin sodium therapy on excretion of 4-carboxy-L-glutamic acid in scleroderma, dermatomyositis, and myositis ossificans progressiva. Arthritis Rheum 29:344–351.

33. Brantus J-F, Meunier PJ 1998 Effects of intravenous etidronate and oral corticosteroids in fibrodysplasia ossificans progressiva. Clin Orthop **346:**117–120.

34. Zasloff MA, Rocke DM, Crofford LJ, Hahn GV, Kaplan FS 1998 Treatment of patients who have fibrodysplasia ossificans progressiva with isotretinoin. Clin Orthop **346:**121–129.

35. Glaser DM, Rocke DM, Kaplan FS 1998 Catastrophic falls in patients who have fibrodysplasia ossificans progressiva. Clin Orthop **346:**110–116.

36. Kaplan FS, Craver R, MacEwen GD, Gannon FH, Finkel G, Hahn G, Tabas J, Gardner RJ, Zasloff MA 1994 Progressive osseous heteroplasia: A distinct developmental disorder of heterotopic ossification. J Bone Joint Surg Am **76:**425–436.

37. Rosenfeld SR, Kaplan FS 1995 Progressive osseous heteroplasia in male patients. Clin Orthop **317:**243–245.

38. Kaplan FS, Shore EM 2000 Progressive osseous heteroplasia. J Bone Miner Res **15:**2084–2094.

39. Eddy MC, Jan De Beur SM, Yandow SM, McAlister WH, Shore EM, Kaplan FS, Whyte MP, Levine MA 2000 Deficiency of the alpha-subunit of the stimulatory G protein and severe extraskeletal ossification. J Bone Miner Res **15:**2074–2083.

40. Yeh GL, Mathur S, Wivel A, Li M, Gannon FH, Ulied A, Audi L, Olmstead EA, Kaplan FS, Shore EM 2000 GNAS1 mutation and Cbfa1 misexpression in a child with severe congenital platelike osteoma cutis. J Bone Miner Res **15:**2063–2073.

41. Shore EM, Ahn J, Jan de Beur S, Li M, Xu M, Gardner RJ, Zasloff MA, Whyte MP, Levine MA, Kaplan FS 2002 Paternally-inherited inactivating mutations of the GNAS1 gene in progressive osseous heteroplasia. N Engl J Med **346:**99–106.

Hypercalciuria and Kidney Stones

Chapter 86.   Nephrolithiasis

Fredric L. Coe and Joan H. Parks

Nephrology Section, Department of Medicine and Kidney Stone Program, The University of Chicago, Chicago, Illinois

INTRODUCTION

All kidney stones are aggregates of crystals mixed with a protein matrix, and all cause disease because of obstruction of urine flow in the renal collecting system, ureters, or urethra; bleeding; or local erosion into the kidney tissue. The common stone is calcium oxalate; this stone is small, recurrent, a cause of pain from passage and obstruction, and caused by metabolic disorders that mostly are treatable.[1] Uric acid stones are uncommon (about 5% of all stones) and radiolucent but otherwise like calcium oxalate stones. Struvite stones, from infection, fill renal collecting systems, erode into the renal tissue, and cause obvious renal functional impairment. Cystine stones have only one cause, hereditary cystinuria. They grow large enough to fill the renal collecting system, begin in childhood, and can cause renal failure. Kidney stones are expensive, and it has been shown that it is cost effective to prevent them.

All stones need crystallographic analysis by simple polarization microscopy or X-ray diffraction. Even if the first few stones are shown to contain uric acid, for example, the next may contain calcium oxalate or struvite. Radiographs are not helpful for identification except in the case of uric acid stones, which are lucent; the rest are similar, although some generalizations can be made. Calcium oxalate stones resemble stars in the night sky, cystine stones are like eggs or staghorns and seem sculpted of a soft stone or wax, and struvite stones are mostly rugged, ringed staghorns that look like tree roots. We use flat plates to count stones; tomograms without prior radiocontrast injections are ideal but expensive. Laboratory evaluation detects causes; therefore, measuring 24-h urine calcium, oxalate, uric acid, citrate, pH, volume, and creatinine estimates completeness of collection. How many urine samples are best? One is certainly minimal; we favor three for better surety, and if we found stones, we would measure four. Blood tests are for hypercalcemia; the rest is vague and unsure. Hormone measurements are never proper for initial evaluation; a parathyroid hormone (PTH) measurement is obtained for patients who are hypercalcemic.

CALCIUM STONES

Just as bone mineral forms when a supersaturated extracellular fluid contacts an appropriate nucleation site, kidney stones form when urine, or more probably, tubule fluid becomes highly supersaturated with a calcium salt such as calcium oxalate or a calcium phosphate phase. What distinguishes the two processes are the greater levels of supersaturation in urine compared with plasma, the presence in urine, and tubule fluid of powerful inhibitors of the crystallization process, and the fact that calcium oxalate, not calcium phosphate, is the main constituent of stones. The causes of calcium stones can have other effects. They increase urine calcium or oxalate concentration; lower urine volume, so concentrations of all solutes increase; lower urine citrate, which normally forms a soluble salt with calcium and prevents crystallization; increase levels of molecules (uric acid in particular) that can promote calcium oxalate nucleation; or cause abnormally high urine pH, which promotes calcium phosphate crystallization, or low urine pH, which promotes uric acid crystallization.

HYPERCALCIURIC STATES

Idiopathic hypercalciuria (IH),[2] the most common hypercalciuric state, occurs in families, affects both sexes equally, and has a pattern of horizontal and vertical transmission like that of a mendelian dominant trait. About 50% of patients with calcium oxalate stones have IH and are detected by a daily urine calcium excretion rate above the usual normal limits of 300 mg (for men) and 250 mg (for women); by normal serum calcium level; and by the absence of other hypercalciuric conditions such as sarcoidosis, vitamin D intoxication, immobilization, hyperthyroidism, glucocorticoid excess, rapidly progressive osteoporosis, Paget's disease, and Cushing's disease.[3] Hypercalciuria increases urine calcium oxalate supersaturation,[4] especially after eating. The mechanism of the hypercalciuria is surely intestinal calcium absorption at an abnormally high rate,[5] and what controversy exists concerns the cause of the high absorption rate. The most satisfactory view is that 1,25-dihydroxyvitamin D or calcitriol levels in the serum are high as a primary defect; in eight studies, hypercalciuric patients had higher levels than normal subjects.[6–13] The high calcitriol levels can increase calcium absorption and suppress PTH secretion, leading to reduced renal tubule

---

The authors have no conflict of interest.

calcium reabsorption. After eating, calcium will enter the blood at a more rapid rate than normal, and tubule reabsorption will be low, so serum calcium levels can remain near normal despite high absorption rates, and the calcium can be excreted rapidly into the urine. Alternative theories include a primary renal tubule leak of calcium and a primary increase in intestinal calcium absorption. Neither would explain the common pattern of low PTH[10] and high calcitriol levels, but they could account for hypercalciuria in some selected patients with high PTH levels or normal calcitriol levels.

In addition to hyperabsorption of calcium, hypercalciuric patients conserve calcium less well than normal people when given a low calcium intake in the range of 200–500 mg daily. In balance studies, when total calcium absorption can be measured, their urine calcium clearly exceeds net calcium absorption on such diets, meaning that bone mineral is being mobilized into the urine. The reason for their labile bone mineral stores may partly be an excessive action of calcitriol. When given to normal men, this hormone promotes the same behavior as seen among patients with infectious hepatitis, a loss of bone mineral during low-calcium diet.[12,13] High levels of serum calcitriol are by no means universal among the patients, despite almost universal calcium hyperabsorption, suggesting that not only high serum levels but possibly also high levels of the calcitriol receptor could mediate excessive calcitriol effects. In rats bred for hypercalciuria, increased calcitriol receptor number is an established cause of increased calcitriol action.[14]

Given the lability of bone mineral and the natural tendency of doctors to use low-calcium diets for treatment of hypercalciuria, one might expect reduced bone mineral density (BMD) among IH patients, and to date, five studies documented just this.[15] In particular, the patients whose hypercalciuria persists during low-calcium diet show decisively low BMDs, whereas those with normal or near-normal calcium retention during low-calcium diet (a minority) have normal BMD. A clinical corollary of this finding is that caution must be used concerning a low-calcium diet as a treatment except among patients clearly able to respond to it with normal calcium conservation. Among patients otherwise prone to osteoporosis, a low-calcium diet has an additional and obvious disadvantage. For these reasons, we favor its use in only very restricted circumstances.[16]

Thiazide diuretic agents reduce urine calcium excretion, calcium oxalate supersaturation,[4] and the rate of stone production.[17] Thiazide affects the connecting segment of the nephron,[18] increasing calcium reabsorption rate, and presumably reduces calcium excretion in patients by a direct renal action. The drugs reduce intestinal calcium absorption in patients who have severe hypercalciuria[19] but less than they lower urine calcium excretion, so calcium balance becomes more positive. Alternative treatments include a low-calcium diet, sodium cellulose phosphate, and orthophosphate, all of which reduce intestinal calcium absorption. The long-term effects of reduced calcium absorption, especially from a low-calcium diet, may include reduced bone mineral stores, because hypercalciuric patients do not reduce their urine calcium excretion rates to values as low as those in normal people when both are given a very low calcium intake.[10] Men who are given calcitriol in excess but at a dose that does not increase serum calcium above normal[12,13] also fail to reduce urine calcium normally while eating a low-calcium diet.

Primary hyperparathyroidism causes hypercalciuria in about 5% of calcium stone formers[20]; 85% have single enlarged glands, so-called adenoma; the rest have at least two enlarged glands, so-called hyperplasia. Serum calcium level is always increased, although the increase commonly is so mild that many values are needed to be sure hypercalcemia is present. Upper limits for our normal subjects are serum calcium levels of 10 mg/dl in women and 10.1 mg/dl in men. Serum levels of at least one-half of our patients who had curative surgery were all below 10.5 mg/dl.[20] Urine calcium excretion is very high, despite the modest hypercalcemia, so a casual analysis can be misleading; extreme hypercalciuria and serum calcium levels of, for example, 10.1 to 10.3 mg/dl, can lead one to think of idiopathic hypercalciuria and probably account for misleading accounts of normocalcemia primary hyperparathyroidism,[21–23] each of which, in retrospect, was almost certainly an instance of mild hypercalcemia.

Among patients who have had curative surgery, serum PTH levels have been elevated between 80% and 100% with a carboxy-terminal assay and between 60% and 80% with amino-terminal or mild molecule assays[20]; therefore, PTH assay is more confirmatory than a structural basis of diagnosis. The best course is to establish whether hypercalcemia is present and then to exclude other causes such as malignant tumors, sarcoidosis, and other granulomatous diseases, vitamin D intoxication, thiazide use, lithium use, and the uncommon or rare disorders.[20] Familial hypocalciuric hypercalcemia is a mendelian dominant disorder, not a cause of stones, best diagnosed by family studies.[20] Low PTH levels are especially valuable to detect states of primary calcitriol excess.[21] Serum calcitriol is increased in most patients[24–26] as a consequence of high PTH and low serum phosphorus level, and the calcitriol stimulates intestinal calcium absorption, causing most of the hypercalciuria. Bone mineral loss into the urine also occurs.

Treatment is surgical in patients with stone disease. Stone formation is greatly reduced, because urine calcium excretion decreases promptly. We follow-up on our patients to be sure that residual hypercalciuria is not present and that serum calcium levels remain normal.

Renal tubular acidosis (RTA) is ostensibly a cause of hypercalciuria,[27] but we suspect that it is as often a consequence as a cause. The defect associated with stones is reduced ability to reduce urine pH; urine citrate excretion is very low, as a rule, and urine calcium is high. It is true that metabolic acidosis is a consequence of sever reductions of tubule ability to reduce pH, because a pH lower that that of blood is needed to titrate urine buffers with protons and to trap ammonia as ammonium ion, for excretion. Metabolic acidosis reduces urine citrate excretion and raises urine calcium, so one is tempted to consider the high pH, high urine calcium, and low urine pH as an expected clustering based on known physiology.

However, we have found[28] that alkali treatment, which should reduce urine calcium excretion, usually does not, although it may raise urine citrate excretion. Metabolic acidosis is not discernible in most patients. Early reports of

RTA[29] included, as a majority, patients such as we have encountered and labeled them as having incomplete RTA. In families, idiopathic hypercalciuria and RTA both appear,[30] and the hypercalciuria of our patients usually responds to thiazide. We are inclined to believe that the hypercalciuria comes first and that nephrocalcinosis, perhaps hypercalciuria itself, damages collecting ducts and causes the incomplete RTA.

The patients form stones composed mainly of calcium phosphate salts. High urine pH increases urine levels of dissociated phosphate, which forms brushite calcium monohydrogen phosphate and apatite. The stones are larger than calcium oxalate stones, and they grow faster. Apart from sporadic and familial incomplete RTA, in rare cases, patients have complete RTA, usually inherited as an autosomal dominant trait. They have metabolic acidosis; their urine calcium excretions decrease with alkali treatment. Diamox (acetazolamide) reduces bicarbonate reabsorption by the proximal tubule and causes alkaline urine and stones. The urine is alkaline because the drug is given in multiple doses, so bicarbonate levels decrease, increase between doses, and decrease again as the bicarbonate is excreted. Inherited or acquired proximal RTA is a steady defect and causes neither stones nor alkaline urine. Hyperkalemic type 4 RTA resulting from obstruction, low rennin or aldosterone secretion rates, or renal disease[31] causes an acid urine pH and not stones.

HYPEROXALURIC STATES

Primary hyperoxaluria always comes from one of two hereditary enzyme defects that increase oxalate production.[32] Oxalate is an end product, excreted only by the kidneys, which filter and secrete it.[33] Urine oxalate excretion is above the usual normal limit of 40 mg daily,[34] in the range of 80–120 mg. The oxalate crystallizes with calcium, causing stones that begin in childhood, and tubulointerstitial nephropathy, which leads to chronic renal failure. Renal tubular acidosis may be an early sign of nephropathy, causing an anion gap, metabolic acidosis that increases the serum chloride level and lowers the bicarbonate level. Renal transplantation requires extensive dialytic preparation so that stored oxalate does not flood the graft and destroy it. Overproduction occurs from pyridoxine deficiency (in animals) and methoxyflurane anesthetic and occurs if one is so foolish or mistaken as to drink ethylene glycol (antifreeze) as a beverage. Treatment is with fluids, citrate (to reduce calcium ion levels), and pyridoxine, which may be helpful in low doses of 20–40 mg daily in some people. Others respond only to 300–400 mg daily, and some do not respond at all.

Enteric hyperoxaluria means that the colon absorbs oxalate excessively because small bowel malabsorption permits undigested fatty acids and bile acids to reach the colon epithelium and increase its permeability.[35] Small-bowel resection, intestinal bypass for obesity, and small-bowel diseases such as Crohn's disease are common causes.[36] Colectomy or ileostomy prevents the oxaluria. Urine oxalate is above normal, in the range of 75–150 mg daily. Urine citrate is low because of the alkali loss from the small bowel, and urine pH is low. Urine calcium usually is low, not high. A low-oxalate diet and a low-fat diet reduce oxaluria; low fat reduces delivery of fatty acids to the colon. Oral calcium, 1–4 g as calcium carbonate, taken with meals, crystallizes with oxalate in the gut lumen. Cholestyramine, 1–4 g with meals, adsorbs oxalate and also bile salts. The four treatments are synergistic and should be used together. Cholestyramine has important side effects of vitamin K depletion and reduced absorption of drugs.

In a way, dietary oxalate excess is an enteric oxaluria. Usual food culprits are nuts, pepper, chocolate, rhubarb, and spinach for a few devotees, and for the rest, mixtures of dark green vegetables and fruits. Vitamin C in large doses may increase urine oxalate, and ascorbic acid itself may, in urine, break down to oxalic acid, giving a wrong impression of hyperoxaluria. Treatments are simply dietary.

HYPERURICOSURIC STATES

About 25% of calcium stone formers excrete more than 800 mg daily of uric acid (750 mg in women) and have no other apparent causes of their stones.[37] Their urine pH is lower than the normal of 6.0, averaging 5.6,[38] so the uric acid can crystallize.[39] Uric acid crystals can promote calcium oxalate crystallization[40] because they share structural features. Treatment with allopurinol reduced stone recurrence in a prospective, controlled trial,[41] and neither allopurinol nor its metabolites affect calcium oxalate crystallization. The hyperuricosuria results from high purine intake[42] and from meats, and dietary treatment should be effective, although it has not been tested. We recommend reducing diet purine intake and reserving allopurinol for those who produce more stones, unless stone disease has been so severe that maximal certainty of treatment is desired despite the risk of drug side effects.

LOW URINE CITRATE

Women with stones excrete only 550 mg of citrate daily compared with 750 mg daily for normal women.[43] This decisive abnormality ought to increase the risk of stones because citrate forms a soluble calcium salt, and what calcium is in the salt is not free to combine with oxalic acid. Normal men excrete no more citrate than women with stones, and men who form stones excrete about the same amount of citrate, so low urine citrate in men is not so much an abnormality as it is a trait that explains why four out of five people with stones are men. Any oral alkali can increase urine citrate. We prefer citrate to sodium bicarbonate for its longer duration of action, and we use 25–50 mEq, two or three times daily. Citrate treatment has been tested in one prospective controlled trial.[44] Barcelo et al.[44] found that of the 38 patients who completed the 36-month trial, the stone formation rate was lower in the treated than in the placebo group ($p < 0.0$) compared with that before treatment.

URIC ACID STONES

Mixed

About 12% of all calcium stones contain some uric acid,[45] and patients form the mixed stones from urine that is supersaturated with uric acid because its pH is below the normal level of 6.0. Hyperuricosuria also is common. The urine of mixed stone formers is like that of patients with hyperuricosuric calcium oxalate stones, and what distinguishes the two groups is simply that in one, uric acid is inferred as a promoter of calcium oxalate stones, and in the other, the uric acid crystals are seen in the stones themselves. Probably if all of the stones of the former group were studied, uric acid would be found in some; the distinction is not so intrinsic as it is based on accident of how patients are studied and the relative proportions of uric acid to calcium oxalate in their stones.

Treatment includes reduced diet purine for hyperuricosuria, oral alkali to raise urine pH to 6 or 6.5, and thiazide for hypercalciuria, which may occur in some patients. The hyperuricosuric calcium oxalate stone formers are defined by absence of hypercalciuria or other causes of stones, so thiazide is not usually needed or appropriate.

Pure

Only about 5% of stone formers produce pure uric acid stones. Their urine is very acid, with pH values below 5.3, which is the pK of uric acid, and frequently below 5.0. Uric acid solubility in urine is just below 100 mg/liter, whereas the salts of monohydrogen urate are relatively much more soluble, so urine pH values near the pK raise uric acid supersaturation drastically by raising the fraction of the total urate that is fully protonated. For example, average normal men excrete 650 mg of uric acid in 1.2 liters of urine,[40] a concentration of 540 mg/liter; at pK 6.0, less than 10% is undissociated, whereas at pH 5.3, 50% (270 mg/liter) is undissociated (2.7 times above the solubility). Uric acid stones occur in people with gout and in others with familial uric acid stones. All have low urine pH, and the reason is unclear. Patients with ileostomy or who work in hot and dry places form scanty and acid urine and uric acid stones. Treatment is always alkali to raise urine pH to 6 and reduced purine intake or allopurinol for hypericosuria.

STRUVITE STONES

Only microorganisms that have urease enzyme can produce struvite stones, by hydrolyzing urine urea to carbon dioxide and ammonia; therefore, urinary infection is the only clinical cause of these infection stones. Struvite forms as the ammonia raises local pH to above 9; phosphate is fully dissociated and combines with urine magnesium and ammonium ion. Carbonate apatite also is formed from the carbonate and calcium because of high pH, so pure struvite stones always contain both crystals. Mixed stones also contain calcium oxalate, which is not particularly favored to form under the same circumstances as struvite and denotes the combination of metabolic and infection stone in the same patient.

Mixed

We find that about one-third of struvite stones are mixed; patients begin their stone careers with passage, and their prognosis for renal function and nephrectomy is excellent. Men are nearly one-half of this group, and almost all men with struvite stones form mixed stones. Urine calcium excretion is above normal for the group in both sexes. Mean serum creatinine is normal. A few patients do have reduced creatinine clearance, which is rare among calcium stone formers.[46]

Pure

More than one-half of this group are women. Stones are frequently staghorns that fill the renal collecting systems. Infection, bleeding, or flank pain, rather than stone passage, calls attention to the stones. Serum creatinine levels are above normal on average, creatinine clearance is low, and hypercalciuria is not usual. Thus, struvite stones seem to be a primary problem, not a complication of metabolic stones.

Treatment

Mixed or pure, these infected stones are treated with removal. Current practice is percutaneous nephrolithotomy if the stones are over 2 cm in diameter, followed by extracorporeal shock wave lithotripsy (ESWL) to fragment what is left, and then a second look with percutaneous nephrolithotomy to remover all debris. If stones are less than 2 cm in diameter, ESWL is an adequate monotherapy. Antibiotic agents are best used before and after removal to sterilize the urinary tract.

CYSTINE STONES

Cysteine, lysine, ornithine, and citrulline share a common set of transporters in gut and kidney that can be deficient by heredity, as one of at least three autosomal recessive diseases.[47] Only cysteine causes disease, and only because it is insoluble enough to crystallize into stones. The stones begin in childhood, may be staghorns, and recur throughout life unless treated well.

The solubility of cysteine in urine is about 1 mM and varies about 2-fold from person to person. Excretion rates in normal people and also in heterozygotes are micromolar, so neither forms cysteine stones. In homozygous cystinuric people, excretion rates range from 1 to 15 mM daily, usual values being about 3–6 mM, so high fluid intake, of 3–6 liters daily, is adequate for most people. Nocturia is mandatory because cystine is excreted constantly. Alkaline pH increases cystine solubility, but only above pH 7.4, and to raise urine pH above serum pH requires a high dose of alkali, enough to overbalance total daily acid production. Calcium phosphate stones could be fostered. Even so, alkali is generally recommended.

If water and alkali fail to prevent stones, adding a drug that forms a soluble disulfide with cysteine, such as d-penicillamine, may be helpful.[47] Cystine is itself the cysteine disulfide and is in equilibrium with cysteine; the drug forms its own cysteine disulfide and reduces free cysteine concentration, and cystine dissociates into cysteine. All available drugs cause allergic side effects such as skin rash and serum-sickness reactions and reduce smell and taste; the latter symptoms respond to zinc repletion. Tiopronin (Thiola; Mission Pharmaceutical, San Antonio, TX, USA), long in European use, is now also available in the United States.

REFERENCES

1. Parks JH, Coe FL 1996 The financial effects of kidney stone prevention. Kidney Int **50:**1706–1712.
2. Coe Fl, Parks JH, Moore EM 1979 Familial idiopathic hypercalciuria. N Engl J Med **300:**337–340.
3. Coe FL, Parks JH 1988 Familial (idiopathic) hypercalciuria. In: Coe FL, Parks JH (eds.) Nephrolithiasis: Pathogenesis and Treatment, 2nd ed. Yearbook Medical Publishers, Chicago, IL, USA, pp. 108–138.
4. Weber DV, Coe FL, Parks JH, Dunn MS, Tembe V 1979 Urinary saturation measurements in calcium nephrolithiasis. Ann Intern Med **90:**180–184.
5. Coe FL, Bushinsky DA 1984 Pathophysiology of hypercalciuria. Am J Physiol **247:**F1–F13.
6. Haussler MR, Baylink DJ, Hughes MR, Brumbaugh PF, Wergedal JE, Shen FH, Nielsen RL, Counts SJ, Bursac KM, McCain TA 1976 The assay of 1,25-dihydroxyvitamin D3; physiologic and pathologic modulation of circulating hormone levels. Clin Endocrinol (Oxf) **5:**151S–165S.
7. Kaplan RA, Haussler MR, Deftos LJ, Bone H, Pak CY 1977 The role of 1-alpha, 25-diydroxyvitamin D in the mediation of intestinal hyperabsorption of calcium in primary hyperparathyroidism and absorptive hypercalciuria. J Clin Invest **59:**756–760.
8. Gray RW, Wilz DR, Caldas AE, Leman J Jr 1977 The importance of phosphate in regulating plasma 1,25-(OH)2-vitamin D levels in humans: Studies in healthy subjects in calcium-stone formers and in patients with primary hyperparathyroidism. J Clin Endocrinol Metab **45:**299–306.
9. Shen FH, Baylink DJ, Neilsen RL 1977 Increased serum 1,25-dihydroxyvitamin D in idiopathic hypercalciuria. J Lab Clin Med **90:**955–962.
10. Coe FL, Favus MJ, Crockett T, Strauss AL, Parks JH, Porat A, Gantt CL, Sherwood LM 1982 Effects of low-calcium diet on urine calcium excretion, parathyroid function and serum 1,25(OH)₂D₃ levels in patients with idiopathic hypercalciuria and in normal subjects. Am J Med **72:**25–31.
11. Broadus AE, Insogna KL, Lang R, Ellison EF, Dreyer BE 1984 Evidence for disordered control of 1,25-dihydroxyvitamin D production in absorptive hypercalciuria. N Engl J Med **311:**73–80.
12. Adams ND, Gray RW, Lemann J Jr 1979 The effects of oral CaCO3 loading and dietary calcium deprivation on plasma 1,25-dihydroxyvitamin D concentrations in healthy adults. J Clin Endocrinol Metab **48:**1008–1016.
13. Maierhofer WJ, Lemann J Jr, Gray RW, Cheung HS 1984 Dietary calcium and serum 1,25-(OH)2-vitamin D concentrations as determinants of calcium balance in healthy men. **26:**752–759.
14. Coe L, Parks JH, Asplin JR 1992 The pathogenesis and treatment of kidney stones, medical progress. N Engl J Med **327:**1141–1152.
15. Li XQ, Tembe V, Horwitz GM, Bushinsky DA, Favus MJ 1993 Increased intestinal vitamin D receptor in genetic hypercalciuric rats: A cause of intestinal calcium reabsorption. J Clin Invest **91:**661–667.
16. Coe FL, Parks JH, Favus MJ 1997 Diet and calcium: The end of an era? Ann Intern Med **126:**553–554.
17. Coe FL 1977 Treated and untreated recurrent calcium nephrolithiasis in patients with idiopathic hypercalciuria, hypericosuria, or no metabolic disorder. Ann Intern Med **87:**404–410.
18. Costanzo LS 1985 Localization of diuretic action in microperfused rat distal tubules: Ca and Na transport. Am J Physiol **248:**F524–F535.
19. Coe FL, Parks JH, Bushinsky DA, Langman CV, Favus MJ 1988 Chlorthalidone promotes mineral retention in patients with idiopathic hypercalciuria. Kidney Int **33:**1140–1146.
20. Coe FL, Parks JH 1988 Primary hyperparathyroidism. In: Coe FL, Parks JH (eds.) Nephrolithiasis: Pathogenesis and Treatment, 2nd ed. Yearbook Medical, Chicago, IL, USA, pp. 59–107.
21. Johnson RD, Conn JW 1969 Hyperparathyroidism with a prolonged period of normocalcemia. JAMA **210:**2063–2066.
22. Yendt ER, Gagne RJA 1968 Detection of primary hyperparathyroidism, with special reference to its occurrence in hypercalciuric females with normal or borderline serum calcium. Can Med Assoc J **98:**331–336.
23. Wills MR, Pak CYC, Hammond WG, Bartter FC. 1979 Normocalcemic primary hyperparathyroidism. Am J Med **47:**384–391.
24. Broadus AE, Horst RL, Lang RL, Littledike ET, Rasmussen H 1980 The importance of circulating 1,25-dihydroxyvitamin D in the pathogenesis of hypercalciuria and renal-stone formation in primary hyperparathyroidism. N Engl J Med **302:**421–426.
25. Pak CYC, Nicar MJ, Peterson R, Zerwekh JE, Snyder W 1981 A lack of unique pathophysiologic background for nephrolithiasis of primary hyperparathyroidism. J Clin Endocrinol Metab **55:**536–542.
26. LoCascio V, Adami S, Galvanini G, Ferrari M, Cominacini L, Tartarotti D 1985 Substrate-product relation of 1-hydroxylase activity in primary hyperparathyroidism. N Engl J Med **313:**1123–1130.
27. Lash JP, Cowell G, Arruda JAL 2002 Calcium nephrolithiasis and renal tubular acidosis. In: Coe FL, Favus MJ (eds.) Disorders of Bone and Mineral Metabolism, 2nd ed. Lippincott, Williams, and Wilkins, Philadelphia, PA, USA, pp. 717–740.
28. Coe FL, Parks JH 1980 Stone disease in distal renal tubular acidosis. Ann Intern Med **93:**60–61.
29. Albright F, Burnett CH, Parson W 1946 Osteomalacia and late rickets: The various etiologies met in the United States with emphasis on that resulting from a specific form of renal acidosis, the therapeutic indications for each sub-group, and the relationship between osteomalacia and Milkmans syndrome. Medicine (Baltimore) **25:**399–479.
30. Buckalew VM Jr, Purvis ML, Shulman MG, Herndon CN, Rudman D 1974 Hereditary renal tubular acidosis. Medicine (Baltimore) **53:**229–254.
31. Wrong O, Davies HEF 1959 The excretion of acid in renal disease. Q J Med **28:**259–311.
32. Williams HE, Smith LH Jr 1968 Disorders of oxalate metabolism. Am J Med **45:**715–735.
33. Hagler L, Herman RH 1973 Oxalate metabolism. Am J Clin Nutr **26:**758–765.
34. Hodgkinson A, Wilkinson R 1974 Plasma oxalate concentration and renal excretion of oxalate in man. Clin Sci **46:**61–73.
35. Kathpalia SC, Favus MJ, Coe FL 1984 Evidence for size and change permselectivity of rat ascending colon: Effects of ricinoleate and bile salts on oxalic acid and neutral sugar transport. J Clin Invest **74:**805–811.
36. Smith LH, Fromm H, Hoffman AF 1972 Acquired hyperoxaluria, nephrolithiasis and intestinal disease. N Engl J Med **286:**1371–1375.
37. Coe FL, Kavalich AG 1974 Hypercalciuria and hyperuricosuria in patients with calcium nephrolithiasis. N Engl J Med **291:**1344–1350.
38. Coe FL, Strauss AL, Tembe V, Le Dun S 1980 Uric acid saturation in calcium nephrolithiasis. Kidney Int **17:**662–668.
39. Coe FL 1983 Uric acid and calcium oxalate nephrolithiasis. Kidney Int **24:**392–403.
40. Deganello S, Coe FL 1983 Epitaxy between uric acid and whewellite: Experimental verification. Am J Physiol **6:**270–276.
41. Ettinger B, Tang A, Citron JT, Livermore B, Williams T 1986 Randomized trial of allopurinol in the prevention of calcium oxalate calculi. N Engl J Med **315:**1386–1389.
42. Kavalich AG, Moran E, Coe FL 1976 Dietary purine consumption by hyperuricosiuric calcium oxalate kidney stone formers and normal subjects. J Chronic Dis **29:**793–800.
43. Parks JH, Coe FL 1986 A urinary calcium-citrate index for the evaluation of nephrolithiasis. Kidney Int **30:**85–90.
44. Barcelo P, Wuhl O, Servitge E, Rousaund A, Pak CYC 1993 Randomized double-blind study of potassium citrate in idiopathic hypocitraturic calcium nephrolithiasis. J Urol **150:**1761–1764.
45. Herring LC 1962 Observations on the analysis of ten thousand urinary renal calculi. J Urol **88:**545–562.
46. Kristensen C, Parks JH, Lindheimer M, Coe FL 1987 Reduced glomerular filtration rate, hypercalciuria and clinical morbidity in primary struvite nephrolithiasis. Kidney Int **32:**749–753.
47. Segal S, Their SO 1983 Cystinuria. In: Stanbury JB, Wyngaarden JB, Fredrickson DS (eds.) The Metabolic Basis of Inherited Disease, 5th ed. McGraw-Hill, New York, NY, USA, pp. 1774–1791.

Chapter 87.   Urologic Aspects of Nephrolithiasis Management

Samuel C. Kim, Ramsay L. Kuo, Ryan F. Paterson, and James E. Lingeman

Methodist Hospital Institute for Kidney Stone Disease and Indiana University School of Medicine, Indianapolis, Indiana

INTRODUCTION

Urologic management of nephrolithiasis has steadily evolved with the introduction of shock wave lithotripsy (SWL) and advances in endoscopic technology. Presently, SWL and other endourological procedures, such as ureteroscopy (URS) and percutaneous nephrolithotomy (PNL), have supplanted the use of open stone surgery. These minimally invasive techniques currently allow the safe removal of urinary calculi regardless of composition, location, or stone burden.

Although there are many surgical options for the treatment of urolithiasis, the fundamental principle that ultimately guides decision-making is the goal of maximizing stone clearance while minimizing patient morbidity. Most of the recommendations delineated by the National Institutes of Health (NIH) Consensus Conference in 1988, the American Urological Association (AUA) Nephrolithiasis Clinical Guidelines Panel in 1994, and the AUA Ureteral Stones Clinical Guidelines Panel in 1997 still apply today.[1–3] Recent advances in endoscopic equipment and the development of adjunctive technologies, such as the holmium laser, have expanded the role of flexible URS in the treatment paradigm for patients with urinary calculi, especially for patients with comorbidities precluding alternate surgical therapy.

When treating nephrolithiasis, surgical decisions can be simplified by stratifying stones into clinical categories that direct treatment selection (Table 1). The initial distinction is identifying the general location of the stone burden—renal or ureteral.

RENAL CALCULI

Stone-related characteristics (size, number, location, and composition), renal anatomy, and patient clinical factors, should all be considered, in conjunction with equipment availability and procedural morbidity, when selecting a surgical approach for renal calculi (Table 2). In addition, multiple minimally invasive techniques are available for the treatment of kidney stones: SWL, URS, PNL, and laparoscopic stone surgery. The current challenge for the urologist is not whether the calculus can be removed endoscopically but selecting the appropriate minimally invasive approach.

SIMPLE RENAL CALCULI

SWL has streamlined the treatment protocol for nephrolithiasis, as the majority of simple renal calculi (80–85%) can be successfully treated with SWL.[4–6] Multiple studies

have examined the effect of stone burden on SWL outcomes. Clearly, larger stone burdens increase the number of treatment sessions and ancillary procedures, while decreasing stone-free rates.[7–9]

PNL, a more invasive approach, results in a significantly higher stone-free rate and lower retreatment rate than that of SWL.[8] However, because of increased patient morbidity, PNL should be limited to kidneys with a larger stone burden (>2.0 cm) or those stones known to be resistant to SWL, including cystine, brushite, and, to a lesser extent, calcium oxalate monohydrate.[7,9,10] As a result, the 1988 NIH Consensus Conference recommendations that simple renal calculi (see Table 1) can be effectively treated with SWL and that complex renal calculi are better managed with PNL still hold true.[1]

Advances in endoscopic technology and equipment have been introduced since publication of the above guideline panels. Currently, retrograde endoscopic procedures with the new generation of flexible ureteroscopes are increasingly used. URS, in conjunction with laser lithotripsy, has been successfully used in settings of SWL failure, complex renal calculi, and lower pole renal calculi.[11–13] URS is especially attractive when patient factors, such as coagulopathy or morbid obesity, preclude alternate approaches.

TABLE 1. CLASSIFICATION SYSTEM FOR PATIENTS WITH NEPHROLITHIASIS

Renal calculi
Simple
Stone burden < 2 cm
Normal renal anatomy
Complex
Stone burden > 2 cm
Staghorn stone
Lower pole calculus
Abnormal renal anatomy
Dilated calyx
Ureteropelvic junction obstruction
Horseshoe kidney
Pelvic kidney
Calyceal diverticulum
Infection and obstruction
Stones difficult to fragment
Cystine
Brushite
Calcium oxalate monohydrate
Ureteral calculi
Proximal/Mid
Less than 1 cm
Greater than 1 cm
Distal
Less than 1 cm
Greater than 1 cm

The authors have no conflict of interest.

TABLE 2. FACTORS AFFECTING THE MANAGEMENT OF RENAL STONES[34]

Stone	Renal anatomy	Clinical
Size	Obstruction/stasis	Infection
Number	Hydronephrosis	Body habitus
Composition	Ureteropelvic junction obstruction	Renal failure
Location (lower pole)	Calyceal diverticulum	Coagulopathy
	Horseshoe kidney/ectopic/ fusion abnormality	Age (pediatric/ elderly)
		Hypertension

(Adapted from Campbell's Urology, vol. 4, Walsh PC, Retik AB, Vaughan ED, Wein AJ, Surgical management of urinan lithiasis, pp. 3361–3451, 2002 with permission from Elsevier.)

COMPLEX RENAL CALCULI

Complex renal calculi (Table 1) present a greater challenge than simple calculi. This category includes not only stones of large size, such as staghorn stones, but also encompasses kidneys with abnormal anatomy and stones that are difficult to fragment. Ureteroscopic techniques can be used in upper urinary tract stones larger than 2 cm; however, stone clearance is significantly less than with PNL and stone recurrence is rapid (16% over 6 months).[11] For this reason, PNL still remains the treatment of choice for most complex renal stones.[1,2,7,14] The combination of PNL and SWL for complex stones was commonplace in the 1990s.[2] PNL techniques have improved, and the need for SWL during percutaneous procedures has declined.[15,16] Even the largest of staghorn calculi can be cleared percutaneously with the aid of secondary PNL and/or multiple accesses as needed (Table 3).

SPECIAL CONSIDERATIONS

An area of controversy continues to be the management of lower pole calyceal calculi. SWL results in significantly lower clearance of lower pole calyceal stones compared with PNL.[9,17] A recent prospective randomized multicenter trial clearly showed the superiority of PNL over SWL in clearance of lower pole calculi greater than 10 mm (stone free rates of 91% versus 21% for PNL and SWL, respectively).[18] Retreatment rates (16% versus 9%) and ancillary treatment rates (14% versus 2%) were also higher for the SWL group. The impact of various lower pole anatomic features on stone clearance after SWL (infundibulopelvic angle, infundibular length, and infundibular width) is unclear at present.[19–27]

Aberrant renal anatomy merits special consideration when addressing urinary calculi. Horseshoe and pelvic kidneys, ureteropelvic junction obstructions (UPJO), and calyceal diverticuli are often associated with nephrolithiasis and can present a treatment challenge. Although SWL may be used as initial treatment for renal calculi in horseshoe kidneys, stone free rates vary greatly.[28–33] Because stone burden and urinary drainage play important roles in stone clearance, SWL is appropriate only for horseshoe kidneys with smaller renal calculi with normal urinary drainage;

PNL produces better results for larger stones or when impaired drainage is present.[34]

Pelvic kidneys can create positioning difficulties for SWL. The retroperitoneal position of the kidney and blockage by the bony pelvis may require SWL to be performed prone.[30] If SWL fails or the stone burden is large, laparoscopic-assisted percutaneous procedures or flexible URS are options.[35–39]

Ureteropelvic junction obstruction can cause urinary stasis in the renal collecting system and can thus contribute to stone formation. Metabolic issues must also be addressed because patients with concomitant UPJO and calcium nephrolithiasis commonly have metabolic abnormalities.[40,41] When UPJO and renal calculi are present, PNL with endopyelotomy is a successful approach to remove the stone burden and endoscopically treat the UPJO.[42–44] Laparoscopic pyeloplasty with pyelolithotomy may be appropriate for some patients.[45,46]

Calyceal diverticula are non–urine-producing congenital urothelium-lined outpouchings that are commonly complicated by urinary calculi. Often, the neck of the diverticulum is quite small and does not allow passage of fragments after SWL.[47–49] For this reason, stone-free rates after SWL are poor.[47,50,51] On the other hand, PNL accomplishes both stone removal and ablation of the diverticular cavity—an option unavailable with SWL.[52]

Although SWL is quite versatile, certain clinical scenarios are not amenable to SWL. The presence of obstruction and/or infection requires prompt attention and precludes primary SWL. Immediate intervention is compulsory if obstruction occurs in a solitary kidney or concomitant obstruction and infection secondary to a calculus occur in any kidney. Once the obstruction and/or infection has been appropriately treated with a combination of decompression and antimicrobial therapy, the offending calculus can be definitively treated as per the above guidelines.

URETERAL CALCULI

For ureteral calculi, stone-related factors, clinical parameters, and other technical issues differ considerably from those for renal calculi because ureteral stones tend to be more resistant to SWL and can be easily treated with flex-

TABLE 3. ADAPTED FROM THE AUA GUIDELINES PANEL SUMMARY FOR STAGHORN STONES[1]

Recommendations
Newly diagnosed struvite staghorn calculi require active treatment intervention
Percutaneous stone removal is preferred (includes secondary percutaneous procedure and/or multiple accesses)
SWL monotherapy and open surgery should not be used as initial therapy
Nephrectomy may be appropriate for a nonfunctioning kidney

Adapted with permission from Segura JW, Preminger GM, Assimos DG, et al. 1994 Nephrolithiasis Clinical Guidelines Panel summary report on the management of staghorn calculi. The American Urological Association Nephrolithiasis Clinical Guidelines Panel. J Urol **151**:1648–1651.

TABLE 4. FACTORS AFFECTING THE MANAGEMENT
OF URETERAL STONES[34]

Stone	Renal anatomy	Clinical
Size	Solitary kidney	Symptom severity
Location	Abnormal ureteral anatomy (i.e., strictures)	Infection
		Equipment availability
Composition	Obstruction	

(Adapted from Campbell's Urology, vol. 4, Walsh PC, Retik AB, Vaughan ED, Wein AJ, Surgical management of urinan lithiasis, pp. 3361–3451, 2002 with permission from Elsevier.)

TABLE 6. INDICATIONS FOR URETEROSCOPY

Bleeding diathesis precluding PNL/SWL
Morbid obesity
Renal anomalies not amenable to SWL (horseshoe kidney, pelvic kidney)
SWL failure
Stones difficult to fragment (cystine, brushite, calcium oxalate monohydrate)
Inability to properly position patient for PNL/SWL (i.e., contractures)
Impacted ureteral stones
Failure of ureteral stone passage with conservative measures

ible URS (Table 4).[53,54] Most ureteral calculi are less than 5 mm in diameter and have a high likelihood of spontaneous passage if symptoms are tolerable.[3] When ureteral stones are larger in size, become increasingly symptomatic, or are unable to pass spontaneously, appropriate surgical intervention can be undertaken.

PROXIMAL URETERAL CALCULI

Multiple endourological options are available for the treatment of proximal ureteral stones: SWL with or without stone manipulation, URS, and PNL. The AUA Ureteral Stones Guidelines Panel in 1997 recommended SWL (in situ or push back) as the treatment of choice for stones 1 cm or smaller in the proximal ureter.[3] Because SWL is non-invasive and can achieve up to 85% stone-free rates for ureteral calculi, SWL remains a reasonable treatment option for proximal and distal ureteral stones less than 1 cm in size.[3,55]

Flexible URS has become increasingly popular as primary therapy for proximal ureteral stones less than 1 cm because of its higher stone-free rates than with SWL (Table 5). Furthermore, URS is effective for patients with stones difficult to fragment, distal ureteral obstruction, impacted stones, and medical conditions precluding other approaches (such as obesity and coagulopathy).[56–58] Current endoscopic equipment, in conjunction with holmium laser lithotripsy and stone baskets, allows the urologist to treat proximal ureteral stones of all sizes.[11,56]

As in renal stone disease, stone burden affects SWL results when treating ureteral stones. Proximal ureteral stones larger than 1 cm undergoing SWL have lower stone-free rates than those less than 1 cm.[55,59] The development of flexible ureteroscopes and adjunctive laser lithotripsy has

allowed proximal ureteral stones, even those larger than 1 cm, to be successfully treated with minimal morbidity; PNL is reserved for large or impacted proximal ureteral stones.[11,13,60]

DISTAL URETERAL CALCULI

Although the likelihood of spontaneous passage of stones is highest in the distal ureter, intervention with URS or SWL often is necessary. For symptomatic ureteral calculi less than 1 cm, both SWL and URS are excellent options. Previous randomized control trials comparing SWL and URS have reached conflicting conclusions.[61–63] URS is not influenced by stone size and can effectively treat distal ureteral calculi larger than 1 cm, a size that would be ineffectively treated by SWL.[55,60,64] Many institutions have limited access to a lithotriptor and therefore patient treatment may be delayed; URS is widely available and treatment can be promptly instituted.

The indications for URS (Table 6) are ever increasing, and the number of URS performed annually is steadily on the rise.[6] URS is effective in treating impacted ureteral stones and as salvage therapy for failed ESWL of ureteral or renal stones. The low success rate of repeat SWL for ureteral stones after failed initial SWL makes URS a particularly attractive option.[59]

CONCLUSIONS

Although most urinary calculi are best treated initially with SWL, endourological techniques play an important adjunctive role. Percutaneous procedures are instrumental in eliminating complex renal calculi, and URS is increasingly used for the treatment of ureteral and renal stones. As endoscopic technology and equipment continue to improve, the role of URS in treating ureteral and renal calculi is likely to further expand. Although multiple minimally invasive procedures can safely treat urinary calculi, prevention of future stone events through appropriate metabolic testing and medical treatment remains paramount.

TABLE 5. RECOMMENDATIONS FOR URETERAL STONES

Ureteral stones 5 mm or less
  Good chance of spontaneous passage
Ureteral stones 1 cm or less
  URS or SWL
    Need for stent placement greater with URS
    Higher likelihood of secondary procedures with SWL
Ureteral stones greater than 1 cm
  Proximal: URS, SWL, or PNL
  Distal: URS or SWL

REFERENCES

1. Consensus Conference 1988 Prevention and treatment of kidney stones. JAMA 260:977–981.
2. Segura JW, Preminger GM, Assimos DG, Dretler SP, Kahn RI, Lin-

geman JE, Macaluso JN Jr, McCullough DL 1994 Nephrolithiasis Clinical Guidelines Panel summary report on the management of staghorn calculi. The American Urological Association Nephrolithiasis Clinical Guidelines Panel. J Urol 151:1648–1651.

3. Segura JW, Preminger GM, Assimos DG, Dretler SP, Kahn RI, Lingeman JE, Macaluso JN Jr 1997 Ureteral Stones Clinical Guidelines Panel summary report on the management of ureteral calculi. The American Urological Association. J Urol 158:1915–1921

4. Krings F, Tuerk C, Steinkogler I, Marberger M 1992 Extracorporeal shock wave lithotripsy retreatment ("stir-up") promotes discharge of persistent caliceal stone fragments after primary extracorporeal shock wave lithotripsy. J Urol 148:1040–1041.

5. Wickham JE 1993 Treatment of urinary tract stones. BMJ 307:1414–1417.

6. Kerbl K, Rehman J, Landman J, Lee D, Sundaram C, Clayman RV 2002 Current management of urolithiasis: Progress or regress? J Endourol 16:281–288.

7. Lam HS, Lingeman JE, Barron M, Newman DM, Mosbaugh PG, Steele RE, Knapp PM, Scott JW, Nyhuis A, Woods JR 1992 Staghorn calculi: Analysis of treatment results between initial percutaneous nephrostolithotomy and extracorporeal shock wave lithotripsy monotherapy with reference to surface area. J Urol 147:1219–1225.

8. Lingeman JE, Coury TA, Newman DM, Kahnoski RJ, Mertz JH, Mosbaugh PG, Steele RE, Woods JR 1987 Comparison of results and morbidity of percutaneous nephrostolithotomy and extracorporeal shock wave lithotripsy. J Urol 138:485–490.

9. Wolf JS Jr, Clayman RV 1997 Percutaneous nephrostolithotomy. What is its role in 1997? Urol Clin North Am 24:43–58.

10. Klee LW, Brito CG, Lingeman JE 1991 The clinical implications of brushite calculi. J Urol 145:715–718.

11. Grasso M, Conlin M, Bagley D 1998 Retrograde ureteropyeloscopic treatment of 2 cm. or greater upper urinary tract and minor Staghorn calculi. J Urol 160:346–351.

12. Grasso M, Ficazzola M 1999 Retrograde ureteropyeloscopy for lower pole caliceal calculi. J Urol 162:1904–1908.

13. Grasso M, Loisides P, Beaghler M, Bagley D 1995 The case for primary endoscopic management of upper urinary tract calculi: I. A critical review of 121 extracorporeal shock-wave lithotripsy failures. Urology 45:363–371.

14. Segura JW 1997 Staghorn calculi. Urol Clin North Am 24:71–80.

15. Wong C, Leveillee RJ 2002 Single upper-pole percutaneous access for treatment of > or = 5-cm complex branched staghorn calculi: Is shockwave lithotripsy necessary? J Endourol 16:477–481.

16. Lam HS, Lingeman JE, Mosbaugh PG, Steele RE, Knapp PM, Scott JW, Newman DM 1992 Evolution of the technique of combination therapy for staghorn calculi: A decreasing role for extracorporeal shock wave lithotripsy. J Urol 148:1058–1062.

17. Lingeman JE, Siegel YI, Steele B, Nyhuis AW, Woods JR 1994 Management of lower pole nephrolithiasis: A critical analysis. J Urol 151:663–667.

18. Albala DM, Assimos DG, Clayman RV, Denstedt JD, Grasso M, Gutierrez-Aceves J, Kahn RI, Leveillee RJ, Lingeman JE, Macaluso JN Jr, Munch LC, Nakada SY, Newman RC, Pearle MS, Preminger GM, Teichman J, Woods JR 2001 Lower pole I: A prospective randomized trial of extracorporeal shock wave lithotripsy and percutaneous nephrostolithotomy for lower pole nephrolithiasis-initial results. J Urol 166:2072–2080.

19. Sabnis RB, Naik K, Patel SH, Desai MR, Bapat SD 1997 Extracorporeal shock wave lithotripsy for lower calyceal stones: Can clearance be predicted? Br J Urol 80:853–857.

20. Elbahnasy AM, Clayman RV, Shalhav AL, Hoenig DM, Chandhoke P, Lingeman JE, Denstedt JD, Kahn R, Assimos DG, Nakada SY 1998 Lower caliceal stone clearance after shock wave lithotripsy or ureteroscopy: The impact of lower pole radiographic anatomy. J Urol 159:676–682.

21. Lojanapiwat B, Soonthornpun S, Wudhikarn S 1999 Lower pole caliceal stone clearance after ESWL: The effect of infundibulopelvic angle. J Med Assoc Thai 82:891–894.

22. Keeley FX Jr, Moussa SA, Smith G, Tolley DA 1999 Clearance of lower-pole stones following shock wave lithotripsy: Effect of the infundibulopelvic angle. Eur Urol 36:371–375.

23. Gupta NP, Singh DV, Hemal AK, Mandal S 2000 Infundibulopelvic anatomy and clearance of inferior caliceal calculi with shock wave lithotripsy. J Urol 163:24–27.

24. Tuckey J, Devasia A, Murthy L, Ramsden P, Thomas D 2000 Is there a simpler method for predicting lower pole stone clearance after

25. Sumino Y, Mimata H, Tasaki Y, Ohno H, Hoshino T, Nomura T, Nomura Y 2002 Predictors of lower pole renal stone clearance after extracorporeal shock wave lithotripsy. J Urol 168:1344–1347.

26. Madbouly K, Sheir KZ, Elsobky E 2001 Impact of lower pole renal anatomy on stone clearance after shock wave lithotripsy: Fact or fiction? J Urol 165:1415–1418.

27. Sorensen CM, Chandhoke PS 2002 Is lower pole caliceal anatomy predictive of extracorporeal shock wave lithotripsy success for primary lower pole kidney stones? J Urol 168:2377–2382.

28. Smith JE, Van Arsdalen KN, Hanno PM, Pollack HM 1989 Extracorporeal shock wave lithotripsy treatment of calculi in horseshoe kidneys. J Urol 142:683–686.

29. Esuvaranathan K, Tan EC, Tung KH, Foo KT 1991 Stones in horseshoe kidneys: Results of treatment by extracorporeal shock wave lithotripsy and endourology. J Urol 146:1213–1215.

30. Kupeli B, Isen K, Biri H, Sinik Z, Alkibay T, Karaoglan U, Bozkirli I 1999 Extracorporeal shockwave lithotripsy in anomalous kidneys. J Endourol 13:349–352.

31. Lampel A, Hohenfellner M, Schultz-Lampel D, Lazica M, Bohnen K, Thurof JW 1996 Urolithiasis in horseshoe kidneys: Therapeutic management. Urology 47:182–186.

32. Kirkali Z, Esen AA, Mungan MU 1996 Effectiveness of extracorporeal shockwave lithotripsy in the management of stone-bearing horseshoe kidneys. J Endourol 10:13–15.

33. Theiss M, Wirth MP, Frohmuller HG 1993 Extracorporeal shock wave lithotripsy in patients with renal malformations. Br J Urol 72:534–538.

34. Lingeman JE, Lifshitz DA, Evan AP 2002 Surgical management of urinary lithiasis. In: Walsh PC, Retik AB, Vaughan ED, Wein AJ (ed.) Campbell's Urology, 8th ed., vol. 4. Saunders, Philadelphia, PA, USA, pp. 3361–3451.

35. Zafar FS, Lingeman JE 1996 Value of laparoscopy in the management of calculi complicating renal malformations. J Endourol 10:379–383.

36. Toth C, Holman E, Pasztor I, Khan AM 1993 Laparoscopically controlled and assisted percutaneous transperitoneal nephrolithotomy in a pelvic dystopic kidney. J Endourol 7:303–305.

37. Holman E, Toth C 1998 Laparoscopically assisted percutaneous transperitoneal nephrolithotomy in pelvic dystopic kidneys: Experience in 15 successful cases. J Laparoendosc Adv Surg Tech A 8:431–435.

38. Figge M 1988 Percutaneous transperitoneal nephrolithotomy. Eur Urol 14:414–416.

39. Kim SC, Kuo RL, Paterson RF, Lingeman JE 2003 Laparoscopic assisted percutaneous nephrolithotomy: Best done tubeless? J Urol 169:305A.

40. Husmann DA, Milliner DS, Segura JW 1995 Ureteropelvic junction obstruction with a simultaneous renal calculus: Long-term followup. J Urol 153:1399–1402.

41. Matin SF, Streem SB 2000 Metabolic risk factors in patients with ureteropelvic junction obstruction and renal calculi. J Urol 163:1676–1678.

42. Oshinsky GS, Jarrett TW, Smith AD 1996 New technique in managing ureteropelvic junction obstruction: Percutaneous endoscopic pyeloplasty. J Endourol 10:147–151.

43. Kletscher BA, Segura JW, LeRoy AJ, Patterson DE 1995 Percutaneous antegrade endopyelotomy: Review of 50 consecutive cases. J Urol 153:701–703.

44. Motola JA, Badlani GH, Smith AD 1993 Results of 212 consecutive endopyelotomies: An 8-year followup. J Urol 149:453–456.

45. Ramakumar S, Lancini V, Chan DY, Parsons JK, Kavoussi LR, Jarrett TW 2002 Laparoscopic pyeloplasty with concomitant pyelolithotomy. J Urol 167:1378–1380.

46. Siqueira TM Jr, Nadu A, Kuo RL, Paterson RF, Lingeman JE, Shalhav AL 2002 Laparoscopic treatment for ureteropelvic junction obstruction. Urology 60:973–978.

47. Jones JA, Lingeman JE, Steidle CP 1991 The roles of extracorporeal shock wave lithotripsy and percutaneous nephrostolithotomy in the management of pyelocaliceal diverticula. J Urol 146:724–727.

48. Ritchie AW, Parr NJ, Moussa SA, Tolley DA 1990 Lithotripsy for calculi in caliceal diverticula? Br J Urol 66:6–8.

49. Psihramis KE, Dretler SP 1987 Extracorporeal shock wave lithotripsy of caliceal diverticula calculi. J Urol 138:707–711.

50. Streem SB, Yost A 1992 Treatment of caliceal diverticular calculi with extracorporeal shock wave lithotripsy: Patient selection and extended followup. J Urol 148:1043–1046.

51. Shalhav AL, Soble JJ, Nakada SY, Wolf JS Jr, McClennan BL,

Clayman RV 1998 Long-term outcome of caliceal diverticula following percutaneous endosurgical management. J Urol **160:**1635–1639.

52. Cohen TD, Preminger GM 1997 Management of calyceal calculi. Urol Clin North Am **24:**81–96.

52. Strohmaier WL, Schubert G, Rosenkranz T, Weigl A 1999 Comparison of extracorporeal shock wave lithotripsy and ureteroscopy in the treatment of ureteral calculi: A prospective study. Eur Urol **36:**376–379.

54. Turk TM, Jenkins AD 1999 A comparison of ureteroscopy to in situ extracorporeal shock wave lithotripsy for the treatment of distal ureteral calculi. J Urol **161:**45–46.

55. Tan YM, Yip SK, Chong TW, Wong MY, Cheng C, Foo KT 2002 Clinical experience and results of ESWL treatment for 3,093 urinary calculi with the Storz Modulith SL 20 lithotripter at the Singapore general hospital. Scand J Urol Nephrol **36:**363–367.

56. Tawfiek ER, Bagley DH 1999 Management of upper urinary tract calculi with ureteroscopic techniques. Urology **53:**25–31.

57. Liong ML, Clayman RV, Gittes RF, Lingeman JE, Huffman JL, Lyon ES 1989 Treatment options for proximal ureteral urolithiasis: Review and recommendations. J Urol **141:**504–509.

58. Andreoni C, Afane J, Olweny E, Clayman RV 2001 Flexible ureteroscopic lithotripsy: First-line therapy for proximal ureteral and renal calculi in the morbidly obese and superobese patient. J Endourol **15:**493–498.

59. Pace KT, Weir MJ, Tariq N, Honey RJ 2000 Low success rate of repeat shock wave lithotripsy for ureteral stones after failed initial treatment. J Urol **164:**1905–1907.

60. Park H, Park M, Park T 1998 Two-year experience with ureteral stones: Extracorporeal shockwave lithotripsy v ureteroscopic manipulation. J Endourol **12:**501–504.

61. Deliveliotis C, Stavropoulos NI, Koutsokalis G, Kostakopoulos A, Dimopoulos C 1996 Distal ureteral calculi: Ureteroscopy vs. ESWL. A prospective analysis. Int Urol Nephrol **28:**627–631.

62. Pearle MS, Nadler R, Bercowsky E, Chen C, Dunn M, Figenshau RS, Hoenig DM, McDougall EM, Mutz J, Nakada SY, Shalhav AL, Sundaram C, Wolf JS Jr, Clayman RV 2001 Prospective randomized trial comparing shock wave lithotripsy and ureteroscopy for management of distal ureteral calculi. J Urol **166:**1255–1260.

63. Peschel R, Janetschek G, Bartsch G 1999 Extracorporeal shock wave lithotripsy versus ureteroscopy for distal ureteral calculi: A prospective randomized study. J Urol **162:**1909–1912.

64. Pardalidis NP, Kosmaoglou EV, Kapotis CG 1999 Endoscopy vs. extracorporeal shockwave lithotripsy in the treatment of distal ureteral stones: Ten years' experience. J Endourol **13:**161–164.

Chapter 88.   Development and Structure of Teeth and Periodontal Tissues

Sheila J. Jones and Alan Boyde

Department of Anatomy and Developmental Biology, University College London, London, United Kingdom

NORMAL DENTAL DEVELOPMENT

Three of the five distinct types of mineralized tissues found in the human body, enamel, dentine, and cementum, only occur in teeth. Because turnover in these tissues is nonexistent or minimal, they form a valuable, permanent record of conditions prevailing at their time of formation; this extends throughout fetal life and up to adulthood. Moreover, the enamel and dentine of the crowns of the deciduous teeth are available for analysis without surgical intervention when the teeth are shed naturally. Enamel is a surface tissue of epithelial origin, whereas human dentine and cementum are avascular connective tissues of mesenchymal origin. Teeth form at special locations within the jaws mapped out by the overlapping of molecular signals common to many developmental processes.[1] Tooth development is rigorously controlled by regulatory genes determining tooth type (incisor, canine, premolar, or molar) and shape.[2] Sequential local interactions at the interface between epithelium over the facial processes and mesenchyme derived from the cranial neural crest play a crucial role in tooth morphogenesis, the main signaling molecules being members of the hedgehog, bone morphogenetic protein (BMP), fibroblast growth factor (FGF), and Wnt (wingless) families.[3–5]

The embryonic tooth germ passes through three morphological stages, described as bud, cap, and bell, and has three main components, the enamel organ, the dental papilla, and the dental follicle. The epithelial enamel organ differentiates into a four-layered structure, within which the enamel knot is the signaling center that regulates tooth shape and size.[5] A complex sequence of epithelial-mesenchymal interactions results in waves of differentiation that start at the eventual enamel-dentine junction underlying the cusp tips (determined by the spatio-temporal induction of secondary enamel knots) and incisal central mammelons (rounded prominences on biting edges when incisors first erupt) and spread laterally, eventually delineating the whole junction between the tissues as the tooth germ grows. The expression of secretory signal molecules varies continuously in the different cell types during tooth initiation and construction.[6] Odontoblasts, which make dentine, are postmitotic

cells that differentiate from mesenchymal cells of the dental papilla at the interface with the inner enamel epithelial cells of the enamel organ, which themselves differentiate into preameloblasts. Dentine formation triggers the preameloblasts to differentiate into ameloblasts, the cells that produce enamel.[7] A bilayer of epithelial cells, the epithelial root sheath, extends from the enamel organ at the base of the developing crown to map out the dentine-cementum junction and initiate the differentiation of the odontoblasts of the root. The third tissue type, cementum, is the product of both fibroblasts and cementoblasts, which differentiate from mesenchymal cells of the dental follicle adjacent to the dentine once epithelial cells of the root sheath have moved away from the interface.[8] In human teeth, some afibrillar cementum may form on the enamel surface close to the junction between the crown and the root if there are gaps in the covering layer of epithelial cells once enamel formation has been completed. Within the developing tooth, a core of loose connective tissue remains and eventually forms the dental pulp.

The dental follicle, also derived from cells of the cranial neural crest, gives rise to three components of the periodontium: cementum, alveolar bone, and the intervening periodontal ligament. The tooth germs are partially enclosed by the developing alveolar bone, which is initially typical woven bone, formed by osteoblasts with enclosed osteocytes, and remodeled to accommodate the growing teeth by osteoclasts of hematopoietic origin. The follicle, a sac of loose connective tissue that separates the developing tooth from its bony crypt, is essential for eruption and will become the periodontal ligament on tooth eruption.[9] This tissue contributes extrinsic collagen fibers to the cementum and alveolar bone, and its main cell type is fibroblastic. (See Fig. 1 for a diagram of a mature tooth and its components.)

NORMAL DENTAL STRUCTURE

Enamel

Enamel matrix is delicate when first secreted, at which time it is protected by the soft enamel organ. The mature, erupted enamel, the hardest of the hard tissues, is acellular and contains ~98% by weight (or ~93% by volume) of an apatitic calcium phosphate of variable composition.[10,11]

The authors have no conflict of interest.

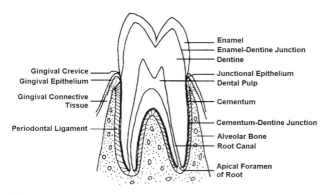

FIG. 1. Organization of dental and periodontal tissues in the erupted tooth.

The final strength of enamel partly derives from the dentine mold on which it is formed. The junction between these tissues is ill-defined and irregular on a microscopic scale, with tongues of dentine projecting into the enamel, crystals of indeterminate provenance at the common boundary, and many fine, short enamel tubules marking where ameloblast processes once contacted odontoblasts. Spindles, expanded continuations of dentine tubules within enamel, most likely result from the envelopment of individual ameloblasts that died as amelogenesis commenced. The extracellular proteinaceous matrix of developing enamel is secreted by ameloblasts that are highly polarized, tall cells. Its main component is amelogenin, a tissue-specific protein rich in proline, leucine, histidine, and glutamyl residues. Other, nonacidic proteins include enamelin, tuftelin, and amelo-

blastin (amelin, sheathlin; see Table 1). This three-dimensional (3-D) protein array is thought to control crystal growth.[12] To achieve enamel's high degree of mineralization, much of its organic matrix is degraded by neutral metalloproteinases and serine proteases and removed, even while ameloblasts are still secretory.[13] Enamel crystals are, even initially, very long and slender, with centers enriched in carbonate, while the net carbonate content falls as they thicken. In humans, relatively large amounts of mineral accumulate at early stages of development, and the enamel has a long post-secretory maturation period during which it becomes hard and the ameloblasts remain active. The maturation phase may last 5 years or more in human third molars. In species with rapid enamel development, cyclical changes in morphology of the maturation ameloblasts are seen to coincide with episodic matrix removal. Enamel's final composition and mechanical properties are not uniform.

The most notable feature of enamel is the organization of the crystals into enamel "prisms" about 6 μm across and up to millimeters long, demarcated by a sharp change in crystal orientation (Fig. 2). Enamel crystals grow mainly with their long c axes nearly parallel to each other, and the larger sides of their flattened hexagonal cross-sections parallel within groups. Where the rate of formation is low, as in the superficial enamel, the secretory interface is nearly flat, and there is little variation in the underlying crystal orientation. However, during most of enamel formation, the secretory (Tomes') process of each ameloblast is lodged in a pit at the interface. Enamel matrix is released between the pits, below a continuous belt of intercellular attachments, and at the pit

TABLE 1. MAIN CONSTITUENTS OF DENTAL TISSUES

	Enamel	Dentine	Cementum

Proteins	Amelogenin:
	    Major protein in immature enamel, secreted by
	    ameloblasts, then degraded and removed.
	Non-amelogenin proteins (enamelins):
	    Includes enamelin and tuftelin; secreted by
	    ameloblasts.
	Ameloblastin:
	    Also known as amelin or sheathlin, secreted by
	    ameloblasts and odontoblasts
		Collagen type 1
		Dentine sialophosphoprotein (DSPP):
		    In predentine, then degraded
		Dentine sialoprotein (DSP):
		    In dentine, processed from DSPP
		Dentine phosphoprotein (DPP):
		    In dentine, processed from DSPP
		Dentine matrix protein 1 (DMP1)
			Collagen type 1
			Bone sialoprotein
			Osteopontin
			Osteocalcin
			α2HS-glycoprotein

Proteoglycans		Decorin:
		    Chondroitin-sulphate-rich
		Biglycan:
		    Chondroitin-sulphate-rich
		Lumican:
		    Keratan-sulphate-rich
		Fibromodulin:
		    Keratan-sulphate-rich
			Decorin:
			    In cellular cementum only
			Biglycan:
			    In cellular cementum only, in
			        incremental lines
			Lumican:
			    In cellular cementum only
			Versican:
			    In cementocyte lacunae only

Proteinases	Enamelysin (MMP-20):
	    Metalloprotease in immature enamel, processes
	        enamel proteins in secretory phase of amelogenesis
	Kallikrein 4 (KLK4):
	    Also known as enamel matrix serine protease-1
	        (EMSP1); in immature enamel, also secreted by
	        odontoblasts, clears enamel proteins during
	        enamel maturation phase
		Matrix metalloproteinases (MMP2)
		    In predentine, degrade and process
		        dentine proteins secreted by
		        odontoblasts	

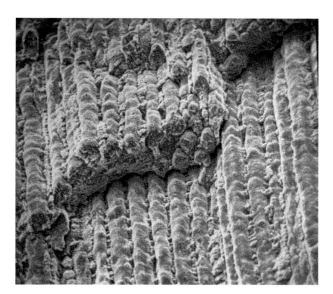

FIG. 2. Human enamel fractured to show the form of the prisms that are about 6 μm across. SEM: field width, 82 μm.

wall/floor.[14] The interpit phase is continuous, and the crystals have their long axes perpendicular to the general plane of the developing enamel surface. In human enamel, the dividing lines of the prism junctions are generally incomplete, and the interlocking prisms are described as keyhole-shaped. The concentration of the cleavage products of the enamel proteins at the discontinuities in crystal orientation is relatively increased during enamel maturation. Tufts and lamellae are other regions that ultimately contain less mineral and higher concentrations of proteins.

As ameloblasts move away from the dentine, they travel in groups across the surface that they make. This results in decussation (crossing in an X fashion) of the enamel prisms, with zones of prisms with contrasting 3-D courses forming the Hunter-Schreger bands. The sides of the prisms show varicosities (Fig. 2) with the same period as cross-striations in the prisms, which are thought to be caused by circadian changes in the composition of the mineral component.[15] A prominence of the cross striations occurs at 7- to 10-day intervals (the regular striae of Retzius), and major life events, such as birth (the neonatal line) or severe illness during enamel formation, may be recorded as conspicuous incremental lines. At the finished enamel surface, perikymata or imbrication lines are outcrops of the internal growth layers. They grade from horizontal bands displaying pits alternating with smoother regions at more incisal or occlusal levels, to small steps at the sharp boundary between the imbricating layers near the neck of the tooth.

The unerupted crown is protected from resorption by a layer of cells termed the reduced enamel epithelium comprising remnants of mature ameloblasts. This is lost once the tooth erupts. As the tooth wears during function, the surfaces features of the enamel become abraded, microcracks develop particularly along developmental faults, and the chemistry of the mineral exposed to the oral environment changes also.

Dentine

Dentine forms the bulk of the tooth and extends within both crown and root. It is pale creamy yellow in color, in contrast to the much whiter, harder enamel. Dentine is tough and elastic, and its prime feature is its penetration by odontoblastic tubules that radiate out from the dental pulp to the periphery (Fig. 3). These are analogous to the canaliculi that house osteocyte processes in bone. The peripheral, first-formed dentine is termed mantle dentine and the inner, circumferential dentine. After differentiating from cells of the dental papilla, the odontoblasts retreat centripetally as a cone-shaped monolayer sheet, depositing a collagenous pre-dentine matrix and leaving elongating cell processes with many side branches that remain in the tubules within the dentine.[16] The curved paths that the cell bodies assume are therefore recorded in the extracellular matrix. This matrix is similar to that of bone, comprised mainly of type I collagen, acidic proteins, and proteoglycans (Table 1). The predominant noncollagenous protein in dentine is the highly phosphorylated dentine phosphoprotein. This and dentine sialo-protein[17] are cleavage products of the dentine sialophosphoprotein gene product and are formed during the maturation of predentine into dentine. Dentine matrix protein 1 and other sialic acid–rich phosphoproteins common to dentine and bone are also present. Decorin, biglycan, lumican, and fibromodulin are the main proteoglycans in predentine.[18] The predentine matrix matures progressively, with the collagen fibrils thickening and compacting, and then mineralizes after a lag time of ~4 days.[19]

Dentine contains ~70% mineral (wet weight). Carbonate-rich calcium hydroxyapatite crystals form in relation to submicroscopic vesicles shed by the odontoblasts in the mantle layer or at sites on collagen fibrils rich in noncollagenous proteins. Mineralization extends radially from initial nucleation sites in the matrix, possibly by a

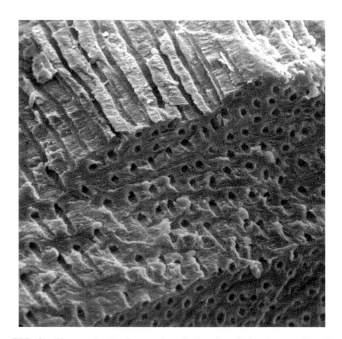

FIG. 3. Human dentine fractured to display the tubules that are about 2 μm across. SEM: field width, 88 μm.

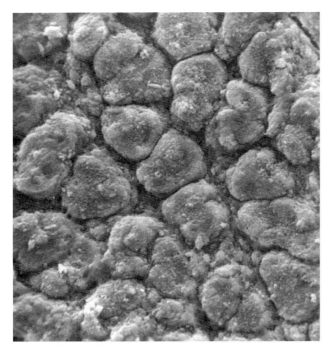

FIG. 4. Human cementum surface, made anorganic, showing mineralized ends of extrinsic fibers, about 6 μm diameter, separated by intrinsic fibers. SEM: field width, 30 μm.

process of secondary nucleation, forming regions of dentine known as calcospherites. These may fail to fuse, leaving unmineralized interglobular dentine between them. In a second, concurrent pattern of mineralization, crystals extend along the fine type I collagen fibrils that lie in a feltwork parallel to the incremental surface. Peritubular dentine is deposited within the tubules, partially or sometimes completely occluding them. It contains a negligible amount of collagen and mineralizes to a higher degree than the surrounding intertubular dentine. Because it is harder and more wear-resistant than intertubular dentine, it stands slightly proud on surfaces of teeth worn through into dentine.

Like enamel, dentine is deposited rhythmically, leaving lines marking daily, and approximately weekly, increments.[20] Major life events, such as birth (the neonatal line) and illness or dietary deficiencies, are recorded as disturbances in the structure of the tissue forming at the time. Once eruption has occurred and root formation is complete, further dentine formation occurs as slowly deposited, regular secondary dentine, or irregularly, as a response of the pulp-dentine complex to attrition or disease. Nerves pass from the dental pulp between odontoblasts and extend into the dentine tubules for variable distances. Dentine is exquisitely painful if touched or subjected to large temperature or osmotic changes.

Like any other loose connective tissue, the dental pulp shows changes with age, but these may include diffuse or local calcifications and the formation of dental stones. In the roots of human teeth, occlusion of the tubules with peritubular dentine extends coronally from the root apex; the resulting transparent dentine can be used as a guide to the age of the tooth.

Cementum

Cementum is a calcified connective tissue that is deposited initially on the newly mineralized dentine matrix of the root by cells derived from the dental follicle.[8] Secretory proteins from the cells of the epithelial root sheath may be included in the matrix formed initially. Cementum is laid down centrifugally from the cementum-dentine junction and is marked by incremental lines that are close together, continuous and evenly spaced where apposition was slow, and patchy and irregular otherwise. The tissue is similar to Sharpey fiber (bundle) bone in that it incorporates extrinsic collagen fibers formed by fibroblasts.[21] These fibers may be very closely packed, comprising the whole tissue in slowly forming acellular cementum, or be separated from each other by intervening intrinsic collagen fibers of cementoblast origin, which lie in the plane of the developing root surface (Fig. 4). Where cementum is deposited very rapidly, it is cellular, containing cementocytes that resemble the osteocytes of Sharpey fiber bone (Fig. 5). In heavily remodeled root apices, there may be patches of cellular cementum without extrinsic fibers. Only in cementum containing intrinsic fibers may a well-defined region of unmineralized precementum, equivalent to osteoid, be present at the surface of the tissue. The collagen of both the extrinsic and intrinsic fibers is type I. The main noncollagenous proteins of cementum identified so far (bone sialoprotein, osteopontin, osteocalcin, and α2 HS-glycoprotein) vary in amount and distribution in the different types of cementum and do not distinguish cementum from other calcified connective tissues[22,23] (Table 1).

Cementum mineralization reflects the rate of formation and the composition of the matrix. In afibrillar coronal cementum, the layer of noncollagenous proteins adsorbed on to the enamel

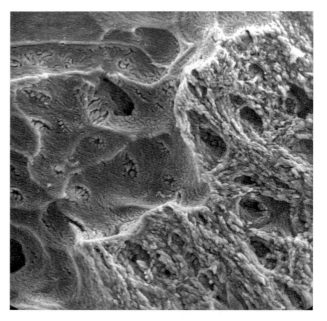

FIG. 5. Human alveolar bone surface made anorganic; the resorption lacunae reveal that the extrinsic (Sharpey's) fibers were only partly mineralized. The remainder of the surface was forming, as evidenced by incomplete mineralization of intrinsic and extrinsic fibers. SEM: field width, 110 μm.

surface mineralizes fully. At the cementum-dentine junction, collagen fibrils and noncollagenous constituents of the two tissues mingle without a regular, distinct border or an osteopontin-rich hypermineralized cement line. The extrinsic fibers of slowly forming cementum mineralize completely, the advancing mineralized front across the fibers being relatively flat and defining a border between cementum and the dental sac or periodontal ligament. This type of cementum is more highly mineralized, more translucent, and paler than dentine. Where only a small proportion of intrinsic fibers exists in acellular cementum, the extrinsic fibers lead the mineralization front. As the rate of deposition of cementum increases and proportionately more intrinsic fibers are deposited, the likelihood that the extrinsic fibers will retain unmineralized cores increases. During periods of fast cellular cementogenesis, even the intrinsic fibers may retain unmineralized sections, and the mineralization front becomes irregular, with the extrinsic component lagging behind the intrinsic. This cementum type is the softest and least well mineralized of the calcified dental tissues. The mineralization front can be read to estimate the current rate of formation, and the degree of mineralization of the fibers within the tissue indicates past rates.[21] The carbonate-rich apatite phase is similar to that in bone.

INTERRELATIONSHIPS OF TEETH, PERIODONTAL TISSUES, AND ALVEOLAR BONE

Teeth are a highly specialized part of an integrated functional unit (see Fig. 1), the primary (but not sole) purpose of which is the mastication of food. Unique among the human calcified tissues, enamel is destined to be exposed to an external environment. As the tooth erupts, the alveolar bone is resorbed to allow its passage, its root develops, and the crown pierces the oral mucosa which finally contributes to a tight ring seal of epithelial cells on the enamel close to the junction of crown and root. The complex molecular signaling cascades in the dental follicle controlling eruption and root growth are unclear.[9] At emergence, the root of the tooth is not yet fully formed, and the pulpal aspect of the root end (apex) resembles a large closing cone in bone. Root completion takes ~18 months in the deciduous teeth and up to 3 years in the permanent teeth. During root development, the follicle becomes organized into the periodontal ligament that supports the tooth, provides nutrient flow and mechanosensation, and allows physiological tooth movement. Through the groups of fibers of the periodontal ligament, comprised of types I and III collagen, functioning teeth are linked to each other, the gingiva, and the alveolar bone. On either side of the ligament, its principal fibers are incorporated within cementum and Sharpey fiber bone. Within the ligament, there is constant adaptive remodeling of the soft tissue.

Cementum in permanent teeth is rarely remodeled, but the surface of alveolar bone (Fig. 5) is continually resorbed and reformed to allow the tooth to move in response to eruption, growth drift, or changing functional forces. Root resorption of deciduous teeth begins shortly after their completion, appearing first and most extensively on the aspect adjacent to the successional permanent tooth. Interspersed between resorptive bursts are occasional short periods of repair by cemento(osteo)blasts. "Odontoclasts" (typical osteoclasts) resorb both cementum and dentine, and in deciduous molars, some enamel.

REFERENCES

1. Thesleff I 2000 Genetic basis of tooth development and dental defects. Acta Odontol Scand **58:**191–194.
2. Jernvall J, Thesleff I 2000 Reiterative signaling and patterning during mammalian tooth morphogenesis. Mech Dev **92:**19–29.
3. James CT, Ohazama A, Tucker AS, Sharpe PT 2002 Tooth development is independent of a Hox patterning programme. Dev Dyn **225:**332–335.
4. Thesleff I, Mikkola M 2002 The role of growth factors in tooth development. Int Rev Cytol **217:**93–135.
5. Mustonen T, Tummers M, Mikami T, Itoh N, Zhang N, Grindley T, Thesleff I 2002 Lunatic fringe, FGF, and BMP regulate the Notch pathway during epithelial morphogenesis of teeth. Dev Biol **248:**281–293.
6. Smith AJ, Lesot H 2001 Induction and regulation of crown dentinogenesis: Embryonic events as a template for dental tissue repair? Crit Rev Oral Biol Med **12:**425–437.
7. Thesleff I, Åberg T 1997 Tooth morphogenesis and the differentiation of ameloblasts. In: Chadwick D, Cardew G (eds.) Dental Enamel. Wiley, Chichester, UK, pp. 1–17.
8. Diekwisch TG 2002 The developmental biology of cementum. Int J Dev Biol **45:**695–706.
9. Wise GE, Frazier-Bowers S, D'Souza RN 2002 Cellular, molecular, and genetic determinants of tooth eruption. Crit Rev Oral Biol Med **13:**323–334.
10. Elliott JC 1997 Structure, crystal chemistry and density of enamel apatites. In: Chadwick D, Cardew G (eds.) Dental Enamel. Wiley, Chichester, UK, pp. 54–67.
11. Elliott JC, Wong FS, Anderson P, Davis GR, Dowker SE 1998 Determination of mineral concentration in dental enamel from X-ray attenuation measurements. Connect Tiss Res **38:**61–79.
12. Diekwisch TGH, Berman BJ, Anderton X, Gurinsky B, Ortega AJ, Satchell PG, Williams M, Arumugham C, Luan X, McIntosh JE, Yamane A, Carlson DS, Sire J-Y, Shuler CF 2002 Membranes, minerals, and proteins of developing vertebrate enamel. Microsc Res Tech **59:**373–395.
13. Simmer JP, Hu JC 2002 Expression, structure, and function of enamel proteinases. Connect Tiss Res **43:**441–449.
14. Boyde A 1997 Microstructure of enamel. In: Chadwick D, Cardew G (eds.) Dental Enamel. Wiley, Chichester, UK, pp. 18–31.
15. Boyde A 1989 Enamel. In: Oksche A, Vollrath L (eds.) Handbook of Microscopic Anatomy, vol. V/6. Springer Verlag, Berlin, Germany, pp. 309–473.
16. Sasaki T, Garant PR 1996 Structure and organization of odontoblasts. Anat Rec **245:**235–249.
17. Butler WT, Brunn JC, Qin C, McKee MD 2002 Extracellular matrix proteins and the dynamics of dentin formation. Connect Tiss Res **43:**301–307.
18. Emberry G, Hall R, Waddington R, Septier D, Goldberg M 2001 Proteoglycans in dentinogenesis. Crit Rev Oral Biol Med **12:**331–349.
19. Linde A, Goldberg M 1993 Dentinogenesis. Crit Rev Oral Biol Med **4:**679–728.
20. Dean MC, Scandrett AE 1996 The relation between long-period incremental markings in dentine and daily cross-striations in enamel in human teeth. Arch Oral Biol **41:**233–241.
21. Jones SJ 1981 Cement. In: Osborn JW (ed.) Dental Anatomy and Embryology. Blackwell Scientific, Boston, MA, USA, pp. 193–205,286–294.
22. McKee MD, Zalzal S, Nanci A 1996 Extracellular matrix in tooth cementum and mantle dentin: Localization of osteopontin and other noncollagenous proteins, plasma proteins and glycoconjugates by electron microscopy. Anat Rec **245:**293–312.
23. Sasano Y, MaruyaY, Sato H, Zhu JX, Takahashi I, Mizoguchi I, Kagayama M 2001 Distinctive expression of extracellular matrix molecules at mRNA and protein levels during formation of cellular and acellular cementum in the rat. Histochem J **33:**91–99.

Chapter 89. Dental Manifestations of Disorders of Bone and Mineral Metabolism

Paul H. Krebsbach and Peter J. Polverini

Department of Oral Medicine, Pathology and Oncology, School of Dentistry, The University of Michigan, Ann Arbor, Michigan

INTRODUCTION

The mammalian tooth is a specialized structure that develops through a series of reciprocal epithelial-mesenchymal interactions culminating in the formation of three distinct mineralized tissues: enamel, dentin, and cementum. Although development of the mammalian dentition differs substantially from that of the skeleton, the cells and the mineralized components of dentin and cementum share many features with those of bone. Localized changes to the teeth and supporting oral structures may occur in response to disorders of mineral metabolism. The clinical presentation may vary from very mild asymptomatic changes to alterations that severely alter the form and function of craniofacial structures. This chapter provides a concise overview of the dental manifestations of selected disorders of bone and mineral metabolism.

ORAL MANIFESTATIONS OF GENETIC SKELETAL DISORDERS

Dentinogenesis Imperfecta

Developmental disorders of the dentition are often found concurrent with osteogenesis imperfecta (OI). Dental abnormalities have been described in several subtypes of OI, but are most prevalent in OI types IB, IC, and IVB.[1] The diverse genetic and clinical presentations that define OI are also hallmarks of the changes observed in dentinogenesis imperfecta (DGI). DGI is an inherited autosomal dominant disorder that affects the development, structure, and function of dentin in both the primary and permanent teeth. The dental defects associated with DGI are specified as type I when they occur concurrent with OI, and type II when only dental defects are observed. It has been reported that 10–50% of patients afflicted with OI also have DGI. This assessment, however, may underestimate the true prevalence because mild forms of DGI may require microscopic analysis for diagnosis.[2] Type III DGI, also known as the Brandywine type for a tri-racial isolate in Brandywine, Maryland, exhibits only dental defects and can vary in the clinical and radiographic presentation.

Clinically, the teeth of individuals with DGI are characterized by an opalescent or amber-like appearance (Fig. 1). The teeth are narrower at the cervical margins and thus exhibit a bulbous or bell-shaped crown. Microscopic anomalies of affected dentin include fewer and irregular dentin tubules containing vesicles and abnormally thick collagen fibers.[3] The mineral content of DGI teeth is ~30% less than normal dentin and intrafibrillar collagen mineralization is absent. The structurally abnormal dentin may not provide adequate support for the overlying enamel. Although enamel is chemically and structurally normal in individuals with DGI, the lack of support from dentin leads to enamel fractures and severe attrition of the teeth. Radiographic analysis may aid in the diagnosis of DGI. The short, conical-shaped roots and cervical constrictions are remarkable. In young individuals, the pulp chambers may appear normal, but with age, the overproduction of abnormal dentin leads to obliteration of the pulp (Fig. 2). A notable radiographic exception is seen in type III DGI in which the pulp chambers and root canals are extraordinarily large.

While patients with OI have mutations in either the *COL1A1* or *COL1A2* genes that encode the subunits of type I collagen, the genetic defect causing dentinogenesis (DGI) have been associated with defects in both the collagen type I genes and the dentin sialophosphoprotein gene (DSPP). The DSPP gene encodes both dentin sialoprotein (DSP) and dentin phosphoprotein (DPP), two proteins that were thought to be expressed only in dentin, but may be transiently expressed in ameloblasts and the inner ear.[4,5] While the function of DSP is unknown, DPP is thought to direct the nucleation of hydroxyapatite crystallites during dentin formation because of its highly repetitive amino acid sequence and high degree of phosphorylation.[6] Three distinct mutations in the *DSPP* gene are associated with the anomalies seen in DGI-1, following the complex, heterogeneous genetic pattern of OI.[5] The DGI type II locus has been mapped to a 2-cM interval at human chromosome 4q21, a region that contains the SIBLING family of proteins, which are associated with mineralized tissues.[7] As in DGI-I, mutations in DSPP are also responsible for the clinical manifestations of DGI-II, but unlike DGI-1, no collagen defects have been described.[8] A nonsense mutation in exon 3 creates a stop codon that blocks the translation of both

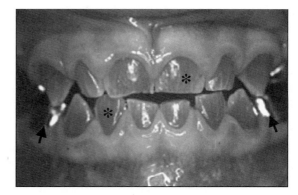

FIG. 1. The permanent teeth of this patient exhibit the characteristic blue-gray or opalescent appearance associated with dentinogenesis imperfecta (asterisks). The enamel of the posterior teeth has fractured and the underlying dentin has undergone severe attrition. Crowns have been made to control further destruction (arrows).

The authors have no conflict of interest.

© 2003 American Society for Bone and Mineral Research

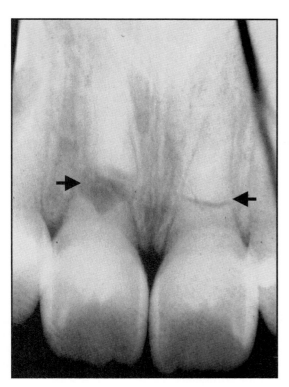

FIG. 2. Radiograph of maxillary central incisors from a patient with dentinogenesis imperfecta. Note the obliterated pulp chambers and the fractures caused by abnormal dentin formation and mineralization (arrows). (Courtesy of Dr. Michael A. Ignelzi, Jr.)

DSP and DPP leading to the structural and functional defects observed with this disorder.[9]

Dentin Dysplasia

Dentin dysplasia (DD) is an autosomal dominant disorder affecting dentin formation, and as in dentinogenesis imperfecta, has been mapped to human chromosome 4q, suggesting that a common gene may be responsible for the altered dentin phenotype. Recently, a candidate gene approach demonstrated that a family with a history of DD exhibited heterozygous substitution of a tyrosine to aspartic acid in the signal domain of DSPP that was present in all affected, but no unaffected, family members.[10] This DSPP mutation inhibits the translation of the protein and suggests that DD and DGI type II are allelic disorders. The clinical appearance of primary teeth is similar in patients with DGI and DD. This similarity is lost, however, once the permanent teeth have erupted. With dentin dysplasia, the permanent teeth are normal in color, have short roots with "thistle-tube" pulp chambers, and contain pulp stones of irregular shape that obliterate the pulp chamber with age.[11,12] The short roots often are associated with periapical radiolucencies that can lead to premature exfoliation of the teeth (Fig. 3).

Osteopetrosis

The lack of appropriate bone resorption observed in osteopetrosis has several implications in the craniofacial re-gion. The jawbones are abnormally dense at the expense of cancellous bone, and these changes may affect normal tooth development. Because normal tooth eruption is dependent on resorption of alveolar bone surrounding the developing tooth germ, inadequate resorptive function in osteopetrosis may limit the eruptive mechanisms and place altered forces on the erupting teeth. Dental findings associated with osteopetrosis include congenitally absent teeth, unerupted and malformed teeth, delayed eruption, and enamel hypoplasia.[13] There is a reduced calcium-phosphorous ratio in both enamel and dentin that may alter hydroxyapatite crystal formation and contribute to an increased caries index, as has been reported in several cases. Additionally, there are deviations in amino acid content, indicative of altered matrix composition.[13] Perhaps the most serious dental complication of osteopetrosis is the propensity to develop osteomyelitis.[14] Because the vascular supply to the jaws is compromised, avascular necrosis and infection after dental extractions may lead to osteomyelitis that is difficult to treat. Therefore, extraction of teeth must be performed as atraumatically as possible.

Mucopolysaccharidoses

The mucopolysaccharidoses (MPS) are a family of related inherited diseases that are characterized by a deficiency in glycosaminoglycan catabolism. These disorders, classified MPS I through MPS VII, are distinguished from each other based on genetic, biochemical, and clinical analyses.[1] Although heterogeneous, several craniofacial characteristics are similar between the different subgroups. The oral manifestations may include a short and broad mandible with abnormal condylar development and limited temporomandibular joint function. The teeth are often peg-shaped and exhibit increased interdental spacing perhaps because of the frequently observed gingival hyperplasia and macroglossia. Some forms of MPS have abnormally thin enamel covering the clinical crowns and radiographic evidence of cystic lesions surrounding the molar teeth that contain excessive dermatan sulfate and collagen.[15–18]

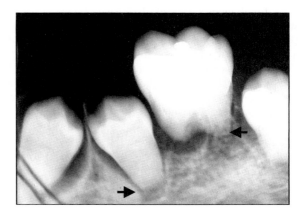

FIG. 3. Radiograph of teeth from a patient with dentin dysplasia. The roots are abnormally short or absent (arrows) and the pulp chamber is obliterated. (Courtesy of Dr. Sharon Brooks.)

Cherubism

Cherubism is an autosomal dominant disorder that manifests as bilateral jaw enlargement primarily involving the mandible of children. The clinical features of cherubism include painless, bilateral expansion of the posterior mandible and upward turning of the eyes that impart the cherubic facies from which this rare developmental jaw condition gets its name. Radiographically, the lesions appear as multilocular, expansile radiolucencies that can interfere with normal tooth eruption. The histopathologic features may not help in the definitive diagnosis of cherubism because the fibrous lesion containing multinucleated giant cells may resemble giant cell granuloma and fibrous dysplasia.[19] However, cherubism can now be distinguished from these other conditions because the mutation that causes cherubism has been identified in the c-Abl-binding protein SH3BP2.[20] Cherubism is also a component of the Noonan-like/multiple giant cell lesion syndrome, which has additional craniofacial and skeletal abnormalities.[21]

ORAL MANIFESTATIONS OF METABOLIC BONE DISEASES

Metabolic diseases of bone are disorders of bone remodeling that characteristically involve the entire skeleton. However, these disorders are often manifest first in the oral cavity and can lead to the diagnosis of the underlying systemic disease. Numerous studies suggest that subclinical derangements in calcium homeostasis and bone metabolism may also contribute to a variety of dental abnormalities including alveolar ridge resorption and periodontal bone loss in susceptible individuals. The significance of this spectrum of diseases and their overall impact on oral health and dental management are likely to increase as the elderly segment of the population increases in the coming decades.[22]

Vitamin D Deficiency

In vitamin D–resistant rickets, the primary oral abnormality is similar to dentin dysplasia. Enamel is usually reported to be normal, but in some instances may be hypoplastic. Patients also suffer from delayed tooth eruption and radiographically, teeth often display enlarged pulp chambers. Other salient radiographic findings include decreased alveolar bone density, thinning of bone trabeculae, loss of lamina dura, and hypomineralized teeth.[19] In familial hypophosphatemia, dental findings are often the first clinically noticeable signs of the disease and resemble those seen in rickets and osteomalacia. Patients may present with abscessed primary or permanent teeth that have no signs of dental caries.[23] Although the enamel is reported to be normal, microbial infection of the pulp is thought to occur though invasion of dentinal tubules exposed by attrition of enamel or through enamel mirofractures.[24]

Hypophosphatasia

Hypophosphatasia is characterized by defective mineralization of the skeletal and dental structures and deficiencies in liver, bone, and kidney isoenzymes of alkaline phosphatase.[25,26] The classic oral presentation of hypophosphatasia is the premature loss of the primary teeth. Tooth loss is presumably caused by hypoplasia of cementum on the root surfaces because periodontal inflammation is often not present. The lack of cementum likely alters the attachment of periodontal ligament fibers between the root and the alveolar bone and contributes to the premature exfoliation of teeth. In the permanent teeth, large pulp spaces, late eruption, and delayed apical closure are often observed.

Paget's Disease

Paget's disease, also known as Osteitis deformans, a disorder of bone remodeling,[27,28] is characterized by the presence of irregular islands of bone with prominent internal cement lines that create a mosaic pattern. In the craniofacial bones, radiographic lesions usually progress from irregular lytic lesions to areas of sclerosis that present with a distinctive cotton-wool appearance. Involvement of the maxilla is more common than the mandible, where patients often present with alveolar ridge enlargement and hypercementosis. In extreme cases, the expanding alveolar ridges can lead to the separation of teeth and poor denture adaptation in the edentulous patient. As the disease progresses, there may be extensive bone deformity with nerve compression and altered blood flow, conditions that can make tooth extraction problematic.

ORAL MANIFESTATIONS OF ACQUIRED DISORDERS

Benign Non-Odontogenic Neoplasms of the Jaws

Benign fibro-osseous lesions of the jaw are a heterogeneous group of disorders characterized by the replacement of normal trabecular bone and marrow with cellular fibrous connective tissue and a disorganized array of randomly oriented mineralized tissue. The most common group of lesions is known collectively as the cemento-osseous dysplasias,[29,30] so named because they contain spherical calcifications believed to be of cemental origin and randomly oriented mineralized structures, sometimes resembling bone. In some cases, these lesions are also associated with long bone fragility (gnatho-diaphyseal dysplasia).[31] Two other conditions included in this category are fibrous dysplasia and cherubism, which are of greater clinical significance because they tend to attain a larger size and have the potential for producing greater facial disfigurement and severe malocclusion.

Among the cemento-osseous dysplasias, the most common is a condition known as periapical cemental dysplasia. This asymptomatic lesion presents radiographically as a mixed radiolucent/radiopaque lesion that involves a single mandibular quadrant in middle-aged women. It is frequently encountered below the apices of the mandibular incisors. The involved teeth are vital and no treatment is required. Florid cemento-osseous dysplasia is a more extensive form of periapical cemental dysplasia that invariably involves multiple jaw quadrants. Fibrous dysplasia is a disorder that can affect single (monostotic) or multiple (polyostotic) bones and can occur as part of the McCune-Albright syndrome, where it is associated with skin pigmentation and endocrinopathies. When it occurs in the absence of endocrine abnormalities, it is referred to as Jaffe syndrome. The underlying cause of fibrous dysplasia and the McCune-Albright syndrome are activating mutations in the *Gsα* gene, resulting in abnormal accumulation and maturation of precursor osteogenic cells to osteoblast cells and formation of sclerotic lesions in craniofacial bones.[32] The condition is commonly found in juveniles and young adults but can be encountered as an adult onset form. Caries prevalence in these patients is higher than in the normal population, and prevalent dental anomalies included malocclusion, tooth rotation, oligodontia, and taurodontism.[33] Other benign expansile lesions of the jaw include the fibro-osseous tumors associated with hyperparathyroidism-jaw tumor syndrome, an autosomal dominant, multi-neoplasia disorder associated with primary parathyroid tumors and caused by mutation of the parafibromin gene, *HRPT2*,[34] and the exostoses seen in torus mandibularis that may be related to loss of function mutations in the gene for low-density lipoprotein receptor-related protein 5.[35]

Malignant Non-Odontogenic Neoplasms of the Jaws

Osteosarcoma is the most common malignant neoplasm derived from bone cells, occurring in 1 of every 100,000 people.[19] The peak incidence when it occurs in the jaws is approximately 10 years later than the peak incidence in the long bones. The radiographic appearance of osteosarcoma varies considerably depending on the histological type. Osteosarcomas that produce large amount of mineralized bone-like tissue will present as large areas of radiopacity within a diffuse radiolucent background. A characteristic finding in jaw lesions is widening of the periodontal ligament in adjacent teeth. Although this finding is not unique to osteosarcoma, it is sufficiently consistent to be of diagnostic value. Occlusal radiographs may also reveal a sunburst pattern of radiopacity radiating from the periosteum and may assist in the diagnosis.

REFERENCES

1. Gorlin RJ, Cohen MMJ, Levin LS 1990 Syndromes of the head and neck. In: Motulsky AG, Harper PS, Bobrow M, Scriver C (eds.) Oxford Monographs on Medical Genetics, 3rd ed. Oxford University Press, New York, NY, USA, pp. 155–166.
2. Waltimo J, Ojanotko-Harri A, Lukinmaa PL 1996 Mild forms of dentinogenesis imperfecta in association with osteogenesis imperfecta as characterized by light and transmission electron microscopy. J Oral Pathol Med 25:256–264.
3. Waltimo J 1994 Hyperfibers and vesicles in dentin matrix in dentinogenesis imperfecta (DI) associated with osteogenesis imperfecta (OI). J Oral Pathol Med 23:389–393.
4. Bronckers AL, D'Souza RN, Butler WT, Lyaruu DM, van Dijk S, Gay S, Woltgens JH 1993 Dentin sialoprotein: Biosynthesis and developmental appearance in rat tooth germs in comparison with amelogenins, osteocalcin and collagen type-I. Cell Tissue Res 272:237–247.
5. Xiao S, Yu C, Chou X, Yuan W, Wang Y, Bu L, Fu G, Qian M, Yang J, Shi Y, Hu L, Han B, Wang Z, Huang W, Liu J, Chen Z, Zhao G, Kong X 2001 Dentinogenesis imperfecta 1 with or without progressive hearing loss is associated with distinct mutations in DSPP. Nat Genet 27:201–204.
6. George A, Bannon L, Sabsay B, Dillon JW, Malone J, Veis A, Jenkins NA, Gilbert DJ, Copeland NG 1996 The carboxyl-terminal domain of phosphophoryn contains unique extended triplet amino acid repeat sequences forming ordered carboxyl-phosphate interaction ridges that may be essential in the biomineralization process. J Biol Chem 271:32869–32873.
7. Aplin HM, Hirst KL, Dixon MJ 1999 Refinement of the dentinogenesis imperfecta type II locus to an interval of less than 2 centiMorgans at chromosome 4q21 and the creation of a yeast artificial chromosome contig of the critical region. J Dent Res 78:1270–1276.
8. Zhang X, Zhao J, Li C, Gao S, Qiu C, Liu P, Wu G, Qiang B, Lo WH, Shen Y 2001 DSPP mutation in dentinogenesis imperfecta Shields type II. Nat Genet 27:151–152.
9. MacDougall M, Simmons D, Luan X, Nydegger J, Feng J, Gu TT 1997 Dentin phosphoprotein and dentin sialoprotein are cleavage products expressed from a single transcript coded by a gene on human chromosome 4. Dentin phosphoprotein DNA sequence determination. J Biol Chem 272:835–842.
10. Rajpar MH, Koch MJ, Davies RM, Mellody KT, Kielty CM, Dixon MJ 2002 Mutation of the signal peptide region of the bicistronic gene DSPP affects translocation to the endoplasmic reticulum and results in defective dentine biomineralization. Hum Mol Genet 11:2559–2565.
11. Giansanti JS, Allen JD 1974 Dentin dysplasia, type II, or dentin dysplasia, coronal type. Oral Surg Oral Med Oral Pathol Oral Radiol Endod 38:911–917.
12. Lukinmaa PL, Ranta H, Ranta K, Kaitila I, Hietanen J 1987 Dental findings in osteogenesis imperfecta: II. Dysplastic and other developmental defects. J Craniofac Genet Dev Biol 7:127–135.
13. Dick HM, Simpson WJ 1972 Dental changes in osteopetrosis. Oral Surg Oral Med Oral Pathol Oral Radiol Endod 34:408–416.
14. Dyson DP 1970 Osteomyelitis of the jaws in Albers-Schonberg disease. Br J Oral Surg 7:178–187.
15. Downs AT, Crisp T, Ferretti G 1995 Hunter's syndrome and oral manifestations: A review. Pediatr Dent 17:98–100.
16. Keith O, Scully C, Weidmann GM 1990 Orofacial features of Scheie (Hurler-Scheie) syndrome (alpha-L- iduronidase deficiency). Oral Surg Oral Med Oral Pathol Oral Radiol Endod 70:70–74.
17. Kinirons MJ, Nelson J 1990 Dental findings in mucopolysaccharidosis type IV A (Morquio's disease type A). Oral Surg Oral Med Oral Pathol Oral Radiol Endod 70:176–179.
18. Smith KS, Hallett KB, Hall RK, Wardrop RW, Firth N 1995 Mucopolysaccharidosis: MPS VI and associated delayed tooth eruption. Int J Oral Maxillofac Surg 24:176–180.
19. Neville BW, Damm DD, Allen CM, Bouquot JE 1995 Abnormalities of the Teeth. In: Oral and Maxillofacial Pathology, 1st ed. W. B. Saunders, New York, NY, USA, pp. 44–79.
20. Ueki Y, Tiziani V, Santanna C, Fukai N, Maulik C, Garfinkle J, Ninomiya C, doAmaral C, Peters H, Habal M, Rhee-Morris L, Doss JB, Kreiborg S, Olsen BR, Reichenberger E 2001 Mutations in the gene encoding c-Abl-binding protein SH3BP2 cause cherubism. Nat Genet 28:125–126.
21. Cohen MM Jr, Gorlin RJ 1991 Noonan-like/multiple giant cell lesion syndrome. Am J Med Genet 40:159–166.
22. Solt DB 1991 The pathogenesis, oral manifestations, and implications for dentistry of metabolic bone disease. Curr Opin Dent 1:783–791.
23. Goodman JR, Gelbier MJ, Bennett JH, Winter GB 1998 Dental problems associated with hypophosphataemic vitamin D resistant rickets. Int J Paediatr Dent 8:19–28.
24. Hillmann G, Geurtsen W 1996 Pathohistology of undecalcified primary teeth in vitamin D-resistant rickets: Review and report of two cases. Oral Surg Oral Med Oral Pathol Oral Radiol Endod 82:218–224.
25. Watanabe H, Hashimoto-Uoshima M, Goseki-Sone M, Orimo H, Ishikawa I 2001 A novel point mutation (C571T) in the tissue-nonspecific alkaline phosphatase gene in a case of adult-type hypophosphatasia. Oral Dis 7:331–335.
26. Chapple IL 1993 Hypophosphatasia: Dental aspects and mode of inheritance. J Clin Periodontol 20:615–622.
27. Carter LC 1991 Paget's disease: Important features for the general practitioner. Comp Contin Edu Dent 11:662–669.
28. Merkow RL, Lane JM 1990 Paget's disease of bone. Orthop Clin North Am 21:171–189.
29. Sapp JP, Eversole LR, Wysocki GP 1997 Bone lesions. In: Contemporary Oral and Maxillofacial Pathology, 1st ed. Mosby-Year Book, Inc., St. Louis, MO, USA, pp. 88–125.
30. Waldron CA 1993 Fibro-osseous lesions of the jaws. J Oral Maxillofac Surg 51:828–835.
31. Riminucci M, Collins MT, Corsi A, Boyde A, Murphey MD, Wientroub S, Kuznetsov SA, Cherman N, Robey PG, Bianco P 2001 Gnathodiaphyseal dysplasia: A syndrome of fibro-osseous lesions of

jawbones, bone fragility, and long bone bowing. J Bone Miner Res **16:**1710–1718.

32. Riminucci M, Liu B, Corsi A, Shenker A, Spiegel AM, Robey PG, Bianco P 1999 The histopathology of fibrous dysplasia of bone in patients with activating mutations of the Gs alpha gene: Site-specific patterns and recurrent histological hallmarks. J Pathol **187:**249–258.

33. Akintoye SO, Lee J, Feimster T, Booher S, Brahim J, Riminucci M, Robey PG, Collins MT 2003 Dental characteristics in fibrous dysplasia and McCune-Albright Syndrome. Oral Surg Oral Med Oral Pathol Oral Radiol Endod (in press).

34. Carpten JD, Robbins CM, Villablanca A, Forsberg L, Presciuttini S, Bailey-Wilson J, Simonds WF, Gillanders EM, Kennedy AM, Chen JD, Agarwal SK, Sood R, Jones MP, Moses TY, Haven C, Petillo D, Leotlela PD, Harding B, Cameron D, Pannett AA, Hoog A, Heath H, James-Newton LA, Robinson B, Zarbo RJ, Cavaco BM, Wassif W, Perrier ND, Rosen IB, Kristoffersson U, Turnpenny PD, Farnebo LO, Besser GM, Jackson CE, Morreau H, Trent JM, Thakker RV, Marx SJ, Teh BT, Larsson C, Hobbs MR 2002 HRPT2, encoding parafibromin, is mutated in hyperparathyroidism-jaw tumor syndrome. Nat Genet **32:**676–680.

35. Boyden LM, Mao J, Belsky J, Mitzner L, Farhi A, Mitnick MA, Wu D, Insogna K, Lifton RP 2002 High bone density due to a mutation in LDL-receptor-related protein 5. N Engl J Med **346:**1513–1521.

Chapter 90.   Periodontal Diseases and Bone

Marjorie K. Jeffcoat

School of Dentistry, University of Alabama at Birmingham, Birmingham, Alabama

INTRODUCTION

Periodontal diseases fall into two broad categories: gingivitis and periodontitis. Gingivitis is characterized by gingival inflammation. Its major etiologic factor is bacterial plaque accumulation on the teeth. The response to the plaque may be modified by systemic or genetic diseases and a myriad of drugs. One of the major features distinguishing gingivitis from periodontitis is the absence of alveolar bone loss in the former. Periodontitis is characterized by loss of soft tissue attachment to the tooth along with alveolar bone loss, resulting in decreased support of the tooth (Fig. 1).

THE DIAGNOSIS

In 1999, the American Academy of Periodontology held a workshop to update the terminology used to distinguish the various forms of periodontitis.[1] Table 1 shows the old terminology as well as the new terminology. This chapter focuses on periodontitis, because one of the hallmarks of periodontitis is alveolar bone loss. Periodontal diseases are classified by clinical syndromes, because to date, there are no definitive tests for periodontitis. Under the old classification system, patients were categorized according to a combination of patient age, response of the disease to therapy, and rate of progression of bone and attachment loss. The new system in the United States uses rate of progression as the key classifying factor. In Europe, the European Academy of Periodontology uses age as the primary classifying factor.

ETIOLOGY

Periodontitis is a multifactorial disease. While the bacteria in the plaque biofilm are considered the major causative agent, susceptibility of the host plays an important role. This interaction is illustrated in Fig. 2. There are approximately 300–400 microbiological species that have been isolated from the oral cavity. At the gingival crevice, there is a shift from a gram-positive aerobic flora in a state of health to gram-negative anaerobic or gram-negative facultative species, which have been implicated in the pathogenesis of periodontal diseases. In a recent report, the bacteria in biofilm were categorized into clusters. The "red cluster" consisting of *P. gingivalis*, *B. forsythus*, and *T. denticola* are most often associated with inflammation and attachment loss.[2]

The pathogenicity of the microbiological biofilm associated with disease is enabled by the virulence factors of the gram-negative and facultative species once they invade the tissue. The predominant virulence factors that play a role in host-interaction are endotoxin, exotoxin, and bacterial enzymes. Gram-negative (LPS) endotoxin produces cytotoxic effects on host tissue, resulting in tissue necrosis and bone resorption through osteoclast stimulation.[3] The exotoxins excreted by the bacteria are metabolic end products such as organic acids, amines, indole, ammonia, and sulfur compounds that produce local cytotoxic and host defense inhib-

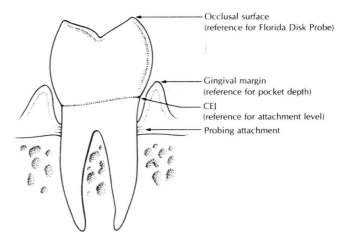

FIG. 1. Anatomy of the tooth. The soft tissue attachment is assessed clinically by measuring the distance from the cemento-enamel junction (CEJ) and pocket base. In health, the alveolar bone crest is no more than 2–3 mm apical of the cemento-enamel junction.

The author has no conflict of interest.

TABLE 1. CLASSIFICATION OF PERIODONTAL DISEASES

Old classification system

Disease	Age	Rate of progression	Responsive to therapy
Juvenile periodontitis	Adolescent	Rapid	Yes
Prepubertal periodontitis	Children	Rapid	Poor
Refractory periodontitis	Any	Rapid	No
Adult periodontitis	35 years and over	Slow to moderate	Yes

New classification system (United States)

Disease	Age	Progression	Replaces old terminology
Chronic periodontitis	Any	Slow	Adult periodontitis
Aggressive periodontitis	Any	Rapid	Juvenile, prepubertal, rapidly progressive periodontitis
Necrotizing ulcerative periodontitis	Any	Rapid	Necrotizing ulcerative periodontitis
Periodontitis as a manifestation of systemic disease	Any	Any rate	Not in older classifications

itory effects.[4,5] The bacterial enzymes such as collagenase, hyaluronidase, and proteinase lead to increased intracellular spaces and permeability and further enable tissue invasion.[6]

Periodontal diseases are initiated by bacteria, and the bacteria may directly interact with the host tissues in mediating the destruction. In general, there is a well-regulated host response mediated through inflammatory cells that control the spread of bacterial infection. However, the host response itself may establish a chronic inflammatory state and may play a role in the local destruction of the supporting structures of the teeth. Mediators produced as part of the inflammatory host response that contribute to tissue destruction include proteinases, cytokines, and prostaglandins. Matrix metalloproteinases are considered the primary proteinases involved in periodontal tissue destruction by degradation of extracellular molecules.[7–9] Two proinflammatory cytokines, interleukin (IL)-1 and tumor necrosis factor (TNF), seem to have a central role in periodontal destruction. The properties of these cytokines that relate to tissue destruction involve the stimulation of bone resorption by IL-1 and induction of tissue-degrading proteinases by TNF.[10] Prostaglandins, especially PGE_2, seem to be partially responsible for the bone loss associated with periodontal diseases.[11] Prostaglandins are arachidonic acid metabolites generated by cyclo-oxygenses. Cyclo-oxygenase (COX2) production of PGE_2 that is associated with inflammation is upregulated by IL-1, TNF, and bacterial LPS.[3,12] Clinical trials have indicated that bone loss associated with periodontitis was partially prevented by administration of inhibitors of prostaglandin synthesis.[13,14]

DIAGNOSTIC TOOLS

The diagnostic tools used today for the diagnosis of periodontal disease are primarily based on the anatomy of the lesions. These are summarized in Table 2. For an extensive review, see Armitage.[15] Visual inspection reveals superficial signs of gingival inflammation such as edema and redness of the tissues. Periodontal probing uses a 0.5-mm probe that is placed between the tooth root and the gingiva in the pocket or sulcus. Probing depth, the distance between the base of the pocket and the gingival margin, provides some indication of prior disease progression and alerts the practitioner to the depth of the anaerobic chamber the pocket provides for growth of gram-negative anaerobic bacteria. This measure is of importance in planning treatment because deep pockets are more difficult to clean. Probing attachment levels (or clinical attachment leads), which measure the distance from the base of the pocket to a fixed landmark such as the cemento-enamel junction, give an estimate of prior soft tissue attachment.

Radiographs are used to determine the extent of alveolar bone loss in teeth at risk. Both radiographs and probing examinations do not provide an indication of current disease activity. Rather, they represent the sum total of disease and healing that has occurred over the lifespan of the tooth. Prior studies have shown, however, that the absence of inflammation, lack of radiographic indication of bone loss, and shallow pockets are associated with a low risk of future progression.

Microbial tests aim to detect the presence of putative periodontal pathogens in a given pocket. In many cases, cultural methods have been replaced by newer ELISA and DNA testing.[2] Only cultural methods can be used to determine which antibiotics may be used to successfully treat a given bacterial infection.[15] At present, these tests are not routinely used in the diagnosis of periodontitis but may be useful for treatment planning in aggressive or refractory disease.

Gingival crevicular fluid is a transudate of plasma. The quantity of gingival crevicular fluid is associated with inflammation. Biochemical profiles of inflammatory markers and mediators have also been studied extensively.[16] Markers such

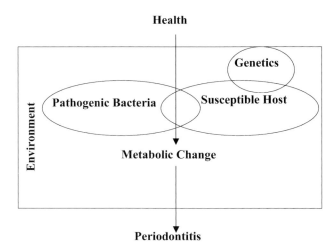

FIG. 2. Etiology of periodontal disease. Periodontal disease occurs when a pathogenic bacterial biofilm is present in a susceptible host. Genetic and environmental factors modify the ultimate response to the bacteria.

© 2003 American Society for Bone and Mineral Research

TABLE 2. DIAGNOSIS

Test	Application	Strengths
Probing pocket depths	All patients	Shallow depths associated with lack of future disease progression
Gingival inflammation	Assessed in all patients	Absence of inflammation is associated with a lack of future progression
Radiographic evidence of bone loss	At-risk patients as determined by PSR screening or periodontal examination	Absence of bone loss is associated with a lower risk of future progression
Microbial/plaque tests	High-risk patients or refractory to treatment	In compromised or refractory patients may be useful in determining the presence of pathogens
Biochemical profiles in gingival crevicular fluid	Not yet determined	A number of biochemical markers may identify individuals at risk

as aspartate aminotransferase, β-glucuronidase, elastase, and many cytokines are elevated in periodontitis and in progressive periodontitis. At present there are no biochemical profiles associated with specific periodontal disease entities.[15]

Genetic testing has become a reality for periodontal disease. Certain IL-1β polymorphisms are associated with a higher risk of periodontitis.[17,18] Other cytokine polymorphisms are under study.

TREATMENT

Treatment of periodontitis is usually divided into two types: surgical and nonsurgical. While this is a helpful categorization for patients, insurance companies, and clinicians, it does not address the mechanism of each treatment modality. Therefore, treatment will be discussed in reference to Fig. 2 (treatment may be directed at the bacteria or the host).

Treatment Directed Against the Bacteria. This mode of treatment includes self-care, such as brushing and flossing,[19] and professionally administered care (Table 3). Professional mechanical therapy, such as scaling and root planing, removes plaque biofilm from the tooth surface, as well as removing calculus (tartar), and it decreases endotoxin on the root surface cementum. Scaling and root planing, when

TABLE 3. NONSURGICAL THERAPY OF PERIODONTITIS

Category of treatment	Treatment	Strengths
	Targeted at bacteria by mechanical means	
Professional mechanical therapy—used in the treatment of gingivitis and periodontitis	Scaling and root planing— with manual instrument and ultrasonics	Decreases gingival inflammation by 40–60% Decreases probing depth Facilitates gain in clinical attachment level
	Targeted at bacteria by chemotherapy	
Chemical plaque control with mouthrinses and tooth pastes	Chlorhexidine Triclosan co-polymer or triclosan zinc-citrate Essential oils Stannous fluoride	Significant reductions in gingival inflammation No evidence that there is a substantial long-term benefit for periodontitis except to control co-existing inflammation
Sustained release antimicrobials	Intrapocket resorbable or nonresorbable delivery systems containing a tetracycline antibiotic, or chlorhexidine	When used as an adjunct to scaling and root planing, gains in clinical attachment level, and decreases in probing depth and bleeding
Systemic antibiotics	Tetracyclines, metranidazole, spiromycin, clindamycin, and combinations such as metronidazole and amoxicillin	Not indicated for most adult periodontitis patients May be useful to treat aggressive destructive periodontitis
	Targeted at host response	
MMP inhibitors low dose tetracyclines	Used in adult or chronic periodontitis	Slows the progression of attachment loss
Nonsteroidal anti-inflammatory drugs	Used in adult or chronic periodontitis in research	Slows the progression of attachment loss
Bisphosphonate	Used in adult or chronic periodontitis research	Increases bone mineral density and slows the progression of attachment loss

TABLE 4. SURGICAL PERIODONTAL THERAPY—SELECTED PROCEDURES

Category and goal	Procedures	Strengths
Pocket therapy—provides access to root surfaces and bony defects, reduces probing depths, facilitates plaque control and enhances restorative and cosmetic dentistry	Gingival flap to provide access to roots and bony defects for debridement	Improvement in clinical attachment level
Regeneration—procedures to facilitate growth of new periodontal ligament, cementum and bone over previously diseased root surfaces	Extraoral autogeneous bone grafts	High potential for bone growth
	Intraoral autogenous grafts (i.e., maxillary tuberosity, healing extraction sites, osseous coagulum)	Case reports indicate bone gain of over 50% Controlled studies compared to non-grafted bone show improved clinical attachment levels and bone, but not as great as in case reports
	Allografts—tissue transferred from one individual to another	Bone fill has been reported in a high proportion of defects, but is variable
	Freeze-dried bone allograft	Osteogenic potential may vary from vial to vial, patient differences, and clinician variability
	Alloplasts—synthetic grafts Absorbable: plaster, calcium carbonates, ceramics such as tricalcium phosphate and absorbable HA Nonabsorbable: dense HA, porous HA, bioglass Calcium coated polymer polymethyl methacrylate and hydroxymethyl methacrylate	Improved probing depth and attachment level
Biologics	Enamel matrix proteins Anorganic bovine derived hydroxyapatite matrix cell-binding peptide	Fill in infrabony osseous defects

performed with hand or ultrasonic instrumentation, decreases gingival inflammation, decreases probing depth, and facilitates gain in clinical attachment levels.[20] This therapy must be distinguished from a dental prophylaxis. The goal of scaling and root planing is to remove plaque, calculus, and endotoxin as far into the periodontal pocket as possible, where a prophylaxis (conventional tooth cleaning) is more superficial. In cases of mild to moderate periodontitis, scaling and root planing may be the definitive therapy for the average patient, as well as for patients with complex medical problems or with end-stage periodontitis.

The bacteria in plaque biofilm may be controlled using chemical agents in mouth rinses, toothpastes, and intrapocket delivery systems. Both antiseptics and antibiotics are available.[21] The antiseptics are the agent of choice for gingivitis because of the unfavorable risk to benefit ratio of antibiotics for the treatment of inflammation. At present, the gold standard antiseptic is chorhexidine gluconate. In the United States, chorhexidine gluconate is available in mouth rinse form. When used in a 30-s rinse, chorhexidine gluconate reduces gingival inflammation up to 60%. Other antiseptics include triclosan copolymer or triclosan zinc-citrate, essential oils, and stannous fluoride.

Sustained release antimicrobial agents are in the forms of gels chips or microspheres. They are placed in the periodontal pocket and deliver antimicrobials (chorhexidine or one of the tetracyclines) from a sustained release matrix.[22–24] When used as an adjunct to scaling and root planing, improvements in clinical attachment levels, decreases in probing depth, and gingival inflammation have been shown. Systemic antibiotics do not automatically kill sensitive plaque bacteria, because the bacteria are in the form of a biofilm necessitating high doses of antimicrobial for efficacy. Tetracyclines, metronidazole, clindamycin, spiramycin, and combinations such as metronidazole and amoxicillin have been tested with mixed results.[25,26] Systemic antibiotics are not indicated for gingivitis in most cases of chronic periodontitis but may be used to treat aggressive destructive periodontitis.

Surgical Techniques. Periodontal surgical therapy aims to facilitate patient plaque control through pocket reduction and improved clinical attachment (Table 4). Simple mucoperiosteal flap elevation provides access to bony defects for more thorough debridement than closed scaling and root planing may provide. The flap may be apically positioned with or without recontouring of the underlying bone.[27] Regenerative techniques may involve grafts that are osteoconductive or osteoinductive.[28–30] Alloplasts or synthetic grafts are generally osteoconductive. Autogenous bone grafts have the highest potential for bone growth. Osteoinductive materials include freeze-dried bone allografts from a tissue bank. Allografts should be tested to avoid transmission of pathogenic viruses from donor to recipient.

Biological agents to promote the growth of new periodontal ligament, cementum, and bone are becoming available. Enamel matrix protein has been shown to increase bone fill in intraosseous defects.[31,32] As well, an anorganic bovine-derived hydroxyapatite matrix cell-binding peptide (P-15) has been shown to increase bone fill in intraosseous defects.[33] The patient's own growth factors are used when a membrane is used to cover the osseous defect and blood clot, thereby promoting osseous fill.

Therapy Directed at the Host Response. A newer concept is therapy directed at the host response (Table 3).[34] Low-dose tetracycline therapy has been shown to improve attachment levels in patients with periodontitis.[35] This therapy is relatively long term, and its mechanism of action is believed to be inhibition of matrix metalloproteinases. Other therapies directed at the host response are used in research. These include nonsteroidal anti-inflammatory drugs that slow the progression of alveolar bone loss.[13,14] Bisphosphonates have also been shown to increase alveolar bone density while slowing the rate of bone loss.[36]

FUTURE DIRECTIONS

Current research is focused on eliminating pathogens and improving host response to bacteria with the aim of moderating bone and attachment loss. As well, bone grafts with allographs, alloplasts, and biologics are under investigation with the aim of improving the predictability of fill of osseous defects.

REFERENCES

1. Armitage GC 1999 Development of a classification system for periodontal diseases and conditions. Ann Periodontol 4:1–6.
2. Socransky SS, Haffajee AD, Cugini MA, Smith C, Kent RL Jr, 1998 Microbial complexes in subgingival plaque. J Clin Periodontol 25:134–144.
3. Offenbacher S, Salvi GE 1999 Induction of prostaglandin release from macrophages by bacterial endotoxin. Clin Infect Dis 28:505–513.
4. Singer RE, Buckner BA 1981 Butyrate and propionate: Important components of toxic dental plaque extracts. Infect Immun 32:458–463.
5. van Steenbergen TJ, van der Mispel LM, de Graaff J 1986 Effects of ammonia and volatile fatty acids produced by oral bacteria on tissue culture cells. J Dent Res 65:909–912.
6. Curtis MA, Kuramitsu HK, Lantz M, Macrina FL, Nakayama K, Potempa J, Reynolds EC, Aduse-Opoku J 1999 Molecular genetics and nomenclature of proteases of *Porphyromonas gingivalis*. J Periodontal Res 34:464–472.
7. Ding Y, Haapasalo M, Kerosuo E, Lounatmaa K, Kotirantice A, Sorsa T 1996 Release and activation of human neutrophil matrix metallo- and serine proteinases during phagocytosis of *Fusobacterium nucleatum*, *Porphyromonas gingivalis*, and *Treponema denticola*. J Clin Periodontol 24:237–248.
8. Ingman T, Tervahartiala T, Ding Y, Tschesche H, Haerian A, Kinane DF 1996 Matrix metalloproteinases and their inhibitors in gingival crevicular fluid and saliva of periodontitis patients. J Clin Periodontol 23:1127–1135.
9. Romanelli R, Mancini S, Laschinger C, Overall CM, Sodek J, McCulloch CA 1999 Activation of neutrophil collagenase in periodontitis. Infect Immun 67:2319–2326.
10. Graves DT 1999 The potential role of chemokines and inflammatory cytokines in periodontal disease progression. Clin Infect Dis 28:482–490.
11. Cavanaugh PF Jr, Meredith MP, Buchanan W, Doyle MJ, Reddy MS, Jeffcoat MK 1998 Coordinate production of PGE2 and IL-1 beta in the gingival crevicular fluid of adults with periodontitis: Its relationship to alveolar bone loss and disruption by twice daily treatment with ketorolac tromethamine oral rinse. J Periodontal Res 33:75–82.
12. Roberts FA, Richardson GJ, Michalek SM 1997 Effects of *Porphyromonas gingivalis* and *Escherichia coli* lipopolysaccharides on mononuclear phagocytes. Infect Immun 65:3248–3254.
13. Williams RC, Jeffcoat MK, Howell TH, Stubb D, Teoh KW, Reddy MS, Goohaber P 1989 Altering the progression of human alveolar bone loss with the non-steroidal anti-inflammatory drug flurbiprofen. J Periodontol 60:485–490.
14. Jeffcoat MK, Reddy MS, Haigh S, Buchanan W, Doyle MJ, Meredith MP, Nelson SL, Goodale MB, Wehmeyer KR 1995 A comparison of topical ketorolac, systemic flurbiprofen, and placebo for the inhibition of bone loss in adult periodontitis. J Periodontol 66:329–338.
15. Armitage GC 1996 Periodontal diseases: Diagnosis. Ann Periodontol 1:37–215.
16. Engebretson SP, Grbic JT, Singer R, Lamster IB 2002 GCF IL-1beta profiles in periodontal disease. J Clin Periodontol 29:48–53.
17. Engebretson SP, Lamster IB, Herrera-Abreu M, Celenti RS, Timms JM, Chaudhary AG, di Giovine FS, Kornman KS 1999 The influence of interleukin gene polymorphism on expression of interleukin-1beta and tumor necrosis factor-alpha in periodontal tissue and gingival crevicular fluid. J Periodontol 70:567–573.
18. Kornman KS, di Giovine FS 1998 Genetic variations in cytokine expression: A risk factor for severity of adult periodontitis. Ann Periodontol 3:327–338.
19. Hancock EB 1996 Prevention. Ann Periodontol 1:223–249.
20. Cobb CM 1996 Non-surgical pocket therapy: Mechanical. Ann Periodontol 1:443–490.
21. Drisko CH 1996 Non-surgical pocket therapy: Pharmacotherapeutics. Ann Periodontol 1:491–566.
22. Jeffcoat MK, Bray KS, Ciancio SG, Dentino AR, Fine DH, Gordon JM, Gunsolley JC, Killoy WJ, Lowenguth RA, Magnusson NI, Offenbacher S, Palcanis KG, Proskin HM, Finkelman RD, Flashner M 1998 Adjunctive use of a subgingival controlled-release chlorhexidine chip reduces probing depth and improves attachment level compared with scaling and root planing alone. J Periodontol 69:989–997.
23. Garrett S, Johnson L, Drisko CH, Adams DF, Bandt C, Beiswanger B, Bogle G, Donly K, Hallmon WW, Hancock EB, Hanes P, Hawley CE, Kiger R, Killoy W, Mellonig JT, Polson A, Raab FJ, Ryder M, Stoller NH, Wang HL, Wolinsky LE, Evans GH, Harrold CQ, Arnold RM, Southard GL, et al 1999 Two multi-center studies evaluating locally delivered doxycycline hyclate, placebo control, oral hygiene, and scaling and root planing in the treatment of periodontitis. J Periodontol 70:490–503.
24. Williams RC, Paquette DW, Offenbacher S, Adams DF, Armitage GC, Bray K, Caton J, Cochran DL, Drisko CH, Fiorellini JP, Giannobile WV, Grossi S, Guerrero DM, Johnson GK, Lamster IB, Magnusson I, Oringer RJ, Persson GR, Van Dyke TE, Wolff LF, Santucci EA, Rodda BE, Lessem J 2001 Treatment of periodontitis by local administration of minocycline microspheres: A controlled trial. J Periodontol 72:1535–1544.
25. Elter JR, Lawrence HP, Offenbacher S, Beck JD 1997 Meta-analysis of the effect of systemic metronidazole as an adjunct to scaling and root planing for adult periodontitis. J Periodontal Res 32:487–496.
26. Bollen CM, Quirynen M 1996 Microbiological response to mechanical treatment in combination with adjunctive therapy. A review of the literature. J Periodontol 67:1143–1158.
27. Palcanis KG 1996 Surgical pocket therapy. Ann Periodontol 1:589–617.
28. Garrett S 1996 Periodontal regeneration around natural teeth. Ann Periodontol 1:621–666.
29. Nasr HF, Aichelmann-Reidy ME, Yukna RA 2000 Bone and bone substitutes. Periodontology 19:74–86.
30. Aichelmann-Reidy ME, Yukna RA 1998 Bone replacement grafts. The bone substitutes. Dent Clin North Am 42:491–503.
31. Kirker-Head CA 2000 Potential applications and delivery strategies for bone morphogenetic proteins. Adv Drug Deliv Rev 43:65–92.
32. Tonetti MS, Land NP, Cortelini P, Suvan JE, Adriaens P, Dubravec D, Fonzar A, Fourmousis I, Mayfield L, Rossi R, Silvestri M, Tiedemann C, Topoll H, Vangsted T, WallKam B 2002 Enamel matrix protein in the regenerative therapy of deep intrabony defects. J Clin Periodontol 29:317–325.
33. Yukna RA, Callan DP, Krauser JT, Evan GH, Aichelmann-Reidy ME, Moore K, Cruz R, Scott JB 1998 Multi-center clinical evaluation of conbiation anorganic bovine derived hydroxyapatite matrix (ABM)/ cell-binding peptide (P-15) as a bone replacement graft material in human periodontal osseous defects: 6 month results. J Periodontol 69:655–663.
34. Kornman KS 1999 Host modulation as a therapeutic strategy in the treatment of periodontal disease. Clin Infect Dis 28:520–526.
35. Caton JG, Ciancio SG, Blieden TM, Bradshaw M, Crout RJ, Hefti AF, Massaro JM, Polson AM, Thomas J, Walker C 2000 Treatment with subantimicrobial dose doxycycline improves the efficacy of scaling and root planing in patients with adult periodontitis. J Periodontol 71:521–532.
36. Jeffcoat MK, Reddy MS 1996 Alveolar bone loss and osteoporosis: Evidence for a common mode of therapy using the bisphosphonate alendronate. In: Biological Mechanisms of Tooth Movement and Craniofacial Adaptation. pp. 365–374.

Chapter 91. Oral Bone Loss and Osteoporosis

Jean Wactawski-Wende

Departments of Social and Preventive Medicine and Gynecology and Obstetrics, University at Buffalo, State of New York, Buffalo, New York

INTRODUCTION

Osteoporosis is a skeletal disorder characterized by compromised bone strength predisposing to increased risk of fracture, with bone strength determined by both bone density and bone quality. Periodontitis is an infection-mediated process characterized by resorption of the alveolar bone as well as loss of the soft tissue attachment to the tooth and is a major cause of tooth loss and edentulism in adults. Tooth loss, in turn, results in the resorption of the remaining residual ridge and continued loss of oral bone. Oral bone loss has been shown to be associated with osteoporosis and low skeletal bone mineral density (BMD). The interaction of host infection and host susceptibility (i.e., osteoporosis) in the incidence and progression of periodontal disease and oral bone loss continues to be an area of intensive investigation, with most published studies supporting a positive association. However, many of these studies are cross-sectional in nature, include relatively small sample sizes and have inadequate control of potential confounding factors, limiting our understanding of the nature of the relationship between these common conditions.

METHODS TO ASSESS ORAL BONE

Interpretation of published findings is complicated by various methods to assess both postcranial and oral bone loss. Techniques used to assess systemic BMD include, single-photon absorptiometry (SPA) and dual-photon absorptiometry (DPA), single-energy absorptiometry (SXA) and DXA, quantitative computerized tomography (QCT), radiographic absorptiometry (RA), and ultrasound (US). Further descriptions of each of these technologies including their precision and accuracy can be found elsewhere. Systemic density can be measured at various skeletal sites, each including differing proportions of cortical and trabecular bone that may more (i.e., wrist) or less (i.e., spine) approximate that found in the oral cavity. Not all studies of oral bone loss and osteoporosis rely on some measure of BMD. Some use clinical observations, such as history of bone fracture.

There are several techniques used to assess oral bone loss; all typically involve use of radiographic measures of the oral bones. The commonly used assessments include measures of loss of alveolar crestal height (ACH), measures of resorption of the residual ridge after tooth loss (RRR), and assessment of oral BMD.

ACH is assessed using oral radiographs (bitewings) taken in regions of the oral cavity that include intact teeth. These radiographs are typically digitized and distance measure-

ments are made from fixed points on the teeth (the cemento-enamel junction or CEJ) to the top of the alveolar bone (crest) adjacent to the tooth (see Fig. 1). ACH is usually measured at two sites per tooth (mesial and distal) and is reported as the average loss of bone height in all teeth measured in the mouth (mean ACH). The larger the mean ACH reported, the worse the bone loss surrounding the teeth. Cross-sectional assessments of bone height can be troublesome because mean ACH values can be impacted by tooth loss. Teeth that have been lost because of periodontal disease no longer contribute to mean ACH assessments. As such, the teeth with the worst periodontal destruction (and presumably the worst oral bone) are lost, no longer contributing to mean ACH measures, resulting in assessments that appear to be better than they actually are. After a tooth is lost, RRR progresses. Most often the extent of RRR is described in edentulous subjects, but RRR can be described in dentate subjects that have lost one or more teeth in the region of tooth loss.

Measurement of oral bone density has been conducted using a variety of techniques that include measurement of absolute bone density (DXA, DPA, QCT, RA) and studies that approximate change in oral density over time, such as computer-assisted densitometric image analysis (CADIA). All techniques used to assess oral bone density are limited to some extent by either cost or precision. QCT provides perhaps the best assessment of oral density because it can measure virtually any region without obstruction by teeth; however, this technique is relatively expensive and includes relatively high exposure to radiation. Both DPA and DXA have been used to assess oral BMD; however, positioning and reproducibility of oral measurements is difficult. RA has been used in several studies using bitewing radiographs taken with a calibrated step-wedge of known density in the field of X-ray. Reproducibility of this method is good when positioning aids are used. Attempts to use radiomorphomet-

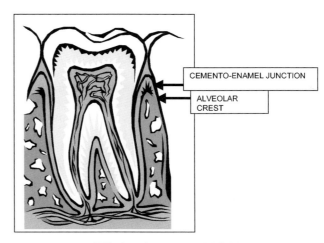

FIG. 1. Alveolar crestal height.

Dr. Wactawski-Wende subcontracted on a grant funded by Wyeth Pharmaceuticals. In addition, she received a speaking honorarium from Merck & Co., Inc. and Wyeth Pharmaceuticals.

ric indices in panoramic radiographs to predict skeletal density have been largely disappointing.[1]

Density assessments in human cadavers have shown variation across regions of the mandible caused by tooth loss and related to age and gender.[2,3] Within the mandible, subregions that may be measured include molar, premolar, or incisor regions. Each region has potential to be of different cortical thickness,[2,3] which may affect density, especially with techniques that are two-dimensional and sensitive to thickness differences.

Although tooth loss is the ultimate endpoint of periodontal destruction, it also has been used as a proxy measure of oral bone loss. Loss of oral bone impacts tooth stability and eventual loss. However, tooth loss can also reflect caries and trauma and is often determined by extraction practices of the dentist. Further discussion on the relationship of measures of the extent of periodontal disease to osteoporosis can be found elsewhere.[4]

Finally, the relationship of oral bone loss and osteoporosis should also consider both the demographic makeup of the population under study (age, gender, race) and control of potential confounding variables,[5] which can vary markedly across studies and impact both the findings and interpretation.

Studies of Osteoporosis and Alveolar Crestal Height Loss and Residual Ridge Resorption

Most, but not all, studies of the relationship between osteoporosis or low skeletal BMD and ACH have shown an association. Loss of ACH and RRR are more predominant in females than males, and most predominant in older subjects.[6–8] Lower BMD of the femur was significantly correlated with worse mean ACH. The significant association between mean ACH and femur BMD has persisted after adjustment for age, years since menopause, estrogen use, body mass index (BMI), and smoking.[9,10] One 2-year longitudinal study in postmenopausal women determined that smokers had a lower spinal BMD, higher frequency of ACH loss, and worse oral density in the crestal and subcrestal regions than nonsmokers.[1]

Osteoporosis and Oral Bone Density

Oral bone density has been found to be associated with postcranial osteoporosis in most studies. Women seem to have significantly lower bone mineral content (BMC) of the forearm and mandible compared with men. In older subjects, mandibular density varies by sex and age, and rates of BMC loss have been found to be greater over time in older women than men.[11–13] Women with a history of osteoporotic fracture were found to have significantly lower mandibular and forearm BMC values than controls.[12] BMC in the mandible and forearm have also been found to decrease at a similar rate (5.6% per year) after glucocorticoid steroid therapy in men and women.[14] The height of the edentulous ridge also has been found to be correlated with total body calcium and mandibular BMD.[15]

Postmortem studies in edentulous female and male subjects found specific gravity of the mandible and radius decreased with increasing age. Females had lower densities than males and mandibular and radius measures were highly correlated.[16] Mandibular density measured by QCT differed between partially and totally edentulous postmenopausal women who had been edentulous more than 12 years, suggesting years edentulous may be important when assessing the relationship between skeletal and mandibular density.[17]

A prospective study to determine the role of hormone therapy in women on the relationship between spinal density (DPA) and mandibular density (RA) found a significant, moderate correlation at baseline and at an average 5-year follow-up.[18] In a small study of estrogen levels among postmenopausal women, alveolar bone density was assessed in crestal and subcrestal regions of posterior interproximal alveolar bone. A net gain in alveolar density was found in E2-sufficient women compared with those E2-deficient; however, the number of sites gaining/losing density were similar. Estrogen deficiency was also found to be associated with greater loss of both oral BMD and ACH in women overall and for crestal region density in osteopenic women.[19] These findings were supported by results of a 3-year double-blind randomized clinical trial of hormone therapy that revealed that both oral and postcranial bone density were increased in postmenopausal women taking oral estrogens compared with placebo. In addition to the positive change in bone density, a significant increase in ACH was observed.[20]

Although there is evidence to support a correlation between systemic and oral bone density, several important questions remain including: determination of normal ranges of mandibular density by age and sex, further comparison of mandibular density in normal and osteoporotic women, assessment of longitudinal progression of mandibular bone loss, comparison of the rate of bone loss in the mandible compared with other skeletal regions, and the effects of different therapies on mandibular density compared with other skeletal sites.[20] Further study of measurement error for various techniques that assess oral density is also needed.

Osteoporosis and Tooth Loss

Numerous studies have looked at the relationship between osteoporosis, tooth loss, and edentulism, and most have found a positive association.[22–24] A strong association between smoking and edentulism was found, and pattern of denture need by age was worse for women with osteoporosis.[25] In males, no relationship was seen between mandibular cortical width and tooth loss; however, in female subjects, a decrease in mandibular cortical bone width was positively correlated with tooth loss.[26] Tooth loss was found to be highly correlated with prevalence of spinal fracture in women.[27] Spinal BMD was significantly lower in the edentulous subjects.[28] Significant correlations were found between fewer number of remaining teeth and bone density of several regions of the femur including the total femur, Ward's triangle, and the intertrochanter region.[9]

A study of estrogen use in women after menopause and tooth retention found estrogen users had more teeth than non-users, and duration of estrogen use independently predicted number of remaining teeth. Long-term users of estrogen had more teeth than never users. Estrogen use was shown to be protective for tooth loss, regardless of type of tooth or location in the mouth.[29]

A 3-year prospective Swedish study of older men and women found that women with the fewest teeth at baseline (lowest tertile) had a risk of hip fracture that was twice that of the women in the highest two tertiles. The association between tooth loss and hip fracture was stronger in the men studied, with the risk of fracture 3-fold higher in men with the fewest teeth at baseline, although the absolute number of hip fractures greatest in women.[30]

Potential Mechanisms and the Biological Basis

Mechanisms by which osteoporosis or systemic bone loss may be associated with periodontal attachment loss, loss of alveolar bone height, and tooth loss continue to be explored. Several potential mechanisms have been proposed.[10] First, low BMD in the oral bones may be associated with low systemic bone. This low bone density or loss of bone density may lead to more rapid resorption of alveolar bone after insult by periodontal bacteria. With less dense oral bone to start with or faster loss of bone, loss of bone surrounding the teeth may occur more rapidly. Although periodontal disease has historically been thought to be the result of an infectious process, others have suggested that periodontal disease may also be an early manifestation of generalized osteopenia.[31] Second, systemic factors affecting bone remodeling may also modify local tissue response to periodontal infection. Persons with systemic bone loss are known to have increased systemic production of cytokines (i.e., interleukin [IL]-1, IL-6) that may have effects on bone throughout the body, including the bones of the oral cavity. Periodontal infection has been shown to increase local cytokine production that, in turn, increases local osteoclast activity, resulting in increased bone resorption. Given the correlation of oral bone loss to osteoporosis, estrogen deficiency may also be involved. A number of studies have assessed the role of hormone therapy in periodontal disease and have found that hormone therapy has a beneficial association with tooth loss,[32–34] mandibular bone density,[17] and gingival bleeding.[35] In addition to the positive change in bone density, a significant increase in ACH has been observed.[20] Third, genetic factors that predispose a person to systemic bone loss also influence or predispose an individual to periodontal destruction. Last, certain lifestyle factors such as cigarette smoking and suboptimal calcium intake, among others, may put individuals at risk for development of both systemic osteopenia and oral bone loss.

Prospective study of the association between osteoporosis and oral bone loss is needed in large cohorts where temporal sequence can be established and where adequate assessment and control of confounding variables can be done. Both osteoporosis and periodontal disease are major health concerns in the United States, especially in older populations. As the population ages, the impact of both osteoporosis and periodontal disease will be more profound. Studies that improve our understanding of the mechanisms by which osteoporosis is associated and oral bone loss are needed and will be increasingly important in the prevention of morbid-

ity and mortality related to these two very prevalent disorders in older Americans.

REFERENCES

1. Devlin H, Horner K 2002 Mandibular radiomorphic indices in the diagnosis of reduced skeletal bone mineral density. Osteoporos Int 13:373–378.
2. Schwartz-Dabney CL, Dechow PC 2002 Edentulation alters material properties of cortical bone in the human mandible. J Dent Res 81:613–617.
3. D'Amelio P, Panattoni GL, DiStefano M, Nassisi R, Violino D, Isaia GC 2002 Densitometric study of dry human mandible. J Clin Densitom 5:363–367.
4. Wactawski-Wende J 2001 Periodontal disease and osteoporosis: Association and mechanisms. Ann Periodontal 6:197–208.
5. Knezovic Zlataric D, Celebic A, Kobler P 2002 Relationship between body mass index and local quality of mandibular bone structure in elderly individuals. J Gerontol A Biol Sci Med Sci 57:M588–M593.
6. Humphries S, Devlin H, Worthington H 1989 A radiographic investigation into bone resorption of mandibular alveolar bone in elderly edentulous adults. J Dent 17:94–96.
7. Ortman LF, Hausmann E, Dunford RG 1989 Skeletal osteopenia and residual ridge resorption. J Prosthet Dent 61:321–325.
8. Hirai T, Ishijima T, Hashikawa Y, Yajima T 1993 Osteoporosis and reduction of residual ridge in edentulous patients. J Prosthet Dent 69:49–56.
9. Wactawski-Wende J, Grossi SG, Trevisan M, Genco RJ, Tezal M, Dunford RG, Ho AW, Hausmann E, Hreshchyshyn MM 1996 The role of osteopenia in oral bone loss and periodontal disease. J Periodontol 67:1076–1084.
10. Tezal M, Wactawski-Wende J, Grossi SG, Ho AW, Dunford R, Genco RJ 2000 The relationship between bone mineral density and periodontitis in postmenopausal women. J Periodontol 71:1492–1498.
11. Payne JB, Reinhardt RA, Nummikoski PV, Dunning DG, Patil KD 2000 The association of cigarette smoking with alveolar bone loss in postmenopausal females. J Clin Periodontol 27:658–664.
12. von Wowern N 1988 Bone mineral content of mandibles: Normal reference values - Rate of age related bone loss. Calcif Tissue Int 43:193–198.
13. von Wowern N, Klausen B, Kollerup G 1994 Osteoporosis: A risk factor in periodontal disease. J Periodontol 65:1134–1138.
14. von Wowern N, Klausen B, Olgaard K 1992 Steroid-induced mandibular bone loss in relation to marginal periodontal changes. J Clin Periodontol 19:182–186.
15. Kribbs PJ, Chesnut CH, Ott SM, Kilcoyne RF 1989 Relationships between mandibular and skeletal bone in an osteoporotic population. J Prosthet Dent 62:703–707.
16. Henrikson P-A, Wallenius K 1974 The mandible and osteoporosis (1). A qualitative comparison between the mandible and the radius. J Oral Rehabil 1:67–74.
17. Klemetti E, Vainio P, Lassila V 1994 Mineral density in the mandibles of partially and totally edentate postmenopausal women. Scand J Dent Res 102:64–67.
18. Jacobs R, Ghyselen J, Koninckx P, van Steenberghe D 1996 Long-term bone mass evaluation of mandible and lumbar spine in a group of women receiving hormone replacement therapy. Eur J Oral Sci 104:10–16.
19. Payne JB, Reinhardt RA, Nummikoski PV, Patil KD 1999 Longitudinal alveolar bone loss in postmenopausal osteoporotic/osteopenic women. Osteoporos Int 10:34–40.
20. Civitelli R, Pilgram TK, Dotson M, Muckerman J, Lewandowski N, Armamento-Villareal R, Yokoyama-Crothers N, Kardaris EE, Hauser J, Cohen S, Hildebolt CF 2002 Alveolar and postcranial bone density in postmenopausal women receiving hormone/estrogen replacement therapy: A randomized, double-blind, placebo-controlled trial. Arch Int Med 162:1409–1415.
21. Kribbs PJ, Chesnut CH 1984 Osteoporosis and dental osteopenia in the elderly. Gerodontology 3:101–106.
22. Kribbs PJ, Chesnut CH, Ott SM, Kilcoyne RF 1990 Relationships between mandibular and skeletal bone in a population of normal women. J Prosthet Dent 63:86–89.
23. Kribbs PJ 1990 Comparison of mandibular bone in normal and osteoporotic women. J Prosthet Dent 63:218–222.
24. Kribbs PJ, Chesnut CH, Ott SM, Kilcoyne RF 1989 Relationships

between mandibular and skeletal bone in an osteoporotic population. J Prosthet Dent **62:**703–707.

25. Daniell HW 1983 Postmenopausal tooth loss. Contributions to edentulism by osteoporosis and cigarette smoking. Arch Intern Med **143:**1678–1682.

26. Taguchi A, Tanimoto K, Suei Y, Wada T 1995 Tooth loss and mandibular osteopenia. Oral Surg Oral Med Oral Pathol Oral Radiol Endod **79:**127–132.

27. Taguchi A, Tanimoto K, Suei Y, Otani K, Wada T 1995 Oral signs as indicators of possible osteoporosis in older women. Oral Surg Oral Med Oral Pathol Oral Radiol Endod **80:**612–616.

28. Bando K, Nitta H, Matsubara M, Ishikawa I 1998 Bone mineral density in periodontally healthy and edentulous postmenopausal women. Ann Periodontol **3:**322–326.

29. Krall EA, Dawson-Hughes B, Hannan MT, Wilson PWF, Kiel DP 1997 Postmenopausal estrogen replacement and tooth retention. Am J Med **102:**536–542.

30. Aström J, Bäckström C, Thidevall G 1990 Tooth loss and hip fractures in the elderly. J Bone Joint Surg Br **72:**324–325.

31. Whalen JP, Krook L 1996 Periodontal disease as the early manifestation of osteoporosis. Nutrition **12:**53–54.

32. Krall EA, Garcia RI, Dawson-Hughes B 1996 Increased risk of tooth loss is related to bone loss at the whole body, hip, and spine. Calcif Tissue Int **59:**433–437.

33. Grodstein F, Colditz GA, Stampfer MJ 1996 Post-menopausal hormone use and tooth loss. A prospective study. J Am Dent Assoc **127:**370–377.

34. Paganini-Hill A 1995 The benefits of estrogen replacement therapy on oral health. The Leisure World Cohort. Arch Intern Med **155:**2325–2329.

35. Norderyd OM, Grossi SG, Machtei EE, Zambon JJ, Hausmann E, Dunford RG, Genco RJ 1993 Periodontal status of women taking postmenopausal estrogen supplementation. J Periodontol **64:**957–962.

Laboratory Values related to Calcium Metabolism/Metabolic Bone Disease [a]

Test	Source of specimen	Reference population	Reference Range	Reference Range (SI units)
Calcium, ionized	Serum or plasma	Cord	5.5±0.3 mg/dL	1.37±0.07 mmol/L
		Newborn 3-24 h	4.3-5.1 mg/dL	1.07-1.27 mmol/L
		Newborn 24-48 h	4.0-4.7 mg/dL	1.00-1.17 mmol/L
		Adult	4.48-4.92 mg/dL	1.12-1.23 mmol/L
		Adult >60 yr		1.13-1.30 mmol/L
Calcium, total	Serum[b]	Child	8.8-10.8 mg/dL	2.2-2.7 mmol/L
		Adult	8.4-10.2 mg/dL	2.1-2.55 mmol/L
	Urine	Ca in diet		
		Free Ca	5-40 mg/dL	0.13-1.0 mmol/d
		Low to average	50-150 mg/dL	1.25-3.8 mmol/d
		Average (20 mmol/d)	100-300 mg/dL	2.1-7.5 mmol/d
Magnesium	Feces	Average 0.64 g/d		16 mmol/d
	Serum	1.3-2.1 mEq/d (higher during menses)		0.65-1.05 mmol/d
	Urine, 24h	6.0-100 mEq/d		3.0-5.0 mmol/d
Phosphatase, acid				
Prostatic (RIA)	Serum		<3.0 ng/ml	<3.0 µg/L
Roy, Brower & Hayden 37C			0.11-0.60 U/L	0.11-0.60 U/L
Phosphatase, acid tartrate resistant (TRAP 5.6) Suomen	Serum		2.5-45 U/L	
Phosphatase, alkaline				
p-Nitrophenyl phosphate, carbonate buffer, 30 C	Serum	Infant		50-165 U/L
		Child		20-150 U/L
		Adult		20-70 U/L
		>60 yr		30-75 U/L
Bowers & McComb IFCC, 30C	Serum	Male		30-90 U/L
		Female		20-80 U/L
Bone-specific alkaline phosphatase				
Hybritech/Beckman IRMA, ELISA	Serum	Male	6.9-20.1 ng/mL	
		Female – premenopausal	4.6-14.3 ng/mL	
		Female -- postmenopausal	7.3-22.4 ng/mL	
Metra Biosystems, ELISA	Serum	Male	15.0-41.3 U/L	
		Female – premenopausal	11.6-29.6 U/L	
Phosphorus, inorganic	Serum	Cord	3.7-8.1 mg/dL	1.2-2.6 nmol/L
		Child	4.5-5.5 mg/dL	1.45-1.78 nmol/L
		Adult	2.7-4.5 mg/dL	0.87-1.45 nmol/L
		>60 year Male	2.3-3.7 mg/dL	0.74-1.2 nmol/L
		>60 year Female	2.8-4.1 mg/dL	0.9-1.3 nmol/L
	Urine	Adult on diet containing .9-1.5 g P and 10 mg Ca/kg: <1.0 g/d		<32 mmol/d
		Unrestricted diet 0.4-1.3 g/d		13-42 mmol/d
Tubular reabsorption of phosphate	Urine, 4-h (0600 – 1200 h), and serum		82-95%	Fraction reabsorbed: 0.82-0.95
Vitamin A (Quest Diagnostics/Nichols)	Serum	Child 1-6 yr	20-43 µg/dL	
		Child 7-12 yr	26-49 µg/dL	
		Child 13-19 yr	26-72 µg/dL	
		Adult >19 yr	38-98 µg/dL	
Retinol (Mayo Medical)	Serum		360-1200 µg/dL	
Retinyl esters (Mayo Medical)			≤10 µg/dL	
Vitamin D3, 25 hydroxy (Mayo Medical Labs)	Serum	Summer (total):	15-80 ng/mL	37-200 nmol/L
		Winter (total):	14-42 ng/mL	
Vitamin D3, 25 hydroxy (RIA, DiaSorin)	Serum/Plasma	Adults	9.0-37.6 ng/mL(mean 23.0 ng/mL)	35-105 nmol/L
Vitamin D3, 1,25 dihydroxy (Mayo)	Serum	Adults	25-45 pg/mL	12-46 µmol/L
VitaminD3,1,25 dihydroxy (RIA DiaSorin)	Serum/Plasma	Adults	15.9-55.6 pg/mL(mean 35.7pg/mL)	
Calcitonin				
Quest Diagn/Nichols two-site ICMA	Serum	Basal Male	≤8 pg/mL	
		Basal Female	≤4 pg/mL	
		Pentagastrin/Ca Male	10-491 pg/mL	
		Pentagastrin/Ca Female	≤70 pg/mL	
CIS Biointernational two-site IRMA	Serum	Basal Male	<10 pg/mL	
		Basal Female	<10 pg/mL	
		Pentagastrin Male	<30 pg/mL	
		Pentagastrin Female	<30 pg/mL	
Mayo Medical Labs	Plasma	Basal Male	<19 pg/mL	
		Basal Female	<14 pg/mL	
		Pentagastrin Male	<110 pg/mL	
		Pentagastrin Female	<30 pg/mL	
RIA, DiaSorin	Serum	Adult	0-95 pg/mL (mean 47 pg/mL)	

Test	Source of specimen	Reference population	Reference Range	Reference Range (SI units)
Parathyroid hormone (Intact) [c]				
Mayo Medical Labs	Serum	Basal		1.0-5.2 pmol/L
Quest Diagnostics/Nichols	Serum	Basal	10-65 pg/mL	
IRMA, DiaSorin	Serum/Plasma		13-54 pg/mL (mean 26 pg/mL)	
Scantibodies	Serum	Basal		0.9-6.3 pmol/L
Osteocalcin [c]				
Quest/Nichols, CIS Bio	Serum	Male	8.0-52.0 ng/mL	
		Female premenopausal	5.8-41.0 ng/mL	
		Female postmenopausal	8.0-56.0 ng/mL	
Mayo Medical Labs, CIA	Serum	Male 20-50 yr	2-15 ng/mL	
		Male 51-70 yr	2-10 ng/mL	
		Female 20-50 yr	2-15 ng/mL	
		Female 51-80 yr	6-22 ng/mL	
IRMA, DiaSorin	Serum	Male	3.2-12.2 ng/mL (mean 6.25ng/mL)	
		Female	2.7-11.5 ng/mL (mean 5.58ng/mL)	
ELISA, Metra Biosystems	Serum	Male	3.4-8.6 ng/mL	
		Female	3.8-10.0 ng/mL	
ELISA, N-Mid,Osteometer BioTech A/S	Serum/Plasma	Male	23.2±7.2 ng/mL	
		Female premenopausal	17.7±6.4 ng/mL	
		Female postmenopausal	28.9±9.7 ng/mL	
IRMA, N-Mid, Osteometer BioTech A/S	Serum/Plasma	Male	23.0±9.7 ng/mL	
		Female premenopausal	18.4±8.9 ng/mL	
		Female postmenopausal	29.9±11.5 ng/mL	
PTHrP [c]				
Quest Diagnostic/Nichols Institute	Serum	Basal		<1.3 pmol/L
IRMA, DiaSorin	Plasma	Adults		<1.5 pmol/L
Collagen cross-links				
Free deoxypyridinoline (DPD)				
Metra Biosystems, ELISA	Urine	Male		2.3-5.4 nmol/mmol creatinine
		Female premenopausal		3.0-7.4 nmol/mmol creatinine
Free pyridinoline (Pyd)				
Metra Biosystems, ELISA	Urine	Male		12.8-25.6 nmol/mmol creatinine
		Female		16.0-37.0 nmol/mmol creatinine
	Serum	Male		1.59±0.38 nmol/L
		Female		1.55±0.26 nmol/L
C-telopeptide (CTx)				
Osteometer Biotech A/S, ELISA	Urine	Male		207±128 µg/mmol creatinine
		Female premenopausal		220±128 µgmmol creatinine
		Female postmenopausal		363±160 µg/mmol creatinine
Osteometer Biotech A/S, RIA	Urine	Male		290±120 µg/mmol creatinine
		Female premenopausal		227±90 µg/mmol creatinine
		Female postmenopausal		429±225 µg/mmol creatinine
N-telopeptide (NTx)				
Ostex International, ELISA	Urine	Male		3-63 nM BCE/mM creatinine
		Female premenopausal		5-65 nM BCE/mM creatinine
		Female postmenopausal		17-188 nM BCE/mM creatinine
	Serum	Male		5.4-24.2 nM BCE
		Female premenopausal		6.2-19.0 nM BCE
		Female postmenopausal		8.1-38.7 nM BCE

ELISA, enzyme-linked immunosorbent assay; RIA, radioimmunoassay; IRMA, immunoradiometric assay; ICMA, immunochemiluminescent assay; IFCC, International Federation of Clinical Chemistry; BCE, bone collagen equivalents

[a] Selected laboratory values in this table were kindly compiled by Barry C. Kress, Ph.D., Hybritech Incorporated, a subsidiary of Beckman Coulter, Inc., San Diego, CA. Every effort was made to include values for all known companies for the various categories.

[b] Divide by 2 to get mEq/L. The total serum calcium can be corrected for alterations in the serum protein concentration by the following formula: Corrected total serum calcium (mg/dL) – observed total serum calcium + [(the normal mean albumin concentration – the observed albumin concentration) x 0.8]. In most situations, the normal mean albumin concentration equals 4 g/dL.

[c] The normal values listed include commercial assays. These are listed not to provide an endorsement for these assays, but because they are representative of values available for daily clinical use. It is likely that normal values in other research or commercial assays will vary to some extent; where ± values are given, the mean plus or minus one standard deviation is given.

Care has been taken to confirm the accuracy of the information presented and to describe generally accepted practices. However, the authors, editors and publisher are not responsible for errors or omissions or for any consequences from application of the information in this book and make no warranty, expressed or implied, with respect to the currency, completeness, or accuracy of the contents of the publication. Application of this information in a particular situation remains the professional responsibility of the practitioner. The authors, editors and publisher have sought to ensure that drug selection and dosage set forth in this text are in accordance with current recommendations and practice at the time of publication. However, in view of ongoing research, changes in government regulations, and the constant flow of information relating to drug therapy and drug reactions, the reader is urged to check the package insert for each drug for any change in indications and dosage and for added warnings and precautions. This is particularly important when the recommended agent is a new or infrequently employed drug. Some drugs and medical devices presented in this publication have Food and Drug Administration (FDA) clearance for limited use in restricted research settings. It is the responsibility of the health care provider to ascertain the FDA status of each drug or device planned for use in their clinical practice.

Formulary of Drugs Commonly Used In Treatment of Mineral Disorders [a]

Drug	Application in treatment of bone and mineral disorders	Dosage (adult) [b]	Rx Cat [c]	Notes
Hormones and Analogs				
1. Calcitonin				
Human (Cibacalcin) im or SQ (0.5-mg vials)	Paget's disease	0.25-0.5 mg im or SQ; q24h	Rx	
Salmon (Calcimar, Miacalcin) im or SQ (100, 200 IU/mL) (SQ preferred)	Paget's disease, osteoporosis, hypercalcemia	50-100 IU, im or SQ; qod or qd for Paget's or osteoporosis; 4-6 IU/kg im or SQ; qid for hypercalcemia	Rx	Modestly effective and short-lived in treatment of hypercalcemia
Nasal spray (200 IU/spray)	Osteoporosis	200 IU nasal qd	Rx	
2. Estrogens				
Estinyl estradiol po (0.02, 0.05, 0.5 mg)	Postmenopausal osteoporosis (prevention and treatment)	0.02 – 0.05 mg; qd 3/4 wk	Rx	To reduce risk of endometrial cancer, estrogens can be cycled with progesterone during last 7-10 days or given concurrent with a progestin throughout the cycle (less breakthrough bleeding). In women who have not had a hysterectomy, a progesterone should be used with the estrogen and does not appear to alter the skeletal effectiveness of estrogen.
17β estradiol (Estrace) po (0.5, 1.2 mg)		0.5 mg qd	Rx	
Transderm patch (Estraderm)		0.05-0.1 mg 2x/wk	Rx	
Esterified estrogens (Estratab) po (0.3, 0.625, 2.5)		0.3-1.25 mg qd	Rx	
Estropipate (Ortho-Est .625) po (0.75, 1.5 mg)		0.75 mg qd	Rx	
Conjugated equine estrogens (Premarin) po (0.3, 0.625, 0.9, 1.25, 2.5 mg)		0.625-1.25 mg qd 3/4 wk	Rx	0.3 mg conjugated equine estrogens (CEE) with calcium also may be effective
Conjugated equine estrogen with medroxyprogesterone acetate (MPA)				
(Premphase)		0.625 mg estrogen qd on days 1-14 and 0.625 mg estrogen with 5 mg MPA qd on days 15-26	Rx	
(Prempro)		0.625 mg estrogen with 2.5 or 5 mg MPA qd	Rx	
3. Selective estrogen-receptor modulators (SERMs)				
Raloxifene (Evista)	Postmenopausal osteoporosis (prevention)	60 mg qd	Rx	Aggravates hot flashes. Decreased risk of endometrial and breast cancer.
4. Glucocorticoids				
Prednisone (Deltasone), po (2.5, 5, 10, 20, 50 mg)	Hypercalcemia due to sarcoidosis, vitamin D intoxication, and certain malignancies such as multiple myeloma and related lymphoproliferative disorders	10-60 mg qd	Rx	Long-term use results in osteoporosis and adrenal suppression. Other glucocorticoids with minimal mineralocorticoid activity can be used.
5. Parathyroid Hormone				
Teriparatide (Forteo)	Osteoporosis	20 µg SQ daily	Rx	
6. Testosterone				
Testosterone cypionate	Male hypogonadism	200-300 mg im q2-3 wk	Rx	
Testosterone enanthate		200-300 mg im q2-3wk	Rx	
Transdermal patch				
Testoderm TTS		5 mg body patch q 24h	Rx	
Androderm		5 mg body patch q 24h	Rx	
Androgel 1%		5 mg topical q day	Rx	
7. Vitamin D preparations				
Cholecalciferol or D_3, p.o (125, 250, 400 U, often in combination with calcium)	Nutritional vitamin D deficiency, osteoporosis, malabsorption, hypoparathyroidism, refractory rickets	400-1000 U; as dietary supplement	OTC	D_2 (or D_3) has been shown to reduce fractures and increase BMD in elderly women in 400-1000 U doses
Ergocalciferol or D2 (Calciferol), po (8000 U/mL drops; 25,000, 50,000 U tabs)		25,000-100,000 U; 3x/wk to qd	Rx	
Calcifediol or 25(OH)D3 (Calderol), (20, 50 mg)	Malabsorption, renal osteodystrophy	20-50 µg; 3x/wk to qd	Rx	25(OH)D_3 may be useful in treatment of steroid-induced osteoporosis

Drug	Application in treatment of bone and mineral disorders	Dosage (adult) [b]	Rx Cat [c]	Notes
Vitamin D preparations (cont.)				
Calcitriol or 1,25(OH)2D3 (Rocaltrol), po (0.25, 0.5 µg); (Calcijex), iv (1 or 2 µg/mL)	Renal osteodystrophy, hypoparathyroidism, refractory rickets	0.25-1.0 µg; qd to bid	Rx	Role of calcitriol in treatment of osteoporosis, psoriasis and certain malignancies is being evaluated, primarily with new analogs
Dihydrotachysterol (DHT), po (0.125, 0.2, 0.4 mg)	Renal osteodystrophy, hypoparathyroidism, refractory rickets	0.2-1.0 mg; qd	Rx	
Poxercalciferol 2.5 µg capsule				
Paricalcitol (Zemplar) 5 µg/mL	Secondary hyperparathyroidism	2.5 µg po 2-3 q wk	Rx	
		Titrate iv; begin at 0.04 µg/kg	Rx	
Bisphosphonates				
1. **Etidronate** (Didronel), po (200, 400 mg); iv (300 mg/6 mL vial)	Paget's disease, heterotopic ossification, hypercalcemia of malignancy	po, 5 mg/kg qd for 6/12 mo for Paget's disease; 20 mg/kg, qd 1 mo before to 3 mo after total hip replacement; 10/20 mg/kg qd for 3 mo after spinal cord injury for heterotopic ossification	Rx	Etidronate is a first-generation bisphosphonate. High doses may cause a mineralization disorder not seen with newer bisphosphonates.
		iv, 7.5 mg/kg, qd for 3 d, given in 250-500 mL normal saline for hypercalcemia of malignancy; 5 mg qd for osteoporosis prevention	Rx	
2. **Alendronate** (Fosamax) po (5, 10, 35, 40, 70 mg)	Osteoporosis prevention and treatment, Paget's disease	5 mg qd or 35 mg q wk for osteoporosis prevention; 10 mg qd or 70 mg q wk for osteoporosis treatment; 40 mg qd for Paget's disease	Rx	Ingest 30 min before breakfast with 1 glass water; remain upright. Esophagitis is a risk.
3. **Pamidronate** (Aredia), iv (30-90 mg/10 mL)	Hypercalcemia of malignancy, Paget's disease	60-90 mg given as a single ivinfusion over 2-4 h for hypercalcemia of malignancy; 30 mg doses over 2 h on 3 consecutive days for a total of 90 mg for Paget's disease	Rx	
4. **Risedronate** (Actonel) (5, 30, 35 mg)	Osteoporosis, Paget's disease	5 mg po qd or 35 mg q wk for osteoporosis; 30 mg qd for 2 mo for Paget's	Rx	
5. **Tiludronate** (Skelid)	Paget's disease	400 mg qd for 3 mo	Rx	
6. **Zoledronate** (Zometa)	Hypercalcemia of malignancy; osteolytic metastases	4 mg iv over 15 min; may repeat in 7 d for hypercalcemia; 4 mg iv over 15 min q 3-4 week for bony metastases	Rx	
Minerals				
1. **Bicarbonate, sodium**, po (325, 527, 650 mg)	Chronic metabolic acidosis leading to bone disease	Must be titrated for each patient	Rx, OTC	
2. **Calcium preparations**				
Calcium carbonate (40% Ca), po (500, 650 mg)	Hypocalcemia (if symptomatic should be treated iv), osteoporosis, rickets, osteomalacia, chronic renal failure, hypoparathyroidism, malabsorption, enteric oxaluria	po 400-2000 mg elemental Ca in divided doses; qd	OTC	Calcium carbonate is the preferred form because it has the highest percentage of calcium and is the least expensive, although calcium citrate may be somewhat better absorbed. In normal subjects, the solubility of the calcium salt has not been shown to affect its absorption from the intestine, in achlorhydric subjects, $CaCO_3$ should be given with meals.
Calcium citrate (21% Ca) po (950-1500 mg)			OTC	
Calcium chloride (36% Ca), iv (100% solution)			Rx	
Calcium bionate (6.5% Ca), po (1.8 g in 5 mL)			Rx	

Drug	Application in treatment of bone and mineral disorders	Dosage (adult) [b]	Rx Cat [c]	Notes
Calcium preparations (cont.)				
Calcium gluconate (9% Ca), po (500, 600, 1000 mg), iv (10% solution, 0.465 mEq/mL)		iv, 2-20 mL 10% calcium gluconate over several hours	Rx	Calcium gluconate is the preferred iv form because, unlike calcium chloride, it does not burn.
Calcium lactate (13% Ca), po (325, 650 mg)			OTC	
Calcium phosphate, dibasic (23% Ca), po (486 mg)			OTC	
Tricalcium phosphate (39% Ca) po (300, 600 mg)			OTC	
3. Magnesium preparations Magnesium oxide (Mag-Ox, Uro-Mag), po (84.5, 241.3 mg Mg)	Hypomagnesemia	240-480 mg elemental Mg	OTC	Low magnesium often coexists with low calcium in alcoholics and malabsorbers. Also found in many antacids and vitamin formulations.
4. Phosphate preparations Neutra-Phos, po (250 mg P, 278 mg K, 164 mg Na)	Hypophosphatemia, vitamin D resistant rickets, hypercalcemia, hypercalciuria	po, 1-3 g in divided doses; qd	Rx, OTC	
Neutra-Phos K, po (250 mg P, 556 mg K)			Rx	
Fleet Phospha-Soda, po (815 mg P, 760 mg Na in 5 mL)			Rx, OTC	
In-Phos, iv (1 g P in 40 mL)		iv, 1.5 g over 6-8 h	Rx	iv phosphorus is seldom necessary and can be toxic if infusion is too rapid
Hyper-Phos-K, iv (1 g P in 15 mL)			Rx	
Diuretics				
1. Thiazides Hydrochlorothiazide, po (25, 50, 100 mg) Chlorhalidone, po (25, 50 mg)	Hypercalciuria, nephrolithiasis	25-50 mg; qd or bid	Rx	Other thiazides may also be effective but are less commonly used for this purpose. These uses are not FDA approved.
2. Loop Diuretics Furosemide, po (20, 40, 80 mg), iv (10 mg/mL)	Hypercalcemia; if symptomatic, use iv	po 20-80 mg, q6h as necessary	Rx	Ethacrynic acid may also be effective but is less commonly used for this purposes. These uses are not FDA approved.
Miscellaneous				
1. Mithramycin or plicamycin (Mithracin), iv (2.5 mg/vial)	Hypercalcemia of malignancy	25 µg in 1 L DSW or normal saline over 4-8 hr	Rx	Has been used in treatment of severe Paget's disease, but toxicity makes it treatment of last resort for this purpose

BMD, bone mineral density; FDA, Food and Drug Administration; PTH, parathyroid hormone

[a] This table is not intended to be an official guideline. See PDR or package insert for more complete information. Selected information kindly provided by Daniel D. Bikle, M.D., Ph.D., Professor, Departments of Medicine and Dermatology, University of California, San Francisco, and Co-Director Special Diagnostic and Treatment Unit, Department of Medicine, Veterans Affairs Medical Center, San Francisco, California.

[b] qd, every day; qo, every other day; bid, twice a day; tid, 3 times a day; qid, 4 times a day; SQ, subcutaneously; im, intramuscularly; po, orally; iv, intravenously; IU, International Units.

[c] Rx Cat, prescription category; Rx, prescriptions required; OTC, over-the-counter preparations available

Summary of Gene Disorders of Serum Mineral Metabolism or Skeleton Formation

Genetic Disorder	OMIM Syndrome #	Gene	Protein	OMIM Gene #
Associated Hypocalcemia				
Albright osteodystrophy	103580	GNAS	G-Protein, α subunit	139320
Autoimmune polendocrinopathy syndrome, type 1	240300	AIRE	Autoimmune regulator	607358
DiGeorge syndrome	188400	DGCR	22q11.2, DiGeorge syndrome region	
Hypocalcemia, autosomal dominant	146200	PTH	Parathyroid hormone	168450
		CaSR	Calcium sensing receptor	601199
Hypoparathyroidism, autosomal dominant	601198	PTH	Parathyroid hormone	168450
		CaSR	Calcium sensing receptor	601199
Hypomagnesemia with 2° hypocalcemia	602014	TRPM6	Receptor cation channel	607009
Hypoparathyroidism-retardation-dysmorphism syndrome	241410	TBCE	Tubulin-specific chaperone E	604934
Hypoparathyroidism, sensorineural deafness renal dysplasia	146255	GATA3	GATA-binding protein	131320
Kenny-Caffey syndrome, type 1	244460	TBCE	Tubulin-specific chaperone E	604934
Osteopetrosis, autosomal recessive	259700	TCIRG1	T-cell immune regulator	604592
Primary hypomagnesemia	248250	PCLN1	Paracellin-1	603959
Pseudohypoparathyroidism, type 1B	603233	GNAS	G-Protein, α subunit	139320
Pseudovitamin D-deficient rickets, type 1	264700	CYP27B1	25(OH)D-1- α -hydroxylase	264700
Renal tubular acidosis, autosomal dominant distal	179800	SLC4A1	Solute carrier 4, anion exchanger	109270
Vitamin D-resistant rickets, type IIA	277440	VDR	Vitamin D receptor	601769
Associated Hypercalcemia				
Familial hypocalciuric hypercalcemia	145980	CaSR	Calcium sensing receptor	601199
Familial isolated hyperparathyroidism, type 1	145000	HPRT2	Parafibromin	607393
		MEN1	Menin	131100
Familial isolated hyperparathyroidism, type 2 (jaw tumor)	145001	HPRT2	Parafibromin	607393
Metaphyseal chondrodysplasia, Jansen type	156400	PTHR1	Parathyroid hormone receptor	168468
Multiple endocrine neoplasia, type 1	131100	MEN1	Menin	131100
Multiple endocrine neoplasia, type 2	171400	RET	RET proto-oncogene	164761
Neonatal hyperparathyroidism	239200	CaSR	Calcium sensing receptor	601199
Williams-Beuren syndrome	194050	ELN	Elastin	130160
		LIMK1	LIM kinase-1	601329
Associated Hypophosphatemia				
Albright osteodystrophy	103580	GNAS	G-Protein, α subunit	139320
Dent disease, Nephrolithiasis, X-linked, type 2	300009	CLCN5	Choride channel 5	300008
Fanconi-Bickel syndrome	227810	SCL2A2	Solute carrier family 2	138160
Hypophosphatasia, Adult type	146300	ALPL	Alkaline phosphatase	171760
Hypophosphatasia, Infantile type	241500	ALPL	Alkaline phosphatase	171760
Hypophosphatemic rickets, autosomal dominant	193100	FGF23	Fibroblast growth factor-23	605380
Hypophosphatemic rickets, X-linked, type 2	307800	PHEX	X-linked endopeptidase	307800
Hypophosphatemic rickets, X-linked, type 3	300008	CLCN5	Choride channel 5	300008
Hypophosphatemic urolithiasis	182309	SLC34A1	Solute carrier family 34, Member 1	182309
Hypophosphatemic osteoporosis	182309	SLC34A1	Solute carrier family 34, Member 1	182309
Metaphyseal chondrodysplasia, Jansen type	156400	PTHR1	Parathyroid hormone receptor	168468
Neonatal hyperparathyroidism	239200	CaSR	Calcium sensing receptor	601199
Nephrolithiasis, X-linked, type 1	310468	CLCN5	Choride channel 5	300008
Nephropathic cystinosis	219800	CTNS	Cystinosin	606272
Pseudovitamin D-deficient rickets, type 1	264700	CYP27B1	25(OH)D-1- α -hydroxylase	264700
Associated Hyperphosphatemia				
Albright osteodystrophy	103580	GNAS	G-Protein, α subunit	139320
Hypoparathyroidism, autosomal dominant	601198	PTH	Parathyroid hormone gene	168450
		CaSR	Calcium sensing receptor	601199
Hypoparathyroidism-retardation-dysmorphism syndrome	241410	TBCE	Tubulin-specific chaperone E	604934
Kenny-Caffey syndrome, type 1	244460	TBCE	Tubulin-specific chaperone E	604934
Paget disease, juvenile	239000	TNFRSF11B	Osteoprotegerin	602643
Pseudohypoparathyroidism, type 1B	603233	GNAS	G-Protein, α subunit	139320

Summary of Gene Disorders of Serum Mineral Metabolism or Skeleton Formation

Genetic Disorder	OMIM Syndrome #	Gene	Protein	OMIM Gene #
Associated Hypomagnesia				
Bartter syndrome, type 1	601678	SLC12A1	Sodium-potassium-chloride cotransporter-2	600839
Bartter syndrome, Gitelman variant	263800	SLC12A3	Thiazide-sensitive Na-Cl cotransporter	600968
Hypomagnesemia with 2° hypocalcemia	602014	TRPM6	Receptor cation channel	607009
Primary hypomagnesemia	248250	PCLN1	Paracellin-1	603959
Renal hypomagnesemia, type 2	154020	FXYD2	Na+,K+-ATPase gamma subunit	601814
Osteochondrodysplasias				
1. Achondroplasias				
Achondroplasia	100800	FGFR3	Fibroblast growth factor receptor-3	134934
Hypochondroplasia	146000	FGFR3	Fibroblast growth factor receptor-3	134934
SADDAN dysplasia	134934	FGFR3	Fibroblast growth factor receptor-3	134934
Thanatophoric dysplasia, type 1	187600	FGFR3	Fibroblast growth factor receptor-3	134934
Thanatophoric dysplasia, type 2	187600	FGFR3	Fibroblast growth factor receptor-3	134934
4. Short-rib dysplasias				
Ellis-van Creveld syndrome	225500	EVC	EVC gene product	604831
		EVC2	EVC2 gene product	607261
5. Atelosteogenesis-omodysplasias				
Neonatal osseous dysplasia	256050	SLC26A2	Diastrophic dysplasia sulfate transporter	606718
6. Diastrophic dysplasias				
Achondrogenesis, type 1B	600972	SLC26A2	Diastrophic dysplasia sulfate transporter	606718
Diastrophic dysplasia	222600	SLC26A2	Diastrophic dysplasia sulfate transporter	606718
Multiple epiphyseal dysplasia, type 4	226900	SLC26A2	Diastrophic dysplasia sulfate transporter	606718
7. Dyssegmental dysplasias				
Dyssegmental dysplasia, Silverman-Handmaker type	224410	HSPG2	Perlecan	142461
Dyssegmental dwarfism	224400	HSPG2	Perlecan	142461
8. Type II collagenopathies				
Achondrogenesis, type II	200610	COL2A1	Collagen-2-A1	120140
Hypochondrogenesis	120140	COL2A1	Collagen-2-A1	120140
Kniest dyplasia	156550	COL2A1	Collagen-2-A1	120140
Spondyloepiphyseal dysplasia, congenital	183900	COL2A1	Collagen-2-A1	120140
Spondyloepimetaphyeal dysplasia, Strudwick type	184250	COL2A1	Collagen-2-A1	120140
Spondylometaphyseal dysplasia	184252	COL2A1	Collagen-2-A1	120140
Spondyloperipheral dysplasia	271700	COL2A1	Collagen-2-A1	120140
Stickler syndrome, type 1	108300	COL2A1	Collagen-2-A1	120140
9. Type XI collagenopathies				
Marshall syndrome	154780	COL11A1	Collagen-11-A1	120280
Otospondylomegaepiphyseal dysplasia	215150	COL11A1	Collagen-11-A2	120290
Stickler syndrome, type 2	604841	COL11A1	Collagen-11-A1	120280
Stickler syndrome, type 3	184840	COL11A1	Collagen-11-A2	120290
10. Other spondyloepi-(meta)-physeal dysplasias				
Dyggve-Melchior-Clausen dysplasia	223800	FLJ90130	Unknown	607461
Progressive pseudorheumatoid dysplasia	208230	WISP3	Wnt1 signalling protein	603400
Immunoosseous dysplasia, Schimke type	242900	SMARCAL1	SMARCA-like protein 1	606622
Schwartz-Jampel syndrome	255800	HSPG2	Perlecan	142461
Smith-McCort dysplasia	607326	FLJ90130	Unknown	607461
Spondyloepimetaphyseal dysplasia, Pakistani	603005	PAPSS2	PAPS synthase	603005
Spondyloepiphyseal dysplasia tarda	313400	SEDL	Sedlin	300202
Wolcott-Rallison syndrome	226980	EIF2AK3	EIF 2A kinase	604032

Summary of Gene Disorders of Serum Mineral Metabolism or Skeleton Formation

Genetic Disorder	OMIM Syndrome #	Gene	Protein	OMIM Gene #
11. Multiple epiphyseal dysplasias & pseudoachondroplasia				
Pseudoachondroplasia	177170	COMP	Cartilage oligomeric matric protein-1	600310
Multiple epiphyseal dysplasia, COL9A1-related	120140	COL9A1	Collagen–9–A1	120140
Multiple epiphyseal dysplasia, type 1	132400	COMP	Cartilage oligomeric matric protein-1	600310
Multiple epiphyseal dysplasia, type 2	600204	COL9A2	Collagen–9–A2	120260
Multiple epiphyseal dysplasia, type 3	600969	COL9A3	Collagen–9–A3	120270
Multiple epiphyseal dysplasia, type 5	607078	MATN3	Matrilin 3	602109
12. Chondrodysplasia punctata (CDP)				
CHILD syndrome	308050	NSDHL	NAD(P)H steroid dehydrogenase-like protein	300275
Chondrodysplasia punctata with coagulation deficiency	277450	GGCX	γ-Glutamyl carboxylase	137167
Chondrodysplasia punctata, X-linked dominant	302960	EBP	Emopamil-binding protein	300205
Chondrodysplasia punctata, X-linked recessive	302950	ARSE	Arylsulfatase E	300180
Desmosterolosis	602398	DHCR24	24-Dehydrocholesterol reductase gene	606418
Moth-eaten skeletal dysplasia	215140	LBR	Lamin B receptor	600024
Rhizomelic chondrodysplasia punctata, type 1	215100	PEX7	Peroxin-7	601757
Rhizomelic chondrodysplasia punctata, type 2	222765	GNPAT	Glyceronephosphate acyltransferase	602744
Rhizomelic chondrodysplasia punctata, type 3	600121	AGPS	Alkyl-DHAP synthase gene	603051
Smith Lemli Opitz syndrome, type 1	270400	DHCR7	Sterol delta-7-reductase gene	602858
Smith Lemli Opitz syndrome, type 2	268670	DHCR7	Sterol delta-7-reductase gene	602858
Zellweger syndrome	214100	PEX1	Peroxin-1	602136
		PEX2	Peroxin-2	170993
		PEX3	Peroxin-3	603164
		PEX5	Peroxin-5	600414
		PEX6	Peroxin-6	601498
		PEX12	Peroxin-12	601758
13. Metaphyseal dysplasias				
Adenosine deaminase deficiency	102700	ADA	Adenosine deaminase	102700
Jansen type	156400	PTHR1	Parathyroid hormone receptor	168468
Schmid type	156500	COL10A1	Collagen-10-A1	120110
Shwachman–Diamond syndrome	260400	SBDS	Unknown	607444
McKusick type (Cartilage-Hair-Hypoplasia)	250250	RMRP	Mitochondrial RNA-processing endoribonuclease	157660
16. Mesomelic dysplasias				
Langer mesomelic dysplasia	249700	SHOX	Short stature homeo box	312865
Leri-Weill dyschondrosteosis	127300	SHOX	Short stature homeo box	312865
Robinow syndrome, recessive	268310	ROR2	NTRKR2/RTK-like orphan receptor 2	602337
Short Stature, idiopathic	604271	SHOX	Short stature homeo box	312865
		SHOXY	Short stature homeo box	400020
17. Acromelic dysplasias				
Albright osteodystrophy	103580	GNAS	G-Protein, α subunit	139320
Brachydactyly, type A1	112500	IHH	Indian hedgehog	600726
Brachydactyly, type B1	113000	ROR2	NTRKR2/RTK-like orphan receptor 2	602337
Brachydactyly, type C	113100	GDF5	Cartilage-derived morphogenetic protein	601146
Brachydactyly, type D	113200	HOXD13	Homeo box 4I	142989
Brachydactyly, type E	113300	HOXD13	Homeo box 4I	142989
Noonan syndrome	163950	PTPN11	Protein tyrosine phosphatase	176876
Trichorhinophalangeal syndrome, type 1	190350	TRPS1	Putative transcription factor	605386
Trichorhinophalangeal syndrome, type 2	150230	TRPS1/EXT1	Putative transcription factor/Exostosin-1	605386/133700
Trichorhinophalangeal syndrome, type 3	190351	TRPS1	Putative transcription factor	605386
18. Acromesomelic dysplasias				
Grebe chondrodysplasia	200700	GDF5	Cartilage-derived morphogenetic protein	601146
Hunter-Thompson type chondrodysplasia	201250	GDF5	Cartilage-derived morphogenetic protein	601146
Du Pan syndrome	228900	GDF5	Cartilage-derived morphogenetic protein	601146

Summary of Gene Disorders of Serum Mineral Metabolism or Skeleton Formation

Genetic Disorder	OMIM Syndrome #	Gene	Protein	OMIM Gene #
19. Dysplasias with predominant membranous bone involvement				
Cleidocranial dysplasia syndrome	119600	RUNX2	Core-binding factor, α subunit 1	600211
Parietal foramina, type 1	168500	MSX2	Muscle segment homeo box	123101
Parietal foramina, type 2	168500	ALX4	Aristaless-like 4	605420
20. Bent-bone dysplasia				
Campomelic dysplasia	114290	SOX9	SRY box-related-9	211970
22. Dysostosis multiplex				
Aspartylglucosaminuria	208400	AGA	Aspartylglucosaminidase	208400
Fucosidosis	230000	FUCA1	α-L-fucosidase	230000
Galactosialidosis	256540	PPGB	β-galactosidase protective protein	256540
α-Mannosidosis	248500	MAN2B1	α-D-Mannosidase	248500
β-Mannosidosis	248510	MANBA	β-D-Mannosidase	248510
Mucopolysaccharidosis, type I	252800	IDUA	α-L-iduronidase	252800
Mucopolysaccharidosis, type II	309900	IDS	Iduronate sulfatase	309900
Mucopolysaccharidosis, type IIIA	252900	SGSH	Heparan sulfate sulfatase	605270
Mucopolysaccharidosis, type IIID	252940	GNS	N-acetylglucosamine-6-sulfatase	607664
Mucopolysaccharidosis, type IVA	253000	GALNS	Galactosamine-6-sulfatase	253000
Mucopolysaccharidosis, type IVB/Gangliosidosis	253010	GLB1	β-galactosidase	230500
Mucopolysaccharidosis, type VI	253200	ARSB	Arylsulfatase B	253200
Mucopolysaccharidosis, type VII	253220	GUSB	β-glucuronidase	253220
Sialidosis	256550	NEU1	α-neuraminidase	256550
Sialuria, infantile	269920	SLC17A5	Sialin	604322
Sialuria, Finnish type	604369	SLC17A5	Sialin	604322
Sialuria, French type	269921	GNE	UDP-GlcNAc 2-epimerase	603824
24. Dysplasias with decreased bone density				
Gaucher disease	230800	GBA	Acid-beta glucosidase	606463
Homocystinuria	236200	CBS	Cystathionine beta-synthase	236200
Osteogenesis imperfecta, type I	166200	COL1A1	Collagen-1-A1	120150
		COL1A1	Collagen-1-A2	120160
Osteogenesis imperfecta, type II	166210	COL1A1	Collagen-1-A1	120150
		COL1A1	Collagen-1-A2	120160
Osteogenesis imperfecta, type III	259420	COL1A1	Collagen-1-A1	120150
		COL1A1	Collagen-1-A2	120160
Osteogenesis imperfecta, type IV	166220	COL1A1	Collagen-1-A1	120150
		COL1A1	Collagen-1-A2	120160
Osteoporosis-pseudoglioma syndrome	259770	LRP5	Lipoprotein receptor-related protein 5	603506
25. Dysplasias with defective mineralization				
Familial hypocalciuric hypercalcemia	145980	CaSR	Calcium sensing receptor	601199
Hypophosphatasia, Adult type	146300	ALPL	Alkaline phosphatase	171760
Hypophosphatasia, Infantile type	241500	ALPL	Alkaline phosphatase	171760
Hypophosphatemic rickets, autosomal dominant	193100	FGF23	Fibroblast growth factor-23	605380
Hypophosphatemic rickets, X-linked, type 2	307800	PHEX	X-linked endopeptidase	307800
Hypophosphatemic rickets, X-linked, type 3	300008	CLCN5	Choride channel 5	300008
Neonatal hyperparathyroidism	239200	CaSR	Calcium sensing receptor	601199
26. Increase bone density without modification of bone shape				
High bone mass trait, autosomal dominant	601884	LRP5	Lipoprotein receptor-related protein 5	603506
Netherton syndrome	256500	SPINK5	LEKTI	605010
OLEDAID syndrome	300301	IKBKG	NEMO	300248
Osteopetrosis, autosomal recessive	259700	CLCN7	Chloride channel 7	602727
		GL	Grey-lethal	607649
		TCIRG1	T-cell immune regulator	604592
Osteopetrosis with renal tubular acidosis	259730	CA2	Carbonic anhydrase II	259730
Osteopetrosis, type I	607634	LRP5	Lipoprotein receptor-related protein 5	603506

Summary of Gene Disorders of Serum Mineral Metabolism or Skeleton Formation

Genetic Disorder	OMIM Syndrome #	Gene	Protein	OMIM Gene #
Osteopetrosis, type II	166600	CLCN7	Chloride channel 7	602727
Pycnodysostosis	265800	CTSK	Cathepsin-K	601105
27. Increased bone density with diaphyseal involvement				
Diaphyseal dysplasia (Camurati-Engelmann disease)	131300	TGFB1	Transforming growth factor-β-1	190180
Kenny-Caffey syndrome, type 1	244460	TBCE	Tubulin-specific chaperone E	604934
Oculodentodigital dysplasia	164200	GJA1	Gap junction protein 1	121014
Osteosclerosis, autosomal dominant	144750	LRP5	Lipoprotein receptor-related protein 5	603506
Paget disease, juvenile	239000	TNFRSF11B	Osteoprotegerin	602643
Paget disease, type 2	602080	TNFRSF11A	RANK	603499
Paget disease, type 3	602080	SQSTM1	Sequestosome 1	601530
Sclerosteosis	269500	SOST	Sclerostin	605740
Trichodentoosseous dysplasia	190320	DLX3	Distal-less homeo box 3	600525
Van Buchem, type 2	607363	LRP5	Lipoprotein receptor-related protein 5	603506
28. Increased bone density with metaphyseal involvement				
Craniometaphyseal dysplasia, autosomal dominant	123000	ANKH	Ankylosis gene	605145
29. Craniotubular digital dysplasias				
Frontometaphyseal dysplasia	305620	FLNA	Filamin A	300017
Osteodysplasty, Melnick-Needles	309350	FLNA	Filamin A	300017
Otopalatodigital syndrome, type I	311300	FLNA	Filamin A	300017
Otopalatodigital syndrome, type II	304120	FLNA	Filamin A	300017
30. Neonatal severe osteosclerotic dysplasias				
Chondrodysplasia, Blomstrand type	215045	PTHR1	Parathyroid hormone receptor	168468
31. Disorganized development of cartilaginous and fibrous components of the skeleton				
Cherubism	118400	SH3BP2	SH3 domain-binding protein	602104
Fibromatosis, gingival	135300	SOS1	SOS homolog 1	182530
McCune-Albright syndrome	174800	GNAS	G-Protein, α subunit	139320
Multiple endochondromatosis	166000	PTHR1	Parathyroid hormone receptor	168468
Multiple exostoses, type 1	133700	EXT1	Exostosin-1	133700
Multiple exostoses, type 2	133701	EXT2	Exostosin-2	133701
Osseous heteroplasia	166350	GNAS	G-Protein, α subunit	139320
32. Osteolyses				
Familial expansile osteolysis	174810	TNFRSF11A	RANK	603499
Mandibuloacral dysplasia	248370	LMNA	Lamin A/C	150330
Osteolysis, idiopathic, Saudi type	605156	MMP2	Matrix metalloproteinase-2	120360
33. Patella dysplasias				
Nail-patella	161200	LMX1B	Lim homeodomain	602575

Localized Skeletal Malformations (Dysotoses)

A. Localized disorders with predominant cranial and facial involvement

Genetic Disorder	OMIM Syndrome #	Gene	Protein	OMIM Gene #
Antley-Bixler syndrome	207410	FGFR2	Fibroblast growth factor receptor-2	176943
Apert syndrome	101200	FGFR2	Fibroblast growth factor receptor-2	176943
Beare-Stevenson cutis gyrata syndrome	123790	FGFR2	Fibroblast growth factor receptor-2	176943
Craniofacial-deafness-hand syndrome	122880	PAX3	Paired homeo box 3	606597
Craniosynostosis, Boston type	604757	MSX2	MSX2 homeo box gene	123101
Craniosynostosis, Muenke type	602849	FGFR3	Fibroblast growth factor receptor-3	134934
Crouzon syndrome	123500	FGFR2	Fibroblast growth factor receptor-2	176943
Greig cephalopolysyndactyly syndrome	175700	GLI3	GLI-Kruppel member 3	165240
Jackson-Weiss syndrome	123150	FGFR2	Fibroblast growth factor receptor-2	176943
Orofaciodigital syndrome I	311200	CXORF5	X open reading frame	300170
Pfeiffer syndrome	101600	FGFR1	Fibroblast growth factor receptor-1	136350
		FGFR2	Fibroblast growth factor receptor-2	176943

Summary of Gene Disorders of Serum Mineral Metabolism or Skeleton Formation

Genetic Disorder	OMIM Syndrome #	Gene	Protein	OMIM Gene #
Robinow-Sorauf syndrome	180750	TWIST	Twist	601622
Saethre-Chotzen syndrome	101400	TWIST	Twist	601622
Shprintzen-Goldberg syndrome	182212	FBN1	Fibrillin-1	134797
Treacher Collins syndrome	154500	TCOF1	Treacle	606847
Waardenburg syndrome, type 1	193500	PAX3	Paired homeo box 3	606597
Waardenburg syndrome, type 2A	193510	MITF	Microphtalmia-associated transcription factor	156845
Waardenburg syndrome, type 3	148820	PAX3	Paired homeo box 3	606597

B. Localized disorders with predominant axial involvement

Genetic Disorder	OMIM Syndrome #	Gene	Protein	OMIM Gene #
Robinow syndrome, recessive also in 16	268310	ROR2	NTRKR2/RTK-like orphan receptor 2	602337
Spondylocostal dysostosis	277300	DLL3	Delta-like 3	602768
Weyers acrodental dysostosis	193530	EVC	EVC gene product	604831

C. Localized disorders with predominant involvement of the extremities

Genetic Disorder	OMIM Syndrome #	Gene	Protein	OMIM Gene #
Bardet-Biedl syndrome, type 1	209900	BBS1	Unknown	209901
Bardet-Biedl syndrome, type 2	209900	BBS2	Unknown	606151
Bardet-Biedl syndrome, type 4	209900	BBS4	Unknown	600374
Bardet-Biedl syndrome, type 6	209900	MKKS	Unknown	604896
Contractural arachnodactyly	121050	FBN2	Fibrillin-2	121050
Fanconi Anemia	227650	FANCA	FA complement	607139
		FANCB	FA complement	227660
		FANCC	FA complement	227645
		FANCD1	FA complement	605724
		FANCD2	FA complement	227646
		FANCE	FA complement	600901
		FANCF	FA complement	603467
		FANCG	FA complement	602956
Guttmacher syndrome	176305	HOXA13	Homeo box A13	142959
Hand foot uterus syndrome	140000	HOXA13	Homeo box A13	142959
Heart-hand syndrome	142900	TBX5	T-Box 5	601620
McKusick-Kaufman syndrome	236700	MKKS	Unknown	604896
Multiple synostosis syndrome 1	186500	NOG	Noggin	602991
Pallister-Hall syndrome	146510	GLI3	GLI-Kruppel member 3	165240
Postaxial polydactyly, type A	174200	GLI3	GLI-Kruppel member 3	165240
Preaxial polydactyly type IV	174700	GLI3	GLI-Kruppel member 3	165240
Rubinstein syndrome	180849	CREBBP	CREB-binding protein	600140
Split-hand malformation 4	605289	TP73L	p63	603273
Syndactyly, type 2	186000	HOXD13	Homeo box 4l	142989
Tarsal-carpal coalition syndrome	186570	NOG	Noggin	602991
Ulnar-mammary syndrome	181450	TBX3	T-Box 3	601621

Information identifying the disorders and their respective affected genes was obtained by a key-word search of the Online Mendelian Inheritance in Man, OMIM(TM), Center for Medical Genetics, Johns Hopkins University (Baltimore, MD) and National Center for Biotechnology Information, National Library of Medicine (Bethesda, MD), 1997. World Wide Web URL: http://www.ncbi.nlm.nih.gov/omim. The classification into groups based on associated serum mineral defects is based on the OMIM clinical synopsis provided for each disorder. The remaining classifications are in part based on the International Nosology and Classification of Constitutive Disorders of Bone (2001)(Hall. C.M. Amer. J. Med. Genet. 113:65-77, 2002). Disorders are separated into two major classifications, osteochondrodysplasias, which comprise 33 numbered groups, and dysostoses, which comprise 3 groups identified alphabetically. The absence of Groups 2, 3, 14, 15, 21 and 23 is due to the lack of defined genetic mutations for disorders in these groups. More detailed information on individual disorders or genes can be obtained by using the OMIM numbers provided to perform a key-word search (http://www.ncbi.nlm.nih.gov/Omim/searchomim.html).

Subject Index